Techniques in Small Animal Soft Tissue, Orthopedic, and Ophthalmic Surgery

Techniques in Small Animal Soft Tissue, Orthopedic, and Ophthalmic Surgery

Edited by

Kristin A. Coleman
Small Animal Surgeon
Gulf Coast Veterinary Specialists
Houston, TX
USA

WILEY Blackwell

Published by John Wiley & Sons, Inc., Hoboken, New Jersey.
Published simultaneously in Canada.

For general information on our other products and services or for technical support, please contact our Customer Care Department within the United States at (800) 762-2974, outside the United States at (317) 572-3993 or fax (317) 572-4002.

Wiley also publishes its books in a variety of electronic formats. Some content that appears in print may not be available in electronic formats. For more information about Wiley products, visit our web site at www.wiley.com.

Library of Congress Cataloging-in-Publication Data applied for:
ISBN 9781394159949 (hardback)

Cover Design: Wiley
Cover Images: © Kristin Coleman

Set in 9.5/12.5pt STIXTwoText by Straive, Pondicherry, India

Printed in Singapore
M006474_120724

We dedicate this book to the families, friends, and animals who supported our hard work in writing these book chapters during free time from our day jobs. My own animals, Kelev (sweet tiny brown dog), Ludwig (obnoxious Maine Coon), Miel (meek ginger cat), and Lilliputian (mischievous apple-headed Siamese Munchkin), were essential to my own sanity when writing chapters for and editing this book.

I personally dedicate this book in memory of my mom, who encouraged my love for and need to care for animals from a young age, and in memory of my dad, who passed away within an hour of the phone call during which I accepted the invitation to write this textbook and who was the one always pushing me to exceed what I thought were my own limits. The dedication, determination, and long hours that went into creating and editing this manuscript were always with the memory of them in my heart and mind. This one was for you, Mama and Daddy.

Contents

List of Contributors

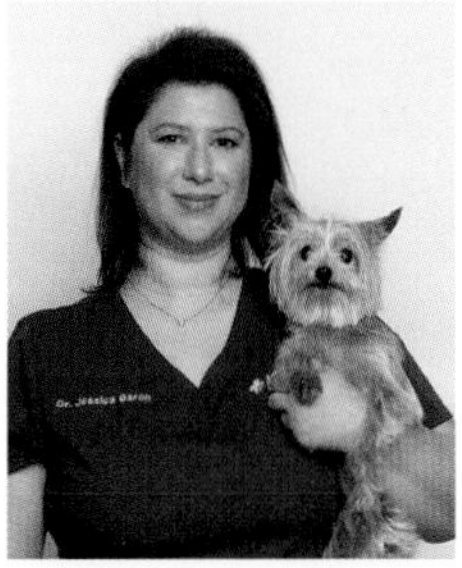

Jessica Baron, DVM, DACVS-SA
Small Animal Surgeon
MedVet Norwalk
Norwalk, CT
USA

Laryngeal Paralysis

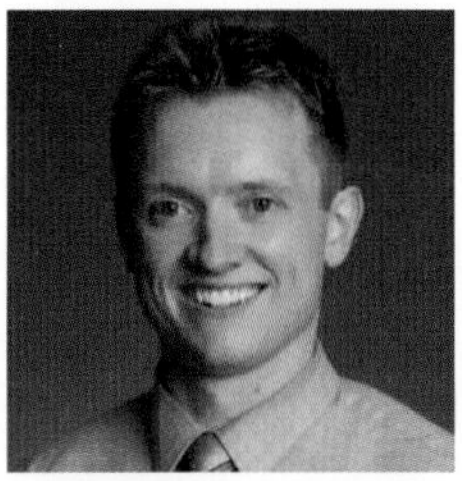

Seth Bleakley, MVB, MS, DACVS-SA, DECVS, MRCVS, CCRT
Small Animal Surgeon
CARE Surgery Center
Phoenix, AZ
USA

Principles of Fracture Repair
Principles of External Coaptation

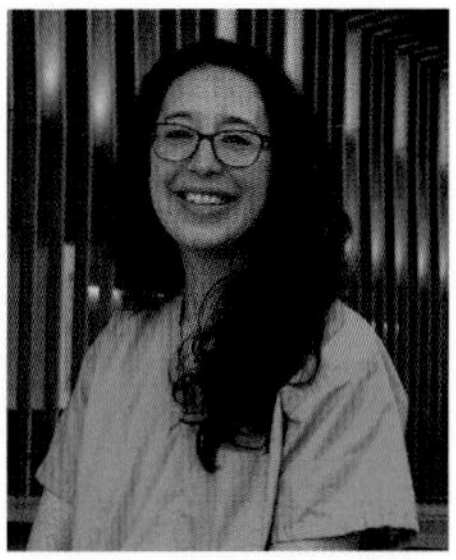

Nicole J. Buote, DVM, DACVS-SA
ACVS Founding Fellow in Minimally Invasive Surgery (Soft Tissue)
Associate Professor, Small Animal Surgery
Cornell University, College of Veterinary Medicine
Ithaca, NY
USA

Nosectomy in Cats
Liver Biopsies

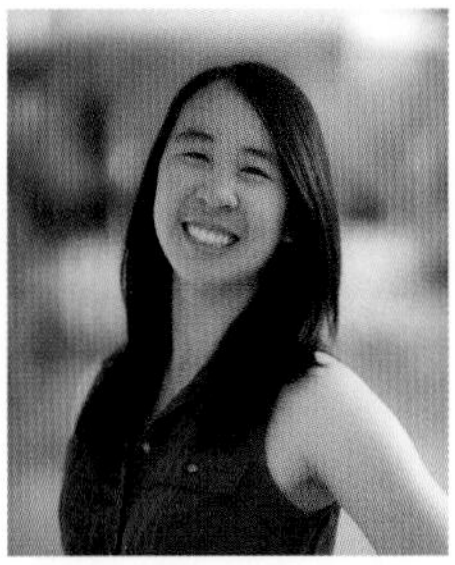

Carolyn L. Chen, DVM
Small Animal Surgery Resident
University of Georgia
Athens, GA
USA

Arthrocentesis

Karen L. Cherrone, DVM, DACVS
Small Animal Surgeon
KLC Veterinary Surgical Services
New York, NY
USA
Pinnectomy

Grayson Cole, DVM, CCRP, DACVS-SA
Small Animal Surgeon
Gulf Coast Veterinary Specialists
Houston, TX
USA
*Total Ear Canal Ablation and Lateral Bulla Osteotomy
(TECA-LBO)*
Sialoadenectomy

Kristin A. Coleman, DVM, MS, DACVS-SA
Small Animal Surgeon
Gulf Coast Veterinary Specialists
Houston, TX
USA
Gastropexy
Caudectomy
Femoral Head and Neck Ostectomy (FHO)

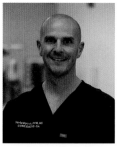

David Dycus, DVM, MS, CCRP, DACVS-SA
Director of Orthopedic Surgery, Nexus Veterinary
Bone & Joint Center
Founder, Ortho Vet Consulting
Severn, MD
USA
Humeral Condylar Fractures (co-author)

Trent T. Gall, DVM, MS, DACVS-SA
Small Animal Surgeon
Gall Mobile Veterinary Surgery
Longmont, CO
USA
*Extracapsular Stabilization for the Cranial Cruciate
Ligament-Deficient Stifle*
Caudectomy (co-author)

Janet A. Grimes, DVM, MS, DACVS-SA
Associate Professor, Small Animal Surgery
University of Georgia, College of Veterinary Medicine
Athens, GA
USA
Cystotomy and Partial Cystectomy
Feline Perineal Urethrostomy

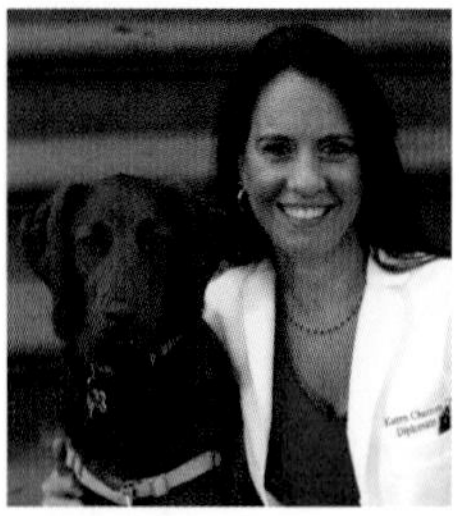

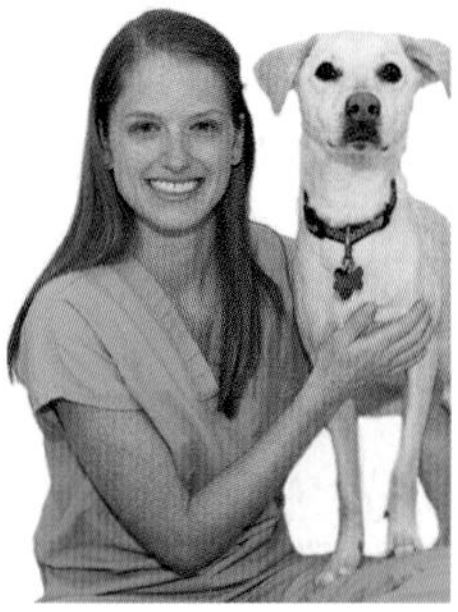

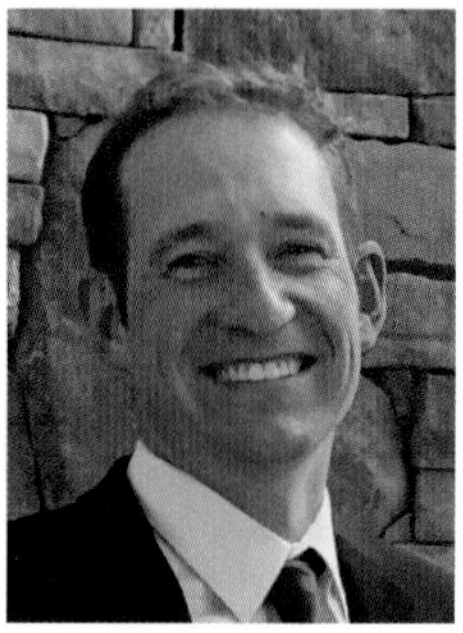

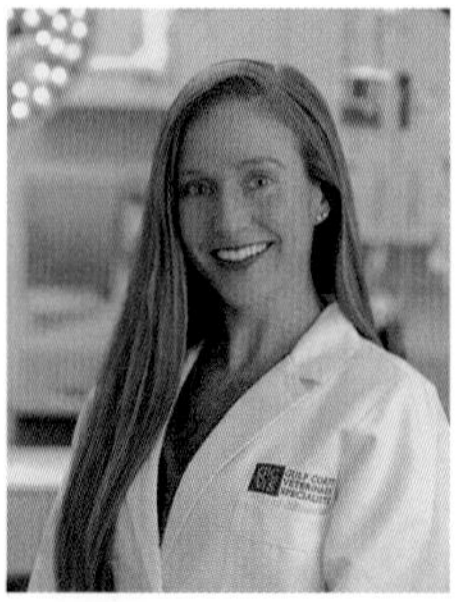

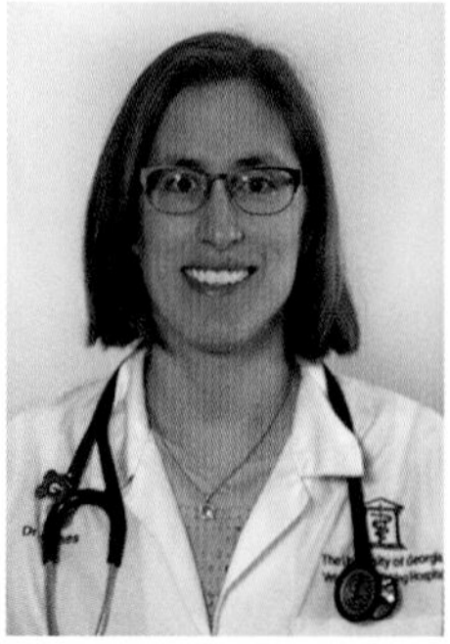

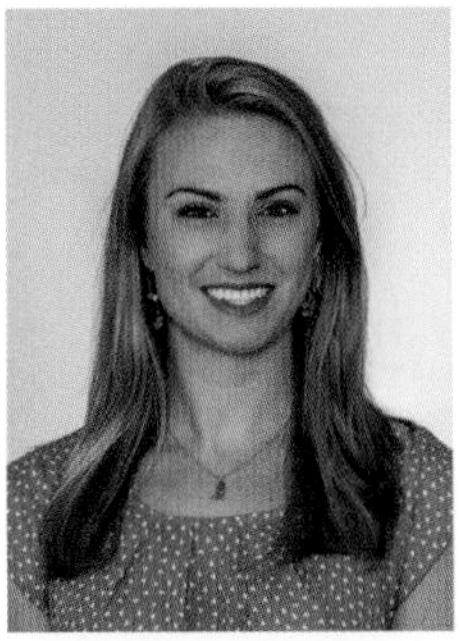

Leah P. Hixon, DVM
Residency-Trained Small Animal Surgeon
Colorado Canine Orthopedics
Colorado Springs, CO
USA
Arthrocentesis (co-author)

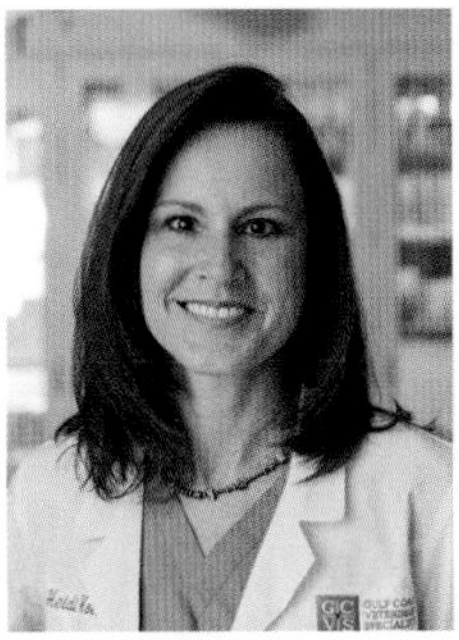

Heidi Hottinger, DVM, DACVS
Small Animal Surgeon
Gulf Coast Veterinary Specialists
Houston, TX
USA
The Art of the Abdominal Explore

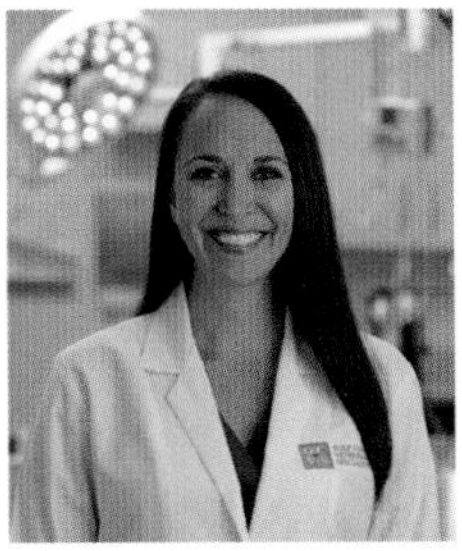

Audrey C. Hudson, DVM, DACVO
Veterinary Ophthalmologist
Gulf Coast Veterinary Specialists
Houston, TX
USA
Surgery for the Prolapsed Third Eyelid Gland

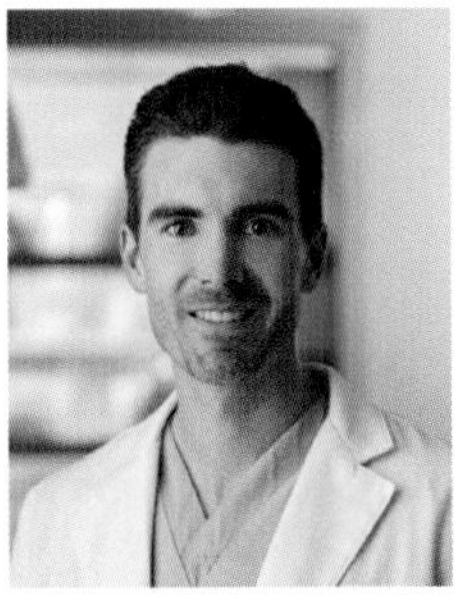

Caleb Hudson, DVM, MS, DACVS-SA
ACVS Founding Fellow in Minimally Invasive Surgery (SA Orthopedics)
ACVS Founding Fellow, Joint Replacement Surgery
Small Animal Surgeon
Nexus Veterinary Specialists
Victoria, TX
USA
Surgery for the Prolapsed Third Eyelid Gland (co-author)
Mandibular Fractures
Osteochondrosis (co-author)

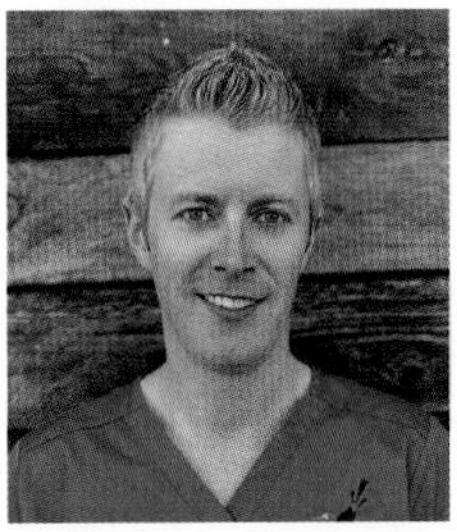

Stephen C. Jones, MVB, MS, DACVS-SA, DECVS
Small Animal Surgeon
Bark City Veterinary Specialists
Park City, UT
USA
Mandibular Fractures (co-author)
Osteochondrosis

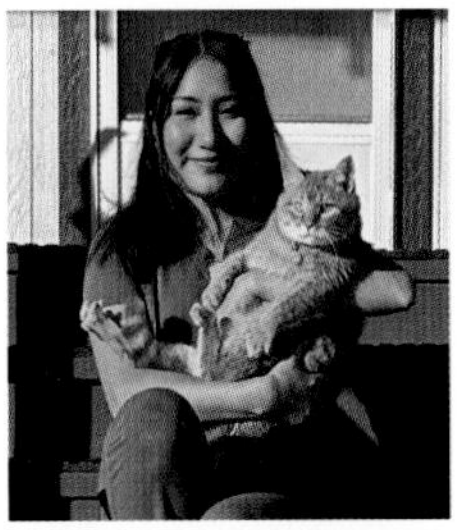

Ivette Juarez, LVT
Operating Room Technician
Gulf Coast Veterinary Specialists
Houston, TX
USA
Preparing for an Abdominal Procedure
Preparing for Orthopedic Procedures

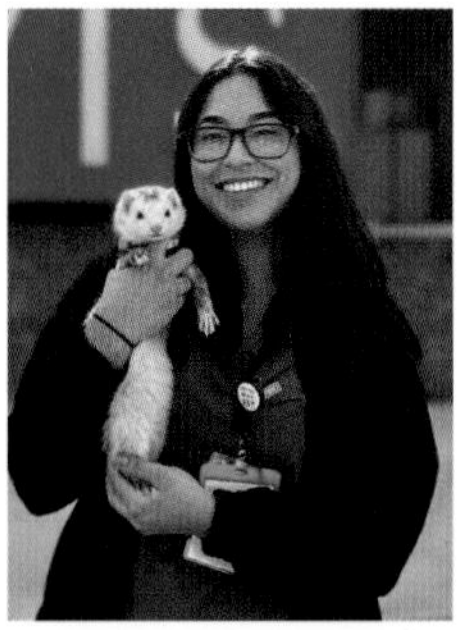

Marbella Lopez, LVT
Operating Room Technician
Gulf Coast Veterinary Specialists
Houston, TX
USA
Preparing for an Abdominal Procedure (co-author)
Preparing for Orthopedic Procedures (co-author)

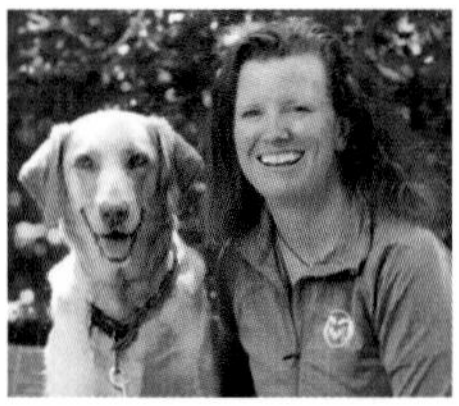

Catriona M. MacPhail, DVM, PhD, DACVS
Small Animal Surgeon
Colorado State University, Veterinary Teaching Hospital
Fort Collins, CO
USA
Prostatic Abscessation
Rectal Prolapse
Perineal Hernia

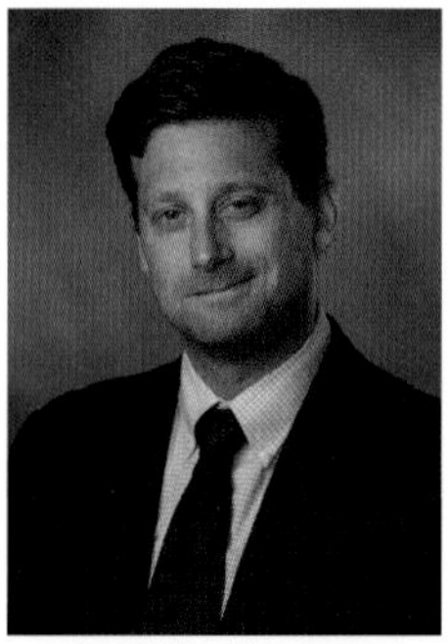

Brad M. Matz, DVM, MS, DACVS-SA
ACVS Fellow, Surgical Oncology
Robert and Charlotte Lowder Distinguished Professor in Oncology
Associate Professor of Small Animal Soft Tissue Surgery
Auburn University, College of Veterinary Medicine
Auburn, AL
USA
Ovariohysterectomy/Ovariectomy
Pyometra

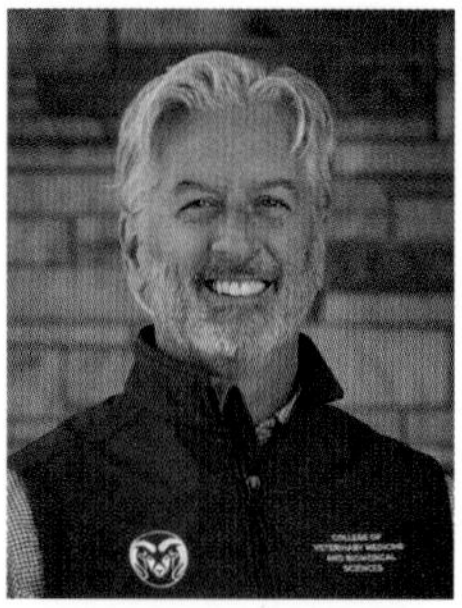

Ross H. Palmer, DVM, MS, DACVS
Professor of Orthopedic Surgery
Associate Director of Education
Colorado State University, Translational Medicine Institute
Fort Collins, CO
USA
Medial Patellar Luxation Repair

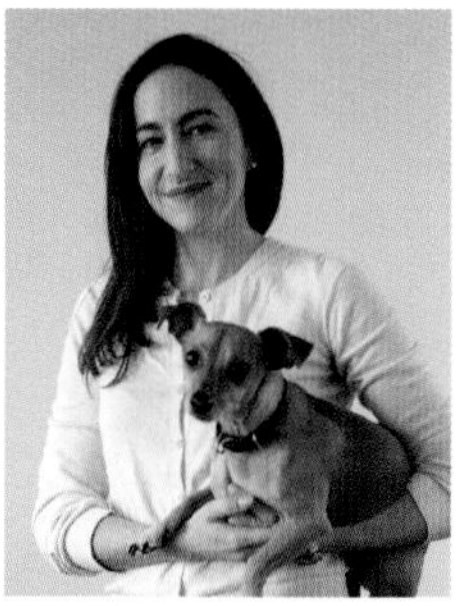

Philippa R. Pavia, VMD, DACVS-SA
Vice President of Medical Operations
Thrive Pet Healthcare
New York, NY
USA
Ventral Bulla Osteotomy (VBO)

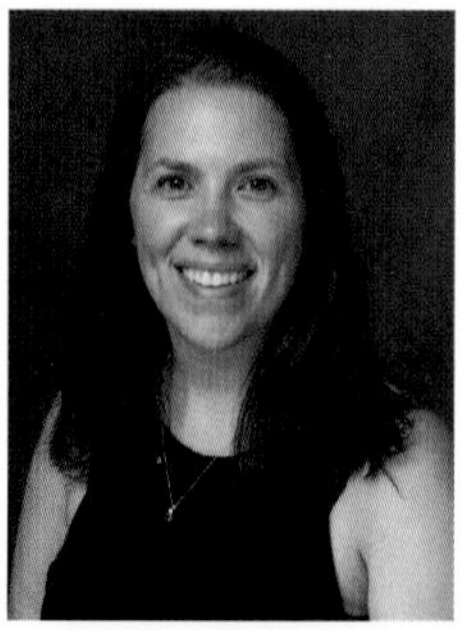

Penny J. Regier, DVM, MS, DACVS-SA
ACVS Minimally Invasive Surgery Fellow, Soft Tissue Surgery
Associate Professor of Small Animal Surgery
University of Florida, College of Veterinary Medicine
Gainesville, FL
USA
Gastrointestinal Procedures

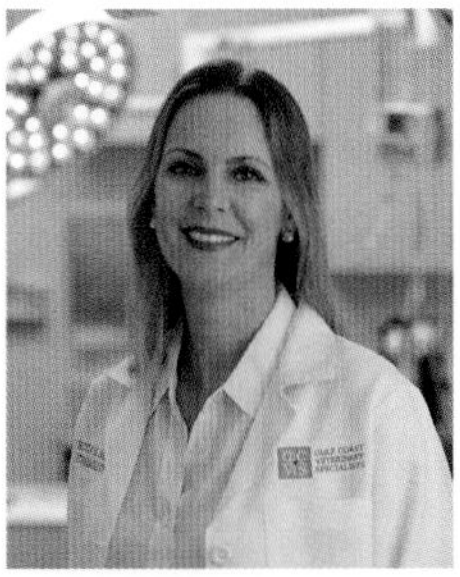

Rebecca S. Salazar, DVM, DACVAA
Anesthesiologist, Department Lead of Anesthesia and Pain Management
Gulf Coast Veterinary Specialists
Houston, TX
USA
Lumbosacral Steroid Epidural

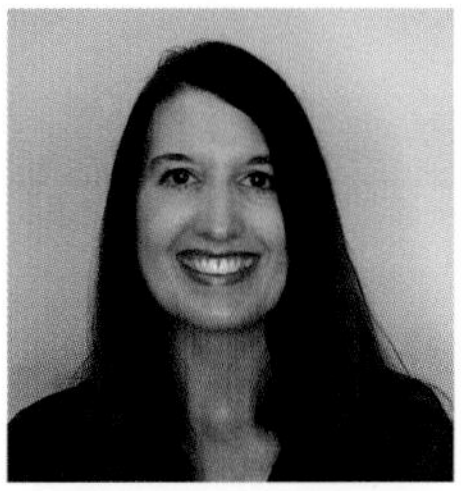

Robin Sankey, DVM, DACVO
Veterinary Ophthalmologist
North Houston Veterinary Ophthalmology
Spring, TX
USA
Steps for Simple Eyelid Mass Removal
Tips and Tricks for Successful Entropion Repair
A Guide to Enucleation

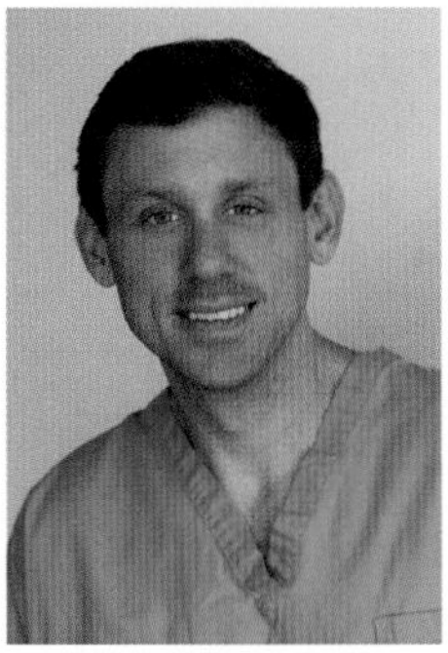

Joey A. Sapora, DVM, MS, DACVS-SA
Clinical Orthopedic Surgeon
Colorado State University, Veterinary Teaching Hospital
Fort Collins, CO
USA
Canine Scrotal Ablation and Scrotal Urethrostomy
Canine Elbow Dysplasia

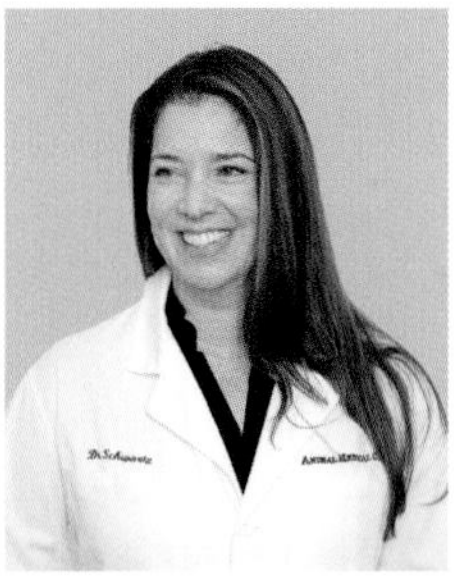

Pamela Schwartz, DVM, DACVS-SA, CCRP
Small Animal Surgeon
Chair, Department of Surgery (Soft Tissue & Orthopedics)
Schwarzman Animal Medical Center
New York, NY
USA
Brachycephalic Obstructive Airway Syndrome in Dogs and Cats
Splenectomy

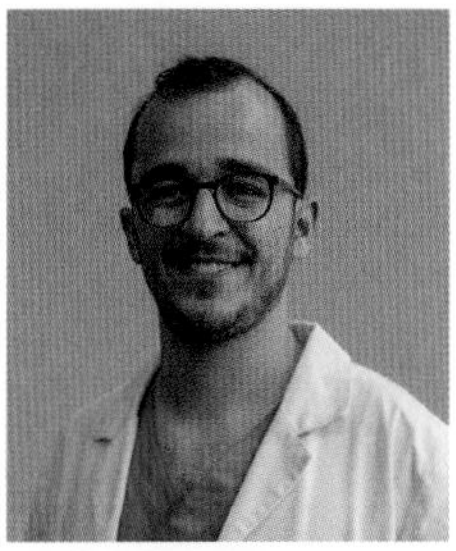

Paul Schwarzmann, Mag. med. vet.
Veterinarian
Tierklinik Schwarzmann
Rankweil, Austria
3D-Printing in Orthopedics

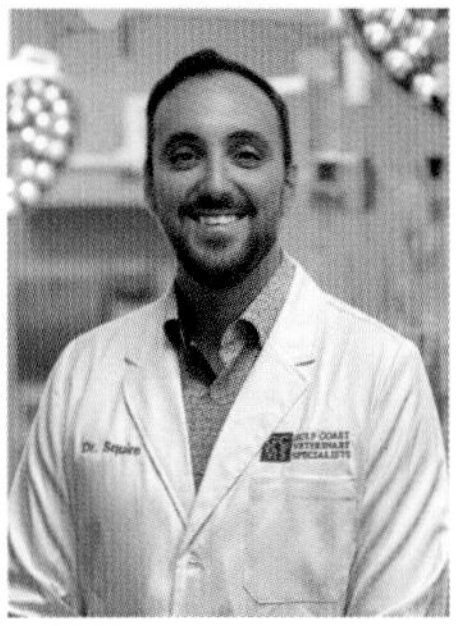

Nathan T. Squire, VMD, MS, DACVS-SA
Small Animal Surgeon
Gulf Coast Veterinary Specialists
Houston, TX
USA
Humeral Condylar Fractures

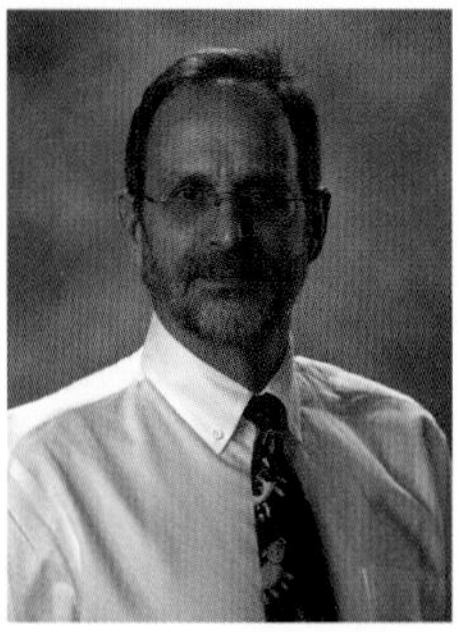

David Michael Tillson, DVM, MS, DACVS
Small Animal Surgeon
Arthur & Louise Oriole Professor in the College
of Veterinary Medicine
Auburn University, College of Veterinary Medicine
Auburn, AL
USA
Summary of Skin Reconstruction Options
Digit Amputation
Cesarean Section
Inguinal, Umbilical, and Diaphragmatic Hernias

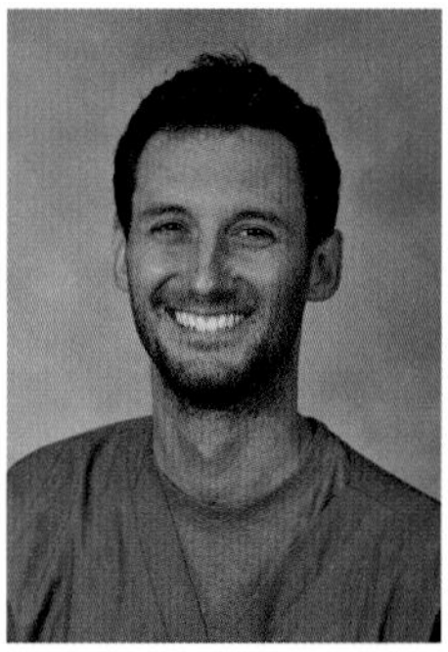

Giovanni Tremolada, DVM, MS, Ph.D, DACVS-SA, DECVS
ACVS Fellow, Surgical Oncology
Clinical Assistant Professor, Surgical Oncology
Colorado State University, Flint Animal Cancer Center
Fort Collins, CO
USA
Mandibulectomy
Thyroidectomy

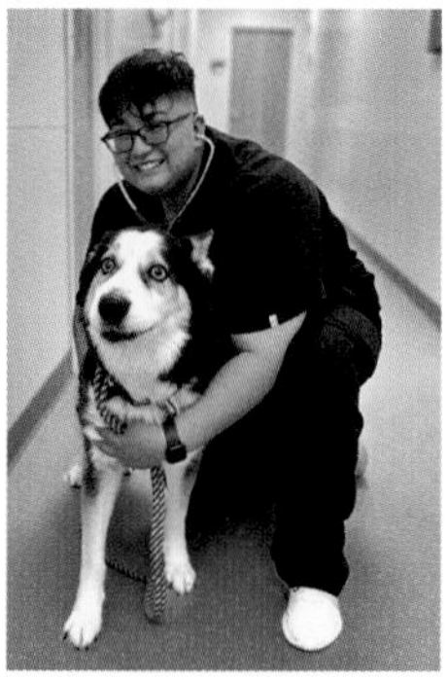

Christine A. Valdez, LVT
Operating Room Technician
Gulf Coast Veterinary Specialists
Houston, TX
USA
Preparing for an Abdominal Procedure (co-author)
Preparing for Orthopedic Procedures (co-author)

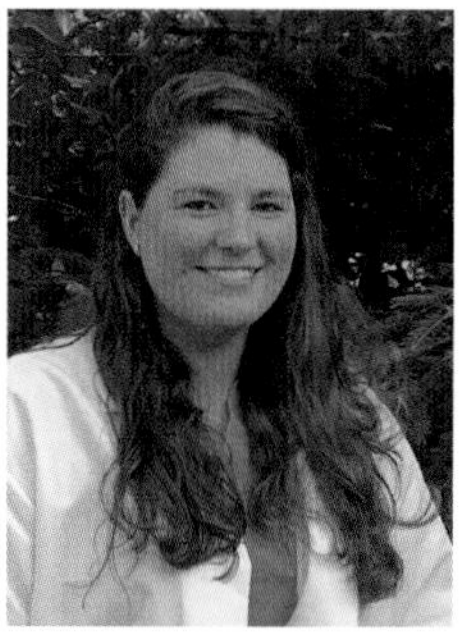

Emily C. Viani, DVM
Residency-Trained Small Animal Surgeon
Tufts Veterinary Emergency Treatment & Specialties
Walpole, MA
USA
Arthrocentesis (co-author)

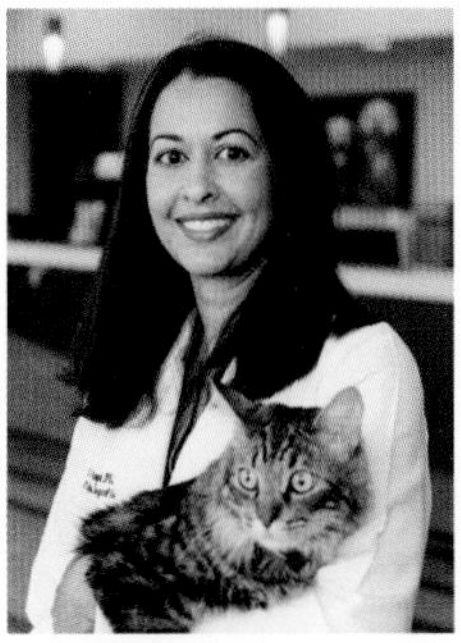

Arathi Vinayak, DVM, DACVS-SA
ACVS Fellow, Surgical Oncology
Small Animal Surgeon
VCA West Coast Animal Emergency and Specialty Hospital
Fountain Valley, CA
USA
Peripheral Lymph Node Extirpation in the Dog and Cat
Limb Amputation in Companion Animals: Thoracic and Pelvic Limb Amputations
Anal Sacculectomy in Dogs and Cats

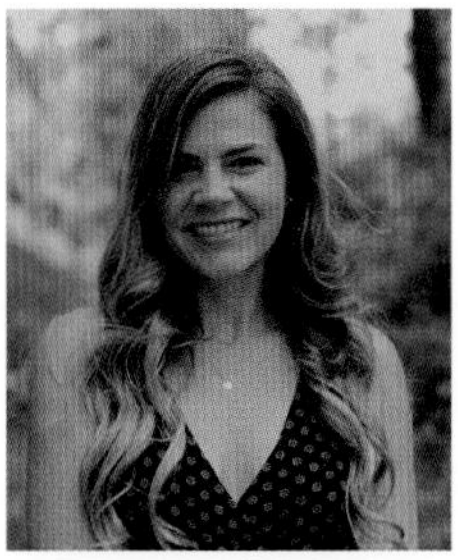

Jess D. Work, DVM
Mixed Animal Practitioner
Deer Park Veterinary Clinic
Deer Park, WA
USA
Aural Hematoma

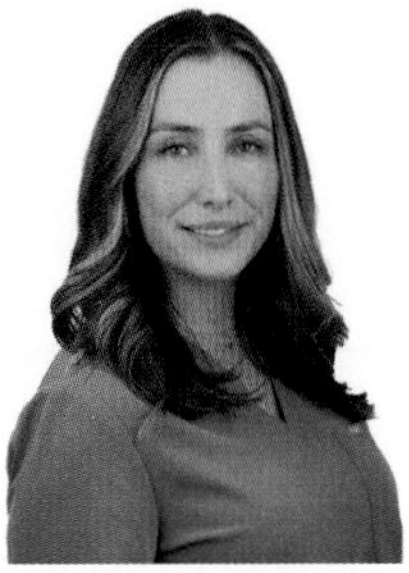

Rebecca J. Webb, BVSc (Hons), MS, MANZCVS, DACVS-SA
Small Animal Surgeon
VetSurg
Ventura, CA
USA
Orthopedic Implants
Metacarpal and Metatarsal Fractures
Pelvic Fractures
Tendon Lacerations
Bone Grafts

Foreword

The year was 2010 at the end of spring semester. As a professor of surgery, I was engaged in one of the most important but lifeless and mundane tasks of giving practical skills exams to sophomore students. I remember so distinctly the young woman who leaned in before tying her first knot and declared, "I want to be a surgeon." Such a statement was not rare, and when I perceived it to be sincere, I often offered to have the student come to the clinic operating rooms and scrub in as a table nurse. Most students would show up a few times and disappear. This young woman checked the schedule daily and came after class or during lunch - changing into scrubs, scrubbing in and then out, changing back into classroom clothing, and returning to class as time demanded - for the entire semester and following year. She also requested a letter of reference for a scholarship and I asked for a CV to work from. Surprisingly then (not now), her CV revealed a person of intensity, excellence, and uncommon achievement (many new assistant professors would have been proud of such a CV), and of course, this was my introduction to the Editor of this surgical textbook, Kristin Ashley Coleman.

Although Dr. Coleman's partial biography is online, it is my prerogative to detail it a bit more in this Foreword. Dr. Coleman externed at the Animal Medical Center in the Interventional Radiology Department, which was a catalyst for her love of MIS. She preceptored before graduation at a clinic in which I occasionally consulted. The owner reported that although Kristin was not antisocial, she was "hard put to spend time having fun since she had not finished reading both volumes of Slatter's Textbook of Small Animal Surgery." That clinic also served the veterinary needs of an oceanarium and through these connections, then student Coleman and I (with others) had an opportunity to design and perform the first reported mastectomy on a sea lion for mammary cancer. She returned to the AMC for an internship and then on to Colorado State University for residency and her master's degree.

Post residency, Dr. Coleman joined a private practice in New York City and became board-certified by the American College of Veterinary Surgeons (SA, March 2017). She then moved to Houston with the Gulf Coast Veterinary Specialists in 2019. Succinctly stated, she has had the opportunity to travel very broadly and witness the human condition. As a practitioner specialist, her interests continued in minimally invasive techniques and development of practitioner / generalist continuing education. At least partially motivated by altruism, she knows the pressure on owners and their veterinarians when specialty care exceeds an owner's ability to pay. The burden falls back to their veterinarian. When the managing editor of Wiley suggested that Dr. Coleman assemble authors for a photo-rich, broad-base manual somewhere between a text and an atlas, filled with 'tips and tricks' of soft tissue, orthopedic and ophthalmic surgical techniques, I knew it would be well done. Congratulations reader on your purchase.

Ralph A Henderson Jr, DVM, MS
Professor Emeritus, Auburn University
College of Veterinary Medicine
Diplomate and Founding Fellow of Surgical Oncology,
American College of Veterinary Surgeons
Charter Diplomate, American College of
Veterinary Internal Medicine, Clinical Oncology (retired)

Preface

Once upon a time in vet school, I believed that only board-certified surgeons could perform surgery on animals beyond a sterilization procedure. It was not until I was under the guidance of some of the amazing surgeons from my residency at CSU VTH, Dr. Clara Goh, Dr. Howie Seim, and Dr. Ross Palmer, who invited me to participate in teaching CE events and opened my eyes to the possibility of teaching general practitioners some of the more complicated surgical procedures. The philosophy was that the world is changing; there is an ever-increasing pet population, and board-certified surgeons are not always within traveling distance to a pet in need of surgical intervention, are not always affordable, and are not always available in a timely manner. For these reasons, general practitioners might be asked by their clientele to perform surgeries with which they may not be familiar or may find that they are uncomfortable with the procedures they are already doing. We all know what it feels like to want to help a patient even when we need significant guidance to do so.

This book is for those practitioners: the ones who want to help their clients, who are asked to perform a surgery they have never performed before, or who simply want a book in hand with a step-by-step guide for how to perform certain commonly encountered procedures for their valued patients and clients. Throughout these 54 chapters, you will find step-by-step instructions with 'tips and tricks' for how to increase the chances of a successful surgical outcome and high-quality pictures and videos to help with understanding the components of each surgery. We have also included ample, relevant pre- and postoperative considerations to ensure that not only is a given surgery carried out in the best possible manner but also that the right decisions can be made both leading up to and following surgery to optimize patient care.

Techniques in Small Animal Soft Tissue, Orthopedic, and Ophthalmic Surgery was written by 35 incredible individuals (mostly board-certified surgeons), who are specialists and experts in their field as well as life-long learners dedicated to educating others to advance the field of veterinary medicine. Although these authors are passionate about surgery and the topics they were invited to write, this book is not all-inclusive. Thanks to other great books already in print with highly detailed pathophysiology of disease processes requiring surgical intervention and with complex anatomy as the primary focus of the text, this book is meant to include a review of these concepts to provide a helpful guide with advice on how to do many surgeries. The reader is strongly encouraged to read other texts, understand the indications for certain surgeries, and perhaps even practice on a cadaver, take a short weekend course for a hands-on training lab, or review videos of these procedures (recommendation: videovet.org) prior to performing them on a client-owned animal.

Even though all chapters in this book were deemed relevant for a general practitioner or a surgeon just out of residency who may not have seen all surgeries being required of them in the real world, we would like feedback on how we did and what you want from a "tips on surgical techniques" book. Which techniques would you like to learn about that we did not include in this edition? Which techniques need more detail or better pictures? We intend for this book to morph over time as procedures, perioperative care, or other recommendations change with updated peer-reviewed literature, and input from our readers is the only way we can create the best guide to practical techniques in surgery as possible.

When I got the phone call from the publishing company inviting me to write a textbook like this, I knew that I could not say 'no', and I knew it meant a lot of hard work. But, just under 2 years after that initial call, we did it. With blood (from the patients, carefully controlled with electrosurgery), sweat, tears, and the creative genius of over 30 incredible colleagues and friends, the "labor of love" is done.

Enough babbling – we hope you enjoy our book! Happy reading!

Acknowledgments

To all of the authors of this book: **thank you**! Being a part of this textbook from ideation to implementation of a handheld book will remain one of my proudest professional accomplishments and is only possible thanks to every one of you.

To those who are going to read this book: **thank you**! I think I speak for all of us when I extend my deepest appreciation to all of you for being the inspiration behind this creation.

About the Companion Website

This book is accompanied by a companion website.

www.wiley.com/go/coleman/surgeries

This website includes:

- Videos
- Figures from the book as PPTs

1

Preparing for an Abdominal Procedure

Ivette Juarez, Christine A. Valdez, and Marbella Lopez

Department of Small Animal Surgery, Gulf Coast Veterinary Specialists, Houston, TX, USA

Key Points

- Learn thorough preparation of an operating room for a standard abdominal exploratory procedure.
- Learn appropriate preparation of the patient, including surgical clip, scrubbing, positioning, and draping.
- Learn about setting up instrumentation for a standard abdominal procedure.

Introduction

This chapter focuses on the detailed preparation of the patient, operating room setup, instrumentation setup, and intraoperative and postoperative considerations when managing an abdominal exploratory procedure.

Preoperative Steps

Equipment Preparation

Immediately prior to an abdominal procedure, the operating room is set up with the appropriate equipment and instrumentation depending on the type of abdominal procedure (Box 1.1, Figure 1.1). Creating a list of commonly used instruments and surgeon's preferences for a variety of procedures may help with efficiency when setting up an operating room (Figure 1.2). Heating systems should be turned on. Intravenous fluids are spiked and primed. Anesthetic machines are checked for leaks (Figure 1.3), and an induction area is prepared (Figure 1.4) with the necessary materials (Box 1.1).

At this point, the patient has had the appropriate diagnostic imaging and the required blood work, and an intravenous catheter has been placed. Once general anesthesia is induced, the patient is positioned in dorsal recumbency. Monitoring equipment may then be attached, including but not limited to electrocardiogram, pulse oximetry, noninvasive blood pressure, and a capnometer. If a patient's position needs to be adjusted at any point, it is ideal to disconnect the breathing circuit from the patient's endotracheal tube to prevent extubation or tracheal damage.

Skin Preparation

Since the duration of anesthesia correlates with infection rates, preoperative preparation should be thorough but efficient. Clipping should be performed outside of the operating room to minimize contamination. The technician should wear exam gloves while clipping. With a #40 clipper blade, shave the patient's ventrum cranial to the xiphoid (mid-thorax), caudal to the pubis, and lateral to the mammary chain (Figure 1.5). Be sure to watch the temperature of the clipper blade. If the blade becomes palpably hot, either replace the blade or spray it with a cooling lubricant. In areas with friable, thin skin, it is advised to have steady movements to reduce the risk of unwanted abrasions. After clipping is completed, a vacuum can be used to pick up loose hair.

Techniques in Small Animal Soft Tissue, Orthopedic, and Ophthalmic Surgery, First Edition. Edited by Kristin A. Coleman.

Companion website: www.wiley.com/go/coleman/surgeries

Box 1.1 Examples of Equipment and Instrumentation Needed for an Abdominal Surgical Procedure

- Suction unit, hose, and canister
- Electrosurgical unit with equipment (e.g., monopolar cautery pen, bipolar cautery pen, foot switch, ground plate, cautery tip cleaner)
- Vessel-sealing device (e.g., LigaSure™ Atlas or Precise)
- General surgery pack (e.g., surgical gowns, large patient drape, towel drapes, bulb syringe, needle counter box, radiopaque gauze)
- Soft tissue instrument tray (e.g., towel clamps, scalpel handles, needle holders, thumb forceps, dissecting scissors, suture cutting scissors, tissue forceps, hemostatic forceps, bowl)
- Suction tip (e.g., Poole, Frazier, Yankauer)
- Retractors (e.g., Balfour, Senn, malleable)
- Stapling equipment (image within this box) (e.g., hemoclip staples, thoracoabdominal (TA) stapler with cartridge, gastrointestinal anastomosis (GIA) stapler with cartridge, skin staples)
- Laparotomy sponges
- Kick bucket
- Light handles
- Sterile gloves
- Suture
- Blades (#10, #11, and #15)

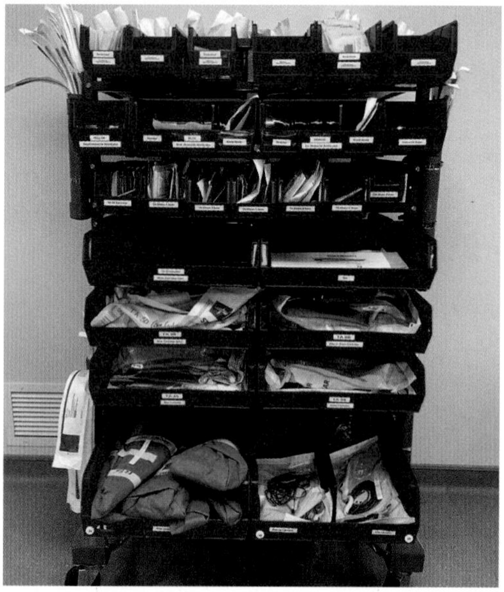

Stapling equipment cart

- Other instruments (e.g., antimicrobial incise drape, biopsy punch, hemostatic products, surgical drain, bladder cystotomy spoon, urethral catheters, sterile lube, sterile syringes, needles, stomach tube)
- Specimen collection (e.g., Formalin, culture, glass slides)

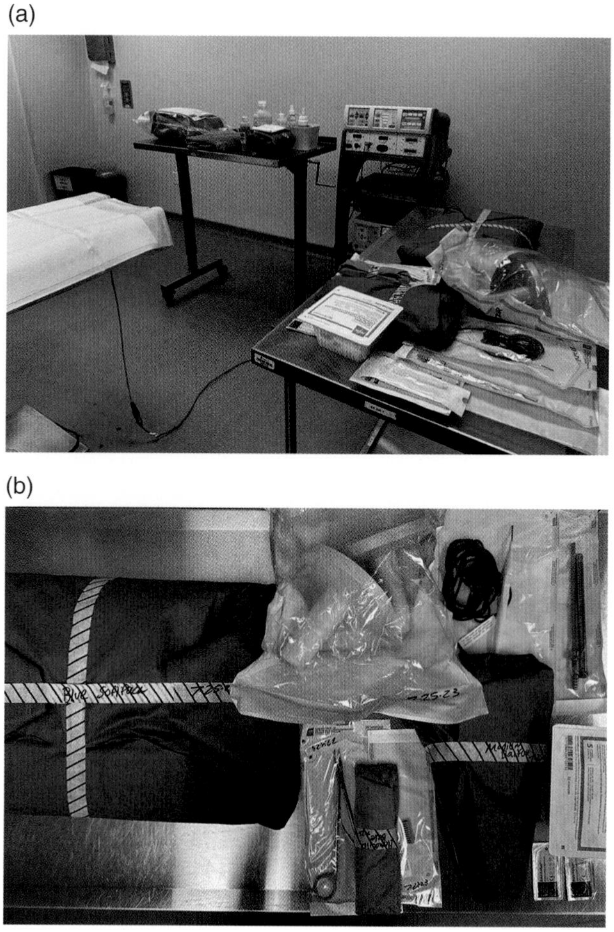

Figure 1.1 (a) Equipment and instrumentation in the operating room. (b) Instrumentation for an exploratory laparotomy laid out.

Male

The cranial and lateral shave margins will remain the same. The caudal clip should extend to the scrotal region in dogs, and if a urology procedure is being performed in cats, the caudal clip should extend dorsal to the prepuce. When shaving around the prepuce, care should be taken near the mucocutaneous junction to not nick the edges. After the clipping is complete, the prepuce should be flushed with diluted povidone-iodine using a syringe. This is done by grasping the edge of the prepuce, inserting the syringe tip, pinching the prepuce, and then injecting the povidone-iodine (Figure 1.6). While still pinching with one hand, massage the prepuce with the other hand to loosen any debris. Place an absorbent pad over the prepuce and expel the flush. This is repeated three times or until the flush is clear.

Female

In urology procedures, include the vulva in your shaving margins for intraoperative catheterization.

Splenectomy/Pyometra

- Soft pack/cautery/light handles
- (2) Poole suction tip
- Balfour
- Blue hemoclip set
- Ligasure
- ABD pads
- 4 mm biopsy punch
- Vetspon
- Extra brown tray

Dr. [redacted]
- LigaSure instrument tray
- Soft Gauze

Dr. [redacted]
- [redacted] Ligasure
- Left-Handed needle drivers

Dr. [redacted]
- Duraprep/Ioban

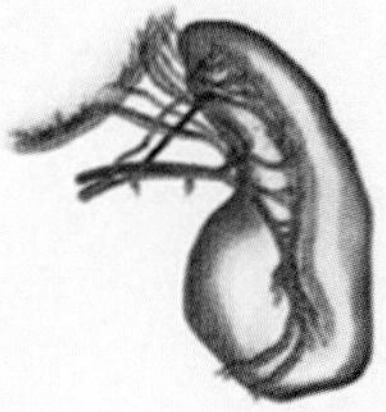

Position: Dorsal recumbency

Subcutaneous Ureteral Bypass (SUB Port)

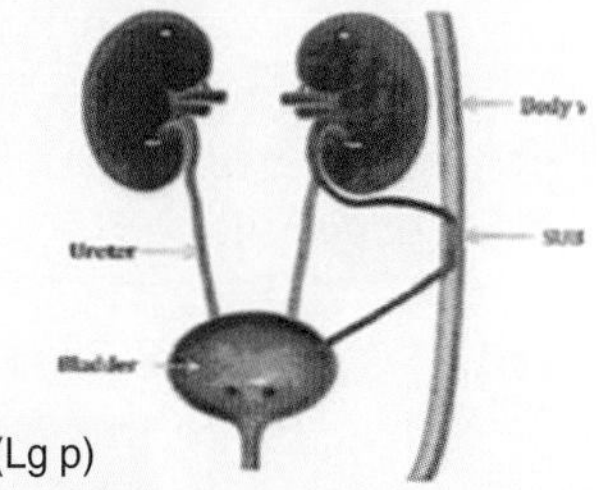

- Soft pack/cautery/light handles
- Poole suction tip
- Balfour
- Sharp senn
- Micro-Cooley needle driver
- Extra Sm towel clamps
- Malleables
- Patient drape
- C-arm drape
- Sterile skin glue
- Sub-port kit system per surgeon
- ABD pads
- CTA's
- 3-Way stop-cock
- Luer lock T-Port (Ax room)
- (3) 6 cc syringe
- 22 g IV catheter (Sm p) or 18g (Lg p)
- 3–0 Monocryl
- 3–0 Prolene
- Omnipaque - Please let O.R Tech know
- Syringe and needle (P dependent 1 ml/pound

Ex: P 10 pounds = 12 cc Syringe)

Position: Dorsal recumbency
Reminder: Normal Ex-Lap shave/need ***C-Arm & Table***

Figure 1.2 Example of a procedure instrument list.

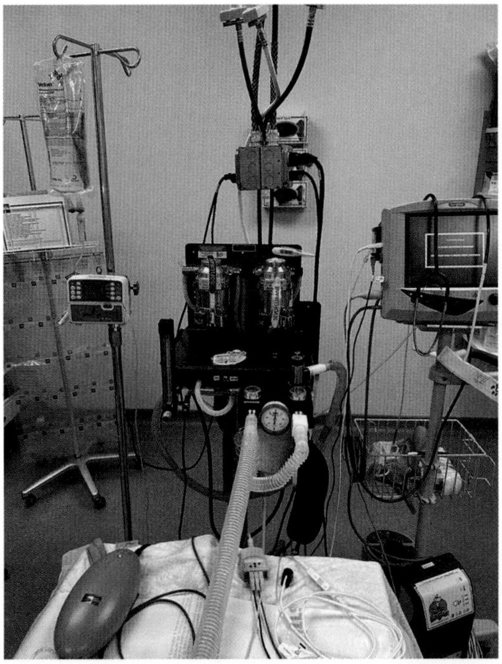

Figure 1.3 Anesthetic machine, intravenous fluids, monitoring equipment, and heating systems ready to be used.

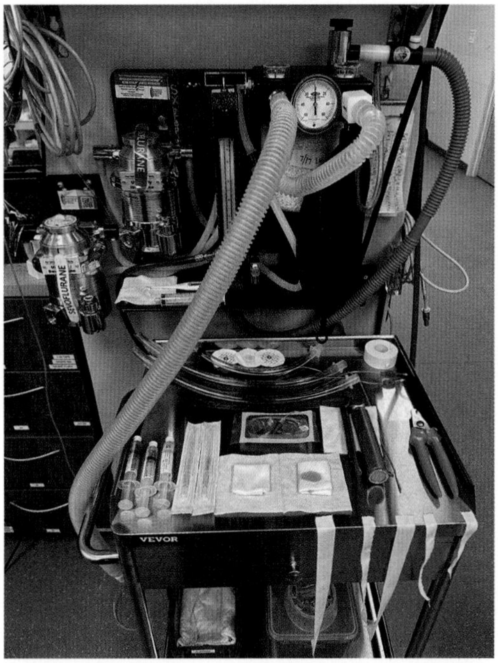

Figure 1.4 Induction area prepared.

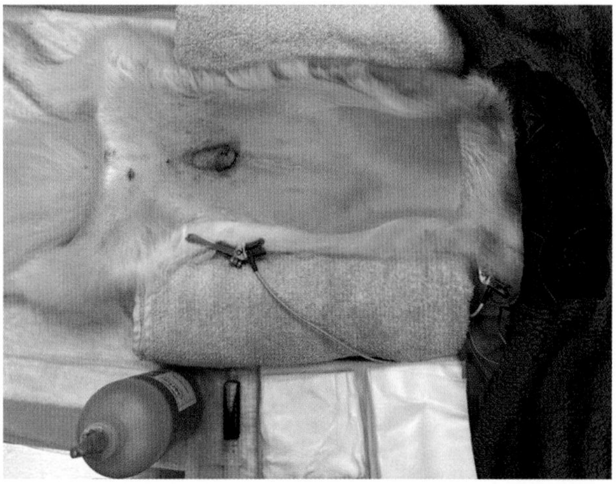

Figure 1.5 Patient has been shaved. Supplies for a "dirty" scrub are laid out.

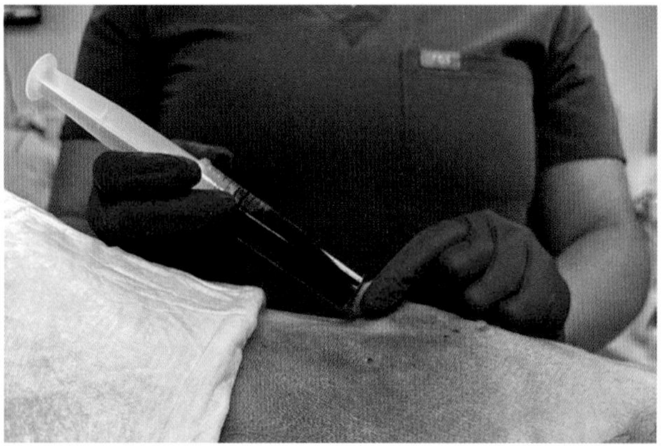

Figure 1.6 A syringe filled with diluted povidone-iodine being inserted inside the prepuce.

The technician should replace their gloves for the "dirty" scrub. Have two stacks of nonwoven gauze set aside. Keep one stack dry and the other one mildly dampened with water (Figure 1.5). Lightly pour chlorhexidine scrub onto the dampened gauze. Begin scrubbing from the center of the abdomen and continue moving outward in a spiral course until the shaved region has been covered. Avoid an aggressive scrubbing motion to reduce the risk of skin irritation and inflammation. Follow it with the dry gauze to clear excess lather. This combination is repeated a minimum of three times or until the gauze no longer contains visible debris. For long-haired patients, water or ultrasonic gel can be used to push the hair down to keep it away from the surgical field.

Transportation into the Operating Room

It is recommended to use a gurney as it is considered the safest method of patient transportation. The patient is moved onto the operating table and is placed in dorsal recumbency. The breathing circuit is once again connected to the patient, with oxygen and anesthetic gas turned back

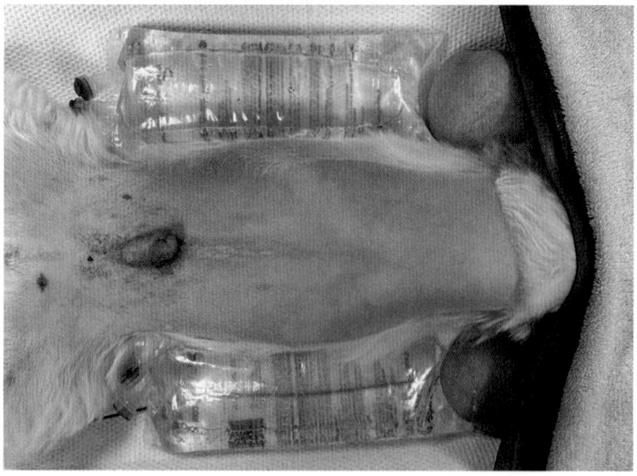

Figure 1.7 Patient is positioned on the operating room table with additional heat support provided by warmed bags of fluids and rice.

on. If the anesthesia machine has both sevoflurane and isoflurane capabilities, be sure that the correct gas is selected. Monitoring equipment, intravenous fluids, and heat support are applied to the patient (Figure 1.7). The anesthetist can administer the prophylactic antibiotic injection around this step or 30–60 minutes before the incision is made.

Positioning

Using a V-top operating table can help keep patients in dorsal recumbency. If using a flat-top table, a V-trough or sandbags can be used to assist in patient stabilization. To keep the sternum centered and prevent shifting, the patient's limbs should be secured with tape, ropes, or leashes. Distal limb perfusion is improved by spreading the forces applied circumferentially to the extremities. Caution should be exercised to prevent overtightening of the limb (Figure 1.8).

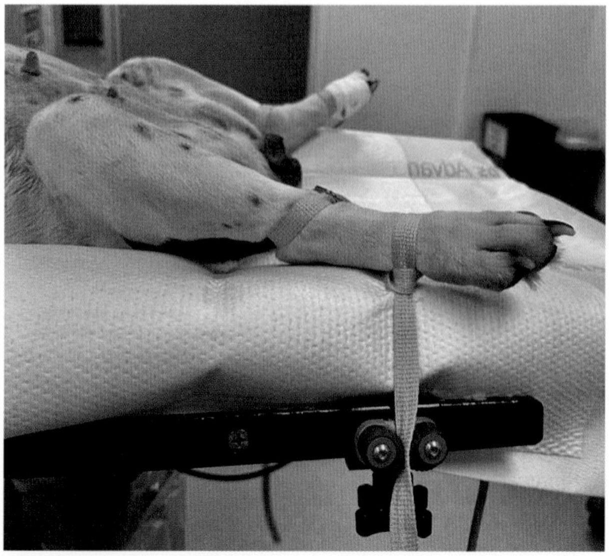

Figure 1.8 Patient's limbs safely secured.

Sterile Scrub

Patient is now ready for sterile preparation. Remove the cap from the sterile saline bottle and have chlorhexidine scrub set to the side. Open a sterile bowl containing a stack of sterile nonwoven gauze. Apply a sterile glove to the dominant hand only. Split the sterile gauze into two stacks with the dominant hand, leaving one stack inside the bowl and keeping the other stack dry outside of the bowl (Figure 1.9). With the nonsterile hand, pour sterile saline into the bowl until the gauze is well dampened. Lightly pour chlorhexidine scrub onto the dampened gauze. With the dominant hand, begin scrubbing from the center of the abdomen and continue moving outward in a spiral course until the shaved region has been covered. Do not scrub toward the center of the abdomen after touching any hair on the periphery; simply throw away that gauze after contacting the hair. Each chlorhexidine swipe should last approximately 60 seconds to allow adequate contact time, before wiping off with the sterile dry gauze. This combination is repeated a minimum of three times. If hair is touched, restart the count. Ensure the abdomen is completely dry prior to the surgeon starting surgery, especially if using alcohol-based scrub.

Draping

Open the general surgery pack (Figure 1.10) and the soft tissue instrument tray (Figure 1.11). Lay out a sterile gown and gloves for the person scrubbing in (Figure 1.12). From this point, each of the following tasks should be performed with the intent of avoiding contamination. Utilize a "four-quarter-drape" technique using the sterile surgical towels on the abdomen. Stepping away from the sterile field, open and hold a surgical towel. Use both hands to fold the top of the longest side away from the sterile assistant. Position each hand on the corners and wrap the towel around them, creating a cuff.

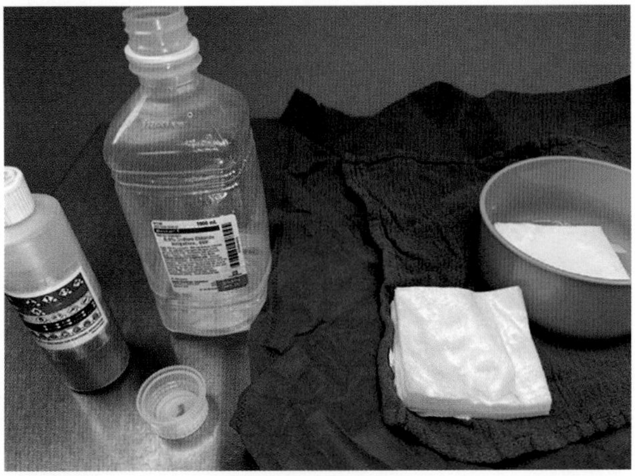

Figure 1.9 Supplies for a sterile scrub.

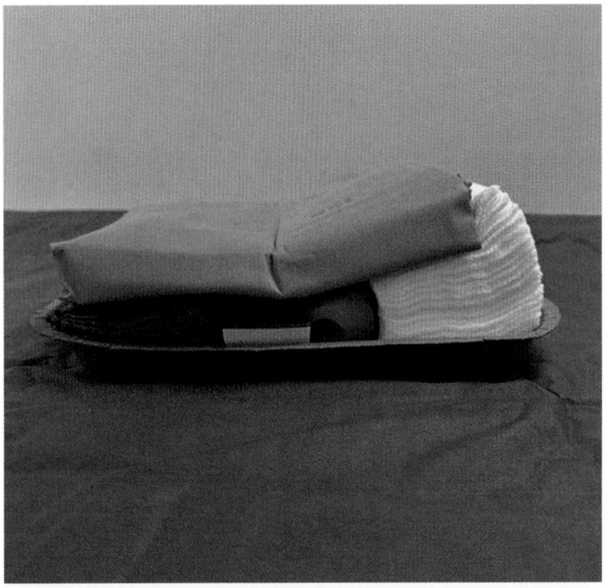

Figure 1.10 General surgery pack.

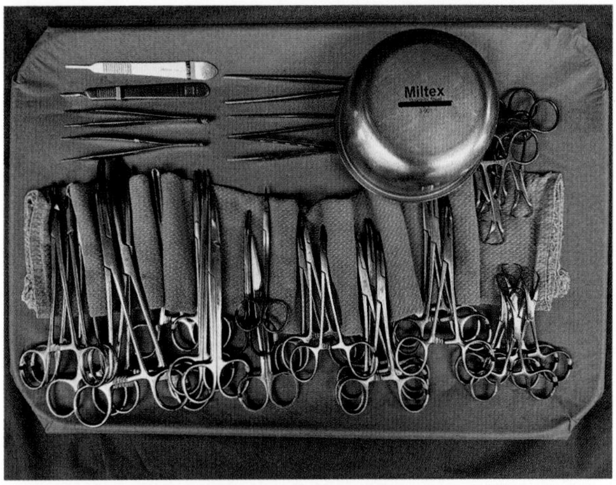

Figure 1.11 A soft tissue instrument tray.

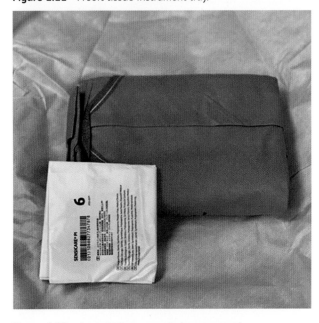

Figure 1.12 A surgical gown and gloves opened.

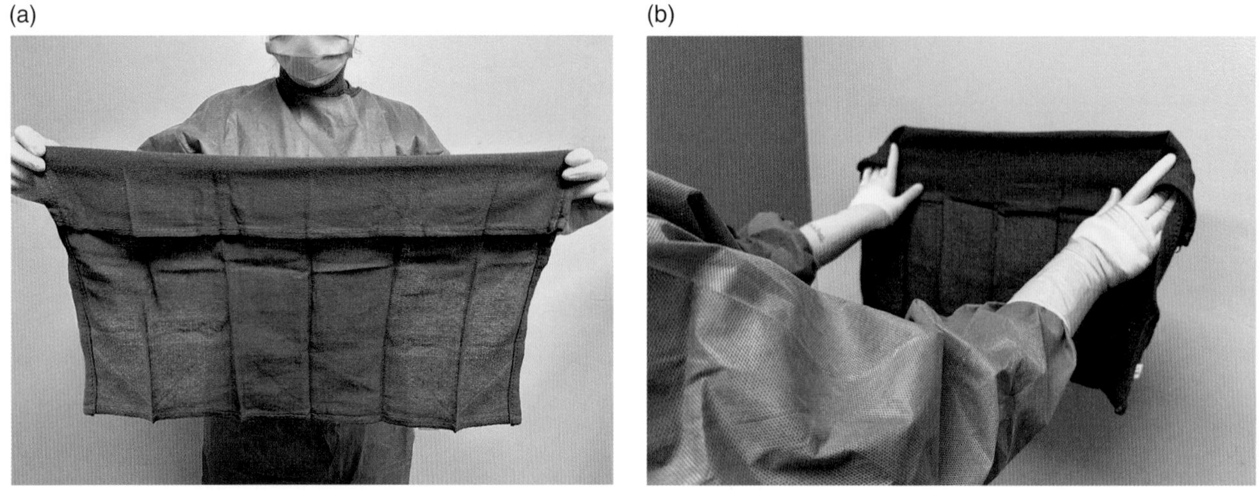

Figure 1.13 Folding of a towel drape. (a) Top of the drape is folded. (b) Drape is wrapped around each hand.

This will protect the sterile glove from contacting the patient while draping (Figure 1.13). While making sure the surgical gown does not touch the unsterile part of the table, place a towel cranially, caudally, then on the side nearest to the sterile assistant first, before placing a towel on the farthest side away from the assistant. Placement of the towels should be approximately 1-inch from the clipped hair. Sterile towels should not be dragged inward after being laid down, as this would no longer be considered sterile due to cross contamination. The corners where the towels meet should overlap each other. Next, place the towel clamps about 5 mm from the lateral aspects of the towel, penetrating both the towel and epidermis. Each towel clamp should only be tightened to the first ridge. Towels should be even and taut to prevent hair from entering the sterile field. For male patients, use a towel clamp to move the prepuce out of the surgical field away from the surgeon's side (Figure 1.14), unless the surgery involves assessing the urinary tract.

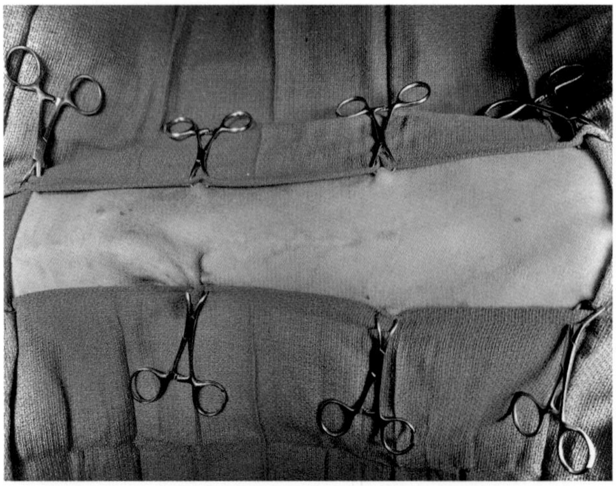

Figure 1.14 The prepuce is moved out of the surgical field using a Backhaus towel clamp.

A large patient drape sheet is then placed on top of the patient. Keeping one hand on the patient drape, start unfolding cranially and caudally, including the sterile instrument table to create one big sterile field. Open the drape toward the sterile assistant. Next, use both hands to spread open the rest of the drape while avoiding contact with the non-sterile table with the front of the sterile gown (Figure 1.15). Refrain from cutting a hole on the patient drape until instrumentation has been set up to reduce skin exposure.

Surgical Instrument Table

The patient and surgical instrument table should now be draped. Before an extra protective layer is added on top of the instrument table with a huck towel, any cord (e.g., monopolar or bipolar cautery and LigaSure) can be laid out and passed off to the circulating technician toward the back of the table to be plugged into their respective power sources. The towel drape will help the cords stay hidden and prevent them from getting in the way intraoperatively (Figure 1.16). If suction or any other connections are at the front end of the patient table, secure them with a spare traumatic forcep, like an Allis tissue forcep. Avoid using an atraumatic forcep, like a mosquito hemostatic forcep, to prevent the more delicate instruments from being damaged.

The soft tissue tray can now be placed on the instrument table with the rings of the instruments facing the surgeon. Instrumentation should be set out in the order that it will be utilized, and the dexterity of the surgeon should be considered (i.e., left- versus right-handed). A set of spare clean instruments (e.g., needle drivers, tissue forceps, and suture scissors) with new sterile gloves for the surgeon should be set to the side in "clean-contaminated" cases, such as gastrointestinal procedures, to reduce cross contamination (Figure 1.17). The circulating technician may begin

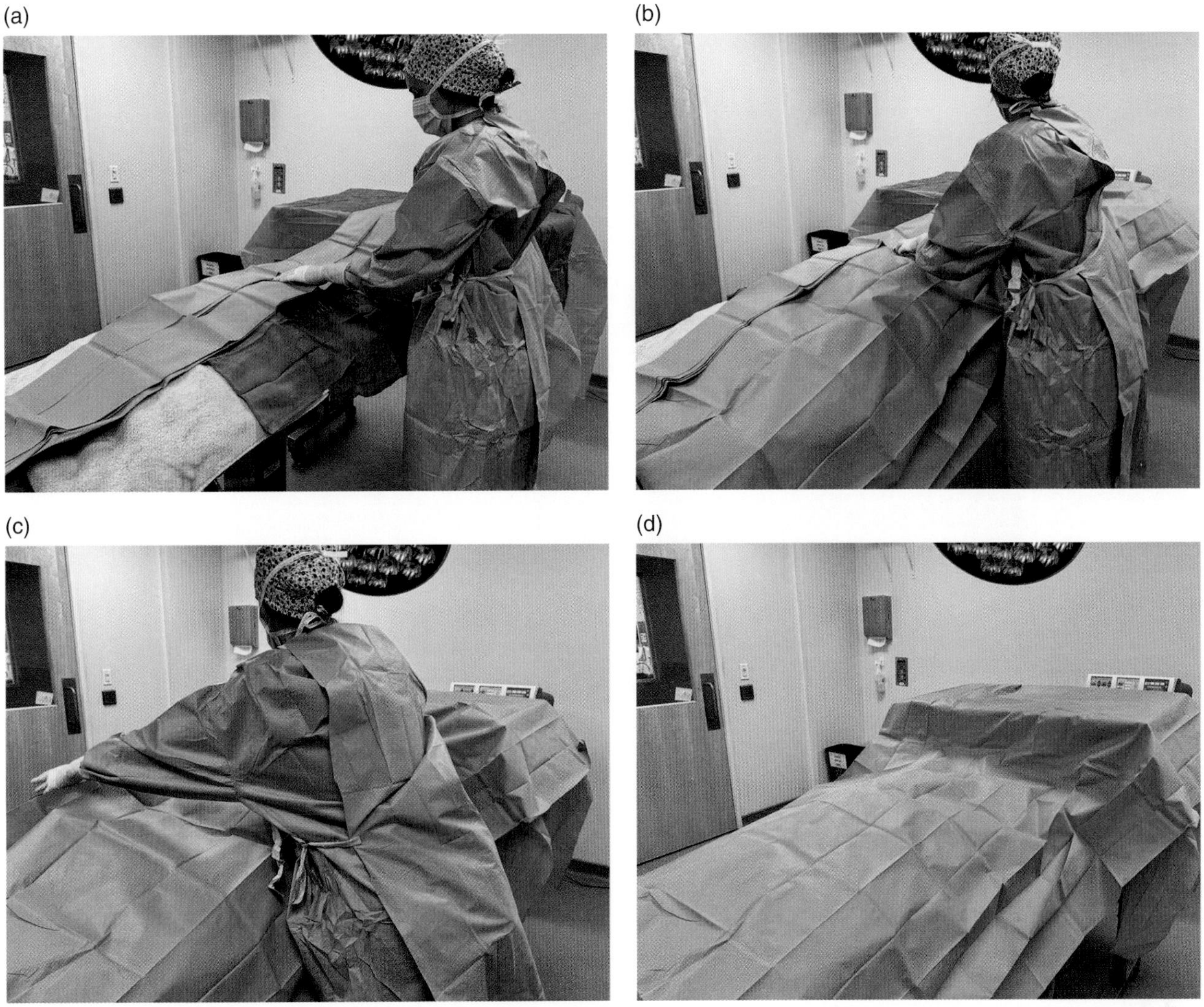

Figure 1.15 (a) A large drape is extended cranially and caudally. (b) The drape is unfolded toward the sterile assistant. (c) Both hands are used to spread open the rest of the drape. (d) One large sterile field is created.

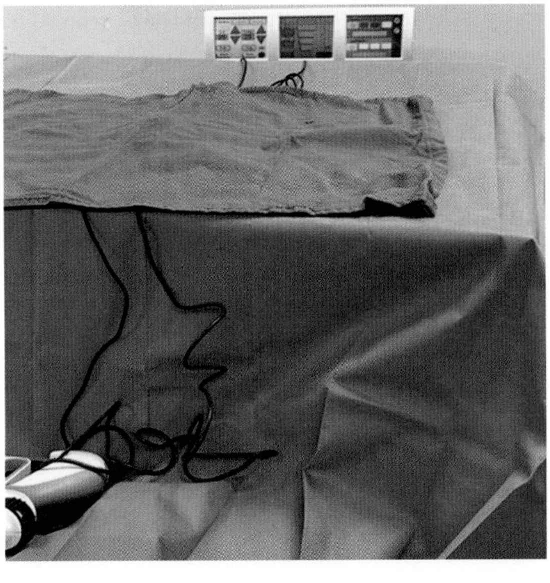

Figure 1.16 Sterile towel placed over excess cords to maintain a clean workspace.

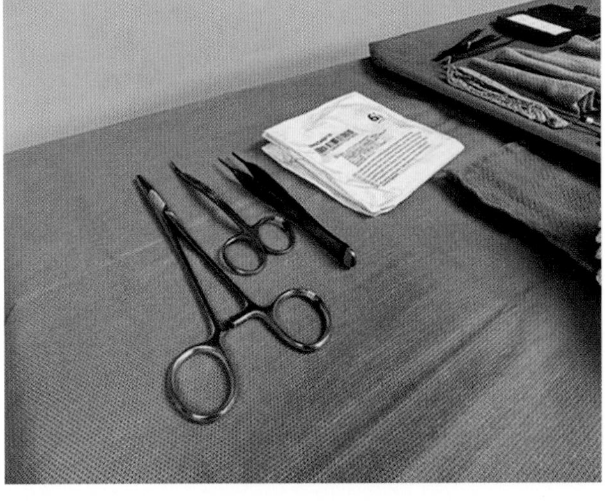

Figure 1.17 Sterile closing instruments saved at the back of the table during a clean-contaminated procedure.

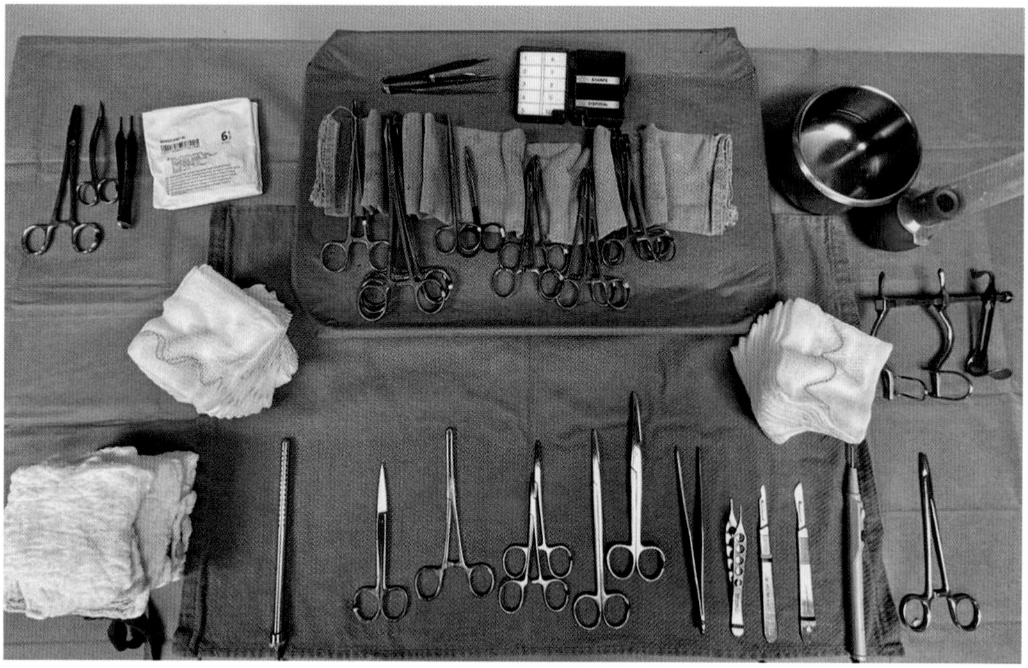

Figure 1.18 Complete instrument set-up.

opening more instruments (e.g., Balfour retractor, abdominal pads, and light handles). A sponge count should be completed, and scalpel blades are to be dropped last (Figure 1.18). Create a hole in the patient drape in a rectangular shape to expose the abdomen. Additional towel clamps on top of the patient drape may be used for extra security to prevent it from sliding and should ideally be non-penetrating through the patient drape (e.g., Lorna towel clamps) (Figure 1.19). The surgeon may want to place an incise drape (e.g., 3M™ Ioban™) over the abdomen. Ioban is an antimicrobial incise drape that adheres securely to the skin, designed to reduce the risk of surgical site infection. Another advantage of using an adhesive incise drape is that it allows the patient to stay warm and dry during lavaging of the abdomen.

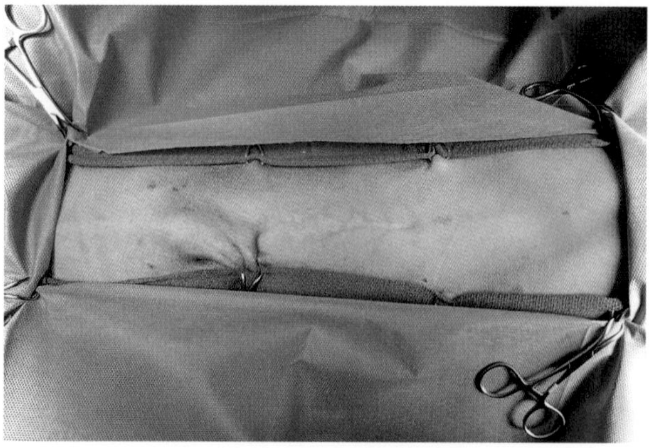

Figure 1.19 Towel clamps securing patient drape over the previously placed towel clamps for the quarter-draping. While the clamps pictured are Backhaus, the most appropriate clamps for securing the patient drape are nonpenetrating clamps, such as Lorna.

This completes the instrument table and patient setup.

Intraoperative Considerations

Checklist

Before the surgeon starts the incision, people in the operating room should introduce themselves and a technician will recite a safety checklist. A checklist helps ensure that important information has been gathered and reduces the potential for medical errors, thus, improving patient care (Figure 1.20).

The operating table should be adjusted to the surgeon's height to ensure good posture (Figure 1.21). The technician circulating should pay attention to the procedure and proactively anticipate the surgeon's needs throughout the entire surgery. Gauze, stapling equipment, or saline may need to be refilled, and the circulating technician should be prepared to refill these items or to obtain additional instrumentation if needed. All personnel should be cognizant of the operating room and respect the sterile field. The room should be kept clean and organized.

The scrub assistant should ensure tidiness of the instrument table. All used gauze should be placed into a designated counting area to ensure nothing is left behind inside

SURGERY SAFETY CHECKLIST

PRE-OP (Before Surgeon arrives)	INTRA-OP (To be read to surgeon)	POST-OP
☐ CPR ___ DNR ___ ☐ CPR sheet ☐ Confirm patient / Procedure / Positioning	Date: Procedure: ___ Surgeon: ___ Anesthetist: ___	☐ Sponge count complete or N/A Hemoclips used: #___ ☐ Marked stapling equipment
☐ Print signed est. ___ $? ___	☐ Anesthetic monitoring devices	☐ Scope/C-arm images iPad ___ Server ___
☐ Allergies? ___ Owner food?___	☐ Specific equipment available	☐ Scope Tower: Buttercup / Blossom / Bubbles
☐ Owner Meds?___	☐ Essential imaging displayed	☐ Confirm charges / Implants
☐ Radiograph request submitted: Pre-op___ Post-op ___ ☐ BW Requested ___ Submitted ___	☐ Gauze: #___ Soft: #___ or N/A Sponge: # ___ Hemoclips: #___	☐ Sharps safely removed ☐ Equipment problems recorded
☐ Reviewed By: ___	☐ Patient name/ Procedure/ Site/State	☐ Remove surgical footwrap or N/A
☐ Anesthetic protocol complete?	☐ Inform surgeon of CPR status	☐ Purse string/ Tampon removed or N/A
☐ Confirm surgical site: ___ ☐ Check skin or N/A	☐ Blades dropped	☐ Recovery concerns: ___ or none IMC vs ICU
Anesthesia machine check ☐ Prep ___ OR ___		☐ Express bladder or N/A (i.e. Epidural) ☐ Nail trim
☐ Antibiotic given or HOLD ☐ Pre-op Text sent		☐ 1st IVC Plan: IVF ___ CRI ___ Flush ___ 2nd Flush ___ Pull___
☐ RTC Time ___	Patient Label	☐ Specimens submitted to: ___ by:___ EVP-Ezyvet charge___
☐ Open Dr. WW Operating Report		☐ Remove ART line / Pressure wrap ☐ Cage card/Smartflow reflects patient's CPR status

Figure 1.20 An example of a surgery safety checklist.

the abdomen before the incision is closed. A kick bucket and a sponge counter bag are two examples of a designated counting area (Figure 1.22).

Anesthetist should monitor and record vital signs on a medical record every 5 min (Figure 1.23). It is important to communicate with the surgeon if a patient's vital signs are abnormal or if the patient's plane of anesthesia changes and intervention is needed. An emergency drug sheet tailored to the patient's weight should be readily available in the case of an emergency (Figure 1.24). The anesthetist may repeat the administration of antibiotic injection if needed. The patient's eyes should be lubed every 30 minutes to reduce the risk of corneal ulceration.

Postoperative Considerations

After the surgery is finished, sharp objects should be removed from the surgical field and all dirty instruments put away for cleaning. Gently remove the large patient drape and huck towels while being mindful of towel clamps. Clean around the incision site with saline. Once

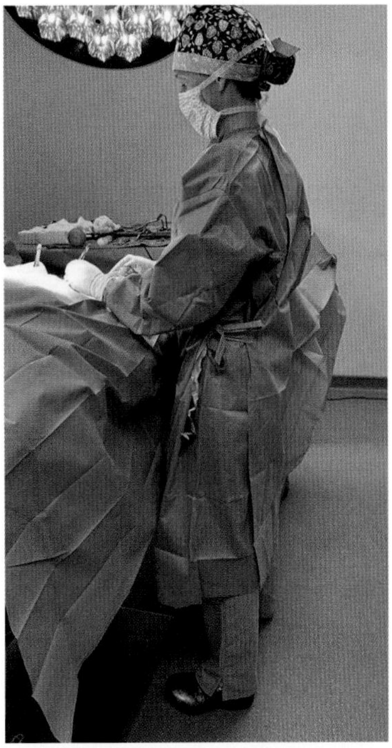

Figure 1.21 Table height is adequate for the surgeon. Arms are at an appropriate working angle of 90°.

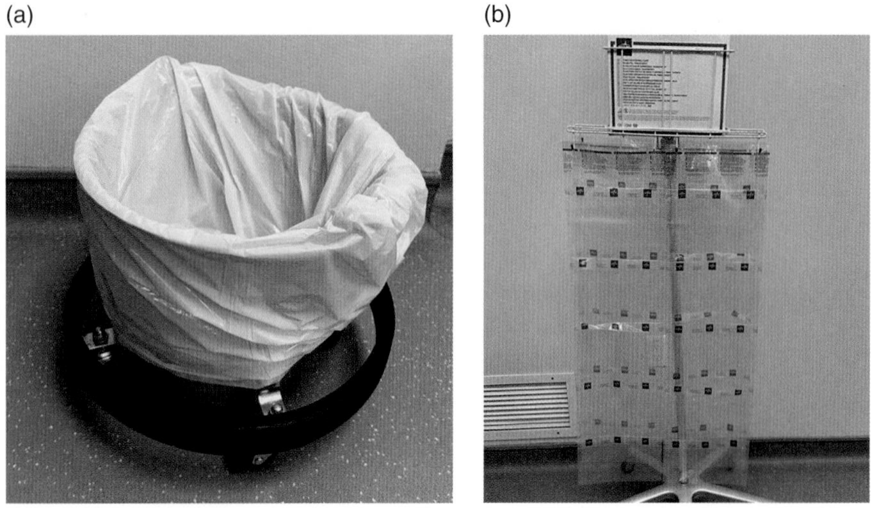

Figure 1.22 Example of a (a) kick bucket and a (b) sponge counter bag.

dry, apply an adhesive wound dressing (e.g., Primapore) to protect the incision for the first 24 hours after surgery (Figure 1.25). Before the patient is moved out of the operating room, ensure there is a recovery area ready for extubation and monitoring.

Recovery period can vary per patient, and it should never be rushed. Keep the patient warm, moisten the tongue, and apply lube to the eyes one more time. Before the anesthetic gas is completely off, ensure the patient has not regurgitated and needs attention. At this point, the patient's nails can be trimmed, anal sacs expressed, and ears cleaned if the patient is not in a critical state. Oxygenate the patient for 5 min after inhalant gas has been turned off. To prepare for extubation, the endotracheal tube's cuff should be completely deflated and untied. The technician should be prompt to react if the patient wakes up in a dysphoric state and needs protection from hurting themselves. The patient should be kept in the recovery area until the doctor is comfortable with the postoperative vital signs.

Before the patient is moved to its recovery kennel, ensure the kennel is prepared. Examples of a well-prepared kennel include having clean and comfortable bedding, heat support, infusion pumps, and an Elizabethan collar (Figure 1.26). The doctor's postoperative treatment plan should be followed and monitoring continued until the patient is discharged into their owner's care.

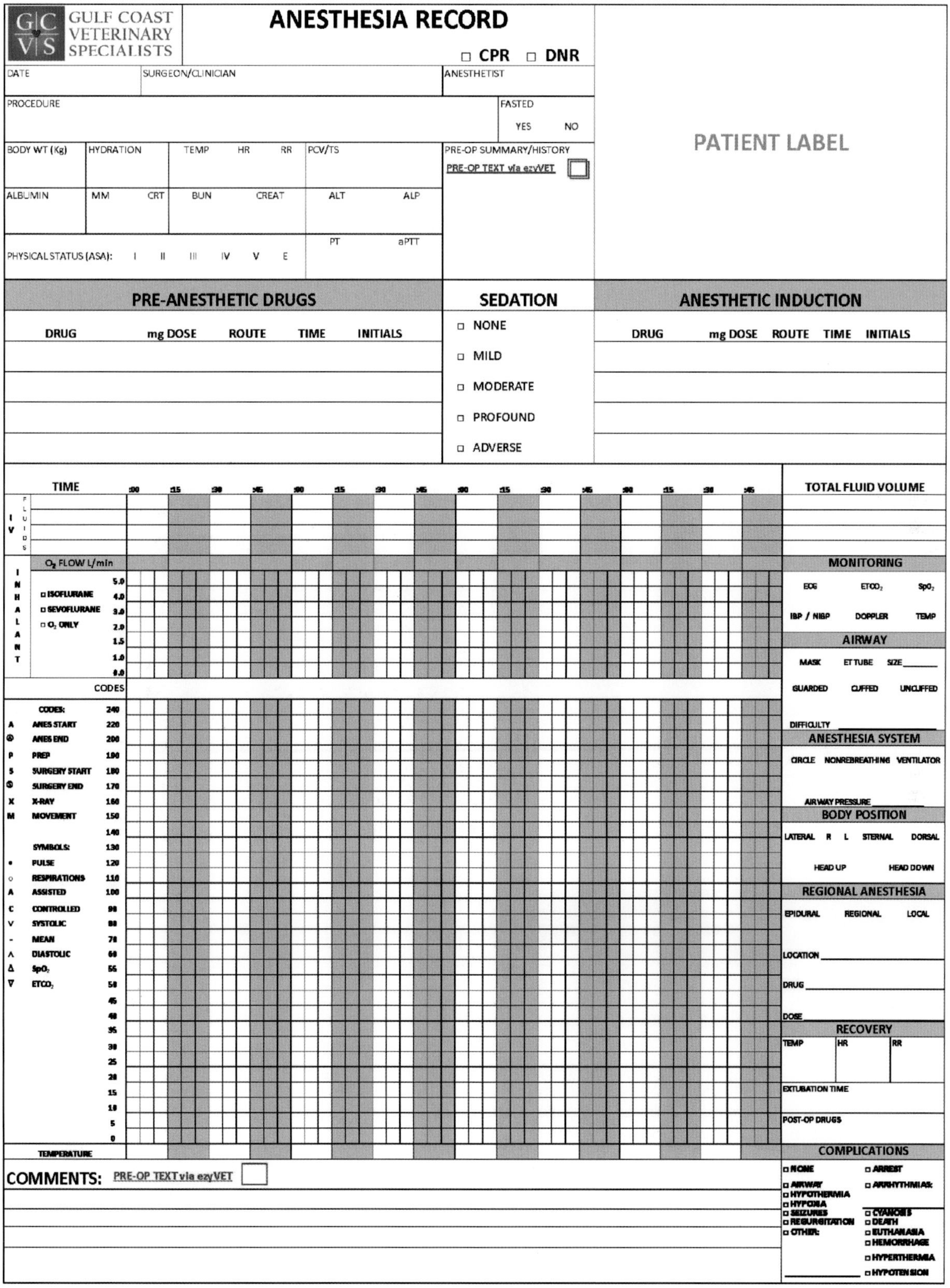

GULF COAST VETERINARY SPECIALISTS

ANESTHESIA RECORD

□ CPR □ DNR

DATE	SURGEON/CLINICIAN	ANESTHETIST

PROCEDURE	FASTED YES NO

BODY WT (Kg)	HYDRATION	TEMP HR RR	PCV/TS	PRE-OP SUMMARY/HISTORY PRE-OP TEXT via ezyVET □
ALBUMIN	MM CRT	BUN CREAT	ALT ALP	
PHYSICAL STATUS (ASA): I II III IV V E			PT aPTT	

PATIENT LABEL

PRE-ANESTHETIC DRUGS				
DRUG	mg DOSE	ROUTE	TIME	INITIALS

SEDATION

□ NONE
□ MILD
□ MODERATE
□ PROFOUND
□ ADVERSE

ANESTHETIC INDUCTION				
DRUG	mg DOSE	ROUTE	TIME	INITIALS

TIME :00 :15 :30 :45 :00 :15 :30 :45 :00 :15 :30 :45 :00 :15 :30 :45

IV FLUIDS

INHALANT: O_2 FLOW L/min; □ ISOFLURANE; □ SEVOFLURANE; □ O_2 ONLY; 5.0 4.0 3.0 2.0 1.5 1.0 0.0

CODES

CODES: A ANES START; ⊗ ANES END; P PREP; S SURGERY START; Ⓢ SURGERY END; X X-RAY; M MOVEMENT

SYMBOLS: • PULSE; ○ RESPIRATIONS; A ASSISTED; C CONTROLLED; V SYSTOLIC; - MEAN; Λ DIASTOLIC; Δ SpO_2; ∇ $ETCO_2$

240 220 200 190 180 170 160 150 140 130 120 110 100 90 80 70 60 55 50 45 40 35 30 25 20 15 10 5 0

TEMPERATURE

TOTAL FLUID VOLUME

MONITORING
ECG $ETCO_2$ SpO_2
IBP / NIBP DOPPLER TEMP

AIRWAY
MASK ET TUBE SIZE______
GUARDED CUFFED UNCUFFED
DIFFICULTY ______

ANESTHESIA SYSTEM
CIRCLE NONREBREATHING VENTILATOR
AIRWAY PRESSURE ______

BODY POSITION
LATERAL R L STERNAL DORSAL
HEAD UP HEAD DOWN

REGIONAL ANESTHESIA
EPIDURAL REGIONAL LOCAL
LOCATION ______
DRUG ______
DOSE ______

RECOVERY
TEMP | HR | RR
EXTUBATION TIME
POST-OP DRUGS

COMPLICATIONS
□ NONE □ ARREST
□ AIRWAY □ ARRHYTHMIAS:
□ HYPOTHERMIA
□ HYPOXIA
□ SEIZURES □ CYANOSIS
□ REGURGITATION □ DEATH
□ OTHER: □ EUTHANASIA
□ HEMORRHAGE
□ HYPERTHERMIA
______ □ HYPOTENSION

COMMENTS: PRE-OP TEXT via ezyVET □

Figure 1.23 A blank anesthesia medical record. See Chapter 37 (Figure 37.25) for an example of a filled in anesthesia record.

Patient name	Clyde Lopez	
Doctor	K.Coleman	
Weight		**5 kg**

Arrest	**Dose/kg**	**Patient dose**		**Concentration**	**Final dose in mL**	
Atropine	0.04 mg/kg	0.2 mg		0.4 mg/mL	0.5 mL	Atropine
Epinephrine (low dose)	0.01 mg/kg	0.05 mg		1 mg/mL	0.05 mL	Epinephrine
Epinephrine (high dose)	0.1 mg/kg	0.5 mg		1 mg/mL	0.5 mL	
Vasopressin	0.8 U/kg	4 U		20 U/mL	0.2 mL	
Diazepam	0.5 mg/kg	2.5 mg		5 mg/mL	0.5 mL	
Antiarrhythmic						
Amiodarone	5 mg/kg	2.5 mg		50 mg/mL	0.5 mL	
Lidocaine	2 mg/kg	10 mg		20 mg/mL	0.5 mL	
Reversal						
Atipamezole	100 mcg/kg	500 mcg		### mcg/mL	0.1 mL	
Flumazenil	0.01 mg/kg	0.05 mg		0.1 mg/mL	0.5 mL	
Naloxone	0.04 mg/kg	0.2 mg		0.4 mg/mL	0.5 mL	
Defibrillation						
Monophasic (external)	4–6 J/kg				20 J to	30J
Biphasic (external)	2–4 J/kg				10 J to	20J
Monophasic (internal)	0.5–1 J/kg				2.5 J to	5J
Biphasic (internal)	0.2–0.4 J/kg				1 J to	2J
Post Arrest						
7.2% NaCl	4 mL/kg (D) 2 mL/kg	20 ml Do 10 mL CAT			20 mL DO	10 mLCat
Mannitol	0.5 g/kg 15–20 min	2.5 g		0.2 g/mL	12.5 mL	
Dobutamine	1–10 mcg/kg/min	5 mcg	100 mcg			
Dopamine (CRI, low)	1–10 mcg/kg/min	25 mcg	50 mcg			
Dopamine (CRI, high)	10–15 mcg/kg/min	50 mcg	75 mcg			
Norepinephrine	0.05–0.1 mcg/kg/min	0.25 mcg	0.5 mcg			
Vasopressin (CRI)	0.5–5 mU/kg/min	2.5 mU	2.5 mU			
Glycopyrrolate	0.011 mg/kg/min	0.06 mg		0.2 g/mL	0.28 mL	

Figure 1.24 An emergency drug sheet.

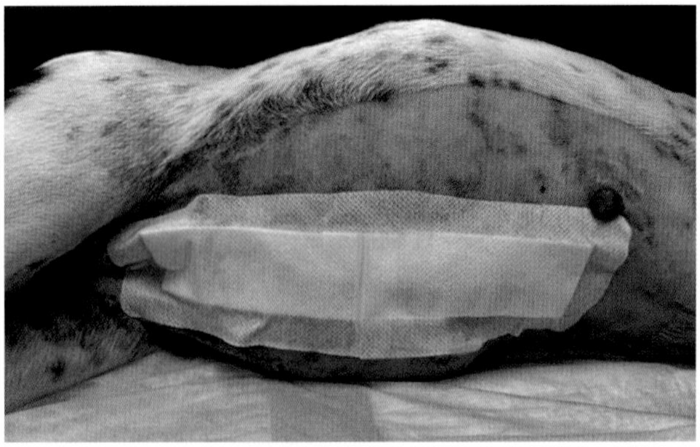

Figure 1.25 A Primapore applied along the incision.

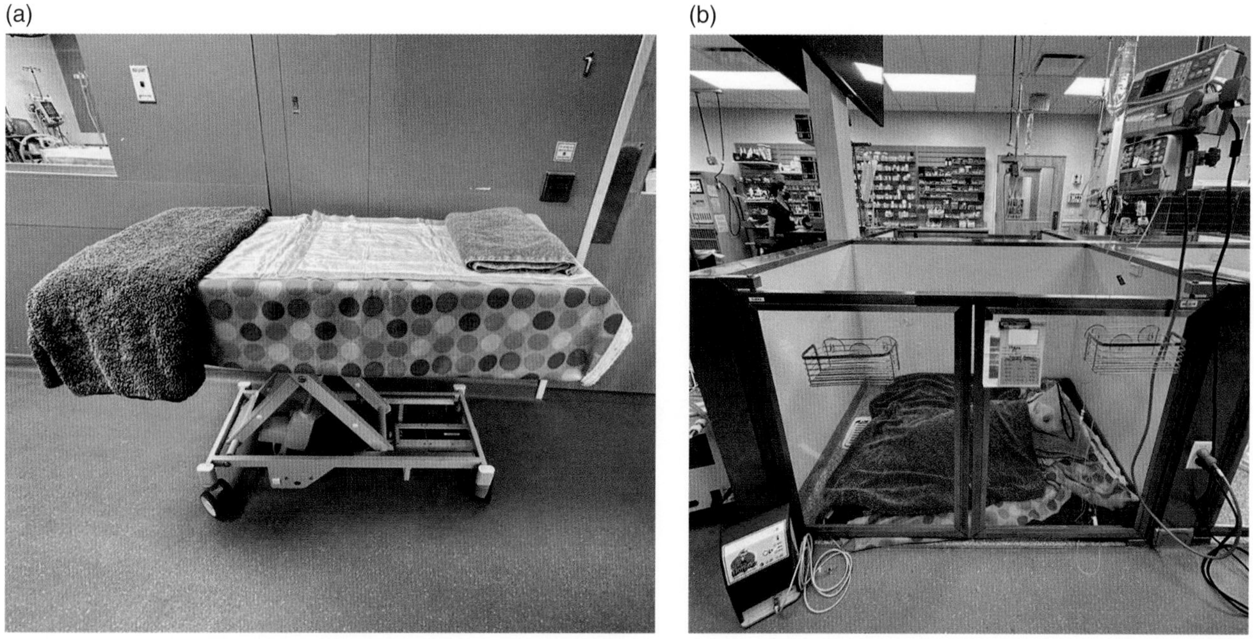

Figure 1.26 Moving patient to recovery. (a) Gurney for transportation. (b) Patient inside the kennel.

2

Steps for Simple Eyelid Mass Removal

Robin Sankey

North Houston Veterinary Ophthalmology, Spring, TX, USA

Key Points

- Eyelid anatomy is important to consider before removal of eyelid masses since anatomical apposition of the eyelids is crucial for proper eyelid function.
- The majority of eyelid masses are benign in dogs, but if an eyelid mass is affecting more than a quarter of the eyelid margin, the patient has cancer elsewhere in the body, a mass has been removed in the same area before, or if the mass is ulcerated, a preoperative biopsy or fine needle aspirate is recommended for proper surgical planning.
- The majority of eyelid masses in cats are malignant, so a presurgical fine needle aspirate or biopsy is recommended.
- Either a V-lid or pentagonal-shaped blepharoplasty is appropriate for removal of masses that affect less than ⅓ of the eyelid margin.
- Debulking eyelid masses with adjunct cryotherapy is another technique that is often successful in the treatment of larger eyelid masses.
- Healing of the eyelid takes 10–14 days following full-thickness mass excision, and a hard plastic cone collar is recommended during this time.

Function and Anatomy

The eyelids are very important for ocular health and have many important functions, including protection of the globe, entrapment and removal of corneal and conjunctival debris, distribution of the tear film, and the production of glandular secretions that prevent the tear film from prematurely evaporating.[1] The upper and lower eyelids are lined by 30–40 small openings of the meibomian gland, which are not only important because they secrete the outer oily layer of the tear film but are also an important landmark used to ensure proper apposition of the eyelid following mass removal (Figure 2.1). The meibomian glands form the "gray line" along the eyelid margin.

Histologically, the eyelids consist of four parts. The outermost layer is continuous with the adjacent skin. The orbicularis oculi muscle layer is just deep to the skin, followed internally by a tarsal plate and stromal layer, and the innermost layer, the palpebral conjunctiva.[2] The tarsal plate is formed of fibrous connective tissue and gives the eyelid its structure. The palpebral conjunctiva refers to the conjunctiva that lines the eyelids, whereas the bulbar conjunctiva is the conjunctiva that covers the globe (or eyeball).

Indications

There are many reasons eyelid masses should be removed, including suspected or confirmed neoplasia, local or corneal irritation or ulceration, or growth of the mass that may interfere with a straightforward removal in the future. In dogs, eyelid tumors are very common, but most are benign. However, if a mass is severely ulcerated, excessively large, or appears highly invasive, then a presurgical biopsy is recommended. Eyelid tumors are much less common in cats and are more likely to be malignant. Up to 91%

Techniques in Small Animal Soft Tissue, Orthopedic, and Ophthalmic Surgery, First Edition. Edited by Kristin A. Coleman.

Companion website: www.wiley.com/go/coleman/surgeries

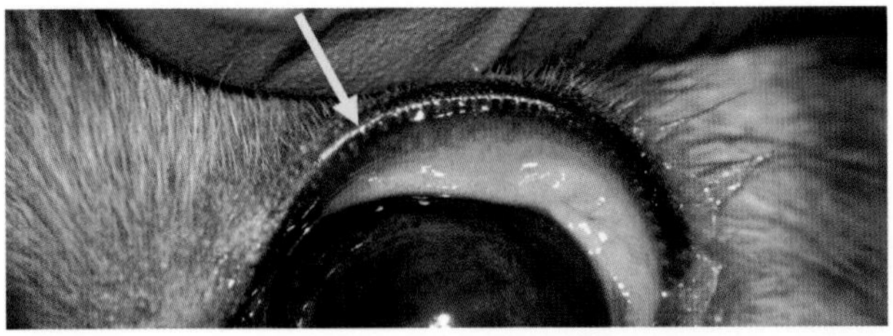

Figure 2.1 One of the many meibomian gland openings indicated by the yellow arrow used as a guide for suture placement with eyelid reconstruction. *Source:* © Robin Sankey.

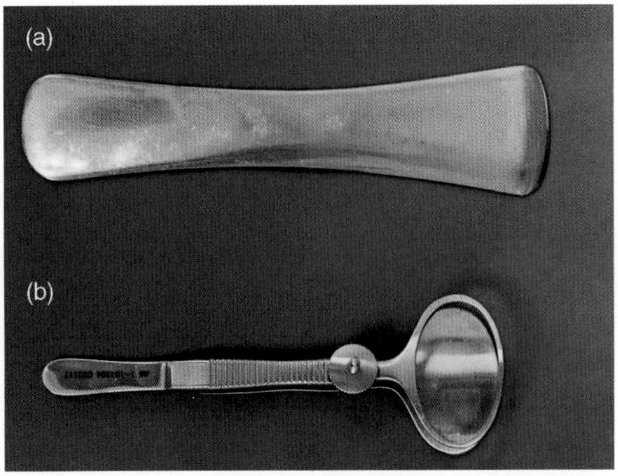

Figure 2.2 Two instruments used to stabilize the eyelid margin during mass excision. (a) Jaeger eyelid plate; (b) chalazion clamp. *Source:* © Robin Sankey.

of eyelid tumors in cats are malignant, so biopsy or a fine needle aspirate is recommended for cats with eyelid tumors so a surgical plan can be formulated before full-thickness surgical excision.[3] The high rate of malignancy in cats is compared with that in dogs, where 92.4% of eyelid masses were benign.[4]

Techniques

There are multiple methods in the literature utilized for eyelid mass removal including, hyperthermic therapy, carbon dioxide laser therapy, radiation therapy, chemotherapy, immunotherapy, and photodynamic therapy, in addition to the surgical techniques discussed in this chapter. However, these methods often require expensive equipment and have not proven to offer better results than surgical methods.[5] Two main surgical techniques for removing eyelid masses affecting less than one-third of the eyelid margin are a V-shaped blepharoplasty and a pentagonal (house-shaped) blepharoplasty. According to current literature, as long as the excised portion of the eyelid margin does not exceed 1/4–1/3 of the affected eyelid length, it can be removed by one of these techniques.[5] If a mass approaches one-third or more of the eyelid margin, it is better to consider referral to an ophthalmologist for a grafting procedure that will prevent excessive shortening of the eyelid margin length. Many grafting techniques are described, but that is beyond the scope of this chapter.

V-Lid Blepharoplasty

This technique is very straightforward to perform for masses that affect less than one-third of the eyelid margin. General anesthesia is typically needed, and the patient is prepped by clipping the hair from the surgical area and cleaning the area with a dilute betadine solution. A 1:50 solution is prepared by diluting betadine solution with a sterile fluid, such as 0.9% sodium chloride or sterile water. Avoid the use of betadine scrub, chlorhexidine, or agents containing alcohol, as these products cause corneal injury.[6] A small amount (0.1–0.3 mL) of local anesthetic, such as lidocaine, bupivacaine, or ropivacaine, injected subdermally around the mass to be excised allows the patient to be maintained under a lighter plane of anesthesia.

A Jaeger Eyelid Plate or chalazion clamp is used to stabilize the eyelid margin (Figure 2.2), while calipers are used to measure the length of the eyelid margin that will be removed, which is most easily done while the eyelid is stabilized. The height of the excision should be twice that of the length of the eyelid margin to be excised. This can be marked using a sterile surgical marker, or a mental note can be made based on the measurement. Next, while holding the eyelid taut over the eyelid plate or within the chalazion clamp, a half-thickness skin incision is made with a surgical blade (usually a #15 Bard-Parker blade, a #64 Beaver blade, or a #69 Beaver blade) in the shape of a V, which is inverted for the removal of upper eyelid masses. Remember, the height of the V should be twice that of the length of the eyelid margin to be removed. This is important to prevent puckering of the skin when the incision is closed. For example, if the length of the area of the eyelid margin to be removed is 4 mm, then the height of the incision would be 8 mm (Figure 2.3). As long as the eyelid mass is expected to be benign, 0.5–1 mm of the eyelid should be removed on either side of the mass. After the partial-thickness cut has been made using the blade, the lid plate or chalazion clamp is removed, the eyelid is stabilized with forceps, and scissors are used to create the full-thickness incision of the incised area. Steven's tenotomy scissors or delicate Metzenbaum scissors are ideal for this step.

There are a few ways to effectively close the defect. The most effective way to close the eyelid margin is with a figure-of-8 suture, which is named because it is shaped like the number eight. The eyelid margin is closed first with a figure-of-8 suture leaving the suture tails long (Figure 2.4).

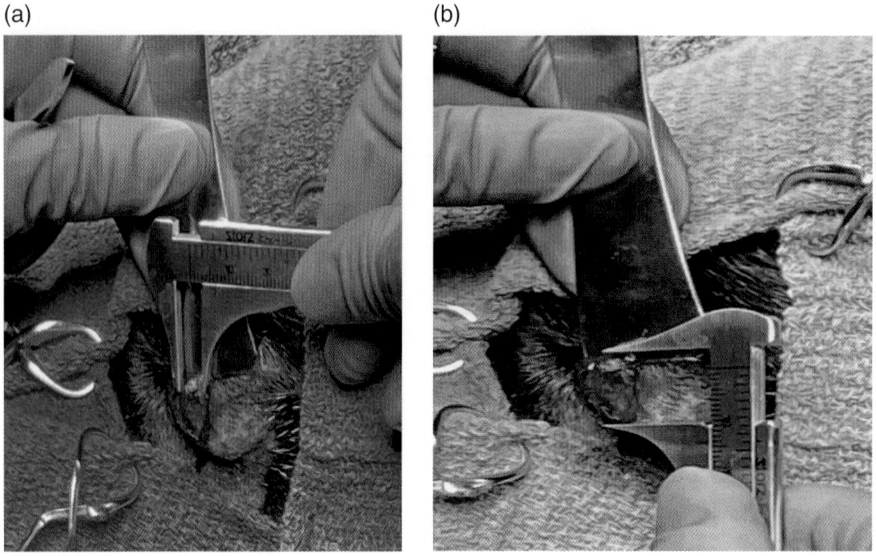

Figure 2.3 Determination of eyelid tissue to be removed. (a) Calipers are used to measure the length in millimeters of the eyelid margin that needs to be removed; (b) the height of the incision should be twice the width. *Source:* © Robin Sankey.

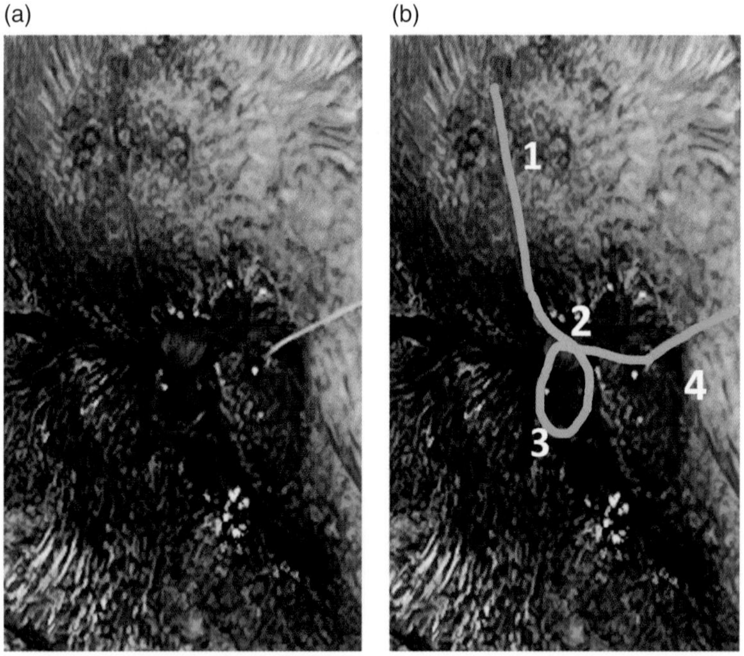

Figure 2.4 How to place a figure-of-8 suture at the eyelid margin. (a) Intra-operative picture of the figure-of-8 suture being placed; (b) using the same image as (a) with color drawn onto the suture, the numbers indicate the order in which the suture bites are taken through the eyelid to create the figure-of-8 suture pattern. The blue line indicates the external portion of the pattern, while the yellow lines indicate the buried portion of the suture pattern. Once the final knot is tied, it resembles a number eight. *Source:* © Robin Sankey.

This is where the gray line of the meibomian glands can be very useful. Use the meibomian gland openings to guide the placement of the suture evenly across the eyelid margin on both sides of the defect. The suture is passed through a meibomian gland opening, and the meibomian gland openings are used to confirm equidistant suture placement on both sides of the incision (Figure 2.5). Some advocate placing an interrupted suture adjacent to the eyelid margin and not across the new eyelid margin, as is done with the figure-of-8 sutures, but this often results in a stair-stepped appearance to the eyelid, which can interfere with normal eyelid function.[5]

The eyelid margin is closed with a 5-0 or 6-0 absorbable braided suture in a simple interrupted pattern. The author

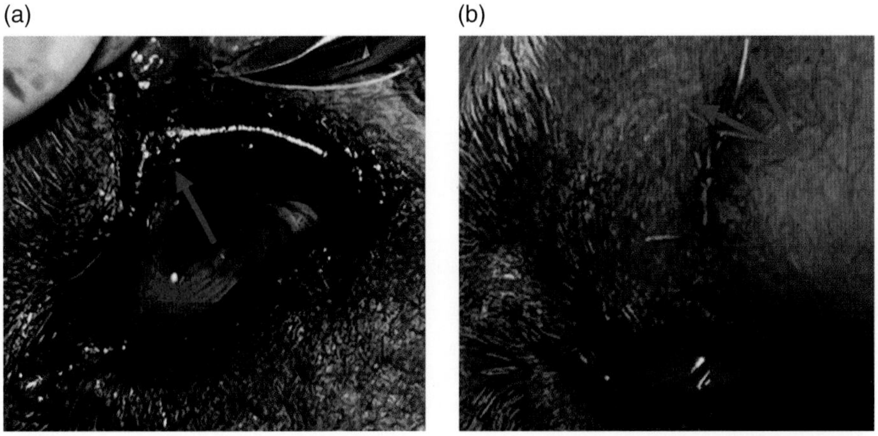

Figure 2.5 Figure-of-8 suture. (a) Proper placement of figure-of-8 suture at the eyelid margin. Note the edges of the newly formed eyelid margin line up; (b) completed closure. Note that the suture tails from the figure-of-8 suture have been trapped away from the eye in additional interrupted sutures placed to close the skin defect. *Source:* © Robin Sankey.

prefers 6-0 polyglactin 910 with a 10 mm ½ circle reverse cutting needle, partially due to the relatively soft texture of the multifilament suture considering the close proximity to the eye. Next, the remaining defect is closed with additional interrupted sutures. This can be done with either 5-0 or 6-0 suture and should be based on the eyelid thickness. For dogs with delicate eyelids, such as Poodles, Shih Tzus, and cats, typically 6-0 polyglactin 910 is used. However, in bulldogs and larger breeds, 5-0 polyglactin 910 is preferable due to the increased thickness of the eyelid. The deeper tarsoconjunctival layer can be closed first with either interrupted sutures or a single horizontal mattress suture, but it is important that the suture material be entirely within the tarsoconjunctival plane and should not be placed full-thickness due to the risk of corneal irritation or ulceration. The knots should be buried within this tarsoconjunctival layer. The skin and associated muscle layer should be closed with additional interrupted sutures, trapping the suture tails from the figure-of-8 suture away from the ocular surface to decrease the risk of corneal ulceration (Figure 2.5). A study performed to evaluate one- versus two-layered closure after eyelid mass resection with a V-shaped blepharoplasty did not find a significant difference in eyelid function and cosmetic outcome between the one- and two-layer closure techniques. Personally, if the defect is large, a two-layer closure is utilized by placing a single horizontal mattress suture in the tarsoconjunctival layer before the closure of the more superficial muscle and skin layer, but for smaller defects, a single-layer closure method is utilized.[5]

Pentagonal (House-Shaped) Blepharoplasty

This technique is another way an eyelid mass can be effectively removed, and the decision on whether to use the V-lid technique or the pentagonal technique is based on surgeon preference. The author tends to base it on the shape that will fit best around the mass. If the mass is small, the author utilizes the V-lid technique, but if the mass has a wide base, the pentagonal blepharoplasty technique is used. With this technique, the eyelid margin is stabilized with a Jaeger lid plate or chalazion clamp, while a pentagonal or house-shaped incision is made surrounding the mass (Figure 2.6). The same rules apply to the incision height being twice that of the length removed at the eyelid margin. The defect is first incised to partial thickness and then removed to full thickness with either tenotomy or fine Metzenbaum scissors as described for the V-lid blepharoplasty. The closure is the same as for the V-lid blepharoplasty. It is always recommended that histopathology be performed even if a benign mass is expected.

Cryotherapy

Cryotherapy is typically used as an adjunct therapy after debulking of an eyelid mass. Cryotherapy typically involves the use of liquid nitrogen transferred from a storage dewar into a portable canister for use. Liquid nitrogen liquefies at −196 °C, so it can cause rapid tissue death.[7] Cryotherapy works well for small, pedunculated masses that affect the eyelid margin or for some larger masses in which owners will not consider referral for a full-thickness excision and grafting procedure with a veterinary ophthalmologist. Since eyelid masses are more common in older patients, debulking and cryotherapy may be the preferred option for patients with increased risk under general anesthesia since sedation and local anesthetic are sometimes sufficient. Following prepping of the area as described for full-thickness removal, subdermal injection of 0.1–0.3 mL of a local anesthetic, such as lidocaine, bupivacaine, or ropivacaine, using a

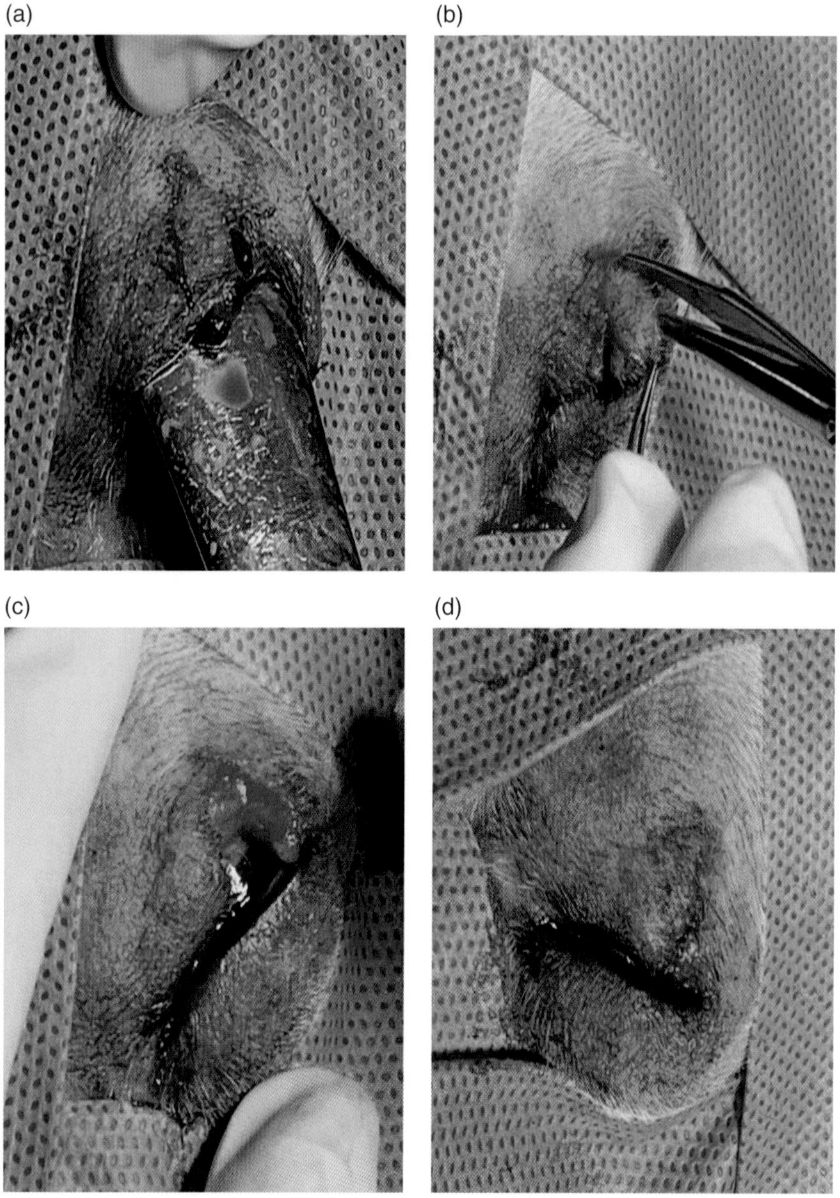

Figure 2.6 Steps for pentagonal (house-shaped) blepharoplasty. (a) The eyelid margin is stabilized with an eyelid plate and a partial-thickness incision is made around the mass and associated eyelid margin in a house-shape; (b,c) full-thickness excision of the eyelid mass and periocular skin; (d) post-closure after the figure-of-8 suture has been placed at the eyelid margin and three additional interrupted sutures have been placed to close the defect and trap the figure-of-8 suture tails away from the eyelid margin. *Source:* © Robin Sankey.

25-gauge needle is recommended (Figure 2.7). If the mass is small and pedunculated and does not extend to the palpebral conjunctival surface of the eyelid, the mass can be cut flush with the eyelid margin using Steven's tenotomy scissors or other delicate scissors, and any inspissated contents expressed with Alabama forceps, between two sterile cotton-tipped applicators, or with digital pressure (Figure 2.8). If the mass extends through to the palpebral conjunctiva, it is recommended to make a small stab incision over the mass on the palpebral conjunctival surface of the eyelid, and the contents can then be either expressed and/or debulked with a small curette or scissors.

Once the external portion of the mass has been excised and the internal contents removed, it is important to protect the corneal and periocular area before cryotherapy. Towels are placed around the patient, and a corneal shield is used to protect the cornea. Corneal shields come in different sizes, and an artificial tear or antibiotic ointment should be applied to the inside of the shield before placing it against the cornea (Figure 2.9). If you do not have a

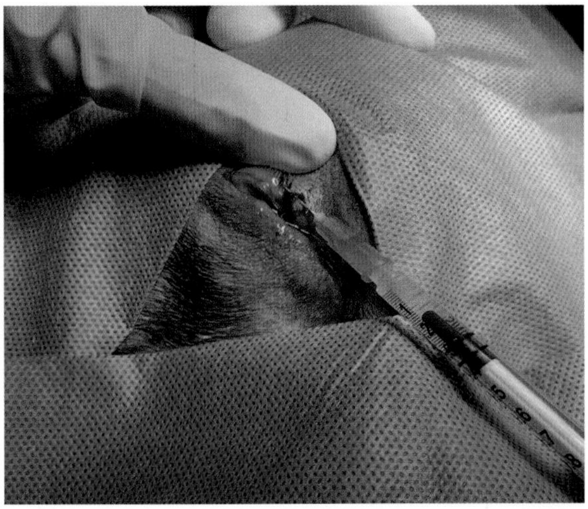

Figure 2.7 Local anesthetic injected subdermally beneath the mass(es) to be removed. *Source:* © Robin Sankey.

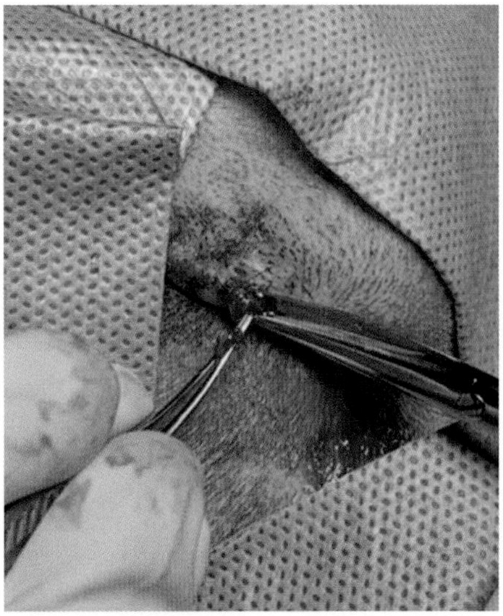

Figure 2.8 Debulking of eyelid mass flush with the eyelid margin. *Source:* © Robin Sankey.

(a) (b)

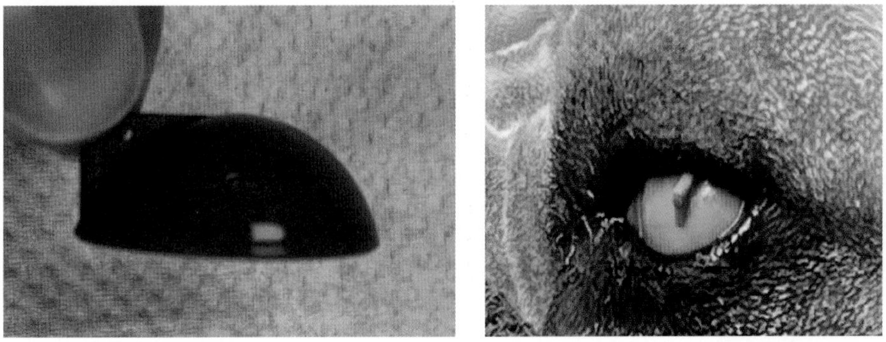

Figure 2.9 (a) Corneal shield; (b) corneal shield placed on a dog's eye after filling the shield with a lubricating ointment or gel. Corneal shields are available in different sizes. *Source:* © Robin Sankey.

corneal shield, a piece of a styrofoam cup can also be used and placed over a well-lubricated cornea within the palpebral fissure in lieu of the corneal shield (Figure 2.11). A probe tip can be used for smaller, well-circumscribed masses, whereas a spray tip for the liquid nitrogen canister can be used in lieu of the probe tip for application following the debulking of larger masses (Figures 2.10 and 2.11). Liquid nitrogen is applied in two to three freeze, slow thaw cycles, depending on if the animal has thin eyelids (Poodles, Shih Tzus, etc.) or if the animal has thicker eyelids (Bulldogs, giant breeds, etc.). If using a probe tip, liquid nitrogen can be applied either 3 mm below the eyelid margin for larger masses or at the eyelid margin for smaller masses and is held in place until an ice ball forms and extends 2–3 mm beyond the probe. Freezing is repeated once the area has completely thawed, which typically takes 45–60 seconds.[8] When using a spray, the tip is held about 1/8 in. from the eyelid surface and the liquid nitrogen is sprayed for 10–20 seconds, depending on the size of the area to be frozen. The area is then allowed to thaw completely before the cycle is repeated. Typically, the defect is left to heal by second intention. However, if the defect is large, the defect can be primarily closed with 5-0 or 6-0 suture (Figure 2.12).

Postoperative Care

For full-thickness eyelid mass excisions, all animals should be sent home with a hard plastic Elizabethan collar to be worn until their follow-up recheck two weeks later to protect the delicate eyelid margin. Typically, the Elizabethan collar is not needed as long for debulking procedures as long as sutures are not placed. The length of time the

(a) (b)

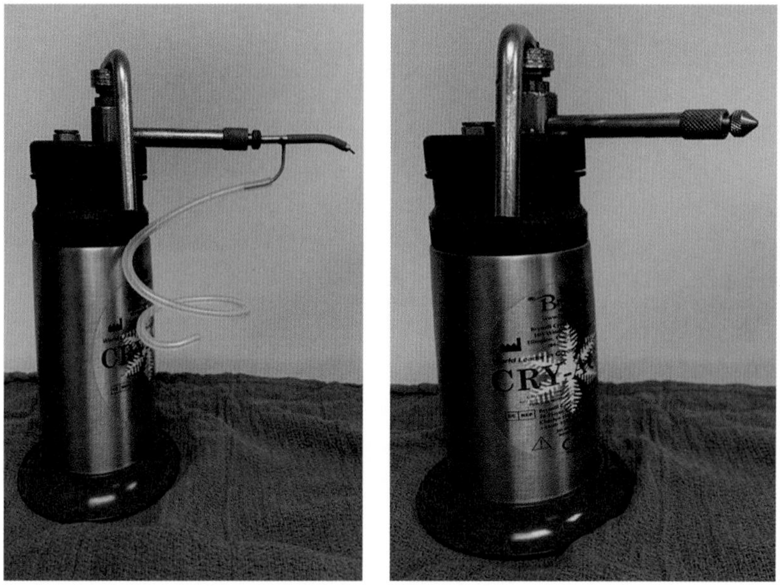

Figure 2.10 Liquid nitrogen canister with attached tips. (a) Probe tip, which is applied directly to the eyelid surface; (b) spray tip for liquid nitrogen canister, which is held about 1/8″ from the eyelid surface during the application of liquid nitrogen. *Source:* © Robin Sankey.

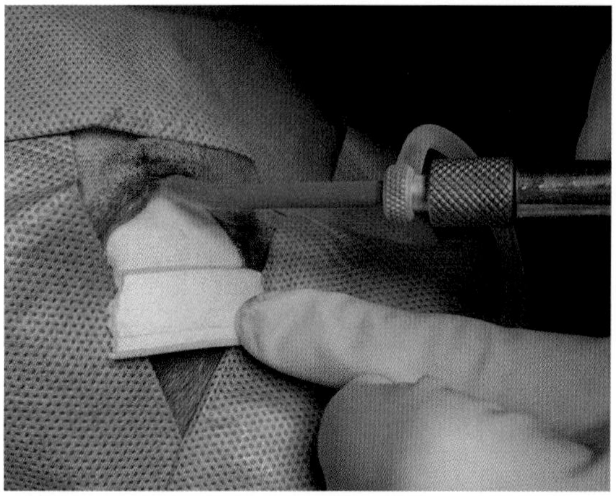

Figure 2.11 Probe tip used for application of liquid nitrogen directly to the eyelid following debulking of the mass. A piece of a styrofoam cup is being used to protect the cornea after coating the corneal surface with a lubricant ointment. *Source:* © Robin Sankey.

E-collar needs to be worn is based on the expected healing time for debulking procedures. Topical ointment antibiotics, such as neomycin, polymyxin, and bacitracin, are dispensed. The author typically avoids topical steroids when eyelid sutures are placed due to the small inherent risk of corneal ulceration due to the proximity of the eyelid sutures to the corneal surface. The owner is instructed not to apply excessive tension on the newly formed eyelid margin when placing the ointment into the eye since the sutured area is very delicate. It is recommended that the owner manipulate the eyelid that did not have surgery to apply the ointment to the ocular surface to decrease the risk of disrupting the delicate eyelid reconstruction. This is not as critical if eyelid sutures were not placed, as is common with most debulking and cryotherapy procedures. Typically, oral anti-inflammatory medications are also dispensed along with a few days of pain medication as needed. The sutures are typically removed after 14 days.

Potential Complications

The most common potential complications include wound dehiscence, mass regrowth, and corneal ulceration due to a suture rubbing. Also, if the newly formed eyelid margin does not have nearly perfect apposition, it can result in disruption of the tear film and trichiasis.[5] When using cryotherapy, it will cause blepharoedema for three to seven days and focal depigmentation, which usually resolves within a few weeks to a few months, but permanent depigmentation or scarring is possible. Occasionally, it can also cause sloughing of the periocular skin and eyelid, which typically occurs with prolonged freezing; however, these cases typically still heal with additional time and medical therapy. Also, if large areas are frozen, there is a risk of a qualitative tear film deficiency secondary to damage to the meibomian glands, since the secretions from these glands are important for preventing premature tear film evaporation. All masses should be submitted for histopathology to get an etiological diagnosis and ensure clean margins.

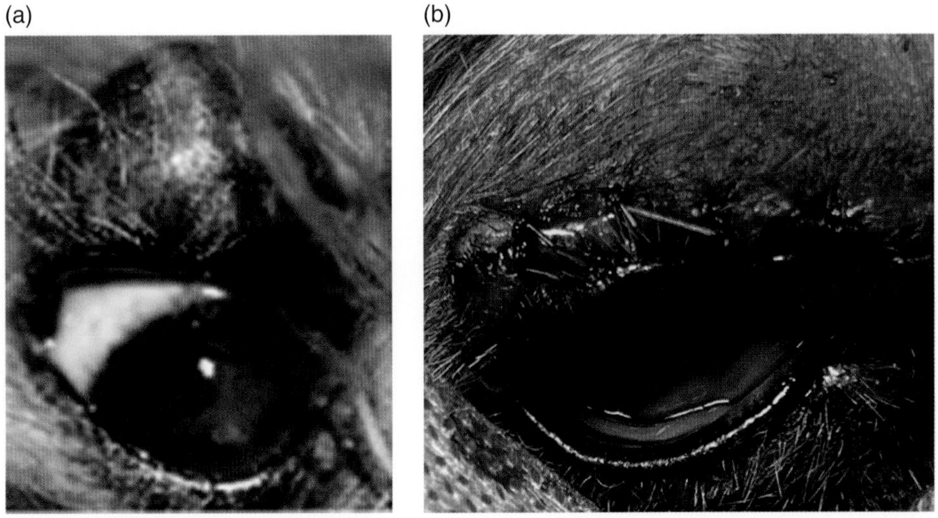

Figure 2.12 Debulking and cryotherapy of a large eyelid mass. (a) Preoperative appearance of the eyelid mass, which is too large for a V-lid or pentagonal blepharoplasty; (b) immediately postoperative picture following debulking, spray cryotherapy, and suturing. Most of the time, the area is left to heal by second intention, but due to the size of the defect, the skin was closed primarily with 6-0 polyglactin 910. *Source:* © Robin Sankey.

Prognosis

The prognosis for eyelid masses is typically good in dogs since most are benign. However, the prognosis is more guarded in cats. In the author's experience, the success rate of preventing regrowth with full-thickness excision is 95%. With debulking and cryotherapy, the success rate of preventing regrowth can still be quite successful in many cases with an 85% success rate in dogs. This is in line with a published study by Zibura et al. that found an average recurrence rate in dogs of 15.2% within 367.9 days after debulking and cryotherapy.[8]

References

1. Stades, F.C. and van der Woerdt, A. (2013). Diseases and surgery of the canine eyelid. In: *Veterinary Ophthalmology* (ed. T. Page), 834. Ames, IA: Wiley-Blackwell.
2. Meekins, J.M., Rankin, A.J., and Samuelson, D.A. (2021). Ophthalmic anatomy. In: *Veterinary Ophthalmology* (ed. T. Page), 46. Hoboken, NJ: Wiley-Blackwell.
3. Foot, B.C. (2022). Diagnosis and treatment of eyelid tumors. *Today's Vet. Pract.* 12 (1): 1–9. https://todaysveterinarypractice.com/ophthalmology/eyelid-tumors-dogs-cats.
4. Wang, S., Dawson, C., Wei, L. et al. (2019). The investigation of histopathology and locations of excised eyelid masses in dogs. *Vet. Rec. Open* 6 (1): e000344, 9.
5. Romkes, G., Klopfleisch, R., and Eule, J.C. (2014). Evaluation of one vs. two-layered closure after wedge excision of 43 eyelid tumors in dogs. *J. Vet. Ophthalmol.* 17 (1): 32–40.
6. Pot, S.A., Voelter, K., and Kircher, P.R. (2021). Surgery of the canine orbit. In: *Veterinary Ophthalmology* (ed. T. Page), 905. Hoboken, NJ: Wiley-Blackwell.
7. Williams, D. (2019). Cryosurgery in veterinary ophthalmology. Improve Veterinary Practice. https://www.veterinary-practice.com/article/cryosurgery-in-veterinary-ophthalmology.
8. Zibura, A.E., Henriksen, M., Rendahl, A. et al. (2019). Retrospective evaluation of palpebral masses treated with debulking and cryotherapy: 46 cases. *J. Vet. Ophthalmol.* 22 (3): 256–264.

3

Surgery for the Prolapsed Third Eyelid Gland

Audrey C. Hudson[1] *and Caleb Hudson*[2]

[1] *Gulf Coast Veterinary Specialists, Houston, TX, USA*
[2] *Nexus Veterinary Specialists, Victoria, TX, USA*

Key Points

- Being familiar with the presentation of TEL gland prolapses including common signalment, laterality, and concurrent conditions is important for acurate diagnosis and client communication.
- Because of the delicate structure of the TEL, understanding of the anatomy and specific location of associated structures is important for precision during surgery.
- Familiarizing oneself with differentials mimicking TEL gland prolapse is important for accurate diagnosis.
- Preoperative screening and postoperative monitoring for keratoconjunctivitis (KCS) is recommended given the risk of KCS in patients with TEL gland disease.
- Preoperative planning of the surgical technique is needed to determine instrumentation and suture material required.
- Reprolapse of the TEL gland after surgery is a common complication. Diligent adherence to the surgical techniques described including the accurate placement and depth of incisions and suture can help decrease the incidence of reprolapse.

Introduction

Prolapse of the gland of the nictitating membrane (NM), or "cherry eye," is the most commonly diagnosed condition of the third eyelid (TEL).[1] Nomenclature to describe this disorder varies among the literature, including "nictitating membrane gland prolapse," "TEL gland prolapse," and "cherry eye." For the purposes of this chapter, we will use the term "TEL gland prolapse." While the exact cause of TEL gland prolapse is unknown, laxity in the attachment of gland to the periorbita is thought to lead to the development of this condition.[2] It is also theorized that young dogs exposed to new, environmental antigens can develop antigenic stimulation of the conjunctival lymphoid tissue, leading to TEL gland prolapse.[3]

Development of TEL gland prolapse typically occurs at an early age in dogs with 75% of cases diagnosed at less than a year of age.[4] Presentation is commonly unilateral initially; however, contralateral gland prolapse can be present simultaneously or occur within months in many cases.[4,5] Conversely, age and laterality of presentation are variable in cats.[6,7] Commonly affected canine breeds include the American Cocker Spaniel, English Bulldog, French Bulldog, Lhasa Apso, Pekingese, Beagle, Shar Pei, Great Dane, and Cane Corso.[4,5,8–10] Reported breeds of cats include the Burmese, Persian, and domestic short hair cat with the Burmese being overrepresented.[7,11,12] A genetic basis has yet to be established.[1,5]

Seated in the ventromedial orbit, the TEL is a thin, reinforced membranous tissue that contributes to tear production, tear film distribution, and protection of the globe.[1] Two connected pieces of cartilage forming a T-shape within the TEL provide structural support to the membrane.[13] The TEL cartilage is composed of hyaline cartilage in the dog but is primarily elastic in the cat.[14] The thicker, vertically oriented cartilage forms the base and primary support of

Techniques in Small Animal Soft Tissue, Orthopedic, and Ophthalmic Surgery, First Edition. Edited by Kristin A. Coleman.

Companion website: www.wiley.com/go/coleman/surgeries

the TEL. It is oriented parallel to the direction of normal TEL excursions, which course ventromedially to dorsolaterally. The cartilage of the leading margin is thinner and positioned horizontally. Crescent-shaped in the dog and reverse-S in shape in the cat, the horizontal cartilage is connected perpendicularly to the vertical cartilaginous base.[14] Both pieces of cartilage are concave, allowing for close apposition to the globe and smooth motion of the TEL over the corneal surface.[13,14] Conjunctiva lining the globe courses anteriorly, forming a conjunctival sac, or bulbar conjunctival fornix, between the globe and TEL. This conjunctiva continues anteriorly lining both the posterior (bulbar) and anterior (palpebral) aspect of the TEL. The palpebral conjunctival fornix is formed by the junction of the palpebral conjunctiva of the TEL and the palpebral conjunctiva of the lower eyelid.[14] While the overlying conjunctiva is loosely attached to the underlying structures of the TEL, the conjunctiva becomes firmly attached to the cartilage at the leading edge. The often-pigmented leading edge of the TEL is the only visible portion of this structure in the awake dog and cat and can be seen adjacent to the ventromedial limbus.[13,14] Surrounding the cartilaginous base of the TEL lies an accessory lacrimal gland that produces 30%–60% of the precorneal tear film.[15] This gland produces seromucous secretions in the dog and serous secretions in the cat.[13,14] The gland communicates with the bulbar conjunctival fornix via numerous small ductules, which transmit and release the glandular secretions into the fornix.[13] A second accessory gland, the Harder's gland or Harderian gland, can be present in addition to or in place of the TEL gland in many small mammals.[14] Diseases and surgery of the Harderian gland are outside of the scope of this chapter. The bulbar conjunctiva of the TEL contains lymphoid tissue. Antigenic stimulation of the lymphoid tissue can cause hyperplastic changes resulting in a raised cobblestoned-appearing swelling, which can be visible on external examination.[13,16] Lymphoid hyperplasia can be differentiated from a prolapsed gland of the TEL, as the follicles are smaller, multifocal, and reside superficially within the bulbar conjunctiva of the TEL.[13] A supportive ligament attached to the base of the TEL is formed by both the superficial and middle muscular fascia. Both of the fascial layers envelope the extraocular muscles and provide stabilization of the TEL as they attach to the orbital septum and limbus of the eye.[13]

Normally retracted in the ventromedial orbit, movement of the TEL is mainly passive secondary to globe positioning. TEL excursions are initiated upon blinking, contraction of the retractor bulbi muscle, and retraction of the globe causing TEL movement in a dorsolateral direction across the surface of the cornea.[14] In the cat, the TEL has additional smooth muscle fiber attachments that are thought to cause active excursions of the TEL.[1,14] The TEL remains retracted within the ventromedial orbit due to resting sympathetic innervation of periocular smooth muscles. Contraction of these smooth muscle fibers maintains the anterior positioning of the globe within the orbit along with retraction of the base of the TEL.[13,14,17] Abnormal protrusion of the TEL can occur when resting enophthalmos is present, such as with the loss of sympathetic tone to the periocular structures, phthisis bulbi, or active contraction of the retractor bulbi muscle seen with ocular discomfort. Because of the finite orbital volume, orbital cellulitis secondary to periocular neoplasia, salivary gland disease, foreign bodies, and retrobulbar abscesses can cause abnormal protrusion of the globe along with protrusion of the TEL and its gland.[1]

Indications/Pre-operative Considerations

Historically, prolapsed TEL glands were treated by surgical excision to resolve the unsightly appearance.[18] In the 1980s, surgical gland repositioning was described and has become the recommended treatment for TEL gland prolapse. Surgical excision of the TEL gland significantly reduces precorneal tear film in both cats[19] and dogs,[20] in addition to degradation of the health of the corneal surface cells.[21] Dogs with prolapsed TEL glands removed or left untreated have been shown to be more likely to develop keratoconjunctivitis sicca (KCS) months to years later.[8,10] However, KCS can still occur after gland repositioning, especially in at-risk dog breeds, including the American Cocker Spaniel, English Bulldog, and Lhasa Apso.[8] Therefore, thorough client communication prior to surgery and continued monitoring of tear production postoperatively are important.[8]

Medical Management

Early in the disease process, massaging the displaced gland proximally into the ventromedial orbit can result in temporary repositioning. However, this technique only results in temporary correction, and long-term success has not been reported.[3] Topical anti-inflammatories can serve as adjunctive therapy to help reduce secondary inflammation of the gland and conjunctiva that occurs with chronic gland prolapse. However, anti-inflammatory therapy alone will not result in gland repositioning.[3]

Surgical Management

Surgical repositioning techniques are the mainstay of therapy and include reinforcing the gland's attachment to deeper structures or creating a pocket in which to bury the prolapsed gland.[1,3] The attempt to find a cosmetically acceptable surgery with a low risk of TEL gland reprolapse has led to the development of a myriad of surgical techniques. An exhaustive review of all reported procedures is beyond the scope of this chapter. Some of the more notable reported procedures will be mentioned with further explanation of the common pocket and tacking techniques.

Pre-operative Considerations: *Diagnosis*

Pre-operative assessment of the TEL and prolapsed gland is necessary for accurate diagnosis and surgical planning. While the TEL gland is likely to be visible, the remainder of the TEL remains seated in the ventromedial orbit. Thorough assessment of the TEL and gland requires retropulsion of the globe and can be performed by applying gentle digital pressure to the globe. Digital pressure is applied over a closed upper eyelid, protecting the cornea from direct contact during this maneuver. The globe should retropulse easily and the TEL elevate passively. The gland will typically prolapse further, allowing a more thorough examination. Additional assessment of the TEL structures, including the leading edge and associated cartilage, the (vertical) cartilaginous base, and bulbar and palpebral conjunctival surfaces can also be performed. Globe resistance to retropulsion, TEL-associated swelling not consistent with a soft, subconjunctival glandular structure, or inflammation not localized to the bulbar aspect of the TEL should be further evaluated for etiologies other than a prolapsed gland. After instillation of a topical anesthetic, such as proparacaine or tetracaine, a cotton-tipped applicator or fine-toothed forceps can be used for additional manipulation of the TEL and associated tissue.[22] In middle-aged and older patients that present with an acute TEL gland prolapse, careful assessment for other underlying causes of TEL gland protrusion is recommended.[4]

Pre-operative Considerations: *Instrumentation*

Given the delicate tissue and need for small movements with instrumentation, ophthalmic surgery is best performed sitting in a chair, with forearms resting on the surgical table and elbows bent at 90°.[22] This positioning provides hand stabilization and improves fine motor control. In addition, specific ophthalmic instrumentation is recommended to prevent damage to the delicate, periocular structures and assure accurate technique.

Recommended Surgical Instrumentation

Barraquer eyelid wire speculum
Bishop-Harmon 0.8 mm 1 × 2 teeth forceps (Figure 3.1a)
Colibri 0.3 mm 1 × 2 teeth forceps (Figure 3.1a)
#15 blade on a Bard-Parker handle (Figure 3.1b)
6400 Beaver blade with handle (Figure 3.1b)
Steven's tenotomy scissors (Figure 3.1c)
Westcott tenotomy scissors (Figure 3.1c)
Derf needle holders (Figure 3.1d)
Castroviejo needle holders (Figure 3.1d)
6-0 Vicryl (polyglactin 910 or polyglycolic acid)
4-0 nonabsorbable suture (e.g., nylon or polypropylene)
Gauze or surgical cellulose spears (Weck-Cel®)
Magnification with head-mounted loupes if needed

For all surgical procedures, the patient is placed in sternal recumbency with the head tilted 45°, rotating the surgical eye upward and positioning it near-parallel with the surgical table. The fur is clipped in the periocular region, and the periocular region and conjunctival fornices are prepped with 5% betadine solution. Quarter-draping with huck towels and towel clamps is performed to sterilely isolate the affected eye.

Various anchoring procedures have been described in which the prolapsed gland is sutured to the episclera,[23] sclera,[24] extraocular muscle attachments,[12,25] cartilage of the TEL,[18] and ventral orbital periosteum.[26–28] Many of the tacking procedures that require the gland to be sutured to the globe can be technically challenging, are associated with an increased rate of gland prolapse recurrence, and risk trauma to the eye. Therefore, tacking the gland to the orbital rim is one of the preferred anchoring techniques and will be described in more detail below (Surgical Techniques: Periosteal Anchoring Technique).[3]

Repositioning the gland within a conjunctival pocket has also been explored as an alternative to gland excision.[8,29,30] Creation of a conjunctival pocket to contain the gland without residual postoperative protrusion proved to be challenging.[8] A novel technique reported by Morgan et al.[8] attempted to mitigate these complications while also improving postoperative cosmesis and maintaining normal TEL anatomy. The theoretical concern of TEL gland ductal occlusion associated with the use of a pocket technique has proved to be an uncommon occurrence.[8,31] With an easy surgical learning curve and an excellent reported success rate, this procedure has become one of the most commonly utilized techniques for treating TEL gland prolapse in both the dog and cat and will be discussed in detail below (Surgical Techniques: Morgan Pocket Technique).[1,8]

Surgical Techniques

Periosteal Anchoring Technique

Anchoring to the periosteum of the orbital rim can be performed through the periocular skin or through the conjunctiva. Because the periosteal tissue is quite tough and significant tissue purchase is needed for this technique to be successful, larger instrumentation is used. Fine-toothed Bishop-Harmon 0.8 mm 1 × 2 teeth forceps are used in place of Colibri 0.3 mm 1 × 2 teeth forceps. Derf needle holders are used in place of Castroviejo needle holders. In contrast to the pocket technique, nonabsorbable sutures, such as nylon or polypropylene, are used to anchor the gland. A larger, 13 mm or longer, 3/8 circle needle can be

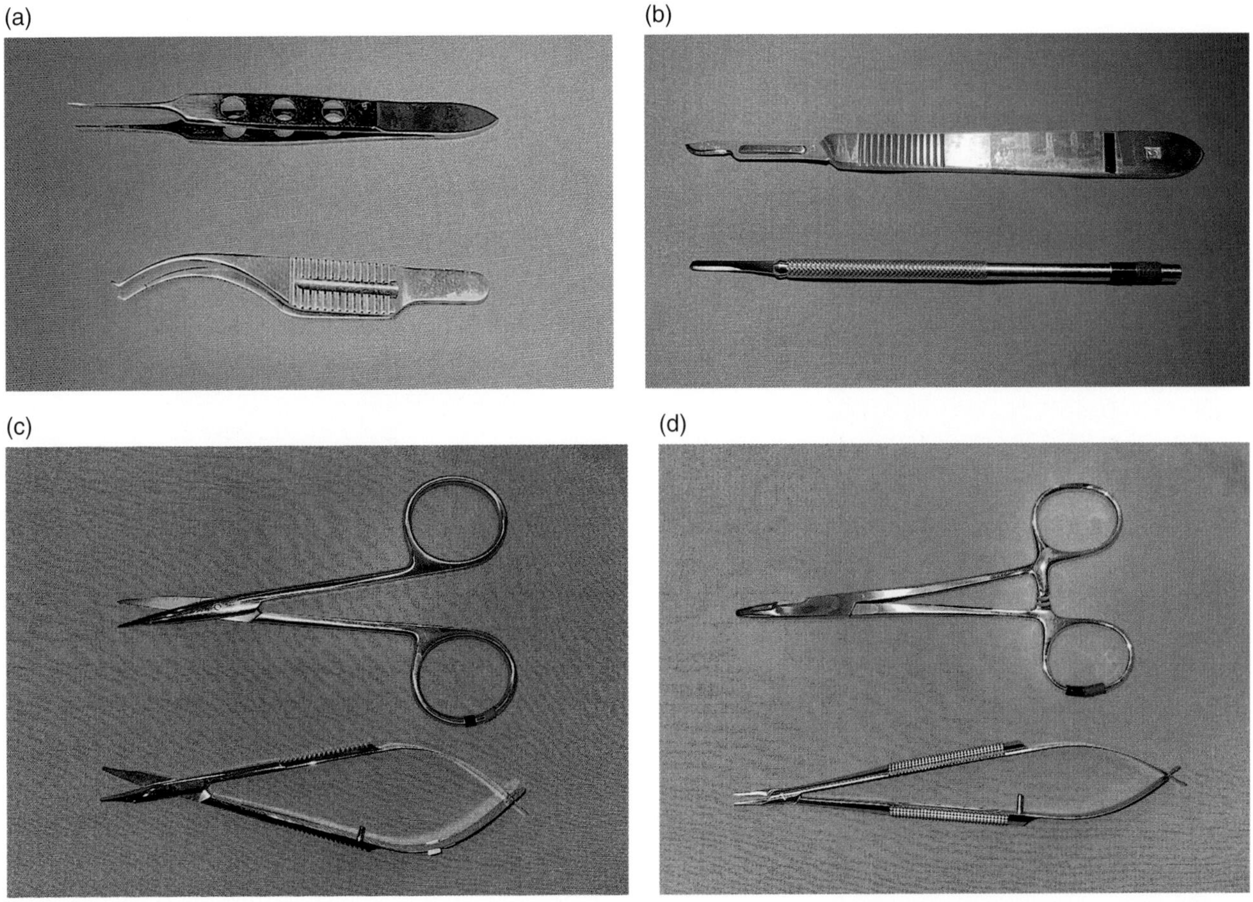

Figure 3.1 Instrumentation commonly utilized during TEL gland repositioning surgery. (a) Ophthalmic forceps, including Bishop-Harmon 0.8 mm, 1 × 2 teeth thumb forceps (top) and Colibri 0.3 mm, 1 × 2 teeth forceps (bottom). (b) Ophthalmic blades including #15 Blade on a Bard-Parker handle (top) and 6400 Beaver blade with handle (bottom). (c) Ophthalmic scissors including Steven's tenotomy scissors (top) and Westcott tenotomy scissors (bottom). (d) Ophthalmic needle holders, including Derf needle holders (top) and Castroviejo needle holders (bottom). *Source:* © Audrey Hudson.

used to accommodate the longer suture bites needed to pass between the periosteum and the gland.

Position and sterilely prepare the patient as described above. After palpating the inferior orbital rim, use a #15 scalpel blade on a Bard-Parker handle to make a skin incision along the ventral, bony orbit. The initial incision is parallel to and 2–3 cm inferior to the lower eyelid margin (Figure 3.2). Bluntly dissect the subcutaneous tissue to expose the periosteum with Steven's tenotomy scissors. The periosteum can be identified by a lighter pink-to-white color, distinct from the glossier surrounding subcutaneous tissue (Figure 3.3). Take a suture bite through the periosteum using 4-0 nonabsorbable suture (Figure 3.4). Because of the firm adherence of the periosteum to the orbital rim, you can confirm accurate placement of your suture within the periosteum by grasping the suture and pulling firmly. A periosteal suture purchase will result in the movement of the head (Figure 3.5). Incorrect suture placement within the subcutaneous tissue alone will result in movement of the overlying skin. Insert the needle through the subconjunctival tissue of the inferior eyelid and TEL, exiting the medial aspect of

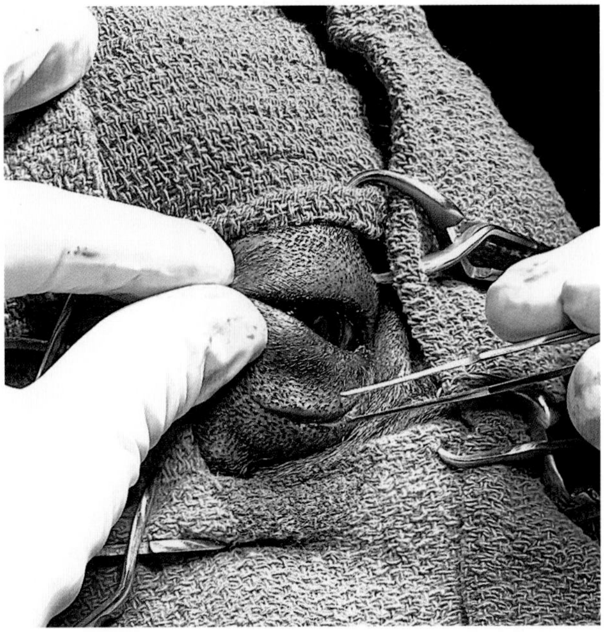

Figure 3.2 Periosteal anchoring technique: incision. The incision is made over the orbital rim, 2–3 cm inferior to the lower eyelid margin. *Source:* © Audrey Hudson.

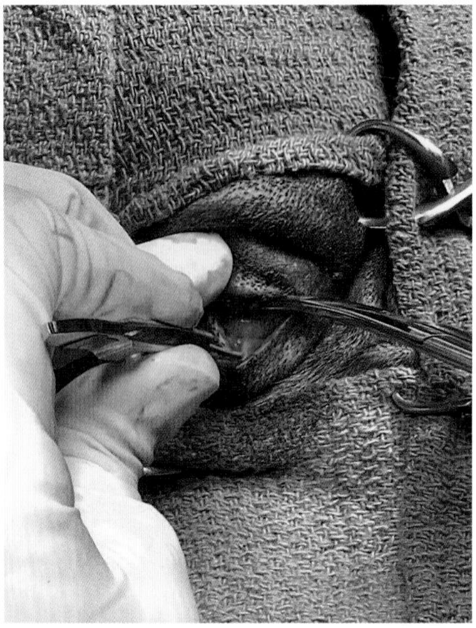

Figure 3.3 Periosteal anchoring technique: exposure of the periosteum. The periosteum is seen deep to the subcutaneous tissue, appears lighter pink, and is duller in appearance compared to the subcutaneous layer. The periosteum is seen grasped in the Bishop-Harmon tissue forceps. *Source:* © Audrey Hudson.

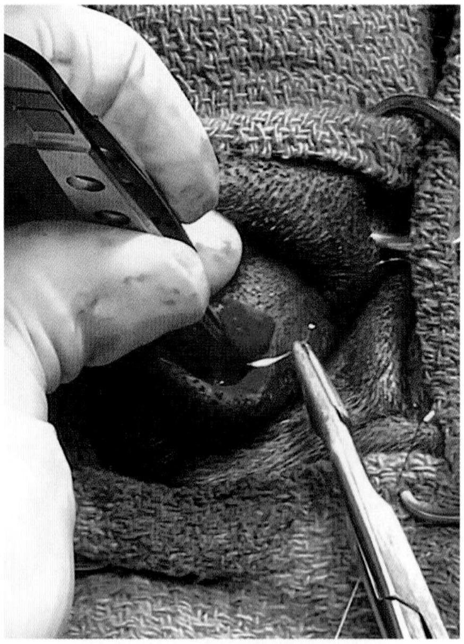

Figure 3.4 Periosteal anchoring technique. Initial periosteal suture is placed (right hand) by grasping the periosteum with forceps (left hand). *Source:* © Audrey Hudson.

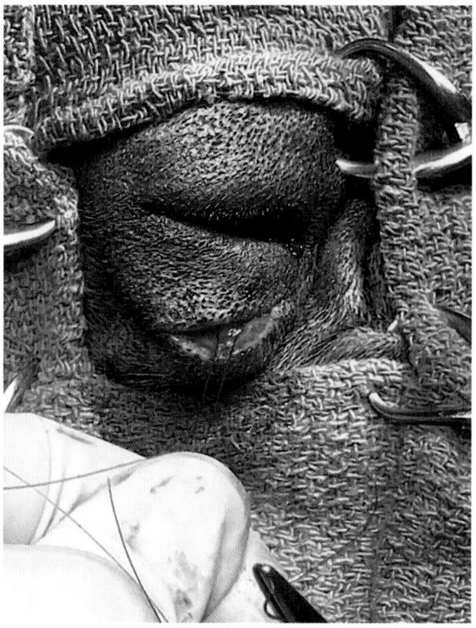

Figure 3.5 Periosteal anchoring technique. Periosteal suture placement confirmation can be achieved by eliciting head movement when gently pulling on the placed suture. *Source:* © Audrey Hudson.

the prolapsed gland's apex (Figure 3.6a–d). Reinsert the needle and suture immediately next to the initial exit site. Tunnel the needle and suture horizontally through the gland exiting the conjunctiva on the lateral aspect of the apex of the prolapsed gland. Reinsert the needle immediately next to this second exit site on the bulbar conjunctiva and direct it inferiorly toward the initial periosteal bite. (When placing anchoring sutures within the prolapsed gland, reinserting the needle immediately next to the preceding exit point serves to minimize non-absorbable suture exposure on the bulbar conjunctiva.) Advance the needle and suture from within the subconjunctival tissue of the gland through the subconjunctival tissue of the TEL and inferior eyelid until the needle and suture exit at the orbital rim (Figure 3.7a,b). A second suture bite is taken through the periosteum as the needle is driven in a downward direction. This second periosteal suture pass should be 3–5 mm from the initial suture insertion through the periosteum. The gland is pulled downward into the normal position in the ventral orbit by tying the ends of the suture over the periosteum (Figure 3.8). The skin is closed in typical fashion.

Morgan Pocket Technique

In contrast to the periosteal anchoring technique, the Morgan pocket technique utilizes surgical manipulation of the thin conjunctiva to reposition and secure the prolapsed gland into its normal position. Misplaced incisions, overhandling of the tissue, and incorrect suture selection or placement can damage the delicate conjunctiva and surrounding ocular tissue. Therefore, appropriate instrumentation is necessary to prevent needless tissue damage. Colibri 0.3 mm 1 × 2 teeth forceps are used in place of fine-toothed Bishop-Harmon 0.8 mm 1 × 2 teeth forceps. Castroviejo needle holders are used in place of Derf needle holders. Handling of the conjunctiva should be minimized, as damage to the incised conjunctival edges and the blood supply can prevent healing of the incision and increase the chance of conjunctival wound dehiscence and reprolapse

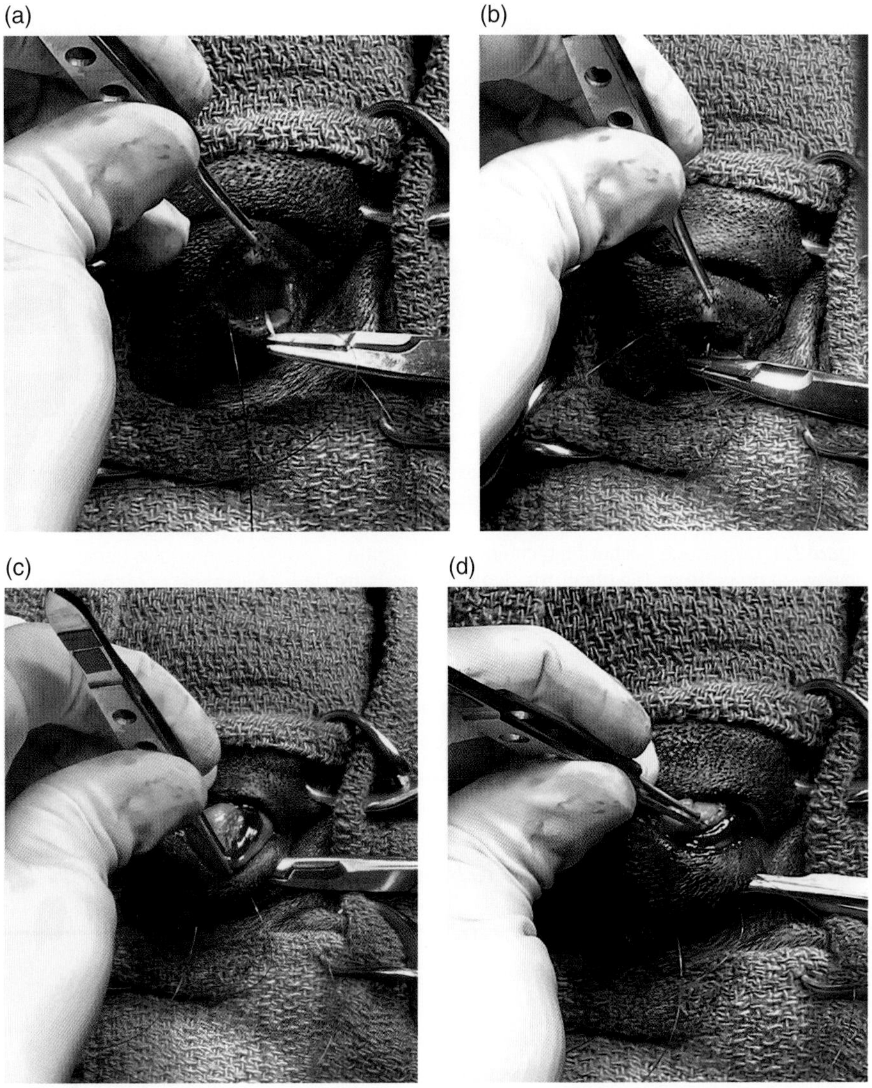

Figure 3.6 Periosteal anchoring technique. Once secured in the periosteum, the suture is aimed upward (a) and passed through the subcutaneous tissue toward the prolapsed gland (b). Pushing upward with the needle holders in the right hand while gently retracting the TEL margin with forceps in the left hand (c), the needle is initially passed through the medial aspect of the apex of the prolapsed gland (d). *Source:* © Audrey Hudson.

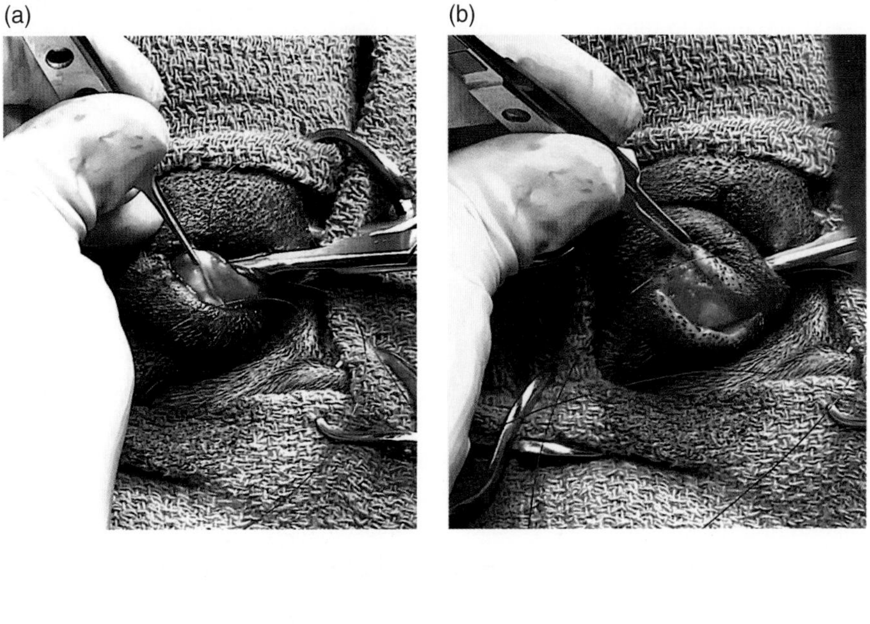

Figure 3.7 Periosteal anchoring technique. Pulling upward on the third eyelid, the needle is pushed through the gland and subconjunctival tissue of the third eyelid (a). Once through the third eyelid, the needle is passed through the subcutaneous eyelid tissue exiting the periosteum (b). *Source:* © Audrey Hudson.

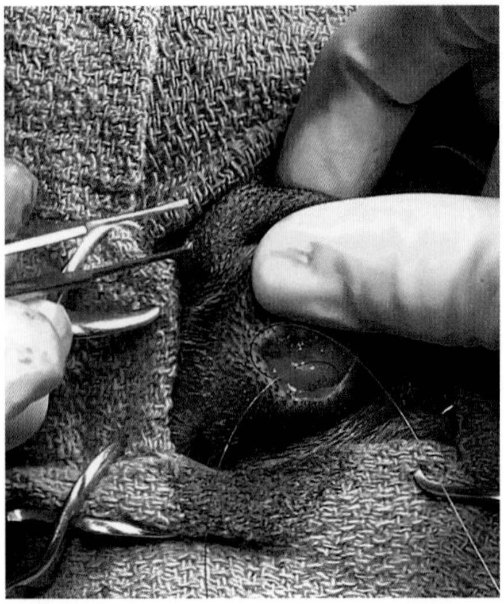

Figure 3.8 Periosteal anchoring technique. With gentle downward pressure on the gland, the two suture ends are tied in the periosteum, pulling the gland into the ventral orbit. *Source:* © Audrey Hudson.

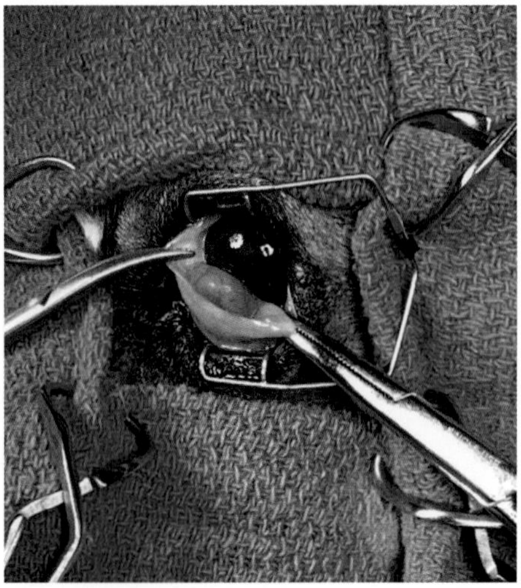

Figure 3.9 Morgan pocket technique: positioning. Two small mosquito hemostats are used to hold the nasal and temporal aspects of the TEL, exposing the prolapsed gland and stabilizing the TEL. *Source:* © Audrey Hudson.

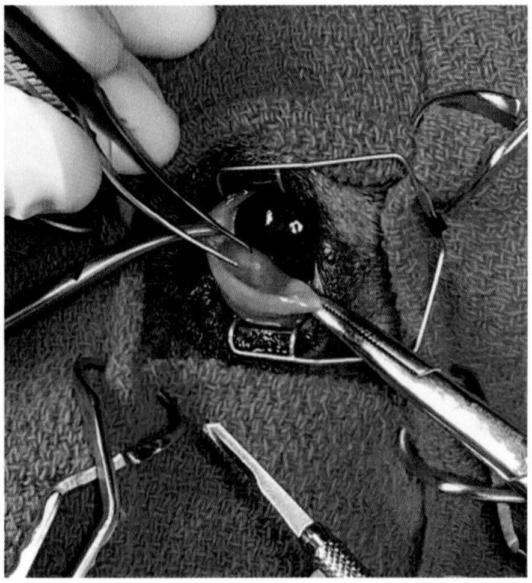

Figure 3.10 Morgan pocket technique. Grasping TEL gland apex with Colibri 0.3 mm 1 × 2 teeth thumb forceps (left hand), a 6400 Beaver blade (right hand) is held ventrally. *Source:* © Audrey Hudson.

of the gland. Smaller diameter (6-0), braided, absorbable suture, such as polyglactin 910 or polyglycolic acid, is preferred, as the softer nature of braided suture decreases the likelihood of abrading the cornea. Because suturing is performed in a small space between the globe and TEL, a small, 10 mm, 1/2 circle needle is recommended. When using the needle's natural curvature as a guide, the 1/2 circle's smaller radius of curvature provides a shorter path for the needle to travel, which reduces the risk of damage to the cornea and globe. This smaller surgical area is maintained by gently grasping the needle holders like a pencil and using the wrist to rotate the needle drivers along the needle's natural curvature.

After positioning and sterilely preparing the patient as described above, place an appropriately sized Barraquer eyelid speculum to retract both the upper and lower eyelids. Two small mosquito hemostats or Allis tissue forceps are used to hold the nasal and temporal aspects of the TEL, exposing the prolapsed gland and stabilizing the TEL (Figure 3.9). Grasp the apex of the prolapsed gland with Colibri 0.3 mm 1×2 teeth forceps in the non-dominant hand and the 6400 Beaver microsurgical blade in the dominant hand (Figure 3.10). Use the 6400 Beaver microsurgical blade to make two elliptical incisions through the bulbar conjunctiva around the base of the prolapsed gland. The first and second incisions should not connect, but should slightly encircle the respective sides of the gland for 120–140°. The first incision is made proximally (halfway between the gland apex and the bulbar conjunctival fornix). The movement and elasticity of the TEL gland and surrounding tissue can make precise, conjunctival incisions challenging. To perform the elliptical incisions efficiently, use the Colibri 0.3 mm 1×2 teeth forceps to apply gentle traction on the apex of the prolapsed gland. Using moderate downward pressure, incise the conjunctiva in a deliberate, linear motion (Figure 3.11a,b). There is a small, centrally located blood vessel running perpendicular to the initial incision (Figure 3.11c). The correct depth of the incision is confirmed when the vessel is well visualized, but not incised. Incision of this prominent vessel will lead to increased hemorrhage during the procedure and decreased visualization of the surgical field. The second incision is made distally (halfway between the gland apex and the leading margin of the TEL) (Figure 3.12a). Adequate tension of the tissue can be achieved by

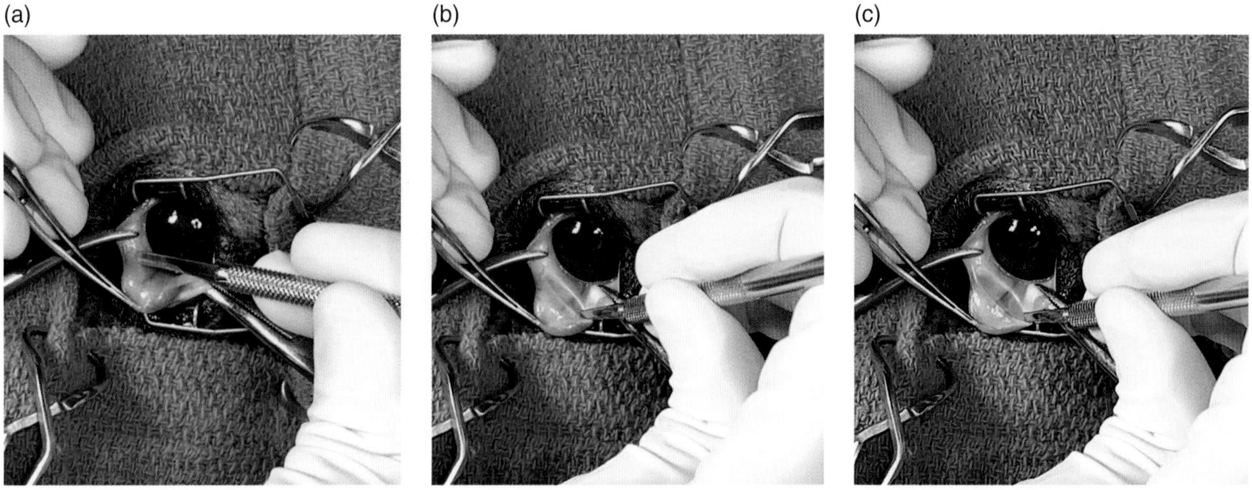

Figure 3.11 Morgan pocket technique: initial incision. (a) Grasping the apex of the TEL gland with Colibri forceps, start the incision on the bulbar aspect of the conjunctiva. (b) Given the elastic nature of the TEL gland, deliberate pressure is needed. (c) Once through the bulbar conjunctiva and subconjunctival tissue, a prominent vessel will be well visualized. *Source:* © Audrey Hudson.

retracting the TEL gland upwards with the Colibri 0.3 mm 1×2 teeth forceps during the incision (Figure 3.12b). However, retraction of the gland in this orientation places the gland in close proximity to the cornea. Therefore, make this incision in a slow and methodical manner. Burying 1–2 mm of the cutting edge of the 6400 Beaver blade while making the incision will typically result in an appropriate depth through the conjunctiva (Figure 3.12c). While described as elliptical incisions, the incisions will look more linear in appearance when tension on the gland is applied (Figure 3.12d). Hemostasis can be controlled with a drop of 1%–2.5% phenylephrine, sterile gauze, or small surgical spears, such as Weck-Cel® sponges (Figure 3.13). Use Steven's tenotomy scissors to bluntly dissect the subconjunctival tissue starting from the proximal incision toward the bulbar conjunctival fornix (Figure 3.14a,b). This pocket is formed within the subconjunctival space by undermining a thin layer of connective tissue in addition to the bulbar conjunctiva. If only the conjunctiva is undermined, the pocket integrity may be compromised, leading to reprolapse of the gland. Removing the overlying conjunctival epithelium of the gland has been reported to expose a larger area of subconjunctival tissue, improving the adhesions between the two incisions and further stabilizing the repair.[30] While removal of the entire conjunctival epithelium can be challenging given the tight adherence of the epithelium to the gland,[8] a modification can be performed by sharply excising a 2–5 mm wide elliptical section of bulbar conjunctival epithelium directly adjacent to the distal incision with Steven's or Westcott tenotomy scissors (Figure 3.15a–e). To close the conjunctival incisions, the conjunctival edge of the first incision closest to the fornix is apposed to the conjunctival edge of the second incision that is closest to the leading edge of the TEL. The conjunctival edges are sutured together using 6-0 absorbable suture.

Starting from the palpebral aspect of the TEL, drive the needle from the intact palpebral conjunctiva through the body of the TEL, exiting in the subconjunctival tissue in the distal elliptical incision on the TEL's bulbar aspect (Figure 3.16a,b). Then, insert the needle in the distal incision, entering the subconjunctival tissue a few millimeters from the incised conjunctiva and exiting the distal conjunctival surface, nearest the leading edge of the TEL (Figure 3.16c). Take the next bite in the most proximal conjunctival edge of the proximal incision, exiting in the subconjunctival space (Figure 3.16d). As the suture is pulled through the tissue, follow the curvature of the needle, rolling it away from the cornea. Continue this pattern by passing the suture over the gland and inserting the needle in the subconjunctival tissue in the distal incision, exiting through the bulbar conjunctiva nearest the leading margin of the TEL. These steps are repeated, and the simple continuous pattern is continued lengthwise traversing the gland until nearly connecting the end of both incisions (Figure 3.16e). Gently pull on both ends of the suture to tighten the pattern and pull the conjunctival edges over the gland (Figure 3.16f). The simple continuous pattern is then repeated back along the incision line to oversew the initial suture pattern (Figure 3.16g,h). During this second pass along the incision, the gland should remain buried and the suture taut across the conjunctival closure. It is not until reaching the initial starting point that the needle is passed back through the subconjunctival tissue of the distal incision (Figure 3.16i) and exited through the palpebral conjunctiva of the TEL 2–4 mm from the initial entry (Figure 3.16j). The suture knot is tied after tightening the suture line (Figures 3.17 and 3.18). This process will result

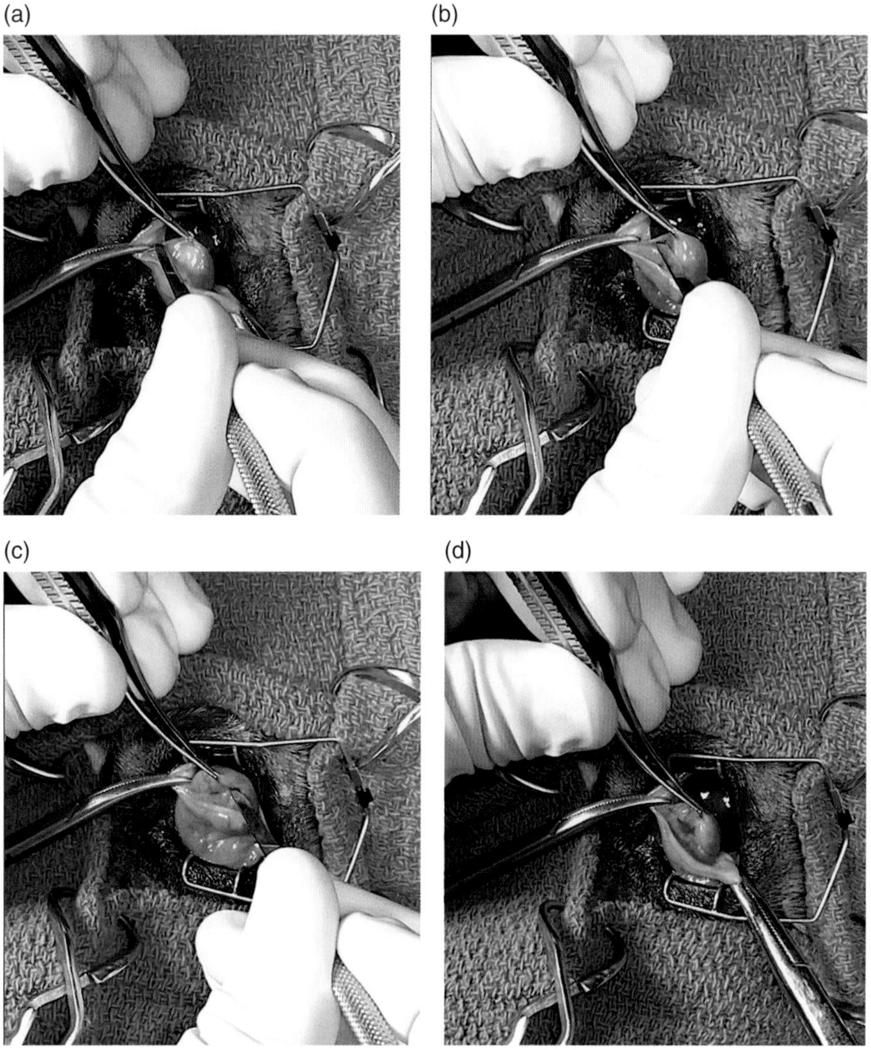

Figure 3.12 Morgan pocket technique: distal incision. (a) Begin the distal incision halfway between the grasped apex of the gland and the leading margin of the third eyelid. (b) Incise the conjunctival and partial subconjunctival tissue with the 6400 Beaver blade. (c) Given the elastic nature of the gland, adequate tension of tissue is necessary and achieved by placing traction on the gland grasped with Colibri forceps in the left hand and firm pressure of the 6400 Beaver blade in the right eye. Appropriate pressure is typically achieved when 1–2 mm of the blade edge disappears within the incision. (d) The resulting conjunctival incision. *Source:* © Audrey Hudson.

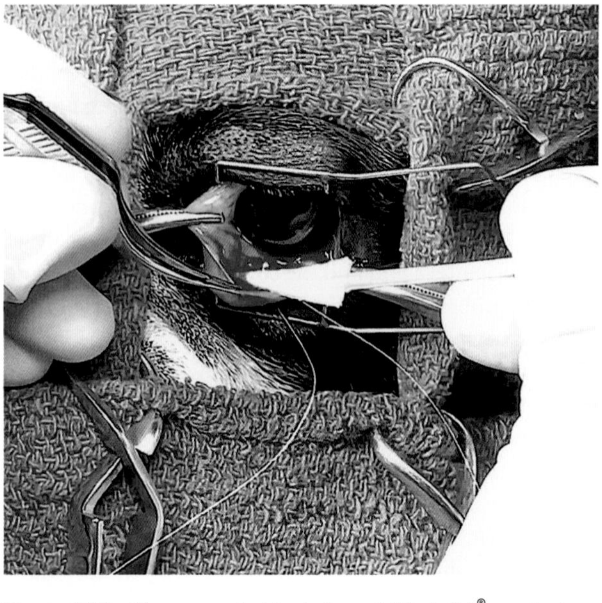

Figure 3.13 Morgan pocket technique. A Weck-Cel® surgical spear being used for hemostasis. *Source:* © Audrey Hudson.

in repositioning of the gland. Small openings are left at both ends of the apposed incisions, rather than fully suturing the entire length of the incisions together. It is thought that this allows normal outflow for the TEL gland's lacrimal ducts. While mild swelling will be present, the gland should no longer be visible.

Combination Procedures

Several combination procedures have been described during which an anchoring technique is performed followed by a pocket procedure.[32] Success rates reported in this study were similar between both the combination procedure and pocket procedure alone. However, the combination procedure was performed in patients with large TEL glands and chronic TEL gland prolapses, as these characteristics pose a higher risk of reprolapse. This discrepancy in case selection may have led to the similar success rates reported between the two protocols. Other described combination procedures include partial removal of the vertical cartilage of the TEL

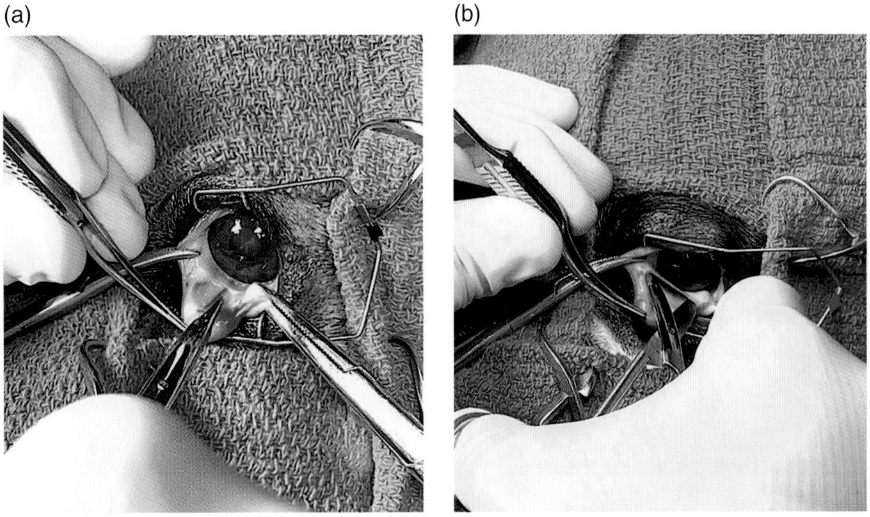

Figure 3.14 Morgan pocket technique: subconjunctival pocket creation. (a) Use Steven's tenotomy scissors to bluntly dissect the subconjunctival tissue, avoiding the prominent vasculature. (b) Assure the pocket is both deep and wide enough for gland replacement. *Source:* © Audrey Hudson.

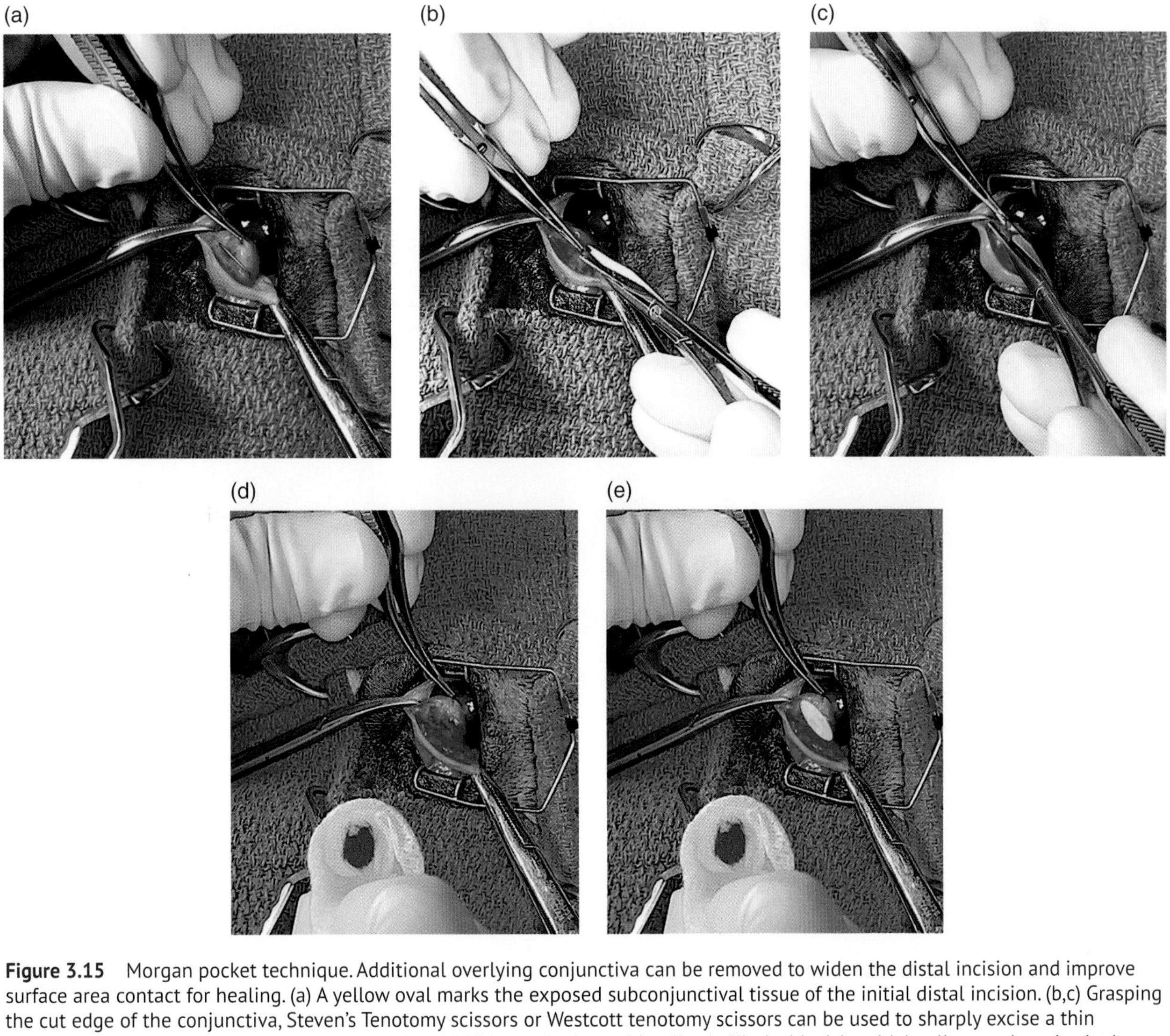

Figure 3.15 Morgan pocket technique. Additional overlying conjunctiva can be removed to widen the distal incision and improve surface area contact for healing. (a) A yellow oval marks the exposed subconjunctival tissue of the initial distal incision. (b,c) Grasping the cut edge of the conjunctiva, Steven's Tenotomy scissors or Westcott tenotomy scissors can be used to sharply excise a thin elliptical piece of tissue along the initial incision. (d) This results in a wider distal elliptical incision. (e) A yellow oval marks the larger surface area of the exposed subconjunctival tissue and can be compared to the subconjunctival surface area of the initial incision (a). *Source:* © Audrey Hudson.

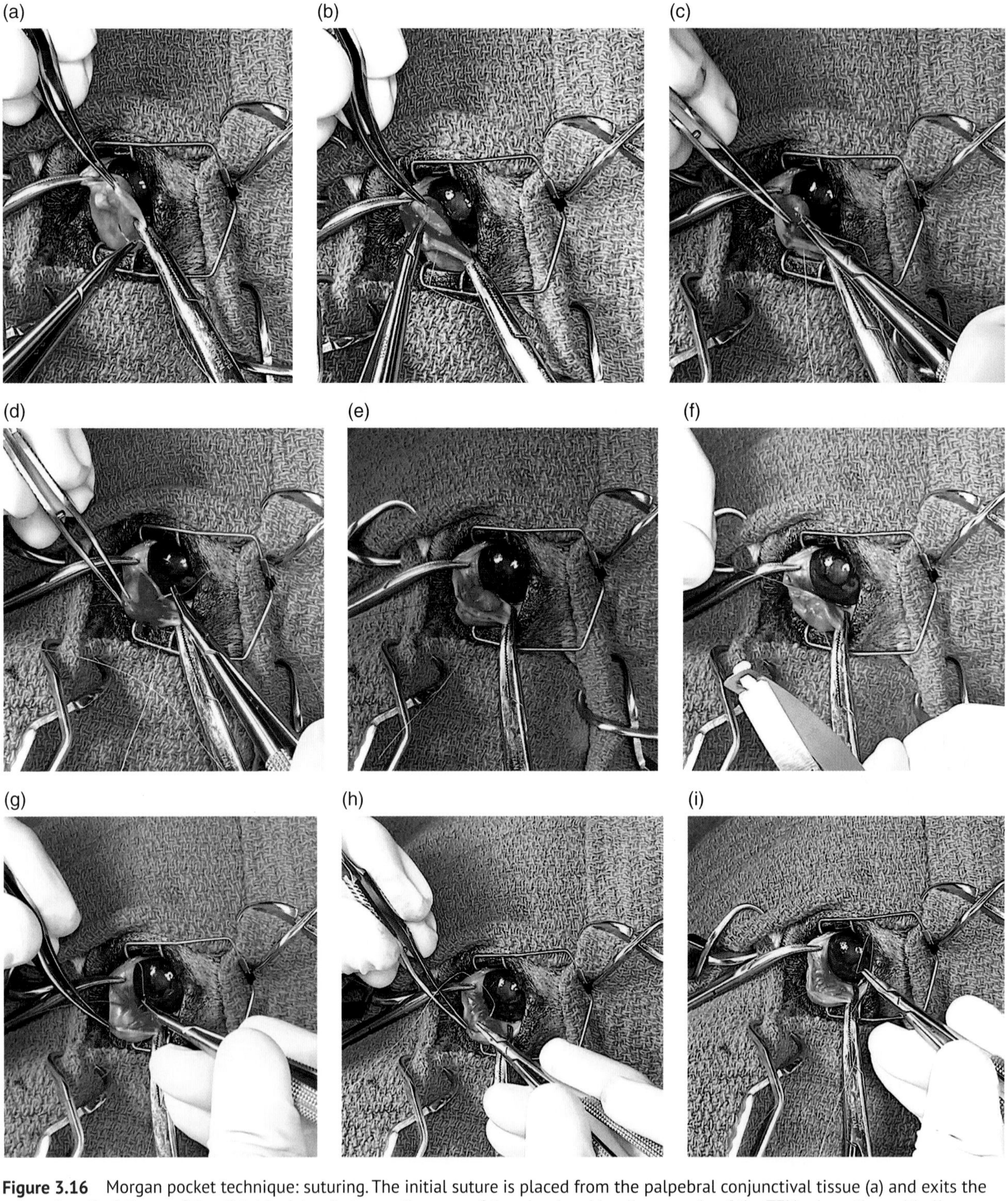

Figure 3.16 Morgan pocket technique: suturing. The initial suture is placed from the palpebral conjunctival tissue (a) and exits the subconjunctival tissue of the distal incision (between the apex of the gland and leading margin of the TEL) where the epithelium was removed. (b) A yellow oval marks the exposed subconjunctival tissue. (c) The second purchase is placed in the subconjunctival tissue of the distal incision and exits the bulbar conjunctiva adjacent to the TEL leading margin. (d) Gently pulling the gland away from the globe, the needle is passed through the conjunctiva of the proximal incision. (e) Allowing the suture to cross over the top of the gland with minimal tension, the suture pattern is continued until the final pass of suture is made at the end of the incisions being confident to leave an opening without completely connecting the proximal and distal incisions. (f) The suture line is then tightened securing the gland in place. (g,h) Oversewing the incision, the simple continuous pattern is continued back toward the suture origin. (i,j) The suture is passed through the subcutaneous tissue of the distal incision and exits through the palpebral conjunctiva. *Source:* © Audrey Hudson.

(j)

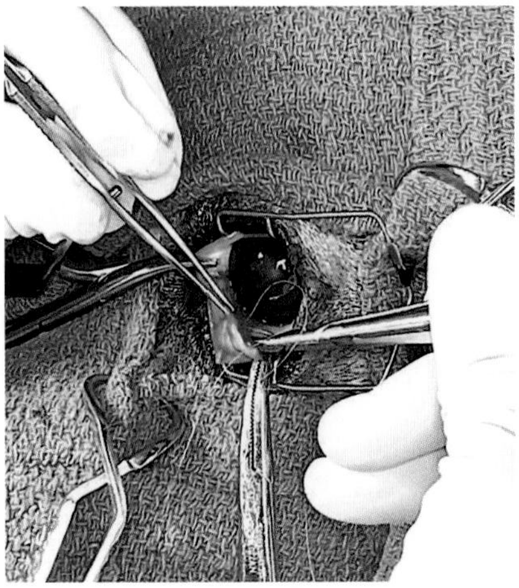

Figure 3.16 (Continued)

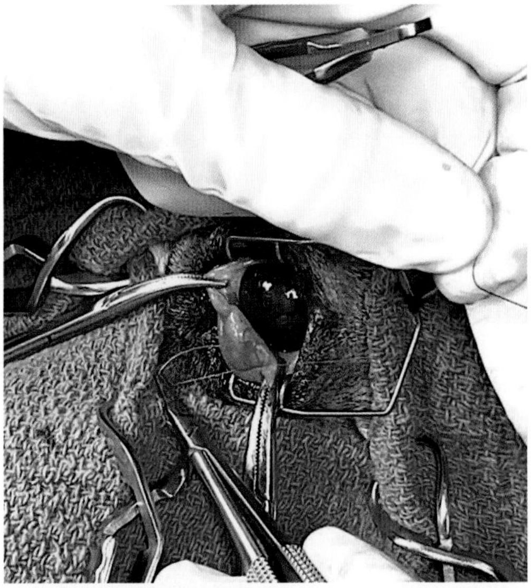

Figure 3.17 Morgan pocket technique: tying knot. The knot is tied on the palpebral aspect of the TEL to avoid corneal abrasions from the suture. *Source:* © Audrey Hudson.

and wedge resection of the TEL.[33] These techniques have been developed in an attempt to decrease reprolapse, which is commonly reported in 10% of patients, and to improve postoperative cosmesis.

Postoperative Considerations

Topical antibiotic therapy is recommended to prevent secondary infection of the surgical site. A degree of inflammation is required to induce the scarring necessary for secure gland repositioning. Therefore, topical antibiotics containing an anti-inflammatory remain controversial.[34] Systemic

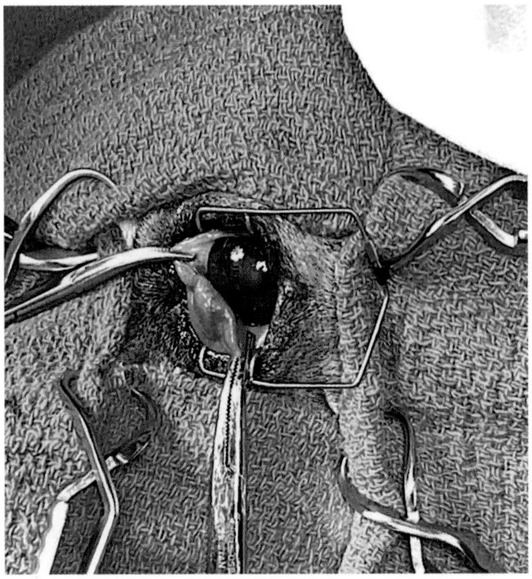

Figure 3.18 Morgan pocket technique: trim suture tags. The suture is trimmed close to the knot. *Source:* © Audrey Hudson.

anti-inflammatory therapy should be used modestly and primarily for immediate postoperative analgesia. Broad-spectrum systemic antibiotics are also administered in the postoperative period.

Complications

Reprolapse

Reprolapse rates vary between techniques, between surgeons, and between patients based on signalment. However, increased reprolapse rates are seen with severe pre-operative inflammation.[18] Both topical and systemic anti-inflammatory therapy can be used for one to two weeks prior to surgery to help decrease the associated swelling. When the gland reprolapses after surgery, the reprolapse typically occurs within the first two months postoperatively.[8] If reprolapse occurs, a repeat procedure utilizing meticulous surgical technique or a combination procedure is recommended.

Residual Conjunctivitis

Given the highly vascular nature of the conjunctiva and incorporated lymphatic tissue, surgical manipulation of the TEL and gland can result in unsightly swelling and chronic protrusion of the TEL.[1,8] This does not represent a true reprolapse but can be cosmetically unappealing to owners. Assessing the TEL for infection, lacrimal cyst formation, and conjunctival suture reaction is recommended in these patients.

Corneal Ulceration

Any suture material that is exposed on the bulbar conjunctival surface of the TEL is in close proximity to the corneal surface and can pose a risk for corneal abrasions. Small diameter braided suture is used to decrease the risk of corneal ulceration if suture becomes exposed. Postoperative topical antibiotics can be dosed in ointment form to add further protection to the cornea. However, patients that display ocular discomfort as evidenced by squinting for longer than 72 hours postoperatively should be rechecked for corneal ulcers.

TEL Gland Cyst Formation

While rare, lacrimal cysts can form if the TEL gland's excretory ducts are buried within a conjunctival pocket. Diagnosis is achieved by aspiration of transparent fluid consistent with lacrimal secretions from the swollen region. Marsupialization of the cyst has been described and is an effective treatment for this complication.[31]

Other Considerations

Neoplasias of the TEL vary widely in type and location arising from the TEL gland, vascular and lymphatic cells of the TEL, and the overlying conjunctiva.[1] In both the dog and cat, adenocarcinoma is the most common type of neoplasia associated with the TEL gland. Recurrence and metastasis rates of TEL neoplasia have been reported but are somewhat variable based on cancer type.[35] It is important to differentiate neoplasia associated with the TEL from a gland prolapse, as the treatment and prognosis vary widely. After initial prolapse, the TEL gland is a soft, pink, rounded structure covered with smooth conjunctiva arising from the bulbar aspect of the TEL. This early presentation can often be readily distinguished from other TEL pathology given the appearance and texture. With chronicity of the prolapsed gland, overlying conjunctival lymphoid hyperplasia, conjunctivitis secondary to exposure, and a change in tear film dynamics lead to periocular inflammation, making the differentiation more challenging. If TEL neoplasia is considered a differential, additional diagnostics, including conjunctival cytology, fine needle aspiration, incisional biopsy, and/or advanced imaging, should be performed prior to attempting a gland repositioning technique.

Other ophthalmic conditions presenting as ventral swellings around the TEL can mimic a TEL gland prolapse. These include non-neoplastic inflammatory masses, most notably nodular granulomatous episcleritis,[36] retrobulbar fat prolapse,[37] parasitic granulomas,[38] and periocular cysts.[39]

Eversion, or bending, of the cartilage within the TEL is common and thought to be due to disproportional growth of the TEL structures.[1,2] Typically seen in younger, larger breed dogs, the anterior bending of the vertical TEL cartilage can resemble a prolapsed gland when it occurs alone or can be accompanied by a prolapse of the gland as well.[1] Surgical correction of the abnormal cartilaginous structure with or without gland repositioning is needed; however, a description of these techniques is beyond the scope of this chapter.

Conclusion

Given the frequent presentation of TEL gland prolapse and the increasing popularity of at-risk breeds, TEL gland repositioning is a frequently performed surgery. Challenges with this procedure include difficulties with tissue handling given the elasticity of the TEL, the redundant conjunctiva and its predilection to inflammation, and both surgeon and owner frustration with gland reprolapses. However, with practice, appropriate instrumentation, and refinement of surgical skills, TEL gland repositioning can be a reliable and rewarding surgery.

References

1 Hartley, C. and Hendrix, D. (2021). Diseases and surgery of the canine conjunctiva and nictitating membrane. In: *Veterinary Ophthalmology*, 6e (ed. K. Gelatt), 1045–1081. Hoboken, NJ: Wiley.

2 Moore, C. and Constantinescu, G. (1997). Surgery of the adnexa. *Vet. Clin. North Am. Small Anim. Pract.* 27 (5): 1011–1065.

3 Maggs, D. (2008). Third eyelid. In: *Slatter's Fundamentals of Veterinary Ophthalmology*, 4e (ed. D. Maggs, P. Miller, and R. Ofri), 152–154. St. Louis, MO: Saunders Elsevier.

4 Mazzucchelli, S., Vaillant, M.D., Weverbrerg, F. et al. (2012). Retrospective study of 155 cases of prolapse of the nictitating membrane gland in dogs. *Vet. Rec.* 170 (17): 443.

5 Edelmann, M.L., Miyadera, K., Iwabe, S. et al. (2013). Investigating the inheritance of prolapsed nictitating membrane glands in a large canine pedigree. *Vet. Ophthalmol.* 16 (6): 416–422.

6 Glaze, M.B., Maggs, D., and Plummer, C. (2021). Feline ophthalmology. In: *Veterinary Ophthalmology*, 6e (ed. K. Gelatt), 1665–1840. Hoboken, NJ: Wiley.

7 Chahory, S., Crasta, M., Trio, S. et al. (2004). Three cases of prolapse of the nictitans gland in cats. *Vet. Ophthalmol.* 7 (6): 417–419.

8 Morgan, R.V., Duddy, J.M., and McClurg, K. (1993). Prolapse of the gland of the third eyelid in dogs: a retrospective study of 89 cases (1980 to 1990). *J. Am. Anim. Hosp. Assoc.* 29 (1): 56–60.

9 Allgower, I. (2019). Ocular disorders of 809 French bulldogs. *Abstracts: Annual Scientific Meeting of the European College of Veterinary Ophthalmologists*, P2. Antwerp.

10 Dugan, S., Severin, G., Hungerford, L. et al. (1992). Clinical and histologic evaluation of the prolapsed third eyelid gland in dogs. *J. Am. Vet. Med. Assoc.* 201 (12): 1861–1867.

11 Christmas, R. (1992). Surgical correction of congenital ocular and nasal dermoids and third eyelid gland prolapse in related Burmese kittens. *Can. Vet. J.* 33: 265–266.

12 Albert, R., Garrett, P., and Whitley, D. (1982). Surgical correction of everted third eyelid in 2 cats. *J. Am. Vet. Med. Assoc.* 180: 763–766.

13 Murphy C, Gutierrez JC. The eye. In: Hermanson J, de Lahunta A, and Evans H (eds.) Miller and Evan's Anatomy of the Dog. 5 St. Louis, MO: Elsevier; 2020. p. 858–911

14 Meekins, J., Rankin, A., and Samuelson, D. (2021). Ophthalmic anatomy. In: *Veterinary Ophthalmology*, 6e (ed. K. Gelatt), 41–123. Hoboken, NJ: Wiley.

15 Helper, L. (1970). The effect of lacrimal gland removal on the conjunctiva and cornea of the dog. *J. Am. Vet. Med. Assoc.* 157: 72–75.

16 Hermanson, J., de Lahunta, A., and Evans, H. (2020). The lymphatic system. In: *Miller and Evan's Anatomy of the Dog*, 5e, 616–649. St. Louis, MO: Elsevier.

17 Hermanson, J., de Lahunta, A., and Evans, H. (2020). Cranial nerves. In: *Miller and Evan's Anatomy of the Dog*, 5e, 814–838. St. Louis, MO: Elsevier.

18 Plummer, C., Kallberg, M., Gelatt, K. et al. (2008). Intranictitans tacking for replacement of prolapsed gland of the third eyelid in dogs. *Vet. Ophthalmol.* 11 (4): 228–233.

19 McLaughlin, S., Brightman, A., Helper, L. et al. (1988). Effect of removal of lacrimal and third eyelid glands on Schirmer tear test results in cats. *J. Am. Vet. Med. Assoc.* 193 (7): 820–822.

20 Saito, A., Izumisawa, Y., Yamashita, K., and Kotani, T. (2001). The effect of third eyelid gland removal on the ocular surface of dogs. *Vet. Ophthalmol.* 4: 13–18.

21 Saito, A., Watanabe, Y., and Kotani, T. (2004). Morphologic changes of the anterior corneal epithelium caused by third eyelid removal in dogs. *Vet. Ophthalmol.* 7 (2): 113–119.

22 Wilkie, D. (2021). Fundamentals of microsurgery. In: *Veterinary Ophthalmology*, 6e (ed. K. Gelatt), 787–814. Hoboken, NJ: Wiley.

23 Blogg, J. (1980). Diseases of the eyelids. In: *The Eye in Veterinary Practice (Extraocular Disease)* (ed. J. Blogg), 295–346. Philadelphia, PA: W.B. Saunders.

24 Gross, S. (1983). Effectiveness of a modification of the Blogg technique for replacing the prolapsed gland of the canine third eyelid. *Proceedings of the American College of Veterinary Ophthalmologists 14th Annual Conference*. Chicago, IL pp. 38–42. ACVO.

25 Sapienza, J., Mayordomo, A., and Beyer, A. (2014). Suture anchor placement technique around the insertion of the ventral rectus muscle for the replacement of the prolapsed gland of the third eyelid in dogs: 100 dogs. *Vet. Ophthalmol.* 17 (2): 81–86.

26 Kaswan, R. and Martin, C. (1985). Surgical correction of third eyelid prolapse in dogs. *J. Am. Vet. Med. Assoc.* 186 (1): 83.

27 Stanley, K. and Kaswan, R. (1994). Modification of the orbital rim anchorage method for surgical replacement of the gland of the third eyelid in dogs. *J. Am. Vet. Med. Assoc.* 205: 1412–1414.

28 Gelatt, K. and Brooks, D. (2011). Surgical procedures for the conjunctiva and the nictitating membrane. In: *Veterinary Ophthalmic Surgery*, 1e. Printed in China (ed. K. Gelatt and J. Gelatt), 181–182. Saunders Elsevier.

29 Twitchell, M. (1984). Surgical repair of a prolapsed gland of the 3rd eyelid in the dog. *Modern Vet. Pract.* 65 (3): 223.

30 Moore, C. (1983). Alternate technique for prolapsed gland of the third eyelid (replacement technique). In: *Current Techniques in Small Animal Surgery* (ed. M. Bojrab), 52–53. Philadelphia, PA: Lea & Febiger.

31 Barbe, C., Raymon-Letron, I., Mias, G. et al. (2017). Case report: marsupialization of a cyst of the nictitating membrane in three dogs. *Vet. Ophthalmol.* 20 (2): 181–188.

32 Multari, D., Perazzi, A., Contiero, B. et al. (2016). Pocket technique or pocket technique combined with modified orbital rim anchorage for the replacement of a prolapsed gland of the third eyelid in dogs: 353 dogs. *Vet. Ophthalmol.* 19 (3): 214–219.

33 Michel, J., Lazard, P., Vigan, M., and Albaric, O. (2020). Treatment of prolapsed gland and cartilage deformity of the nictitating membrane with pocket technique and chondrectomy alone, or combined with a wedge conjunctivectomy: 132 dogs (1998-2018). *Vet. Ophthalmol.* 23 (2): 305–331.

34 White, C. and Brennan, M. (2018). Review: an evidence-based rapid review of surgical techniques for correction of prolapsed nictitans glands in dogs. *Vet. Sci.* 5 (75): 1–16.

35 Dees, D., Schobert, C., Dubielzig, R., and Stein, T. (2016). Third eyelid gland neoplasms of dogs and cats: a retrospective histopathologic study of 145 cases. *Vet. Ophthalmol.* 19 (2): 138–143.

36 Paulsen, M., Lavach, J., Snyder, S. et al. (1987). Nodular granulomatous episclerokeratitis in dogs: 19 cases (1973–1985). *J. Am. Vet. Med. Assoc.* 190 (12): 1581–1587.

37 Allevi, G., Bevere, N., and Boydell, P. (2003). Ventral subconjunctival orbital fat hernia in the dog: a case report. *Vet. Cremona* 17 (3): 85–88.

38 Komnenou, A., Eberhard, M., Kaldrymidou, E. et al. (2002). Subconjunctival filariasis due to *Onchocerca* sp. in dogs: report of 23 cases in Greece. *Vet. Ophthalmol.* 5 (2): 119–126.

39 Lamagna, B., Peruccio, C., Guardascione, A. et al. (2012). Conjunctival dacryops in two golden retrievers. *Vet. Ophthalmol.* 15 (3): 194–199.

4

Tips and Tricks for Successful Entropion Repair

Robin Sankey

North Houston Veterinary Ophthalmology, Spring, TX, USA

Key Points

- Developmental entropion is the most common type of entropion and is likely hereditary, but the mechanism of inheritance is not known.
- Eyelid tacking is recommended until the animal is as close to maturity as possible, which varies by breed, but typically one year of age is an acceptable age to plan for surgical entropion repair.
- A macropalpebral fissure is a common contributing factor of entropion in many large and giant breed dogs and needs to be addressed when presented with entropion in these breeds.
- A Hotz-Celsus combined with eyelid shortening, when needed, will correct most cases of entropion in canine and feline patients.
- Always warn owners that additional correction may be needed at some point following the initial surgery. It is better to undercorrect than it is to overcorrect.
- Postoperative care involves the use of a hard plastic cone collar, oral antibiotics, anti-inflammatories, and pain medications. Sutures should be removed 10–14 days after surgery.

Introduction

Entropion refers to an inward rolling of the eyelids or inversion toward the cornea, whereas ectropion refers to an outward or eversion of the eyelids away from the cornea. Entropion is one of the most common ocular problems encountered by general practitioners. Although entropion can occur in any breed, there are breeds that more commonly experience this condition and different causes of entropion. Determining why the patient has entropion is important to successful repair, so this chapter will discuss the most common reasons for entropion and how these causes are prevalent among certain breeds. There are numerous ways to correct entropion, but this chapter will focus on the Hotz-Celsus technique and reduction in the size of the palpebral fissure when indicated, since this will correct most cases of entropion that are encountered in general practice.

Predisposed Breeds and Entropion Types

Entropion is much more common in dogs than in cats at a ratio of 7.12–1, so most of this discussion will pertain to the canine species.[1] As mentioned, entropion can occur in any breed, but it is most commonly found in breeds including the Shar Pei, Chow Chow, Rottweiler, Labrador, Bulldog, Great Dane, St. Bernard, Mastiff, Shih Tzu, Pekinese, and Pug. In our feline species, Maine Coons and Persians appear to be most commonly affected.[1]

There are several causes of entropion, which include primary (also called developmental), spastic, conformational changes secondary to age or disease, and cicatricial. Primary, also called developmental entropion, is the most common cause of entropion encountered in dogs. Developmental entropion appears to be hereditary, but the exact mechanism appears to be quite complex. It is often associated with factors that affect the length of the eyelid

Techniques in Small Animal Soft Tissue, Orthopedic, and Ophthalmic Surgery, First Edition. Edited by Kristin A. Coleman.

Companion website: www.wiley.com/go/coleman/surgeries

opening, the skull conformation, the orbital anatomy, gender, and how extensive and heavy the folds are in the periocular region.[2] The age of onset varies by breed, with the Shar Pei and Chow Chow breeds often being affected as early as two to six weeks of age. Other breeds are often affected at four to seven months of age.[2] The Shar Pei and Chow Chow breeds typically need eyelid tacking performed early and may require multiple eyelid tacking procedures performed before they are old enough to consider surgical correction. These two breeds commonly have all four eyelids affected by entropion. Brachycephalic breeds, such as the Pug, Shih Tzu, and Pekinese, often have medial lower eyelid entropion. Giant breeds, such as the Great Dane, St. Bernard, and Mastiff, as well as the English and American Bulldogs, commonly have an exceptionally large eyelid opening called a macropalpebral fissure. This often results in a "diamond eye" shape, causing entropion of the medial and lateral portions of the eyelids and ectropion of the central portion of the eyelids. Shortening of the palpebral fissure along with a Hotz-Celsus procedure is often required for successful correction. In breeds with excessive numbers of wrinkles or heavy brows, a brow sling procedure may need to be considered. However, since this chapter focuses on the most common cases encountered in general practice, this procedure will not be discussed, since it is rarely required for successful entropion correction.

Spastic entropion is the second most common type of entropion encountered in canines, while it is the most common cause of entropion encountered in our feline patients.[1] Spastic entropion refers to entropion that occurs when an animal retracts the globe secondary to pain. Most commonly, this is due to ulcerative keratitis, distichiasis, and conjunctivitis.[3] Using proparacaine temporarily relieves this type of entropion, and the entropion typically resolves once the source of the pain resolves, at least in dogs. In cats, spastic entropion is more likely to require surgical correction, as it is a vicious cycle of ongoing ocular surface irritation and entropion.[1]

Age-related changes, disease, trauma, or surgery are also causes of entropion. For example, loss of lid support, atrophy of the retrobulbar fat pad, phthisis bulbi, and atrophy of periocular muscles due to age or diseases, such as myositis, can result in entropion.[2] Age-related changes are the second most common cause of entropion in felines.[1] Cicatricial entropion refers to entropion that occurs from scarring following trauma, surgery, or eyelid disease. Any of these additional causes of entropion can necessitate the need for surgical intervention.

Clinical Signs

There are several clinical signs associated with entropion. Typically, patients will present with blepharospasm, conjunctival hyperemia, increased lacrimation, mucoid discharge, and a moist appearance to the entropic portion of the eyelid(s). The portion of the cornea that is irritated by the hairs adjacent to the eyelids often has edema, vascularization, pigmentation, granulation tissue, and/or corneal ulceration. Cats may also develop a corneal sequestrum, which is an area of corneal stromal necrosis that presents light brown in color to a dense black scab on the corneal surface. In most cases, the corneal changes can be drastically improved with correction of the entropion, but they cannot always be completely resolved. A corneal sequestrum is best treated with a keratectomy, so referral to a veterinary ophthalmologist is recommended in these cases. To try to prevent long-standing changes from entropion, early intervention is the best practice.

Diagnosis

Diagnosing entropion is typically straightforward, but some cases are difficult, especially when the entropion is mild. Examination of the patient at a distance with no distortion of the face from an assistant holding should first be performed before moving in for an up-close look. When examining up close, be sure the assistant is not restraining too tightly around the neck, since this can place too much traction on the skin and distort the appearance of the eyelids.[2] Looking closely for corneal changes in the suspected or the obviously entropic area can help the clinician decide when intervention is warranted. Applying proparacaine to relieve any spastic component after the initial examination also can be an especially useful diagnostic tool. Another useful tool can be to gently pinch the skin adjacent to the eyelid starting about 10 mm below the eyelid margin, apply gentle traction to force the eyelid to roll inward against the cornea, then release the pinched portion of the skin. The eyelid should correct itself into a normal position with one blink. If it remains entropic, the patient suffers from habitual entropion[2] (Video 4.1). This technique can be especially useful if there is a question as to whether a patient has entropion. If it is still not clear if entropion is the cause of the presenting ocular abnormalities, temporary eyelid tacking can be a useful diagnostic tool to monitor for improvement of corneal changes, squinting, conjunctival hyperemia, and ocular discharge, which often accompany entropion with varying severity. These signs should improve within a few weeks if the entropion is temporarily relieved by the tacking.

The normal palpebral fissure opening, when measured in a stretched horizontal position from the medial to the lateral canthus, is about 33 mm in medium to large-breed dogs. However, in dogs with a macropalpebral fissure, the palpebral fissure is often 39 mm or more in length when measured horizontally in the same stretched position.[2]

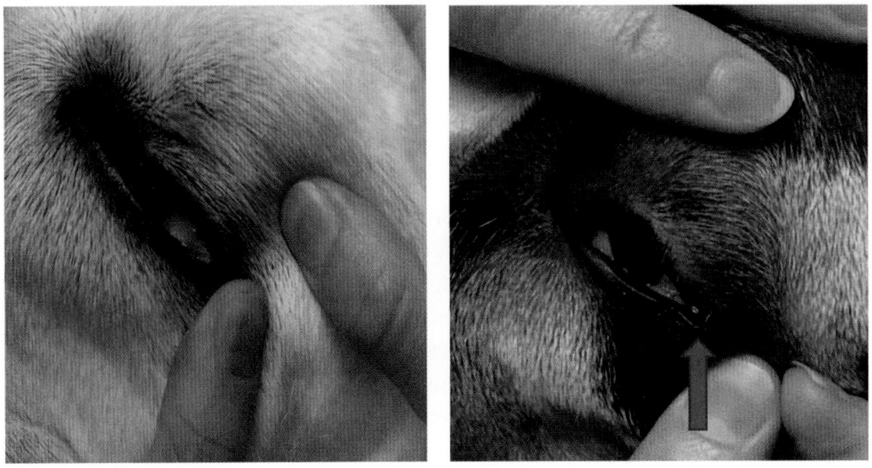

Figure 4.1 Diagnosing if an entropic pet would benefit from eyelid shortening. (a) No notching is seen when lateral tension is applied on the eyelid margin with a normal eyelid; (b) an excessively long inferior eyelid indicated by notching of the eyelid when lateral tension is applied (blue arrow). *Source:* © Robin Sankey.

The horizontal length of the palpebral fissure can be measured with a pair of calipers, but in some patients, this can be difficult. There are a few things the author has found to help determine if the patient would benefit from a reduction in the size of the palpebral fissure. First, if the patient has a diamond eye shape or the eyelids obviously do not fit closely to the normal corneal curvature or are ectropic in places, they will likely benefit from eyelid shorting. Also, in the entropic patient, if an outward notch of the eyelid appears in the lateral portion of the eyelid when it is tensed and stretched in a lateral direction, the eyelid will benefit from shortening (Figure 4.1).

Treatment

If the entropion is mild, corneal lubrication may provide adequate protection. However, if corneal changes are present, intervention is recommended sooner than later to try to prevent chronic corneal changes, ulceration, and even corneal rupture. Ideally, permanent correction should be delayed until the patient is fully grown, which is 1.5–2 years of age. However, in many patients, this is not possible due to the severity and persistence of the entropion, so typically, the author's goal is to get them as close to one year of age as possible. The author always discusses with the owners that waiting until the patient is fully grown is ideal because the amount of correction can change, and some cases will resolve or at least significantly improve as they reach maturity, which can affect the surgical plan and the outcome. However, if the entropion is severe or requires multiple eyelid tackings, most owners are anxious to get them in for surgical correction as soon as possible.

Temporary eyelid tacking is performed with 4-0 or 5-0 nonabsorbable suture material. Interrupted sutures are placed by taking two, roughly 5 mm "bites" of skin perpendicular to and starting about 2 mm from the eyelid margin while directing the needle away from the eye. Each interrupted suture should evert the eyelid margin away from the eye to prevent inversion. The number of sutures placed varies by the amount of the eyelid that is needed to be everted, but typically three to five sutures are needed if just one eyelid is affected (Figure 4.2). Sutures are typically left in place for two to six weeks, depending on the reason for the suture placement. For developmental entropion, the author recommends leaving the sutures in place until they are no longer holding the tissue, the patient develops a suture reaction, or they fall out on their own. For suspected spastic entropion, the tacking sutures are left in place for one to two weeks beyond the resolution of the painful stimulus.

There are numerous techniques used for the surgical repair of entropion, but the Hotz-Celsus is the most used and is appropriate in most situations and will be the

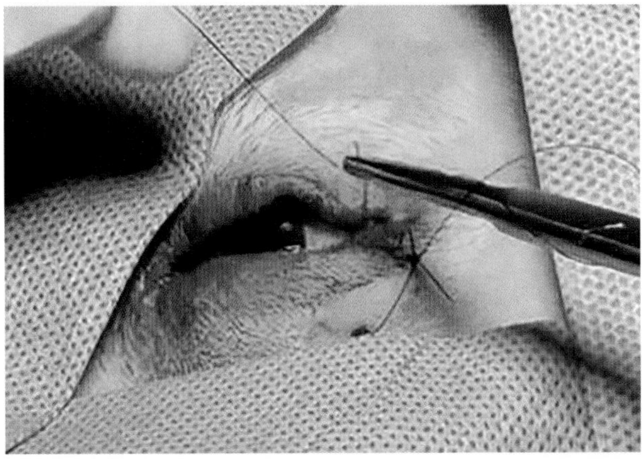

Figure 4.2 Eyelid Tacking. Two "bites" of skin are taken for each interrupted suture placed. The size of each "bite" of skin is based on the amount of eversion needed so the eyelid is no longer entropic. Often, two 5 mm "bites" of skin are adequate. *Source:* © Robin Sankey.

technique focused upon in this chapter. If the patient has a macropalpebral fissure and would benefit from a reduction in the size of the eyelid opening, this should either be performed first with a plan to perform a Hotz-Celsus if additional correction is needed, or it can be combined with a Hotz-Celsus to save time if the surgeon is sure both procedures will be needed for a successful repair. It is important not to overcorrect because this could result in iatrogenic ectropion and the need for additional surgery. Remember, Bulldogs and many giant breeds often need a combo procedure.

If it has been determined that the patient needs correction, the surgeon must decide how much tissue needs to be removed. There are multiple ways to decide, but this chapter will focus on the technique that seems the most straightforward. First, decide which eyelid is most affected (superior or inferior) and which portion(s) of the eyelids are affected. Sometimes, it is the entire eyelid, while other times, it is just the nasal (i.e., medial) or temporal (i.e., lateral) portion of the eyelid that is entropic. The most common area affected is the inferior temporal portion of the eyelid. With the eyelid in its entropic state, starting about 2–2.5 mm from the eyelid margin, forceps are used to pinch the amount of skin adjacent to the eyelid margin that is needed to evert the eyelid into a normal position. Toothed forceps work best for this and will leave two marks on the skin, indicating the placement of the dorsal and ventral aspects of the incision (Figure 4.3). Next, an eyelid plate is used to stabilize the eyelid margin, and calipers can be used to measure the width between the teeth marks of the forceps, and the calipers should be locked in place. A #15 Bard-Parker surgical blade is used to make the first incision parallel to the eyelid margin starting 2–2.5 mm from the eyelid margin (at the junction of the haired and nonhaired portion of the eyelids) and is extended 1 mm beyond the medial and lateral extent of the entropion.[2] With a little bit of blood from the incision on the dorsal blade of the caliper, invert it and run it across the skin where the second parallel incision will be made (Figure 4.4). The surgical blade is then used to create the second partial-thickness parallel incision that has been outlined with the blood from the dorsal incision. The ventral incision is typically tapered toward the first incision at the temporal and nasal aspects until the dorsal and ventral parallel incisions meet (Figure 4.5). The author prefers a #15 Bard-Parker surgery blade, but the use of a #69 or #64 Beaver blade for small patients is also acceptable if preferred. The skin between the two parallel incisions is removed using tenotomy or Metzenbaum scissors.

Some ophthalmologists advocate for the removal of a thin strip of the exposed orbicularis oculi muscle while others do not, as it causes more bleeding.[2,4,5] Many ophthalmologists do not feel this makes a difference in the surgical outcome. Hemostasis is controlled with pressure, cautery, or clamping small bleeders with mosquito forceps, but typically bleeding is minimal and easily controlled with

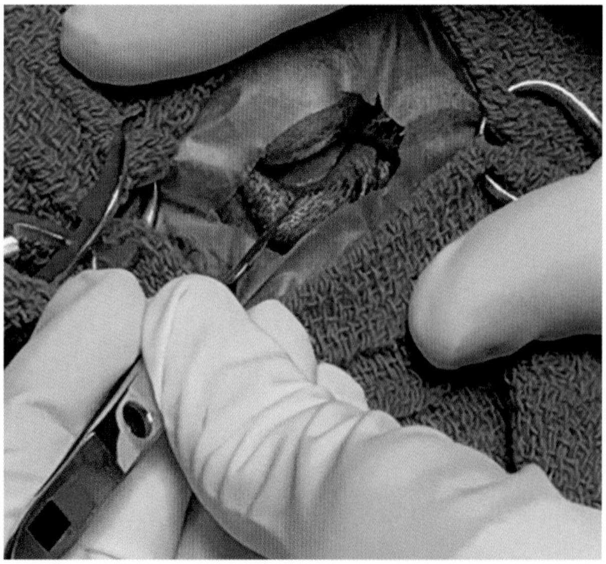

Figure 4.3 Deciding how much tissue to remove with the Hotz-Celsus procedure. Using toothed forceps to pinch the amount of tissue needed to evert the eyelid. The tissue between the teeth marks denotes the amount of tissue to be removed to evert the eyelid margin. *Source:* © Robin Sankey.

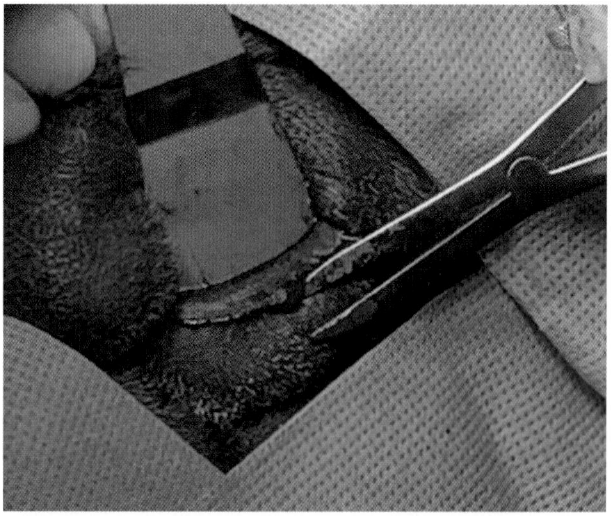

Figure 4.4 Castroviejo caliper used to mark the placement of the parallel elliptical incision for the Hotz-Celsus procedure. First, a toothed forcep was used to mark the amount of tissue removal needed for eyelid eversion (as depicted in Figure 4.3). The calipers are used to measure the distance between the two marks and are then locked in place. The first incision is made parallel to and 2.0–2.5 mm from the eyelid margin. The upper tooth of the locked caliper is then wiped through the blood of the initial parallel incision and inverted to then create a line where the second parallel incision of the Hotz-Celsus will be made. *Source:* © Robin Sankey.

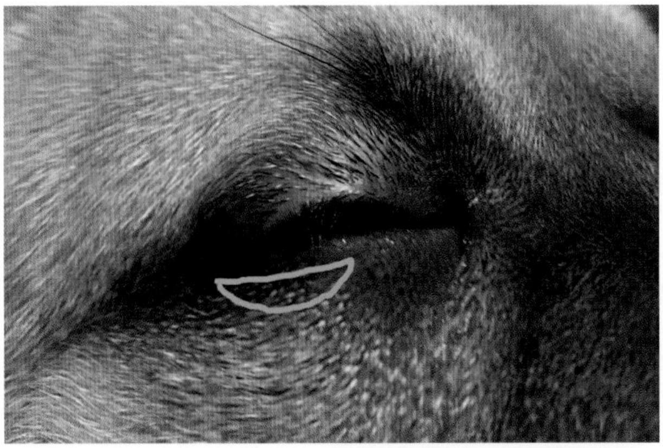

Figure 4.5 Hotz-Celsus drawn on an anesthetized dog. The dorsal incision is made parallel to the eyelid margin starting about 2–2.5 mm from the eyelid margin. The ventral incision is then tapered toward the medial and lateral aspects of the dorsal incision. The outlined area will then be removed with tenotomy or Metzenbaum scissors. *Source:* © Robin Sankey.

intermittent pressure. The skin is then closed in a single layer with interrupted sutures with proper alignment being crucial. The author prefers to place the first suture in the middle of the incised area, followed by sutures placed to split the medial and lateral aspects in half again. The remaining incision is closed using the law of bisection by splitting the distance needing to be closed in half until a suture is placed every two to three millimeters. Suture-sized 4-0 to 6-0 with 10–16 mm, 3/8–1/2 circle, extra sharp-pointed round, micropoint, or extra-fine-cutting needles are used.[6] The author prefers absorbable sutures, even though the sutures are typically removed at 14 days to reduce the risk of skin irritation or a suture reaction. However, sometimes a suture gets missed or the patient is too aggressive to allow suture removal, so the author likes having the flexibility that absorbable suture allows. After the first few sutures are placed, evaluate if the eyelid eversion is sufficient. If additional correction is needed, a little bit more skin from the Hotz-Celsus can be removed. Figure 4.6 shows a severe case of entropion in a Shar Pei. As severely as this patient was affected, just performing a Hotz-Celsus was enough to properly evert the eyelid margins and provide relief for this patient.

There are certain breeds that almost always need to have their eyelids shortened, such as Bulldogs and giant breeds (Figure 4.7), but the eyelid length should be evaluated for each patient individually because there are exceptions to every rule. If the eyelids have a diamond shape, such as in most Bulldogs and many giant breeds, shortening is recommended because if just a Hotz-Celsus is performed, the excessively long eyelid will still be prone to entropion. Reduction in the size of the palpebral fissure can be performed alone or in combination with the Hotz-Celsus procedure. The amount the eyelid needs to be shortened can be estimated at the time of surgery by retracting the eyelid laterally and looking for a notch in the eyelid to form (as shown in Figure 4.1).

Using the toothed forceps, pinch the excess eyelid margin to mark the area of the eyelid margin that needs to be shortened. Next, stabilize the eyelid margin with the lid plate, and using your surgical blade, create a V-shaped partial-thickness wedge through the skin. The wedge of eyelid margin and associated periocular skin to be removed should be twice as high as it is wide (see Chapter 2 for more details on this). The author prefers to reduce the size of the palpebral fissure by removing the "V-shaped" piece of eyelid margin where it is ectropic or the loosest, which is typically centrally for dogs with the diamond eye conformation or temporally in most other patients. The partial thickness Hotz-Celsus is then made as previously directed to help evert the entropic portion of the eyelid. The skin between the parallel cuts of the Hotz-Celsus is removed first, followed by full-thickness excision of the incised outline of the eyelid wedge. In dogs with the diamond eye configuration with central ectropion and medial and lateral entropion, the Hotz-Celsus can be narrowed centrally and then widened temporally and medially to remove an appropriate amount of eyelid. Alternatively, an elliptical-shaped wedge of skin can be removed medially and laterally and not connected along the central portion of the eyelid. Hemostasis is controlled with pressure, cautery, or clamping small bleeders with mosquito forceps. The eyelid margin is closed first with a figure-of-8 suture pattern, leaving the suture tails long to trap the suture tails away from the eye to prevent them from rubbing the cornea as discussed in Chapter 2 of this book on eyelid mass removal.

If correction of only one eyelid on an eye is planned, the author recommends that the opposite eyelid be evaluated during surgery to be sure it still appears to be in a normal position, as sometimes the eyelid position changes when the opposite eyelid is surgically altered.

Postoperative Care

A hard, plastic Elizabethan collar is needed for at least 10–14 days until the sutures are removed, but the author often recommends that the patient continues to wear it for a few days following suture removal due to residual mild skin irritation. A topical antibiotic ointment is sent home and applied TID to QID to the corneal surface. This provides a topical antibiotic source to help prevent infection. It also helps prevent corneal irritation if a suture should shift and start to rub the cornea during healing. The author prescribes systemic antibiotics due to the numerous sutures

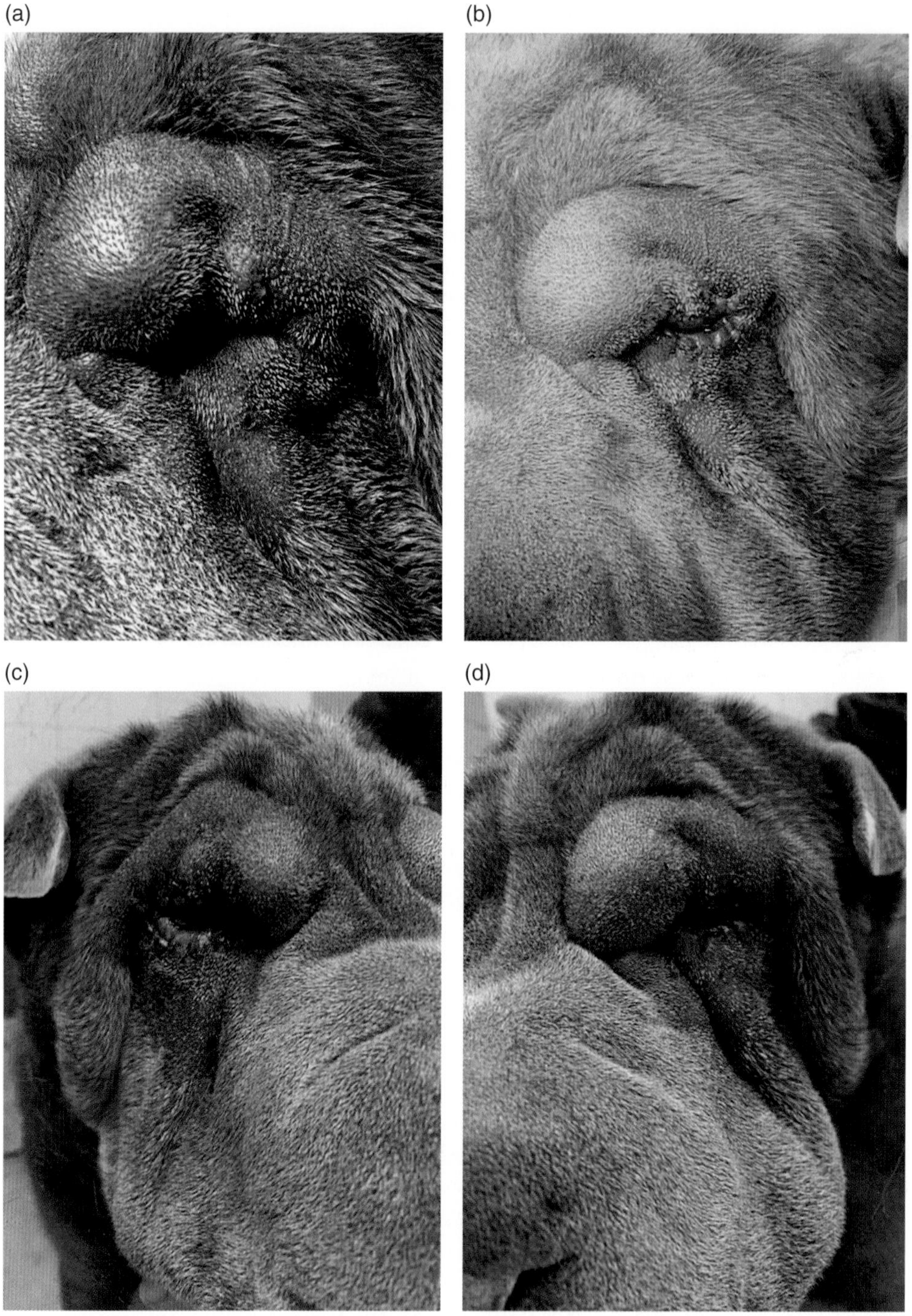

Figure 4.6 Severe entropion in a Shar Pei. (a) preoperative picture; (b–d) immediate postoperative after Hotz-Celsus repair. *Source:* © Robin Sankey.

present and the tendency for pre-existing or post-surgical moist dermatitis. Topical Optixcare is great for sending home with owners to aid in soaking discharge that accumulates on the skin sutures. This can be applied liberally over the discharge, left to soak for a few minutes, and then gently removed with a moist cotton ball. Oral anti-inflammatory and pain medications are also dispensed.

Complications

Complications are typically minimal with swelling, moist dermatitis, and suture reaction being the most common potential complications. There is a risk of corneal ulceration if a suture should shift and start rubbing the cornea, so the author advises owners to contact the clinic right

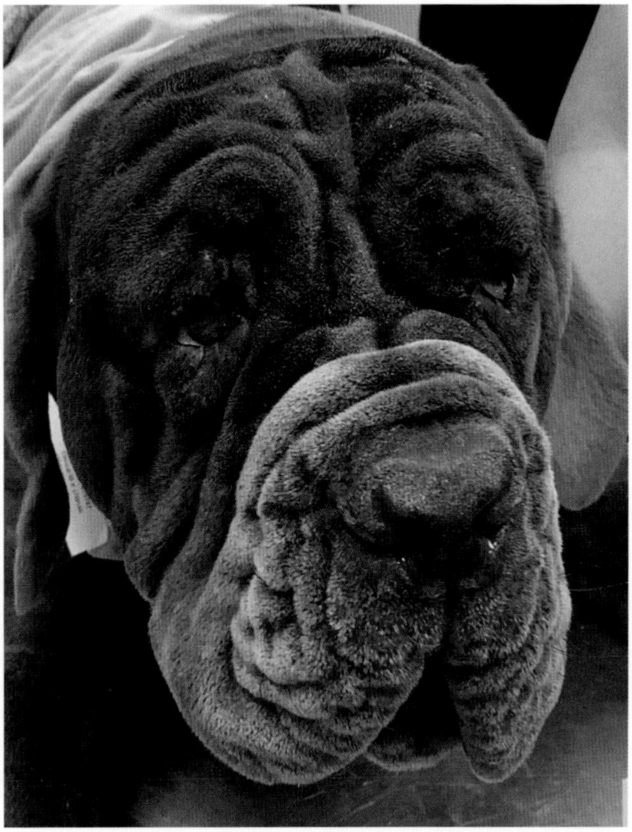

Figure 4.7 Neapolitan Mastiff. Note the macropalpebral fissure. For this patient, first, the upper and lower eyelids should be shortened. A Hotz-Celsus would then be performed if entropion is noted once the eyelids are appropriately shortened. With this degree of eyelid abnormality, there is an increased risk of needing a second surgery to obtain the optimal eyelid position. Remember, it is better to slightly undercorrect than to overcorrect. *Source:* © Robin Sankey.

away if a sudden increase in squinting is noticed. The author always warns owners that additional correction may be required either shortly after surgery or at some point in the future, since it is ultimately not known what the animal will look like until they are fully healed. Also, aging, trauma, myositis, and corneal pain can result in additional changes in eyelid conformation that warrant additional correction.

To access the videos for this chapter, please go to

www.wiley.com/go/coleman/surgeries

VIDEO 4.1 This video shows another way to determine if a patient has entropion. The video depicts a normal dog without entropion. Note how the inverted eyelid corrects itself in one blink. If the lid were to remain inverted after a single blink, that would support a diagnosis of habitual entropion. *Source:* © Robin Sankey.

References

1 Williams, D.L. and Kim, J.Y. (2009). Feline entropion: a case series of 50 affected animals (2003–2008). *Vet. Ophthalmol.* 12 (4): 221–226.

2 Gelatt, K.N., Gilger, B.C., and Kern, T.J. (ed.) (2013). *Veterinary Ophthalmology*, 844–847. Ames, IA: Wiley-Blackwell.

3 Read, R.A. and Hugh, C.B. (2007). Entropion correction in dogs and cats using a combination Hotz-Celsus and lateral eyelid wedge resection: results in 311 cats. *Vet. Ophthalmol.* 10 (1): 6–11.

4 Moore, C.P. and Constantinescu, G.M. (1997). Surgery of the adnexa. *Vet. Clin. North Am. Small Anim. Pract.* 27 (5): 1020.

5 Maggs, D.J., Miller, P.E., and Ofri, R. (ed.) (2013). *Slatter's Fundamentals of Veterinary Ophthalmology*, 120. St. Louis, MO: Elsevier-Saunders.

6 Gelatt, K.N., Ben-Shlomo, G., Gilger, B.C. et al. (2021). *Veterinary Ophthalmology*, 927. Hoboken, NJ: Wiley-Blackwell.

5

A Guide to Enucleation

Robin Sankey

North Houston Veterinary Ophthalmology, Spring, TX, USA

Key Points

- The two main approaches for enucleation include transconjunctival and transpalpebral.
- The transpalpebral approach is recommended over the transconjunctival approach in cases where infection or neoplasia is present.
- Manipulation of the globe or eyelids can cause an oculocardiac reflex, which leads to a sudden, potentially life-threatening decrease in the heart rate and blood pressure. Typically, this can be corrected with cessation of the stimulus and administration of an intravenous dose of an anticholinergic drug.
- An orbital prosthesis can be placed following enucleation to prevent a concave depression in the skin overlying the orbit. However, there is a 5–10% risk of the prosthesis becoming infected, which could necessitate removal of the prosthesis with additional surgery.
- Complications from routine enucleation without the placement of an orbital prosthesis are uncommon. Retention of conjunctival tissue, medial caruncle, nictitans, or any part of the nictitans gland can result in a draining fistula or cyst formation and often necessitates removal of the retained tissue to achieve resolution.
- Healing of the enucleation surgical site will take 10–14 days. A rigid cone collar, along with oral anti-inflammatory and pain medications, is recommended.

Introduction

Enucleation refers to the removal of the globe and is a commonly performed surgery in our animal companions for a variety of reasons. There are two main approaches to enucleation: the transconjunctival approach (also called the subconjunctival approach) and the transpalpebral approach. The author prefers the transconjunctival approach, however, that is a purely personal preference, and there are occasions when the transpalpebral approach is optimal. Both techniques will be discussed in this chapter.

Anatomy

As with any surgery, it is important to consider globe and orbital anatomy before performing a procedure. The globe refers to the spherical portion of the eye and is enclosed within the orbit and covered externally by the eyelids. The orbit surrounds and protects the globe, and in dogs and cats is made up of portions of the frontal, lacrimal, zygomatic, maxillary, sphenoid, and palatine bones. The orbit in these species is incomplete, meaning it is not fully surrounded by bone.[1] Instead, the temporal orbit and part of the ventral aspect of the orbit are covered by dense

Techniques in Small Animal Soft Tissue, Orthopedic, and Ophthalmic Surgery, First Edition. Edited by Kristin A. Coleman.

Companion website: www.wiley.com/go/coleman/surgeries

periorbital tissue that encloses the globe along with the orbital ligament that spans the caudolateral opening from the frontal process of the zygomatic bone to the zygomatic process of the frontal bone.[2] The surrounding muscles also provide additional support and structure for the orbit and include the temporalis, masseter, and pterygoid muscles. The incomplete orbit in carnivores allows them to open their jaws wider than herbivores, making consuming prey easier.[1] Also within the orbit is the zygomatic salivary gland, which lies dorsal and lateral to the pterygoid muscle and ventral to the globe.[3]

The bony orbit is lined by orbital facia, which is a dense connective tissue that is made up of the periorbita, Tenon's capsule, and the facial sheaths that surround the extraocular muscles. The periorbita is a cone-shaped fibrous membrane that lines the orbit and encloses the globe, extraocular muscles, nerves, and blood vessels.[1] Tenon's capsule is a thin, fibrous capsule that envelops the globe from the level of the limbus to the optic nerve. The limbus is the point where the cornea meets the sclera. Tenon's capsule is separated from the sclera by a thin space known as the episcleral space.[3] There are six extraocular muscles enclosed in the facial sheath, including the dorsal and ventral oblique muscles and the dorsal, ventral, medial, and lateral recti muscles. These muscles are attached directly to the globe and are responsible for the suspension and centralization of the globe within the orbit and the movement of the globe.[1] These muscles are severed during enucleation.

The main arterial supply to the eye is primarily from the maxillary and the external ophthalmic arteries and their branches that arise from the external carotid artery.[3] The main arteries to avoid course along the ventral and ventromedial aspect of the orbit, and these can be avoided by remaining close to the ventral aspect of the globe during dissection. Also, the angularis oculi vein should be avoided when removing the eyelids. It lies at the dorsomedial aspect of the orbital rim (Figure 5.1) and can be avoided by not removing more than ~5 mm of the superior eyelid in this area.

There is inherent bleeding that occurs during enucleation due to the many arterial and venous branches that supply blood to and drain blood from the many intraocular and extraocular structures within the orbit, and as long as the main vessels are not punctured or transected, the smaller branches should vasoconstrict without ligation. The venous supply to the globe largely parallels the arterial supply.[3]

The optic nerves from the right and left eyes join at the optic chiasm, which is the site where there is a significant cross-over of the nerve fibers to the contralateral optic tract. There is a 75% crossover in the dog and 65% in the cat. This is significant because too much tension on the globe during removal prior to severing the optic nerve could result in blindness in the contralateral eye. This is of greatest concern in the feline species due to anatomical differences between dogs and cats. Mammalian optic nerves have a sigmoid flexure within their optic nerves, presumably allowing for ocular motility and some globe protrusion without traction on the optic nerve. However, cats lack the degree of sigmoid flexure present in dogs, thus, they are more prone to tractional injuries of the optic nerve due to the shortened space between the posterior aspect of the globe and the optic chiasm. Also, the feline globe is only slightly smaller than the orbit, making exposure of the optic nerve more difficult during enucleation and increasing the risk of excessive traction on the optic nerve during globe removal.[5]

Something else to be aware of is the risk of the oculocardiac reflex (OCR) when manipulating the globe or periocular tissues. The OCR occurs due to stimulation of the ophthalmic branch of the trigeminal nerve, which in turn results in stimulation of the vagus nerve to then cause inhibitory effects on the cardiac myocardium. This can result in a significant decrease in heart rate and blood pressure, which could compromise organ perfusion and lead to death if not corrected immediately. Typically, temporary cessation of surgical manipulation along with administration of an anticholinergic allows the heart rate and blood pressure to return to normal. The incidence of the OCR in a multicenter retrospective study showed an incidence of 4.8% during enucleation, which is overall low, but a retrobulbar block can prevent the OCR from being an issue and can improve intraoperative comfort, thus,

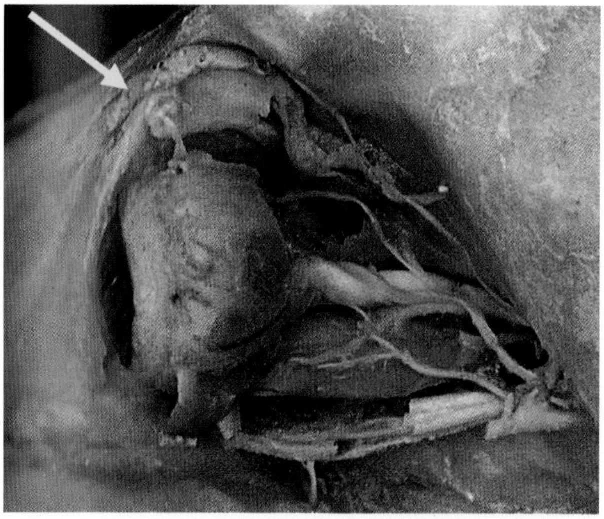

Figure 5.1 Angularis oculi vein (yellow arrow). Lateral view of the globe to show the vascular supply of the eye. The angularis oculi vein lies in the dorsal medial aspect of the orbit and is typically avoided by not removing too much of the superior eyelid in this area. *Source:* Stanley et al.[4]/Reproduced with permission from ELSEVIER.

allowing a lighter plane of anesthesia.[6] How to perform this block is beyond the scope of this chapter; however, it is a useful skill to reduce the risk of the OCR and to improve patient comfort.

Indications for Enucleation

Enucleation is performed for many different reasons including trauma, ocular congenital defects, intraocular infection, blindness, pain, neoplasia, and the inability to treat a chronic condition that would cause discomfort to the animal if left untreated.[7] See Figure 5.2 for a picture of a globe proptosis, which is one of the most common globe-threatening ocular emergencies seen in practice.

Techniques

The transconjunctival and transpalpebral approaches are the two techniques primarily used for enucleation. The periocular hair and eyelids should be shaved, and the skin, eyelids, and conjunctival sac of the globe should be antiseptically prepped. Use dilute povidone-iodine (Betadine®) solution (1:50) around the eyes and be sure to use the povidone-iodine *solution* and not the *scrub*. Povidone-iodine scrub, chlorhexidine products, or products containing alcohol should be avoided near the corneal surface, as they can result in excessive tissue inflammation and damage. A gel ocular lubricant placed over the cornea and palpebral fissure before clipping the patient can help prevent hair from embedding into the palpebral fissure. The hair can then be easily rinsed from the surface with sterile water or saline during the antiseptic prep. Dilute Betadine-soaked sterile cotton-tipped applicators are ideal for aseptically prepping the conjunctival sac and removing any residual hair or debris.

The patient is positioned in sternal recumbency. The head can either be positioned with the head straight with the eyes parallel to the table or the head can be tilted to expose the affected eye (affected side more dorsal) if the surgeon prefers. The head is secured in place with a vacuum pillow, sandbags, or towels. Surgical tape can also be secured to the table across the top of the head if additional support is needed to keep the head in the desired position. The anesthesia equipment should be placed at the aboral end of the animal to prevent equipment and staff from needing to be directly in the surgical field. Also, the placement of an IV catheter in the pelvic limb is helpful to allow for ongoing access to the catheter, since a thoracic limb catheter will be in the surgical field and will be more difficult to access during the procedure.

An elbow adapter placed between the endotracheal tube and the anesthesia breathing circuit tubing helps with positioning the equipment so that it does not get in the way of the procedure. The adapter also helps decrease tension on the endotracheal tube, since the tubing has to span the distance of the table when the gas anesthesia machine is placed at the aboral end of the patient. Also, the endotracheal tube is secured to the mandible instead of the maxilla to prevent the ET tube tie from being in the way during the surgical procedure (Figure 5.3).

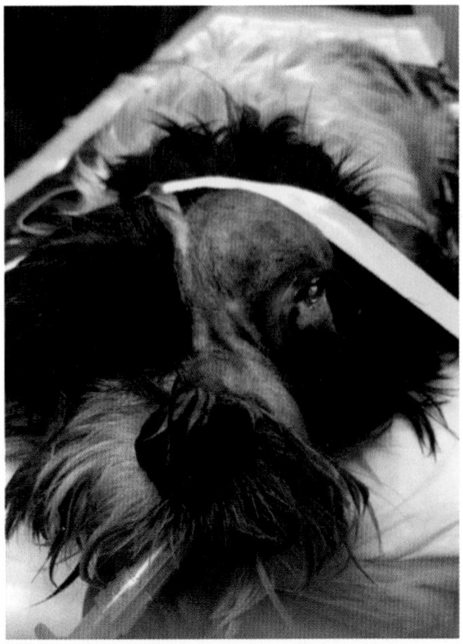

Figure 5.2 Proptosed left globe. *Source:* © Kristin Coleman.

Transconjunctival Enucleation

The transconjunctival technique can be performed if it is your technique of choice in most situations, except when infection or neoplasia of the cornea or conjunctiva is present, or if there is concern that a corneal perforation could contaminate the surgical area. Then, the transpalpebral technique is a better option for globe removal.

For transconjunctival enucleation, first, a lateral skin canthotomy is performed. The author typically makes this incision about 8–10 mm long. It is used to provide more room for dissection around the globe and provides improved visualization of the periorbital tissues. Metzenbaum scissors or lightweight Mayo scissors are used, starting in the lateral canthotomy incision, to remove the superior and inferior eyelids along with about 5 mm of the periocular skin, being careful to avoid the angularis oculi vein as discussed above. Removal of the superior and inferior eyelids is joined at the medial canthus, and the medial caruncle is removed. The medial caruncle is

(a) (b)

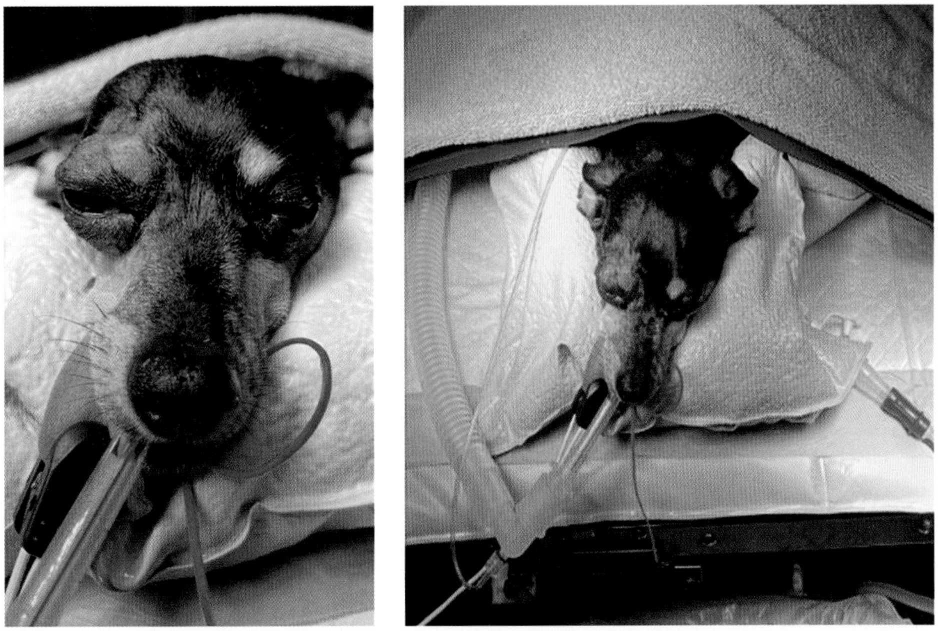

Figure 5.3 (a) Positioning of the head using a vacuum pillow. The orange tie used to secure the endotracheal tube is tied to the mandible to prevent the tie from being in the way during the procedure; (b) view of the elbow connector attached to the endotracheal tube used to aid in positioning the anesthesia tubing and equipment. *Source:* © Kristin Coleman.

a slightly raised nodule of conjunctival tissue and sits in the corner of the eye adjacent to the medial canthus.

The third eyelid and associated gland are then removed. The author finds it helpful to grasp the third eyelid with forceps and apply gentle dorsal traction on the third eyelid, which allows resection of the third eyelid at the base. The third eyelid can then be palpated to be sure the ventral portion of the gland is completely excised. Next, starting about 5 mm posterior to the limbus, heavily curved enucleation scissors (Figure 5.4) are used to resect the conjunctival tissue and to transect the extraocular muscles at their insertions onto the globe. The curved nature of these scissors is especially useful for the transection of the extraocular muscles close to the globe during this step of transconjunctival enucleation, but any curved Metzenbaum scissors can be used.

Once the conjunctival tissue and extraocular muscle attachments have been severed, gentle forward traction on the globe using forceps (Bishop Harmon or Brown-Adson Forceps) is used while the curved scissors transect the optic nerve and associated artery and vein on the posterior aspect of the globe. The optic nerve and vessels are not clamped or ligated before severing them. Clamping or ligating will potentially cause more tension on the optic nerve, the ligature often does not stay in place, it prolongs surgery time, and it is not necessary for hemostasis.

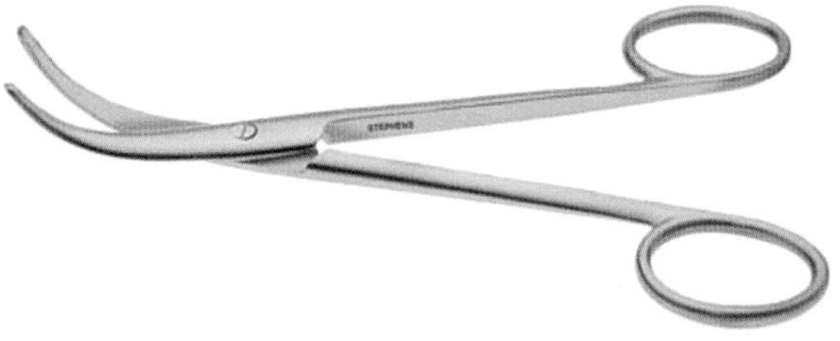

Figure 5.4 Heavy curved enucleation scissors. *Source:* Stephens instruments.

Once the globe is removed, the orbit is packed with gauze, and all remaining conjunctival tissue is removed (Figure 5.5). The gauze-packing in the orbit is then removed, and hemostatic sponges or sleeves are placed within the orbit as needed for additional hemostasis (Figure 5.6). The periorbital tissue is then closed in a continuous pattern with 4-0 or 5-0 synthetic absorbable suture. The author prefers 5-0 polyglactin 910 due to the ease of suture handling, adequate strength, and the cosmetic outcome associated with using this small suture. However, others may prefer a monofilament absorbable suture to decrease tissue drag, but in the author's opinion, this is not a significant issue with the 5-0 polyglactin 910.

Following the closure of the periorbital tissue, the subcutaneous layer is then closed. At this point, the skin is evaluated to see if additional removal of the skin edges is needed to facilitate cosmetic closure. Ideally, the skin edges should be well apposed with minimal tension or excessive overlap of tissues. If too much skin is left in place, there is an increased risk of puckering of the skin edges, which can affect the cosmetic outcome in the postoperative period. However, if extra skin is left, the result after healing is often

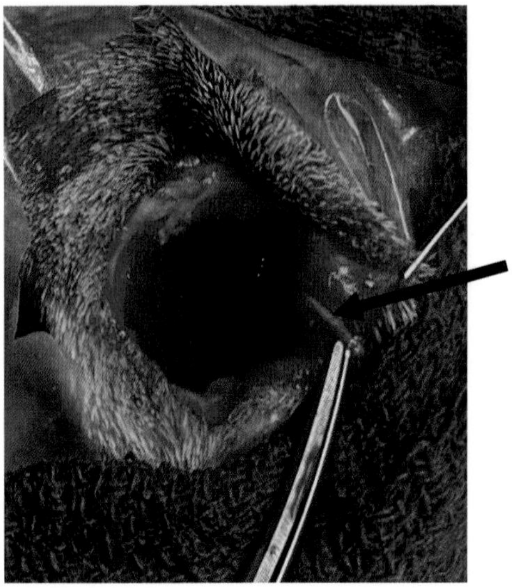

Figure 5.5 Conjunctival tissue. The conjunctival tissue has a distinct look and needs to be removed completely to reduce the risk of chronic drainage from the enucleation site. The black arrow points to a thin, shiny strip of conjunctival tissue. *Source:* © Robin Sankey.

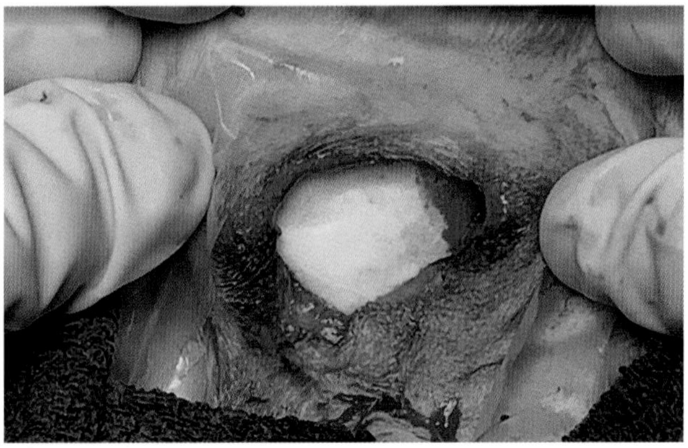

Figure 5.6 Packing orbit with gauze to achieve hemostasis prior to closure. Be sure to remove the gauze before closing the orbit. Hemostatic sponges or sleeves can be placed in the orbit as needed for additional hemostasis. *Source:* © Robin Sankey.

still cosmetically appealing. Finally, the skin layer is closed according to the surgeon's preference. The author typically closes the subcutaneous layer in a continuous pattern followed by the skin in an intradermal pattern with 5-0 polyglactin 910. If any small gaps or suture line imperfections are present, tissue glue can be applied to the skin or additional interrupted skin sutures can be placed. Others may prefer a nonabsorbable monofilament suture, such as nylon, for external skin closure in a cruciate mattress, simple continuous, or an interrupted pattern, which is also fine to use.

Postoperatively, a pressure bandage is placed to reduce swelling and postoperative bleeding. A rolled-up piece of gauze is secured in place over the suture line using a 3-0 or 4-0 suture of your choice. A "bite" of skin above and below the incision line is taken either on the nasal or temporal aspect of the incision, and the knot is then tied on top of the rolled gauze. A second suture is placed in the same way along the opposite side of the enucleation site to secure the gauze across the incision line (Figure 5.7). The bandage is removed just before the patient is discharged from the hospital. The bandage aids in hemostasis and helps diminish immediate postoperative swelling.

Transconjunctival enucleation tends to be faster due to fewer steps, offers better visualization of the tissues, and typically involves the removal of less periorbital tissue compared to the transpalpebral method, which leads to less skin depression around the orbit and a better cosmetic outcome. However, there is a higher risk of leaving conjunctival tissue, the medial caruncle, the nictitans, or the nictitans glandular tissue behind. Removal of these tissues is imperative since retained tissues can result in draining fistulas from the orbit.[8] Also, if surface infection is present, there is an increased risk of seeding the infection into the orbit.

Transpalpebral Enucleation

Transpalpebral enucleation is preferable to know if you only want to learn one technique since it can be used for all routine enucleation cases. As stated above, transpalpebral enucleation is best used for cases with infection or neoplasia of the cornea or conjunctiva or when there is concern that corneal perforation could result in the spread of infection or neoplastic cells into the orbit.

With this method, the eyelids, nictitans with gland, conjunctival tissue, and globe are removed en bloc. First, the eyelids are sutured together in a continuous pattern using a suture material of your choice. Leaving a small loop of suture or a long suture tail at the medial and/or lateral aspects of the sutured eyelids is useful so a hemostat can be attached to the suture and used to stabilize and manipulate the ocular tissue as needed during dissection and removal. In lieu of sutures, the eyelids can be apposed using towel clamps or hemostats, but the suture method is less cumbersome in the author's opinion.

An elliptical skin incision is then made approximately 5 mm proximal to the eyelid margin and joined near the medial and lateral canthi. The subcutaneous tissue is bluntly dissected, and the medial and lateral canthal ligaments are severed using Metzenbaum scissors. Gentle forward traction on the eyelids with either the preplaced hemostats on the simple continuous line of suture apposing the eyelids or the forceps placed in the incised eyelid skin will help with the dissection of the subcutaneous and conjunctival tissue to the level of the conjunctiva just posterior to the limbus. Then, the extraocular muscles can be

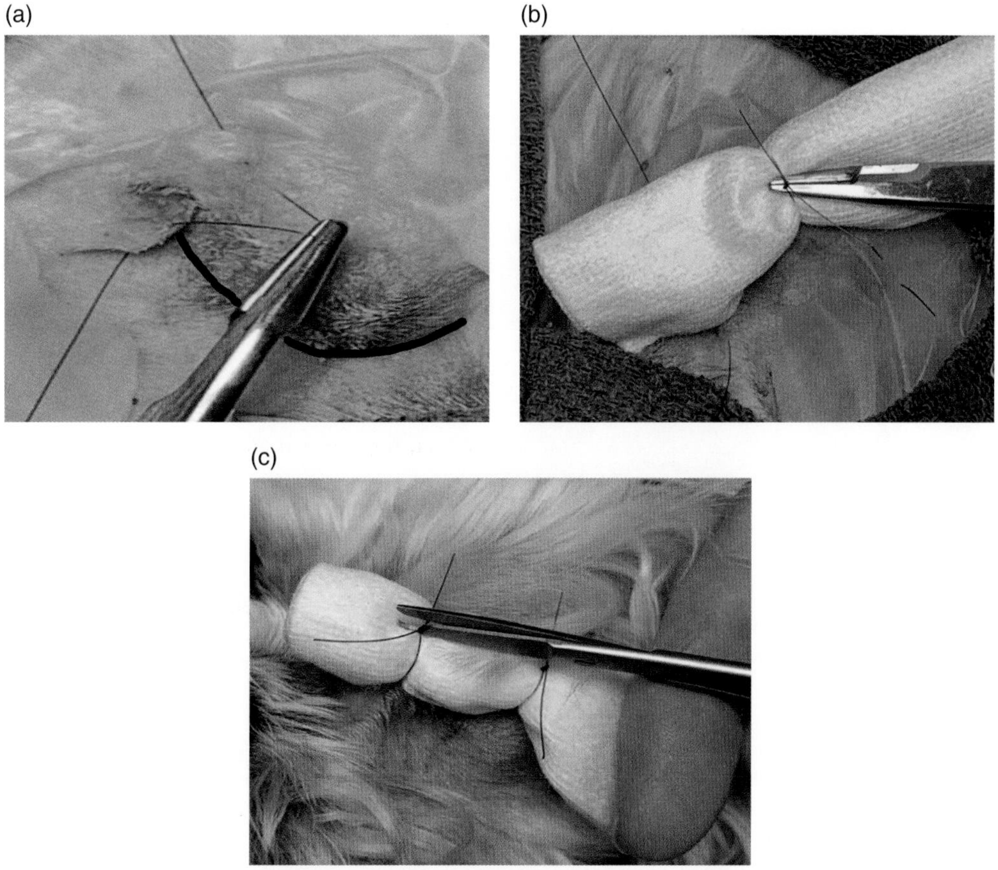

Figure 5.7 Placement of the postoperative gauze bandage. (a) A bite of skin (~4 mm in width) is taken dorsal and ventral to the incision line (black line) before placement of a rolled piece of gauze; (b) two sutures are tied in place to secure the bandage; (c) removal is easy by slipping a pair of suture scissors between the knot and gauze at the time of the patient's discharge. *Source:* © Robin Sankey.

severed along with the optic nerve as described for the transconjunctival approach (Figure 5.8). The closure is performed in the same way as the transconjunctival approach.[8] If you inadvertently expose the cornea by cutting through the conjunctiva, the hole can be closed with a suture, a hemostat, or an Allis tissue forcep.

Orbital Prosthesis

An orbital prosthesis is an optional addition that is purely used for cosmetic purposes since it prevents depression over the anterior surface of the orbit as is common after enucleation. Silicone spheres come in many sizes and must be sterilized before use. No alteration to the sphere is needed prior to placement within the orbit. The goal when selecting an orbital prosthesis is to select a sphere that fits snugly into the orbit but does not protrude beyond the orbital rim and does not cause compression of the orbital tissue.[1] The existing globe can be used to estimate the size of the prosthesis if the globe has not been altered in size by disease processes, such as glaucoma, phthisis bulbi, or intraocular tumors, and was not inadvertently ruptured during removal. It is ideal to control hemorrhage before placement of the prosthesis since hemorrhage can result in displacement of the prosthesis. Potential complications with the placement of an orbital prosthesis include seroma formation, displacement of the implant, intraorbital infection, and implant extrusion.[7] The author warns clients that infection is estimated to occur in 5–10% of cases and is the most common cause of implant extrusion and the need to remove the implant with a second surgery. An orbital prosthetic is not recommended with endophthalmitis, significant surface or periocular infection, or when neoplasia is suspected that could or does extend into the orbit due to the increased risk of implant extrusion.

Postoperative Care

Postoperative care involves a hard, plastic E-collar for 10–14 days, systemic anti-inflammatories and pain

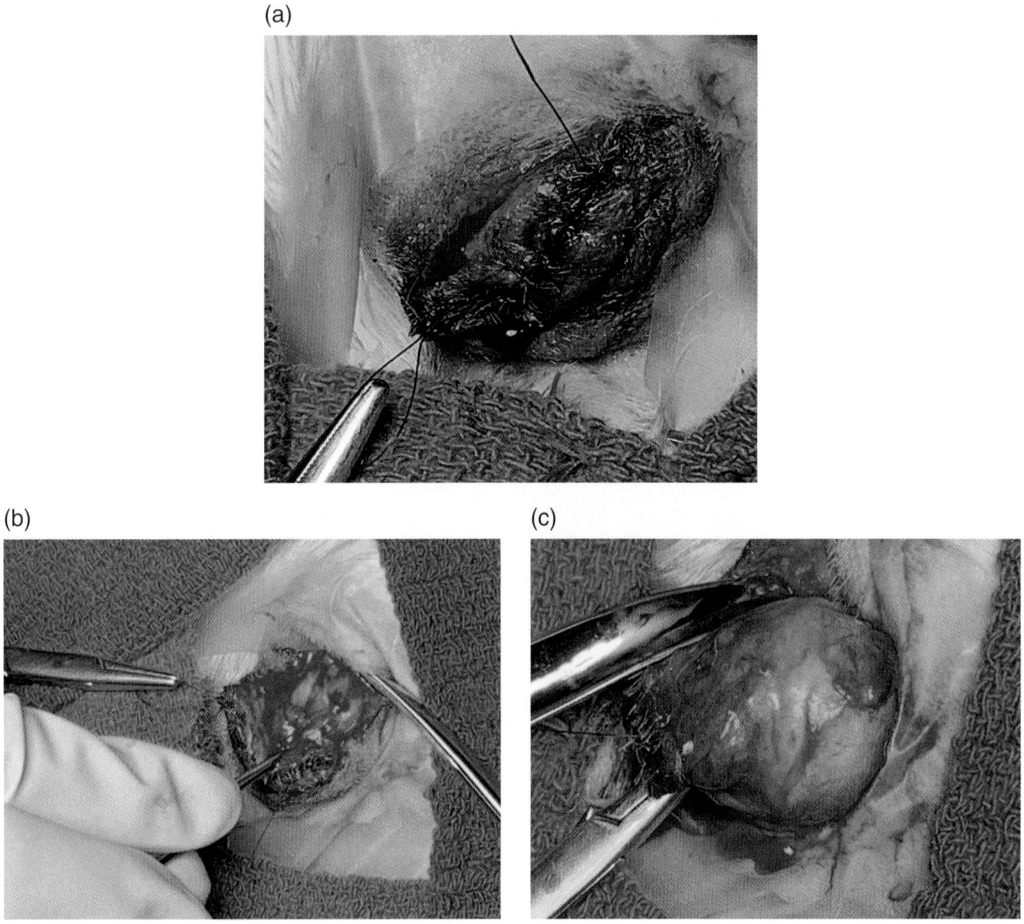

Figure 5.8 (a) Elliptical incision around sutured eyelid opening with hemostats placed on suture ends to facilitate skin manipulation and eventually globe manipulation during enucleation; (b) the subcutaneous tissue is bluntly dissected to the level of the bulbar conjunctiva just posterior to the limbus using Metzenbaum scissors; (c) subcutaneous dissection is continued until just posterior to the limbus. The tissue is then dissected down to the level of the sclera to allow for the transection of the extraocular muscles. *Source:* © Robin Sankey.

medication in all cases unless contraindicated, and systemic antibiotics in some cases. An enucleation procedure should be sterile, so postoperative antibiotics are not necessary in routine cases. However, if an orbital implant is placed or there is a preoperative infection present, systemic antibiotics are recommended. External skin sutures, if placed, are removed after 10–14 days. It is common for there to be a small amount of bleeding from the incision site and the ipsilateral nostril for one to two days postoperatively until the patent nasolacrimal puncta seals. Gentle cleaning of the incision area to remove dried blood or discharge is recommended to prevent a skin infection and/or premature loss of skin sutures. However, discharge accumulation is often minimal and cleaning is often not needed. Cold compresses for 5–10 minutes three times daily for the first 48 hours can help with postoperative swelling and bruising. Activity is also limited for the first few days following enucleation to decrease the risk of postoperative bleeding.

Complications

Thankfully, enucleation is about 95% successful overall, so most patients do not have complications. The most common complications are suture line infection or suture reaction, and the use of systemic antibiotics often resolves this complication. Retention of conjunctival tissue, medial caruncle, nictitans, or any part of the nictitans gland can result in a draining fistula or cyst formation and often necessitates removal of the retained tissue to achieve resolution. Infection of an orbital prosthesis could necessitate removal if culturing followed by appropriate systemic antibiotic therapy does not resolve the infection. In the author's experience, infection is the most common cause of spontaneous orbital prosthetic extrusion, but traumatic extrusion can also occur, which is typically from failure to utilize the E-collar as instructed. Orbital emphysema is an exceedingly rare complication of enucleation. Should this rare complication occur, referral to a veterinary ophthalmologist or investigation into current treatment options is recommended.

References

1 Samuelson, D.A. (2013). Ophthalmic anatomy. In: *Veterinary Ophthalmology* (ed. T. Page), 41–42. Ames, IA: Wiley-Blackwell.
2 Cook, C.S., Peiffer, R.L., and Landis, M.L. (2009). Clinical basic science. In: *Small Animal Ophthalmology, a Problem-Oriented Approach* (ed. T. Page). Edinburgh, London, New York, Oxford, Philadelphia, St. Louis, Sydney, Toronto: Elsevier-Saunders.
3 Murphy, C.J., Samuelson, D.A., and Pollock, R.V.H. (2013). The eye. In: *Miller's Anatomy of the Dog* (ed. T. Page). St. Louis, MO: Elsevier.
4 Stanley, H.D., Goody, P.C., Stickland, N.C. et al. (2009). Color atlas of veterinary anatomy. In: *The Dog and Cat*, vol. 3, 47. Edinburgh, London, New York, Oxford, Philadelphia, St. Louis, Sydney, Toronto: Mosby-Elsevier.
5 Donaldson, D., Riera, M.M., Holloway, A. et al. (2014). Contralateral optic neuropathy and retinopathy associated with visual and afferent pupillomotor dysfunction following enucleation in six cats. *Vet. Ophthalmol.* 17 (5): 373–384.
6 Vezina-Audette, R. (2020). Anesthesia case of the month. *J. Am. Vet. Med. Assoc.* 256 (2): 176–178.
7 Spiess, B.M. and Pot, A.S. (2013). Diseases and surgery of the canine orbit. In: *Veterinary Ophthalmology* (ed. T. Page), 816–819. Ames, IA: Wiley-Blackwell.
8 Pot, S.A., Voelter, K., and Kircher, P.R. (2021). Diseases and surgery of the canine orbit. In: *Veterinary Ophthalmology* (ed. T. Page), 907. Hoboken, NJ: Wiley-Blackwell.

6

Nosectomy in Cats

Nicole J. Buote

Department of Clinical Sciences, Cornell University, Ithaca, NY, USA

Key Points

- Nosectomy is only indicated for injuries or lesions confined to the nasal planum, philtrum or alar folds.
- Meticulous surgical technique to control hemorrhage and appose the skin to the nasal mucosa decreases the chance of postoperative complications.
- Postoperative care is not demanding but the postoperative appearance of the pet should be thoroughly discussed with the owners before the procedure is performed.

Introduction

Nosectomy can provide feline patients with relief from painful ulcerative conditions as well as supply owners with important prognostic information if a neoplastic process is considered for their pet. Nosectomy is an easy-to-perform procedure even with minimal surgical experience, but certain technique recommendations should be followed (e.g., meticulous suturing of skin to mucosa).[1,2] While trauma to the nose and brachycephalic nasal stenosis or stricture from previous interventions can be indications for nosectomy in cats, neoplasia is the most common reason for the performance of this procedure.

Indications/Pre-operative Considerations

The most common cause for a nosectomy in feline patients is the appearance of cancer along the nasal philtrum, alar folds, or nasal planum (Figure 6.1). Squamous cell carcinoma (SCC) is the most common cancer affecting this area in cats and dogs.[1] In cats, SCC originates from the cornified external surface of the nasal planum, which is different than in dogs where it usually grows from the mucous membrane of the nostril or nasal planum.[3] Light pigmentation (i.e., white hair coat) has long been identified as a predisposing cause for SCC in animals, as have short hair coats and chronic exposure to ultraviolet light. In one study, white-haired cats had a 13.4 times higher risk of developing head and neck SCC compared to darker colored cats.[4] Other tumors, such as mast cell tumors, lymphoma, fibrosarcoma, malignant melanoma, hemangioma, and fibroma, can be found on the nose as well.[1] Noncancerous diseases, such as eosinophilic granulomas and immune-mediated diseases, can involve the nasal planum and present with a similar erosive or proliferative appearance (Figure 6.2).

While rare, trauma to the nasal planum or complications from nasal surgery (e.g., alar fold resections for stenotic nares) can also require nosectomy in cats.[2] Complications from nasal surgery in brachycephalic feline breeds are occasionally seen, and while surgeries including ala vestibuloplasty and pedicle flaps can be performed, nosectomy is a simple technique to remove nasal obstructions.

Preoperative considerations and diagnostics depend on the primary differential or cause for surgery. If the patient presents with an ulcerative or proliferative lesion on the nose, neoplasia should be the first consideration. Usually,

Techniques in Small Animal Soft Tissue, Orthopedic, and Ophthalmic Surgery, First Edition. Edited by Kristin A. Coleman.

Companion website: www.wiley.com/go/coleman/surgeries

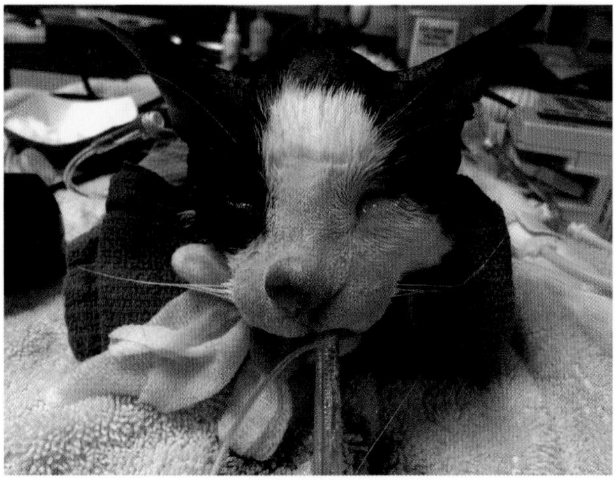

Figure 6.1 Photograph of a squamous cell carcinoma on a feline patient. It is evident that a biopsy has been taken from this patient, as a defect and suture are visible. This patient also had ulcerative lesions on both pinna, so those have also been clipped for surgery.

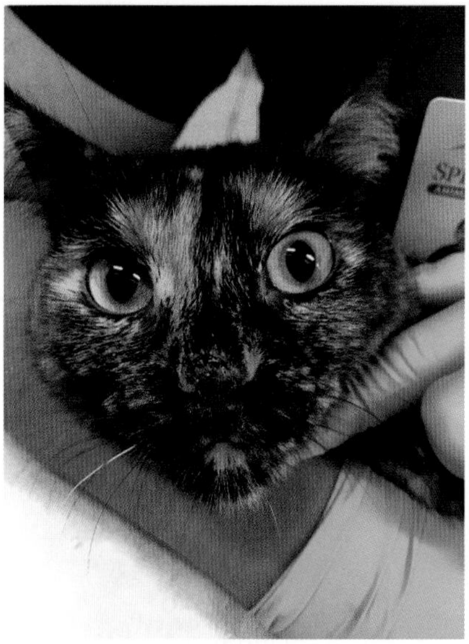

Figure 6.2 Photograph of an eosinophilic granuloma lesion on a feline patient.

SCC starts as a benign crusting or erythema, which is easily overlooked by owners, but it will eventually advance to a deeper ulcerative lesion. A sharp veterinarian should pursue any lesion in this area aggressively because time wasted leads to lost opportunities for treatment. In cats with SCC, 30% of patients will have SCC in multiple head and neck locations, so a thorough examination of the pinna, periocular region, and neck is recommended.[1] If SCC or another neoplasia is suspected, a biopsy of the lesion is recommended before nosectomy is performed. Cytology (fine needle aspiration) or impression smears are not usually accurate because inflammatory cells and hemorrhage are commonly present in both cancerous and noncancerous lesions.

Staging tests for any presumed neoplasia include chest radiographs and lymph node examination. If lesions are proliferative and/or concern exists regarding their invasiveness, advanced imaging of the head can be performed to ensure a nosectomy will remove the entire lesion. Computed tomography can also provide information about the size and character of the regional lymph nodes, in case they need to be sampled or removed.

Surgical Procedure

Nosectomy or nasal planum resection can provide excellent local tumor control if the lesion is superficial and/or small in size. This procedure is easy to perform and does not require specialized surgical equipment. More aggressive surgical procedures or medical treatments (e.g., radiation, photodynamic therapy) can always be pursued after nosectomy if necessary. Preoperatively, bilateral infraorbital nerve blocks can be performed to aid in postoperative analgesia. For nosectomy, the procedure is as follows:

1) The hair around the nose is clipped with a 2–3 cm margin around the planned incision.
2) The patient is placed in sternal recumbency with the head elevated on a towel. Be sure to confirm head is straight so that the incision can be made as symmetrically as possible (Figure 6.1).
3) If the nosectomy is being performed for a presumed/diagnosed cancerous lesion, a lateral margin of 5 mm is recommended.[5] The deep margin will be the junction between the cartilaginous and bony nasal tissue.
4) The incision through the skin and underlying turbinates should be made with a #15 blade. Brisk hemorrhage will occur but can be controlled with digital pressure until the nasal planum is removed.
5) Once the nasal planum is removed, hemorrhage can be controlled with the sensible use of electrosurgery (i.e., monopolar cautery) along the edges of the incision. Be careful not to create char on the tissue, as this may impede wound healing (Figure 6.3).
6) Closure of the incision should be performed by suturing the skin to the nasal mucosa with simple interrupted sutures of absorbable (e.g., Monocryl™) monofilament 4-0 to 5-0 suture material (Figure 6.4).

Potential Complications

While complications are uncommon with this procedure, stenosis of the nasal opening can be seen if an appropriate surgical technique is not employed. Previously, some

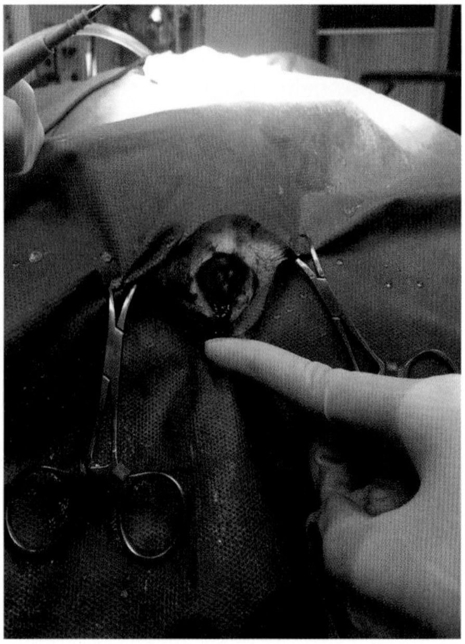

Figure 6.3 Intraoperative photograph of patient from Figure 6.1 after nasal planum resection. The cartilaginous turbinates are visible.

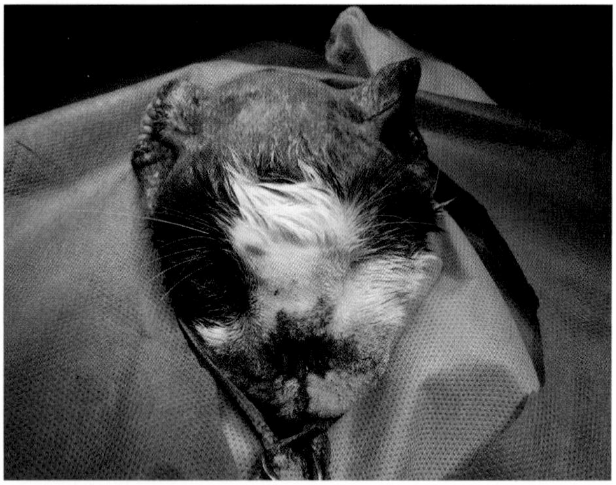

Figure 6.4 Immediate postoperative appearance after nosectomy of patient from Figure 6.1. A skin to mucosa closure has been performed with simple interrupted sutures using an absorbable suture material. Partial pinnectomies have also been performed in this patient.

surgeons performed closure with a purse-string technique, but this created more stenosis postoperatively than the technique described above and is not recommended. With appropriate skin-to-mucosa suturing, the risk of stenosis is very low. If stenosis is diagnosed and the patient is clinical (open mouth breathing or stertorous), re-resection of skin and underlying turbinates can be performed. More advanced skin reconstructions or stenting (temporary or permanent) can also be pursued but have more variable outcomes.[6,7] Other complications include mild postoperative hemorrhage or discharge, sneezing, and a transient decrease in appetite.

Post-operative Care/Prognosis

Postoperative care for feline nosectomies is straightforward and centers around appropriate pain management and incision care. The patient should be provided with an E-collar to prevent rubbing or scratching at the incision site. Intravenous fluids and analgesia should be continued for 12–24 hours after the procedure or until the patient is eating on their own. Some cats will not eat for multiple days due to congestion at the site decreasing their sense of smell. Offer them wet food, and their favorite foods and consider the use of appetite stimulants if needed. A feeding tube has not ever been necessary in the author's experience. While some clinicians recommend removal of scabs from the incision site to decrease congestion, the author does not unless the patient has become an obligate mouth-breather. Removal of this scab, especially within the first few postoperative days, can lead to trauma to the incision and increase the risk of postoperative complications (e.g., stenosis). If a scab must be removed, it should be done gently with warm water-soaked cotton-tipped applicators, and the patient may need to be sedated. Patients are discharged with nonsteroidal anti-inflammatories if appropriate and gabapentin (10 mg/kg PO q 8–12 h for 5 days) (Figure 6.5).

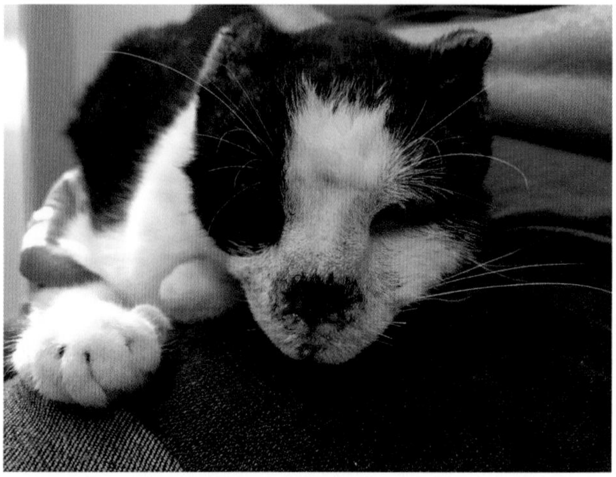

Figure 6.5 Photograph of patient from Figure 6.1 two days postoperatively at time of discharge. Patient is comfortable and is eating on his own. There is no hemorrhage but minimal nasal discharge. No scab is present along the suture line.

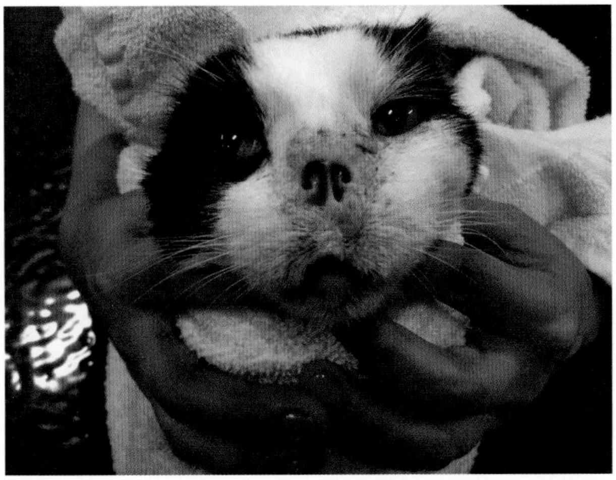

Figure 6.6 Photograph of patient from Figure 6.1 that is 1.3 years postoperative. There is mild stenosis on the left side of the nasal opening, but the patient was not clinical.

The author uses absorbable sutures to avoid the necessary sedation for suture removal, but a recheck at 10–14 days is still recommended to assess the incision and ensure the patient is healing well.

The cosmetic appearance of cats is considered good by most owners, especially as the incision heals and the nasal opening decreases slightly (Figure 6.6). The prognosis depends solely on the cause for nosectomy (trauma, stenosis, cancer). If the nosectomy was performed for presumed cancer, the biopsy results will supply information regarding life span and necessary adjunctive treatments. Follow-up treatments for SCC are rare if clean margins are attained and most times cats are considered cured after this procedure.[1] With SCC, local recurrence with incomplete margins has been reported in 29% of cats and was seen in no cats with completely resected tumors.[8]

References

1 Ayres, S.A. and Liptak, J.M. (2012). Head and neck tumors. In: *Veterinary Surgical Oncology*, 1e (ed. S.T. Kudnig and B. Seguin), 81–117. Wiley https://doi.org/10.1002/9781118729038.

2 Fossum, T.W. (2018). Surgery of the upper respiratory system. In: *Small Animal Surgery*, 5e (ed. T.W. Fossum), 833–883. Elsevier Health Sciences (US).

3 Withrow, S.J. (2007). Tumors of the respiratory system: cancer of the nasal planum. In: *Withrow & MacEwen's Small Animal Clinical Oncology*, 4e (ed. S.J. Withrow and D.M. Vail), 511–515. St. Louis, MO: Saunders Elsevier.

4 Dorn, C.R., Taylor, D.O., and Schneider, R. (1971). Sunlight exposure and risk of developing cutaneous and oral squamous cell carcinomas in white cats. *J. Natl. Cancer Inst.* 46 (5): 1073–1078.

5 Thomson, M. (2007). Squamous cell carcinoma of the nasal planum in cats and dogs. *Clin. Tech. Small Anim. Pract.* 22 (2): 42–45.

6 Novo, R.E. and Kramek, B. (1999). Surgical repair of nasopharyngeal stenosis in a cat using a stent. *J. Am. Anim. Hosp. Assoc.* 35 (3): 251–256.

7 Berns, C.N., Schmiedt, C.W., Dickerson, V.M. et al. (2020). Single pedicle advancement flap for treatment of feline stenotic nares: technique and results in five cases. *J. Feline Med. Surg.* 22 (12): 1238–1242.

8 Lana, S.E., Ogilvie, G.K., Withrow, S.J. et al. (1997). Feline cutaneous squamous cell carcinoma of the nasal planum and the pinnae: 61 cases. *J. Am. Anim. Hosp. Assoc.* 33 (4): 329–332.

7

Brachycephalic Obstructive Airway Syndrome in Dogs and Cats

Pamela Schwartz

Schwarzman Animal Medical Center, New York, NY, USA

Key Points

- There are three extreme brachycephalic breeds of dog: Pugs, English Bulldogs, and French Bulldogs.
- Medical management is essential in combination with corrective surgery to regulate pre-existing gastrointestinal disease as well as decrease gastrointestinal clinical signs secondary to brachycephalic obstructive airway syndrome (BOAS).
- Early surgical intervention of BOAS is paramount, as chronic, irreversible changes can occur in dogs younger than 1 year of age.
- A preoperative brachycephalic risk (BRisk) score has been developed to predict the risk of major complications or death objectively and accurately in dogs undergoing corrective surgery for BOAS.
- Surgery to address all identified abnormalities (e.g., elongated and/or thickened soft palate, stenotic nares, everted laryngeal saccules, and/or everted and enlarged tonsils) appears to have the best outcome, although the anatomy is never normalized with surgery, and many dogs continue to have clinical signs.
- Decreasing risk factors that can be controlled and lifelong lifestyle changes are warranted in dogs affected by BOAS, such as weight management and avoidance of extreme heat.

Introduction

The popularity of brachycephalic breeds has risen significantly in recent years. In particular, French Bulldogs have increased by 300% through kennel club registrations over the past 10 years in the United Kingdom.[1]

The English Bulldog, French Bulldog, and Pug have especially increased in popularity and are classified as "extreme brachycephalic breeds."[2,3] Extreme brachycephalic breeds have been noted to die at a younger age than other breeds, with a higher proportion of deaths related to upper respiratory disorders.[2] Despite the increase in popularity of brachycephalic breeds, many owners are unaware of the conformation-associated health risks related with these breeds, which may result in unrealistic expectations when pursuing treatment.[1,4–6]

Brachycephalic obstructive airway syndrome (BOAS) is a term that describes several conformational abnormalities leading to respiratory distress, which often requires surgical intervention to alleviate clinical signs.[5,7,8] Several anatomical changes have been documented to be associated with brachycephalic breeds. Anatomic abnormalities associated with BOAS include macroglossia, stenotic nares, aberrant nasopharyngeal turbinates, elongated soft palate, excessively thickened soft palate, hypoplastic trachea, and redundant pharyngeal folds.[7,9–11] Macroglossia in brachycephalic breeds creates lower air-to-soft tissue ratios within the oropharyngeal and nasopharyngeal regions, which can contribute to upper airway obstruction.[12] Although one study documents increased nasal mucosal contact points and more prevalent aberrant turbinates in brachycephalic dogs, no correlation could be made between these findings

Techniques in Small Animal Soft Tissue, Orthopedic, and Ophthalmic Surgery, First Edition. Edited by Kristin A. Coleman.

Companion website: www.wiley.com/go/coleman/surgeries

and brachycephalic airway syndrome due to lack of knowledge of these dogs' clinical signs.[11] It is also unknown if the thickening of the soft palate is a primary structural abnormality or a secondary change; however, it is considered a component in severe BOAS.[9,10] Combinations of this altered anatomy lead to increased resistance during inspiration.[10] Brachycephalic dogs must create a higher negative pressure distal to the resistance, through labored breathing, to maintain appropriate oxygen levels.[10] Secondary manifestations of increased airway resistance include everted laryngeal saccules, tonsillar eversion and hyperplasia, and laryngeal collapse.[7,10] Gastrointestinal disease is common in many brachycephalic breeds and is likely associated with negative intra-thoracic pressure generated during inspiration.[7,13,14] It is not completely understood which anatomic change or a combination thereof leads to the most severe clinical signs.

Clinical signs in dogs with BOAS may include both respiratory and gastrointestinal signs. Reported clinical signs may include exercise intolerance, heat intolerance, sleep apnea, increased respiratory rate and effort, stertor or stridor, regurgitation, gagging, vomiting, nausea, dyspnea, and when severe, may progress to syncope, collapse, heat stroke, and death[1,3,5–7,10,13] (Video 7.1). A correlation has been established between BOAS and gastrointestinal signs in the extreme brachycephalic breeds, with French Bulldogs having the highest prevalence of presurgical regurgitation and vomiting.[13] It is important that veterinarians recognize that gastrointestinal signs are often a sequela of BOAS, requiring surgical intervention through corrective upper airway surgery. Gastroesophageal reflux, vomiting, or regurgitation can lead to aspiration pneumonia.[7] There are clinical signs spanning from "normal" or a "normal variant" for a brachycephalic dog to a dog clinically affected with BOAS.[3] A normalization phenomenon exists that describes the acceptance of some chronic and highly breed-associated conditions as normal.[6] In a questionnaire-based study, 58% of owners reported a high frequency and severity of clinical signs in their dogs without perceiving them to have a breathing problem.[6] Lack of recognition of clinical signs indicating disease may result in a lack of treatment until clinical signs progress and negatively affect an animal's welfare and outcome.[6] Since clinical signs are progressive, it is paramount that veterinarians recommend brachycephalic breeds seek early surgical intervention, even if not mentioned by the client as a concern, prior to the development of chronic and irreversible negative effects of BOAS or a respiratory crisis.[3,6,7]

A thorough clinical history should be obtained, which can provide significant insight into any underlying problems. It is imperative to identify signs of both respiratory and gastrointestinal disease. It should be noted that lack of clinical signs does not equate to lack of conformational changes. One study evaluating brachycephalic dogs without clinical signs of upper airway disease found that all dogs had obvious redundancy or moderate to severe elongation of the soft palate.[15] Another study found that the degree of nasopharyngeal occlusion by the soft palate evaluated by computed tomography (CT) was not correlated to the severity of clinical signs.[16] The severity of respiratory signs influences the severity of gastrointestinal signs and vice versa. Brachycephalic dogs exhibiting respiratory signs have evidence of gastrointestinal disease (esophageal, gastric, or duodenal) on histologic evaluation whether or not gastrointestinal signs or endoscopically visible lesions are present. Gastroesophageal reflux can contribute to upper respiratory problems by producing upper esophageal, pharyngeal, and laryngeal inflammation.[17] It is shown that treatment of upper gastrointestinal disease prior to anesthesia can decrease the complication rate associated with corrective upper respiratory surgery and improve prognosis.[18]

Due to the progressive nature of BOAS and increased risk of post-operative complications when dogs present for surgery on an emergent basis, it is paramount that dogs have early surgical intervention, prior to severe clinical signs and development of irreversible secondary changes.[7,19] Studies document the presence of severe secondary changes in dogs younger than one year of age.[20] One study, where all dogs were at least one year of age, documented that performing surgery at a younger age was associated with an increased likelihood of a poorer prognosis after surgery.[8] This is likely related to more severe disease in this population and supports performing surgery as early as possible. Dogs that have surgery at a younger age have significantly fewer complications, with the odds of developing complications increasing with each year of age.[7] Although the benefit of prophylactic surgery is not fully known, the author recommends and routinely performs laryngeal examination, and if warranted, corrective airway surgery, under the same anesthetic episode of surgical sterilization. The author recommends surgical intervention prior to obvious clinical signs to improve quality of life and to attempt to slow the progression of diseases, between the age of six months and one year.

How to determine which patient would benefit from corrective surgery, including which procedures, remains controversial. This is generally based on clinical signs and laryngeal examination findings. The prognosis appears to be related to the severity of airway pathology present and not the surgical procedure(s) performed. The author routinely performs surgical correction of all identifiable abnormalities of the nares, palate, saccules, and tonsils. Although most dogs improve after surgery, it is known that clinical signs, such as snoring while sleeping, stertor/stridor while awake, and dyspnea, can persist after surgery.[21] Decreasing risk factors that can be controlled, such as obesity, are paramount.[4,17,22] Therefore, lifelong lifestyle changes are warranted despite surgery, such as weight management to maintain a slim body condition and avoidance of extreme heat.

A numeric scoring system, the BOAS index, has been established in three breeds (Pug, French Bulldog, and Bulldog) to reflect the severity of the disease and to assess the outcome after surgery.[22] This requires whole-body barometric plethysmography (WBBP), which is noninvasive, but may not be available to most clinicians. A preoperative brachycephalic risk (BRisk) score has been developed to predict the risk of major complications or death objectively and accurately in dogs undergoing corrective surgery for BOAS. There are six variables that are each independent predictors of outcome that make up the BRisk score: breed, history of airway surgery, additional planned procedures (other than airway surgery), body condition score, admission clinical findings regarding the severity of airway compromise, and admission rectal temperature. Dogs with a BRisk score >3 are 9.1 times greater risk for a negative outcome than dogs with a low score (<3). This score can help clinicians set realistic expectations and assist owners in their decision-making process.[4]

Diagnostics

A general physical examination and a minimum database should be performed. Blood samples should be collected for complete blood count and serum biochemical analysis to screen overall health. Venous or arterial blood gas samples provide important information about pH, blood oxygen, and carbon dioxide (pv-/paCO_2) concentrations prior to general anesthesia, which can be serially monitored during surgery and in the postoperative period. Brachycephalic dogs are noted to have lower arterial blood oxygen and higher arterial CO_2 levels than non-brachycephalic breeds.[23]

Three-view thoracic radiographs are obtained to evaluate for the presence of pneumonia, pulmonary edema, hypoplastic trachea, and/or hiatal hernia.[14] French Bulldogs appear to have a high prevalence of hiatal hernia.[24] The author routinely performs thoracic radiographs on the day of surgery, so the lungs are determined to be free of pneumonia prior to anesthesia (Figure 7.1). Pneumonia can complicate the balance between ventilation and perfusion and potentially worsen with anesthesia,[25] therefore, consideration should be given to postponing corrective surgery in the presence of pneumonia.

More advanced imaging, such as CT and endoscopy, can be considered but are likely limited to specialty hospitals, and cost may be prohibitive for some. The majority of anatomic abnormalities to be evaluated for surgery will be based on a lightly sedated oropharyngeal-laryngeal examination. The author prefers to perform the pharyngeal-laryngeal examination on the day of surgery, preventing a separate sedative episode, for which untreated brachycephalic patients may have difficulty recovering. Aberrant nasopharyngeal turbinates require CT and endoscopy for diagnosis and treatment, respectively.[26,27] Upper gastrointestinal endoscopy may be considered for dogs with persistent gastrointestinal signs after corrective BOAS surgery if medical management techniques are considered unsuccessful.

Perioperative Considerations

Medical treatment is recommended to decrease the risk of gastroesophageal reflux and aspiration pneumonia by decreasing perioperative upper gastrointestinal signs of nausea, vomiting, and regurgitation. There is an increased frequency of regurgitation after surgical treatment of BOAS, especially in dogs with preoperative regurgitation.[28] Multimodal treatment with combinations of antiemetics, prokinetics, antiacid gastroprotectants, opioids, anxiolytics, and anti-inflammatories are recommended. There is no known ideal protocol, and the combination of medications will depend on the severity of clinical signs, patient temperament, drug availability, and clinician comfort with certain protocols[14] (Table 7.1).

The effect of maropitant[i] in preventing nausea and vomiting when administered one hour prior to pre-medication is well established.[29,30] Maropitant also has the added value of reducing the minimum alveolar concentration of sevoflurane in dogs.[31] The author administers maropitant prior to pre-medication then every 24 hours while hospitalized and only if needed after the patient is discharged.

Although reflux can be influenced by anesthesia, the high prevalence of presurgical gastrointestinal signs in addition to endoscopic changes suggests a chronic gastroesophageal reflux in brachycephalic breeds.[13,17,32] Pre- and postoperative antiacid treatment improves digestive clinical signs and lesions in dogs undergoing corrective surgery for BOAS and is recommended in dogs without obvious clinical signs.[32] The author typically gives omeprazole on the morning of surgery if no gastrointestinal signs are noted. If preoperative regurgitation is noted or suspected to occur frequently (multiple times weekly or daily), the author treats with omeprazole and cisapride for a minimum of two to four weeks prior to surgery until gastrointestinal signs are minimized or resolved.

The postoperative effects of ileus, such as vomiting, decreased tolerance of oral diets, and prolonged recovery from surgery, can be considered detrimental in a brachycephalic patient. Because the side effects of ileus are similar to upper gastrointestinal signs in brachycephalic breeds, it

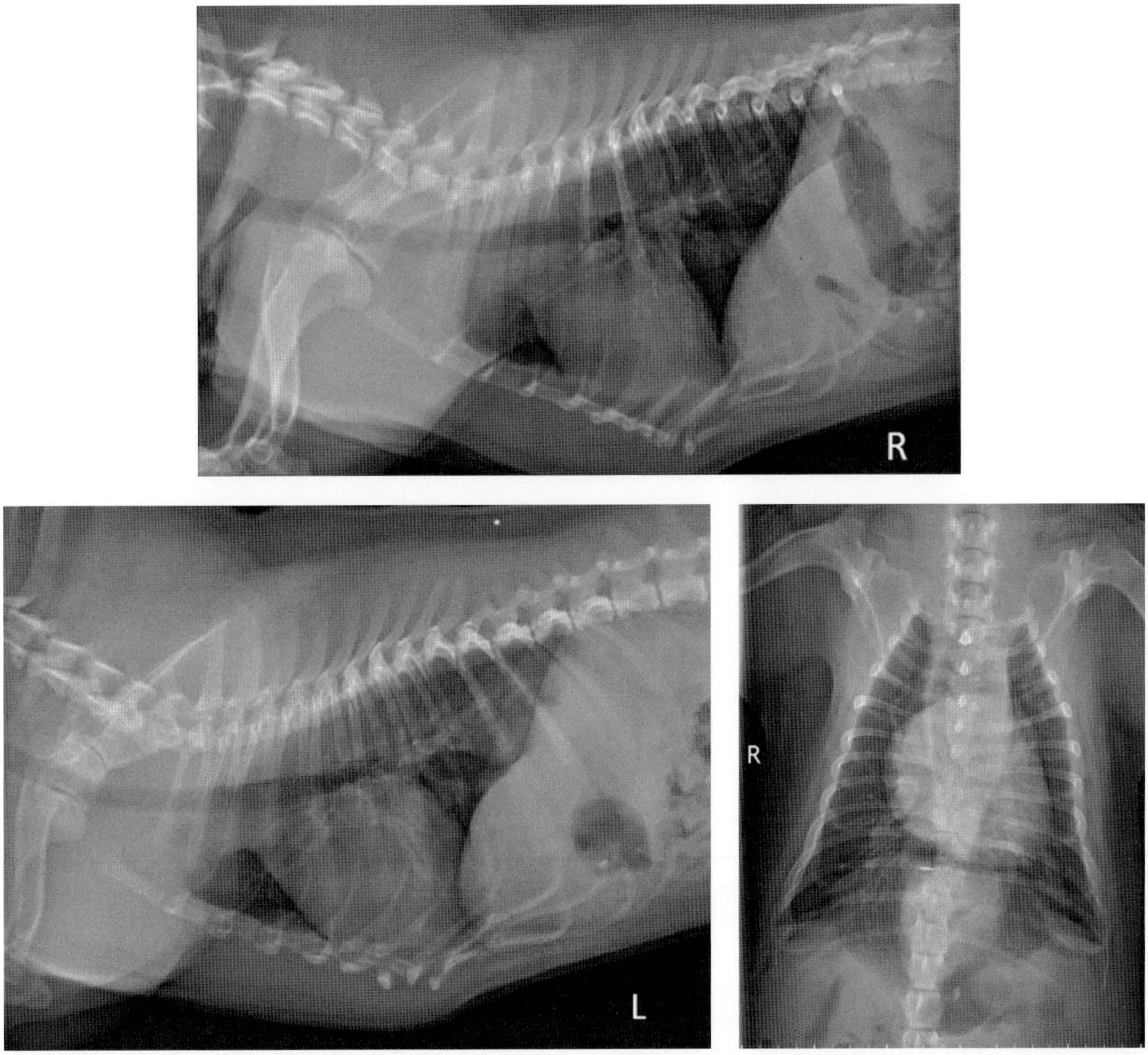

Figure 7.1 Right and left lateral and ventrodorsal (VD) radiographic views of a French Bulldog obtained prior to BOAS surgery. Within the mediastinum there is a rounded soft-tissue opacity present caudodorsally on the left lateral image and along the midline on the VD image. This is not visualized well on the right lateral image. This is consistent with a sliding hiatal hernia. There is scant fluid within the caudal esophagus on the right lateral image, which may indicate gastroesophageal reflux. There is no evidence of pneumonia detected.

may be difficult to distinguish between the worsening of preexisting GOR and the effects of postoperative ileus. Therefore, efforts should be made to mitigate any effects of postoperative ileus. Administration of both a gastroprotectant and prokinetic postoperatively minimized vomiting, regurgitation, and reflux in one study.[18] Ultrasound can be utilized to evaluate intestinal motility in dogs with suspected ileus.[33] The author administers omeprazole and cisapride for two to four weeks postoperative if frequent (multiple times daily) regurgitation is noted after surgery.

Nebulized epinephrine causes a clinically significant reduction in the BOAS index in preoperative dogs with a BOAS index of >70% and in dogs recovering from BOAS surgery purportedly through reduction of mucosal edema.[34] While WBBP needed to measure the BOAS index may not be readily available to most, epinephrine nebulization has minimal side effects, so it can be performed without knowledge of the patient's BOAS index. The most notable side effect in one study was nausea, which could be due to the medication itself or from stress during administration.[34] Although nausea could be due to stress, it is also recognized as a clinical sign with underlying gastroesophageal reflux and may be associated with the brachycephalic population at hand. Nebulization should be discontinued

Table 7.1 A list of multimodal medications used most frequently in the perioperative period.

Perioperative treatment		
Medication	**Dosage**	**Timing and frequency**
Maropitant	1 mg/kg IV or SQ	30–60 min prior to pre-medication, then every 24 h
Metoclopromide	1 mg/kg IV bolus over 10 min	Once 30–60 min prior to pre-medication
	1 mg/kg/h IV CRI	During surgery and for 24 h postoperatively
Cisapride	0.25–0.5 mg/kg orally	Give every 8–12 h preopertively to minimize gastrointestinal signs. Continue postoperatively if regurgitation persists or worsens.
Pantoprozole	1 mg/kg IV	Every 12 h
Ondansetron	0.5–1 mg/kg IV (slowly)	Every 8–12 h postoperatively as needed
Dexamethasone SP	0.1 mg/kg IV	Given 20 min prior to surgery. This can be given again postoperatively if pharyngeal swelling is a concern.
Butorphanol	0.4 mg/kg IM or IV	Once as a premedication
	0.2–0.4 mg/kg IV bolus	Postoperatively as needed
	0.1–0.4 mg/kg/h IV CRI	Intraoperatively and postoperatively
Epinephrine	0.05 mg/kg epinephrine is added to 0.9% saline to make a 5-mL nebulization solution delivered as a flow by for 10 min	After extubation, then every 6 h for 24 h
Acepromazine	0.005–0.05 mg/kg IM or IV	As a pre-medication only if needed, then as needed postoperatively
Trazodone	3–10 mg/kg PO	After extubation as needed every 6 h
Dexmedetomidine	1–3 mcg/kg IV bolus	Postoperatively as needed
	1–3 mcg/kg/h IV CRI	Postoperatively as needed

should it present obvious stress to the patient. The author typically initiates epinephrine nebulization in the postoperative period immediately after extubation then every 6 hours for 24 hours, which is when most patients are being discharged. Some clinicians do not continue this treatment after 24 hours because of a rebound phenomenon of worsening stridor in children with croup after treatment with nebulized adrenaline. Although a rebound phenomenon has been suggested in children, a review of the literature established that no study has reported the symptoms as being worse than baseline, and the re-emergence of symptoms is less marked when children receive nebulization concurrently with steroids.[35]

Most literature suggests the use of corticosteroids during the perioperative period to reduce surgery-induced and postoperative (panting) pharyngeal swelling and edema, however, controlled evidence is lacking. The author administers one dose of corticosteroids 20 minutes prior to surgery, and if postoperative obstruction is a concern related to pharyngeal edema, additional doses are repeated as needed.

Sedative-anxiolytic drugs in combination with opioids are recommended, however, the desired effect can also relax the smooth muscle of the nasopharyngeal and oropharyngeal region risking further obstruction.[36] The author prefers drugs that are reversible with a short duration of action and can be administered as a constant infusion (butorphanol and dexmedetomidine), which allows for these drugs to be titrated quickly up or down to achieve the lowest dose required without excessive sedation.

Brachycephalic breeds have lower than normal arterial oxygen concentrations at rest compared to non-brachycephalic dogs.[23] Preoxygenation for three minutes prior to general anesthesia increases the time to desaturation.[37] Brachycephalic dogs may particularly benefit from preoxygenation as upper airway obstruction is common and intubation can be more difficult, delaying a patent airway.[14] If a face mask to deliver oxygen is stressful, the mask can be removed to deliver oxygen from the end of the anesthetic tubing, allowing some distance between the pet and the oxygen delivery system if needed. Anxiolytic drugs are administered as needed preoperatively and induction should occur rapidly.

The initial 12–24 hours of recovery is considered the high-risk period for the brachycephalic patient, particularly because of the possibility of airway obstruction.[7,25] Brachycephalic patients recovering from surgery should be placed in sternal recumbency, with the head slightly elevated, and remain intubated until their endotracheal tube is no longer tolerated.[14,25,38] Opioids and anxiolytics should be used to obtain a calm state without excessive sedation (Table 7.1). Oxygen should be provided to any patient that shows increased respiratory effort. Clinicians should be prepared with induction drugs, endotracheal tubes, and a laryngoscope for emergency reintubation in the presence of upper airway obstruction. If a postoperative obstruction occurs after BOAS corrective surgery, the author typically reintubates, assessing the larynx for the cause of obstruction. The author will treat with additional corticosteroids and anxiolytics, allowing a more prolonged recovery. Temporary tracheostomy should be considered if additional treatment for postoperative swelling, pain, and anxiety is considered ineffective after re-attempting extubation.

Stenotic Nares

Stenotic nares are a congenital malformation of the nasal cartilage, resulting in medial collapse and narrowing of the external nares[39,40] (Figure 7.2). The decrease in the transverse diameter of the nares leads to increased negative upper airway pressures to overcome the increased resistance in airflow.[40] There are several surgical techniques that have been described for the management of stenotic nares.

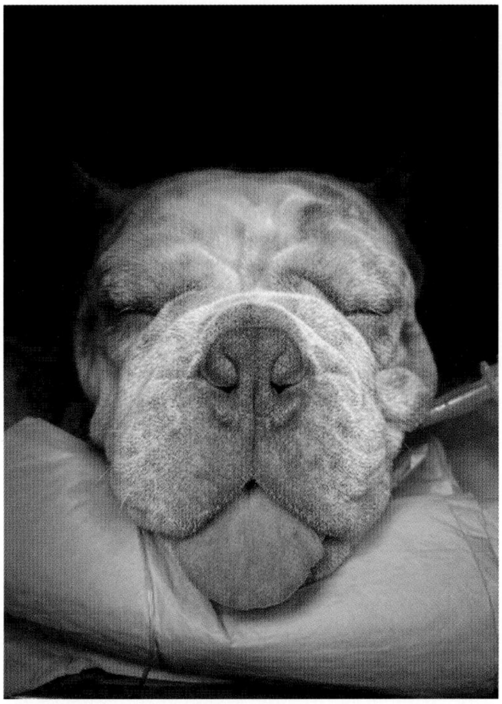

Figure 7.2 Stenotic nares. *Source:* © Pamela Schwartz.

All techniques can be performed with a scalpel blade, electrocautery, or CO_2 laser.

Several wedge resection (alarplasty or alaplasty) techniques (vertical, horizontal, lateral) have been described, removing wedge-shaped portions of the wing of the nostril and underlying alar fold, requiring suture to appose the nasal epithelium[39,40] (Figure 7.3a,b). When using a blade for these techniques, hemorrhage occurs rapidly, which may impair visibility.[41] Hemorrhage is controlled during surgery with direct pressure using a sterile cotton-tipped applicator or gauze and typically resolves once the wound is sutured. A punch resection alarplasty is similar to the wedge techniques but utilizes a dermatological punch biopsy tool[ii] to remove a circular plug of tissue in the ala nasi, which is then sutured closed. With each of these techniques, the nares are widened by narrowing the thickness of the alar nasi, removing tissue to the level of the alar fold.[42,43]

Vertical Alar Wedge Resection – Surgical Technique

The patient is placed in sternal recumbency with the chin elevated slightly. The most ventromedial aspect of the alar wing (alar fold) is grasped at the level of the proposed tissue to be removed (Figure 7.4). The author uses a rat tooth or Bishop Harmon forceps to hold this tissue in place, making a cut on either side using an 11-blade to subsequently remove this triangular section of tissue. The author recommends starting a minimum of 1–2 mm from the edge of the alar fold, as the wedge can be difficult to close if there is not a substantial amount of tissue to move laterally to close. Hemostasis is obtained using a sterile cotton-tipped applicator; however, bleeding will persist until the edges are sutured. The author prefers 4-0 PDS on an RB-1 needle (the editor prefers 4-0 Monocryl on a reverse cutting needle) for closure, placing the most distal/ventral suture first, initially holding the edges closed without tying the knot, to ensure adequate patency of the nostril prior to closure. If needed, an additional wedge of tissue can be removed prior to closure. Two to three interrupted sutures are placed to appose the cut surfaces.

Alapexy is a surgical technique used to fix the alae in an abducted position. This technique involves creating two elliptical incisions, one at the ventrolateral aspect of the alar skin and a corresponding incision in the skin lateral to the ala. These paired incised surfaces are then apposed using suture. This technique may be more time-consuming than other alarplasty techniques due to the need for two incisions and a two-layer closure.[43] It is difficult to make comparisons regarding the effectiveness of different surgical techniques for stenotic nares since most are performed in combination with additional upper airway corrective surgery.

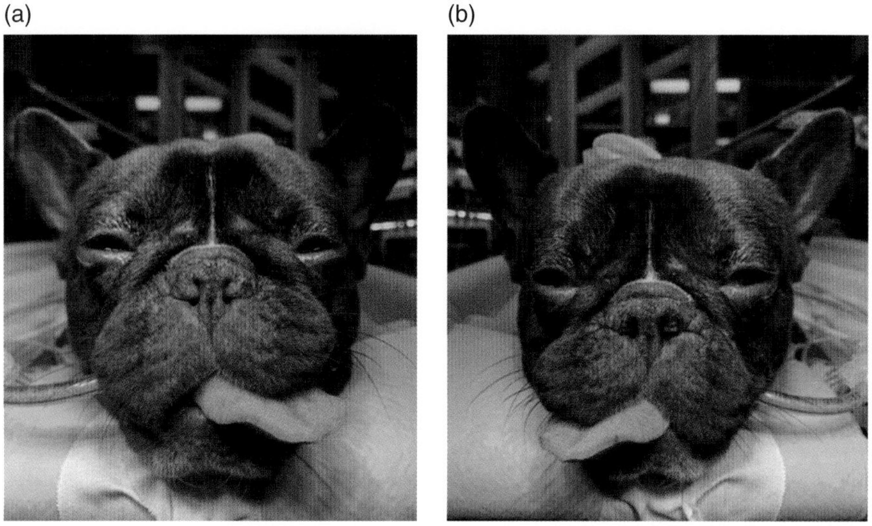

Figure 7.3 (a) Preoperative image of stenotic nares. (b) Postoperative image of the same dog immediately after vertical alar wedge resection. *Source:* © Pamela Schwartz.

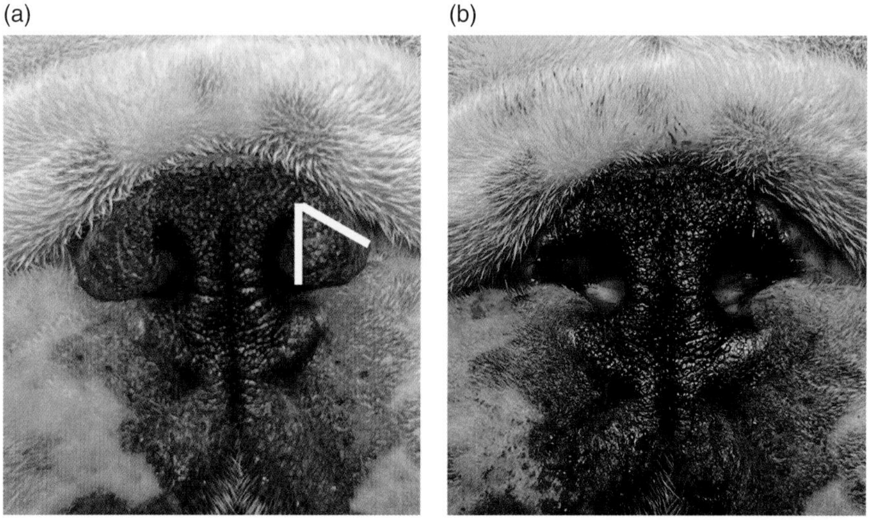

Figure 7.4 The white lines outline the proposed vertical wedge to be resected in the preoperative image (a) and the resulting widening of the nares in the postoperative image (b). *Source:* © Kristin Coleman.

Amputation of the alar skin and underlying cartilage (Trader's technique) is the first noted corrective surgery for stenotic nares described by Trader in 1949.[44] This technique may not be favored by some presumably due to hemorrhage associated with the technique, a resulting open wound, and the plethora of other techniques that are available. An advantage of this surgery is the larger amount of tissue that can be removed with the amputation technique compared to alarplasty techniques.[40] A study revisited the Trader's technique in immature Shih Tzus documenting the complete resolution of all clinical signs associated with stenotic nares, as well as a cosmetic outcome in all dogs.[40] The author performs a modified Trader's technique, utilizing a carbon dioxide laser instead of a blade, preventing the need to control hemorrhage with epinephrine-soaked gauze strips in the immediate postoperative period. In the author's opinion, this technique allows the most significant widening of the nares with cosmetic results (Figure 7.5).

Modified Trader's Technique – Surgical Technique

Safety glasses specific to the laser are required to be worn by all staff within the operating suite if laser is utilized. The patient is placed in sternal recumbency with the chin elevated slightly. The most ventromedial aspect of the alar wing (alar fold) is grasped with rat-toothed forceps and pulled ventromedially. A sterile cotton-tipped applicator is placed ventral to the alar fold within the nostril as a barrier to the blade or laser to protect the underlying nasal skin from inadvertent damage. The laser or electrocautery is used to mark the planned region of alar amputation. The proposed line is evaluated and can be adjusted as needed prior to incising. A #11 blade or CO_2 laser is used to excise the alar fold holding the blade or laser at an approximately 40–45° angle from the coronal plane (Figure 7.6; Video 7.2). The same procedure is repeated on the opposite side to make the resulting nares symmetrical. If a blade is utilized, hemostasis is achieved with direct pressure or electrocautery.

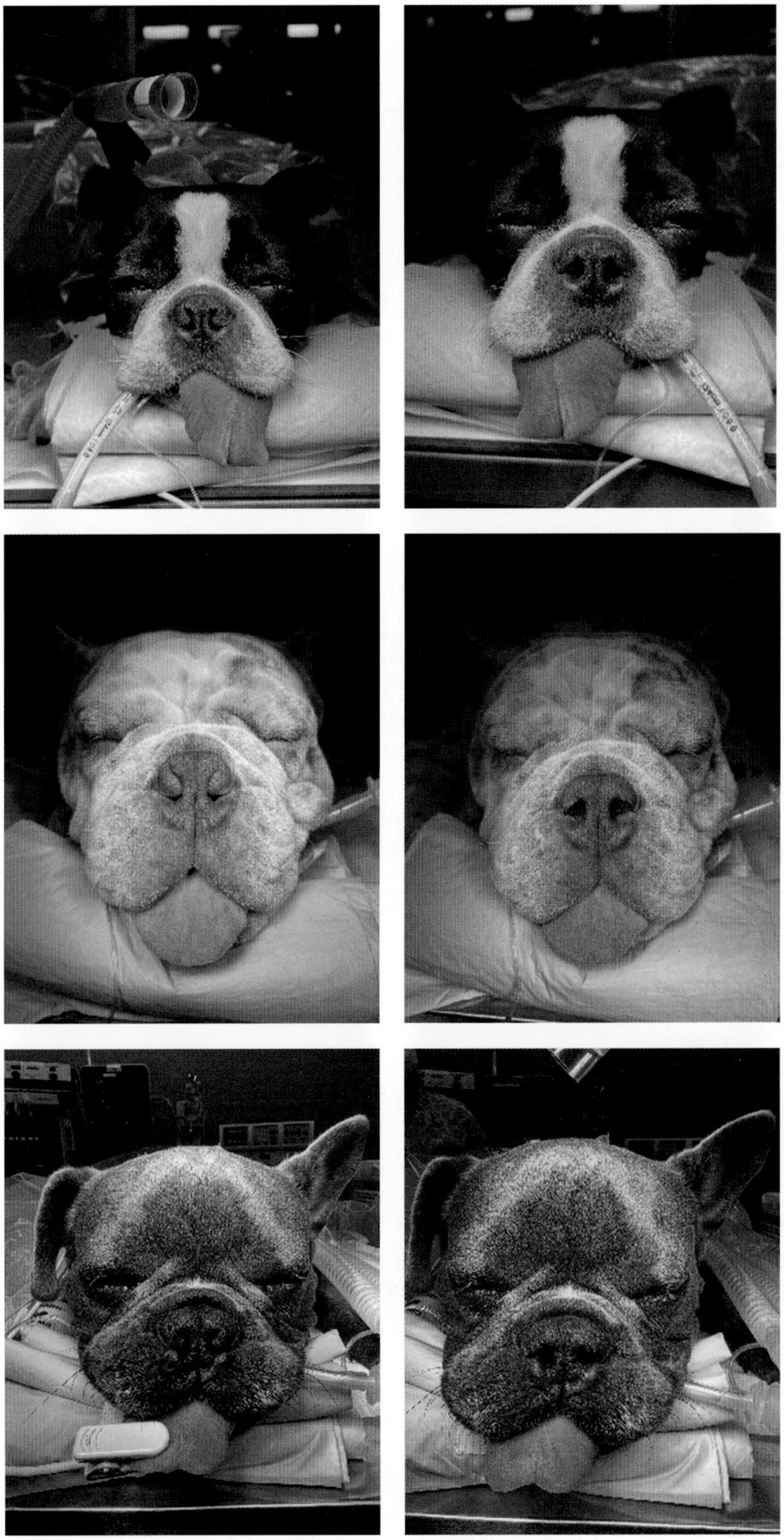

Figure 7.5 Preoperative stenotic nares and immediate postoperative photo after Trader's technique using CO_2 laser in three separate breeds. *Source:* © Pamela Schwartz.

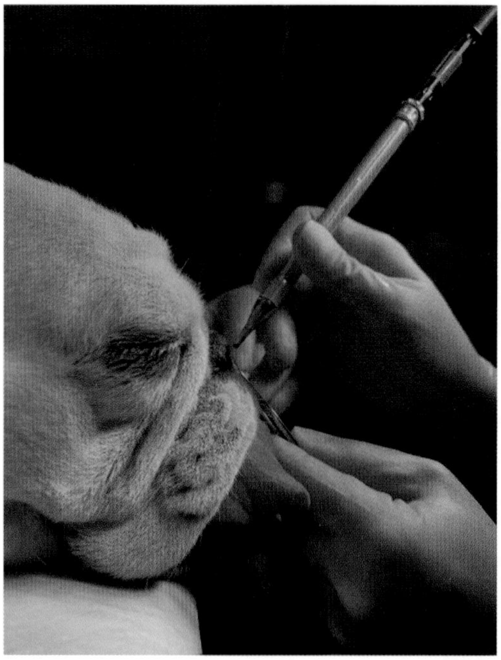

Figure 7.6 The CO_2 laser is used to excise the alar fold holding the handpiece at an approximately 40–45° angle from the coronal plane. *Source:* © Pamela Schwartz.

Laser-Assisted Turbinectomy (LATE)

The laser-assisted turbinectomy (LATE) is an endosurgical procedure developed for the removal of obstructive turbinate tissue to improve endonasal airway patency in brachycephalic dogs.[27] CT and anterior and posterior rhinoscopy have identified intranasal anatomical variations in three brachycephalic breeds (Pug, French Bulldog, and English Bulldog).[26] Abnormal configuration of the nasal conchal tissue is classified as rostral aberrant turbinates and caudal aberrant turbinates (Figure 7.7).[26,27] Direct intraconchal contact points are responsible for obstruction of the intranasal passageway.[26] The surgery results in decreased mucosal contact points in the nasal passages.

The most common complication is transient intraoperative hemorrhage in 32.3% of dogs. Regrowth of turbinates requiring another surgical procedure has been noted in 15.8%.[27] Postoperative complications include dyspnea, which may require temporary tracheostomy, especially when laryngeal collapse is present, postoperative regurgitation, and reverse sneezing which is self-limiting.[45] At the time of follow-up, 40% of dogs had intermittent nasal noise when sniffing and excited, which was a different noise than noted preoperatively, and 20% of dogs had a BOAS index that remained >50%.[45]

The outcome of the LATE procedure, performed two to six months after conventional multilevel surgery, was assessed using the median BOAS index based on WBBP. The median BOAS index decreased from 66.7% to 42.3% after LATE.[45]

There can be several disadvantages when considering the LATE procedure. Specialty equipment for diagnostics and treatment (CT, endoscopy, diode laser), advanced training, and additional time are required, especially if being performed as part of a multilevel surgery strategy. The mean surgical time for the LATE procedure is 18 minutes with a range of 7–59 minutes.[27] Due to the need for advanced training and specialty equipment required for this technique, it is not described here and can be referenced in Oechtering et al.[27]

(a) (b)

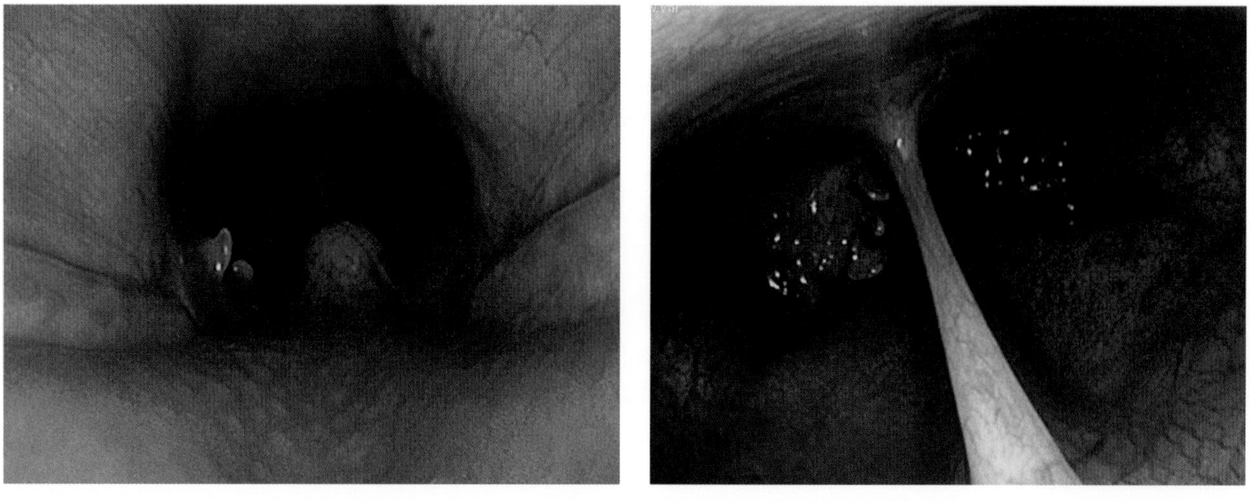

Figure 7.7 (a) Retroflex endoscopy of a normal nonobstructed nasopharynx in a mesaticephalic breed of dog. (b) The appearance of obstructive caudal aberrant nasal turbinates in a brachycephalic breed of dog. *Source:* © Dr. Sarah Marvel.

Soft Palate

Traditional surgical correction objectives are aimed at trimming the length of the soft palate when the palate is elongated (staphylectomy), thus, relieving obstruction of the rima glottis.[46] Staphylectomy may be performed using scissors (cut-and-sew technique), an energy-sealing device, or CO_2 laser. Staphylectomy using Harmonic Focus Shears[iii] is associated with less hemorrhage and a shorter average surgical time compared to traditional sharp resection with sewing.[46] CO_2 laser also allows a shorter surgical time compared to incisional palate resection, however, a similar comparison was not made regarding its effect on hemorrhage.[15] CO_2 laser allows shorter surgical time and less use of an additional sealing device, suggestive of less bleeding compared to diode laser or electrocautery.[47]

Traditional landmarks for shortening the soft palate are the tip of the epiglottis and the middle to caudal third of the tonsillar crypt.[15,48] Although some have suggested that trimming shorter than the traditional landmarks can lead to complications such as nasal regurgitation and rhinitis, more recent literature suggests otherwise.[16,47,49] The author trims the soft palate shorter than the traditional recommendations. An extended palatoplasty described by Dunié-Mérigot et al. and H-pharyngoplasty described by Carabalona et al. are techniques to trim the soft palate beyond the traditional landmarks.[47,49]

CO_2 Laser Staphylectomy – Surgical Technique

Safety glasses specific to the laser are required to be worn by all staff within the operating suite. The patient should be positioned in sternal recumbency with the mouth opened by suspending the maxilla (Figure 7.8). The soft palate should be evaluated while the head and tongue are in a neutral position. Normally, the soft palate should not extend past the tip of the epiglottis or the mid-to caudal aspect of the tonsillar crypt[38] (Figure 7.9a). The tongue is grasped with a gauze sponge and pulled cranially by an assistant as needed throughout the surgery. A DeBakey forcep is used to grasp and retract the tip of the soft palate ventrally toward the base of the tongue to visualize the planned location of the incision (Figure 7.9b; Video 7.3). The DeBakey forcep is changed out for an Allis tissue forceps for continual traction, which will cause less hand fatigue than the DeBakey forceps. One or more saline-soaked gauze are placed caudal to the soft palate covering the endotracheal tube to prevent damage from the laser (Figure 7.9c). A sterile tongue depressor is also used just caudal to the soft palate during laser used as an additional barrier to protect the endotracheal tube from inadvertent damage (Figure 7.9d).

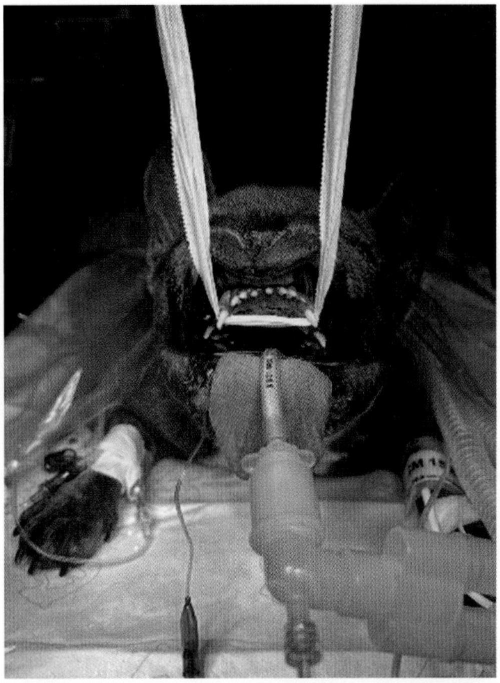

Figure 7.8 Patient positioning with the maxilla suspended with tape. *Source:* © Pamela Schwartz.

The laser is used to mark the planned region of the staphylectomy site starting at and preserving the medial aspect of the tonsillar crypt. A curved line is drawn toward the pterygoid process then back down toward the opposite tonsillar crypt (Figure 7.9d). The soft palate with the proposed staphylectomy line can then be evaluated and adjusted as needed prior to cutting. Once this line is deemed satisfactory, the laser is used to perform the staphylectomy, placing the laser beam as perpendicular as possible to the tissue to avoid splitting the palate in a cranial to caudal direction, until the excess soft palate is excised (Figure 7.10). The saline-soaked gauze is removed to assess the soft palate length. The procedure can be repeated if additional tissue needs to be excised until the shortness of the palate is deemed satisfactory (Figure 7.11). The author only sutures the oral and nasal mucosal surfaces if the distance between the two is subjectively too wide (>4 mm). If closure is performed, the author typically places as few simple interrupted sutures as needed using of 4-0 Monocryl (Figure 7.12; Video 7.4).

Cut-and-Sew Staphylectomy Technique

The positioning is as described for the laser staphylectomy. The editor prefers to have an assistant press ventrally on the endotracheal tube for additional working space in the oropharynx. The distal aspect of the soft palate is grasped with an Allis tissue forceps, or a stay suture can be used to

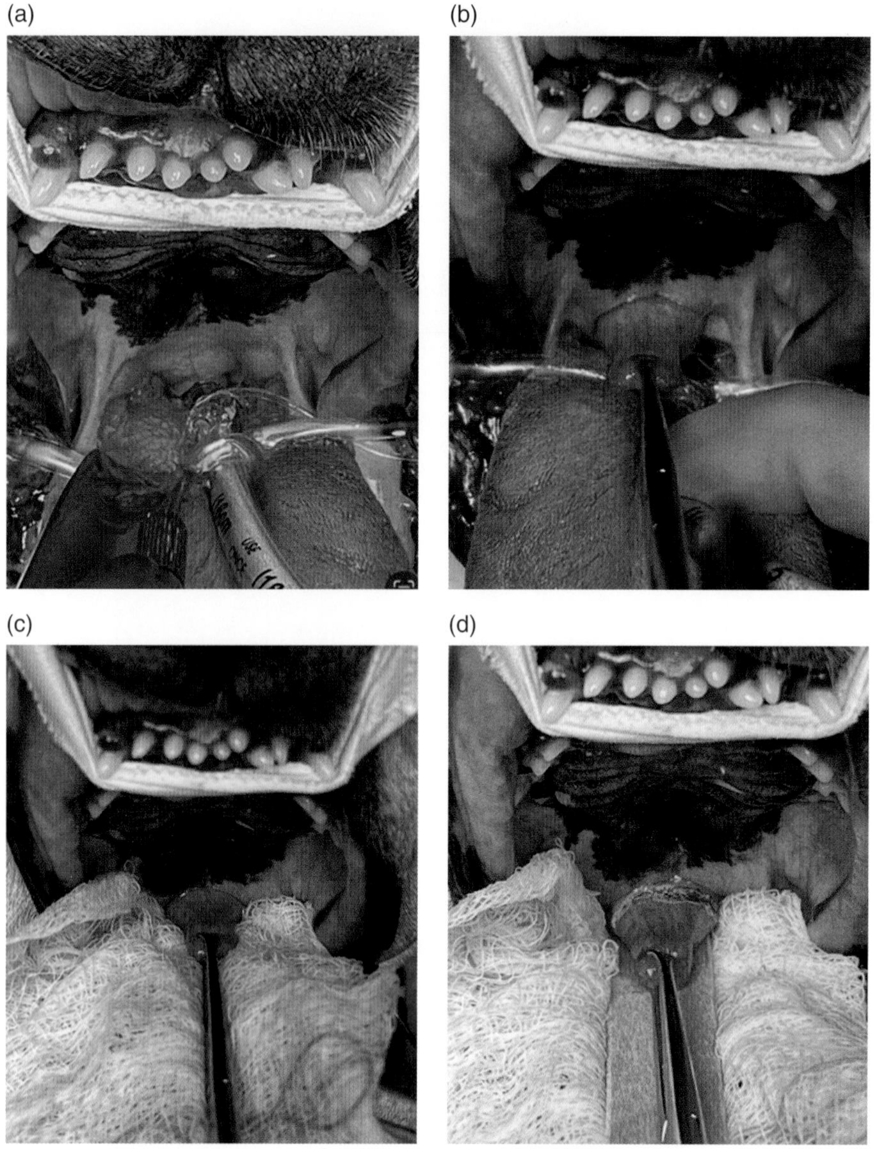

Figure 7.9 (a) Note the soft palate drapes over the endotracheal tube. (b) The tip of soft palate is grasped with Allis tissue forceps and retracted rostrally toward the base of the tongue for surgical planning. (c) A saline-soaked gauze is placed caudal to the soft palate, covering the endotracheal tube. (d) During the use of the CO_2 laser, a sterile tongue depressor is placed between the soft palate and the gauze as an additional barrier to protect against inadvertent damage to the endotracheal tube or surrounding soft tissue structures. Note the planned mark for staphylectomy made with the CO_2 laser. *Source:* © Pamela Schwartz.

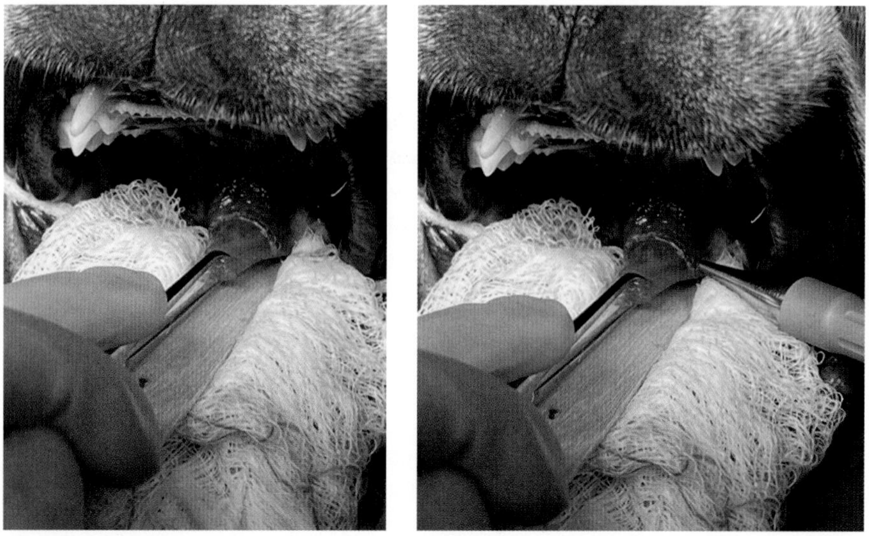

Figure 7.10 The laser is used to mark the planned region of the staphylectomy site starting at the medial aspect of the tonsillar crypt. A curved line is drawn toward the pterygoid process then back down toward the opposite tonsillar crypt. Note the position of the laser is perpendicular to the soft palate at the pre-determined line as opposed to a 45° angle from cranial to caudal, which would create more separation between the oral and nasopharyngeal mucosal surfaces. *Source:* © Pamela Schwartz.

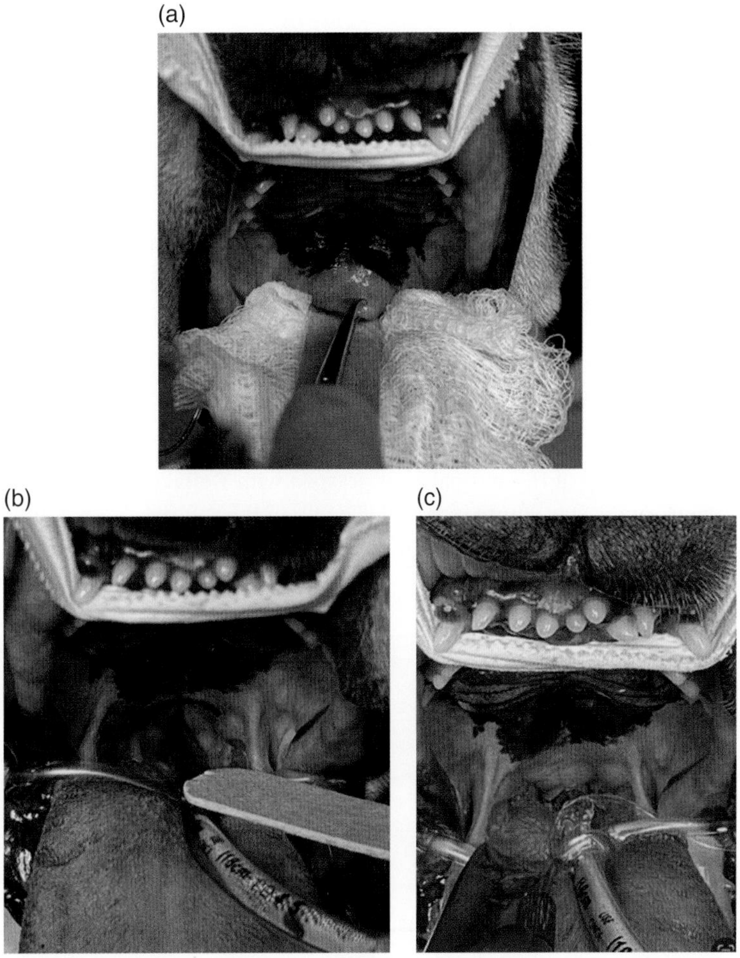

Figure 7.11 (a) After the first pass with the laser, the soft palate was deemed too long, and the procedure was repeated to remove the additional soft palate. (b) Immediately postoperative staphylectomy showing the level of the soft palate falling at the top of the arytenoid cartilage. Note the oral and nasal mucosal surfaces are not sutured. (c) The preoperative photo is included for direct comparison. *Source:* © Pamela Schwartz.

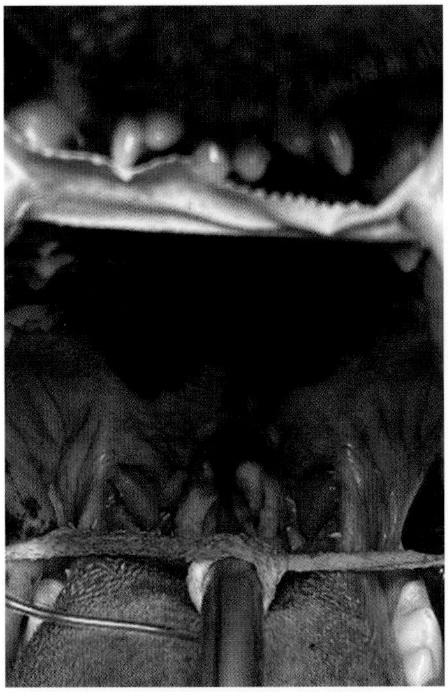

Figure 7.12 Staphylectomy with the oral and nasal mucosal surfaces sutured. *Source:* © Pamela Schwartz.

retract the soft palate rostrally. Stay sutures are placed at the proposed start and end points of the soft palate at the level of the mid-point of the tonsillar crypts, which are ideally two packs of 4-0 Monocryl or Biosyn with a hemostat to elevate the site for suturing. The author prefers to place the first throw for the continuous suture and the end of the suture that is normally cut is left long as a stay suture. Curved Metzenbaum scissors are used to make small cuts across the soft palate, followed closely by suturing. This technique prevents the oral and nasopharyngeal mucosa from becoming widely separated from one another, which can be more challenging to manipulate within the small surgical field. This is continued until the entire amount of desired soft palate is excised. Hemorrhage is controlled using hemostats or electrocautery, and any bleeding will ultimately tamponade once the edges of the palate are closed.

As staphylectomy does not address the thickness of the soft palate, additional techniques, such as the split staphylectomy and folded flap palatoplasty (FFP), have been designed to address both shortening and thinning of the soft palate simultaneously.[50] Palatoplasty may be performed using electrocautery, CO_2 laser, or diode laser; however, dogs have a more favorable outcome and fewer complications with CO_2 or monopolar electrocautery in comparison to use with a diode laser.[47] Compared with traditional staphylectomies, the suture placement associated with FFP is more rostral, and therefore, further away from the pharynx, which may result in less postoperative irritation and subsequently less pharyngeal inflammation and edema.[41] The author prefers FFP when the soft palate is subjectively excessively thickened in addition to elongated.

Folded Flap Palatoplasty Technique Using Monopolar Electrocautery – Surgical Technique

The ventral tip of the soft palate is grasped with DeBakey forceps, and a stay suture is placed. The tip of the soft palate is pulled rostrally until the caudal opening of the nasopharynx is visible. The ventral mucosa of the soft palate is marked with monopolar electrocautery where the ventral tip of the soft palate meets it. Two additional stay sutures are then placed on either side of the most ventral stay suture for manipulation of the soft palate during dissection (Figure 7.13a). The stay sutures are pulled rostrally to help facilitate the area of tissue to be removed and subsequent cautery marks are made on the ventral mucosa to correspond with these stay sutures. The cautery marks are connected to make a triangular or trapezoidal shape marking the area to be incised (Figure 7.13b). Caution is used to spare the tonsillar crypts, making the most lateral aspect of the incision 2–4 mm axial to either tonsillar crypt. The ventral mucosa and associated soft tissues of the soft palate (connective tissue, part of the palatinus and levator veli palatini muscles) are excised until the oropharyngeal mucosa is approached (Figure 7.13c). If the nasopharyngeal

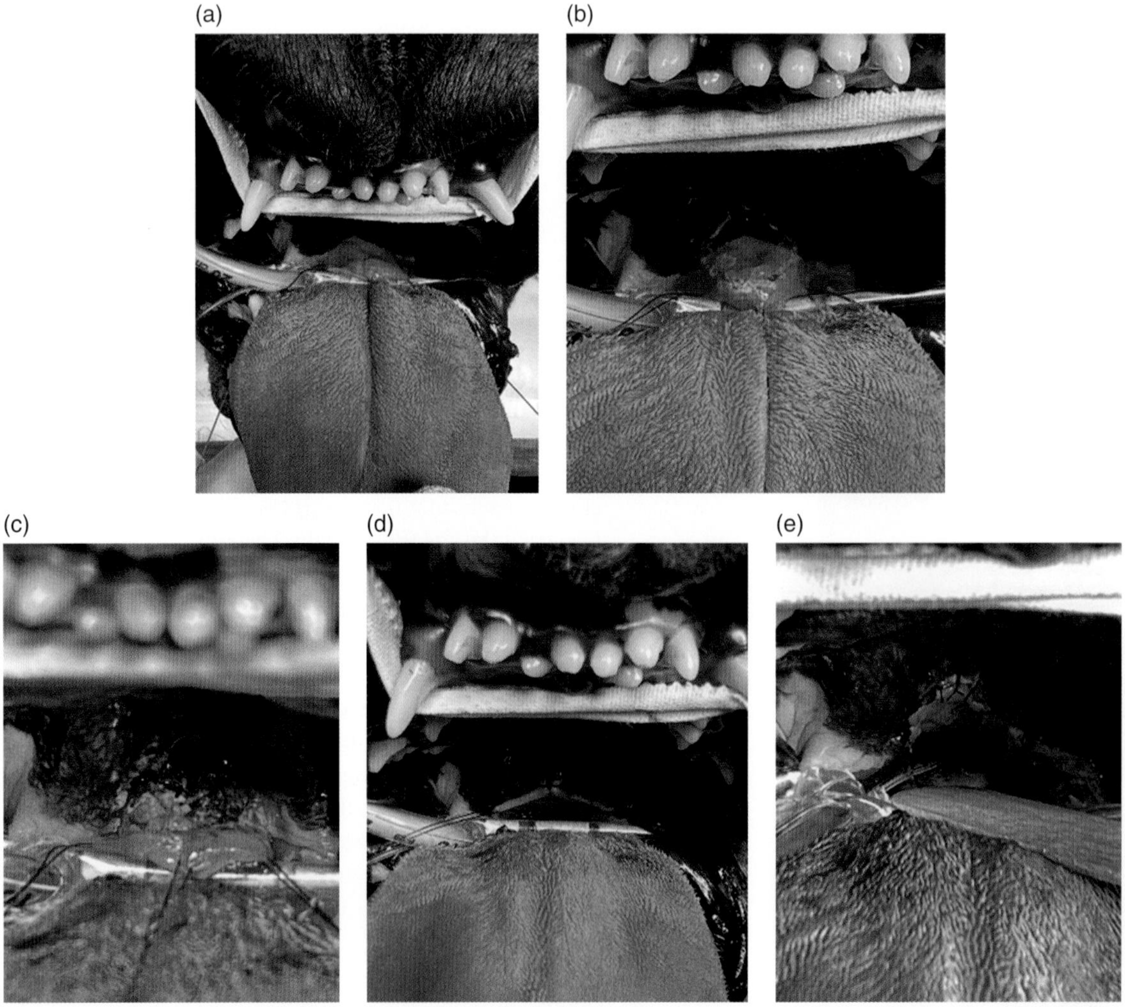

Figure 7.13 (a) Note three stay sutures at the distal end of the soft palate, one at the tip and two on either side of the first. (b) Monopolar electrocautery is used to mark a triangular or trapezoidal area to be incised. (c) The ventral mucosa and associated soft tissues of the soft palate are excised until the nasopharyngeal mucosa is approached. A small defect can be seen in the nasopharyngeal mucosa, which is sutured prior to closure. (d) The stay sutures are advanced rostrally, and the mucosal surfaces apposed. (e) Finished palatoplasty. *Source:* © Pamela Schwartz.

mucosa is entered, dissection cannot continue further caudally and any defect within the nasopharyngeal mucosa should be closed. Once the planned excision is complete, the stay sutures are advanced, and the palate's free edges can be trimmed as deemed necessary prior to closure. The most distal stay suture on the free end of the soft palate is brought up to the most rostral aspect of the ventral mucosa and sutured (Figure 7.13d; Video 7.5). Each mucosal surface lateral to this is then apposed using interrupted sutures (Figure 7.13e).

Eversion of the Laryngeal Saccules

Eversion of the laryngeal saccules is recognized as the first stage of laryngeal collapse[20] (Figure 7.14). Everted saccules are positioned just rostral to the vocal folds.[39] During the laryngeal examination, light anesthesia is important, as saccule eversion can be a dynamic process, and eversion can be missed if the patient is not breathing during the examination. If the saccules have been everted more chronically, it is possible that they will remain everted after general anesthesia, due to secondary changes such as elongation and thickening from fibrosis. The saccules can be removed using Metzenbaum scissors, a blade, or CO_2 laser. The author prefers using scissors, due to ease and avoiding concerns related to using CO_2 laser close to the endotracheal tube and vocal folds. One study reports a minimum of stage I laryngeal collapse in all dogs aged six months or less, further supporting the recommendation that dogs undergo surgical treatment as early as possible.[20]

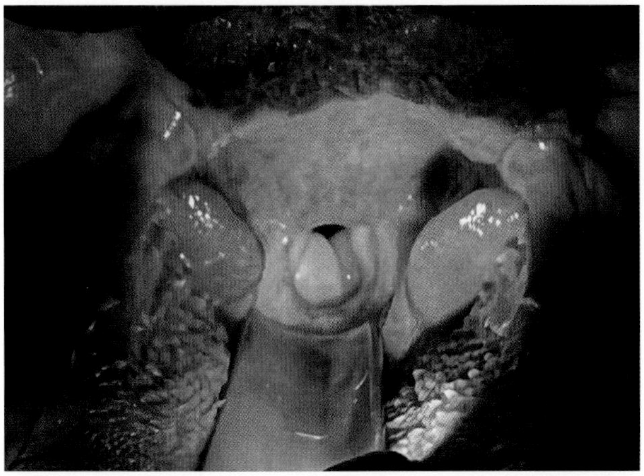

Figure 7.14 The laryngeal saccules are bilaterally everted causing partial obstruction to the rima glottis. Eversion and enlargement of the palatine tonsils are also noted. *Source:* © Pamela Schwartz.

Laryngeal Sacculectomy – Surgical Technique

The author prefers the patient remain intubated for removal of the saccules, having an assistant displace the endotracheal tube dorsally using an instrument, finger, or tongue depressor. Alternatively, the patient can be extubated briefly or the endotracheal tube can be temporarily replaced with a feeding tube to allow oxygen insufflation.[20] The saccule is grasped at the most distal aspect (toward the rima glottis) and retracted rostrally using caution so as not to cause any inadvertent damage to the vocal folds, which are immediately caudal and in close proximity. The saccule is excised using curved Metzenbaum scissors starting ventrally and advancing dorsally using small cutting motions, which helps avoid inadvertent damage to the vocal folds (Figure 7.15a–c; Video 7.6). If hemorrhage is noted, it is controlled by direct pressure using a sterile cotton-tipped applicator.

Advanced Laryngeal Collapse

Laryngeal collapse is commonly noted in dogs with BOAS and is described as a loss of cartilage rigidity, which allows medial deviation of the rostral laryngeal cartilages. Increased airway resistance and velocity and increased negative intraglottic luminal pressure lead to a gradual collapse of the rostral laryngeal opening.[20,21,51,52] Three stages of laryngeal collapse have been described: stage I is eversion of the laryngeal saccules, stage II is loss of rigidity and medial displacement of the cuneiform process of the arytenoid cartilages, and stage III is collapse of the corniculate process of the arytenoid cartilages and subsequent loss of the dorsal arch of the rima glottis with consistent crossing of the cuneiform cartilages medially.[20,52,53]

Grade II or III laryngeal collapse has been diagnosed commonly with percentages as high as 63.9%[8,21,54] (Figure 7.16; Video 7.7). Postoperative BOAS indices in dogs with advanced laryngeal collapse are higher than in dogs with only everted saccules, further supporting earlier surgical intervention.[8] Multilevel corrective BOAS surgery should always be considered as the first choice for treatment, as long-term outcome in dogs with laryngeal collapse is considered good, although clinical signs rarely resolve.[21] Treatment for more advanced laryngeal collapse should only be considered if clinical signs worsen after multilevel surgery for BOAS.

The best management of stage II or III laryngeal collapse is still controversial.[52] Reported options for treatment of stage III collapse include arytenoid lateralization, permanent tracheotomy, and subtotal epiglottectomy in association with ablation of unilateral cartilage.[52,55–57] Arytenoid lateralization may be a useful treatment for stage II and III collapse in brachycephalic dogs with one

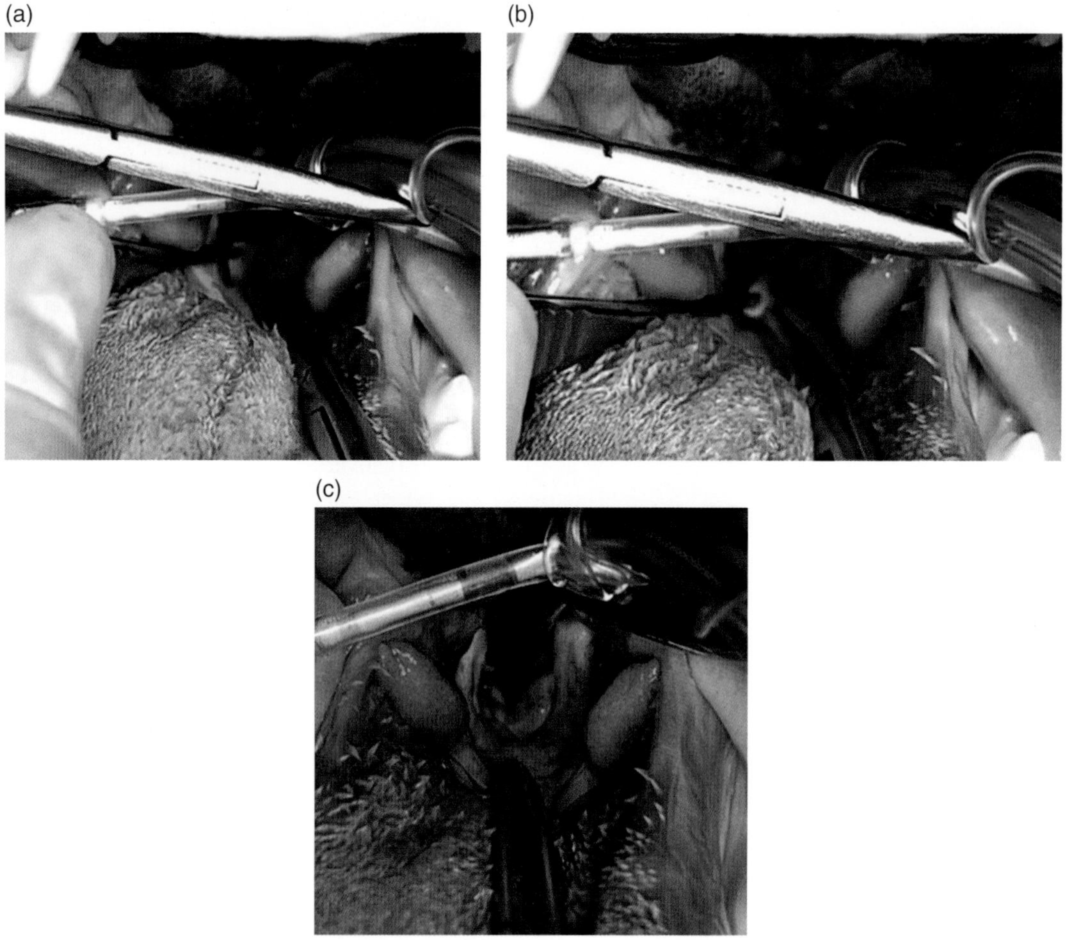

Figure 7.15 (a) The left laryngeal saccule is exteriorized away from the vocal fold. (b) The laryngeal saccule is excised using Metzenbaum scissors cutting from ventral to dorsal. (c) Photo immediately after bilateral laryngeal saccule removal. The edges of the vocal folds can be visualized just caudal to the cut edges of the laryngeal saccules. *Source:* © Pamela Schwartz.

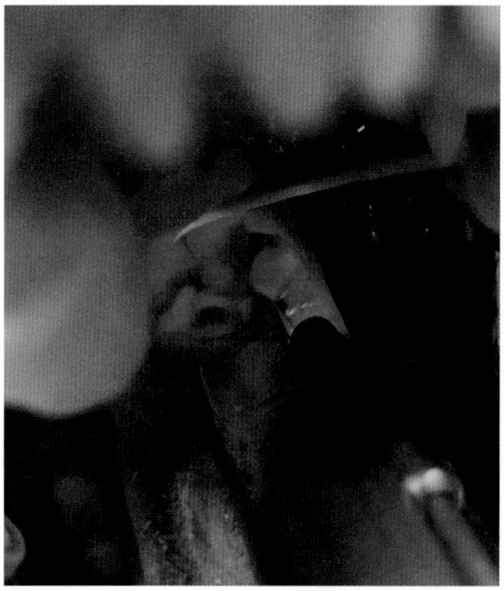

Figure 7.16 Stage III laryngeal collapse is noted with the left cuneiform process of the arytenoid cartilage folded inward toward and crossing slightly rostral to the right cuneiform process. *Source:* © Pamela Schwartz.

study showing good long-term results in dogs that survive; two dogs (16.7%) were euthanized postoperatively due to dyspnea secondary to minimal enlargement of the rima glottis.[51] One study identified degenerative histologic characteristics and decreased load to failure and stiffness of the arytenoid cartilage in brachycephalic dogs compared to non-brachycephalic dogs, which could result in failure after arytenoid lateralization, although further studies are warranted.[58] Another study evaluated arytenoid lateralization for the treatment of combined laryngeal paralysis and laryngeal collapse, however, none of the dogs treated were brachycephalic.[57] Subtotal epiglottectomy in association with ablation of unilateral cartilage shows promise with 12.5% requiring a temporary tracheostomy and variable outcome in the 75% of patients that were followed up at one year.[52] Permanent tracheotomy in brachycephalic breeds is associated with major complications (80%) resulting in postoperative death in 53%.[55] Because these are considered salvage procedures with higher complication and mortality rates, referral to a board-certified surgeon is recommended. Temporary tracheostomy can be performed if needed prior to referral.

Tonsillectomy

Historically, tonsillectomy was considered controversial.[10] Eversion and enlargement of the palatine tonsils are suspected secondary changes due to increased negative airway pressure and can contribute to pharyngeal obstruction (Figure 7.14). One study documents everted tonsils in 56% of dogs with BOAS.[59] Although the full advantage is not completely known, tonsillectomy has been documented as part of multilevel BOAS surgery strategy.[8,45] Tonsillectomy can be performed using a blade, scissors, monopolar electrocautery, CO_2 laser, or vessel-sealing devices such as the LigaSure.[iv] Complications after tonsillectomy include hemorrhage, pharyngeal swelling, and postoperative aspiration of blood or fluid.[60] A clamping technique combined with monopolar electrocautery has been associated with a high risk of bleeding compared to energy-based vessel sealing devices.[61,62] The author prefers CO_2 laser, however, knowledge of anatomy is paramount to avoid hemorrhage and inadvertent damage to neighboring structures.

Tonsillectomy – Surgical Technique

The endotracheal tube is protected using saline-soaked sponges and a sterile tongue depressor as needed. Safety glasses specific to the laser are required to be worn by all staff within the operating suite if utilizing CO_2 laser. The tonsil is grasped with DeBakey or Allis tissue forceps and retracted from the tonsillar crypt (Figure 7.17a). Care is taken when manipulating the tonsil, as the tonsil is friable, and excessive manipulation can lead to hemorrhage or tearing of the tonsil. Retracting the edge of the tonsillar crypt dorsally helps to expose the tonsil and its attachments. The tonsil is then dissected free from its attachments while retracting it from the crypt (Figure 7.17b–g). The base of the tonsil is transected with scissors, a scalpel, electrocautery, laser, or vessel-sealing device. The tonsillar artery may need ligation if scissors or a scalpel are utilized. The mucosal crypt is closed with a rapidly absorbable monofilament suture (Figure 7.18). The author prefers simple continuous closure with a small (4-0) rapidly dissolving suture.

Temporary Tracheostomy

Temporary tracheostomy is indicated in dogs that have continued airway obstruction despite corrective surgery for BOAS.[18,63] Continued airway obstruction may be attributable to conformational changes that cannot be corrected (i.e., advanced laryngeal collapse), as well as pharyngeal swelling and edema from manipulation during surgery.

Historically, temporary tubed tracheostomy has been associated with a high complication rate. Complications associated with temporary tubed tracheostomy may include coughing, occlusion of the tube with mucus or debris causing obstruction, inadvertent dislodgement of the tube, dyspnea, vomiting, pneumonia, subcutaneous emphysema, pneumomediastinum, sinus bradycardia, and death.[64–67] One study reports a complication rate of 86%, with unsuccessful tube management in 19% of dogs ultimately leading to death or euthanasia.[64] Another study evaluating temporary tracheostomy tube-placement in dogs following corrective surgery for BOAS noted a high overall complication rate of 95.2% but successful management in 97.5%.[67] Studies note that breed and age are risk factors with Bulldogs being less likely to have a successful outcome with temporary tubed tracheostomy, and the odds that a dog would require a temporary tracheostomy increasing with each year of age.[63,64] An additional study found a correlation between dogs requiring a temporary tracheostomy after surgery and death or euthanasia in the postoperative period.[68] The high complication rate and intensive management required for the successful management of traditional tubed tracheostomies have led to the development of novel techniques. Use of silicone tracheal stents or modified techniques with placement of a Penrose drain dorsal to the trachea continue to have high complication rates.[65,66]

A tubeless temporary tracheostomy technique has been developed by Dr. Heidi Hottinger (publication in progress) to potentially alleviate some of the complications associated with a tube tracheostomy for a variety of airway diseases, including BOAS. The goal of the tubeless temporary tracheostomy is to minimize handling and stress, as there is no tube maintenance. Only the surrounding skin is cared for using baby wipes initially every two hours and Aquaphor to decrease irritation from frequent cleaning of the skin. Suction, which can induce a vasovagal response, is not recommended, and any mucus can be cleaned with a sterile cotton-tipped applicator only as needed. This technique has been used in over 60 patients in Dr. Hottinger's and the editor's clinic with the average time to discharge being one to two days. If pneumonia is present, the average hospital stay is extended to 3.3 days. Reported complications include mild to excessive mucoid discharge for the first one to two weeks (which then subsides) in up to 30% of cases, persistent stoma requiring outpatient surgical closure (usually only sedation needed) (20%), pneumonia, local dermatitis, dehiscence, and death (15%) within one week of surgery. Of the four cats in this population,

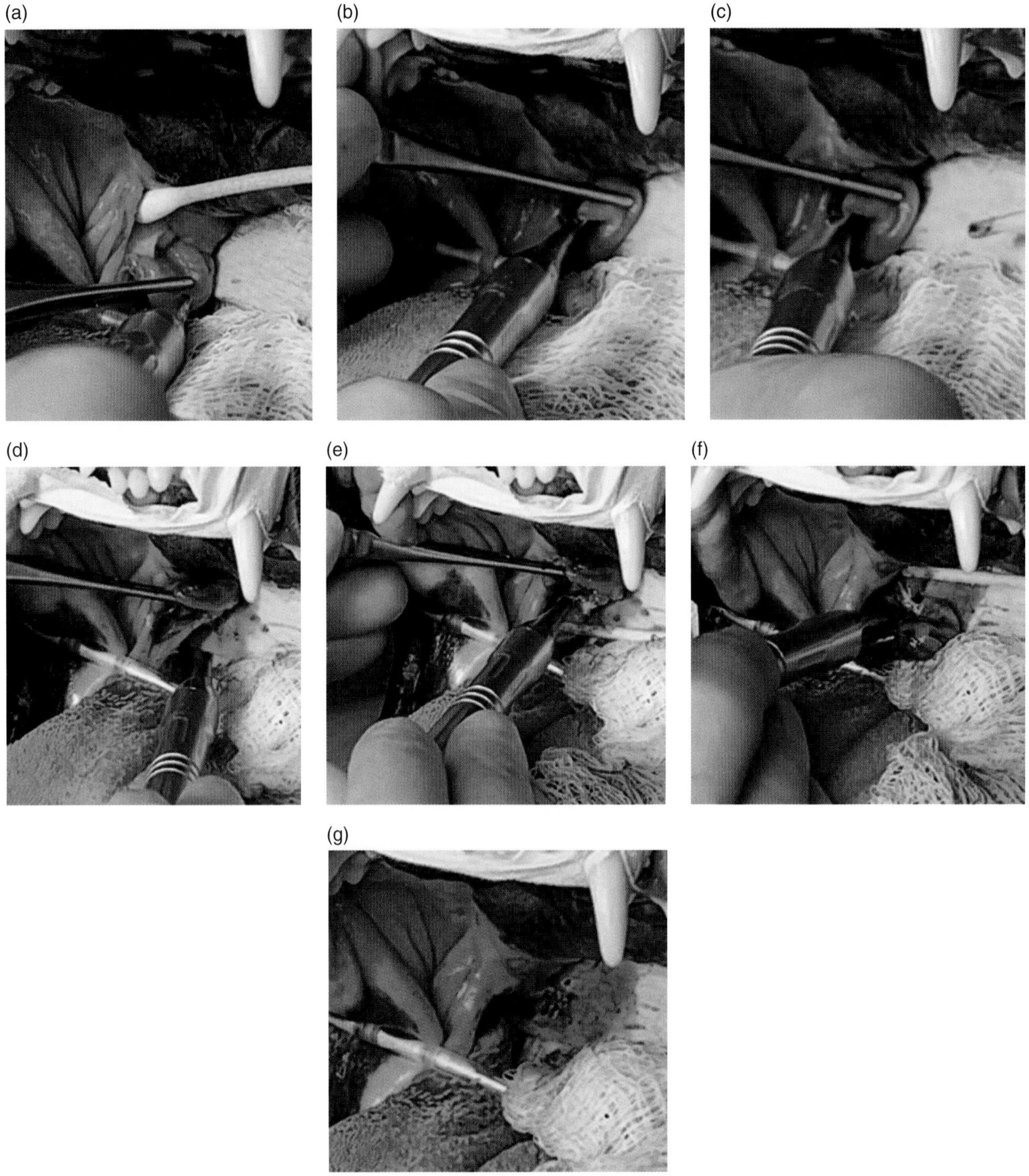

Figure 7.17 (a) The right tonsil is grasped with DeBakey Forceps and retracted. A sterile cotton-tipped applicator is used to retract the tissue dorsally to expose the dorsomedial attachments of the tonsil. (b–f) CO_2 laser is used to dissect the attachments of the tonsil, first rostromedially, retracting the tonsil while advancing more caudally to completely excise the tonsil. (g) The tonsillar crypt can be seen empty after tonsillectomy. *Source:* © Pamela Schwartz.

there was a 25% risk of death (1 out of the 4). Of the cases that died or were euthanized, the majority were due to the primary disease process. A population of cases failed airway normalization (10%) and required conversion to a permanent tracheostomy. A tubed tracheostomy in comparison is much more labor-intensive with some patients requiring interventions as frequently as every 15–60 minutes to combat the formation of mucus plugs. Future studies are warranted to compare this technique to that of the traditional tubed tracheostomy.

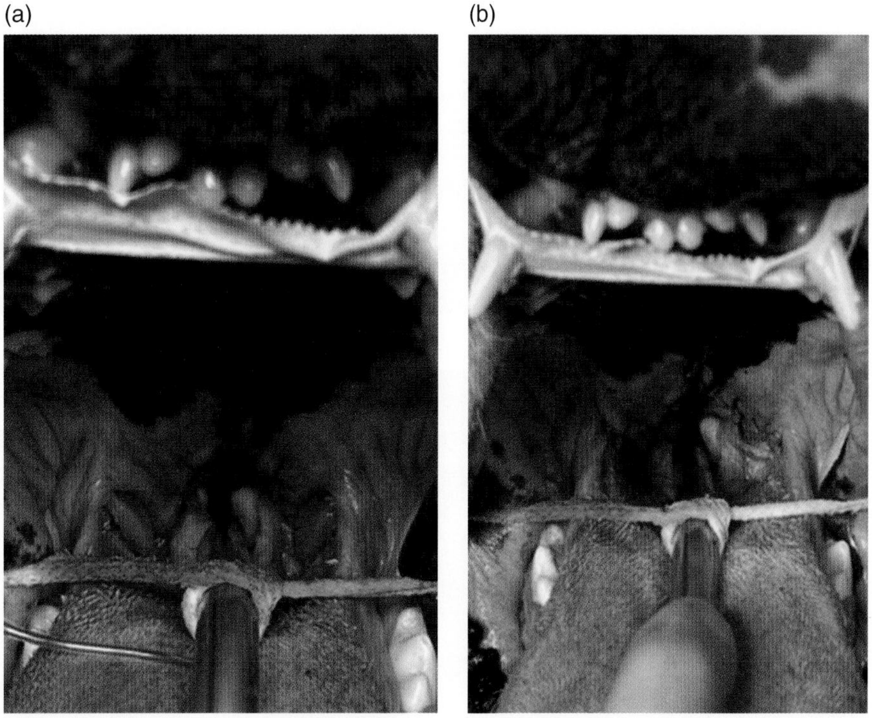

Figure 7.18 (a) Everted tonsils preoperatively. (b) Immediately post bilateral tonsillectomy. Note the crypts are sutured closed. *Source:* © Pamela Schwartz.

Temporary Tracheostomy – Surgical Technique

The patient is placed in dorsal recumbency with the neck extended. Rolled towels can be placed underneath the neck, which moves the trachea to a more superficial position. The fur is clipped from the ramus of the mandible to the thoracic inlet and aseptically prepped and draped (Figure 7.19). A ventral midline incision is made starting caudal to the thyroid cartilage, extending far enough to include the fourth and fifth tracheal rings (Figure 7.20a). Subcutaneous dissection is continued to expose the paired sternohyoid muscles (Figure 7.20b). The sternohyoid muscles are separated at their median raphe to expose the trachea (Figure 7.20c). To improve exposure, elevate the sternohyoid muscles to access the lateral aspects of the trachea, and bluntly dissect the dorsal fascial attachments. Dissection too dorsally could result in iatrogenic injury to the vagosympathetic trunk. If needed, a curved instrument can be placed dorsally to elevate the trachea to a more superficial position (Figure 7.20d). A transverse incision is made through the annular ligament using a blade between the third and fourth or fourth and fifth tracheal rings (Figure 7.20d). This incision should not exceed more than half of the tracheal circumference. Nonabsorbable stay sutures are placed encircling the cartilage cranial and caudal to the tracheostomy site, which can be manipulated to separate the edges during tube insertion. Suction all blood or mucus prior to tube insertion. To facilitate tube insertion

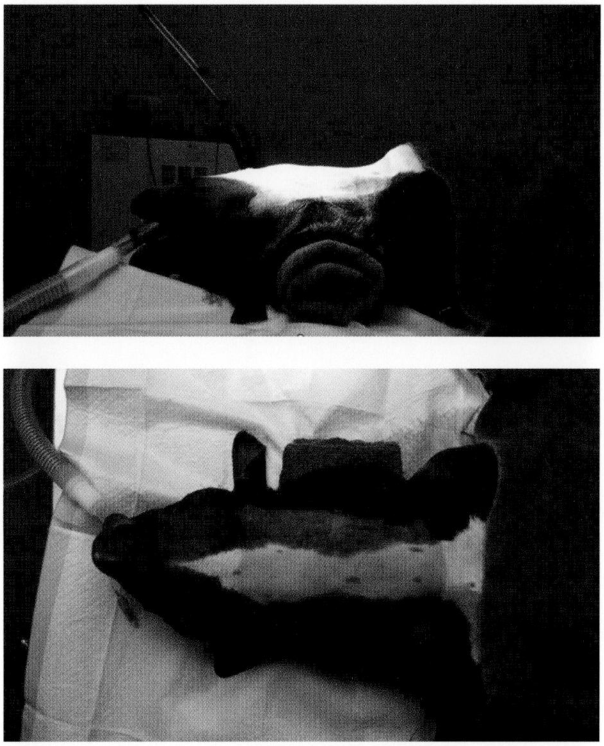

Figure 7.19 Positioning for a temporary tracheostomy. Rolled towels are placed underneath the neck, which moves the trachea to a more superficial position. The fur is clipped from the ramus of the mandible to the thoracic inlet and aseptically prepped and draped. *Source:* © Heidi Hottinger.

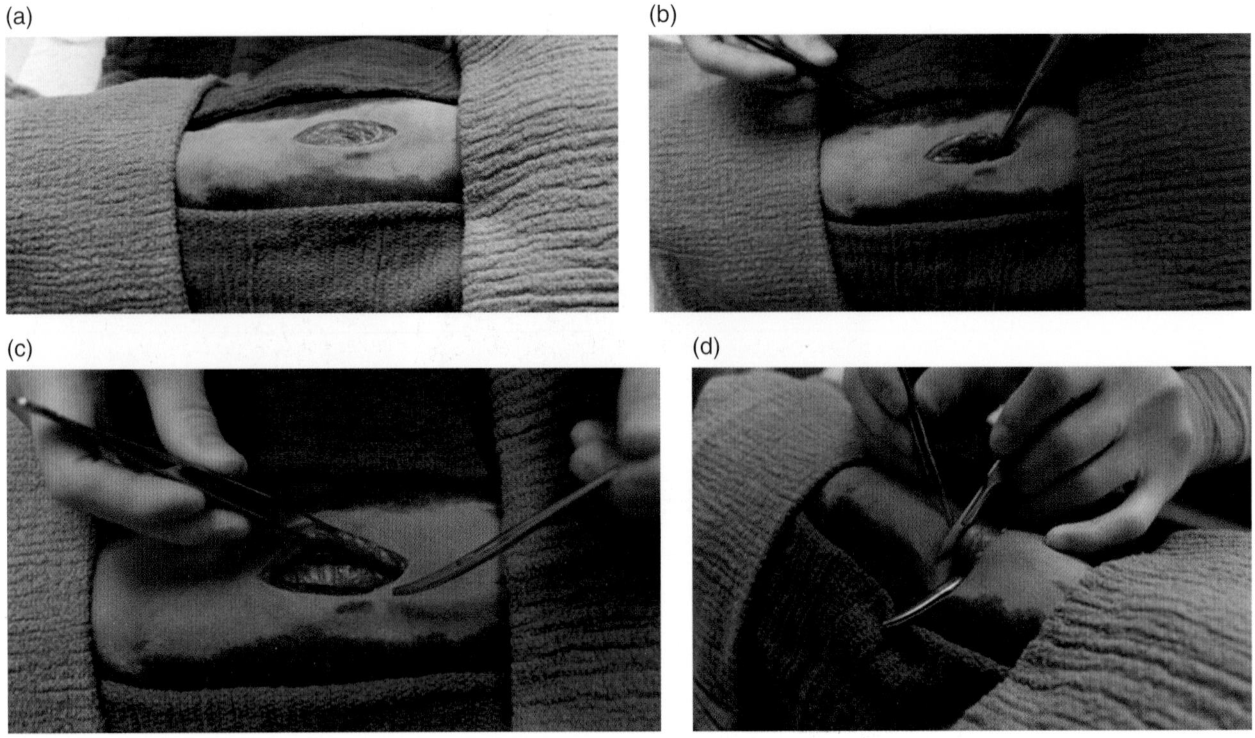

Figure 7.20 (a) A ventral midline incision is made starting caudal to the thyroid cartilage, extending far enough to include the fourth and fifth tracheal rings. (b) The sternohyoid muscles are noted. (c) The trachea is exposed. (d) A curved instrument is placed dorsally to elevate the trachea. A transverse incision is made through the annular ligament between the third and fourth or fourth and fifth tracheal rings, being sure to not transect through more than 50% of the circumference. *Source:* © Heidi Hottinger.

into the caudal trachea, the caudal stay suture is tensioned, and the cranial cartilage can be flattened with a hemostat.

If the tube is difficult to insert, the annular ligament incision can be extended slightly, or an ellipse of cartilage can be resected. Once the tube is placed, the sternohyoid muscles, subcutaneous tissue, and skin are apposed cranial and caudal to the tracheostomy tube. The tube is secured to the neck using umbilical tape, or there is a plethora of commercially available tracheal ties (Figure 7.21).

The author recommends labeling the stay sutures with white tape (i.e., the cranial suture "up" and the caudal suture "down") to easily identify them if a rapid tube

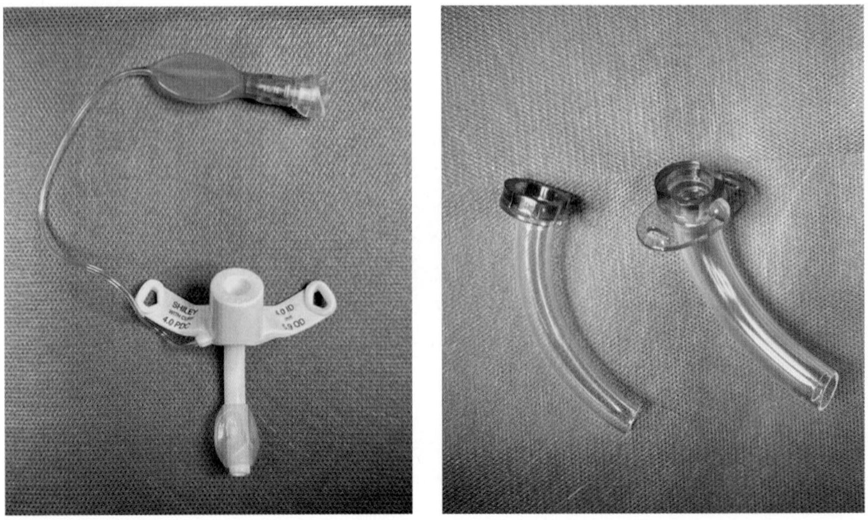

Figure 7.21 Cuffed and noncuffed tracheostomy tubes. Cuffed tubes are typically used if mechanical ventilation is needed. Note the open circles on either end of the flange, which are used to secure the tube around the patient's neck. *Source:* © Pamela Schwartz.

exchange is required. In the postoperative period, the tube can be temporarily occluded to determine if the patient can tolerate breathing through the upper airway. Once the tube is removed, the tracheal stoma can be left open to heal by second intention.

Tubeless Temporary Tracheostomy – Surgical Technique

The patient is placed in dorsal recumbency with the neck extended. A rolled towel is placed underneath the neck to facilitate dorsiflexion, which moves the trachea to a more superficial position. The fur is clipped from the ramus of the mandible to the thoracic inlet and aseptically prepped and draped (Figure 7.19). A ventral midline incision is made starting caudal to the cricoid cartilage, extending far enough to include the fourth and fifth tracheal rings (Figure 7.20a). Subcutaneous dissection is continued to expose the paired sternohyoid muscles (Figure 7.20b). The sternohyoid muscles are separated at their median raphe to expose the trachea (Figure 7.20c). To improve exposure, elevate the sternohyoid muscles to access the lateral aspects of the trachea, and bluntly dissect the dorsal fascial attachments. Dissection too dorsally could result in iatrogenic injury to the vagosympathetic trunk. If needed, a curved instrument can be placed dorsally to elevate the trachea (Figure 7.20d). A transverse incision is made through the annular ligament using a blade between the second and third tracheal rings in brachycephalic dog breeds and between the third and fourth or fourth and fifth rings in normocephalic breeds (Figure 7.20d). This incision should not exceed more than half of the tracheal circumference. A tracheostomy tube is not placed; instead, the closure begins with the first two sutures engaging the commissures of the tracheostomy using a rapidly absorbable suture. The first suture is placed through the subcutis, medial edge of the sternohyoid muscle, and full thickness through the trachea, all in a single interrupted throw (Figure 7.22a–d). This is repeated on the opposite side. This adequately elevates the trachea as well as excludes the sternohyoid muscle from the field (Figure 7.23). Additional sutures are placed on either side of the stoma, engaging full-thickness trachea to subcutis, moving lateral to medial until skin-skin apposition is noted cranial and caudal to the tracheostomy site (Figure 7.24a,b). Suturing the trachea to the subcutis helps apply cranial and caudal tension on the stoma to widen it. The skin is then apposed cranial and caudal to the tracheostomy site, using absorbable interrupted skin sutures (Figure 7.25). Once the patient is extubated, flow-by oxygen can be administered at the stoma site. Intubation of the tubeless tracheostomy site is not preferred, as it can disrupt the sutures. Closure consists of

(a) (b) (c) (d)

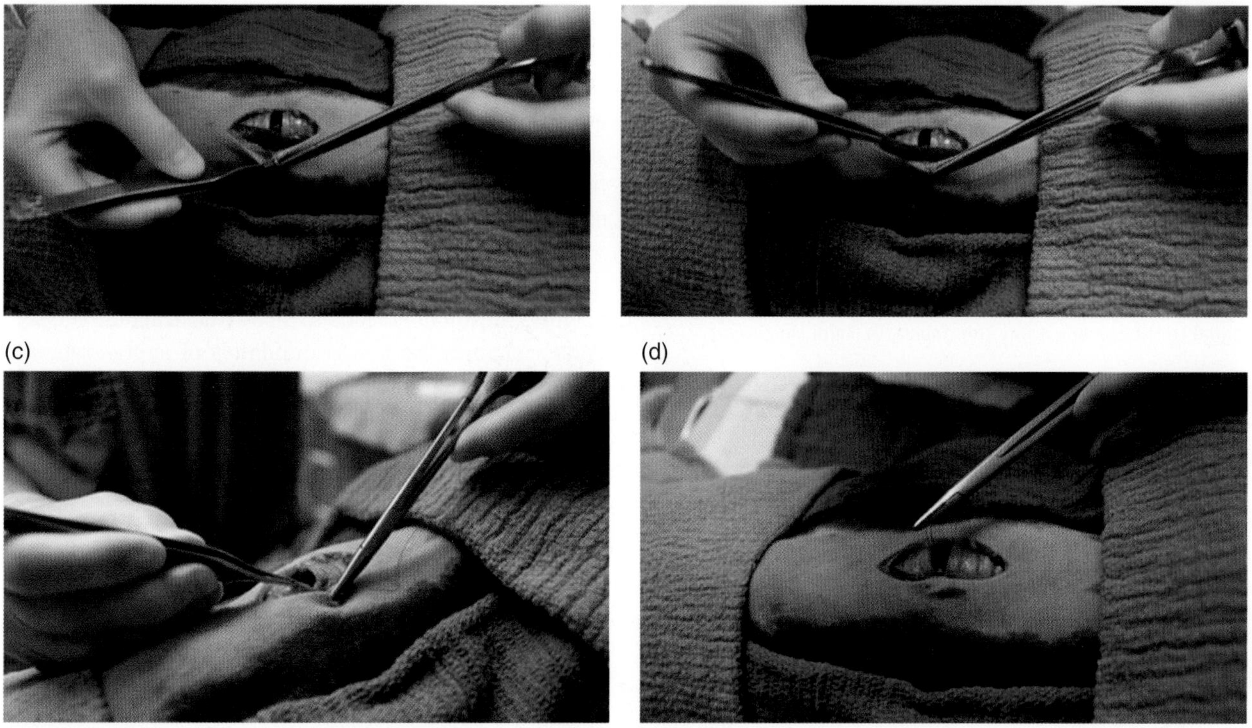

Figure 7.22 The first suture is placed through the skin and subcutis (a), medial edge of the sternohyoid muscle (b), then full thickness through the trachea (c), all in a single interrupted throw (d). *Source:* © Heidi Hottinger.

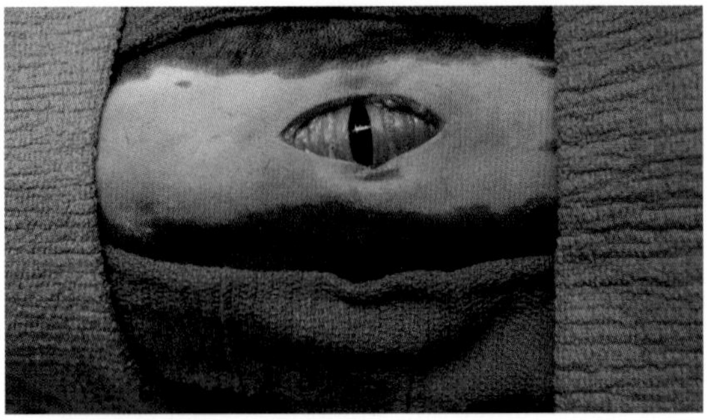

Figure 7.23 Placement of the first two sutures on either side of the tracheostomy site, which elevates the trachea and excludes the sternohyoideus muscles from the field. *Source:* © Heidi Hottinger.

(a)
(b)

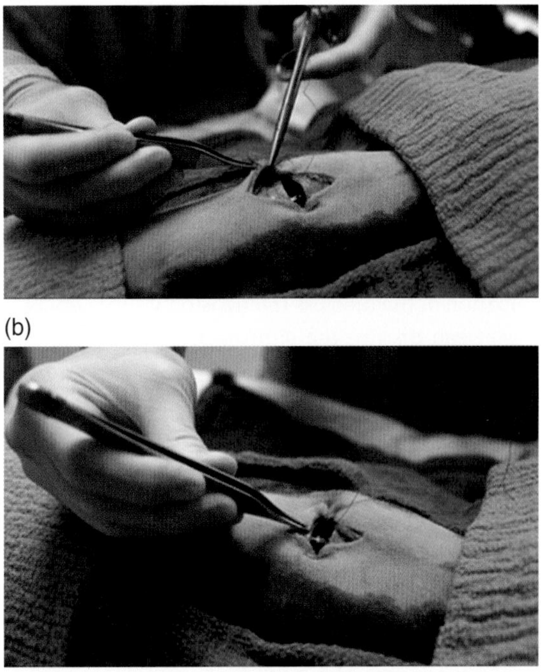

Figure 7.24 (a,b) Additional sutures are placed on either side of the stoma, engaging full-thickness trachea to subcutis, moving lateral to medial until skin-skin apposition is noted cranial and caudal to the tracheostomy site. *Source:* © Heidi Hottinger.

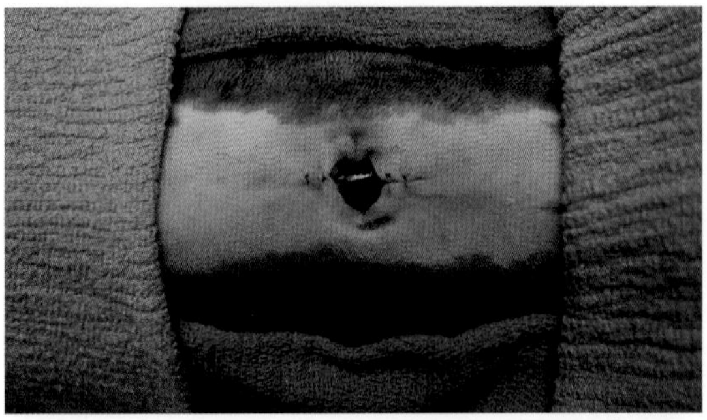

Figure 7.25 The skin is apposed cranial and caudal to the tracheostomy site using absorbable interrupted skin sutures. *Source:* © Heidi Hottinger.

second-intention healing and usually occurs within six to eight weeks postoperatively.

Postoperative Outcome

Brachycephalic breeds have a higher risk of developing complications in the perianesthetic period but even more so in the postanesthetic period.[25] The most common postoperative complications are vomiting, regurgitation, aspiration pneumonia, dyspnea, airway obstruction, and death.[25,28,49] The postoperative mortality rate is generally less than 5% but is reported to be as high as 7%.[7,47,49,67,68] The most common cause of death is secondary to airway obstruction and aspiration pneumonia.

Most dogs that undergo surgical correction of BOAS improve and have a good long-term outcome, but it is important for owners to know that the anatomy cannot be normalized and many dogs will continue to have clinical signs.[8,21,69] The author recommends that owners take normal brachycephalic precautions after surgery (avoiding extreme heat, maintaining a slim body condition) and recheck if a progression in clinical signs is noted or a whistling noise develops, which could indicate laryngeal collapse.

Norwich Terriers

The Norwich Terrier appears to have an obstructive airway syndrome that differs from that encountered by brachycephalic breeds. Similar to some brachycephalic breeds, half of Norwich Terriers lacked clinical signs despite the identification of severe obstruction on laryngeal examination.[70] Differing from brachycephalic breeds, nasal and palate abnormalities are not common. The site of obstruction appears to be at the level of the larynx with narrowing noted caudal to the vocal folds that decreases the luminal diameter.[70] The small size of the laryngeal opening presumably leads to airway obstruction and secondary changes such as redundancy of supra-arytenoid tissue, everted laryngeal saccules, and laryngeal collapse. The role of surgery is unclear, although corrective surgery can be considered if secondary changes are present. The author anecdotally performed staphylectomy in a three-year-old Norwich Terrier with progressive respiratory signs. The elongated soft palate was a presumed secondary change, as CT and laryngeal examination documented a characteristic small laryngeal opening as well as stage II laryngeal collapse. Although the syndrome in Norwich Terriers differs from other brachycephalic breeds, they should be considered similarly challenging anesthetic candidates and should be watched carefully in the postanesthetic period.[70]

Cats

Much less is known regarding BOAS in cats, as it appears to be less common compared to dogs. Abnormalities of the nares appear to be the primary component of BOAS in cats.[71–73] In some cases, stenotic external nares and a narrowed nasal vestibule are the primary causes of obstruction, whereas some cats appear to have ventral nasal obstruction resulting from redundant skin along the floor of the nares.[71,73] One study evaluating Persian and Exotic Shorthair show cats identified moderate to severe stenotic nares in 86% and hypoplasia of the nose leather in 95% with the nose leather top positioned above the level of the lower eyelid in 93%. Despite these conformational abnormalities, few cat owners perceived any problems related to the airways.[74]

Because the obstruction is generally at the level of the nares, signs associated with BOAS in cats are mostly alleviated by the surgical intervention of the alar wings and alar folds. One study shows success in cats using a blade to remove the axial alar wing and alar fold bilaterally as reported for dogs.[73] If obstruction is secondary to redundant skin along the floor of the nares, techniques used in dogs may be insufficient, as this anatomical abnormality is not addressed. In cats with obstruction from redundant skin along the floor of the nares, a single pedicle advancement flap allowed a reduction in stertorous breathing and no episodes of respiratory distress.[71] In cats where the obstruction results from the alar folds and redundant skin, a combined surgery of "alar fold lift-up" and "sulcus pull-down" has been described as successful.[70] Because of the paucity of information on cats, it is difficult to make direct comparisons between surgical techniques. There seems to be a low complication rate regardless of the surgical technique. The author prefers a modified Trader's technique using a CO_2 laser with or without suture as the first stage (Figure 7.26). Although the author has not needed to consider a second surgery on a cat, if the cat's outcome is not perceived as successful once recovered, the author typically prepares owners for a single pedicle advancement flap if additional relief is needed.

Modified Trader's Technique in Cats – Surgical Technique

The cat is positioned in sternal recumbency with the head slightly elevated in a neutral position. Safety glasses specific to the laser are required to be worn by all staff within the operating suite if utilizing CO_2 laser. The alar fold is grasped with Bishop Harmon forceps and retracted ventromedially. A sterile cotton-tipped applicator is placed ventral to the alar fold within the nostril as a barrier to the

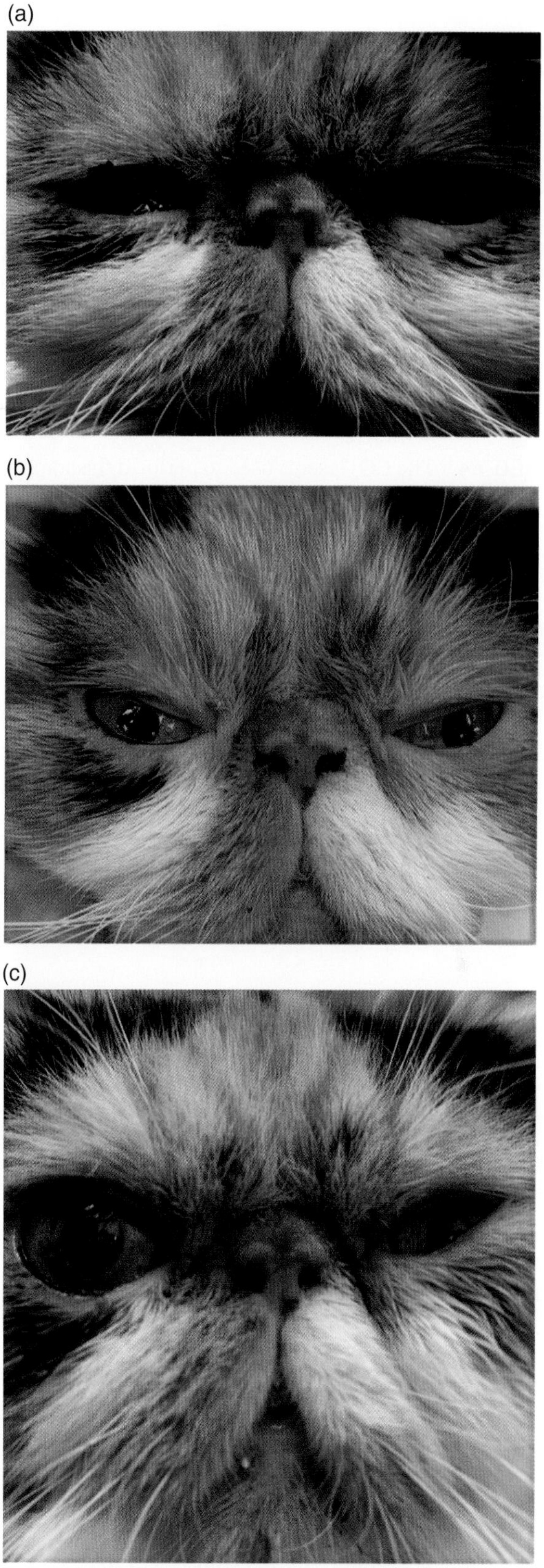

Figure 7.26 Persian cat. (a) Stenotic nares preoperatively. (b) Nares postoperatively after a modified Trader's technique. No sutures are placed. (c) Appearance of the nares after complete healing by second intention. *Source:* © Pamela Schwartz.

blade or laser to protect the underlying nasal skin from inadvertent damage. The laser or blade is used to excise as much of the alar wing and alar fold as possible and, if needed, the skin just adjacent to the alar fold. This is left open to heal by second intention. Alternatively, a rapidly absorbable interrupted suture can be placed to help exteriorize the nasal mucosal surface, although this is rarely needed.

To access the videos for this chapter, please go to

www.wiley.com/go/coleman/surgeries

VIDEO 7.1 Pre-operative video of a Boston Terrier with moderate stertorous breathing at rest. *Source:* © Pamela Schwartz.

VIDEO 7.2 Trader's technique using CO_2 laser. *Source:* © Pamela Schwartz.

VIDEO 7.3 DeBakey forceps are used to grasp and retract the most distal aspect of the soft palate. *Source:* © Pamela Schwartz.

VIDEO 7.4 The CO_2 laser is used to perform the staphylectomy, placing the laser beam as perpendicular as possible to the tissue to avoid splitting the palate in a cranial to caudal direction, until the excess soft palate is excised. *Source:* © Pamela Schwartz.

VIDEO 7.5 Suturing of the folded flap palatoplasty, which begins with assessment at the point of midline to ensure both symmetry and adequate resection. Once satisfied, the clinician should begin apposition at the point of midline with either a simple interrupted suture pattern or two simple continuous suture lines. *Source:* © Heidi Hottinger.

VIDEO 7.6 The saccule is grasped at the most distal aspect and retracted rostrally using caution not to cause inadvertent damage to the vocal folds, which are in close proximity to the saccules. The saccule is excised using Metzenbaum scissors starting ventrally and cutting dorsally. *Source:* © Pamela Schwartz.

VIDEO 7.7 Stage II laryngeal collapse is noted. The cuneiform processes are medially displaced. *Source:* © Pamela Schwartz.

Notes

i Cerenia, Zoetis, Florham Park, NJ, USA.
ii Miltex sterile disposable biopsy punch; Miltex Instrument Co., Inc., Bethpage, NY, USA.
iii Ethicon, Wthicon Inc., Johnson & Johnson Medtech, Cincinnati, OH, USA.
iv Covidien Inc., USA.

References

1 Ladlow, J., Liu, N.C., Kalmar, L. et al. (2018). Brachycephalic obstructive airway syndrome. *Vet. Rec.* 182 (13): 375–378.
2 O'Neill, D.G., Jackson, C., Guy, J.H. et al. (2015). Epidemiological associations between brachycephaly and upper respiratory tract disorders in dogs attending veterinary practices in England. *Canine Genet. Epidemiol.* 2: 10.
3 Emmerson, T. (2014). Brachycephalic obstructive airway syndrome: a growing problem. *J. Small Anim. Pract.* 55 (11): 543–544.
4 Tarricone, J., Hayes, G.M., Singh, A. et al. (2019). Development and validation of a brachycephalic risk (BRisk) score to predict the risk of complications in dogs presenting for surgical treatment of brachycephalic obstructive airway syndrome. *Vet. Surg.* 48 (7): 1253–1261.
5 Kenny, D.D., Freemantle, R., Jeffery, A. et al. (2022). Impact of an educational intervention on public perception of brachycephalic obstructive airway syndrome in brachycephalic dogs. *Vet. Rec.* 190 (11): e1430.
6 Packer, R., Hendricks, A., and Burn, C. (2012). Do dog owners perceive the clinical signs related to conformational inherited disorders as 'normal' for the breed? A potential constraint to improving canine welfare. *Anim. Welfare* 21: 81.
7 Lindsay, B., Cook, D., Wetzel, J.M. et al. (2020). Brachycephalic airway syndrome: management of post-operative respiratory complications in 248 dogs. *Aust. Vet. J.* 98 (5): 173–180.
8 Liu, N.C., Oechtering, G.U., Adams, V.J. et al. (2017). Outcomes and prognostic factors of surgical treatments for

brachycephalic obstructive airway syndrome in 3 breeds. *Vet. Surg.* 46 (2): 271–280.

9 Grand, J.G. and Bureau, S. (2011). Structural characteristics of the soft palate and meatus nasopharyngeus in brachycephalic and non-brachycephalic dogs analysed by CT. *J. Small Anim. Pract.* 52 (5): 232–239.

10 Daniel Koch, S.A., Hubler, M., and Montavon, P.M. (2003). Brachycephalic syndrome in dogs. *Compendium* 25 (1): 48–54.

11 Auger, M., Alexander, K., Beauchamp, G. et al. (2016). Use of CT to evaluate and compare intranasal features in brachycephalic and normocephalic dogs. *J. Small Anim. Pract.* 57 (10): 529–536.

12 Jones, B.A., Stanley, B.J., and Nelson, N.C. (2020). The impact of tongue dimension on air volume in brachycephalic dogs. *Vet. Surg.* 49 (3): 512–520.

13 Kaye, B.M., Rutherford, L., Perridge, D.J. et al. (2018). Relationship between brachycephalic airway syndrome and gastrointestinal signs in three breeds of dog. *J. Small Anim. Pract.* 59 (11): 670–673.

14 Downing, F. and Gibson, S. (2018). Anaesthesia of brachycephalic dogs. *J. Small Anim. Pract.* 59 (12): 725–733.

15 Davidson, E.B., Davis, M.S., Campbell, G.A. et al. (2001). Evaluation of carbon dioxide laser and conventional incisional techniques for resection of soft palates in brachycephalic dogs. *J. Am. Vet. Med. Assoc.* 219 (6): 776–781.

16 Sarran, D., Caron, A., Testault, I. et al. (2018). Position of maximal nasopharyngeal maximal occlusion in relation to hamuli pterygoidei: use of hamuli pterygoidei as landmarks for palatoplasty in brachycephalic airway obstruction syndrome surgical treatment. *J. Small Anim. Pract.* 59 (10): 625–633.

17 Poncet, C.M., Dupre, G.P., Freiche, V.G. et al. (2005). Prevalence of gastrointestinal tract lesions in 73 brachycephalic dogs with upper respiratory syndrome. *J. Small Anim. Pract.* 46 (6): 273–279.

18 Poncet, C.M., Dupre, G.P., Freiche, V.G. et al. (2006). Long-term results of upper respiratory syndrome surgery and gastrointestinal tract medical treatment in 51 brachycephalic dogs. *J. Small Anim. Pract.* 47 (3): 137–142.

19 Phillips, H. (2022). Updates in upper respiratory surgery. *Vet. Clin. North Am. Small Anim. Pract.* 52 (2): 339–368.

20 Pink, J.J., Doyle, R.S., Hughes, J.M.L. et al. (2006). Laryngeal collapse in seven brachycephalic puppies. *J. Small Anim. Pract.* 47 (3): 131–135.

21 Torrez, C.V. and Hunt, G.B. (2006). Results of surgical correction of abnormalities associated with brachycephalic airway obstruction syndrome in dogs in Australia. *J. Small Anim. Pract.* 47 (3): 150–154.

22 Liu, N.-C., Adams, V.J., Kalmar, L. et al. (2016). Whole-body barometric plethysmography characterizes upper airway obstruction in 3 brachycephalic breeds of dogs. *J. Vet. Intern. Med.* 30 (3): 853–865.

23 Hoareau, G.L., Jourdan, G., Mellema, M. et al. (2012). Evaluation of arterial blood gases and arterial blood pressures in brachycephalic dogs. *J. Vet. Intern. Med.* 26 (4): 897–904.

24 Reeve, E.J., Sutton, D., Friend, E.J. et al. (2017). Documenting the prevalence of hiatal hernia and oesophageal abnormalities in brachycephalic dogs using fluoroscopy. *J. Small Anim. Pract.* 58 (12): 703–708.

25 Gruenheid, M., Aarnes, T.K., McLoughlin, M.A. et al. (2018). Risk of anesthesia-related complications in brachycephalic dogs. *J. Am. Vet. Med. Assoc.* 253 (3): 301–306.

26 Oechtering, G.U., Pohl, S., Schlueter, C. et al. (2016). A novel approach to brachycephalic syndrome. 1. Evaluation of anatomical intranasal airway obstruction. *Vet. Surg.* 45 (2): 165–172.

27 Oechtering, G.U., Pohl, S., Schlueter, C. et al. (2016). A novel approach to brachycephalic syndrome. 2. Laser-assisted turbinectomy (LATE). *Vet. Surg.* 45 (2): 173–181.

28 Fenner, J.V.H., Quinn, R.J., and Demetriou, J.L. (2020). Postoperative regurgitation in dogs after upper airway surgery to treat brachycephalic obstructive airway syndrome: 258 cases (2013–2017). *Vet. Surg.* 49 (1): 53–60.

29 Hay Kraus, B.L. (2013). Efficacy of maropitant in preventing vomiting in dogs premedicated with hydromorphone. *Vet. Anaesth. Analg.* 40 (1): 28–34.

30 Hay Kraus, B.L. (2014). Effect of dosing interval on efficacy of maropitant for prevention of hydromorphone-induced vomiting and signs of nausea in dogs. *J. Am. Vet. Med. Assoc.* 245 (9): 1015–1020.

31 Fukui, S., Ooyama, N., Tamura, J. et al. (2017). Interaction between maropitant and carprofen on sparing of the minimum alveolar concentration for blunting adrenergic response (MAC-BAR) of sevoflurane in dogs. *J. Vet. Med. Sci.* 79 (3): 502–508.

32 Vangrinsven, E., Broux, O., Massart, L. et al. (2021). Diagnosis and treatment of gastro-oesophageal junction abnormalities in dogs with brachycephalic syndrome. *J. Small Anim. Pract.* 62 (3): 200–208.

33 Sanderson, J.J., Boysen, S.R., McMurray, J.M. et al. (2017). The effect of fasting on gastrointestinal motility in healthy dogs as assessed by sonography. *J. Vet. Emerg. Crit. Care* 27 (6): 645–650.

34 Franklin, P.H., Liu, N.C., and Ladlow, J.F. (2021). Nebulization of epinephrine to reduce the severity of brachycephalic obstructive airway syndrome in dogs. *Vet. Surg.* 50 (1): 62–70.

35 Sakthivel, M., Elkashif, S., Al Ansari, K., and Powell, C.V.E. (2019). Rebound stridor in children with drop after nebulised adrenaline: does it really exist? *Breathe* 15 (1): e1–e7.

36 Packer, R.M. and Tivers, M.S. (2015). Strategies for the management and prevention of conformation-related respiratory disorders in brachycephalic dogs. *Vet. Med.* 6: 219–232.
37 McNally, E.M., Robertson, S.A., and Pablo, L.S. (2009). Comparison of time to desaturation between preoxygenated and nonpreoxygenated dogs following sedation with acepromazine maleate and morphine and induction of anesthesia with propofol. *Am. J. Vet. Res.* 70 (11): 1333–1338.
38 Trappler, M. and Moore, K. (2011). Canine brachycephalic airway syndrome: surgical management. *Compend. Contin. Educ. Vet.* 33 (5): E1–E7; quiz E8.
39 Fossum, T.W. (2012). *Small Animal Surgery*, 4e. Elsevier Health Sciences.
40 Huck, J.L., Stanley, B.J., and Hauptman, J.G. (2008). Technique and outcome of nares amputation (Trader's technique) in immature shih tzus. *J. Am. Anim. Hosp. Assoc.* 44 (2): 82–85.
41 Findji, L., Dupré, G. (2013). Brachycephalic syndrome: innovative surgical techniques. *Clinicians Brief*, 79–85.
42 Trostel, C.T. and Frankel, D.J. (2010). Punch resection alaplasty technique in dogs and cats with stenotic nares: 14 cases. *J. Am. Anim. Hosp. Assoc.* 46 (1): 5–11.
43 Ellison, G.W. (2004). Alapexy: an alternative technique for repair of stenotic nares in dogs. *J. Am. Anim. Hosp. Assoc.* 40 (6): 484–489.
44 Trader, R. (1949). Nose operation. *J. Am. Vet. Med. Assoc.* 114: 210–211.
45 Liu, N.C., Genain, M.A., Kalmar, L. et al. (2019). Objective effectiveness of and indications for laser-assisted turbinectomy in brachycephalic obstructive airway syndrome. *Vet. Surg.* 48 (1): 79–87.
46 Gilman, O., Moreira, L., Dobromylskyj, M. et al. (2023). A comparison of harmonic and traditional sharp staphylectomy techniques in 15 brachycephalic dogs. *J. Small Anim. Pract.* 64 (1): 31–34.
47 Dunié-Mérigot, A., Bouvy, B., and Poncet, C. (2010). Comparative use of CO_2 laser, diode laser and monopolar electrocautery for resection of the soft palate in dogs with brachycephalic airway obstructive syndrome. *Vet. Rec.* 167 (18): 700–704.
48 Fossum, T.W., Cho, J., Dewey, C.W. et al. (2019). Surgery of the upper respiratory system. In: *Small Animal Surgery* (ed. T.W. Fossum), 833–883. Elsevier.
49 Carabalona, J.P.R., Le Boedec, K., and Poncet, C.M. (2021). Complications, prognostic factors, and long-term outcomes for dogs with brachycephalic obstructive airway syndrome that underwent H-pharyngoplasty and ala-vestibuloplasty: 423 cases (2011–2017). *J. Am. Vet. Med. Assoc.* 260 (S1): s65–s73.
50 Holloway, G.L., Higgins, J., and Beranek, J.P. (2022). Split staphylectomy to address soft palate thickness in brachycephalic dogs: 75 cases (2016–2018). *J. Small Anim. Pract.* 63 (6): 460–467.
51 White, R.N. (2012). Surgical management of laryngeal collapse associated with brachycephalic airway obstruction syndrome in dogs. *J. Small Anim. Pract.* 53 (1): 44–50.
52 Collivignarelli, F., Bianchi, A., Vignoli, M. et al. (2022). Subtotal epiglottectomy and ablation of unilateral arytenoid cartilage as surgical treatments for grade III laryngeal collapse in dogs. *Animals* 12 (9): 1118.
53 Leonard, H.C. (1960). Collapse of the larynx and adjacent structures in the dog. *J. Am. Vet. Med. Assoc.* 137: 360–363.
54 Haimel, G. and Dupré, G. (2015). Brachycephalic airway syndrome: a comparative study between pugs and French bulldogs. *J. Small Anim. Pract.* 56 (12): 714–719.
55 Gobbetti, M., Romussi, S., Buracco, P. et al. (2018). Long-term outcome of permanent tracheostomy in 15 dogs with severe laryngeal collapse secondary to brachycephalic airway obstructive syndrome. *Vet. Surg.* 47 (5): 648–653.
56 Krainer, D. and Dupré, G. (2022). Brachycephalic obstructive airway syndrome. *Vet. Clin. North Am. Small Anim. Pract.* 52 (3): 749–780.
57 Nelissen, P. and White, R.A. (2012). Arytenoid lateralization for management of combined laryngeal paralysis and laryngeal collapse in small dogs. *Vet. Surg.* 41 (2): 261–265.
58 Tokunaga, S., Ehrhart, E.J., and Monnet, E. (2020). Histological and mechanical comparisons of arytenoid cartilage between 4 brachycephalic and 8 non-brachycephalic dogs: a pilot study. *PLoS One* 15 (9): e0239223.
59 Fasanella, F.J., Shivley, J.M., Wardlaw, J.L. et al. (2010). Brachycephalic airway obstructive syndrome in dogs: 90 cases (1991–2008). *J. Am. Vet. Med. Assoc.* 237 (9): 1048–1051.
60 Anderson, G.M. (2012). Soft tissues of the oral cavity. In: *Veterinary Surgery: Small Animal* (ed. K.N. Tobias and S.A. Johnston), 1425–1438. Elsevier.
61 Turkki, O.M., Bergman, C.E., Lee, M.H. et al. (2022). Complications of canine tonsillectomy by clamping technique combined with monopolar electrosurgery - a retrospective study of 39 cases. *BMC Vet. Res.* 18 (1): 242.
62 Belch, A., Matiasovic, M., Rasotto, R. et al. (2017). Comparison of the use of LigaSure versus a standard technique for tonsillectomy in dogs. *Vet. Rec.* 180 (8): 196.
63 Worth, D.B., Grimes, J.A., Jiménez, D.A. et al. (2018). Risk factors for temporary tracheostomy tube placement following surgery to alleviate signs of brachycephalic obstructive airway syndrome in dogs. *J. Am. Vet. Med. Assoc.* 253 (9): 1158–1163.

64 Nicholson, I. and Baines, S. (2012). Complications associated with temporary tracheostomy tubes in 42 dogs (1998 to 2007). *J. Small Anim. Pract.* 53 (2): 108–114.

65 Trinterud, T., Nelissen, P., and White, R.A. (2014). Use of silicone tracheal stoma stents for temporary tracheostomy in dogs with upper airway obstruction. *J. Small Anim. Pract.* 55 (11): 551–559.

66 Bird, F.G., Vallefuoco, R., Dupré, G. et al. (2018). A modified temporary tracheostomy in dogs: outcome and complications in 21 dogs (2012 to 2017). *J. Small Anim. Pract.* 59 (12): 769–776.

67 Stordalen, M.B., Silveira, F., Fenner, J.V.H. et al. (2020). Outcome of temporary tracheostomy tube-placement following surgery for brachycephalic obstructive airway syndrome in 42 dogs. *J. Small Anim. Pract.* 61 (5): 292–299.

68 Ree, J.J., Milovancev, M., MacIntyre, L.A. et al. (2016). Factors associated with major complications in the short-term postoperative period in dogs undergoing surgery for brachycephalic airway syndrome. *Can. Vet. J.* 57 (9): 976–980.

69 Riecks, T.W., Birchard, S.J., and Stephens, J.A. (2007). Surgical correction of brachycephalic syndrome in dogs: 62 cases (1991–2004). *J. Am. Vet. Med. Assoc.* 230 (9): 1324–1328.

70 Johnson, L.R., Mayhew, P.D., Steffey, M.A. et al. (2013). Upper airway obstruction in Norwich terriers: 16 cases. *J. Vet. Intern. Med.* 27 (6): 1409–1415.

71 Berns, C.N., Schmiedt, C.W., Dickerson, V.M. et al. (2020). Single pedicle advancement flap for treatment of feline stenotic nares: technique and results in five cases. *J. Feline Med. Surg.* 22 (12): 1238–1242.

72 Pavletic, M.M. and Trout, N.J. (2023). Successful correction of stenotic nares using combined alar fold lift-up and sulcus pull-down techniques in brachycephalic cats: 8 cases (2017–2022). *J. Am. Vet. Med. Assoc.* 1: 1–5.

73 Gleason, H.E., Phillips, H., Fries, R. et al. (2023). Ala vestibuloplasty improves cardiopulmonary and activity-related parameters in brachycephalic cats. *Vet. Surg.* 52 (4): 575–586.

74 Anagrius, K.L., Dimopoulou, M., Moe, A.N. et al. (2021). Facial conformation characteristics in Persian and Exotic shorthair cats. *J. Feline Med. Surg.* 23 (12): 1089–1097.

8

Aural Hematoma

Jess D. Work

Deer Park Veterinary Clinic, Deer Park, WA, USA

Key Points

- Aural hematoma is usually a condition associated with self-inflicted trauma (e.g., head shaking).
- Recurrence of the hematoma is common if underlying etiologies are not properly addressed.
- Aural hematoma can be managed both medically and surgically.

Introduction and Pathophysiology

A common condition encountered in small animal practice, the aural hematoma is one seen across a variety of species and may be associated with an array of underlying causes or trauma. Management of the hematoma itself will be the author's primary focus of this chapter, though care should be taken to evaluate the history and underlying etiology or contributing factors to each case in an effort to minimize complications and local recurrence.

The aural hematoma most often develops following trauma to the auricle, or pinna, resulting in vascular damage and subsequent hemorrhage within the subcutaneous space of its ventral/concave surface (Figure 8.1). Aural hematomas may be unilateral or bilateral in presentation. Direct trauma to the pinna, such as from an animal bite, may result in the initial hematoma formation in the dog or cat, though most cases are the result of self-trauma associated with some other underlying pathology or infection. More often, the repeated trauma of the pinna slapping against the sides of the head, associated with pruritus and head shaking, creates the lesion. Etiologies associated with otic pruritus and head shaking include parasitic infestations (*Otodectes* sp.), bacterial or fungal infections, chronic otic foreign bodies (grass awns), or underlying allergic disorders, such as atopy, flea allergy dermatitis, or food adverse reactions. Less common etiologies may include inflammatory polyps, otic neoplasms, coagulopathies, or endocrine disorders.[1]

While the size and shape of the pinna may play a role in the size and extent of the lesion formed, aural hematomas can be seen in all ear types of dogs and cats. Left unattended, the general progression of the lesion and associated clinical signs will often result in enlargement of the initial hematoma (associated with head shaking) followed by varying degrees of auricular scarring and contracture. In humans, this crumpled appearance of the ear is referred to as a "cauliflower ear," which is an aural hematoma between the cartilage and perichondrium of the pinna often secondary to trauma. Untreated hematomas in animals are also at higher risk for abscess formation or cellulitis. Failure to treat these lesions most often results in prolonging the discomfort experienced by the patient and a poor cosmetic outcome for the conformation of the pinna (Figure 8.2).

Treatment options for aural hematoma include both conservative, medical management strategies and surgical techniques, which are further described within this chapter.

Techniques in Small Animal Soft Tissue, Orthopedic, and Ophthalmic Surgery, First Edition. Edited by Kristin A. Coleman.

Companion website: www.wiley.com/go/coleman/surgeries

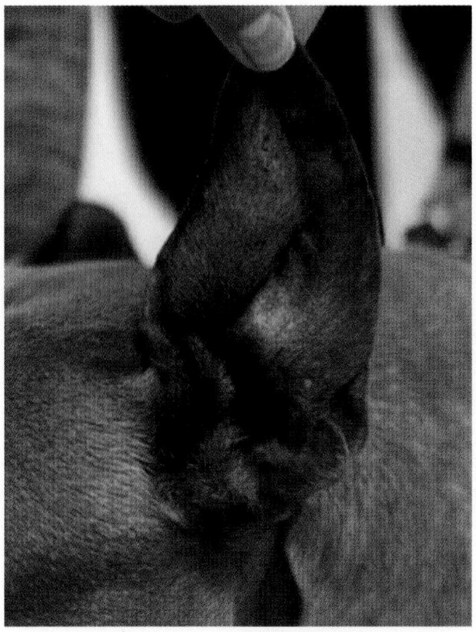

Figure 8.1 Typical canine aural hematoma. Note the fluffy appearance on the inner pinna. *Source:* © Jess Work.

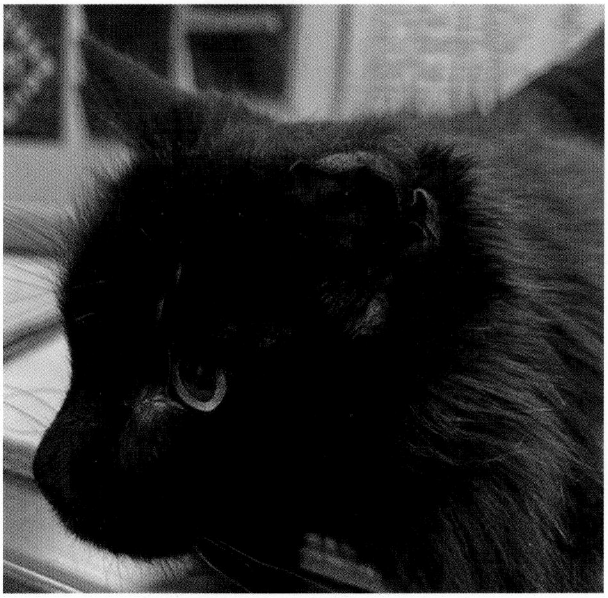

Figure 8.2 Scarring and contracture of the pinna as results of aural hematoma in a cat. *Source:* © Jess Work.

Indications/Pre-op Considerations

The primary goals of aural hematoma treatment are to reduce the hematoma and prevent recurrence. An additional goal is to maintain a cosmetic or natural appearance to the pinna; however, this may still be difficult to achieve depending on the severity and chronicity of the lesion.

Medical management of the aural hematoma is favored by many practitioners due to both anecdotal and reported successful outcomes,[2] minimally invasive office visits, avoidance of sedation/general anesthesia, and possible financial constraints voiced by patient owners. The potential drawbacks of a strictly medical approach to treatment often include a longer overall duration of treatment to time of lesion resolution, patients in which the use of corticosteroids may be contraindicated, and the need for continued bandage placement, which may not be well-tolerated in some patients.

Table 8.1 Corticosteroids commonly used in the treatment of aural hematomas.[3–5]

Medication	Route	Dosing
Dexamethasone	Intralesional	0.2–0.4 mg (diluted in saline) q 24 h for 1–5 d
Methylprednisolone	Intralesional	10–40 mg q 7 d for 1–3 wk
Triamcinolone	Intralesional	1–10 mg q 7 d for 1–3 wk
Prednisone	Oral	0.5 mg/kg body weight q 12 h tapering after 3–7 d

The most common medical approach to treatment of the aural hematoma includes addressing the underlying cause of head shaking, stabilizing the ear with a head bandage or wrap, and steroid therapy; with or without drainage of the hematoma. Steroid therapy may include either intralesional injections, systemic/oral treatment, or a combination of both (Table 8.1). Triamcinolone, dexamethasone, and methylprednisolone acetate have all been reported as successful intralesional options. In the author's experience, these treatments are easily performed using a butterfly catheter, which may also be utilized to drain the hematoma prior to depositing medication.

A surgical approach is indicated in any patient presenting with an aural hematoma that is an acceptable candidate for sedation/anesthesia and general surgery and is often the favored approach for larger hematomas or recurrent lesions that have failed to respond to medical therapy.

Preoperative evaluation and diagnostics to consider include a full otic exam and visualization of the horizontal canal and tympanic membrane (if possible), CBC, general chemistry, otic cytology (both stained and wet mount to assess for underlying etiologies), and otic culture if complicated infections are suspected. Coagulopathy and endocrine evaluations may also be pursued if thought to be contributing causes.

Following sedation, local anesthetic administration, or induction of general anesthesia, the affected pinna should be prepped as required for the procedure being performed. Care should be taken to cleanse and evaluate the ear canal following preoperative sampling then pack the ear canal gently with cotton balls or sponges to prevent hair clippings, surgical scrub, and contents of the hematoma from filling the canal. Both the convex and concave surfaces of the pinna should be prepared aseptically to facilitate manipulation throughout the procedure.[6]

Surgical Procedures

Incisional Drainage and Pinnal Tacking

This method is performed under general anesthesia (Figures 8.3, 8.4, 8.5, and 8.6).

A longitudinal, S-shaped, or elliptical incision is made on the concave surface of the pinna, directly over the hematoma, to facilitate drainage of the serosanguinous fluid as well as blood and fibrin clots often seen in more chronic lesions. Though less common, hematomas that extend to the convex side of the pinna may be accessed by incising through the cartilage if needed. The lesion is lavaged with sterile saline.

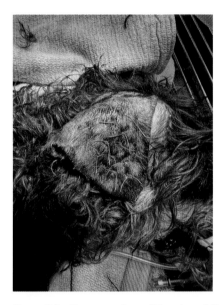

Figure 8.3 Convex surface of the pinna following surgical-tacking. *Source:* © Jess Work.

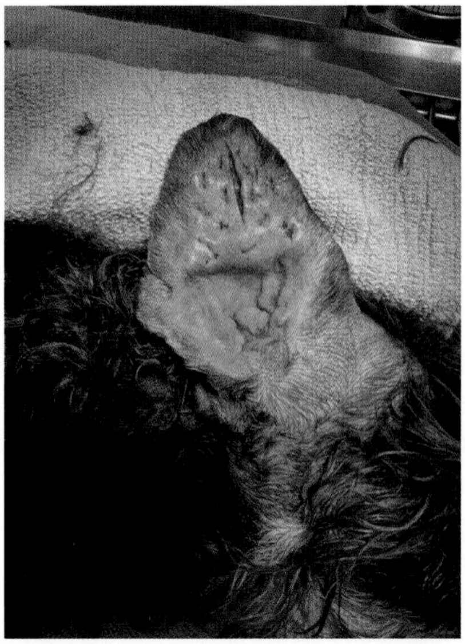

Figure 8.4 Concave surface of same patient. *Source:* © Jess Work.

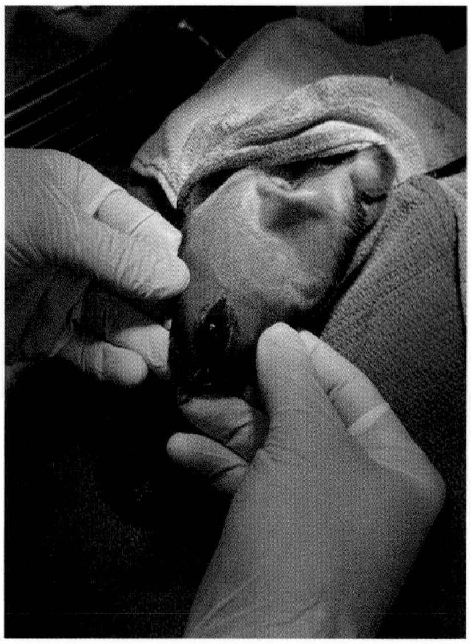

Figure 8.5 Removal of clot from incision. *Source:* © Jess Work.

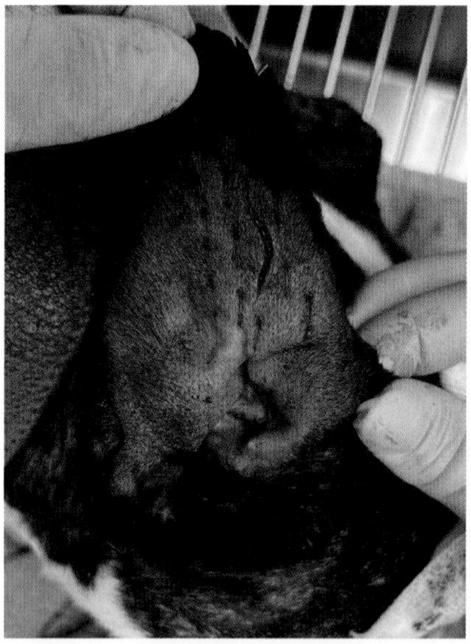

Figure 8.6 S-shaped incision on concave surface of pinna. *Source:* © Jess Work.

The subcutaneous defect is then reduced by placing a series of full-thickness, interrupted tacking sutures to secure the skin to the cartilage and aid in preventing the defect from refilling with blood immediately after surgery. Ideally, sutures should be placed in a longitudinal fashion, making them parallel to the majority of larger blood vessels within the pinna. Care should be taken not to overtighten

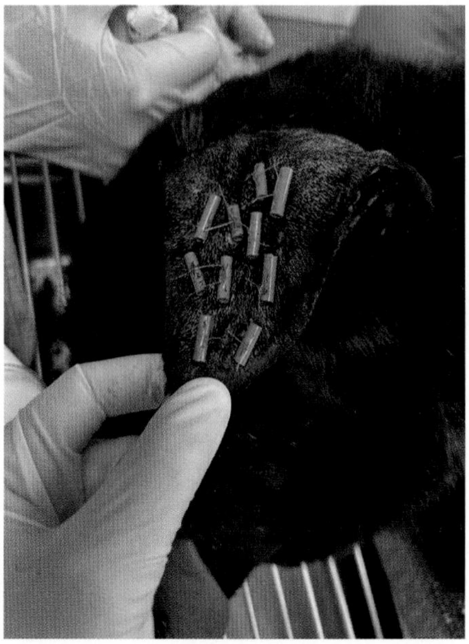

Figure 8.7 Use of red rubber feeding tube as stenting material for tacking. *Source:* © Jess Work.

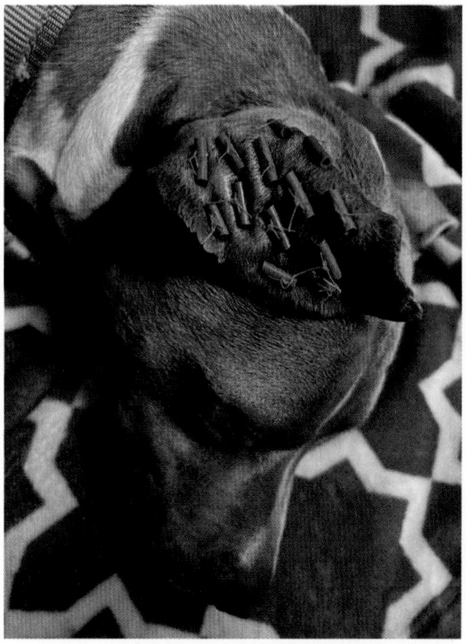

Figure 8.8 Use of red rubber feeding tube as stenting material for tacking. *Source:* © Jess Work.

these sutures and avoid placement directly over easily visualized vasculature to reduce the risk of tissue necrosis. The incision is left open to heal by second intention.

Tips/Tricks

The use of a straight needle may be preferred by the surgeon to facilitate accurate placement of the tacking sutures and more quickly pass the suture full thickness through the ear.

Preferred suture materials for tacking include 3-0 and 2-0 nonabsorbable monofilament. Stenting material may be used to help prevent overtightening of the tacking sutures. Small (1.0–1.5 cm) pieces of IV tubing or red rubber catheters work well (Figures 8.7 and 8.8).

Placement of tacking sutures should ensure the knot (and stent material if applicable) are on the convex/dorsal aspect of the pinna. This facilitates patient comfort during healing as well as ease during the removal of the material at the end of the postoperative period.

Punch Biopsy Technique

This method is typically performed under general anesthesia. If reducing a small lesion and tacking sutures are not to be utilized, sedation, and local anesthetic may be considered for some patients.

A 4.0 or 6.0 mm punch biopsy tool is used to create one or more circular drainage incisions through the skin and subcutaneous layers on the concave surface of the pinna, directly over the hematoma. If multiple punches are made, they should be spaced approximately 1.0 cm or more apart. The lesion is lavaged with sterile saline. Based on practitioner preference and depth of anesthesia, tacking sutures (3-0 or 2-0 nonabsorbable monofilament) may or may not be used as described in the preceding method. The punch incisions are left open to heal by second intention.

Carbon Dioxide Laser

This method is performed under general anesthesia.[7]

Much like the punch biopsy technique described above, the CO_2 laser is used to create multiple skin incisions over the surface of the hematoma to facilitate drainage and encourage adhesion formation between the separated layers of tissue. The lesion is lavaged with sterile saline. The incisions are left open to heal by second intention.

Temporary Cannula Placement

This method is typically performed in an awake or sedated patient with local anesthetic (Figures 8.9 and 8.10).

A small stab incision (1.0–2.0 mm) is made into the most gravity-dependent aspect of the hematoma on the concave surface of the pinna using a #11 blade, #15 blade, or 16-ga hypodermic needle. Contents of the hematoma are drained, and the lesion lavaged with sterile saline. A disposable, plastic, bovine teat cannula is manually introduced into the lesion to facilitate continued drainage in the postoperative period. Depending on the product used and the practitioner's preference, the cannula may be further secured using

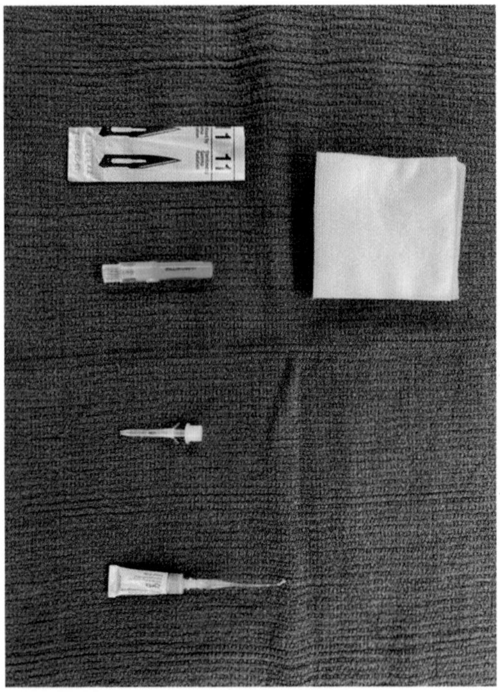

Figure 8.9 Materials needed for teat cannula procedure. *Source:* © Jess Work.

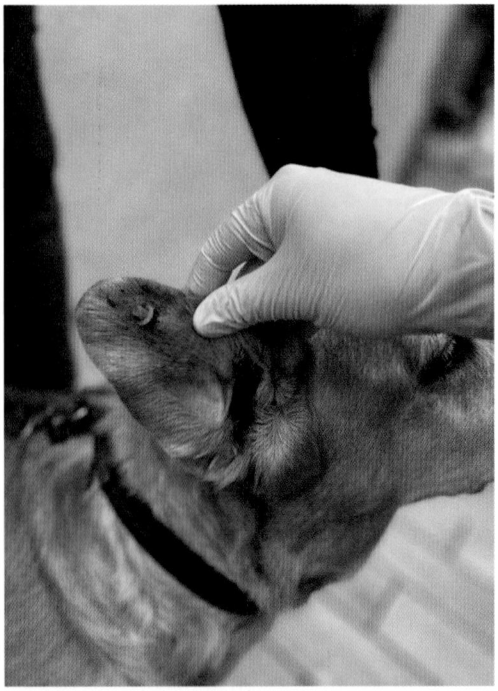

Figure 8.10 Teat cannula placement in a mildly sedated patient. *Source:* © Jess Work.

tissue adhesive or suture material (3-0 or 2-0 nonabsorbable monofilament).

The cannula is removed in two to three weeks when the lesion is reduced and fluid is no longer draining from the cannula opening. Practitioner preference and patient attitude may dictate whether or not the manufacturer-provided cap is utilized in the postoperative period. If patient and owner compliance allows, the cap may be left on at the time of hospital discharge and removed several times daily by the owner throughout recovery to facilitate controlled drainage.

Active Drain System Placement

This method is typically performed on a sedated patient with local anesthetic or under general anesthesia.[6]

An active drain system is created using a modified butterfly catheter system. The plastic hub is removed from the system and discarded. The cut end of the tubing is then fenestrated to create several holes, taking care not to weaken the tubing to the point that breakage may occur. A small stab incision (2.0 mm) is made into the most gravity-dependent aspect of the hematoma on the concave surface of the pinna using a #11 blade or #15 blade. Contents of the hematoma are drained, and the lesion lavaged with sterile saline. The fenestrated tubing is then inserted into the incision and secured with a purse-string suture using 3-0 or 2-0 nonabsorbable monofilament, followed by a finger trap pattern. The pinna and tubing are secured to the head with a bandage or head wrap, and active suction is achieved by inserting the butterfly catheter needle into a plain, red-top Vacutainer tube. The tube should also be secured to the patient with bandage material or stockinette wrap.

The Vacutainer tube should be replaced two to three times daily at a minimum throughout the first week of the postoperative period. The suture and system may be removed once the active drain is no longer productive and the skin of the pinna has adhered to the underlying cartilage. This typically occurs five to seven days post-procedure. Continued bandaging or head wrap is recommended for an additional one to two weeks.

Potential Complications

The most common complication following treatment of the aural hematoma is a recurrence of the lesion within the first four weeks of the postoperative period. This is most often associated with failure to fully address the underlying etiology of the hematoma, as well as continued self-trauma by the patient. Tissue necrosis may be seen in cases where tacking sutures have been overtightened or if bandages/wraps have been placed too tightly. Stenting (as described above) may help to reduce the risk of this complication. Other complications may include infection, chronic draining tract formation, and tissue contracture resulting in a misshapen or cauliflower-appearance to the pinna.

Post-op Care/Prognosis

General postoperative care for all of the described procedures should include appropriate systemic analgesic, antipruritic, antimicrobial, and topical otic therapies as indicated by each case. Patients should be confined, and the use of an Elizabethan collar should be encouraged to prevent further self-trauma throughout the recovery period.

Most techniques described in the prior sections benefit from postoperative use of bandages or head wraps. Depending on the size of the hematoma and practitioner preference, these dressings may be utilized for the first 48–72 hours after surgery to protect the surgical site and facilitate cleanliness and hygiene. Dressings may be continued up to one- or two-weeks post-op to aid in promoting adhesions between tissue layers.

If bandages or head wraps are utilized, these should be changed daily or as indicated by strikethrough, soiling, or topical therapy administration frequency. Care should be taken in the removal of disposable bandages to avoid accidental lacerations to the pinna by bandage scissors. Methods to prevent accidental trauma include drawing an outline of the pinna location on the outer surface of the bandage and the instruction to those removing the dressing to only cut material on the ventral aspect of the head and neck. More recently, commercial products, such as the "No Flap Ear Wrap" have become available as a washable, reusable alternative to wrapping and securing the pinna to the head during the postoperative period.

For procedures that utilize them, tacking sutures and stents are typically removed two to three weeks post-op.

In general, the postoperative prognosis for most cases of aural hematomas is good to excellent, provided that the underlying cause of the hematoma has also been addressed. Client expectations in regards to cosmesis should be approached with caution, as there may be some cases that develop long-term conformation changes of the pinna despite all medical or surgical efforts to avoid tissue contracture.

References

1. Hnilica, K.A. (2010). *Small Animal Dermatology: A Color Atlas and Therapeutic Guide*, 3e. St. Louis, MO: Elsevier.
2. Cordero, A.M.C., Marquez, C.L., Nunez, C.R. et al. (2020). Non-surgical treatment of canine auricular hematoma with intralesional and systemic corticosteroids, a pilot study. *Vet. Sci. Med.* 3: 1–4.
3. Hewitt, J. and Bajwa, J. (2020). Aural hematoma and its treatment: a review. *Can. Vet. J.* 61 (3): 313–315.
4. MacPhail, C. (2016). Current treatment options for auricular hematomas. *Vet. Clin. North Am. Small Anim. Pract.* 46: 635–641.
5. Kuwahara, J. (1986). Canine and feline aural hematomas: results of treatment with corticosteroids. *J. Am. Anim. Hosp. Assoc.* 22: 641–647.
6. Seibert, R. and Tobias, K.M. (2013). Surgical treatment for aural hematoma. *Clinician's Brief* (March), 29–32.
7. Dye, T.L., Teague, H.D., Ostwald, D.A. et al. (2002). Evaluation of a technique using the carbon dioxide laser for the treatment of aural hematomas. *J. Am. Anim. Hosp. Assoc.* 38 (4): 385–390.

9

Pinnectomy

Karen L. Cherrone

KLC Veterinary Surgical Services, New York, NY, USA

Key Points

- Most common indications for pinnectomy are trauma, lacerations, and neoplasia. The underlying cause will determine the extent of pinnectomy.
- The most common indication for feline pinnectomy is squamous cell carcinoma.
- The region should be appropriately clipped, prepped, and sterilely draped for surgery.
- It is easiest to amputate the pinna using sharp, serrated Mayo scissors.
- Cauterize bleeding vessels.
- Do not suture the auricular cartilage.

Anatomy

The pinna directs sound toward the middle ear. The size and shape of the auricular cartilage (scapha) determines if the pinna is erect or hanging. The lateral surface is convex, and the medial surface (conchal cavity) is concave. The cartilage contains many foramina where blood vessels and nerves enter.

Within the concave surface, there is a protuberance (anthelix) that separates the concha from the more distally located and flat scapha. The basal portion of the concha twists as it rolls to form a tube. A separate cartilaginous band, the annular cartilage, fits within the base of this tube.

Opposite the anthelix is a cartilage plate called the tragus, delineated by the lateral margin of the opening of the ear canal. Caudal to this, delineating the caudal margin of the ear canal, is the antitragus. There is a gradual decrease in the amount of hair from the apex to the base of the pinna.

The external carotid artery branches into the caudal auricular artery, which forms the lateral, intermediate, and medial vascular rami on the convex surface of the pinna. Branches of these vessels enter the foramina of the pinna and supply the concave surface. Sensory innervation is supplied by the second cervical nerve (convex surface) and the auriculotemporal branches of the trigeminal nerve (concave surface).[1]

Indications for Pinnectomy

Trauma and Lacerations

The most common indications for pinnectomy are trauma, lacerations, and neoplasia. Cosmetic forms of pinnectomy (e.g., ear-cropping) are not supported by the author or editor and will not be discussed in this chapter. Acute, minor fresh wounds to the pinna (<6 hours since injury) may be able to be copiously lavaged and primarily repaired. Chronic, minor wounds should have any infection managed first prior to consideration of delayed primary closure. If the wounds or lacerations are severe, subtotal or total pinnectomy may be indicated.[1]

Neoplasia

Any neoplasia that occurs on the skin may occur on the pinna.

Actinic lesions are caused by ultraviolet B light (UBV). They begin as erythematous areas and progress to crusts and plaques over time. These lesions are considered

Techniques in Small Animal Soft Tissue, Orthopedic, and Ophthalmic Surgery, First Edition. Edited by Kristin A. Coleman.

Companion website: www.wiley.com/go/coleman/surgeries

pre-malignant but may develop into carcinoma in situ if left untreated. White cats and poorly pigmented dog breeds (e.g., Dalmatians and Bull Terriers) are at greater risk of these lesions. Avoidance of the sun and sunscreen are recommended to reduce the risk of developing these lesions and other forms of dermal neoplasia.[1,2]

Squamous cell carcinoma (SCC) of the pinna occurs most commonly in white-coated, older cats causing an erosive, painful lesion that is invasive into the auricular cartilage. Metastasis is uncommon. When they do metastasize, it is usually to the lungs and regional lymph nodes. Tumors may also be noted on the eyelids and nares. Diagnosis may be obtained via fine needle aspirate or incisional biopsy.[1]

Hemangioma and hemangiosarcoma of the pinna are considered UVB-induced. They are most common in white or light-colored cats and rare in dogs. Hemangiomas are generally small, raised, blue, or purple-tinged lesions. Hemangiosarcomas tend to be large, ulcerated, invasive, and painful.[1]

Basal cell carcinomas are the most common feline cutaneous neoplasm and are often found on the pinna. They tend to be raised, slow-growing, and white or hyperpigmented. The pigmented lesions are often mistaken for melanoma. Siamese, Himalayan, and Persian cats may be predisposed. Excision with a narrow margin is often curative, although a much more aggressive form invading adjacent structures and the pinnal vascular and lymphatic supply has been described.[1,3]

Mast cell tumors are the second most common feline cutaneous neoplasm. Those of the pinna account for 59% of all cutaneous mast cell tumors of the head region (Figure 9.1).[1,4] Siamese cats are predisposed. Excision with a narrow margin is often curative.

Mast cell tumors on the pinna in dogs tend to be a more aggressive type and higher grade, and they often involve other areas of the body and can metastasize to regional lymph nodes (42.8% in one study).[1,5] Regional lymph nodes should be aspirated even if they are normal on palpation. These canine pinnal mast cell tumors need a wide excision for a cure (>2 cm and one fascial plane in most cases), which may be accomplished in most patients with a pinnectomy. Radiation therapy or re-excision of the scar could be considered if the margins are dirty or incomplete. Follow-up with an oncologist for mast cell tumors is highly recommended since mast cell tumors on the head and pinna are considered to behave more aggressively.[1]

Histiocytomas are often seen in young dogs (mean age 3.5 years). An attempt should be made to differentiate them from other malignant round-cell tumors. Most will resolve spontaneously over several months. Surgery should be avoided for this benign juvenile disease, which is often diagnosed on fine needle aspirate. For palliation of scratching and pruritis, conservative surgical resection or cryotherapy could be considered.[1]

Sebaceous adenomas are benign tumors. They are common on the head, neck, pinna, and feet in older dogs and are raised, white to yellow masses that are often pedunculated and cauliflower-like (Figure 9.2). Surgical excision is generally curative. **Sebaceous adenocarcinomas** are more invasive, can metastasize, and require a more extensive surgical excision and potentially other adjunctive treatment modalities.[1]

Other reported infectious or inflammatory conditions of the pinna are generally medically managed. Surgery is rarely indicated unless palliative excision of the severely affected pinna is required.

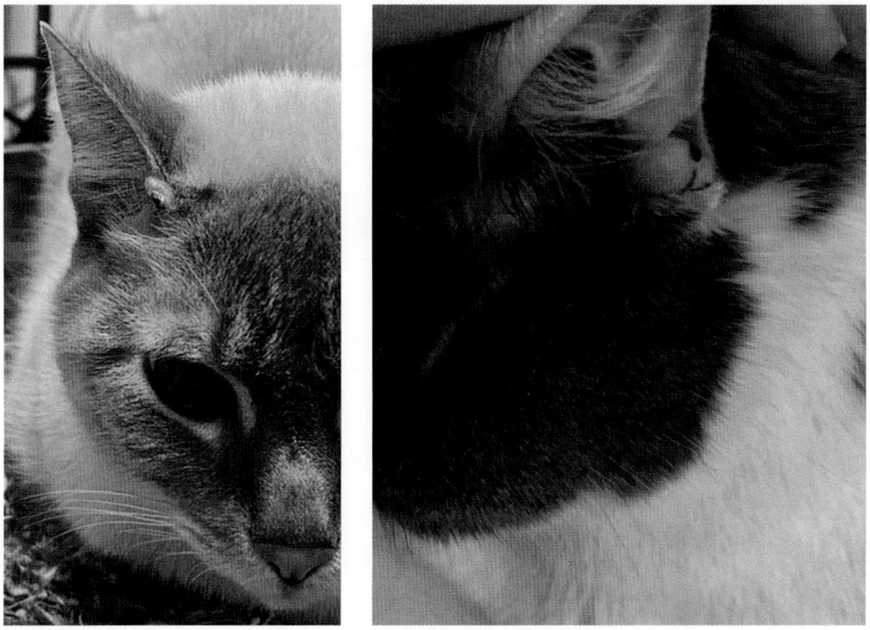

Figure 9.1 Examples of MCTs on the pinnae of cats.

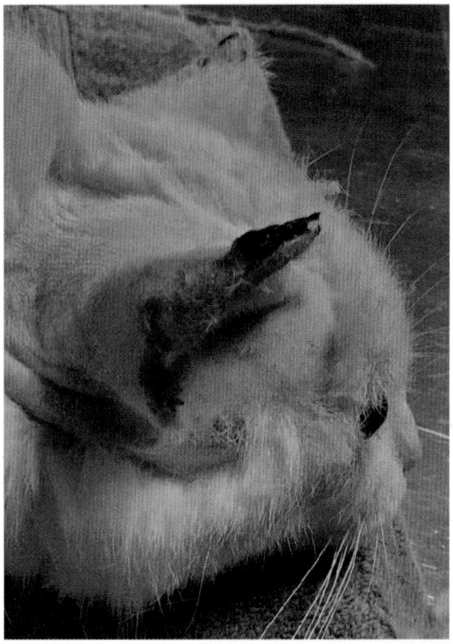

Figure 9.2 Squamous cell carcinoma in a feline patient's right distal pinna. Cranial is to the right of the image.

Subtotal and Total Pinnectomy

Pinnectomy is a simple procedure for the management of trauma, lacerations, or neoplasia of the pinna in dogs and cats. The underlying reason for performing a subtotal or total pinnectomy will determine how extensive of a pinnectomy will need to be performed. The most common indication for feline pinnectomy is squamous cell carcinoma.[1,6] For SCC, the pinna should be amputated at least 1–2 cm from the margin of crusting. For other neoplasia, a wide margin is also indicated (see above or other texts for recommendations on ideal margins for various cancers). For lacerations or trauma, a narrow margin of normal tissue is indicated. For unilateral pinnectomy, the patient should be positioned in lateral recumbency with the affected ear in the upward position. For bilateral pinnectomy, the patient should be positioned in sternal recumbency (Figure 9.3). The entire pinna (or pinnae, if bilateral) should be clipped free of hair and surgically prepped. Care should be taken not to get chlorhexidine or alcohol down

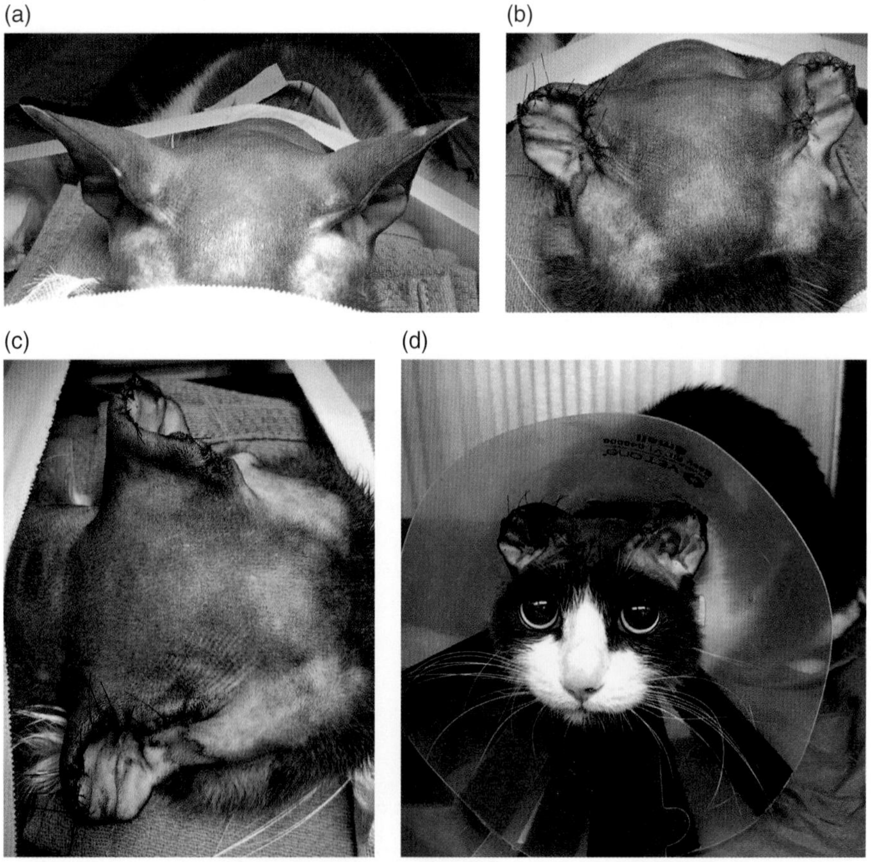

Figure 9.3 Bilateral pinnectomy for distal pinnal MCT in a feline patient. (a) Patient is positioned in sternal recumbency with both pinnae and the dorsal head clipped and prepped. (b) While achieving margins for the particular tumor type, symmetry may be considered, and the edges are rounded in this case. (c) An important part of the closure is ensuring that the dorsal pinnal skin is pulled over the transected cartilage and sutured to the inner pinnal skin. Tags from the cruciate mattress sutures are left long to make suture removal easier at the two-week post-op recheck. (d) A cone collar should be discharged with the patient to prevent scratching of the incision(s). *Source:* (c) Kristin Coleman.

into the canals. The region should be draped sterilely using four corner utility drapes and a surgical patient drape. It is easiest to amputate the pinna using sharp, serrated Mayo scissors. Do not dissect the skin off of the cartilage, as this increases the incidence of seroma or hematoma formation. Bleeding vessels should be cauterized. The skin on the convex surface is pulled over the cut edge of the auricular cartilage and sutured to the skin on the concave surface using a simple continuous or simple interrupted suture pattern with nonabsorbable, monofilament suture material, such as 3-0 or 4-0 nylon or polypropylene (Figure 9.4). Larger gauge sutures should be avoided, for this can cause

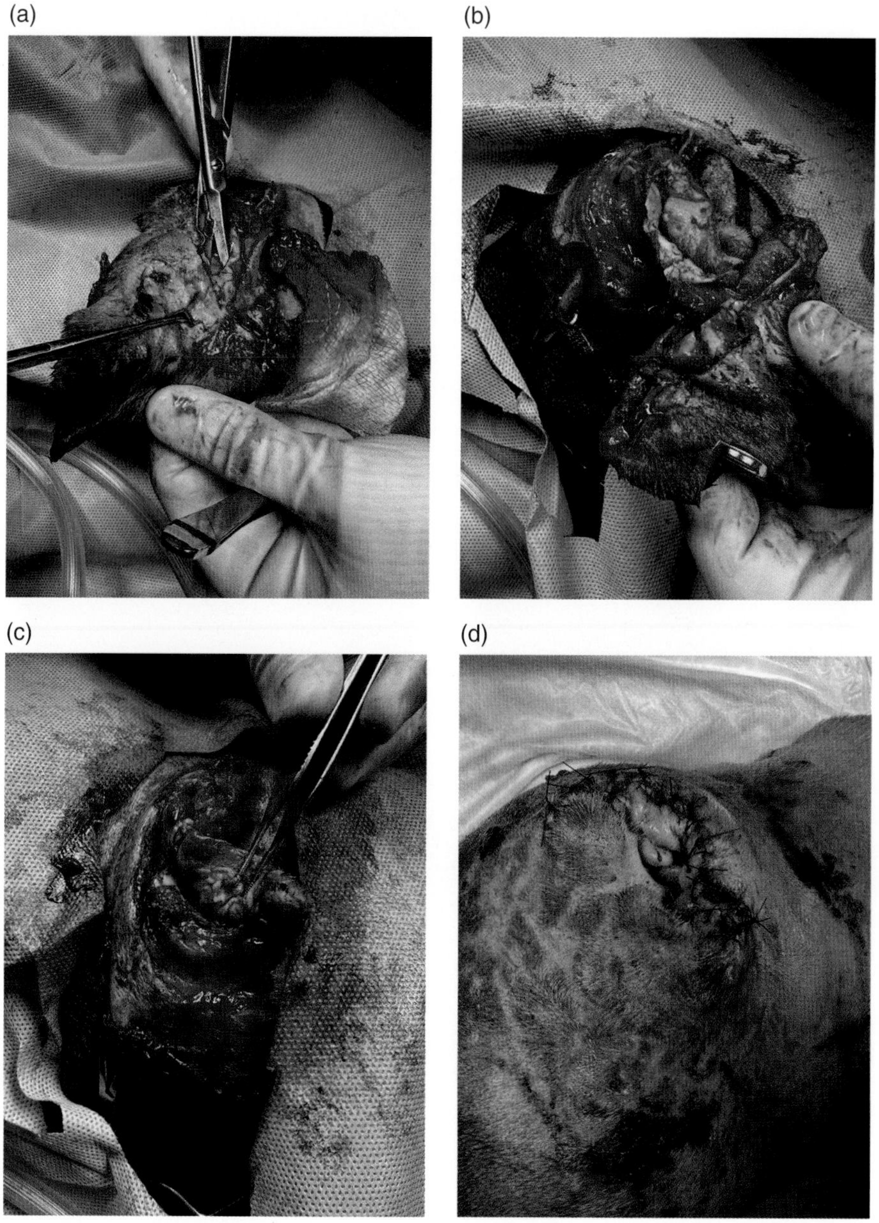

Figure 9.4 Right total pinnectomy performed due to trauma in a canine patient that is positioned in left lateral recumbency. (a) Incision is made through the skin and subcutaneous layer with a scalpel blade, and Mayo scissors are used to transect the pinnal cartilage at the site of planned pinnectomy. (b) The main blood vessels to ligate and transect during pinnectomy are on the dorsal or caudal aspect of the pinna. (c) Prior to closure, the transected cartilage is assessed to ensure skin closure over the cut edge will be without tension. If tension is suspected, additional cartilage may be removed. (d) Closure in this particular patient: buried simple interrupted sutures are placed in the rostral and caudal subcutaneous tissues, followed by 3-0 nylon cruciate mattress sutures for the entirety of the incision. *Source:* Photo courtesy of Dr. Nathan Squire.

more trauma to the pinna and delayed healing. Do not place sutures through the cartilage. For small tumors on the convex surface, resect the neoplasm, mobilize the already loose skin around the defect by undermining the cartilage and skin and suture the skin margins. If a large defect is present with a large amount of tension with primary closure, various types of skin flaps have been described for closure. For small tumors on the concave surface, repair the skin defect by elevating a flap of skin and rotating it into the defect.[1]

Postoperative Care

An Elizabethan collar should be used to prevent self-mutilation. Head wraps for sites closed with sutures should only be used in cases of aggressive head-shakers. Any larger defects that are healing via the second intention method should be lightly bandaged. The ear is very sensitive. Perioperative analgesics are recommended, and the patient should be sent home with oral analgesics. Sutures are generally removed from the pinna after two weeks.

References

1 Tobias, K.M. and Johnston, S.A. (2017). Pinna and external ear canal. *Vet. Surg.* 122: 2309–2312, 2320–2321.
2 Matousek, J.L. (2004). Diseases of the ear pinna. *Vet. Clin. North Am. Small Anim. Pract.* 34: 511–540.
3 Day, D.G., Couto, C.G., Weisbrode, S.E. et al. (1994). Basal cell carcinoma in two cats. *J. Am. Anim. Hosp. Assoc.* 30: 265–269.
4 Miller, M.A., Nelson, S.L., Turk, J.R. et al. (1991). Cutaneous neoplasia in 340 cats. *Vet. Pathol.* 28 (5): 389–395.
5 Higginbotham, M.L., Henry, C.J., Watson, Z. et al. (2000). Biological behavior of canine aural mast cell tumors. *Proceedings of the 20th Annual Meeting of the Veterinary Cancer Society*, Pacific Grove, CA. p. 52.
6 Fan, T.M. and de Lorimier, L.P. (2004). Inflammatory polyps and aural neoplasia. *Vet. Clin. North Am. Small Anim. Pract.* 34: 489–509.

10

Total Ear Canal Ablation and Lateral Bulla Osteotomy (TECA-LBO)

Grayson Cole

Gulf Coast Veterinary Specialists, Houston, TX, USA

Key Points

- Knowledge of regional anatomy is critical to successful surgery.
- TECA-LBO is the treatment of choice for aural neoplasia or end-stage otitis externa.
- Removal of all secretory tissue is mandatory for a positive long-term prognosis.
- Appropriate client communication of possible complications should be performed prior to surgery.

Introduction

A total ear canal ablation (TECA) refers to complete removal of the external ear canal. As there is no longer an egress for the middle ear, this surgery requires the evacuation of diseased tissue, fluid, and epithelium from the middle ear within the osseous tympanic bulla. The middle ear procedure most often performed adjunctly with the TECA is a lateral bulla osteotomy (LBO). The procedure will be referred to as total ear canal ablation and lateral bulla osteotomy (TECA-LBO) for the remainder of the chapter.

Indications and Pre-operative Considerations

The most common indications for TECA-LBO are severe or end-stage otitis externa and neoplasia or polyps of the external ear canal. In many cases, the lumen of the ear canal is completely obliterated, rendering the likelihood of successful medical management unlikely (Figure 10.1). Less common indications include otitis media, neoplasia near to the ear canal, such that an appropriate margin would include the ear canal, trauma to the ear canal, such as rupture or avulsion, congenital anomalies of the ear, such as a patulous eustachian tube, stenotic canal, or segmental external auditory canal atresia.[1] A TECA-LBO could also be considered to utilize the skin of the pinna for facial wound reconstruction[2] (Figure 10.2) or for severe disease of the parotid salivary gland in which dissection results in denuding of the external ear canal. Finally, it is the treatment of choice for ears that have failed less invasive procedures, such as a lateral ear canal resection.

As with any procedure requiring general anesthesia, a minimum database (e.g., complete blood cell count and serum chemistry) is recommended prior to the procedure. Thoracic radiographs are indicated for geriatric patients or patients for which neoplasia is a differential diagnosis for their ear disease. Patients with the significant systemic disease should be worked up and treated prior to surgery due to the elective nature of TECA-LBO, except for certain trauma cases, which require more immediate surgical intervention.

The gold standard of diagnostic imaging for the tympanic bulla is computed tomography (CT); however, it is feasible to perform TECA-LBO without imaging of the bulla or with guidance from open-mouth bulla radiography, magnetic resonance imaging (MRI), or video-otoscopy. Cross-sectional imaging is especially helpful in cases of suspected or confirmed neoplasia due to the ability to determine if the disease has led to rupture of the external

Techniques in Small Animal Soft Tissue, Orthopedic, and Ophthalmic Surgery, First Edition. Edited by Kristin A. Coleman.

Companion website: www.wiley.com/go/coleman/surgeries

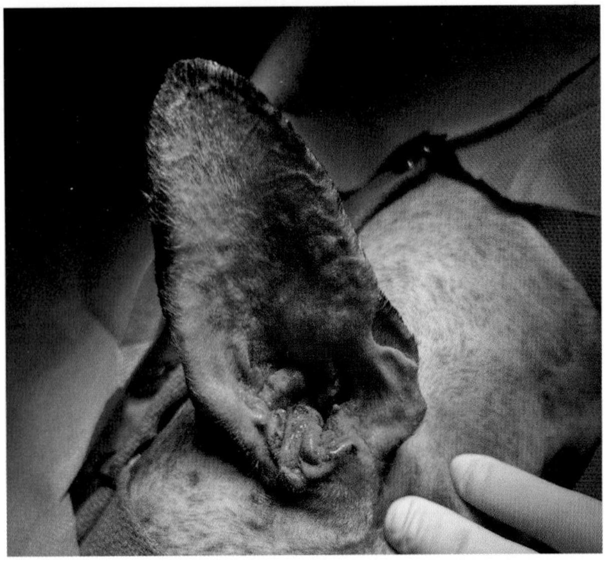

Figure 10.1 Dorsal is at the top of the image and the rostral is to the left of the image. An end-stage ear with no appreciable opening to the external ear canal.

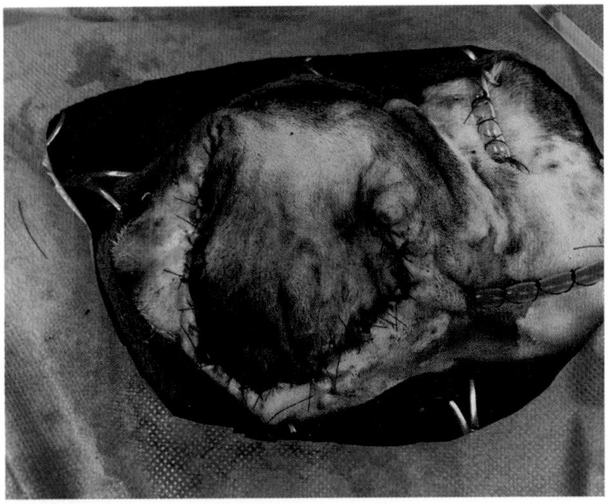

Figure 10.2 Dorsal is at the top of the image and the rostral is to the left of the image. An image of a dog who underwent a left TECA-LBO and then a left pinna flap to reconstruct a wound on the side of the face.

or middle ear and to evaluate local lymph nodes. CT can be helpful for surgical planning, especially when disease exists outside of the confines of the external and middle ear (Figure 10.3).

Infection can also result in rupture of the external ear or lysis of the tympanic bulla, which can increase the difficulty of the procedure. It can also be helpful to evaluate the contralateral middle ear, which allows the clinician to inform the client of future treatment recommendations if indicated.

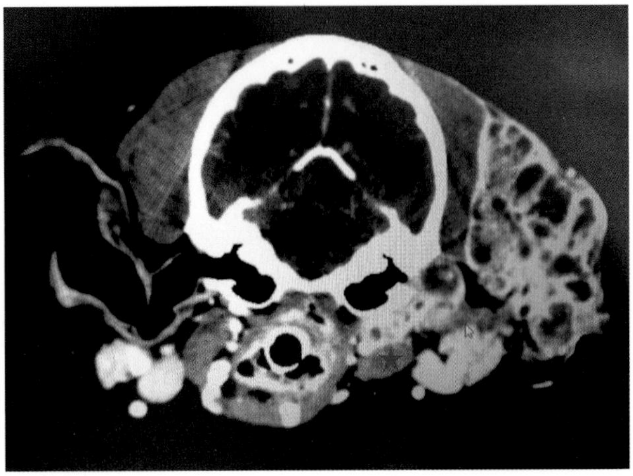

Figure 10.3 An axial CT image of a dog diagnosed with ceruminous gland adenocarcinoma. Note the extent of the disease ventral to the right bulla (red star).

For patients with chronic or recurrent otitis, a common consideration is whether to continue medical management or to proceed with surgery. Consultation with a board-certified veterinary dermatologist is often helpful in determining the likely success of future medical management, as well as obtaining diagnostic information in the form of video-otoscopic images, culture, cytology, histopathology, and CT of the bulla(e) prior to surgery. Ultimately, the decision to proceed with surgery or continued medical management is best made by the client after a thorough explanation of the risks of and postoperative care required from surgery, the at-home care required with either route, and prognosis of medical compared with surgical management. In the author's experience, ears that may not appear obviously end-stage on otic exam may still fail medical management, or the client may reach a point of not being able to administer topical medication to their pet's external ear canal due to the patient's temperament. Delaying surgery to meet specific criteria, such as palpable canal mineralization or stenosis, is often not in the best interest of the patient or client.

Once surgical management is elected, another consideration is whether to perform TECA-LBO or other reported surgical procedures, such as lateral wall resection (LWR) or ventral bulla osteotomy (VBO). A LWR procedure does not treat the underlying cause of otitis (typically, atopy) and may need to be converted to TECA-LBO in the future. Therefore, the procedure is rarely indicated. A possible indication would be benign neoplasia with no history of significant ear infection in which a resection with an appropriate margin can be performed with LWR. In the author's opinion, the benefit of the LWR procedure most often does not outweigh the risk of the need to perform yet another surgery to convert to TECA-LBO and will not be discussed further. A VBO is indicated in cases in which there is middle ear disease but no significant external ear pathology. Again, consultation with a board-certified veterinary dermatologist can be pivotal in making the decision between TECA-LBO and VBO in cases that have primarily middle ear pathology. VBO as a solo procedure should be reserved for patients without external ear pathology.

Brachycephalic patients offer unique challenges in the execution of TECA-LBO. Pharyngeal swelling can occur after TECA-LBO, which can further compromise the already abnormal airways of brachycephalic patients. Although bilateral single-session TECA-LBO is a commonly performed and generally well-tolerated procedure in meso- or dolichocephalic breeds,[3] the author does not perform bilateral single-session TECA-LBO in brachycephalic breeds with respiratory clinical signs who have not already undergone airway surgery, primarily due to the concern for postoperative airway compromise. In the author's experience, combining upper airway surgery with unilateral TECA-LBO, followed by the contralateral TECA-LBO at least four weeks postoperatively or aggressive medical management supervised by a board-certified veterinary dermatologist, is a preferred and anecdotally successful strategy.

In addition to concerns regarding postoperative upper airway obstruction, the skull anatomy of the brachycephalic dog can make the approach to the LBO more challenging than that of meso- or dolichocephalic skulls, as the ostium is often obscured by the mandible. Utilization of a burr or Kerrison rongeurs can be helpful to accomplish the surgery through this approach in the author's experience. If the approach to the LBO does not yield appropriate visualization, a TECA can be combined with a VBO. Alternatively, bulla endoscopy can be performed to improve middle ear visualization intra-operatively.[4] To the author's knowledge, no specific literature on TECA-LBO in brachycephalic cats exists; however, similar concerns would apply for postoperative pharyngeal swelling. The surgeon should be prepared to perform a temporary tracheostomy on any postoperative TECA-LBO patient; however, this will be more commonly indicated in brachycephalic patients. Regardless of the breed and laterality of the procedure, the same goals remain: to completely remove all of the external ear canal and to debride the middle ear to prevent a chronic draining tract and recurrent infection.

A full discussion of appropriate anesthesia and analgesia techniques is outside the scope of this chapter. However, a premedication with a full mu agonist opioid is appropriate with intra- and postoperative opioid administration, either through continuous rate infusion (CRI) or boluses. The surgery can be stimulating and painful; therefore, the use of lidocaine or ketamine CRIs can also be used for their minimal alveolar concentration (MAC) sparing effects and for additional analgesia. A preoperative greater auricular and auriculotemporal nerve block can also be performed for intra-operative and postoperative analgesia.[5] Current research at the author's institution is evaluating these nerve blocks with liposome-encapsulated bupivacaine to provide up to 72 hours of analgesia. These results are pending; however, anecdotal experience is encouraging.

The most common reports of TECA-LBO are in the dog and cat. Other species that have been reported in the veterinary literature include rabbits,[6] chinchillas,[7] harbor seals,[8] and North American bison.[9] The author has anecdotal experience of performing a TECA-LBO in an ocelot, which did not differ significantly from the procedure in a domestic cat.

Surgical Procedure

Skin Incision

Several different skin incisions have been described for TECA-LBO procedures. In dogs, a T-shaped skin incision has been described. With this technique, an incision is made circumferentially around the external auditory meatus. In addition, a linear incision is made from dorsal to ventral at the level of the palpable vertical ear canal. An alternative is to simply make a circumferential incision around the external auditory meatus. As per the author's opinion, this provides adequate exposure of the external ear canal and avoids both the need to make an additional incision and the perils of closing a T-shaped incision (Figure 10.4). In cats, a U-shaped incision has been reported in an effort to restore symmetry to the ear carriage

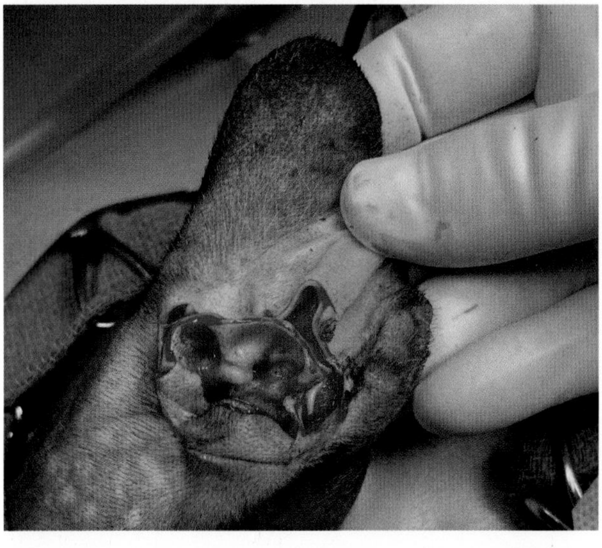

Figure 10.4 A circumferential incision is made around the external auditory meatus through the skin, thin subcutaneous layer, and cartilage.

after surgery (for unilateral TECA-LBO).[10] In the author's experience, a simple circumferential incision works well for cats, too.

Auricular Muscle Dissection

The auricular muscles will need to be transected circumferentially around the external ear canal. This can be accomplished with blunt or sharp dissection or with monopolar electrosurgery (Figure 10.5). There is often increased vasculature in chronically infected or neoplastic ears, so dissection with monopolar cautery is helpful to alleviate hemorrhage. Grasping the external ear canal with an Allis tissue forceps after establishing a dissection plane between the perichondrium and auricular muscle attachments can be helpful for counter-traction during the procedure.

Some surgeons utilize a Lone Star retractor or two small-tipped Gelpi retractors placed perpendicular to each other during this portion of the procedure. The author prefers a surgical assistant and a Senn retractor due to the frequency in which the retraction requires adjustment as the dissection proceeds from superficial to deep toward the bulla. Due to concern for damage to the facial nerve from the thermal spread of monopolar cautery, the author discontinues monopolar cautery after dissection of the vertical canal once the cartilage changes from auricular to annular with the horizontal canal.

For continued external ear canal dissection between the cartilage and muscular insertions, sharp dissection with tenotomy scissors with curved tips pointing toward the ear canal and taking tiny bites in a circumferential trajectory combined with bipolar cautery for hemostasis when needed is preferred by the author (Figure 10.6). The facial nerve exits the stylomastoid foramen and becomes visible during the TECA-LBO procedure caudal and ventral to the external ear canal near the junction between the vertical and horizontal canals (Figure 10.7). In chronically inflamed ears, the facial nerve may be adhered to the ear canal and require gentle dissection of the cartilage prior to ear canal transection.

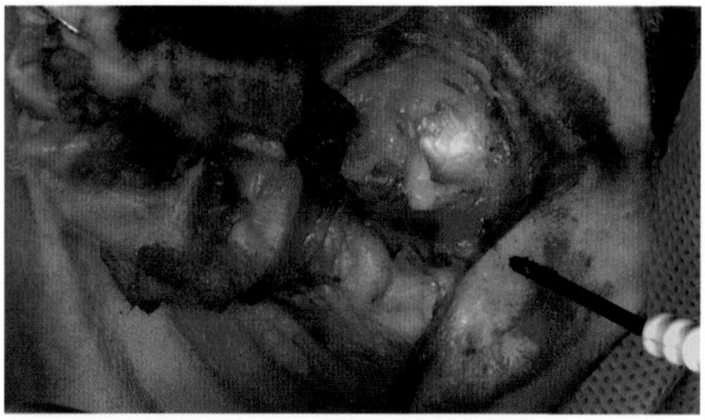

Figure 10.5 Dorsal is at the top of the image and the rostral is to the right of the image. The auricular musculature is dissected from the vertical ear canal.

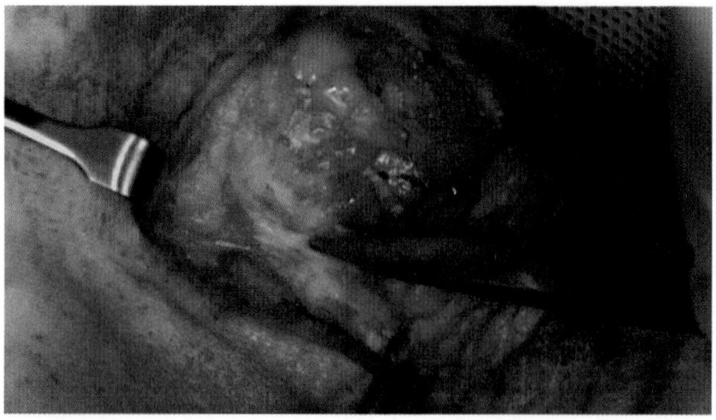

Figure 10.6 Dorsal is at the top of the image and the rostral is to the right of the image. Dissection with tenotomy scissors at the insertion of the auricular muscles onto the external ear canal. A Senn retractor is being used to provide visualization.

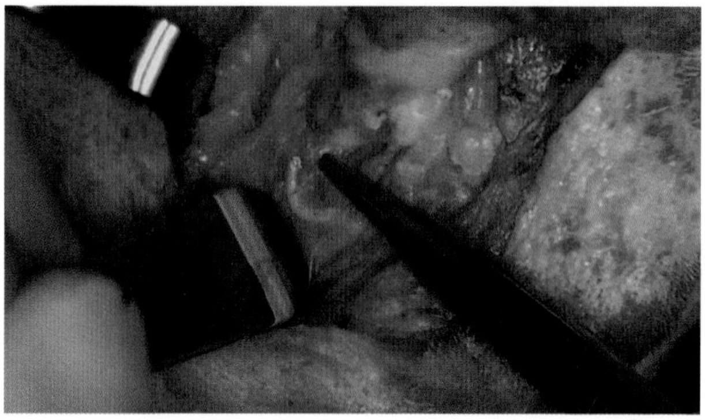

Figure 10.7 Dorsal is at the top of the image and rostral is to the right of the image. The facial nerve can be seen caudal and ventral to the ear canal, between the two instruments.

External Ear Transection

When the ear canal has been dissected from the surrounding auricular musculature to the level of the bulla, the ear will need to be transected from the bulla as it attaches to the external acoustic meatus. The author prefers to palpate 360° around the canal to determine that the dissection has progressed to the level of the bone prior to canal transection. Curved Mayo scissors are typically sufficient to transect the canal, and the cut can be made from caudal to cranial while a Freer periosteal elevator or other instrument protects the facial nerve (Figures 10.8 and 10.9). Mineralized ear canals may require a scalpel or bone-cutting forceps for transection. The external ear canal should be submitted for histopathology.

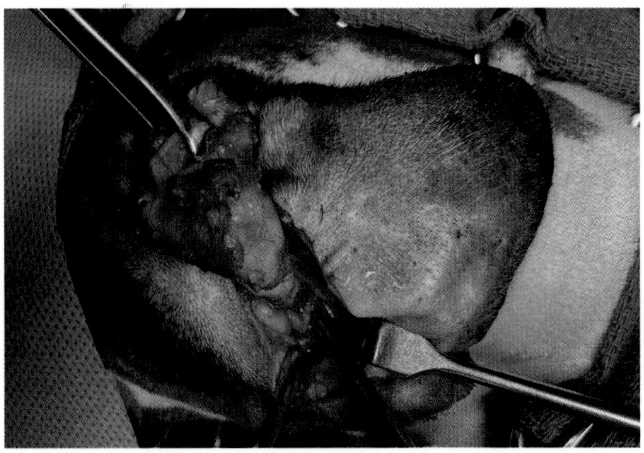

Figure 10.8 The Patient is positioned in the right lateral recumbency, and the rostral is to the left of the image. An additional view of the left facial nerve, which is mildly erythematous in this patient, is located just dorsal to the DeBakey forcep tips.

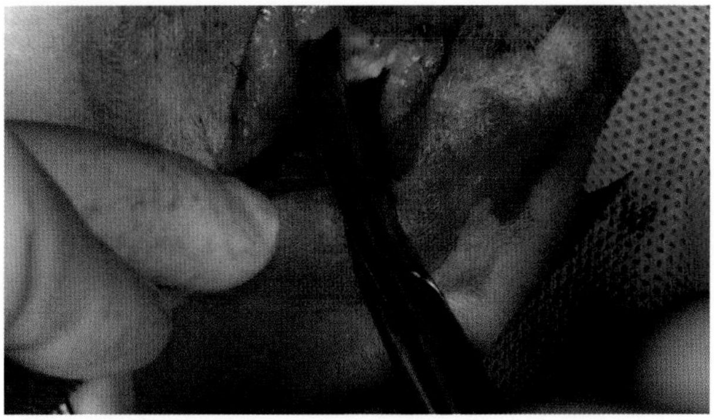

Figure 10.9 Curved Mayo scissors are used to transect the canal at the attachment to the external acoustic meatus starting from the caudal aspect as a Freer periosteal elevator is held over the facial nerve. The direction of scissor placement is chosen to reduce the risk of iatrogenic nerve transection at this stage.

Lateral Bulla Osteotomy

After transection and removal of the external ear canal, the ostium should be visible. Invariably, remnants of the external ear canal cartilage will be present around the opening to the bulla (Figure 10.10). Digital palpation or palpation using a Freer elevator can be helpful in distinguishing cartilage remnants from the bone of the bulla and surrounding musculature. All external ear and cartilage remnants should be removed. Lempert or double-action rongeurs are helpful for this portion of the procedure. The canal remnants may be very tightly attached to bone, and utilization of a Freer elevator or other instrument to provide downward pressure on the bulla as the rongeur applies upward force to the remnants, as well as removing the remnants via tiny bites with the rongeurs, can prevent lifting the patient's head during the procedure (Figure 10.10).

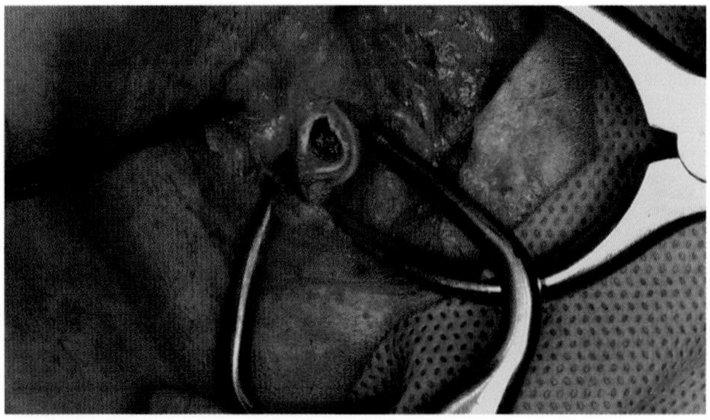

Figure 10.10 Visible ear canal remnants remain on the external acoustic meatus after canal transection with the Mayo scissors and will need to be removed. Debris is obscuring the view of the tympanum.

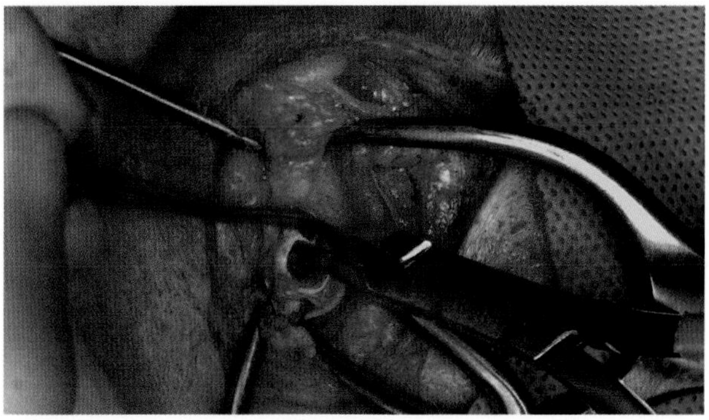

Figure 10.11 Removal of external ear remnants is performed with Lempert rongeurs using counter-traction with a Freer periosteal elevator positioned on the bulla. Visualization is improved with Gelpi perineal retractors with short tips placed perpendicular to each other in the surgical site. Care is taken when placing the retractors to avoid the region of the facial nerve.

Once the bulla is free from external ear canal remnants, the bone at the level of the ostium should be removed to improve visualization of the bulla contents and provide adequate entry for the curette to debride (Figure 10.11). This can be done using Lempert or Kerrison rongeurs. In addition, a high-speed burr can be helpful in accurately removing bone to aid in middle ear entry, especially when significant bulla remodeling has occurred or the anatomy is challenging, as previously described with brachycephalic patients. The surgeon should be very careful to keep the burr inside or immediately adjacent to the middle ear until it has come to a complete stop to avoid iatrogenic damage to the rostroventrally located retroarticular (also known as the retroglenoid or emissary) vein (branch of maxillary vein), the caudally located facial nerve, the ventrally located external carotid artery, or surrounding musculature. There is no reported quantity of bone that should be removed based on the current veterinary literature;

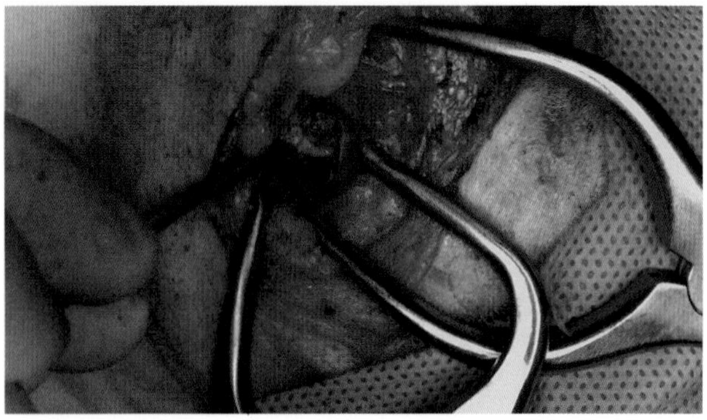

Figure 10.12 Appearance of bulla after removal of some bone of the ventral and caudal bulla rims. Debris is still present in the bulla.

however, sufficient bone should be removed such that the bulla can be thoroughly debrided (Figure 10.12).

Often, after the initial entry into the bulla, copious amounts of infected tissue, debris, or tumor are present. This should be removed via traction or gentle curettage. Cup biopsy forceps can be helpful in this endeavor. The ossicles may be damaged or diseased with chronic otitis media and may be inadvertently removed during debridement. Healthy ossicles should be left intact. Care should be taken when debriding the mesotympanum and epitympanum to avoid iatrogenic damage to the dorsomedially located round window and vestibular apparatus. The caudoventrally located hypotympanum can be curetted with relative safety.

In cats, there is a bony shelf that separates the larger ventromedial compartment (hypotympanum) from the smaller rostrolateral compartment housing the epitympanum and mesotympanum. When performing an LBO, this bony shelf will need to be penetrated to appropriately evacuate the hypotympanum (Figure 10.13). Unless there is significant bony remodeling, this is a relatively thin shelf and can be disrupted with a curette or curved hemostats. The bony shelf can be further removed with a curette or Lempert or Kerrison rongeurs until sufficient bone has been removed to debride the middle ear.

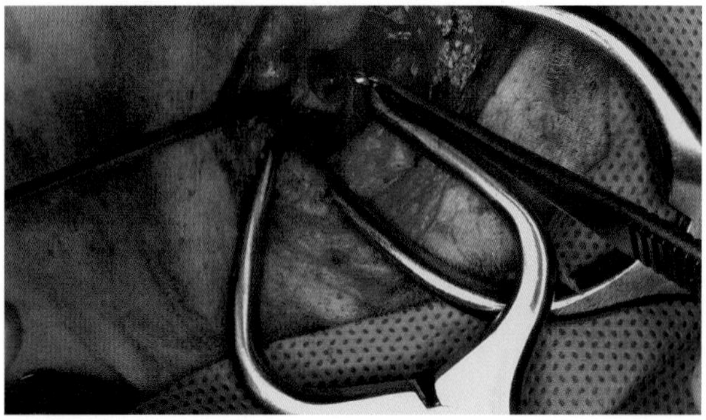

Figure 10.13 The bony separation of the mesotympanum and hypotympanum has been disrupted to lavage and debride the whole middle ear in this feline patient. The more ventromedially located hypotympanum is in the center of the bulla, beneath the disrupted bony shelf.

After evacuation, debridement, and lavage of the bulla, a sample should be obtained for bacterial culture and sensitivity. A culturette from a commercial laboratory with an attached cotton swab is convenient for this indication. According to one study, cultures obtained before and after middle ear debridement can differ in 70% of cases, and cultures taken prior to debridement and lavage of the tympanum are more likely to grow several different isolates.[11] However, post-lavage middle ear cultures are often recommended due to the likelihood of isolating an organism that may remain in the middle ear after surgery.

Closure

A three-layer closure is often performed. The auricular muscles can be apposed routinely. No attempt should be made to tack down deeper structures due to concern for facial nerve trauma. A subcuticular layer inclusive or exclusive of auricular cartilage can also be performed. The skin in this location is often thin and tightly overlying the cartilage and can make perfect skin apposition challenging. The author prefers skin sutures rather than an intradermal closure to try to address this challenge. Patients typically tolerate suture removal; however, aggressive patients can be closed with fine monofilament synthetic absorbable skin sutures, such as 5-0 Monocryl, which do not require removal.

No significant difference in postoperative complication rate was found in patients in which passive drains were placed versus patients without a drain in one study.[12] A drain may still be selected on a case-by-case basis in patients with concern for infected tissues in the remaining auricular musculature, which most commonly occurs in patients with ear canal rupture. Further, a drain may help to mitigate the buildup of fluid in the pharyngeal region and may be selected in patients with concern for pharyngeal swelling. If a passive drain is placed, it should be always covered with a sterile dressing, and a stockinette can be helpful to secure a dressing to the head without a tight bandage. A closed suction drain can also be utilized. A standard Jackson-Pratt closed suction drain is often too large for this location, so a closed suction drain can be made from a butterfly catheter and vacutainer tubing as described by Heiser et al.[13] Drains should be used with caution in surgical oncology patients. A full discussion of the pros and cons of drains and different types is outside the scope of this chapter, as the author very rarely places any type of drain after TECA-LBO.

Potential Complications

A thorough discussion of complications related to general anesthesia is outside the scope of this chapter; however, these should be discussed with clients prior to scheduling the procedure.

Hemorrhage

The retroglenoid (also known as retroarticular or emissary) vein courses the rostral and ventral to the tympanic bulla. This can be inadvertently damaged during entrance, osteotomy, and debridement of the tympanic bulla. Due to its depth and proximity to the bone, it is difficult to attenuate via suture ligation or hemoclips. Bipolar cautery or topical pressure with Gelfoam or Vetspon is preferred by the author, and after a few minutes intra-operatively, the hemorrhage from this low-pressure vein will cease to the point of allowing continuation of the procedure.

The internal carotid artery lies deep to the medial wall of the tympanum. If the medial wall of the bulla is disrupted during bulla debridement, hemorrhage can be severe. Preoperative CT is helpful in this regard to alert the surgeon to the presence of osteolysis of the bulla, which may make medial wall penetration more likely. Should severe bleeding occur in this location, the surgical site may need to be packed and the site closed to tamponade the hemorrhage. If this is the case prior to complete bulla debridement, an additional surgery may be required to fully debride the epithelium. Ligation of the common carotid artery in the neck could also be considered.

Maintaining an incision close to the ear canal can prevent hemorrhage from the lateral and medial auricular veins and the greater auricular artery. Staying close to the horizontal ear canal cartilage during dissection will also avoid encountering and accidental laceration of the ventrally located external carotid artery; however, if hemorrhage from this artery occurs, ligation may be performed to complete the procedure. The remainder of the vasculature is commonly easily attenuated with cautery.

Pinna Necrosis

As discussed above, maintaining an incision close to the ear canal cartilage will prevent damage to the medial and lateral auricular veins and the greater auricular artery. Damage to either may result in pinnal necrosis, which is more commonly seen 5–14 days after surgery than immediately postoperatively. Pinna necrosis should be treated via partial pinnectomy once the tissues have completely declared themselves (typically at least 14 days after surgery). A pinnectomy can easily be performed in combination with TECA-LBO if there is a concern for tumor extension into the pinna, if there is extensive soft tissue trauma of both pinna and external ear canal, or if there is pinnal disease from self-trauma or other reasons (Figure 10.14).

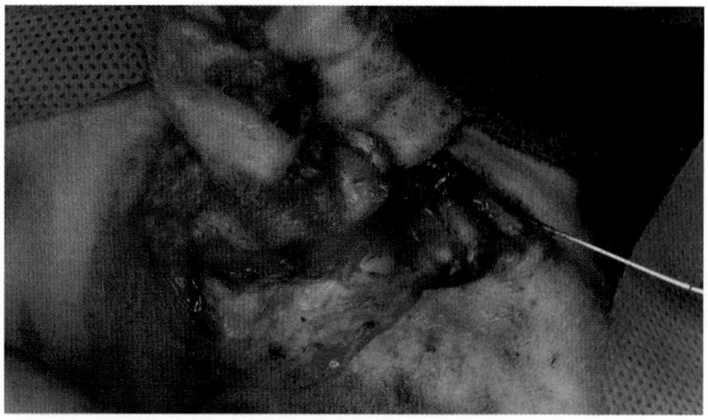

Figure 10.14 A TECA-LBO and pinnectomy combination for significant pinnal pathology.

Infection

As it is often impossible to completely resolve ear infections preoperatively, owners should be counseled on the possibility of surgical site infections. It is recommended to perform a middle ear culture after transection and removal of the external ear and debridement of the middle ear. Different organisms are often grown from middle and external ear cultures in chronically infected ears with 96% of middle ears in one study revealing positive culture growth[3]; therefore, a middle ear culture is a better indicator of what residual bacterial populations require continued treatment compared with samples from the now-removed external ear canal. According to a recent paper, approximately 10% of patients undergoing TECA-LBO require revision surgery due to infection.[14] Further, not treating postoperatively with antibiotics based on a middle ear culture made patients 10 times more likely to develop postoperative infections, which required revision surgery.[14] The author prefers to treat with empirical antibiotics pending the middle ear culture results, and once the results are final, treat with an antibiotic to which the bacteria are susceptible for four to six weeks. The antibiotic selection is based on previous ear cultures for that particular patient; otherwise, a broad-spectrum antibiotic with good bone penetration, such as amoxicillin-clavulanic acid, is selected.

Dehiscence

Minor dehiscence of a TECA-LBO incision is not uncommon. A few millimeters of dehiscence can often be managed conservatively with additional time with the patient in an E-collar. Dehiscence can be associated with necrosis of the pinna, which was addressed above. Should a surgical revision be required due to the extent of dehiscence, or necrosis, it is recommended to wait approximately 14 days to ensure that tissues have declared themselves and that the results have been evaluated from the original bacterial culture.

Upper Airway Obstruction

TECA-LBO, especially bilateral in brachycephalic breeds of dogs, could potentially lead to pharyngeal swelling, which can exacerbate pre-existing upper airway pathology. This is most commonly seen in brachycephalic patients; however, infectious or neoplastic disease can rupture out of the external or medial ear and lead to more pharyngeal swelling than a typical patient. As discussed above, bilateral single-session TECA-LBO should be pursued with caution in brachycephalic patients. In addition, a temporary tracheotomy may be required postoperatively, and patients should be monitored closely after extubation.

Facial Nerve Paresis or Paralysis

Facial nerve paralysis or paresis is one of the most common complications after TECA-LBO in dogs and cats.[3] Incidence of facial nerve paresis, which typically resolves within one month of surgery, is between 27% and 56% in the literature with some reports indicating a higher rate in cats, and others revealing no significant difference between dogs and cats.[3,15,16] Facial nerve paralysis, or permanent facial nerve deficits, occur less commonly with reported ranges between 13% and 28%.[3,15,16] As the inflammatory process tends to peak at 72 hours for any surgical procedure, it may be advisable to send patients home with eye lubricant for one to two weeks regardless of the presence of a blink reflex the morning following surgery. To the author's knowledge, there is no long-term literature documenting the outcomes of dogs and cats with facial nerve paralysis. It is the author's anecdotal experience that the nictitans can help to lubricate the eye due to the function of the abducens nerve to retract the globe. In these situations, the patient may be able to be weaned slowly off of supplemental eye lubrication with careful observation for clinical signs related to eye ulceration. Patients with facial nerve paralysis can also be administered eye lubricant indefinitely in the affected eye(s).

Vestibular Signs

As the middle ear helps to regulate balance, otitis media can result in vestibular signs. Vestibular ataxia, nystagmus, and a head tilt are all common clinical signs of vestibular signs in dogs and cats. For patients undergoing TECA-LBO, vestibular signs can also be iatrogenic secondary to curettage of the middle ear, specifically the vestibular or oval window. This structure is located in the mesotympanum on the dorsolateral aspect of the bony prominence called the promontory.[17] The third inner ear ossicle (from external to internal), called the stapes, is attached to the oval window. In patients with severe or chronic otitis media, the ossicles may be detached, damaged, or apparently absent. Care should be taken in the curettage of the bulla in the rostromediodorsal aspect to avoid iatrogenic trauma to these structures. In one study, a head tilt was reported in 11% of postoperative TECA-LBO patients with a median duration of two months. Nystagmus was found in 4.5% of patients, all of whom also had a head tilt.[3] Owners of patients with vestibular signs preoperatively should be warned that these signs may not immediately resolve after surgery and can worsen immediately postoperatively. No prospective literature exists regarding the treatment of vestibular signs after TECA-LBO; however, meclizine, maropitant, and supportive care have been used anecdotally. Care should be taken to ensure that the patient is able to eat and drink prior to discharge, as patients with severe vestibular signs are often inappetent.

Horner's Syndrome

Horner's syndrome is also a relatively common complication after TECA-LBO. Clinical signs of Horner's syndrome include ptosis, miosis, enophthalmos, and prolapse of the nictitans. Middle ear curettage may result in iatrogenic damage to the sympathetic plexus, which course over the bony promontory. The incidence of Horner's syndrome for postoperative TECA-LBO patients ranges from 3% to 5% in the dogs.[15] The reported incidence is higher in cats ranging from 42% to 58%, with approximately 14% of cases demonstrating long-term deficits.[16] It is thought that the fragility of the feline sympathetic plexus results in this greater incidence of deficits, as no significant anatomical variations in the promontory have been found. Conveniently, the elevated nictitans and ptosis help to cover the cornea if the patient has concurrent facial nerve paralysis or paresis.

Chronic Draining Tracts

A draining tract can be seen after TECA-LBO surgery. The incidence is between 2% and 10% of cases in the literature; however, it may be underreported due to a lack of follow-up.[18] In some reports, a draining tract was found more than four years after the original surgery.[18] In one report, the need for revisional surgery due to a draining tract is less common when culture-appropriate postoperative antibiotics are administered in the first month postoperatively.[14] It has also been reported when there is residual epithelial tissue or recurrence of neoplasia. Rigid otoscopy has been reported as an adjunct for visualization and debridement of the middle ear in the dog at the time of revision surgery with 100% of ears containing epithelial remnants without the use of otoscopy in one cadaver study.[4] The author prefers surgical loupes with 2.5 times magnification with a headlight to aid in bulla debridement; however, no prospective data is available to compare outcomes with and without a headlight and magnification. Patients who present for a draining tract after TECA-LBO should be evaluated with a CT scan or MRI prior to surgery to appropriately formulate a surgical plan. Resolution of clinical signs without surgery is uncommon, and reoperation via a lateral or ventral approach has been shown to permanently alleviate clinical signs.[19]

Hearing Loss

Hearing loss could be considered more of an expected outcome of TECA-LBO rather than a complication. Nonetheless, it is a concern that is often brought up by owners, and information regarding the pet's hearing ability should be discussed pre-operatively. Many patients have a decrease in their hearing function prior to surgery due to chronic and end-stage otitis externa and/or media. However, the majority of the middle ear and the entire internal ear should be intact after surgery, so their bone-conduction hearing should be unharmed. As such, pets often reportedly maintain some hearing ability after surgery. In one study, approximately 3% of clients reported normal hearing, 49% reported partial hearing, and 48% reported complete deafness in their pets after TECA-LBO.[15] One study evaluating brainstem auditory-evoked responses found that 76% of dogs that responded before surgery also responded after TECA-LBO.[20] Although hearing loss alone is often not a deterrent to pursuing surgery for many clients, some clients require reassurance that unilateral TECA-LBO will not impact contralateral hearing function.

Post-operative Care and Prognosis

A TECA-LBO can be painful surgery, and opioids are commonly utilized in the immediate postoperative period, especially for patients for whom a nerve block is not performed. Eye lubrication is recommended as the blink response is often difficult to evaluate immediately after recovery from surgery. Ideally, patients should be monitored overnight to ensure an appropriate recovery from anesthesia, monitor for respiratory difficulty, and ensure adequate analgesia. Patients should be in a well-padded area, as vestibular signs may result in rolling or exaggerated head motions. Patients are frequently discharged once they are able to eat on their own and their pain level is deemed adequate on oral pain medications. This is often within the first 48 hours after surgery.

The total recovery time is approximately 14 days. During this time, an E-collar is recommended to prevent scratching at the incision, although different apparatuses to cover the surgical incision can be used. In cases of known otitis, an empirical antibiotic is often sent home orally pending bacterial culture and sensitivity results. Secondary infection in cases of neoplasia is not uncommon; therefore, the use of empirical oral postoperative antibiotics is up to the discretion of the surgeon in these cases. The owners should be instructed to either apply eye ointment to the ipsilateral eye or carefully evaluate for a blink reflex and apply eye ointment as needed. Anecdotally, facial nerve function can be present immediately after surgery and then decrease during the inflammatory phase of wound-healing, so owners should be carefully counseled to monitor for appropriate blinking if eye ointment is not dispensed.

At-home analgesia is often accomplished with a non-steroidal anti-inflammatory medication (NSAID). As steroids are commonly used during treatment of otitis, a current medication history should be obtained prior to prescribing NSAIDs, and as a TECA-LBO if often elective, patients can be weaned off of steroids prior to surgery to facilitate the utilization of postoperative NSAIDs. Other oral analgesics can be utilized, such as gabapentin, tramadol, amantadine, and formulations of acetaminophen with codeine. No prospective data is available to compare the efficacy of these oral analgesics in isolation or combination after surgery for TECA-LBO, so clinician preference is typically the deciding factor.

As with any soft tissue surgery, exercise restriction and incisional monitoring are recommended for the first two weeks until a postoperative recheck is performed. If adequate wound-healing is present at the recheck, external sutures are removed, and the patient is allowed to return to normal activity. For patients with benign disease, follow-up typically involves antibiotics if indicated based on culture susceptibility and further consultation with their primary care veterinarian or a dermatologist for care related to generalized skin disease or the contralateral ear canal, if still present.

The incidence of specific complications is described above; however, overall client satisfaction with the procedure is generally high with approximately 90% of clients reporting that they were completely satisfied with the procedure in one report.[15] Anecdotally, many clients report that their pets are more energetic, and they are happy with the lack of need for topical ear medications and cleanings after TECA-LBO.

References

1 Coomer, A.R. and Bacon, N. (2009). Primary anastomosis of segmental external auditory canal atresia in a cat. *J. Feline Med. Surg.* 11 (10): 864–868. https://doi.org/10.1016/j.jfms.2009.02.010.

2 Price, J.B., Wood, C.J., and Liptak, J.M. (2021). The pinna composite flap for wound reconstruction in a dog. *Vet. Surg.* 50 (8): 1704–1708. https://doi.org/10.1111/vsu.13732.

3 Coleman, K.A. and Smeak, D.D. (2016). Complication rates after bilateral versus unilateral total ear canal ablation with lateral bulla osteotomy for end-stage inflammatory ear disease in dogs: 79 ears. *Vet. Surg.* 45 (5): 659–663. https://doi.org/10.1111/vsu.12505.

4 Watt, M.M., Regier, P.J., Ferrigno, C.R.A. et al. (2020). Otoscopic evaluation of epithelial remnants in the tympanic cavity after total ear canal ablation and lateral bulla osteotomy. *Vet. Surg.* 49 (7): 1406–1411. https://doi.org/10.1111/vsu.13492.

5 Stathopoulou, T.-R., Pinelas, R., Haar, G.T. et al. (2018). Description of a new approach for great auricular and auriculotemporal nerve blocks: a cadaveric study in foxes and dogs. *Vet. Med. Sci.* 4 (2): 91–97. https://doi.org/10.1002/vms3.90.

6 Chow, E.P. (2011). Surgical management of rabbit ear disease. *J. Exotic Pet. Med.* 20 (3): 182–187. http://doi.org/10.1053/j.jepm.2011.04.004.

7 Rockwell, K.R., Wells, A., and Dearmin, M. (2019). Total ear canal ablation and temporary bulla fenestration for treatment of otitis media in a chinchilla (*Chinchilla laniger*). *J. Exotic Pet. Med.* 29: 173–177. http://doi.org/10.1053/j.jepm.2018.11.005.

8 Ready, Z.C., Flower, J.E., Collins, J.E. et al. (2021). Total ear canal ablation and lateral bulla osteotomy (TECA-LBO) in Atlantic harbor seals (*Phoca vitulina concolor*) for successful surgical management of otitis media. *J. Zoo Wildl. Med.* 52 (2): 827–837. http://doi.org/10.1638/2020-0060.

9 Ferrell, S.T., Valverde, C., and Phillips, L.G. (2001). Chronic otitis externa/media with total ear canal ablation and bulla curettage in a North American Bison (*Bison bison*). *J. Zoo Wildl. Med.* 32 (3): 393–395. http://doi.org/10.1638/1042-7260(2001)032[0393:COEMWT]2.0.CO;2.

10 McNabb, A.H. and Flanders, J.A. (2004). Cosmetic results of a ventrally based advancement flap for closure of total ear canal ablations in 6 cats: 2002–2003. *Vet. Surg.* 33 (5): 435–439. https://doi.org/10.1111/j.1532-950X.2004.04065.x.

11 Hettlich, B.E., Boothe, H.W., Simpson, R.B. et al. (2005). Effect of tympanic cavity evacuation and flushing on microbial isolates during total ear canal ablation with lateral bulla osteotomy in dogs. *J. Am. Vet. Med. Assoc.* 227 (5): 748–755. https://doi.org/10.2460/javma.2005.227.748.

12 Devitt, C.M., Seim, H.B. 3rd, Willer, R. et al. (1997). Passive drainage versus primary closure after total ear canal ablation-lateral bulla osteotomy in dogs: 59 dogs (1985-1995). *Vet. Surg.* 26 (3): 210–216. http://doi.org/10.1111/j.1532-950X.1997.tb01486.x.

13 Heiser, B., Okrasinski, E.B., Murray, R. et al. (2018). In vitro evaluation of evacuated blood collection tubes as a closed-suction surgical drain reservoir. *J. Am. Anim. Hosp. Assoc.* 54 (1): 30–35. https://doi.org/10.5326/JAAHA-MS-6519.

14 Folk, C.A., Lux, C.N., Sun, X. et al. (2022). Effect of empirical versus definitive antimicrobial selection on postoperative complications in dogs and cats undergoing total ear canal ablation with lateral bulla osteotomy: 120 cases (2009–2019). *J. Am. Vet. Med. Assoc.* 260 (8): 899–910. http://doi.org/10.2460/javma.21.10.0462.

15 Spivack, R.E., Elkins, A.D., Moore, G.E. et al. (2013). Postoperative complications following TECA-LBO in the dog and cat. *J. Am. Anim. Hosp. Assoc.* 49 (3): 160–168. https://doi.org/10.5326/JAAHA-MS-5738.

16 Bacon, N.J., Gilbert, R.L., Bostock, D.E. et al. (2003). Total ear canal ablation in the cat: indications, morbidity and long-term survival. *J. Small Anim. Pract.* 44 (10): 430–434. https://doi.org/10.1111/j.1748-5827.2003.tb00101.x.

17 Cole, L.K. (2009). Anatomy and physiology of the canine ear. *Vet. Dermatol.* 20 (5-6): 412–421. https://doi.org/10.1111/j.1365-3164.2009.00849.x.

18 Haar, G.T. (2016). Ear canal surgery. In: *Complications in Small Animal Surgery* (ed. D. Griffon and A. Hamaide), 155–163. John Wiley & Sons, Inc https://doi.org/10.1002/9781119421344.ch22.

19 Smeak, D.D., Crocker, C.B., and Birchard, S.J. (1996). Treatment of recurrent otitis media that developed after total ear canal ablation and lateral bulla osteotomy in dogs: nine cases (1986-1994). *J. Am. Vet. Med. Assoc.* 209 (5): 937–942.

20 Krahwinkel, D.J., Pardo, A.D., Sims, M.H. et al. (1993). Effect of total ablation of the external acoustic meatus and bulla osteotomy on auditory function in dogs. *J. Am. Vet. Med. Assoc.* 202 (6): 949–952.

11

Ventral Bulla Osteotomy (VBO)

Philippa R. Pavia

Thrive Pet Healthcare, New York, NY, USA

Key Points

- Case selection and appropriate diagnosis are of the utmost importance when deciding upon a VBO, as TECA-LBO may be more appropriate for some conditions.
- Excellent knowledge of the species-specific local anatomy is required to ensure complete removal of abnormal tissue while decreasing the risk of neurological signs post-operatively.
- The most common neurological sequela following VBO include Horner's syndrome and vestibular signs.
- Bilateral single-stage VBO carries a significantly increased risk of respiratory complications in cats; even with bilateral disease, staged unilateral surgeries are often recommended.
- Neoplasia is rarely an indication for VBO, as neoplastic processes are often lytic and/or infiltrative rather than confined to the tympanic bulla.

Indications and Pre-operative Considerations

Indications

Ventral bulla osteotomy (VBO) is indicated for diseases of the middle ear, including chronic otitis media that cannot be resolved medically, inflammatory polyps, cholesteatomas, granulomas, and, rarely, neoplasia.[1] To ensure appropriate case selection, signalment, presenting signs, results of diagnostic testing/imaging, and response to therapy should all be taken into consideration.

Clinical signs of middle ear disease can include head shaking, pain on deep palpation of the ear, head tilt (pain or vestibular), and other signs of vestibular dysfunction if the inner ear is also affected (circling, loss of balance, and nystagmus). Horner's signs and facial nerve paralysis may also be present. Signs of nasopharyngeal polyps can include dysphagia, gagging, dyspnea, sneezing, stridor, and nasal discharge based on location; signs are often unilateral but may be bilateral depending on the size and origin of the polyp. If the polyp extends into the external ear canal, aural discharge may also be present.

Sedation may be required for a complete oral and otoscopic exam to evaluate the nasopharynx and external ear canal for the presence or absence of masses or infection. Otoscopic examination is often used to evaluate the external ear canals and determine if the tympanic membrane is intact. Video otoscopy under anesthesia can be used for evaluation of the horizontal canal, and endoscopy can be used to fully assess the nasopharynx.

Preoperative Imaging

No matter the diagnosis (polyp, otitis media, or mass lesions), preoperative imaging is recommended to confirm the location and extent of disease and better guide treatment. Computed tomography (CT) is the gold standard for identifying masses, presence of fluid in the middle ear, laterality of polyps, bony changes, and extent of disease.[2,3]

Techniques in Small Animal Soft Tissue, Orthopedic, and Ophthalmic Surgery, First Edition. Edited by Kristin A. Coleman.

Companion website: www.wiley.com/go/coleman/surgeries

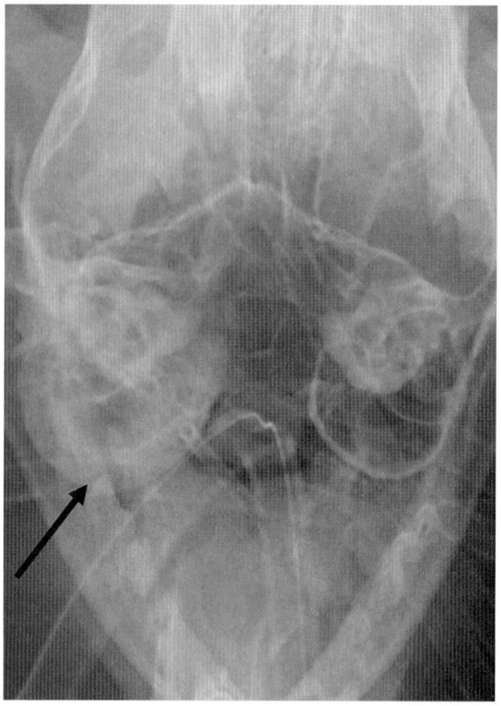

Figure 11.1 Ventrodorsal open-mouth radiographic view of a cat with a nasopharyngeal polyp and secondary right-sided chronic otitis media. Note the markedly thickened bone of the right bulla with the black arrow. *Source:* © Philippa Pavia.

If access to CT is not available, skull radiography may be performed, though it is often not sensitive for detection of middle ear disease. Radiography may show fluid opacity within the bulla and/or thickening of the bone. Lysis of bone is not expected with nonneoplastic disease, though may be present with malignancy (Figure 11.1).[4,5]

Decision-Making, Alternate Techniques, Nonsurgical Options

Depending on the etiology of middle ear disease and the results of imaging, the decision must be made whether VBO or lateral bulla osteotomy would be preferable for access to the middle ear. VBO is the procedure of choice when the external ear canal is unaffected (e.g., the disease is confined to the middle ear) and when superior visualization and access to the bulla (especially in cats) is required. In general, when the external ear canal is involved, total ear canal ablation with lateral bulla osteotomy (TECA-LBO) is indicated (see Chapter 10 for more details on this procedure).[6–10]

However, it has been suggested that VBO combined with total ear canal ablation from a standard lateral approach may be preferable in some brachycephalic dogs in which the bulla lies medial to the mandible, as this anatomy increases the difficulty of a lateral bulla osteotomy and subsequent risk for inadequate bulla debridement.[11,12]

Although VBO may be the ultimate recommendation, nonsurgical and less invasive treatment options should be considered before surgery. We will, therefore, explore differential diagnoses for middle ear disease and alternative options to surgery.

Differential Diagnoses

Polyps

Inflammatory polyps are benign, pedunculated masses originating from the mucosa of the nasopharynx, oropharynx, middle ear, or auditory (eustachian) tube and can be found in the pharynx, external ear canal, or confined to the middle ear. They are also referred to as nasopharyngeal or aural polyps depending on location. They are the most common nasopharyngeal disease of younger cats[13] and the most common nonneoplastic aural mass in cats (Figure 11.2).[14] They are usually found in young cats but have been reported in older cats and, rarely, in dogs.[15–18]

Although inflammation is present histopathologically, it is unknown whether inflammation is the cause or result of polyps. The cause of polyps is unknown despite their frequency; congenital and viral causes have been suggested.[19–21]

Nasopharyngeal inflammatory polyps may be treated with traction-avulsion, traction and corticosteroids, or traction with VBO. One study suggested that post-traction treatment with steroids decreased recurrence from 64% to 0%, though case numbers were small (22 cats).[22] Other studies showed a higher rate of recurrence with traction-avulsion of aural inflammatory polyps (50% with middle ear involvement or growing into the external ear canal) compared to those of nasopharyngeal origin (11%).[21–23] Endoscopic-guided transtympanic excision has also been described for the removal of polyps in two cats.[24] If recurrence is noted, or if there is failure of clinical signs to improve post-traction, VBO becomes indicated.

To perform removal by traction, the animal is placed under general anesthesia or deep sedation. The polyp should then be easily identified at the caudal border of the soft palate (or, less frequently, in the ear canal). The palate can be retracted rostrally (a spay hook is often helpful for this purpose), or the polyp manipulated caudally. The polyp is grasped with Allis tissue forceps or hemostats, as close to the base as possible. Gentle rostroventral tension, with or without a gentle rotation/twisting motion, is placed on the instrument. If necessary, a second instrument is used to grasp the polyp further dorsally as more of the stalk becomes visible. Ideally, the stalk associated with the polyp

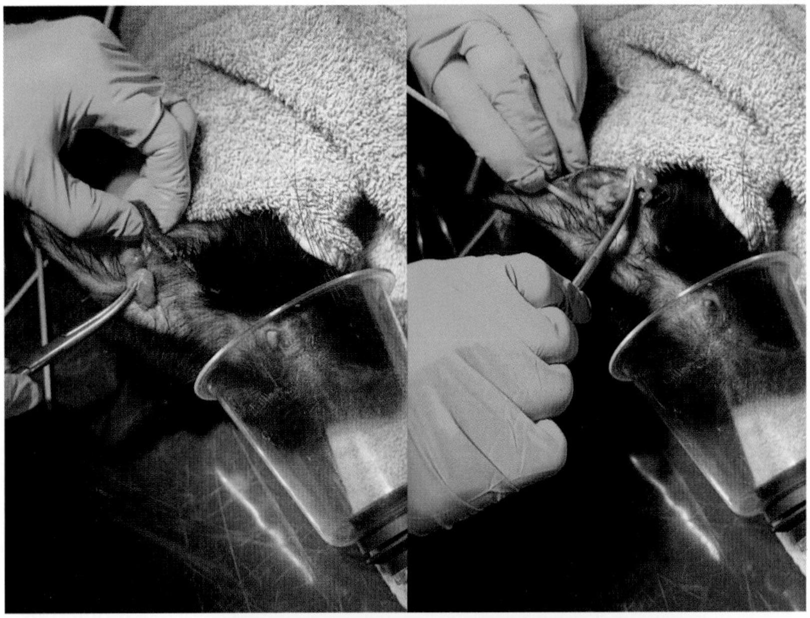

Figure 11.2 A left aural polyp was noted on otoscopic evaluation; due to financial constraints, the client elected traction-avulsion with corticosteroid therapy as an initial therapy. *Source:* © Philippa Pavia.

will also be removed from the auditory tube. In some patients, blood will be evident beneath the tympanic membrane on otoscopic examination, and there is frequently mild pharyngeal bleeding with the removal of nasopharyngeal polyps. Retraction may result in Horner's syndrome or vestibular signs. Rarely, an approach to the nasopharynx via a midline incision in the soft palate is required to facilitate polyp exposure and removal (Figures 11.3 and 11.4).[21,25] One tip to reduce the risk of bleeding into the lower airways and to provide adequate control of the anesthetic depth is to intubate the patient prior to attempting polyp removal.

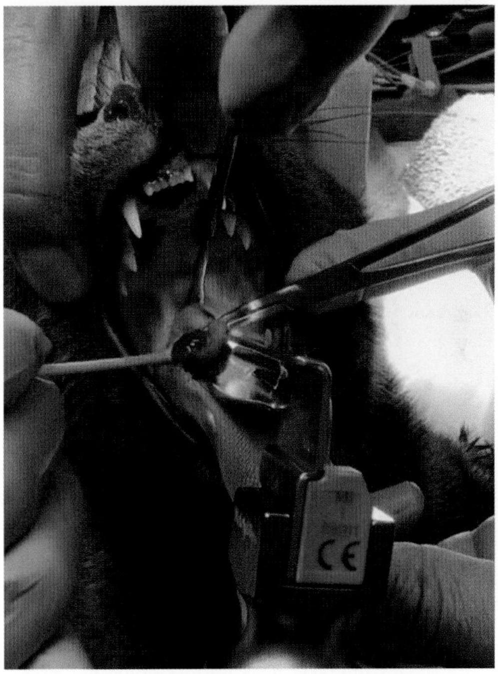

Figure 11.3 A large nasopharyngeal polyp, obstructing the airway of an eight month-old shelter kitten, being removed via traction-avulsion with the aid of a spay hook and laryngoscope. A cotton-tipped applicator is being used to gently dab the area of the stalk to free it from oronasal secretions and ensure proximal placement of the curved Kelly hemostats. *Source:* © Philippa Pavia.

Steatoma/Cholesteatoma

Found in dogs and rarely in cats, aural cholesteatomas are congenital or acquired epidermoid cysts (keratin debris surrounded by keratinizing stratified squamous epithelium) in the middle ear.[26,27] They represent the presence of squamous epithelium within the middle ear; in the congenital presentation, the tympanic membrane is intact; however, the formation of acquired cholesteatomas requires inflammation (chronic otitis media/externa) as well as a defect in the tympanic membrane to allow squamous epithelium entry into the middle ear.

Congenital cholesteatoma is a developmental defect that occurs when a squamous epithelial cyst forms within the middle ear behind an intact tympanic membrane. Acquired cholesteatomas occur when retraction of the tympanic membrane into the middle ear or migration of squamous epithelium through a perforated tympanic membrane leads to cyst formation. Despite their nonneoplastic etiology, severe cholesteatoma may expand rapidly and cause destruction of surrounding structures, including bone (Figure 11.5). Diagnosis is made via a combination of history, clinical signs, changes in imaging (CT), appearance of keratin within a cystic structure at surgery, and histopathology.[26,27]

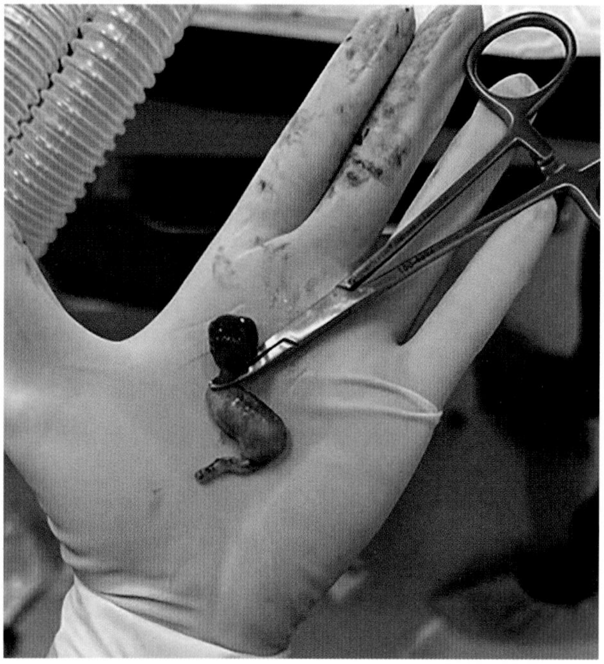

Figure 11.4 The large polyp from Figure 11.3 post-removal. *Source:* © Philippa Pavia.

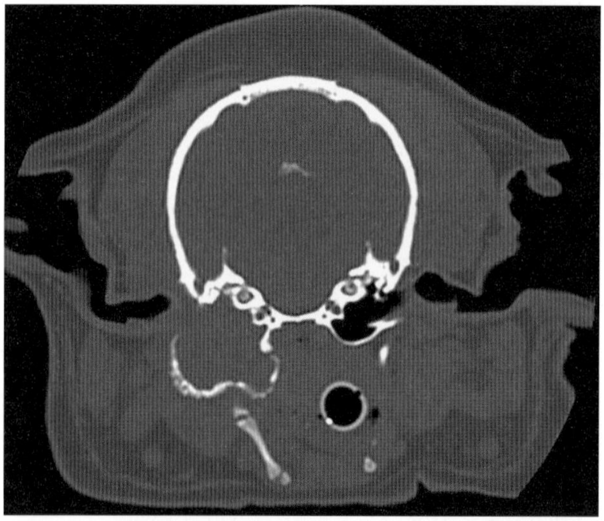

Figure 11.5 Transverse image of a CT scan through the bullae of a 12-year-old castrated male terrier mix. Presented for pain upon opening of the mouth; biopsy of the middle ear contents at the time of right VBO revealed cholesteatoma. *Source:* Courtesy of Dr. Alla Bezhentseva.

Small, noninvasive cholesteatomas may be treated with long-term antibiotics based on culture and bacterial sensitivity, and vitamin A therapy may also be helpful.[28] When the patient is experiencing clinical signs, such as the development of a head tilt, the author also treats with the occasional course of prednisolone (anti-inflammatory dose) or nonsteroidal anti-inflammatory, if not otherwise contraindicated. Depending on the extent of involvement of the external ear canal in the presence of chronic otitis, VBO or total ear canal ablation with lateral bulla osteotomy may be indicated. Prognosis depends on severity of disease (size, invasiveness, tissue destruction); in one study, 52% of dogs undergoing surgery for cholesteatoma removal via VBO or total ear canal ablation with lateral bulla osteotomy had recurrent signs post-operatively.[27]

Clinical signs associated with cholesteatoma are those of chronic otitis externa (discharge, swelling, redness), as well as an inability to fully open the mouth, head tilt, facial nerve paralysis, ataxia, nystagmus, circling, and unilateral atrophy of the temporalis and masseter muscles. If bulla expansion into the nasopharynx and oropharynx occurs, respiratory signs may also be present.[26,27]

Cholesterol Granuloma

Cholesterol granuloma, predominantly found in dogs but also noted in cats, is also the result of chronic inflammation and may be present in the same ear or patient as cholesteatoma. In this disease process, the granulomatous tissue contains cholesterol crystals.[29–31] Cholesterol granulomas may be seen as a complication following total ear canal ablation with lateral bulla osteotomy.[32]

Results of diagnostic imaging may be similar to those of cholesteatoma, and surgical appearance may also be similar, though gross keratinaceous debris will be absent and pathologic findings will be consistent with cholesterol precipitates, acicular clefts, and mononuclear inflammatory cells. Prognosis is expected to mirror that of cholesteatoma; in two reported cases of aural cholesterol granuloma formation in dogs, neoplasia resolved following VBO.[29,30] In a single case report of middle ear cholesterol granuloma in a cat, surgery was not elected due to severity of neurological signs.[31]

Neoplasia

Neoplasia originating in the middle ear has been reported in older cats (over 10 years of age) and dogs over 6 years old. It is not a common diagnosis and is rarely an indication for VBO, as neoplasia can be invasive and surgery would provide only temporary palliation.[33–35] Tumors found in the middle ear in cats can include squamous cell carcinoma, papillary adenoma, ceruminous gland adenocarcinoma, anaplastic carcinoma, lymphoblastic lymphosarcoma, and lymphoma. In dogs, tumors originating in the middle ear are usually benign, but malignant tumors from surrounding structures may secondarily involve the middle ear. These may include basal cell tumor, papilloma, papillary adenoma, ceruminous or sebaceous gland adenocarcinoma, squamous cell, and anaplastic neoplasia.[33,36]

Clinical signs suggestive of neoplasia can overlap with other causes of middle ear disease but may be more likely to include seizures, discomfort, and neurological deficits, such as Horner's syndrome. Diagnostic imaging is helpful to differentiate between potential causes and should be strongly recommended if severity of signs and signalment elevate concern for neoplasia.

Long-term surgical outcomes for the treatment of malignant middle ear tumors are expected to be poor. Since that outcome is anticipated, surgery is rarely performed and data on outcomes is not robust.[33,37]

Chronic Otitis

Chronic middle ear infection without a mechanical or anatomical underlying cause may be treated by video otoscopy-guided myringotomy and flush.[38] With isolated recurrent infection of the middle ear (i.e., minimal involvement of the external ear canal), VBO becomes a reasonable option.

Additional Preoperative Considerations

Once the decision to proceed with VBO has been made, a decision regarding unilateral versus bilateral surgery may be required based on the presence of bilateral disease. Manipulation of pharyngeal tissue during VBO may cause swelling, and bilateral single-stage VBO has been associated with an increased risk of respiratory complications postoperatively. The decision to proceed with single-stage bilateral surgery should, therefore, be made with caution and in close communication with the patient's owner about risk.[39–42]

Surgical Procedure

Prep and Positioning

The patient is intubated and positioned in dorsal recumbency with dorsal cervical support or padding, such as a rolled towel, to gently extend the neck for improved exposure of the surgical region. The ventral cervical and intermandibular regions are prepared. It is best to prepare a wider area than anticipated, as skin may move with final positioning in the operating room, and a novice surgeon may require additional room for sterile palpation to confirm anatomy before making the first incision. An example of an instrument table used for the VBO set-up should at least include retractors, periosteal elevators, rongeurs, and an IM pin (Figure 11.6).

Approach and Bulla Osteotomy

The bulla may be palpated directly caudomedial to the rami of the mandible (Figure 11.7). The incision is made over the bulla in a rostro-caudal orientation (paramedian), extending ~3–5 cm in cats and ~6–10 cm in dogs.

The platysma muscle should be incised, and the mandibular salivary gland and bifurcation of the linguofacial vein are retracted if necessary. The digastricus (lateral) and hyoglossus/styloglossus muscles (medial) are then bluntly divided. The hypoglossal nerve is located on the medial aspect of the hyoglossus muscle, which can be damaged by indelicate retraction, and is retracted medially with this

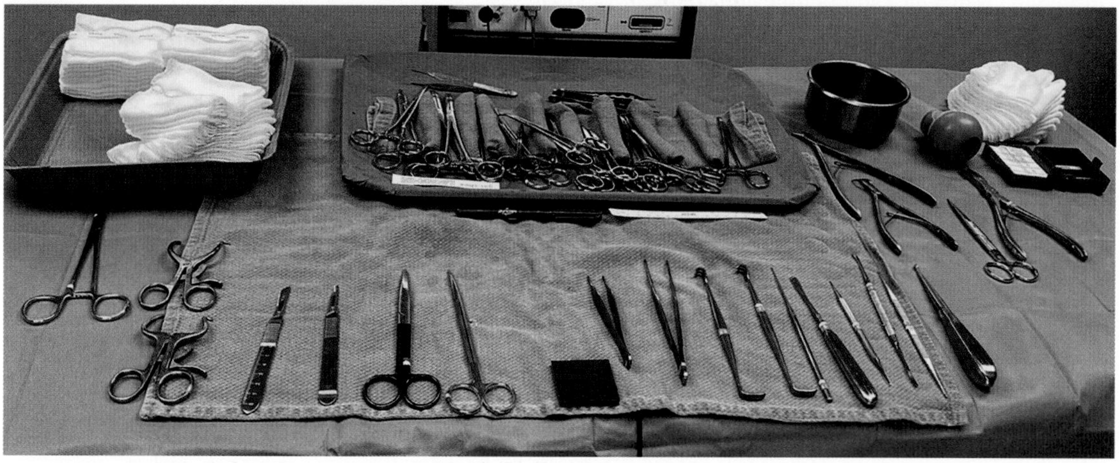

Figure 11.6 Example of sterile instrument table for VBO. Instruments to perform a VBO should ideally include a #10 or #15 blade for initial skin incision, two small Gelpi perineal retractors, Senn retractors (if you have an assistant during surgery), a variety of thumb forceps (Brown-Adson and DeBakey seen here), hemostats, curettes (or dental instruments if available), periosteal elevator(s), bowl for sterile saline, and rongeurs (single- and double-action types seen here). Not shown but necessary: either a burr or IM pin with Jacob's chuck attachment for bulla entry. *Source:* © Kristin Coleman.

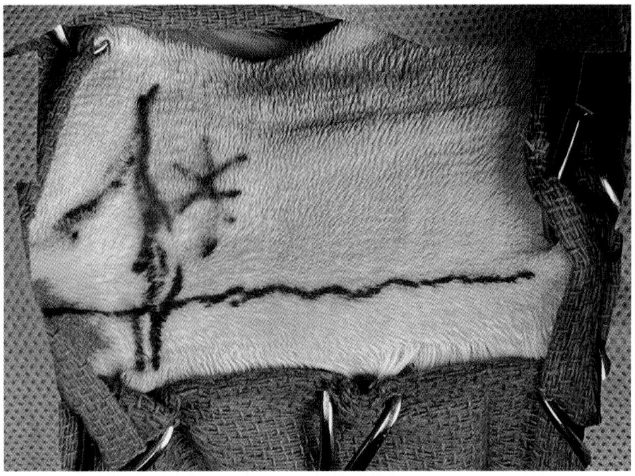

Figure 11.7 Location of feline tympanic bulla. The patient is positioned in dorsal recumbency, the head is to the left of the picture, the side-to-side line is on midline, and the perpendicular line is immediately caudal to the angle of the mandible with a star (*) drawn in the area of the palpable left tympanic bulla. *Source:* © Kristin Coleman.

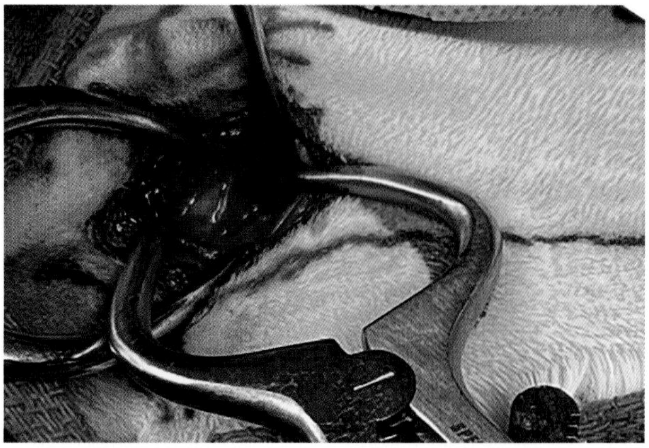

Figure 11.8 Dissection of tissue from bulla with Freer periosteal elevator. Notice that Gelpi retractors are placed in the surgical site perpendicular to each other to aid in visualization. *Source:* © Kristin Coleman.

muscle. Judicious use of self-retaining (Gelpi or Weitlaner) retractors is, therefore, recommended, and be aware of the length of the tips on the ends of the retractors when placing them into the surgical site.

In cats, the bulla may then be palpated and visualized rostromedial to the hyoid and caudomedial to the caudal border of the mandible. Tissue should be dissected from the entire ventral aspect of the bulla with a Freer periosteal elevator (Figure 11.8) until the bulla appears as an egg (Figure 11.9), and a Steinmann pin is used to make a ventral opening (Figure 11.10). A tip for choosing the size of the pin is to "go big": this will decrease the risk of iatrogenic damage by allowing for just one pin penetration through the ventral bulla wall. Once appropriate bulla penetration is confirmed, rongeurs (e.g., Lempert, Love-Kerrison) are used to enlarge the hole. Burrs are rarely required in cats but may be helpful in larger dogs with bony thickening.

Identification of the bulla in dogs may be more difficult than in cats, as the canine bulla is deeper from the skin and there is more soft tissue surrounding it, thus, making it less prominent and not immediately palpable. Anatomical landmarks become more important: the midline of a line between the wing of the atlas and the angle of the mandible is a landmark on the transverse plane. The paracondylar process of the occipital bone is pointed and may also be palpated 5–10 mm caudolateral to the bulla.

Prior to surgery, the anatomy of the middle ear in dogs and cats should be reviewed, as they are not the same. In the dog, the tympanic cavity is composed of the small dorsal epitympanic recess and the larger tympanic cavity proper.

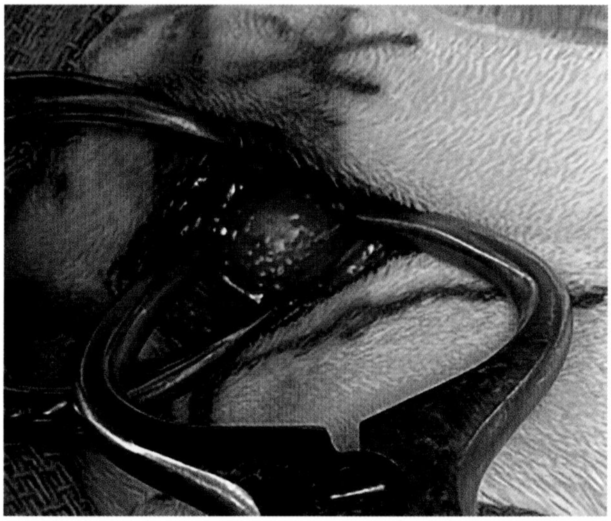

Figure 11.9 Soft tissue has been bluntly dissected from the entire ventral surface of the left tympanic bulla in this feline patient, and small Gelpi retractors are placed deep/dorsal to the tissue at 90° angles to each other for ideal visualization. *Source:* © Kristin Coleman.

The feline bulla is divided by a thin bony septum into a larger ventromedial and smaller dorsolateral compartment, which is further divided into the epitympanum and mesotympanum. The lateral wall of the dorsolateral compartment is formed by the tympanic membrane (Figure 11.11).[43] The larger ventromedial compartment is an air-filled tympanic cavity. The compartments communicate through a small fissure, which is closely associated with the promontory. Postganglionic sympathetic nerves reside on this structure within the tympanic plexus and are vulnerable to trauma during surgery.[6,44] However, it is also important to ensure perforation of the bony septum and

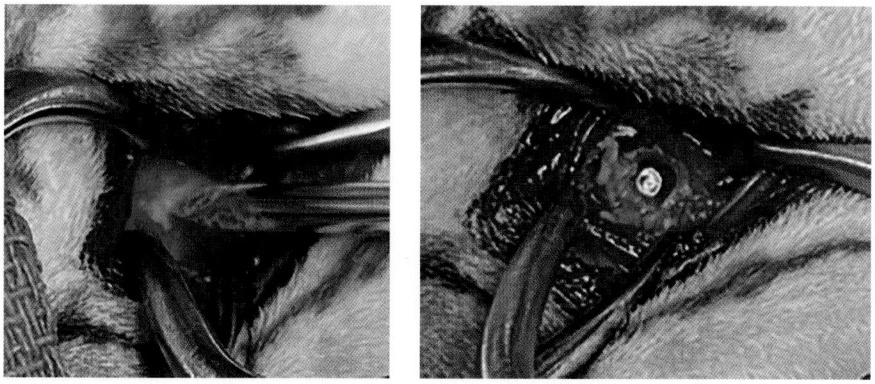

Figure 11.10 Once there is a visualization of the ventral surface of the tympanic bulla, puncturing of the bone with a large-gauge Steinmann pin (either by hand-driven Jacob's chuck or drill) or burr is performed. The image on the left shows the central placement of the 9/64″ Steinmann pin to reduce the risk of slipping from the bone. After rotating the pin, a hole is created in the bone, as shown in the right image. Rongeurs may now be used to chip away small bites of bone until adequate exposure of the middle ear cavity is achieved. *Source:* © Kristin Coleman.

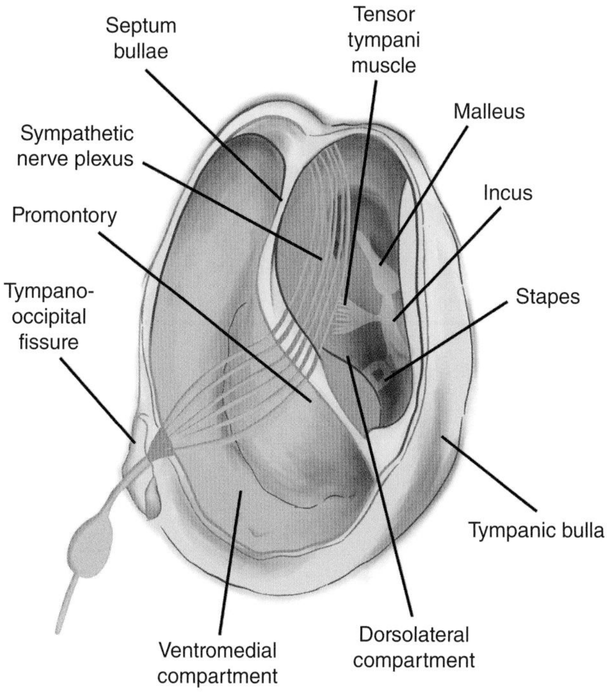

Figure 11.11 Feline tympanic bulla and internal anatomy. *Source:* © Philippa Pavia.

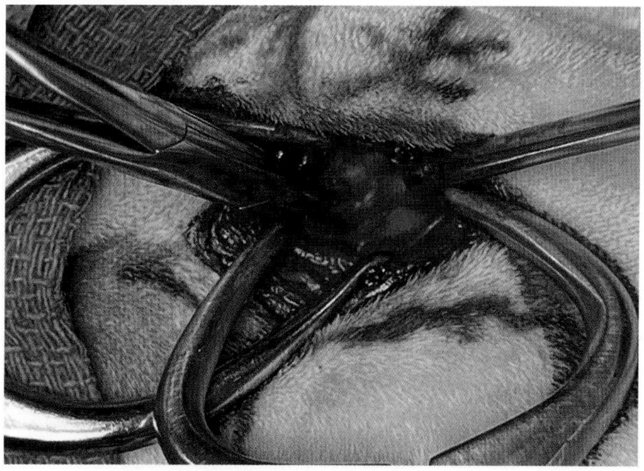

Figure 11.12 Following the removal of the ventral bone of the bulla, samples are collected and contents are cleared. The thin bony septum separating the larger ventromedial and smaller dorsolateral compartments is usually fragile enough to be penetrated by light pressure from the tip of a mosquito hemostat, as seen in this image. A Frazier suction tip is aiding in visualization. *Source:* © Kristin Coleman.

evaluation of the smaller dorsolateral compartment, as this is the origin of many polyps (Figure 11.12).[44,45] If the polyp extends into the external ear canal, the ear may be included in the surgical field to provide traction on the polyp. Traction may be placed on a nasopharyngeal polyp by the anesthetist during surgery, and a forcep should be placed across the polyp before positioning if this option is likely to be desired.

Samples are obtained for culture/sensitivity and histopathology, and the compartments are cleared of inflammatory debris, neoplastic tissue, or foreign material with a small curette, mosquito hemostats, thumb forceps, and copious lavage and suction. The bulla and surrounding tissues are flushed with copious warm sterile saline before closure. If continued drainage is desired, a small closed suction drain (such as a Blake drain) or a small Penrose drain may be placed in the cavity and exited through a separate incision. If there is evidence of gross infection, clean instruments and a glove change are often performed. Soft tissues should be closed in layers with absorbable monofilament suture. Bandaging is not generally required, though may be elected if a drain is placed. The use of Elizabethan collars is up to the surgeon's discretion, though they are rarely required, and may place pressure on the incision. If chosen, a soft cone collar is all that is needed to prevent scratching of the incision.

Complications

Following VBO, transient Horner's syndrome (particularly in cats) and vestibular signs are common (Figure 11.13); facial nerve paralysis may also be seen. Additional risks include polyp regrowth, recurrent otitis media, hemorrhage, infection, hypoglossal nerve damage, damage to auditory ossicles and vascular structures, and respiratory distress.[1,7,10,11,23,25,41,42,45]

Horner's syndrome secondary to iatrogenic sympathetic nerve damage is noted in the majority of cats, up to 94% in some studies; those with pre-existing neurological signs are more likely to have permanent signs postoperatively.[10,25,42,45] One study showed that cats with Horner's syndrome pre-operatively had 2.6, 3.3, and 5.6 times the odds of having permanent Horner's syndrome, head tilt, and facial nerve paralysis, respectively.[42] However, in general, signs are predominantly transient, resolving in weeks to months, with approximately 17–25% showing permanent signs.[25,45] Vestibular signs are also fairly common in cats, occurring in up to 42%, but are also expected to resolve.[45] Decreased hearing is to be expected in dogs and cats but may not be noticed with unilateral disease and subsequent unilateral VBO.[7,10]

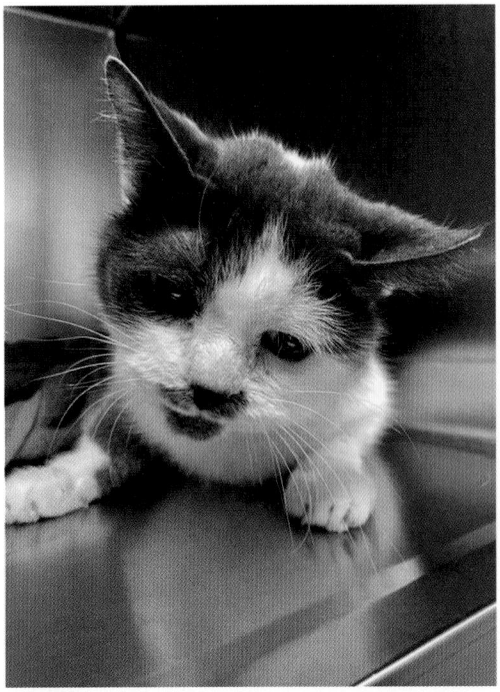

Figure 11.13 Patient with pre-operative vestibular signs in the form of a left head tilt. *Source:* © Kristin Coleman.

As discussed elsewhere in this chapter, manipulation of pharyngeal tissue may cause swelling, and single-stage bilateral VBO, which causes increased/bilateral cervical swelling, may, therefore, be associated with an increased risk of respiratory complications and surgery-related mortality.[39–42] Of cats undergoing unilateral, staged bilateral, and single-stage bilateral VBO in one study population, 9%, 29%, and 47% of these cases had postoperative respiratory complications, suggesting that there is an over fivefold increase in risk over unilateral surgery by performing the procedure bilaterally in a single operative event. The risk is nearly double compared to staged bilateral procedures.[42]

Postoperative Care/Prognosis

Antibiotic therapy is often indicated based on the results of surgical bacterial culture and sensitivity testing, as infection is a common secondary (or inciting) factor for surgical disease of the middle ear. With polyp removal, long-term antibiotics should not be required if all diseased tissue is removed at the time of surgery. The prognosis for polyp removal via VBO is expected to be excellent, and long-term care is generally not required.[44] For polyps requiring treatment via traction in conjunction with VBO, results are similarly promising with recurrence rates between 0% and 8%.[25,45] Outcomes in dogs are less frequently reported but are expected to be similar to those in cats.[15,46] Horner's syndrome, even if permanent, is unlikely to affect quality of life.

For VBO to treat chronic infection and inflammation and secondary processes, such as cholesteatoma in dogs, long-term therapy with antibiotics may be indicated and recurrence is possible.[27] Dogs and cats with neoplasia will likely require additional therapies or palliative care with progression or recurrence.[34,35]

Conclusion

VBO is a delicate procedure requiring technical skill but is an excellent method for access, visualization, and removal of abnormal tissue originating from the middle ear. Diagnosis and decision to treat should be based on history, signalment, clinical signs, and results of diagnostic imaging. Knowledge of the surgical anatomy of the bulla and middle ear will increase success and decrease risk of iatrogenic complications, and long-term outcomes are expected to be excellent for nonneoplastic conditions, such as inflammatory polyps.

References

1 Hardie, E. (2013). Surgical diseases of the middle ear. In: *Small Animal Soft Tissue Surgery* (ed. E. Monnet), 149–156. Ames, IA: Wiley.

2 Detweiler, D.A., Johnson, L.R., Kass, P.H. et al. (2006). Computed tomographic evidence of bulla effusion in cats with Sinonasal disease: 2001–2004. *J. Vet. Intern. Med.* 20 (5): 1080–1084.

3 Rohleder, J.J., Jones, J.C., Duncan, R.B. et al. (2006). Comparative performance of radiography and computed tomography in the diagnosis of middle ear disease in 31 dogs. *Vet. Radiol. Ultrasound* 47 (1): 45–52.

4 King, A.M., Weinrauch, S.A., Doust, R. et al. (2007). Comparison of ultrasonography, radiography and a single computed tomography slice for fluid identification within the feline tympanic bulla. *Vet. J.* 173 (3): 638–644.

5 Hammond, G.J.C., Sullivan, M., Weinrauch, S. et al. (2005). A comparison of the rostrocaudal open mouth and rostro 10° ventro-caudodorsal oblique radiographic views for imaging fluid in the feline tympanic bulla. *Vet. Radiol. Ultrasound* 46 (3): 205–209.

6 Smeak, D. and Inpanbutr, N. (2005). Lateral approach to subtotal bulla osteotomy in dogs: pertinent anatomy and procedural details. *Compend. Contin. Educ. Pract. Vet.* 27 (5): 377–384.

7 McAnulty, J., Hattel, A., and Harvey, C. (1995). Wound healing and brain stem auditory evoked potentials after experimental ventral tympanic bulla osteotomy in dogs. *Vet. Surg.* 24 (1): 9–14.

8 Smeak, D., Crocker, C., and Birchard, S. (1996). Treatment of recurrent otitis media that developed after total ear canal ablation and lateral bulla osteotomy in dogs: nine cases (1986-1994). *J. Am. Vet. Med. Assoc.* 209 (5): 937–942.

9 da Silva, A.M., de Souza, W.M., de Carvalho, R.G. et al. (2009). Morphological aspects of tympanic bulla after ventral osteotomy in cats. *Acta Cir. Bras.* 24 (3): 177–182.

10 Anders, B.B., Hoelzler, M.G., Scavelli, T.D. et al. (2008). Analysis of auditory and neurologic effects associated with ventral bulla osteotomy for removal of inflammatory polyps or nasopharyngeal masses in cats. *J. Am. Vet. Med. Assoc.* 233 (4): 580–585.

11 Sharp, N.J.H. (1990). Chronic otitis externa and otitis media treated by total ear canal ablation and ventral bulla osteotomy in thirteen dogs. *Vet. Surg.* 19 (2): 162–166.

12 Bacon, N. (2018). Pinna and external ear canal. In: *Veterinary Surgery: Small Animal*, 2e (ed. S.A. Johnston and K.M. Tobias), 2059–2077. St. Louis, MO: Elsevier.

13 Allen, H., Broussard, J., and Noone, K. (1999). Nasopharyngeal diseases in cats: a retrospective study of 53 cases (1991-1998). *J. Am. Anim. Hosp. Assoc.* 35 (6): 457–461.

14 Rogers, K.S. (1988). Tumors of the ear canal. *Vet. Clin. North Am. Small Anim. Pract.* 18 (4): 859–868.

15 Fingland, R., Gratzek, A., Vorhies, M. et al. (1993). Nasopharyngeal polyp in a dog. *J. Am. Anim. Hosp. Assoc.* 29 (4): 311–314.

16 Kerr, L. (1989). Pulmonary edema secondary to upper airway obstruction in the dog: a review of nine cases. *J. Am. Anim. Hosp. Assoc.* 25 (2): 207–212.

17 Pollock, S. (1971). Nasopharyngeal polyp in a dog. A case study. *Vet. Med. Small Anim. Clin.* 66 (7): 705–706.

18 Smart, L. and Jandrey, K.E. (2008). Upper airway obstruction caused by a nasopharyngeal polyp and brachycephalic airway syndrome in a Chinese Shar-Pei puppy. *J. Vet. Emerg. Crit. Care* 18 (4): 393–398.

19 Baker, G. (1982). Nasopharyngeal polyps in cats. *Vet. Rec.* 111 (2): 43.

20 Parker, N. and Binnington, A. (1987). Nasopharyngeal polyps in cats: three case reports and a review of the literature. *J. Am. Anim. Hosp. Assoc.* 21 (4): 473–478.

21 Veir, J., Lappin, M., Foley, J. et al. (2002). Feline inflammatory polyps: historical, clinical, and PCR findings for feline Calici virus and Feline herpes virus-1 in 28 cases. *J. Feline Med. Surg.* 4 (4): 195–199.

22 Anderson, D., Robinson, R., and White, R. (2000). Management of inflammatory polyps in 37 cats. *Vet. Rec.* 147 (24): 684–687. https://pubmed.ncbi.nlm.nih.gov/11132674.

23 Muilenburg, R.K. and Fry, T.R. (2002). Feline nasopharyngeal polyps. *Vet. Clin. North Am. Small Anim. Pract.* 32 (4): 839–849.

24 Diel, J. (2008). Removal of an ear polyp via perendoscopic transtympanic excision (PTTE) in two cats. *Der Praktische Tierarzt* 89 (2): 94–98.

25 Kapatkin, A., Matthiesen, D., and Noone, K. (1990). Results of surgery and long-term follow-up in 31 cats with nasopharyngeal polyps. *J. Am. Anim. Hosp. Assoc.* 26 (4): 387–392.

26 Little, C., Lane, J., Gibbs, C. et al. (1991). Inflammatory middle ear disease of the dog: the clinical and pathological features of cholesteatoma, a complication of otitis media. *Vet. Rec.* 128 (14): 319–322.

27 Hardie, E.M., Linder, K.E., and Pease, A.P. (2008). Aural cholesteatoma in twenty dogs. *Vet. Surg.* 37 (8): 763–770.

28 Rao, U.S.V., Srinivas, D.R., Humbarwadi, R.S. et al. (2009). Role of vitamin a in the evolution of cholesteatoma. *Indian J. Otolaryngol. Head Neck Surg.* 61 (2): 150–152.

29 Cox, C.L. and Payne-Johnson, C.E. (1995). Aural cholesterol granuloma in a dog. *J. Small Anim. Pract.* 36 (1): 25–28.

30 Fliegner, R.A., Jubb, K.V.F., and Lording, P.M. (2007). Cholesterol granuloma associated with otitis media and destruction of the tympanic bulla in a dog. *Vet. Pathol.* 44 (4): 547–549.

31 Van der Heyden, S., Butaye, P., and Roels, S. (2013). Cholesterol granuloma associated with otitis media and leptomeningitis in a cat due to a *Streptococcus canis* infection. *Can. Vet. J.* 54 (1): 72–73.

32 Riedinger, B., Albaric, O., and Gauthier, O. (2012). Cholesterol granuloma as long-term complication of total ear canal ablation in a dog. *J. Small Anim. Pract.* 53 (3): 188–191.

33 Little, C., Pearson, G., and Lane, J. (1989). Neoplasia involving the middle ear cavity of dogs. *Vet. Rec.* 124 (3): 54–57.

34 Kirpensteijn, J. (1993). Aural neoplasms. *Semin. Vet. Med. Surg. Small Anim.* 8 (1): 17–23.

35 Fan, T.M. and de Lorimier, L.P. (2004). Inflammatory polyps and aural neoplasia. *Vet. Clin. North Am. Small Anim. Pract.* 34 (2): 489–509.

36 Yoshikawa, H., Mayer, M.N., Linn, K.A. et al. (2008). A dog with squamous cell carcinoma in the middle ear. *Can. Vet. J.* 49 (9): 877–879.

37 Lucroy, M.D., Vernau, K.M., Samii, V.F. et al. (2004). Middle ear tumours with brainstem extension treated by ventral bulla osteotomy and craniectomy in two cats. *Vet. Comp. Oncol.* 2 (4): 234–242.

38 Palmeiro, B.S., Morris, D.O., Wiemelt, S.P. et al. (2004). Evaluation of outcome of otitis media after lavage of the tympanic bulla and long-term antimicrobial drug treatment in dogs: 44 cases (1998–2002). *J. Am. Vet. Med. Assoc.* 225 (4): 548–553.

39 Smeak, D.D. (2011). Management of complications associated with total ear canal ablation and bulla osteotomy in dogs and cats. *Vet. Clin. North Am. Small Anim. Pract.* 41 (5): 981–994.

40 Vlasin, M., Artingstall, R., and Mala, B. (2021). Acute upper airway obstruction as a life-threatening complication of ventral bulla osteotomy: report of two consecutive cases. *J. Feline Med. Surg. Open Rep.* 7 (1): 205511692110059.

41 De Gennaro, C., Vettorato, E., and Corletto, F. (2017). Severe upper airway obstruction following bilateral ventral bulla osteotomy in a cat. *Can. Vet. J.* 58 (12): 1313–1316.

42 Wainberg, S.H., Selmic, S.E., and Haagsma, A.N. (2019). Comparison of complications and outcome following unilateral, staged bilateral, and single-stage bilateral ventral bulla osteotomy in cat. *J. Am. Vet. Med. Assoc.* 255 (7): 828–836.

43 White, R. (2018). Middle and inner ear. In: *Veterinary Surgery: Small Animal*, 2e (ed. S.A. Johnston and K.M. Tobias), 2328–2340. St. Louis, MO: Elsevier.

44 Donnelly, K. and Tillson, D. (2004). Feline inflammatory polyps and ventral bulla osteotomy. *Compendium Continuing Educ. Pract. Vet.* 26 (6): 446–454.

45 Faulkner, J. and Budsberg, S. (1990). Results of ventral bulla osteotomy for treatment of middle ear polyps in cats. *J. Am. Anim. Hosp. Assoc.* 26 (5): 496–499.

46 Pratschke, K.M. (2003). Inflammatory polyps of the middle ear in 5 dogs. *Vet. Surg.* 32 (3): 292–296.

12

Mandibulectomy

Giovanni Tremolada

Department of Clinical Sciences, Colorado State University, Fort Collins, CO, USA

Key Points

- Good knowledge of the mandibular anatomy is imperative when considering surgery.
- In addition to general health screening bloodwork, blood-typing for dogs and both blood-typing and cross-matching for cats should be performed before surgery. Having the availability of blood products is mandatory if hemorrhage is expected.
- Dogs tolerate mandibulectomies very well and will be able to eat within a few hours to a day after surgery.
- Cats have more trouble eating after mandibulectomies, and most will need to have a feeding tube placed at the surgery to help with postoperative management, especially with ease of medication administration. Some cats will not return to eating after mandibulectomies and, thus, will require lifelong management of an esophagostomy tube.
- Cosmetic changes are usually mild to moderate after mandibulectomies. Showing pictures of previous patients who have received a similar surgery to owners will help them understand how their pet will look postoperatively and in deciding if they want to pursue surgery.

Introduction

The inferior jaw of dogs and cats consists of two mandibles (right and left) that are connected rostrally by the intermandibular suture (mandibular symphysis).[1] Each mandible can be divided into a horizontal portion, called the body, and a vertical portion, called the ramus (Figure 12.1). The dorsal aspect of the body of the mandible contains the dental alveoli, including the recessions where the teeth are located, and is called the alveolar border. The rostroventral aspect of the mandible has three foramina (rostral, middle, and caudal); these foramina are the areas where mental vessels and nerves exit from. The larger middle foramen is located at the level of the rostral root of the second premolar in the dog and at the level of the apex of the canine tooth in the cat. The rostrolateral aspect of the mandible, bordered by the lips, is called the labial aspect, while the caudal aspect where the check is located is called the buccal aspect. The medial aspect of each body of the mandible is called the lingual aspect. The ramus of the mandible is the portion of the mandible that does not have teeth, and this is composed of three main areas – the angular process, the condylar process, and the coronoid process (Figure 12.1).

The main blood supply to the mandible is from the inferior alveolar artery. Caudally, this vessel is located on the medial side of the mandible and enters into the mandibular canal at the level of the mandibular foramen (Figure 12.1). Together with the artery and vein travels the inferior alveolar nerve. It is important to be able to identify the location of the mandibular foramen before surgery in case a nerve block of the inferior alveolar nerve needs to be performed as a part of a multimodal analgesic plan. Knowing the location of the mandibular foramen is also important during surgery when a complete unilateral

Techniques in Small Animal Soft Tissue, Orthopedic, and Ophthalmic Surgery, First Edition. Edited by Kristin A. Coleman.

Companion website: www.wiley.com/go/coleman/surgeries

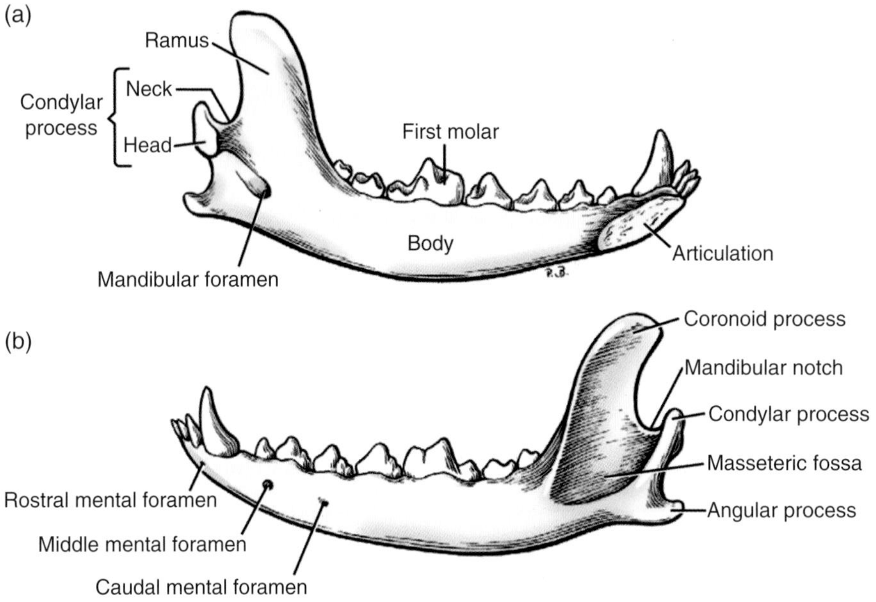

Figure 12.1 Anatomy of the mandible of a dog. (a) Medial view; (b) lateral view. *Source:* Reproduced with permission from Evans and de Lahunta,[1] Elsevier.

mandibulectomy or a caudal mandibulectomy is performed, as inadvertent transection of the structures that traverse this foramen can result in significant hemorrhage.

The inferior labial artery, a branch of the facial artery, is responsible for the vascularization of the lower lip. The ventral buccal branch of the facial nerve provides motor innervation of the lower lip, and the mandibular branch of the trigeminal nerve provides its sensory innervation. The ventral buccal branch of the facial nerve is also responsible for the motor innervation of the masticatory muscles. Most of the muscles of mastication (masseter, pterygoid, and digastricus) are inserted on the ramus of the mandible.

Indications and Preoperative Considerations

Mandibulectomies are usually performed for trauma and benign or malignant tumors involving the oral cavity. Segmental mandibulectomy has also been reported in a dog with advanced-stage cholesteatoma to help with discomfort in opening the mouth.[2]

Different types of mandibulectomies can be performed with different degrees of postoperative cosmetic alteration and surgical challenges. The extension of the resection must be decided based on the size, location, and biological behavior of the tumor. Commonly, mandibulectomies are classified as unilateral rostral mandibulectomy, bilateral rostral mandibulectomy, segmental or central mandibulectomy, rim mandibulectomy (if a segmental or rostral mandibulectomy is performed preserving the ventral margin of the mandible), total unilateral mandibulectomy, caudal mandibulectomy and one and half mandibulectomy (Figure 12.2).[3]

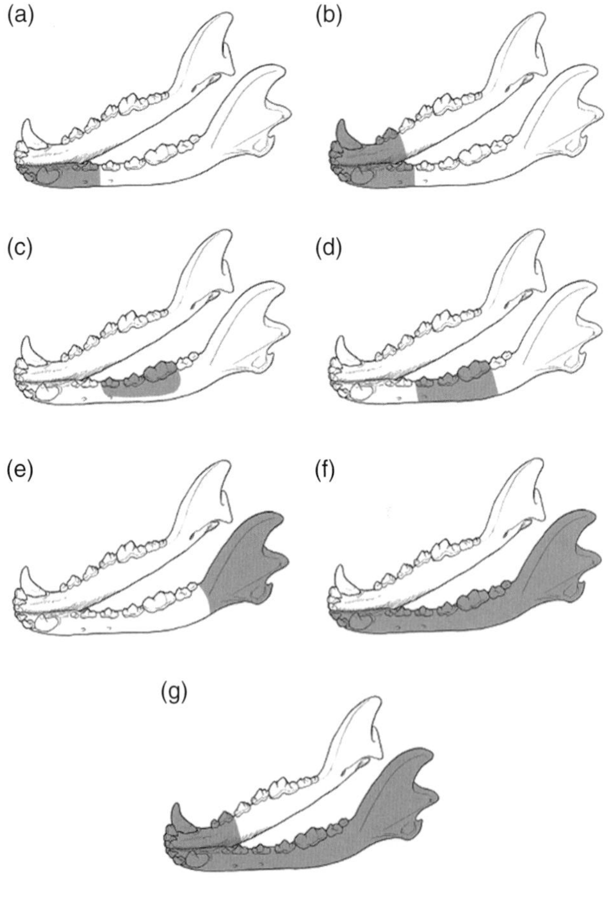

Figure 12.2 Schematics showing the different types of mandibulectomies that can be performed in dogs. (a) Unilateral rostral mandibulectomy; (b) bilateral rostral mandibulectomy; (c) rim mandibulectomy; (d) segmental mandibulectomy; (e) caudal mandibulectomy; (f) hemimandibulectomy; (g) one and half mandibulectomy. *Source:* Reproduced with permission from Monnet, John Wiley & Sons.

A sedated oral exam is an important step in the patient's evaluation, allowing for a better gross evaluation of the extent of the tumor. An awake oral exam may be challenging, as an animal may not allow the clinician to open the mouth due to discomfort related to the presence of an oral mass. During the sedated oral exam, a biopsy of the mass should be obtained. Even if a good correlation exists between cytology and histology for oral tumors in dogs,[4] the author prefers to obtain a deep, large biopsy to maximize the chance of having a definitive diagnosis. Electrosurgery can be used to collect a sample from the mass, but this may create artifacts that alter the sample's quality. Multiple good quality, deep biopsies should be obtained to maximize the chance of obtaining a correct final diagnosis. A core punch or a wedge biopsy are considered appropriate techniques. The bleeding resulting from obtaining the biopsy can usually be stopped by compressing the area with a gauze, using electrosurgery, silver nitrate sticks, or suturing the edges of the biopsy site. It is not uncommon that the sutures placed to close the biopsy tract could cut through the friable neoplastic tissue, and for this reason, the author does not routinely use this technique. Biopsies must be obtained from an intraoral approach and from a location that will be resected with the mass at the time of surgery. If the size of the mass is small (<1 cm), an excisional biopsy can be considered. In this case, it is imperative to obtain pictures before removing the mass. This is because the oral mucosa heals quickly, and, in case of a diagnosis of a malignant tumor and the subsequent need for revision surgery, identifying the area where the mass was located could be extremely challenging. Documentation, especially in recording the teeth closest to the mass's location prior to resection, is also pertinent for the medical record and for future intervention.

Obtaining a preoperative diagnosis is fundamental before considering surgical removal of a large oral mass. This information will help the clinician choose the appropriate surgical dose, suggest alternative treatment options (e.g., radiation therapy, chemotherapy, etc.), and give the owner information about the prognosis. Common malignant oral tumors in dogs are melanoma, squamous cell carcinoma (SCC), osteosarcoma, and fibrosarcoma.[5] Benign tumors, like acanthomatous ameloblastoma and peripheral odontogenic fibroma, are not infrequent. Even if benign, canine acanthomatous ameloblastoma can invade the bone, and a mandibulectomy should be performed to decrease the chance of local recurrence. In cats, the most common tumor type is SCC, accounting for 70% of all oral tumors,[5] but other tumors like osteomas, osteosarcoma, and odontogenic tumors can be encountered.

Skull CT scan, including the cervical region to assess lymph nodes, is the preferred method to assess the extent of oral neoplasia,[6] as bony changes can be seen on radiographs only if 40% of the cortical bone is lost.[7] For small rostral lesions, the use of intraoral radiographs may be adequate. Margins for both benign and malignant tumors should always be measured based on advanced imaging findings and not gross extension of the tumor. Different types of margins have been suggested for benign and malignant tumors. Some authors have suggested obtaining margins of 2–3 cm for malignant tumors affecting the mandible,[7] while others suggested smaller margins (1–2 cm).[3] The author tends to obtain margins of 1–2 cm for most malignant tumors, especially in small dogs and cats where the 2–3 cm margins would not be possible to achieve, and margins of 1 cm or less for benign tumors. Margins of 2–3 cm are usually attempted in dogs affected by oral fibrosarcoma, due to the high chance of local recurrence.[8]

It is important to remember that oral fibrosarcoma can appear as a benign lesion on histology even if it biologically behaves as an aggressive tumor (so-called histological low grade-biological high grade or "high-low" tumors). The histologic diagnosis should always be correlated to the clinical behavior of the mass. Signalment is another important factor to consider, as retrievers seem to be more frequently affected by this type of tumor compared to other breeds. Signalment and biological behavior should always be relayed to the pathologist at the time of the submission of the biopsy sample to help in formulating a correct diagnosis.

Metastasis to locoregional lymph nodes is not uncommon in dogs with malignant oral tumors and is a negative prognostic factor.[9] In dogs with oral melanoma, metastatic lymph nodes can be of normal size in 40% of the cases.[10] Unfortunately, CT appearance of neck lymph nodes in dogs affected by oral and nasal tumors is not predictive of the presence of metastatic disease.[11] Some surgeons routinely perform full neck lymph node dissection for better staging of malignant oral tumors, but the clinical benefit is unknown. A possible alternative to this method is the sentinel lymph node mapping technique. With this technique, it is possible to identify the first lymph node within a lymphocentrum that drains lymph from a tumor. Once identified, a selective lymphadenectomy is performed. Different techniques for preoperative or intraoperative sentinel lymph node mapping have been described.[12–15] A thorough discussion of these techniques is outside the purpose of this chapter.

All malignant oral tumors can metastasize to the lung. Thoracic radiographs or thoracic CT scans should be performed before surgery. The author prefers to obtain a thoracic CT scan at the time of the head and neck CT performed for surgical planning, as this imaging technique has a higher accuracy for detecting pulmonary nodules compared to thoracic radiographs.[16]

Surgical Procedure

More complex mandibulectomies (complete unilateral, complete resection of the ramus, and complete unilateral and one and half mandibulectomies) should be performed by surgeons already proficient with other types of mandibulectomies and will not be discussed in this chapter. Before surgery, all animals should have baseline bloodwork (CBC, serum chemistry), a blood type (plus cross-matching for cats or dogs that have had a previous blood transfusion), and urine analysis. Positioning may vary from lateral to dorsal or even sternal recumbency, depending on the surgeon's preference. Laparotomy sponges or 4×4 gauzes should be packed into the dog's or cat's pharynx to minimize the risk of aspiration pneumonia or blood ingestion. It is imperative to record the number of sponges/gauzes used and make sure that all of them are retrieved before recovering the animal from anesthesia. The author usually positions animals in an obliqued lateral recumbency for unilateral rostral and segmental/rim mandibulectomies and in dorsal for bilateral rostral mandibulectomies.

Bilateral Rostral Mandibulectomy

Hair is clipped from the ventral and lateral aspects of the chin down to the mid-body of the mandible. Clipping is extended to the angle of the mandible if more aggressive bilateral resection is needed or to the thoracic inlet if cervical lymph node extirpation is planned. The dog is positioned in dorsal recumbency. Surgical margins are measured with a ruler and marked with a sterile pencil. A scalpel blade is usually used to incise the oral mucosa, as electrosurgery may delay mucosal healing and predispose to dehiscence. Electrosurgery can be used after incising the mucosa to dissect tissues until bone is reached.

During the dissection on the lateral side of the mandible, the rostral, middle, and caudal mental arteries may be encountered. Those vessels should be identified and cauterized or ligated with an absorbable suture. If the mass is small and rostral enough, a portion of the symphysis can be left intact, leaving the mandible as a single unit, and preventing mandibular drifting.[17] Also, if the mass is small and centered on the incisive teeth, the canines can be preserved, avoiding the risk of postoperative mandibular drift.[18] Preserving the canines should be done only if appropriate margins can be obtained while removing the tumor.

After dissection of the soft tissue, the bone cut can be performed using an oscillating or reciprocating saw, a piezotome, or a burr. The use of an osteotome and mallet is not advised, as this may fracture or fissure the jaw in an uncontrolled, unexpected direction. The bone cut should be done between teeth and not through them. If the root of a tooth is accidentally damaged, the tooth should be extracted to avoid the risk of a tooth root abscess. Osteotomies are made in the interdental space beyond the planned surgical margin. To protect the soft tissues on the medial aspect of the mandible, if the cut is performed caudal to the symphysis, a Freer periosteal elevator, a Hohmann retractor, or a Senn retractor can be interposed between the mandibular bone and the oral soft tissues. If the bone cut is performed caudal to PM_2, the inferior alveolar artery will be transected inside the mandibular canal. This vessel should be grabbed with fine-tipped hemostats or DeBakey forceps and occluded with hemoclips, a ligature, indirect electrosurgery by applying the cautery pen to the forceps grasping the vessel, or, in small dogs and cats, by filling the alveolar canal with bone wax to tamponade the hemorrhage. Having these instruments ready before the bone cut is performed will diminish the amount of bleeding encountered during the procedure. The author commonly uses hemoclips or electrosurgery to address the bleeding from the artery but still uses bone wax to help stop the minor bleeding arising from the cut surface of the bone. The bone cut is performed in the same way on the contralateral side.

A wedge of skin is commonly removed before closure to avoid having a redundant amount of skin that may lead to wound dehiscence, and this is balanced with not having enough skin for closure over the cut edge of the mandible, which could also lead to dehiscence with too much tension. If the tumor involves the skin (skin is not freely movable on top of the mass) this should be removed en bloc. If the most caudal part of the symphysis is preserved, bone tunnels can be drilled and sutures passed through them to allow placement of sutures to decrease the chance of dehiscence. The defect created is closed in three layers forming a "T" when closing the mucosal layer. The labial mucosa is elevated to create a mucosal flap, to achieve a tension-free closure. The author mainly utilizes monofilament absorbable sutures in cruciate mattress patterns for each layer (2-0, 3-0, or 4-0 depending on the patient's size). Some surgeons may prefer using a simple continuous pattern for the mucosal layer closure to decrease the surgical time, and some may elect to use a multifilament absorbable suture, such as polyglactin 910.

Unilateral Rostral Mandibulectomy

Hair is clipped from the ventrolateral aspect of the lip ipsilateral to the mass. The dog is positioned in a lateral, slightly obliqued recumbency. The surgical margins are measured with a sterile marker and pencil, and the mucosa is incised with a scalpel blade. Usually, the rostral mandibular cut is performed at the level of the symphysis or between one of the incisor teeth, depending on the location of the mass. The soft tissue covering the rostral mandible is elevated, and the arteries, veins, and nerves arising from the rostral, middle, and caudal mental foramina are identified, ligated, and transected. The author usually uses electrosurgery for this part of the surgery.

The caudal bone cut is usually done between PM_2 and PM_3 to avoid having to elevate the root of the canine tooth that extends caudally to the level of PM_1. Even if a larger amount of mandible is removed compared with what would have been removed measuring 1–2 cm of margins, this is not a problem, as the cosmetic appearance and function of the mandible are similar. The bone cut should be performed between teeth, and if a tooth root is accidentally damaged, the tooth should be extracted to avoid the risk of tooth root abscess formation. The rostral cut is usually performed first, using an oscillating saw. When transecting the caudal aspect of the mandible, the inferior alveolar artery will be transected. This vessel should be grabbed with fine-tipped hemostats or DeBakey forceps and occluded with hemoclips, a ligature, indirect electrosurgery by applying the cautery pen to the forceps grasping the vessel, or, in small dogs and cats, by filling the alveolar canal with bone wax to tamponade the hemorrhage. Closure of the mandibulectomy is usually performed in two layers with absorbable monofilament sutures in a simple continuous or cruciate mattress pattern (2-0, 3-0, or 4-0 depending on the size of the patient). Bone tunnels can be drilled in the rostral aspect of the mandible with suture passed through the tunnels to help prevent dehiscence if the mucosal bites do not seem to offer enough strength to repair.

Segmental, Rim, and Caudal Mandibulectomy

Hair is clipped from the ventrolateral aspect of the lip ipsilateral to the mass. For masses extending to the caudal aspect of the mandible, the cheek is shaved, too. The dog is positioned in a lateral slightly ventrally obliqued recumbency. The surgical margins of the mucosa are marked with a sterile marker and are incised with a scalpel blade. As much as possible of the labial mucosa is saved, without compromising the surgical margins, as this will be used to close the defect created. If the mass has a large medial component, the author starts the dissection of the mucosa at the rostral aspect of the planned mandibulectomy site and elevates both the buccal and lingual mucosa.

A Freer periosteal elevator, a Hohmann retractor, or a Senn retractor is used to protect the soft tissues on the medial aspect of the mandible, and the bone cut is performed with an oscillating saw. Once this cut is finished, bleeding from the inferior alveolar artery is controlled by grabbing the vessel with fine-tipped hemostats or DeBakey forceps and stopped with a hemoclip, ligature, or electrosurgery. In small dogs and cats, filling the alveolar canal with bone wax can also be done to tamponade the hemorrhage. Now that the mandible has been transected, the caudal segment can be moved abaxially improving the exposure of the lingual mucosa, and therefore, making the dissection easier (Figure 12.3).

For small benign or malignant tumors at the alveolar margin of the mandible with no or minimal bone involvement and not invading the mandibular canal, a rim mandibulectomy can be performed. In this technique, the mucosa is incised with a scalpel blade until the underlying bone is exposed. A piezotome, a sagittal or biradial saw blade, or a burr, depending on the surgeon's preference, is used to perform the bone cut making sure to preserve the ventral aspect of the mandible. Sparing the ventral aspect of the mandible will prevent mandibular drift from happening, avoiding the postoperative alterations in the kinematics of the contralateral temporomandibular joint. Bone cuts for both segmental and rim mandibulectomy should be performed between teeth. If a tooth root is accidentally damaged, the tooth should be extracted to avoid the risk of tooth root abscess formation (Figure 12.4).

Closure is performed by suturing the submucosa and mucosa in two layers in a continuous or cruciate mattress pattern with monofilament (e.g., poliglecaprone 25) or multifilament (e.g., polyglactin 910) absorbable sutures (2-0, 3-0, or 4-0 depending on the size of the dog).

If the mass is affecting the caudal aspect of the mandible, a full-thickness incision of the lip (i.e., cheilotomy) from the oral commissure to the ramus of the mandible should be performed to increase the exposure.[18] This will also help with the proper positioning of the saw blade for the caudal cut, minimizing the risk of an invertedly incomplete excision of the tumor. The author tends to place two stay sutures at the level of the transected lip mucosa to help with orientation during closure.

If a caudal mandibulectomy is performed, it is important to identify and ligate the inferior alveolar artery before it enters the mandibular foramen during the dissection of the medial aspect of the mandible to avoid significant hemorrhage. The mandibulectomy site is closed as previously described, and the lip incision is closed in three layers with 3-0 or 4-0 monofilament absorbable suture in a simple continuous pattern, beginning with the commissure to ensure apposition.

Potential Complications

Changes in cosmetic appearance can vary depending on the extent of the procedure. It is advised to show the owner pictures of dogs that previously received the procedure to help the client understand how their animal will look after the procedure. Especially for the more invasive procedures, it may be advisable to send a picture of the animal to the

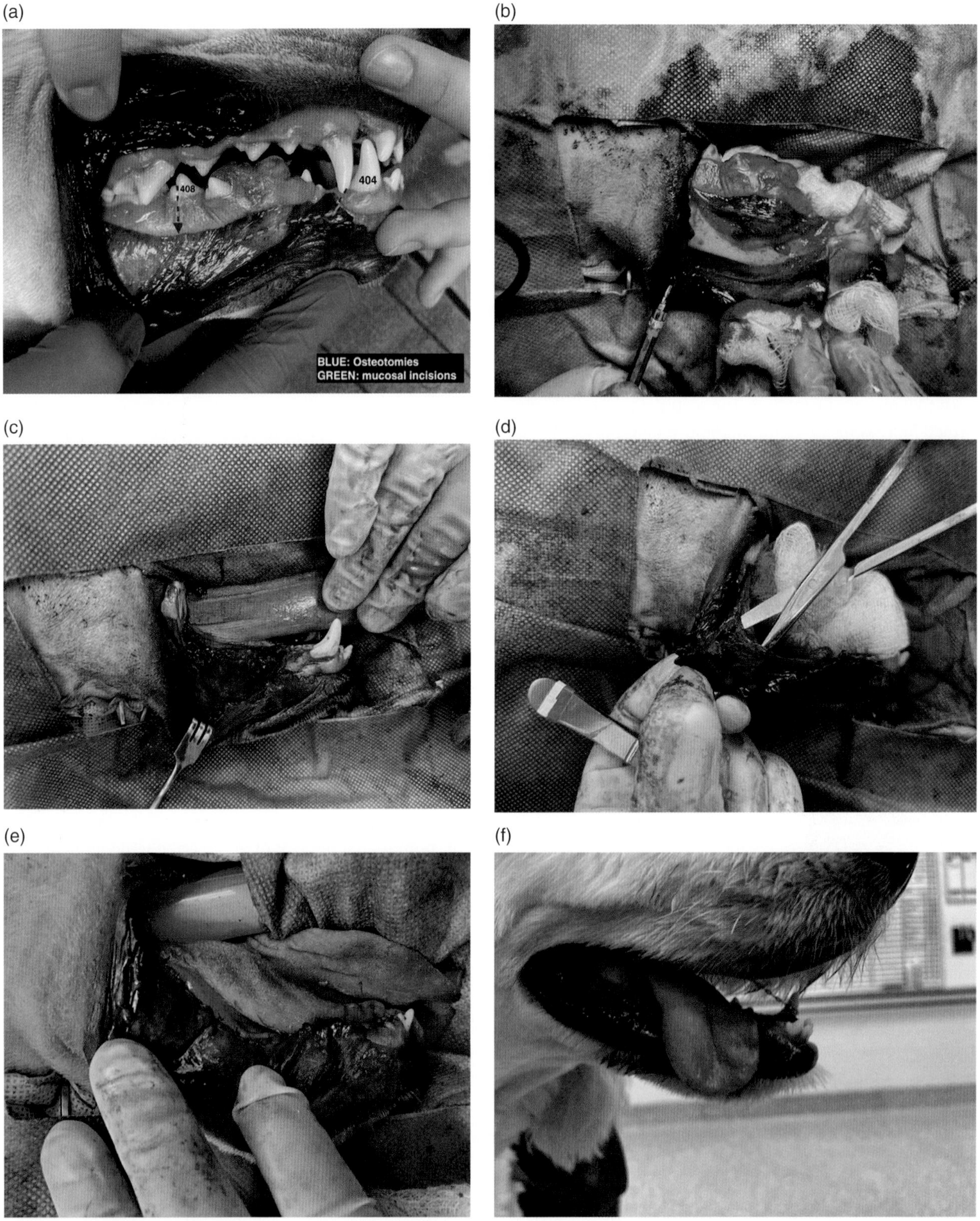

Figure 12.3 Step-by-step surgery description of a segmental mandibulectomy. (a) Soft tissue and bone margins for the mandibulectomy are planned based on the results of preoperative advanced imaging. Blue arrows represent the bone margins; green dotted line represents the soft tissue margin; (b) once the mucosa is incised and elevated, a sagittal saw is used to perform the rostral and caudal mandibular osteotomies. The author usually starts with the rostral osteotomy to help with the medial soft tissue dissection; (c) appearance of the surgical site after the segment of the mandible containing the tumor has been removed; (d) elevation of the labial mucosal flap to obtain a tension-free closure. This step is of paramount importance to prevent dehiscence of the surgical site; (e) immediate postoperative appearance of the surgical site after closure in two layers with monofilament synthetic absorbable suture using a simple interrupted pattern; (f) two weeks postoperative appearance of the surgical site. In this patient, orthodontic buttons and an orthodontic elastic rubber chain were applied to help prevent mandibular drifting, which may require referral to or the aid of a veterinary dentist. *Source:* © Josep Aisa.

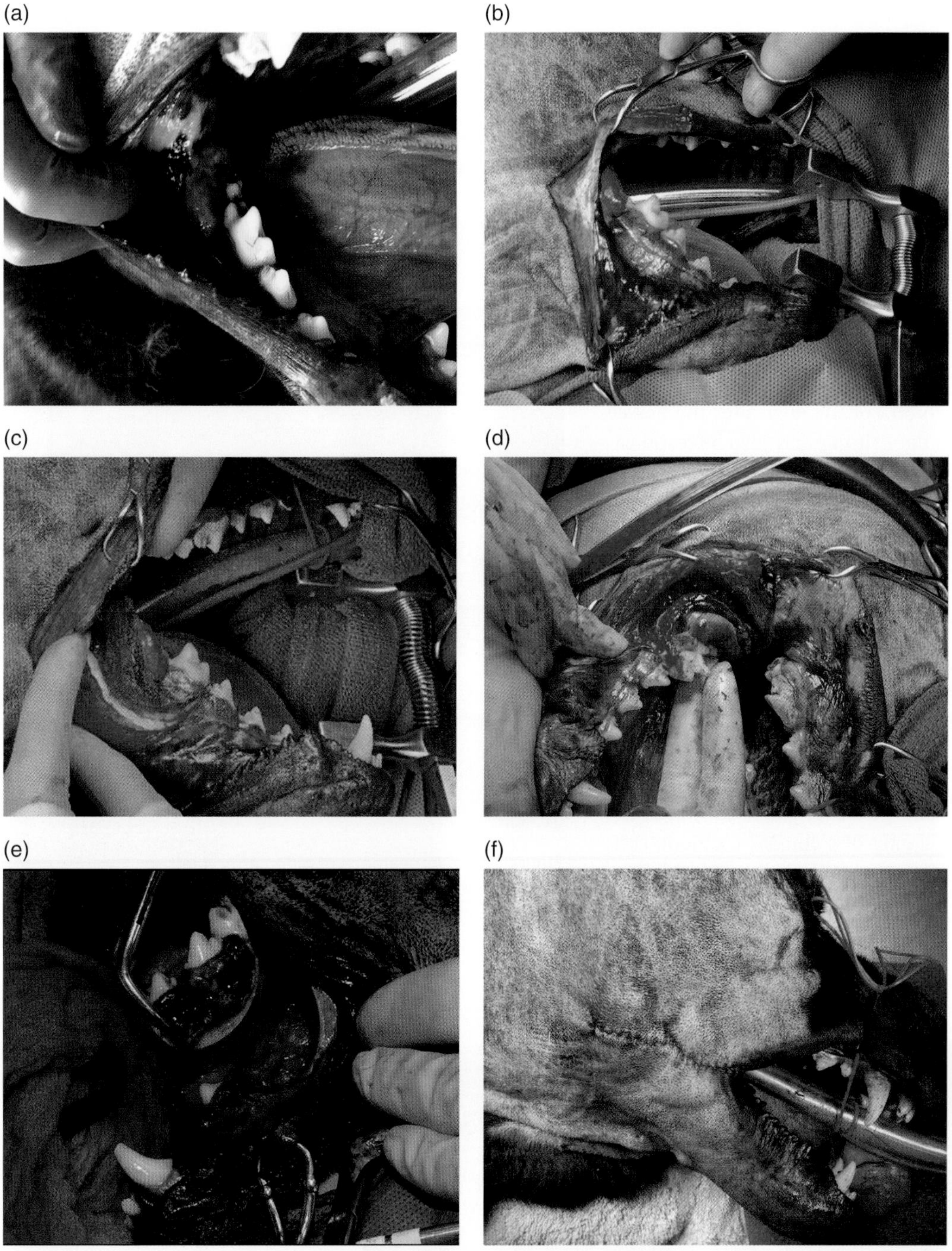

Figure 12.4 Step-by-step surgery description of a rim mandibulectomy. (a) A small oral amelanotic melanoma not invading the bone in the caudal mandible of a dog; (b) to gain better exposure of the mass and caudal mandible, a cheilotomy has been performed; (c) after marking the desired soft tissue margins with a sterile marker, dissection of the gingiva surrounding the tumor has been performed with etching of the desired bone margins made around the mass using monopolar electrosurgery; (d) in this case, the ostectomy was performed by means of a combination of sagittal saw and burr; (e) in a different case, the ostectomy for a small oral melanoma was performed using a biradial saw; (f) appearance of the dog after closure of the cheilotomy site. *Source:* © Kristin Coleman.

owner, once recovered from anesthesia, before the pet is dismissed or discharged from the clinic.

Several complications are described after mandibulectomies. A large retrospective study looking at complications after mandibulectomy and maxillectomies in dogs found an overall 38% complication rate after mandibulectomies. Mandibular drift and malocclusion were the most common (14%), followed by dehiscence (13.3%), pseudo-ranula formation (7.9%), and difficulty prehending food (6.5%).[19] Mandibular drift happens more commonly after segmental mandibulectomies or unilateral rostral mandibulectomies that do not spare the symphysis. This can lead to alteration of the kinematics of the contralateral temporomandibular joint and cause subsequent arthritis. To prevent mandibular drift from happening, the mandibulectomy site can be reconstructed with a compression-resistant matrix and bone morphogenic protein (rh BMP-2) for non-neoplastic[20] and benign odontogenic tumors.[21] Rib autograft is another method described to prevent mandibular drifting.[22] Elastic training, consisting of the application of orthodontic buttons and an orthodontic elastic rubber chain on teeth of the contralateral mandible, can be used instead of reconstructing the defect. Unfortunately, this technique resulted in the recurrence of the drift in 50% of the dogs after the device was removed.[23] Mandibular drifting may also be responsible for upper lip or palatal ulceration due to trauma from the drifting canine tooth. If this is seen, extraction of the canine tooth responsible for the trauma or crown amputation and vital pulpotomy is recommended.[18]

Suture dehiscence often happens at the level of the mucosa at the mandibular osteotomy site. This can be treated with a revision surgery or commonly allowing the area to heal by the second intention. The mouth has great healing potential, and even if the bone is exposed, granulation tissue will cover it quickly (Figure 12.5). Pseudo-ranula, which is a fluid-filled soft balloon-like structure on the lateral aspect of the base of the tongue usually seen the morning after surgery, is only of a limited cosmetic concern and is likely caused by the accumulation of inflammatory fluid caused by surgery in the sublingual mucosa (Figure 12.6). Another possible cause for this type of lesion is the transection of the mandibular/sublingual salivary gland duct that traverses the base of the tongue to exit rostrolateral to the frenulum within the sublingual caruncle. The pseudo-ranula usually resolves within two weeks from surgery and does not require treatment.

In dogs, difficulty in prehending food is mostly seen after aggressive bilateral rostral mandibulectomies (past PM_2). Most of these dogs will adapt to this new condition within

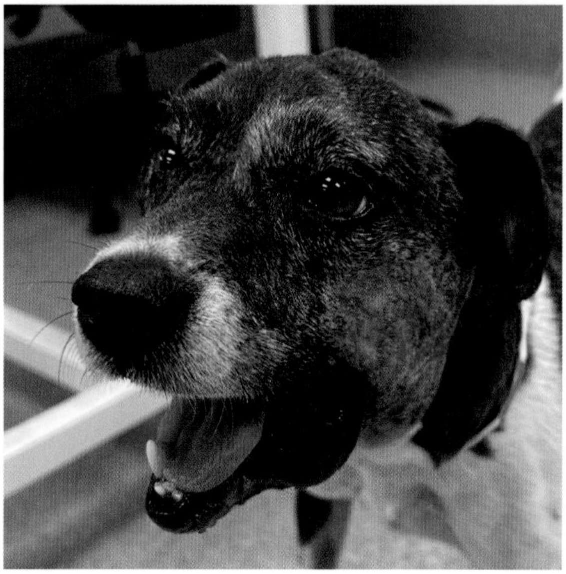

Figure 12.6 Appearance of a dog after a left hemimandibulectomy for a squamous cell carcinoma, notice the pseudoranula formation under the tongue. *Source:* © Giovanni Tremolada.

(a) (b)

Figure 12.5 Bone exposure in a bilateral rostral mandibulectomy after dehiscence. (a) Recheck at one week after the procedure. Note the granulation tissue and the presence of exposed bone. (b) Same dog one week after the recheck. Note the bone has been completely covered by granulation tissue. An attempt to revise the mandibulectomy site was not done in this case for owner's financial concerns and because the dog was asymptomatic for the dehiscence. *Source:* © Giovanni Tremolada.

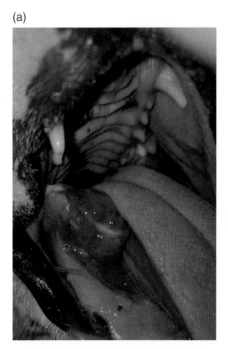

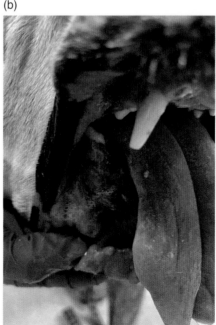

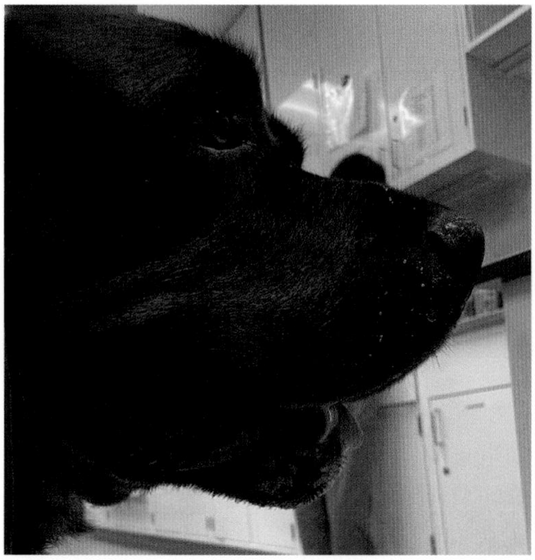

Figure 12.7 Appearance of a dog after bilateral rostral mandibulectomy. Notice the saliva accumulation at the level of the chin. This is a common complication after this procedure. *Source:* © Giovanni Tremolada.

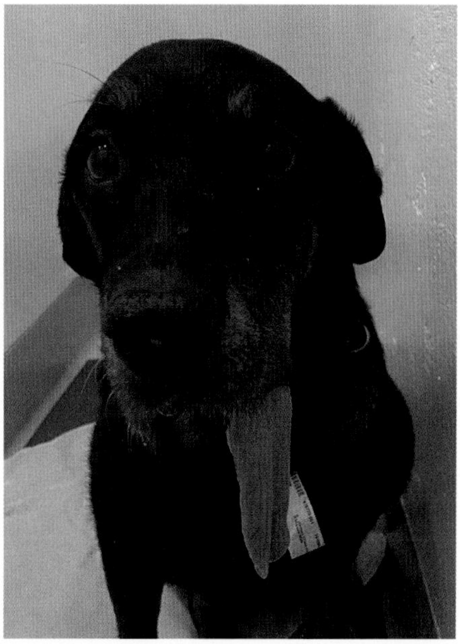

Figure 12.8 Appearance of a dog one year after one and half mandibulectomy for a mandibular osteosarcoma. Note the typical appearance with marked tongue protrusion. *Source:* © Giovanni Tremolada.

a few days from surgery. Dogs after bilateral rostral mandibulectomies frequently also have an accumulation of saliva at the rostral aspect of the mandible (Figure 12.7). This is usually not of concern but can be responsible for lip dermatitis in some cases, and owners should be warned of the extra drooling that may require cleaning of their dog's chin and the surgical site. Tongue protrusion and excessive drooling are commonly seen after large segmental mandibulectomies or unilateral mandibulectomies (Figure 12.8). A commissurorraphy can be performed to reduce the severity of these clinical signs.[24] Surgical site infection is uncommon despite working in a contaminated environment, as the oral cavity has an excellent blood supply and immunoglobulin A (IgA) is the main immune factor in saliva to regulate oral homeostasis and provide protection from common oral pathogens.

Cats are reported not to tolerate mandibular surgery as well as dogs. Short-term inappetence has been reported in 83% of cats following bilateral rostral mandibulectomy and in 74% after unilateral mandibulectomies.[25] In that study, 13% of cats undergoing some type of mandibulectomy never returned to eating spontaneously.[25] Of this 13%, more than half of the cases were cats that received a one and a half (also known as "three quarter") mandibulectomies. In a more recent study on eight cats undergoing radical mandibulectomy, six returned to eating spontaneously within 12 weeks from surgery, with two cats requiring lifelong feeding tubes.[26] The possibility for cats to never return to eating independently should always be discussed before surgery with the client. For this reason, while in dogs, the author does not place routinely esophageal feeding tubes, all cats undergoing mandibulectomies are discharged with an esophageal feeding tube. After mandibulectomies, cats will also have issues grooming, and the owner will need to help with it. Cosmetic appearance is usually good (Figure 12.9).

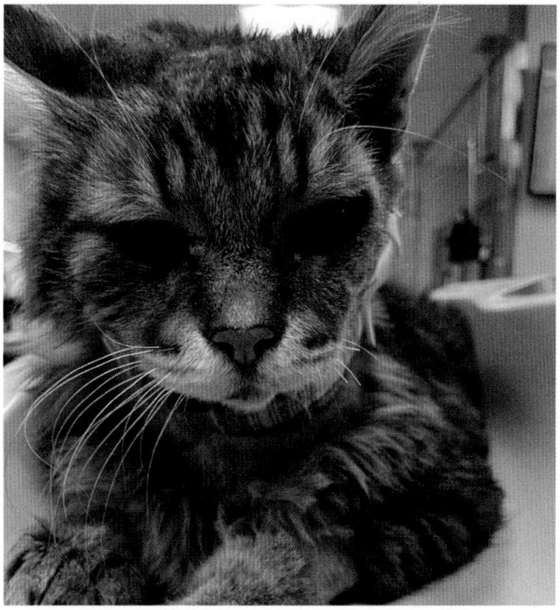

Figure 12.9 Appearance of a cat two days postoperative after a hemimandibulectomy for an odontogenic tumor. Note the good aesthetic appearance and the presence of an esophagostomy feeding tube to support the animal in the first few weeks after surgery. This cat was able to return to spontaneously eating within the first week after surgery. *Source:* © Giovanni Tremolada.

Postoperative Care

Animals are hospitalized on IV fluids and pain medications until they can eat or tolerate tube feeding. Most of the dogs will be able to be discharged from the hospital within 24–48 hours after surgery. Blood-tinged saliva may be noted in the first few days after surgery, and this is considered normal. Pain is controlled immediately after surgery with injectable opioids and an nonsteroidal anti-inflammatory drug (NSAID), if indicated. The author routinely infiltrates the tissues transected with liposomal encapsulated bupivacaine for long-lasting local anesthesia. Preoperative inferior alveolar block can be done with lidocaine or bupivacaine to help with intraoperative pain management. Dogs are usually discharged with a 7–10 day course of an NSAID (if not contraindicated) and gabapentin (5–10 mg/kg PO BID-TID). If infection is suspected, such as a necrotic center of the tumor or osteomyelitis of the mandible, a short course of an antibiotic known for its bone-penetrating ability, such as clindamycin, can be dispensed.

Soft food (either canned or moistening kibble) is prescribed after surgery for two weeks, and chew toys/sticks are not allowed for a month. Sometimes, for more extensive mandibulectomies, hand-feeding meatballs of soft food may be necessary for the first few weeks after surgery until the dog adapts to eating spontaneously. Warm soft food is usually offered to cats to entice them to eat. If they are not eating spontaneously, food should be administered through the feeding tube placed at the time of surgery. Both dogs and cats are discharged with an Elizabethan collar to avoid traumatizing the incision site. The animal should return after two weeks to recheck the incision site, and they should return earlier if the owner notices incisional complications or a foul smell from the mouth. Re-staging should be performed accordingly depending on the final diagnosis of the mandibular mass removed (lymph node palpation, chest radiographs, serial sedated oral exams, etc.).

References

1. Evans, H.E. and de Lahunta, A. (2013). The skull. In: *Miller's Anatomy of the Dog*, 4e, 104–105. St. Louis: Elsevier.
2. Abrams, B.E., Selmic, L.E., Cocca, C.J. et al. (2019). Segmental mandibulectomy as a novel adjunct management strategy for the treatment of an advanced cholesteatoma in a dog. *Can. Vet. J.* 60: 995–1000.
3. Verstraete, F.M.J., Arzi, B., and Lanz, G.C. (2019). *Oral and Maxillofacial Surgery in Dogs and Cats*, 2e, 515–528. St. Louis: Elsevier.
4. Bonfanti, U., Bertazzolo, W., Gracis, M. et al. (2015). Diagnostic value of cytological analysis of tumours and tumour-like lesions of the oral cavity in dogs and cats: a prospective study on 114 cases. *Vet. J.* 205: 322–327.
5. Mikiewicz, M., Pazdzior-Czapula, K., Gesek, M. et al. (2019). Canine and feline oral cavity tumours and tumour-like lesions: a retrospective study of 486 cases (2015-2017). *J. Comp. Pathol.* 172: 80–87.
6. Ghirelli, C.O., Villamizar, L.A., and Pinto, A.C. (2013). Comparison of standard radiography and computed tomography in 21 dogs with maxillary masses. *J. Vet. Dent.* 30: 72–76.
7. Liptak, J.M. and Lascellas, B.D.X. (2022). Oral tumors. In: *Veterinary Surgical Oncology* (ed. S.T. Kudnig and B. Seguin), 182–264. Hoboken, NJ: Wiley-Blackwell.
8. Schwarz, P.D., Withrow, S.J., Curtis, C.R. et al. (1991). Mandibular resection as a treatment for oral cancer in 81 dogs. *J. Am. Anim. Hosp. Assoc.* 27: 601–610.
9. Tuohy, J.L., Selmic, L.E., Worley, D.R. et al. (2014). Outcome following curative-intent surgery for oral melanoma in dogs: 70 cases (1998–2011). *J. Am. Vet. Med. Assoc.* 245: 1266–1273.
10. Williams, L.E. and Packer, R.A. (2003). Association between lymph node size and metastasis in dogs with oral malignant melanoma: 100 cases (1987-2001). *J. Am. Vet. Med. Assoc.* 222: 1234–1236.
11. Skinner, O.T., Boston, S.E., Giglio, R.F. et al. (2018). Diagnostic accuracy of contrast-enhanced computed tomography for assessment of mandibular and medial retropharyngeal lymph node metastasis in dogs with oral and nasal cancer. *Vet. Comp. Oncol.* 16: 562–570.
12. Grimes, J.A., Secrest, S.A., Northrup, N.C. et al. (2017). Indirect computed tomography lymphangiography with aqueous contrast for evaluation of sentinel lymph nodes in dogs with tumors of the head. *Vet. Radiol. Ultrasound* 58: 559–564.
13. Randall, E.K., Jones, M.D., Kraft, S.L. et al. (2020). The development of an indirect computed tomography lymphography protocol for sentinel lymph node detection in head and neck cancer and comparison to other sentinel lymph node mapping techniques. *Vet. Comp. Oncol.* 18: 634–644.
14. Worley, D.R. (2022). Hemolymphatic system. In: *Veterinary Surgical Oncology* (ed. S.T. Kudnig and B. Seguin), 624–638. Hoboken, NJ: Wiley Blackwell.
15. Chiti, L.E., Stefanello, D., and Manfredi, M. (2021). To map or not to map the cN0 neck: impact of sentinel lymph node biopsy in canine head and neck tumours. *Vet. Comp. Oncol.* 19: 661–670.
16. Nemanic, S., London, C.A., and Wisner, E.R. (2006). Comparison of thoracic radiographs and single breath-hold helical CT for detection of pulmonary nodules in dogs with metastatic neoplasia. *J. Vet. Intern. Med.* 20: 508–515.

17 Smithson, C.W. and Taney, K. (2009). Symphyseal sparing rostral mandibulectomy. *J. Vet. Dent.* 26: 264–269.

18 Dernell, W.S., Schwarz, P.D., and Withrow, S.J. (1998). Mandibulectomy. In: *Current Techniques in Small Animal Surgery*, 3e (ed. M.J. Bojrab, G.W. Ellison, and B. Slocum), 132–142. Baltimore, MD: Williams and Wilkins.

19 Cray, M., Selmic, L.E., Kindra, C. et al. (2021). Analysis of risk factors associated with complications following mandibulectomy and maxillectomy in dogs. *J. Am. Vet. Med. Assoc.* 259: 265–274.

20 Boudrieau, R.J. (2015). Initial experience with rhBMP-2 delivered in a compressive resistant matrix for mandibular reconstruction in 5 dogs. *Vet. Surg.* 44: 443–458.

21 Tsugawa, A.J., Arzi, B., Vapniarsky, N. et al. (2022). A retrospective study on mandibular reconstruction following excision of canine acanthomatous ameloblastoma. *Front. Vet. Sci.* 9: 900031. https://doi.org/10.3389/fvets.2022.900031.

22 Bracker, K.E. and Trout, N.J. (2000). Use of a free cortical ulnar autograft following en bloc resection of a mandibular tumor. *J. Am. Anim. Hosp. Assoc.* 36: 76–79.

23 Bar-Am, Y. and Verstraete, F.J. (2010). Elastic training for the prevention of mandibular drift following mandibulectomy in dogs: 18 cases (2005-2008). *Vet. Surg.* 39: 574–580.

24 Durand, C. (2017). Commissurorraphy in the dog. *J. Vet. Dent.* 34: 36–40.

25 Northrup, N.C., Selting, K.A., Rassnick, K.M. et al. (2006). Outcomes of cats with oral tumors treated with mandibulectomy: 42 cases. *J. Am. Anim. Hosp. Assoc.* 42: 350–360.

26 Boston, S.E., van Stee, L.L., Bacon, N.J. et al. (2020). Outcomes of eight cats with oral neoplasia treated with radical mandibulectomy. *Vet. Surg.* 49: 222–232.

13

Sialoadenectomy

Grayson Cole

Gulf Coast Veterinary Specialists, Houston, TX, USA

Key Points

- Knowledge of salivary gland anatomy is critical to successful surgery.
- There are four paired major salivary glands (mandibular, sublingual, parotid, and zygomatic), as well as minor salivary tissue in dogs and cats.
- Removal of all salivary tissue is mandatory for a positive long-term prognosis for surgical treatment of salivary mucoceles.
- Medical management is recommended for sialoadenosis.

Introduction

There are four major salivary glands in the dog and cat. These are the paired mandibular, sublingual, zygomatic, and parotid salivary glands. These major glands secrete saliva into the mouth via ducts that travel from the gland to the oral cavity. There is additional minor salivary gland tissue in the oral cavity of the dog and cat that is named according to its location and includes tissue in the nasopharynx, oropharynx, tongue, palate, cheek, lip, and gingiva.[1] The molar salivary glands are the most prominent of the minor glands in the cat. These glands secrete saliva directly into the mouth. In one anatomical study utilizing advanced imaging, no variation of salivary gland anatomy was seen in the cats that were examined compared to the documented canine anatomy.[2] However, variation of the mandibular gland anatomy was occasionally seen in dogs, which resulted in the gland being located medial to the digastricus and rostral to the medial retropharyngeal lymph node.[2] Salivary gland surgery requires an understanding of local relevant anatomy, as well as physiology and potential pathophysiology.

Indications and Pre-operative Considerations

Sialocele

The most common indication for salivary gland surgery in veterinary medicine is a salivary mucocele, which is also commonly referred to as a sialocele. For consistency, it will be referred to as a sialocele for the remainder of the chapter. A sialocele is defined as an accumulation of salivary fluid due to its leakage into the interstitial space.[3] Although specific underlying causes have been reported, such as trauma, foreign bodies, sialoliths, neoplasia, and even heartworm infection,[4] an underlying cause is rarely found. Thus, an idiopathic sialocele is the most common type seen in veterinary medicine.

Depending upon the gland affected and the deposition of saliva, a sialocele can manifest in different ways. The most common presentation of a sialocele is a submandibular swelling secondary to leakage from the mandibular and sublingual gland complex, which share a capsule.[3] Alternative differential diagnoses for submandibular swellings include

Techniques in Small Animal Soft Tissue, Orthopedic, and Ophthalmic Surgery, First Edition. Edited by Kristin A. Coleman.

Companion website: www.wiley.com/go/coleman/surgeries

branchial cysts, foreign bodies, trauma, and neoplasia. Salivary mucoceles have also been reported in alternate locations, including in the nasopharynx,[5] pharynx,[6] side of the face,[7] and periorbital region. Pharyngeal mucoceles are most commonly seen in miniature and toy poodles. Approximately 50% of patients with a pharyngeal sialocele present for dyspnea, and 43% have a concurrent cervical mucocele. The mandibular–sublingual complex is the most commonly implicated source of pharyngeal mucoceles. In one study, recurrence occurred only in one patient of 14 who had the associated mandibular and sublingual salivary glands excised.[6]

The location of the swelling is generally related to which salivary gland is affected. A mucocele underneath the tongue is also often referred to as a ranula, which is the result of a sublingual sialocele within the polystomatic portion. Sialoceles originating from the parotid salivary gland will typically present with swelling on the side of the face, near the ear canal.[8] Further, sialoceles originating from the zygomatic salivary gland frequently result in exophthalmos; however, there is one report of a zygomatic sialocele resulting in submandibular swelling.[3]

Salivary Neoplasia

Salivary neoplasia can arise from any of the major or minor salivary glands. Approximately 88% of all salivary gland neoplasia are epithelial tumors.[1] The most commonly reported cancers are adenocarcinoma, mucoepidermoid carcinoma, acinar cell carcinoma, squamous cell carcinoma, and carcinosarcomas. Other reported tumors include extraskeletal osteosarcoma,[9] sialolipomas,[10] pleomorphic adenoma,[11] and basal cell carcinoma.[12] As with any neoplastic process, the workup should include FNA or biopsy of the area of concern, as well as appropriate staging. Staging should include thoracic radiographs, abdominal ultrasound, and FNA of the suspected draining lymph node. These diagnostics could also be supplanted by computed tomography (CT) of the thorax, abdomen, and ideally, the head and neck to evaluate the primary tumor and local lymph nodes. Surgical excision is the treatment of choice for most salivary gland tumors; however, due to the anatomic location of all salivary gland tissue, wide excision is not feasible. Therefore, owners should be counseled that radiation or other adjunctive therapy may be recommended after reviewing the histopathology results.

Sialoliths

Although uncommon, sialoliths have also been reported in the dog. The etiology is thought to be due to slow or obstructed salivary flow from a chronic sialocele or secondary to a previously performed parotid duct transposition.

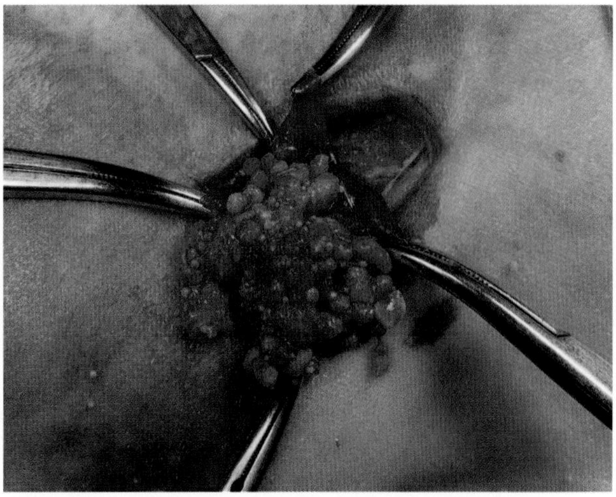

Figure 13.1 Sialoliths seen during sialoadenectomy in a dog (dorsal is at the top and rostral is to the right). *Source:* © Dr. Kristin Coleman.

The stone composition is often calcium oxalate or calcium carbonate.[13] Sialoliths can be incidental findings but can also obstruct salivary ducts and can be seen concurrently with a sialocele.[14] Surgical excision of the affected salivary gland and duct is curative (Figure 13.1).

Sialoadenitis

Sialoadenitis, an immune-mediated inflammatory condition, has been reported in dogs.[15] The predominant clinical finding in this condition is enlargement of the affected salivary gland; however, dogs may also present with pain in the region of the gland, hypersialism, or nausea.[15] Histopathological findings include inflammatory infiltrates of predominately neutrophils, which surround and can replace salivary acini and ducts. Necrosis can also occur, which may be due to pressure necrosis from inflammation within the inflexible capsule of the gland. This condition may respond to corticosteroids and can be differentiated from sialoadenosis on the basis of cytology or histopathology.[15]

Sialoadenosis

Sialoadenosis is a noninflammatory condition of the salivary glands. It is typically associated with bilaterally enlarged and uniform salivary glands that are nonpainful.[16] Surgical excision is not helpful, but dogs will often respond to phenobarbital treatment.[16] Confusingly, this condition has also been described in the literature as necrotizing sialometaplasia and hypersialism. The pathophysiology is poorly understood but thought to be related to a primary abnormality of sympathetic innervation to the associated salivary gland. Besides the palpably enlarged glands, patients can also present with retching, gulping, and vomiting. Cytology and histopathology can reveal inflammation or normal salivary tissue.[16] In one study, all dogs had reported improvement in clinical signs within days of starting typical anti-seizure doses of phenobarbital; however, treatment duration can be prolonged due to relapse of signs after less than a month of treatment.[16] Sialoadenosis should be considered in dogs with bilaterally symmetrical salivary gland enlargement and concurrent gastrointestinal signs. Although cytology and histopathology are not definitive for the diagnosis of this condition, they may be able to rule out neoplastic or inflammatory salivary gland diseases.

Pre-operative Diagnostic Imaging

When preparing for sialoadenectomy of a ventral cervical sialocele that does not trend toward a particular laterality, diagnostic imaging can be helpful in determining which gland is affected; however, the salivary gland in question may appear normal on imaging, as the salivary leakage is often from the duct. Skull and neck radiographs are often non-diagnostic with the exception of radiopaque sialoliths. Ultrasound is a commonly performed diagnostic tool. Ultrasound is helpful in identifying fluid pockets for sampling (if needed in cases of sialoceles), and it may be possible to associate the fluid pocket with a particular salivary gland, aiding in guiding the surgeon to the appropriate gland for surgical excision. Ultrasound can also be utilized to evaluate the surrounding lymph nodes, either for sampling or planned excision if definitive surgery is pursued.

Advanced imaging has also been described for further characterization of salivary gland pathology. Magnetic resonance imaging has been reported but is uncommonly utilized clinically. CT can be utilized to evaluate the salivary glands and associated lymph nodes as well. This is especially helpful in cases of confirmed or suspected neoplasia, as feasibility of resection will depend upon how invasive the tumor is. Common findings for dogs with sialoceles on CT include mineralized foci or osseous metaplasia in the associated salivary gland and frond-like walls of the mucocele itself.[17] If further detail is needed, sialography has also been reported either with traditional radiography[7] or in combination with CT.[18] Even with CT and sialography, the sensitivity in detecting the diseased gland as compared to histopathology was only 67% in one report.[18]

Knowledge of the location of the individual caruncles is essential in performing sialography. The zygomatic caruncle is caudal to the last maxillary molar, the parotid caruncle is adjacent to the maxillary fourth premolar, and the mandibular and sublingual glands share a capsule with both ducts depositing saliva into the mouth via the sublingual caruncle ventral and rostral to the tongue within the frenulum[19]. These caruncles can often be cannulated with an intravenous catheter in order to inject contrast. In one study, non-diluted iodinated contrast at a dose of 2 mL/kg was used for sialography.[18] CT sialography can also be a helpful tool in determining if head and neck swelling of unknown etiology has salivary gland involvement.

Surgical Procedure

Mandibular and Sublingual Salivary Gland Excision

Skin Incision

Both lateral and ventral approaches have been described to approach the mandibular and sublingual salivary gland complex.[20] Generally, this is considered to be secondary to surgeon preference, positioning of the actual mucocele itself if present, and whether or not a unilateral or bilateral approach is to be performed. According to one study, a ventral approach led to higher risk of wound complications but a lower risk of sialocele recurrence.[20] However, tunneling under the digastricus muscle was not performed in all cases in the lateral approach group, which makes comparing recurrence rates between the two groups unreliable. The author prefers a lateral-oblique approach, which allows for approaching the gland itself from a subjectively easier lateral approach, then the dissection can be continued more ventrally as the duct is approached from caudal to rostral (Figure 13.2).

Mandibular Salivary Gland Dissection

The mandibular and sublingual salivary gland complex is typically found just rostral to the bifurcation of the jugular vein into the maxillary and linguofacial veins (Figure 13.3).

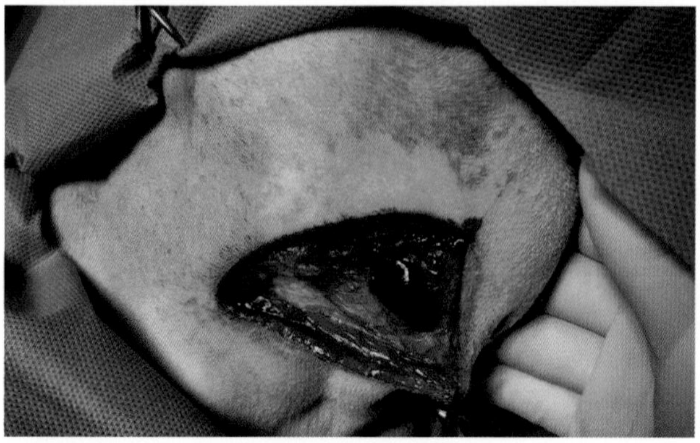

Figure 13.2 An incision is made over the right mandibular region. A small incision was then made into the salivary mucocele, and saliva is seen exiting the area (dorsal is at the top and rostral is to the right).

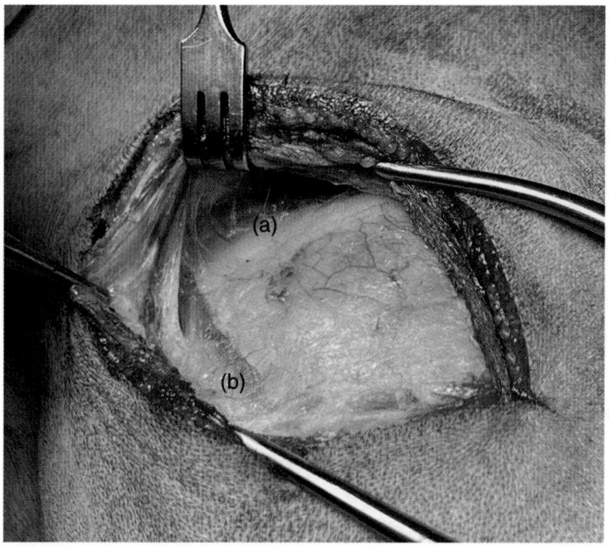

Figure 13.3 The mandibular salivary gland can be seen in the jugular bifurcation prior to dissection: (a) maxillary vein and (b) linguofacial vein (dorsal is at the top and rostral is to the right). *Source:* © Dr. Kristin Coleman.

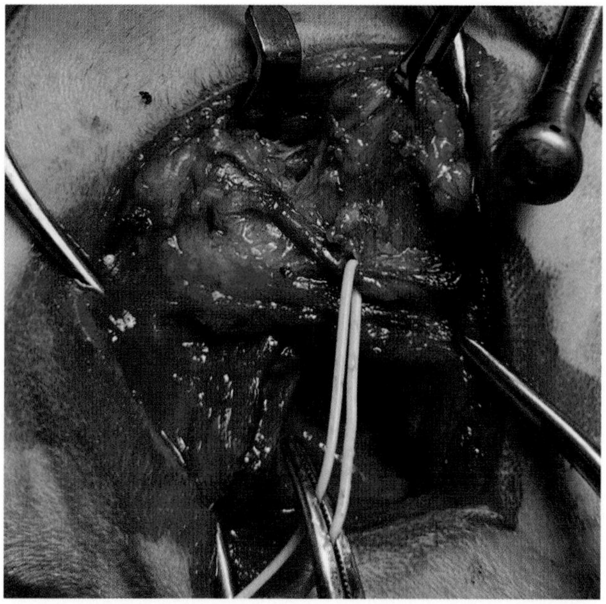

Figure 13.4 The mandibular salivary gland is grasped with an Allis tissue forcep to aid in dissection, as the linguofacial vein is retracted ventrally with vessel loops (dorsal is at the top and rostral is to the right).

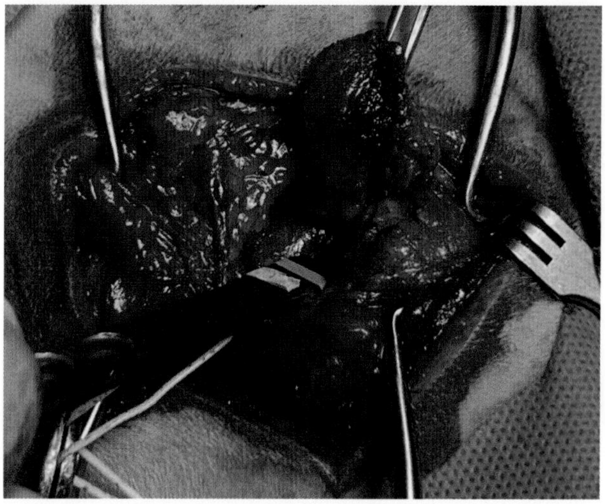

Figure 13.5 The mandibular and sublingual gland complex is dissected free to the level at which the duct dives underneath the digastricus muscle (dorsal is at the top and rostral is to the right).

Incising the capsule is helpful to facilitate dissection of the gland, which proceeds from caudal to rostral (Figure 13.2). Vessel loops can be useful to retract the jugular, maxillary, and/or linguofacial veins away from the surgical site in an atraumatic fashion (Figure 13.4). The mandibular lymph node is frequently just rostral and ventral to the mandibular salivary gland and should be extirpated in cases of suspected neoplasia. In the author's experience, this lymph node is often slightly enlarged and dark in appearance in cases with salivary mucoceles, but histopathology is often unrewarding.

After dissecting the mandibular and sublingual salivary gland complex from surrounding tissues and the surrounding capsule, the salivary duct will pass deep to the digastricus muscle (Figure 13.5). Tunneling under the digastricus muscle has been shown to result in the extraction of additional salivary gland tissue and may result in a lower risk of mucocele recurrence.[21] This additional step is not required if the salivary gland is being excised for a reason other than a mucocele, unless there is concern for disease progression from the gland into the salivary duct. The author prefers to use a large right-angle forceps to pass from medial to lateral, deep to the digastricus muscle (Figure 13.6). At this point, the duct can be clamped rostral to the gland, and the gland can be excised and submitted for histopathology, which will remove the bulk of salivary tissue and will allow for easier manipulation of the duct.

After transecting the gland, the duct can be pulled from lateral to medial, deep to the digastricus muscle in order to facilitate continued rostral dissection (Figure 13.7). The dissection should be continued at least to the level of the lingual nerve (Figure 13.8) or until no additional glandular tissue is seen. At this point in the author's experience, it is common to evert the oral or lingual mucosa by traction, so care should be utilized when excising additional tissue rostral to the lingual nerve.

Mucocele Dissection

By the time the mandibular and sublingual complex and duct have been excised, the surgeon often will have already encountered the mucocele itself. Chronic

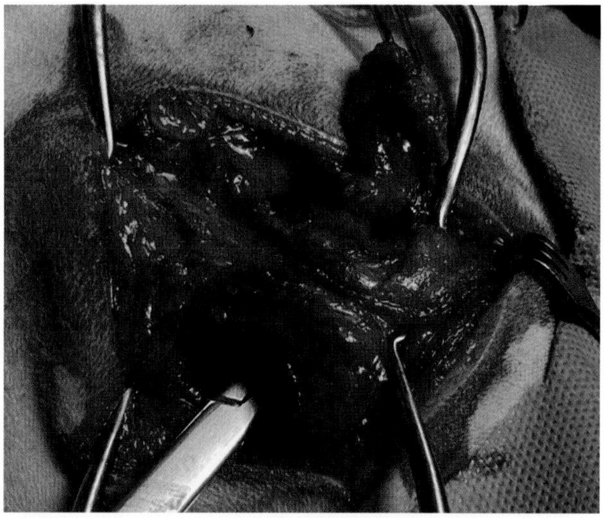

Figure 13.6 While securing the gland complex with an Allis tissue forcep, a large right-angle forceps is used to tunnel from medial to lateral underneath the digastricus muscle (dorsal is at the top and rostral is to the right).

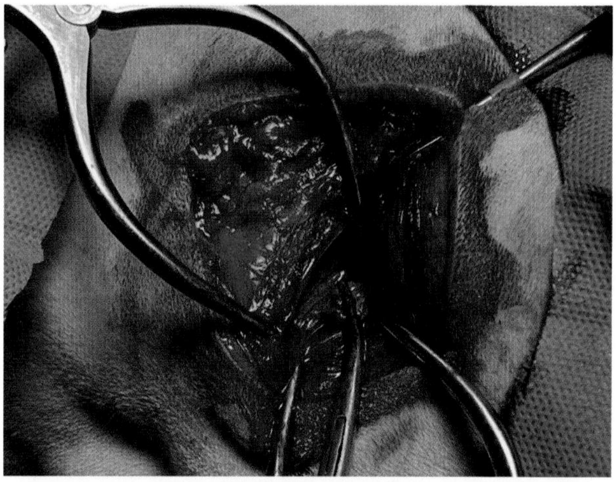

Figure 13.7 After transecting the mandibular and sublingual gland complex from the duct, the duct tissue is pulled from lateral to medial underneath the digastricus, such that the dissection can be continued rostrally. The duct with remaining salivary tissue is grasped with a Kelly hemostat, and a Senn retractor is being used to retract the digastricus laterally to facilitate further dissection (dorsal is at the top and rostral is to the right).

mucoceles may have mineralized or thick debris, and the debris should be lavaged out of the mucocele itself. Sometimes the mucocele can be excised en bloc. In the author's experience, this is only necessary when the wall of the mucocele is thickened from chronicity and well-demarcated; otherwise, the inflammation in the area causing the sialocele should resolve with removal of the diseased salivary tissue, drain placement, and warm compresses postoperatively. These patients still need a drain

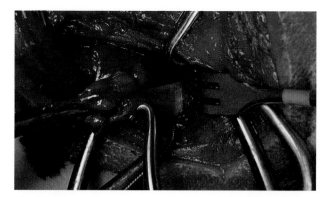

Figure 13.8 Dissection of the duct is continued to the level of the lingual nerve, which is seen in this image just caudal to the Senn retractor with fascial attachments extending to the salivary tissue (dorsal is at the top and rostral is to the right).

postoperatively due to the amount of dissection required and inflammation present in the subcutaneous tissues secondary to the salivary leakage. More often, it is appropriate to leave the mucocele in place and place a drain. Both closed suction and passive drains can be utilized. A butterfly catheter can be fashioned into a closed suction drain since Jackson–Pratt drain is often too large for the surgical site. A sterile dressing should always be placed over any drain exit site. The drain is often removed three to seven days after surgery, and the timing of drain removal is often up to surgeon discretion, or based on monitoring of drain fluid production over time.

Closure

After placing and securing the drain, a routine closure can be performed. The surgeon should ensure that samples have been collected for both histopathology and bacterial culture if indicated prior to closure. Often, these incisions can be closed in three layers with the platysma muscle, subcutaneous tissue, and skin being closed in layers. Depending upon the extent of the oral dissection, closure of the myohyoideus muscle fascia or oral mucosa may be required.

Zygomatic Salivary Gland Excision

Zygomatic salivary gland excision can be technically challenging. The approach is made along the zygomatic arch, and the temporalis fascia needs to be elevated to gain access to the zygomatic arch. A portion of the arch is then transected to gain access to the zygomatic salivary gland, duct, and mucocele. It has been reported to pre-drill holes prior to osteotomy and repair the defect with wire following zygomatic sialoadenectomy[22]. However, the ostectomized zygomatic arch can also be removed and not replaced with no reported adverse events.[3] The gland is typically present just deep to the arch and can be removed without disruption of the orbital ligament.[3] Care should be taken to avoid damage to the globe. The surgical site can then be closed routinely, with a drain if indicated.

Parotid Salivary Gland Excision

Parotid salivary gland excision can also be challenging due to the regional anatomy. There is risk of iatrogenic damage to the external ear canal (since this salivary gland is superficial to the vertical portion), superficial temporary artery, and the facial nerve. The incision is made from dorsal to ventral from the level of the ear canal to the caudal aspect of the ramus of the mandible.[7] The platysma is transected followed by transection of the parotidoauricularis muscle. The gland is then bluntly dissected from the surrounding tissue and fascia. The gland is a Y-shaped structure, and the duct located rostrally should be ligated prior to excising the gland. It has been reported to inject methylene blue into the duct or the gland itself to facilitate dissection and try to avoid iatrogenic damage.[23] In this case series of seven dogs, approximately 2 mL of new methylene blue was used per gland, and there were no postoperative facial nerve deficits. A drain is recommended prior to closure in cases of sialocele.

Alternative Treatment Options for Sialoceles

Radiation therapy has been reported for the treatment of salivary mucoceles in dogs.[24] In one case series, 11 dogs were treated for sialoceles, 2 as the primary treatment method with the remainder undergoing previous surgical intervention. These patients were treated with 4 Gy of radiation per fraction for a total dose of either 12 or 16 Gy. The only recurrence that was reported was in the set of patients receiving 12 Gy, so the authors ultimately recommended the 16 Gy course. Radiation treatment is thought to damage the salivary gland tissue such that saliva production is diminished, thus resulting in the elimination of the sialocele.[24] The radiation was well tolerated with no acute toxicity, but one dog was diagnosed with a late toxic effect of local alopecia around the treatment site. At this time, the information for radiation therapy as a treatment option for sialocele is limited to this short case series; however, it should remain a consideration for sialoceles that are refractory to surgical management.

Injection of N-acetylcysteine (NAC) directly into the salivary duct has also been described for the treatment of some sialoceles.[25] In this series of 23 dogs, approximately 5 mL of 10% commercially available NAC was injected into the corresponding duct through the papilla in the mouth under sedation or anesthesia.[25] Grossly detected sialoceles resolved in all dogs; however, they reported a 22% recurrence rate, which reportedly resolved with additional medical treatment.[25] No significant adverse events were recorded during the duration of the study.[25] As with radiation therapy, no prospective data are available comparing this treatment method to surgery or any other treatment option. However, it could also be considered for patients who are refractory to standard treatment, or patients for whom surgery is not an option.

Potential Complications

As with any surgery, complications associated with general anesthesia are possible, as well as hemorrhage, infection, dehiscence, and seroma formation. For salivary mucoceles specifically, recurrence can be seen, especially if functional salivary tissue is left behind. Recurrence has been reported in approximately 5% of cases.[26] Other complications are specific to the gland being removed. In the case of the mandibular and sublingual salivary gland complex, damage to the hypoglossal nerve can occur, leading to dysfunction of the tongue. This complex is also near the jugular vein bifurcation, which can be traumatized during the dissection. With respect to the parotid salivary gland, iatrogenic damage to the facial nerve or branches of the trigeminal nerve, as well as injury to the superficial temporary artery or other carotid artery branches, can occur. Finally, for the zygomatic salivary gland, damage to the globe is possible. For patients in which the zygomatic arch is repaired with implants, implant infection or failure is possible, in addition to nonunion of the ostectomy. Patients with zygomatic arch ostectomies without primary repair may be more susceptible to orbital trauma in the future; however, damage to the eye from trauma after zygomatic arch ostectomy has not been reported to the author's knowledge in the dog.

Postoperative Care and Prognosis

Patients undergoing salivary gland excision tend to have a postoperative convalescence period of approximately 14 days, similar to other soft tissue surgeries. The author's preference is to keep these patients overnight in the hospital, especially for respiratory monitoring if there was a pharyngeal mucocele present, but they are often feeling well enough to go home the following day. Postoperative care includes appropriate analgesia and incisional monitoring. If a drain is placed, it should be covered by a sterile dressing. For passive drains, owners should be instructed on how to keep the drain exit site clean and how to change dressings. For closed suction drains, owners should be counseled on how to empty the drain and keep the exit area clean and covered. The decision of when to remove a drain is surgeon-dependent; however, most often drains can be removed within three to seven days after surgery. Exercise restrictions are recommended for the first two weeks with a harness and leash, to avoid compressing the neck with a neck lead. Because the incision may be on the neck, an E-collar may not be advisable; however, a soft E-collar can prevent dogs from scratching at the incision. Alternatives to an E-collar include a stockinette or adhesive dressing. Commercially available postoperative head wraps are also available for dogs. Antibiotics beyond perioperative administration are not always required for salivary gland excisions, but if there is an index of suspicion for infection, they may be administered. Antibiotics should be administered based on culture, should a positive culture result be obtained. Patients are generally allowed to return to normal activity after a two-week postoperative recheck.

Prognosis is generally excellent for salivary gland excision with sialoceles, with a small percentage of cases developing recurrence. In the case of neoplasia, the prognosis will be directly related to the specific diagnosis. In cases of infection or necrosis, salivary gland excision is typically curative.

References

1 Lieske, D. and Rissi, D. (2020). A retrospective study of salivary gland diseases in 179 dogs (2010–2018). *J. Vet. Diagn. Invest.* 32 (4): 604–610.

2 Durand, A., Finck, M., Sullivan, M. et al. (2016). Computed tomography and magnetic resonance diagnosis of variations in the anatomical location of the major salivary glands in 1680 dogs and 187 cats. *Vet. J.* 209: 156–162.

3 Landy, S., Peralta, S., and Fiani, N. (2021). An atypical presentation of a zygomatic sialocele in a dog. *J. Vet. Dentistry* 38 (4): 223–230.

4 Henry, C. (1992). Salivary mucocele associated with dirofilariasis in a dog. *J. Am. Vet. Med. Assoc.* 200 (12): 1965–1966.

5 De Lorenzi, D., Bertoncello, D., Mantovani, C. et al. (2018). Nasopharyngeal sialoceles in 11 brachycephalic dogs. *Vet. Surg.* 47 (3): 431–438.

6 Benjamino, K., Birchard, S., Niles, J. et al. (2012). Pharyngeal mucoceles in dogs: 14 cases. *J. Am. Anim. Hosp. Assoc.* 48 (1): 31–35.

7 Guthrie, K. and Hardie, R. (2014). Surgical excision of the parotid salivary gland for treatment of a traumatic Mucocele in a dog. *J. Am. Anim. Hosp. Assoc.* 50 (3): 216–220.

8 Proot, J.L.J., Nelissen, P., Ladlow, J.F. et al. (2016). Parotidectomy for the treatment of parotid sialocoele in 14 dogs. *J. Small Anim. Pract.* 57 (2): 79–83. https://doi.org/10.1111/jsap.12429.

9 Thomsen, B. and Myers, R. (1999). Extraskeletal osteosarcoma of the mandibular salivary gland in a dog. *Vet. Pathol.* 36 (1): 71–73.

10 Clark, K., Hanna, P., and Béraud, R. (2013). Sialolipoma of a minor salivary gland in a dog. *Can. Vet. J.* 54 (5): 467–470.

11 Shimoyama, Y., Yamashita, K., Ohmachi, T. et al. (2006). Pleomorphic adenoma of the salivary gland in two dogs. *J. Compar. Pathol.* 134 (2): 254–259.

12 Sozmen, M., Brown, P., and Eveson, J. (2003). Salivary gland basal cell adenocarcinoma: a report of cases in a cat and two dogs. *J. Vet. Med. Series A* 50 (8): 399–401.

13 Han, H., Mann, F., and Park, J. (2016). Canine sialolithiasis: two case reports with breed, gender, and age distribution of 29 cases (1964–2010). *J. Am. Anim. Hosp. Assoc.* 52 (1): 22–26.

14 Aita, N., Sakawa, Y., and Iso, H. (2006). Sialocele with sialolithiasis in a dog. *J. Jap. Vet. Med. Assoc.* 59: 687–689.

15 McGill, S., Lester, N., McLachlan, A. et al. (2009). Concurrent sialocoele and necrotising sialadenitis in a dog. *J. Small Anim. Pract.* 50 (3): 151–156.

16 Boydell, P., Pike, R., Crossley, D. et al. (2000). Sialadenosis in dogs. *J. Am. Vet. Med. Assoc.* 216 (6): 872–874.

17 Oetelaar, G., Heng, H., Lim, C. et al. (2022). Computed tomographic appearance of sialoceles in 12 dogs. *Vet. Radiol. Ultrasound* 63 (1): 30–37.

18 Tan, Y., Marques, A., Schwarz, T. et al. (2022). Clinical and CT sialography findings in 22 dogs with surgically confirmed sialoceles. *Vet. Radiol. Ultrasound* 63: 699–710.

19 Gaber, W., Shalaan, S., Misk, N. et al. (2020). Surgical anatomy, morphometry, and histochemistry of major salivary glands in dogs: updates and recommendation. *Int. J. Vet. Health Sci. Res.* 8: 252–259.

20 Cinti, F., Rossanese, M., Buracco, P. et al. (2021). Complications between ventral and lateral approach for mandibular and sublingual sialoadenectomy in dogs with sialocele. *Vet. Surg.* 50 (3): 579–587.

21 Marsh, A. and Adin, C. (2013). Tunneling under the digastricus muscle increases salivary duct exposure and completeness of excision in mandibular and sublingual sialoadenectomy in dogs. *Vet. Surg.* 42 (3): 238–242.

22 Bartoe, J, Brightman, A, Davidson, H. (2007). Modified lateral orbitotomy for vision-sparing excision of a zygomatic mucocele in a dog. *Vet. Ophthalmol.* 10 (2):127–131

23 Gordo, I., Camarasa, J., Campmany, M. et al. (2020). The use of methylene blue to assist with parotid sialadenectomy in dogs. *J. Small Anim. Pract.* 61 (11): 689–695.

24 Poirier, V., Mayer-Stankeová, S., Buchholz, J. et al. (2018). Efficacy of radiation therapy for the treatment of sialocele in dogs. *J. Vet. Internal Med.* 32 (1): 107–110.

25 Ortillés, Á., Leiva, M., Allgoewer, I. et al. (2020). Intracanalicular injection of N-acetylcysteine as adjunctive treatment for sialoceles in dogs: 25 cases (2000-2017). *J. Am. Vet. Med. Assoc.* 257 (8): 826–832.

26 Tsioli, V., Papazoglou, L., Basdani, E. et al. (2013). Surgical management of recurrent cervical sialoceles in four dogs. *J. Small Anim. Pract.* 54 (6): 331–333.

14

Thyroidectomy

Giovanni Tremolada

Department of Clinical Sciences, Colorado State University, Fort Collins, CO, USA

Key Points

- The most common reason for thyroidectomy in the dog is neoplasia, and thyroid masses in dogs are more commonly a malignant neoplasia.
- Full patient staging is recommended before surgery.
- Surgery is the treatment of choice for freely movable tumors.
- Hemorrhage is a potentially serious complication, and blood products should be available at the time of surgery.
- Bilateral thyroidectomies can be performed, but the animal may require post-operative long-term supplementation of vitamin D/calcium carbonate and levothyroxine.
- Survival time for dogs with non-metastasized, non-invasive thyroid carcinoma is excellent, and surgery can be curative for some patients.
- Survival time is still good when surgery is performed in dogs with pulmonary metastasis at diagnosis.
- The role of adjuvant chemotherapy is unclear.

Introduction

Basic Thyroid Gland Anatomy and Physiology

In dogs and cats, the thyroid gland is composed of two separate structures, often referred to as lobes. The lobes are rarely connected by a bridge of glandular tissue or isthmus, located ventral to the trachea, called *isthmus glandularis*.[1] The normal thyroid gland lobe appears as an elongated, dark-red structure located laterally and slightly dorsal to the cranial trachea, usually with the cranial aspect near the first tracheal ring or cricoid cartilage and caudal aspect extending to the fifth to eighth tracheal rings. In dogs, the two thyroid gland lobes are not the only source of thyroid tissue, as ectopic tissue can be found in 23–80% of dogs. In cats, the reported percentage of ectopic thyroid tissue is around 4%. This ectopic tissue can be found anywhere from the base of the tongue to the base of the heart.[1]

The main arterial supply to the thyroid gland is provided by the cranial thyroid artery, a branch of the common carotid artery, and the caudal thyroid artery, most commonly arising from the brachiocephalic trunk. The main venous drainage of the gland is supplied by the cranial and caudal thyroid veins, which both empty into the internal jugular vein at different levels. Most cats are missing the caudal thyroid vein.[2] As suggested by their names, these vessels are located at the cranial and caudal poles of each thyroid lobe (Figure 14.1). The lymphatic drainage of the thyroid gland is represented by the cranial deep cervical lymph nodes (if present) or the medial retropharyngeal lymph nodes for the cranial half of the gland and the caudal deep cervical lymph node for the caudal half of the

Techniques in Small Animal Soft Tissue, Orthopedic, and Ophthalmic Surgery, First Edition. Edited by Kristin A. Coleman.

Companion website: www.wiley.com/go/coleman/surgeries

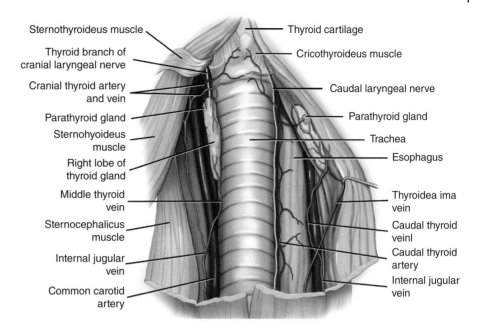

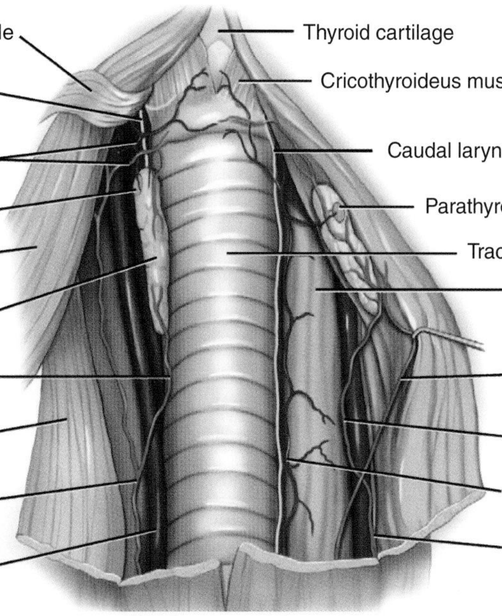

Figure 14.1 Vascular anatomy of the thyroid and parathyroid glands and important structures in the visceral space of the neck. *Source:* Reproduced with permission from Hullinger[1], Elsevier.

gland.[3] Both cranial and caudal deep cervical lymph nodes, if normal, are usually small and may not be identified on imaging or in surgery.

The thyroid lobes are covered by the sternocephalicus and sternohyoideus muscles ventrally and the sternothyroideus muscle laterally. Anatomically, the right thyroid lobe is often located cranial to the left thyroid lobe and is in closer contact with the recurrent laryngeal nerve, which is dorsal and usually medial to the thyroid glands. The distance between the left recurrent laryngeal nerve and the thyroid gland on the left side is greater because of the presence of the esophagus on its dorsolateral border (Figure 14.1). Other important structures in the visceral space of the neck that a surgeon should be familiar with are the vagosympathetic trunk, the internal jugular vein, and the common carotid artery.

The thyroid gland is responsible for the production of thyroid hormones under the regulation of the hypothalamus–hypophysis axis. The thyroid-releasing hormone (THR) produced by the hypothalamus will activate the hypophysis of the pituitary gland to release the thyroid-stimulating hormone (TSH or thyrotropin). TSH will trigger the thyroid gland to produce and secrete thyroxine (T_4) and triiodothyronine (T_3). In the bloodstream, the majority of T_4 and T_3 are bound to plasma protein and are, therefore, inactive. Only a small percentage of the free T_4 and T_3 exert a function on the body, with T_3 being the most biologically active compound. The amount of T_4 and T_3 in the bloodstream acts as negative feedback on the hypophysis and inhibits the secretion of TSH. The mechanism of production and release of TRH by the hypothalamus is not well understood. The thyroid gland is responsible not only for production of T_3 and T_4 but also for secretion of calcitonin through the C-cells to help regulating the body's calcium homeostasis. Other texts covering the pathophysiology of the thyroid gland will have details about this topic.

Basic Parathyroid Anatomy and Physiology

The parathyroid glands in dogs and cats are two paired glands with a total of four glands (two per thyroid gland lobe), located at or near the cranial and caudal poles of the thyroid. The normal parathyroid gland appears as a small (~2–3 mm) tan, flat structure. Parathyroid glands are commonly referred to as external and internal based on their location relative to the thyroid parenchyma. External parathyroid glands are located at the cranial poles of the thyroid gland lobes (one on the right, one on the left) and usually are separated from the thyroid parenchyma, while the internal parathyroid glands are in the caudal poles of the thyroid gland lobes and are commonly embedded in the gland parenchyma. Variation in location of both internal and external parathyroid glands is common; therefore, a thorough exploration of the area surrounding the thyroid gland should be performed to identify them. Ectopic parathyroid tissue is uncommon in dogs, but may be more frequent than previously reported.[4] On the contrary, in cats, the presence of ectopic parathyroid tissue has been reported in 35–50% of cases.[5,6]

The function of parathyroid glands is to secrete parathyroid hormone from their chief cells. Because of its direct effect on bones and indirect effect on GI tract and kidneys, this hormone regulates the body's calcium and phosphorus homeostasis. Increased ionized calcium concentration in the blood acts as negative feedback on the parathyroid's chief cells, decreasing its secretion.

Indications/Pre-op Considerations

The most common reason for unilateral or bilateral thyroidectomy in dogs is neoplasia, with carcinoma being the most common tumor type. Commonly, dogs present to their veterinarian for the presence of a ventral cervical mass without other clinical signs.[7] If the dog is affected by hyperthyroidism, clinical signs, such as tachycardia, restlessness, weight loss, polyphagia, polyuria, and polydipsia, can be present;[7] however, the majority of thyroid carcinomas in dogs are non-functional, meaning excessive thyroid hormone is not being secreted by the neoplastic gland. Thyroid tumors usually affect old, mid- to large breed dogs with Golden retrievers and Beagles being overrepresented.[8] In the cat, thyroidectomy (unilateral or bilateral) is more commonly performed for benign functional lesions causing hyperthyroidism.[9] Bilateral thyroidectomy in cats should only be performed when clinical signs cannot be controlled by medical management or treatment with I^{131} is not available.

Fine needle aspirate, either "blind" or ultrasound-guided, is usually sufficient to obtain a diagnosis of a neuroendocrine neoplasia of a thyroid gland mass. Blood contamination can preclude obtaining a definitive diagnosis. Biopsy of the mass with a Tru-Cut needle is usually discouraged because of the risk of profuse and potentially fatal hemorrhage,[10,11] but a more recent study did not show evidence of a high complication rate when this was performed.[12]

A minimum database including complete blood count, blood type, biochemical profile, and urine analysis should be performed before surgery. A total T_4 measurement is also routinely evaluated at the author's practice. While it is important to treat cats for hyperthyroidism before surgery,[13] this does not seem to be required in dogs.[7,14] Hypercalcemia of malignancy secondary to thyroid carcinoma has been described in a case report and was resolved after surgery.[15]

Before surgery, patients are staged with cervical imaging (ultrasound or CT), thoracic imaging (radiographs or CT), and abdominal imaging (ultrasound or CT). For small masses that are freely movable,[4] cervical ultrasound is considered by the author an acceptable preoperative test. An expert ultrasonographer or radiologist can identify the presence of vascular invasion, the status of the thyroid glands, and the locoregional lymph nodes. In cases of larger or less movable/more "fixed" masses, the author prefers to obtain a CT angiogram of the cervical region to help planning for surgery or radiation therapy. If possible, any abnormal structure identified on imaging should be sampled. Thoracic radiographs or thoracic CT scans can be used to identify the presence of metastatic disease, with CT being a more sensitive test.[16] Abdominal ultrasound or CT scan is usually recommended since thyroid neoplasia affects older animals, and the presence of a concomitant abdominal neoplasia was identified in 33% of dogs in one study.[4]

Surgical Procedure

It is the author's opinion that surgery in a general practice setting should be considered only for small, freely movable thyroid tumors. Additionally, access to blood products should be available if needed due to the risk of hemorrhage with thyroidectomy.

The patient is prepared by clipping the ventral aspect of the neck from the angle of the mandible to the thoracic inlet. The dog is then positioned on the surgical table in dorsal recumbency with the forelimbs retracted caudally. To help with exposure of the thyroid gland, a small towel can be rolled under the patient's neck (Figure 14.2). Particular attention should be paid to positioning the patient's neck straight to avoid distortion of the local anatomy and facilitate the surgical approach. Once the surgical area is aseptically prepared and the patient is draped, a skin incision from just caudal to the larynx, which is easy to locate with the palpable caudal cricoid cartilage of the larynx, to cranial to the manubrium is performed with a scalpel blade or electrosurgery. The exact length of the incision will depend on the size and location of the thyroid mass. After dissecting through skin, subcutaneous tissue, and platysma muscle, the paired sternohyoideus muscles are identified and bluntly separated on midline. To help identify midline, gentle pressure with DeBakey forceps can be applied onto the sternohyoideus muscle bellies, making the median raphe (e.g., aponeurosis) and separation of the muscles more obvious (Figure 14.3). At the caudal aspect of the approach, the sternothyroideus muscles are also separated. Once the trachea is visualized, the paratracheal fascia is bluntly dissected and one or two self-retaining retractors (Weitlaner or Gelpi) are positioned to expose the visceral space of the neck. Care should be taken to not damage the carotid sheath, trachea, or thyroid glands when placing the retractors.

Once the pathologic thyroid gland is identified, its dissection can start, paying particular attention to avoid hemorrhage. Because the thyroid gland is an extremely well-vascularized organ, minor bleeding is to be expected. This is especially true in cases of thyroidectomy for a neoplastic process, since neovascularization is frequently noted. The use of monopolar and/or bipolar electrosurgery, hemoclips, and vessel sealing devices is recommended to decrease the amount of intraoperative bleeding. Minimizing bleeding allows for better identification of the important nearby structures (i.e., recurrent laryngeal

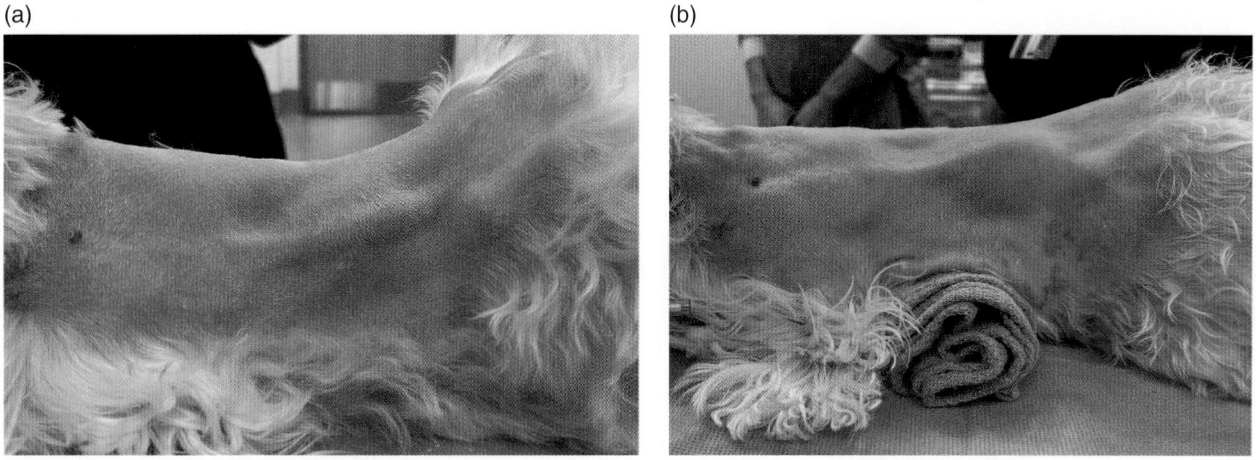

Figure 14.2 Positioning for surgery of a dog affected by a thyroid carcinoma. (a) Patient in dorsal recumbency without a towel underneath the neck; note how the thyroid mass is not readily identifiable. (b) Same patient after positioning a towel underneath the neck; note how the mass can be identified more easily (head to the left of the images). *Source:* © Giovanni Tremolada.

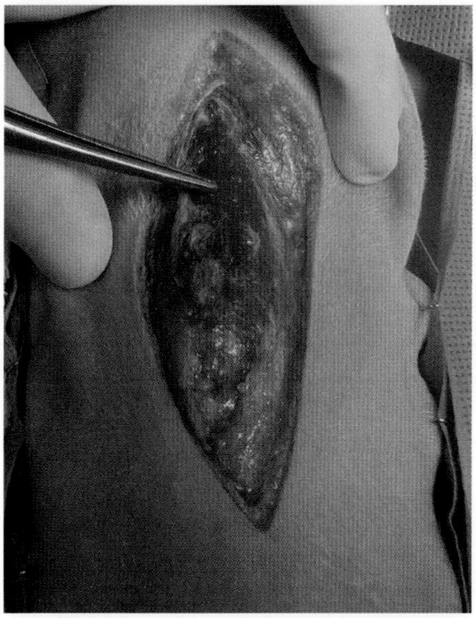

Figure 14.3 Surgical approach to the thyroid glands. The tip of the DeBakey forceps is pointing to the area where the sternohyoideus muscles are connected in a median raphe. Other than the initial platysma muscle incision, all deeper muscles may be simply divided on their median raphe if the approach continues on midline. *Source:* © Giovanni Tremolada.

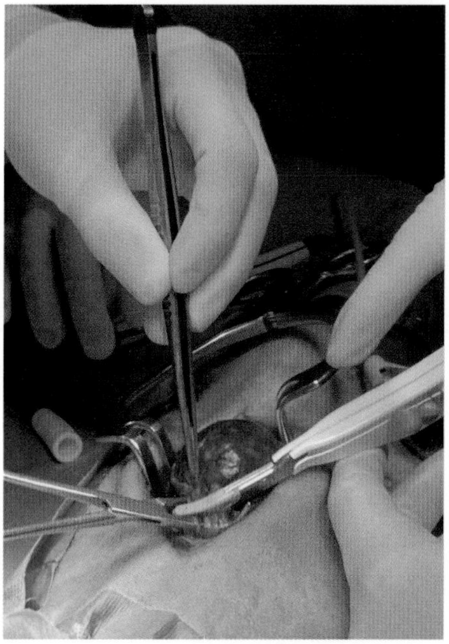

Figure 14.4 Isolation of the caudal thyroid artery and vein with right-angle forceps and position of a vessel sealing device to seal the vascular pedicle. The use of this device has been shown to reduce the amount of hemorrhage and reduce the surgical time. *Source:* © Giovanni Tremolada.

nerve, common carotid artery, and vagosympathetic trunk) and for decreasing surgical time.[17] The main vascular supply to the thyroid gland lobes present at both poles can be ligated with 2-0, 3-0, or 4-0 monofilament absorbable sutures, stapled with hemoclips, or sealed by using a vessel sealing device (Figure 14.4).

To make dissection easier and improve visualization of the surrounding structures, the author usually starts the dissection with a combination of right-angle forceps, electrosurgery, and a vessel sealing device at one of the poles. Once the pole is freed, the gland is reflected cranially or caudally until the thyroid gland can be removed. Attention during the dissection should be posed not to accidentally penetrate the thyroid capsule, as this will result in significant bleeding. For this reason, the thyroid gland should be manipulated by grasping the peri-glandular fascia with DeBakey forceps and not the gland itself (Figure 14.5). In cases of large thyroid masses, especially if left-sided, an orogastric tube can be positioned during surgery to help identify the esophagus.

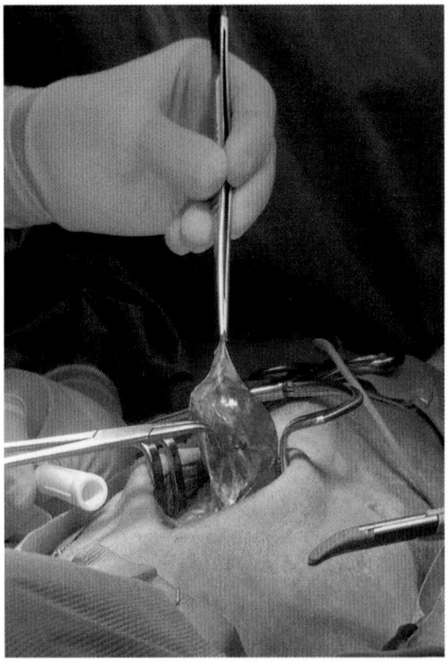

Figure 14.5 After transection of the caudal thyroid artery and vein, the thyroid gland is manipulated by grasping the surrounding fascia. By doing so, the risk of hemorrhage is minimized. The dissection in this case was continued using a combination of right angle forceps and a vessel sealing device. Another tip is to elevate the thyroid mass as it is dissected from the surrounding tissues, which will increase the distance between the mass and the carotid sheath contents, particularly the vagosympathetic trunk, which can be iatrogenically damaged during this surgery. *Source:* © Giovanni Tremolada.

Once the affected thyroid gland lobe is removed, the author usually visually inspects the contralateral side. In cases where a bilateral thyroidectomy is needed, care should be taken to identify and preserve at least one parathyroid gland and one recurrent laryngeal nerve. Usually, when identified, the parathyroid gland can be separated from the thyroid gland lobe using fine instruments like sterile cotton tip applicators, bipolar electrosurgery, and fine-tipped scissors (Figure 14.6a,b). If the blood supply to the parathyroid is damaged, the parathyroid gland can reimplanted in a pouch created in a muscle (usually the sternohyoideus) and closed with 3-0 or 4-0 monofilament absorbable suture.[18,19] In a canine experimental model, mincing or cutting the parathyroid gland into thin slices has been shown to be a superior technique in obtaining a viable parathyroid transplant compared to implanting an intact parathyroid gland.[20] Hypocalcemia is still commonly seen after reimplanting parathyroid glands, as neovascularization of the parathyroid gland can take several days to weeks. For this reason, calcitriol and calcium supplementation may need to be started in the immediate post-operative period.[19] To facilitate frequent biochemical analyses to assess the ionized calcium level for the first few

(a)

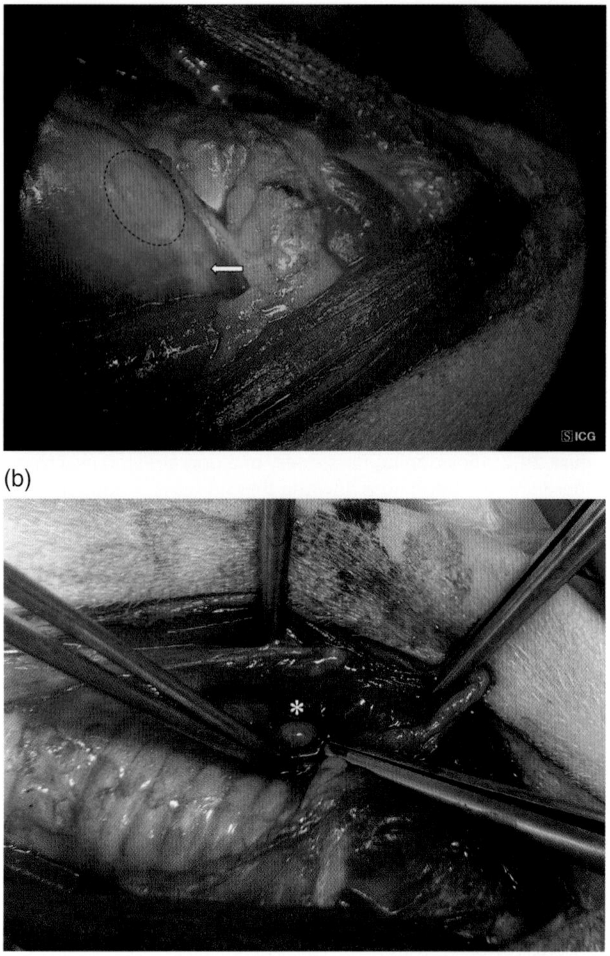

(b)

Figure 14.6 Bilateral thyroidectomy with preservation of a parathyroid gland. (a) Visualization of the parathyroid gland (dotted circle) and its vascular supply (white arrow) after intraoperative injection of indocyanine green. Note how the vascular supply of the parathyroid gland can be readily identified using this technique. (b) The parathyroid gland (directly below asterisk) with its vascular supply was spared and left in situ. This procedure was performed because the dog was affected by a bilateral thyroid carcinoma, so both thyroid gland lobes were entirely removed. This patient never developed clinical post-operative hypocalcemia, so supplementation of vitamin D or calcium carbonate was not started. Thyroid hormone supplementation via levothyroxine is often initiated and titrated as directed by follow-up bloodwork. *Source:* © Giovanni Tremolada.

days in hospital after bilateral thyroidectomy, a single-lumen jugular catheter or similar central line is most easily placed at the time of closure within the sterile field of the ventral cervical region. A possible increased risk of local recurrence exists when a parathyroid gland is saved after intracapsular dissection from a neoplastic thyroid gland.

Any abnormal lymph nodes noted on pre-operative imaging are extirpated during the same procedure. A recent retrospective study reported a higher than expected rate of lymph nodes metastasis (45%) in dogs with thyroid carcinoma. The authors of that study suggested to perform routine extirpation of all the identifiable locoregional lymph nodes for accurate staging, as metastasis was found in lymph nodes contralateral to the thyroid mass.[3] Once the thyroid and/or the lymph nodes have been removed, the surgical area is gently lavaged with warm sterile saline before closure. The sternohyoideus muscle fascia, subcutaneous, and intradermal layers are apposed using 3-0 or 4-0 absorbable monofilament suture. If an intradermal suture layer is not desired, a non-absorbable 3-0 or 4-0 suture may be used to appose the skin. An infiltration block with a long-lasting local anesthetic (bupivacaine or ropivacaine) can be performed at the time of closure as part of multimodal pain management strategy.

Potential Complications

In the largest study to date describing complications after unilateral thyroidectomy, the total complication rate was ~20%. Hemorrhage (7.7%) and aspiration pneumonia (3.2%) were the most common complications,[21] and only 3.2% of the dogs required a blood transfusion. Overall, perioperative mortality for unilateral thyroidectomy was 1.9%.[21] Unilateral laryngeal paralysis may occur after surgery if one of the laryngeal recurrent nerves is iatrogenically compromised. This complication usually does not require intervention if only one nerve is damaged.[4,7] Hypocalcemia and hypothyroidism can develop in cases of bilateral thyroparathyroidectomies.[4] Other possible complications from the surgery are Horner's syndrome, incisional infection, incisional dehiscence, and seroma formation.[21]

Post-operative Care

After a thyroidectomy, patients are usually administered intravenous (IV) fluids at a maintenance rate of 60–90 mL/kg/day until they are able to eat. An infiltration block with a long-lasting local anesthetic (bupivacaine, ropivacaine, liposomal encapsulated bupivacaine) can be performed at time of closure of the incision to help with pain management for the first few hours after surgery. An opioid may be used for the first 24 hours in hospital either as a bolus or as a continuous rate infusion (CRI) combined with the use of a non-steroidal anti-inflammatory drug (NSAID) unless contraindicated. Most patients can be discharged from the hospital within 24–36 hours of surgery on an oral NSAID and/or gabapentin (5–10 mg/kg BID-TID). Because of the location of the incision, an Elizabethan collar may interfere with the surgical site. The author sometimes uses, instead of an Elizabethan collar, a stockinette with a laparotomy sponge or an adhesive bandage to protect the incision site for the first few days after surgery.

Patients that underwent bilateral thyroidectomy are hospitalized for three to five days, and ionized calcium values are monitored every 12 hours. If significant hypocalcemia or clinical signs related to hypocalcemia (tremors, face rubbing, weakness, etc.) are noted, supplementation with calcitriol with or without calcium carbonate is started. In emergency situations (profound neurologic signs with an animal not able to eat or even seizure activity), an IV dose of 0.5–1 mL/kg (50–100 mg/kg) of 10% calcium gluconate is given over 30 minutes while monitoring the ECG for signs of bradycardia. If the dog is stable and able to eat, the author usually starts supplementing liquid calcitriol at a dose of 10–15 ng/kg by mouth BID for the first three to four days and then maintains the dog at 5–7 ng/kg BID for one week. Supplementation of calcium carbonate (50–75 mg/kg by mouth BID) can be started at the same time. If the dog is eating normally, this may not be required, as the amount of calcium contained in a balanced diet may be enough. If TUMS® is used to supplement calcium carbonate, it is imperative to make sure that the product does not contain xylitol to avoid liver toxicity. Ionized calcium is then checked weekly. If the dog is hyper or normo-calcemic, the dose of calcitriol can be reduced by half while the dog is monitored at home for signs of hypocalcemia. Even the dogs that received parathyroid reimplantation should be monitored for hypocalcemia, as neovascularization of the gland may take days to weeks for calcium homeostasis to resume. If no parathyroid glands have been spared at the time of surgery, the dog will likely need to be maintained on supplementation for the rest of its life, as ectopic parathyroid tissue is rare in dogs. Hypothyroidism can occur post-operatively after bilateral thyroidectomy[4] and when functional tumors are removed.[7] Serial thyroid levels should be checked in the post-operative time to assess if supplementation with levothyroxine is indicated (0.02 mg/kg every 12 hours orally, with a maximum initial dose of 0.8 mg BID) and to monitor the response to the therapy.

Prognosis

Dogs affected by a benign thyroid tumor (functional or not) can be considered cured with surgical removal of the mass.[8] In animals affected by thyroid carcinoma, different prognostic factors have been described, including size, mobility, surgical versus non-surgical treatment, histopathologic characteristics, and stage of the disease.[7,8,21–24] Animals with fixed tumors treated with surgery seem to have a shorter survival time (6–12 months) compared to dogs with movable ones (36 months). Dogs surgically treated for unilateral thyroid carcinoma have a reported MST of 911 days.[21] In dogs with tumors with gross vascular invasion noted on histologic analysis following surgical resection or CT scan, the reported overall median survival time (MST) after surgical resection is 621 days.[24] Dogs with bilateral simultaneous thyroid tumors still have an excellent MST (38.3 months)[4] but are at an increased risk for the presence of distant metastasis at presentation.[23] Two studies looked at the survival after thyroidectomy for functional thyroid tumors and found vastly different MSTs of 36 and 72 months.[7,23] Histologic vascular invasion has been shown to be a negative prognostic factor in one study, while the type of carcinoma (follicular versus medullary) does not seem to affect the prognosis.[22]

The value of adjuvant chemotherapy after thyroidectomy for carcinomas is still debated, with one study not being able to show an advantage in survival for dogs treated with surgery and chemotherapy compared to surgery alone.[25] Due to the slow progression of metastatic disease in dogs with thyroid carcinoma, surgical removal of the primary tumor should be considered despite the presence of thoracic metastasis, as clinical signs are usually related to the local invasion of the primary tumor within the cervical region. Tumors that are not amenable to surgical resection can be treated with radiation therapy or I^{131} with reported good survival time.[26–28] Carcinosarcoma is a rare thyroid tumor, and dogs affected by this tumor have a poor prognosis with an overall MST of 156 days.[29]

References

1 Hullinger, R.L. (2013). Endocrine system. In: *Miller's Anatomy of the Dog*, 4e (ed. H.E. Evans and A. de Lahunta), 412–416. St. Louis: Elsevier.

2 Scavelli, T.D. and Peterson, M.E. (1993). The thyroid. In: *Textbook of Small Animal Surgery*, 2e (ed. D. Slatter), 1514–1523. Philadelphia: Saunders.

3 Skinner, O.T., Souza, C.H.M., and Kim, D.Y. (2021). Metastasis to ipsilateral medial retropharyngeal and deep cervical lymph nodes in 22 dogs with thyroid carcinoma. *Vet. Surg.* 50: 150–157.

4 Tuohy, J.L., Worley, D.R., and Withrow, S.J. (2012). Outcome following simultaneous bilateral thyroid lobectomy for treatment of thyroid gland carcinoma in dogs: 15 cases (1994-2010). *J. Am. Vet. Med. Assoc.* 241: 95–103.

5 Flanders, J.A., Neth, S., Erb, H.N. et al. (1991). Functional analysis of ectopic parathyroid activity in cats. *Am. J. Vet. Res.* 52: 1336–1340.

6 Nicholas, J.S. and Swingle, W.W. (1925). An experimental and morphological study of the parathyroid glands of the cat. *Am. J. Anat.* 34: 469–509.

7 Scharf, V.F., Oblak, M.L., Hoffman, K. et al. (2020). Clinical features and outcome of functional thyroid tumours in 70 dogs. *J. Small Anim. Pract.* 61 (8): 504–511.

8 Wucherer, K.L. and Wilke, V. (2010). Thyroid cancer in dogs: an update based on 638 cases (1995-2005). *J. Am. Anim. Hosp. Assoc.* 46 (4): 249–254.

9 Scott-Moncrieff, J.C. (2015). Feline hyperthyroidism. In: *Canine and Feline Endocrinology*, 4e (ed. E.C. Feldman, R.W. Nelson, and C.E. Reusch), 136–195. St. Louis: Elsevier.

10 Ehrhart, N. (2003). Thyroid. In: *Textbook of Small Animal Surgery*, 3e (ed. D. Slatter), 1700–1710. Philadelphia: Saunders.

11 Townsend, K.L. and Ham, K.M. (2022). Current concepts in parathyroid/thyroid surgery. *Vet. Clin. North Am. Small Anim. Pract.* 52: 455–471.

12 Scheemaeker, S., Vandermeulen, E., Ducatelle, R. et al. (2023). Ultrasound-guided core needle biopsy in dogs with thyroid carcinoma. *Vet. Comp. Oncol.* https://doi.org/10.1111/vco.12895.

13 Feldman, E.C. and Nelson, R.W. (2004). Feline hyperthyroidism (thyrotoxicosis). In: *Canine and Feline Endocrinology and Reproduction*, 3e (ed. E.C. Feldman and R.W. Nelson), 152–218. Saunders: St. Louis.

14 Simpson, A.C. and McCown, J.L. (2009). Systemic hypertension in a dog with a functional thyroid gland adenocarcinoma. *J. Am. Vet. Med. Assoc.* 235: 1474–1479.

15 Lane, A.E. and Wyatt, K.M. (2012). Paraneoplastic hypercalcemia in a dog with thyroid carcinoma. *Can. Vet. J.* 53: 1101–1104.

16 Nemanic, S., London, C.A., and Wisner, E.R. (2006). Comparison of thoracic radiographs and single breath-hold helical CT for detection of pulmonary nodules in dogs with metastatic neoplasia. *J. Vet. Intern. Med.* 20: 508–515.

17 Lorange, M., De Arburn Parent, R., Huneault, L. et al. (2019). Use of a vessel-sealing device versus conventional hemostatic techniques in dogs undergoing thyroidectomy because of suspected thyroid carcinoma. *J. Am. Vet. Med. Assoc.* 254: 1186–1191.

18 Halsted, W.S. (1909). Auto- and isotransplantation, in dogs, of the parathyroid glandules. *J. Exp. Med.* 11: 175–199.

19 Tobias, K.M. (2010). Feline thyroidectomy. In: *Manual of Small Animal Soft Tissue Surgery* (ed. K.M. Tobias), 433–440. Ames, IA: Wiley-Blackwell.

20 Matsuura, H., Sako, K., and Marchetta, F.C. (1973). Reimplantation of autogenous parathyroid tissue: an experimental study. *J. Surg. Oncol.* 5: 297–305.

21 Reagan, J.K., Selmic, L.E., Fallon, C. et al. (2019). Complications and outcomes associated with unilateral thyroidectomy in dogs with naturally occurring thyroid tumors: 156 cases (2003-2015). *J. Am. Vet. Med. Assoc.* 255: 926–932.

22 Campos, M., Ducatelle, R., Rutteman, G. et al. (2014). Clinical, pathologic, and immunohistochemical prognostic factors in dogs with thyroid carcinoma. *J. Vet. Intern. Med.* 28: 1805–1813.

23 Frederick, A.N., Pardo, A.D., Schmiedt, C.W. et al. (2020). Outcomes for dogs with functional thyroid tumors treated by surgical excision alone. *J. Am. Vet. Med. Assoc.* 256: 444–448.

24 Latifi, M., Skinner, O.T., Spoldi, E. et al. (2021). Outcome and postoperative complications in 73 dogs with thyroid carcinoma with gross vascular invasion managed with thyroidectomy. *Vet. Comp. Oncol.* 19 (4): 685–696.

25 Nadeau, M.E. and Kitchell, B.E. (2011). Evaluation of the use of chemotherapy and other prognostic variables for surgically excised canine thyroid carcinoma with and without metastasis. *Can. Vet. J.* 52: 994–998.

26 Worth, A.J., Zuber, R.M., and Hocking, M. (2005). Radioiodide (131I) therapy for the treatment of canine thyroid carcinoma. *Aust. Vet. J.* 83: 208–214.

27 Lee, B.I., LaRue, S.M., Seguin, B. et al. (2020). Safety and efficacy of stereotactic body radiation therapy (SBRT) for the treatment of canine thyroid carcinoma. *Vet. Comp. Oncol.* 18: 843–853.

28 Pack, L., Roberts, R.E., Dawson, S.D. et al. (2000). Definitive radiation therapy for infiltrative thyroid carcinoma in dogs. *Vet. Radiol. Ultrasound* 42: 471–474.

29 Cook, M.R., Gasparini, M., Cianciolo, R.E. et al. (2022). Clinical outcomes of thyroid tumours with concurrent epithelial and mesenchymal components in 14 dogs (2006-2020). *Vet. Med. Sci.* 8: 509–516.

15

Laryngeal Paralysis

Jessica Baron

MedVet Norwalk, Norwalk, CT, USA

Key Points

- Acquired laryngeal paralysis is the most common form of the disease and results in a partial or complete loss of function of the larynx.
- Exercise intolerance caused by laryngeal paralysis is more apparent in hot and humid weather, so more cases of patients with laryngeal paralysis may present in the spring and summer.
- The most common surgical intervention for laryngeal paralysis is a unilateral cricoarytenoid lateralization or "tie-back" procedure.
- Aspiration pneumonia is a life-long risk following surgery, but overall, the majority of patients have an improved quality of life.

Introduction

Laryngeal paralysis is caused by a failure of the arytenoid cartilages to abduct during inspiration, causing an airway obstruction. It has been reported in both dogs and cats. Laryngeal paralysis can be congenital or acquired with the latter being the most common. It can be either unilateral or bilateral and results in a partial or complete loss of function of the larynx.[1]

Anatomy

The larynx is located immediately cranial to the trachea and is responsible for controlling breathing, vocalization, and protecting the lower airway.[1] It is comprised of several structures, including the laryngeal cartilages (epiglottis, thyroid, cricoid, inter-arytenoid, sesamoid, and paired arytenoids), vocal folds, and intrinsic and extrinsic musculature. The cricoarytenoideus dorsalis muscle (CAD) is responsible for abducting the arytenoid cartilages to open the glottis during inspiration. This muscle is controlled by the recurrent laryngeal nerves, which originate from the vagus nerve.

Etiology

Congenital laryngeal paralysis can be hereditary or caused by congenital polyneuropathy. Hereditary laryngeal paralysis typically occurs in dogs less than one year old and has been reported in Bouvier de Flandres and Siberian Huskies.[2] Congenital polyneuropathy causing laryngeal paralysis can also be associated with other clinical signs including hypotonia, hyporeflexia, and diffuse muscle atrophy. It has been reported in several breeds, including Rottweilers, Dalmatians, Bouvier de Flandres, Afghan hounds, and Siberian Huskies.[2]

Acquired laryngeal paralysis is mostly commonly idiopathic. Canine geriatric onset laryngeal paralysis polyneuropathy (GOLPP), previously known as idiopathic laryngeal paralysis, is a progressive disease that causes

Techniques in Small Animal Soft Tissue, Orthopedic, and Ophthalmic Surgery, First Edition. Edited by Kristin A. Coleman.

Companion website: www.wiley.com/go/coleman/surgeries

degeneration of nerves that control muscles of the larynx, causing paralysis of the larynx via inability to abduct the arytenoid cartilages.[1,3,4] Acquired laryngeal paralysis occurs most commonly in older large-breed dogs, such as Labrador Retrievers, Golden Retrievers, and St. Bernards. In these cases, laryngeal paralysis is accompanied by esophageal dysfunction (~2/3 cases) and hind end weakness (~1/3 cases).[3,5] The exact cause of GOLPP is unknown, but it is believed to be a combination of environmental and genetic factors.[1,3] Infection, trauma, tumors, iatrogenic causes, and neurological diseases, like myasthenia gravis, can also cause laryngeal paralysis.[1]

History and Clinical Findings

Pets with laryngeal paralysis typically present with respiratory stridor, exercise intolerance, and periods of difficulty breathing, especially when the pet is excited or stressed.[1] Exercise intolerance may become more apparent in hot and humid weather, so more cases may present in the spring and summer. In severe cases, a pet may present urgently when they have become cyanotic or experience an episode of collapse, or an owner may report a change in the sound of a bark, hacking, coughing, gagging during eating/drinking, pelvic limb weakness or scuffing of toes, and generalized muscle atrophy.

Diagnostics

Laryngeal paralysis is diagnosed via sedated laryngeal exam. Prior to sedated laryngeal exam, a complete blood count and chemistry profile should be performed. Blood work is typically unremarkable, although an elevated white blood cell count should raise concern for aspiration pneumonia. Thyroid testing should be considered to rule out the cases of laryngeal dysfunction secondary to hypothyroidism. Three-view thoracic radiographs should also be performed to rule out intrathoracic disease, megaesophagus, aspiration pneumonia, or non-cardiogenic pulmonary edema.[1] Pre-operative aspiration pneumonia is associated with an increased risk of postoperative complications, so, if possible, surgery should be delayed until the pneumonia is resolved.

For laryngeal examination, the patient is placed in sternal recumbency and must be under a light plane of anesthesia. It is the author's preference to administer propofol slowly until the patient allows for opening of the mouth and exam of the larynx without causing apnea, and there are various pre-medication protocols that exist for administration of other drugs, such as the addition of intravenous midazolam, butorphanol, and/or dexmedetomidine in the editor's practice. The oral cavity, oropharynx, and larynx should be thoroughly evaluated for any pathology, including masses. Using a laryngoscope or endoscope, the larynx is observed while the patient is breathing. It is important the anesthetist announces when the pet is inspiring during the exam. In a normal dog, the arytenoid cartilages will abduct during inspiration. In a dog with laryngeal paralysis, the arytenoid cartilages can be erythematous, edematous, and ulcerated, and the arytenoid cartilages fail to abduct during inspiration. Paradoxical motion can also be seen, where the arytenoid cartilages are pulled inward, closing the glottis during inspiration, and then return to a neutral position during expiration. Paradoxical motion can be mistaken for normal motion of the arytenoids; therefore, it is important to know the timing of inspiration and expiration to help differentiate. To improve laryngeal motion during the exam, doxapram should be used (dose: 1–1.5 mg/kg IV given quickly).[3,6,7] Please note that it may worsen paradoxical motion or increase occlusion of the glottis.

Treatment

The treatment of laryngeal paralysis can vary from medical management to surgical intervention. Medical management can include weight loss, reduced stress, sedatives, and environmental changes, like avoidance heat and exercise, especially in hot and humid weather. However, when the patient's quality of life is affected, the symptoms can no longer be managed medically, or the patient experiences a respiratory crisis, surgical intervention is required. If a pet presents in a respiratory crisis, patient stabilization is warranted and includes sedation, patient cooling (if needed), and providing supplemental oxygen either by flow-by, nasal cannula, oxygen cage, or emergent intubation. In the author's opinion, a temporary tracheostomy is rarely needed.[1,2]

The most common surgical intervention for laryngeal paralysis is a unilateral cricoarytenoid lateralization or "tie-back" procedure. Other surgical options include bilateral arytenoid lateralization, transoral partial laryngectomy, ventriculocordectomy, partial arytenoidectomy, modified castellated laryngofissure, and permanent tracheostomy.[1]

Anesthetic Considerations

It is recommended the patient be pre-medicated with antacids, anti-nausea, and promotility medications prior to general anesthesia. Due to the risk for regurgitation and aspiration perioperatively, limited use of opioids is recommended. If opioids are used, it is the author's preference to use partial mu agonists or rapid-acting pure mu agonists, such a fentanyl or remifentanil, following intubation. Local incisional blocks using lidocaine or long-acting liposomal bupivacaine are recommended so that opioids, if used, can be discontinued immediately following surgery.

Unilateral Cricoarytenoid Lateralization

Unilateral cricoarytenoid lateralization is the standard procedure for treating laryngeal paralysis and relieving airway obstruction.[1,8] Unilateral thyroarytenoid lateralization has also been described but is performed less commonly. "Tying open" one side of the larynx (i.e., "tie-back" procedure) resolves clinical signs and is associated with less complications than a bilateral lateralization procedure. The patient is placed in lateral recumbency. If you are right-handed, it is preferred to perform the procedure on the left side of the larynx (patient placed in right lateral recumbency), as it is easier to pass the suture in this direction.[1,9] It is the author's preference to place a rolled towel under the larynx/surgical site and have the patient's head extended slightly to allow for visualization of pertinent anatomy (Figure 15.1).

A 4–6 cm skin incision is made centered over the larynx immediately ventral to the jugular groove. The rostral landmark is the ramus of the mandible. Dorsally, the wings of the atlas can be palpated. The incision is then continued through the subcutaneous tissue and platysma.[1] The deeper fat is then dissected until the dorsal edge of the thyroid cartilage can be palpated and retracted laterally using the surgeon's index finger. The overlying thyropharyngeus muscle is then identified and incised along the caudodorsal edge of the thyroid cartilage (Figure 15.2). A stay suture is then placed through the thyroid cartilage, which allows the cartilage to be retracted laterally throughout the remainder of the procedure (Figure 15.3). Once the thyroid cartilage is retracted, the inner membrane is transected close to the abducted cartilage, the muscular process of the arytenoid cartilage can be palpated, and cricoarytenoideus dorsalis can be identified. This CAD muscle or fibrous connection

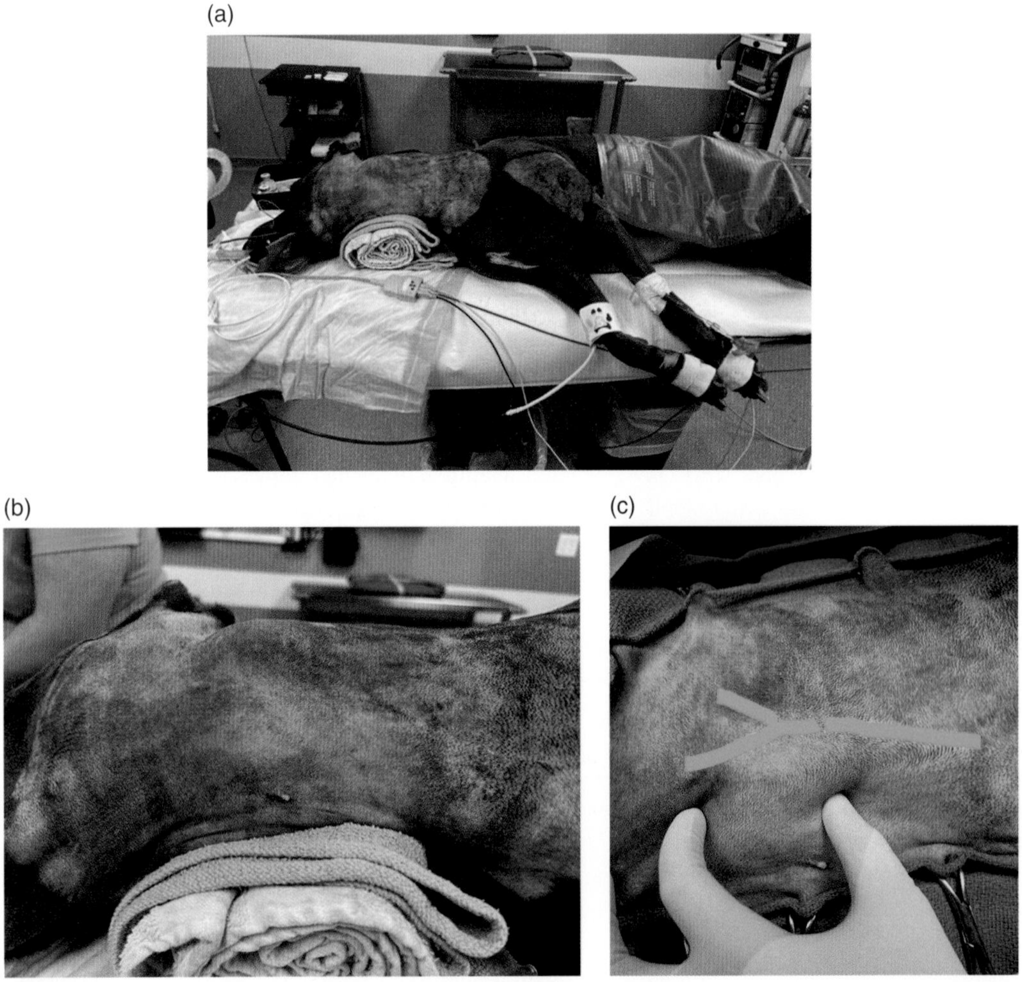

Figure 15.1 Positioning canine patient for left unilateral cricoarytenoid lateralization. (a) Patient is positioned in right lateral recumbency, and the forelimbs are pulled caudally for improved cervical visualization. (b) Rolled towels should be placed under the neck to elevate the larynx. (c) After prepping and draping, the larynx is palpated just cranial to the tracheal rings with the planned incision ventral to the jugular groove. The surgeon's thumb is just caudal to the cricoid cartilage, which is a palpable step from the trachea. The blue line represents the approximate location of the jugular vein and branching into the dorsal maxillary vein and ventral linguofacial vein. *Source:* © Kristin Coleman.

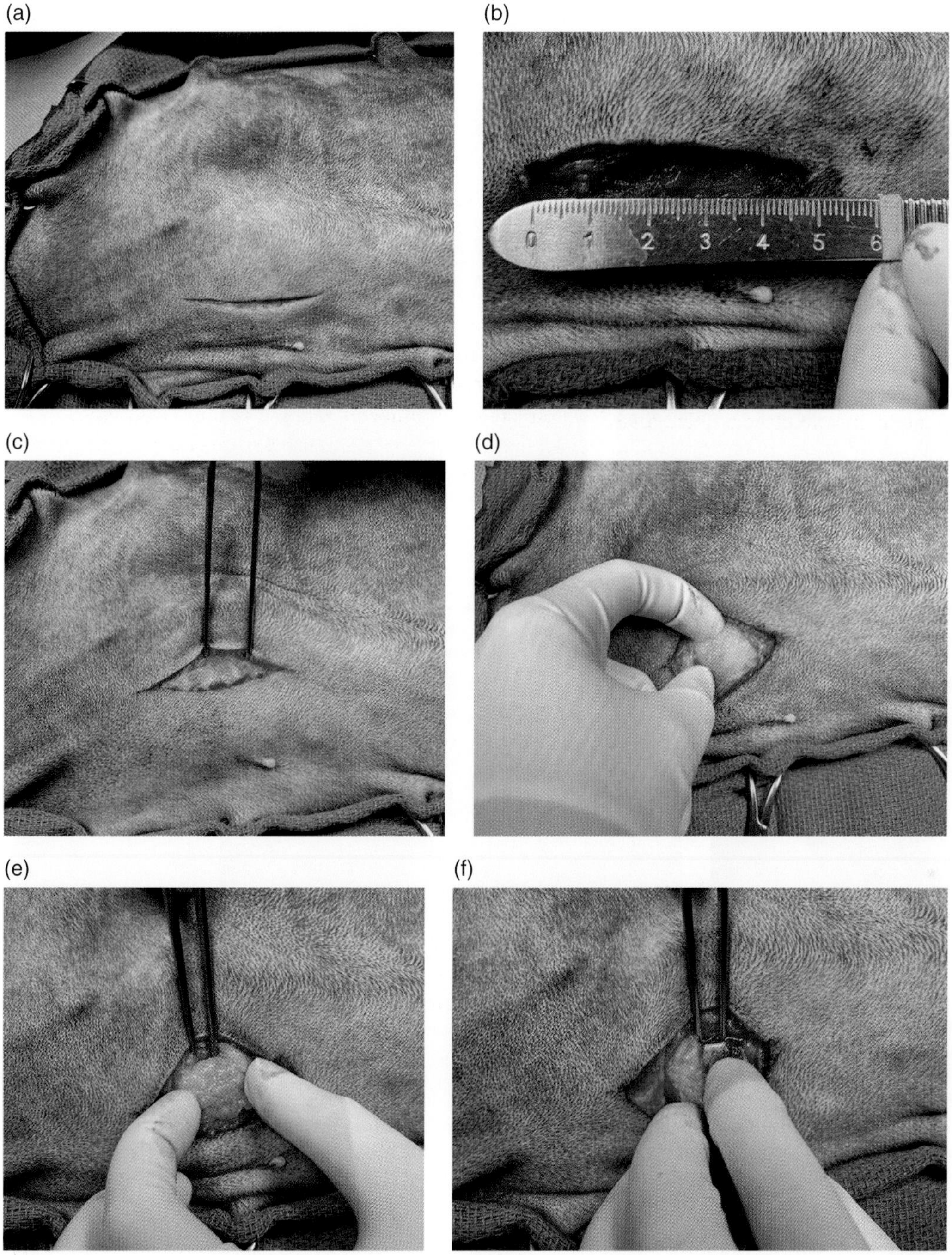

Figure 15.2 Approach to left unilateral cricoarytenoid lateralization on canine patient. Cranial is to the left and dorsal is to the top of the images. (a) Craniocaudal incision is made through the skin and subcutaneous layers over the center of the palpable larynx. (b) Incision should be an approximate length of 4–6 cm to provide adequate visualization during the procedure. (c) The first of two muscles to be transected during the approach is the platysma muscle, which is just deep to the subcutis. (d) After transecting platysma muscle and traversing through a layer of fat, the surgeon should begin feeling for the dorsal ridge of the thyroid cartilage and use their fingertip to grasp the edge for abduction. (e) Once the thyroid cartilage has been abducted with the fingertip, it should be held in place with forceps in order to complete dissection down to the level of the cartilage (e.g., through the remainder of the fat). (f) The second of the two muscles to be transected during the approach is the one overlying the thyroid cartilage and must be re-apposed at the time of closure due to its role in swallowing: the thyropharyngeus muscle. *Source:* © Kristin Coleman.

if the CAD is atrophied can then be transected. Exposure of the cricoarytenoid articulation is performed by making a small window caudal to the muscular process (Figure 15.4).[1,10]

Once the approach is complete, a non-absorbable suture is used to perform the cricoarytenoid lateralization. It is the author's preference to use 0-polypropylene on large to giant breed dogs and 2-0 polypropylene on medium to large breed

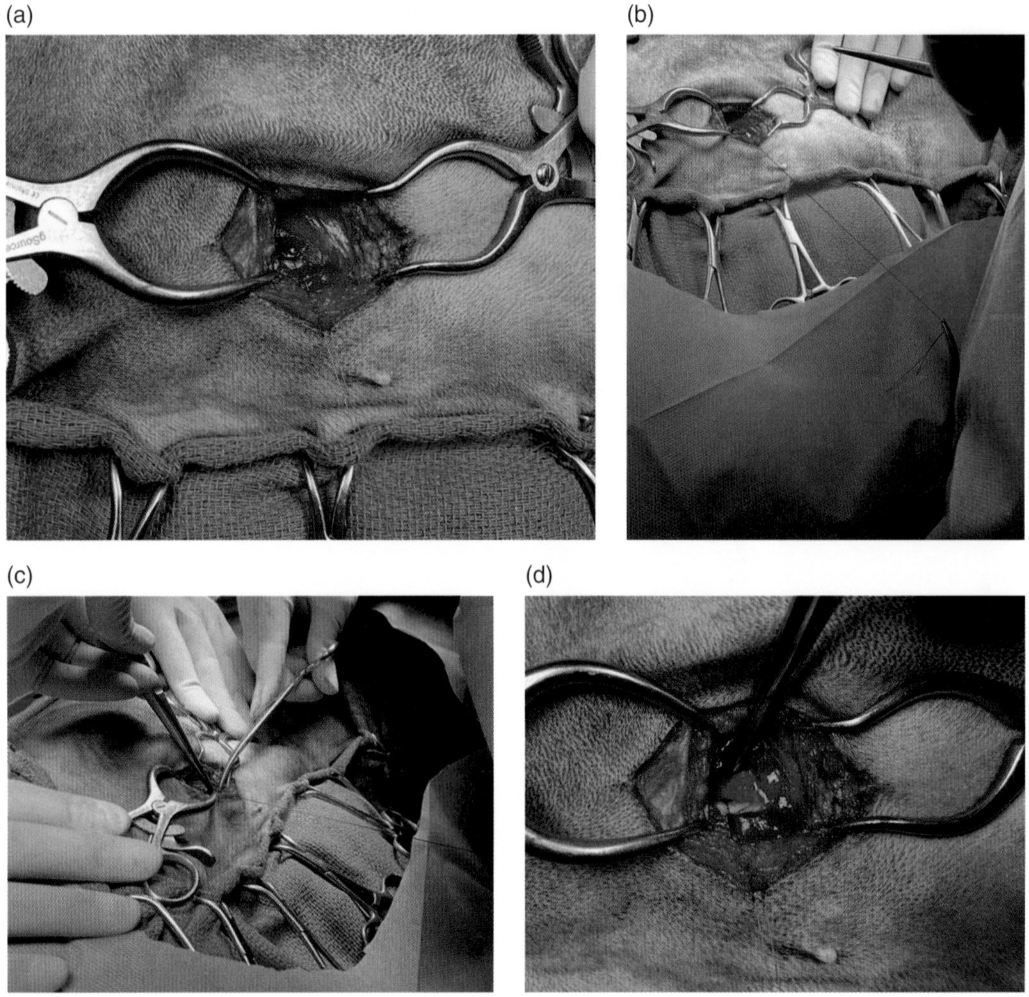

Figure 15.3 Placement of thyroid cartilage stay suture for left unilateral cricoarytenoid lateralization on canine patient. Cranial is to the left and dorsal is to the top of the images. (a) After transecting the thyropharyngeus muscle along the dorsal edge of the caudal thyroid cartilage, a blue (3-0 polypropylene) stay suture is passed from medial to lateral through the exposed cartilage. (b) The stay suture is purposefully left long in order for the surgeon's sterile gowned abdomen to control abduction of the cartilage, which allows for both hands to be used for the remainder of the surgery and prevents the need for a second assistant to hold the stay suture. (c) With the thyroid cartilage abducted with the surgeon's abdomen, both hands may be used for the rest of the procedure, and the one assistant on the dorsal aspect of the patient is all that is needed for retraction, which may be with a combination of Gelpi and Senn retractors, being mindful of the dorsally located jugular vein. (d) With the thyroid cartilage abducted, the next step is to palpate for the muscular process of the arytenoid cartilage, which is the bump just caudal to the tips of the DeBakey forceps. The membrane just medial to the thyroid cartilage should then be incised (close to the thyroid cartilage) to allow access to the muscular process. *Source:* © Kristin Coleman.

dogs, both of which should be on CT or similar needles. The suture is first passed around the caudodorsal border of the cricoid cartilage to exit at a precise location from where the muscular process was separated from the cricoid cartilage at the caudal aspect of the joint capsule.[2] While pulling up or laterally on the suture that was just passed around and the through the cricoid cartilage, the anesthetist may then deflate the endotracheal tube (ET) tube cuff and move the ET tube several inches caudally and cranially to ensure that the suture did not inadvertently grab the tube during passage. The suture is regrasped and then passed through the center of the muscular process via the cricoarytenoid joint surface (Figure 15.5).[11] The suture is tagged using a mosquito forceps, and a second suture is passed in the exact same manner if desired. The sutures are then tied separately. The suture should not be overtightened, as it can be unnecessary if the proper exit and entry points are adhered to or can cause the cartilage or suture to break (Figure 15.6). To ensure adequate glottis opening, the patient can be temporarily extubated for observation of the larynx either during tying the suture or after tying suture, prior to closure. The thyropharyngeus muscle is then closed in a continuous pattern using an absorbable suture. The subcutaneous tissue and skin can then be closed routinely.[1,10,12]

Following surgery, the patient should be recovered in sternal recumbency with the head elevated, and opioids are

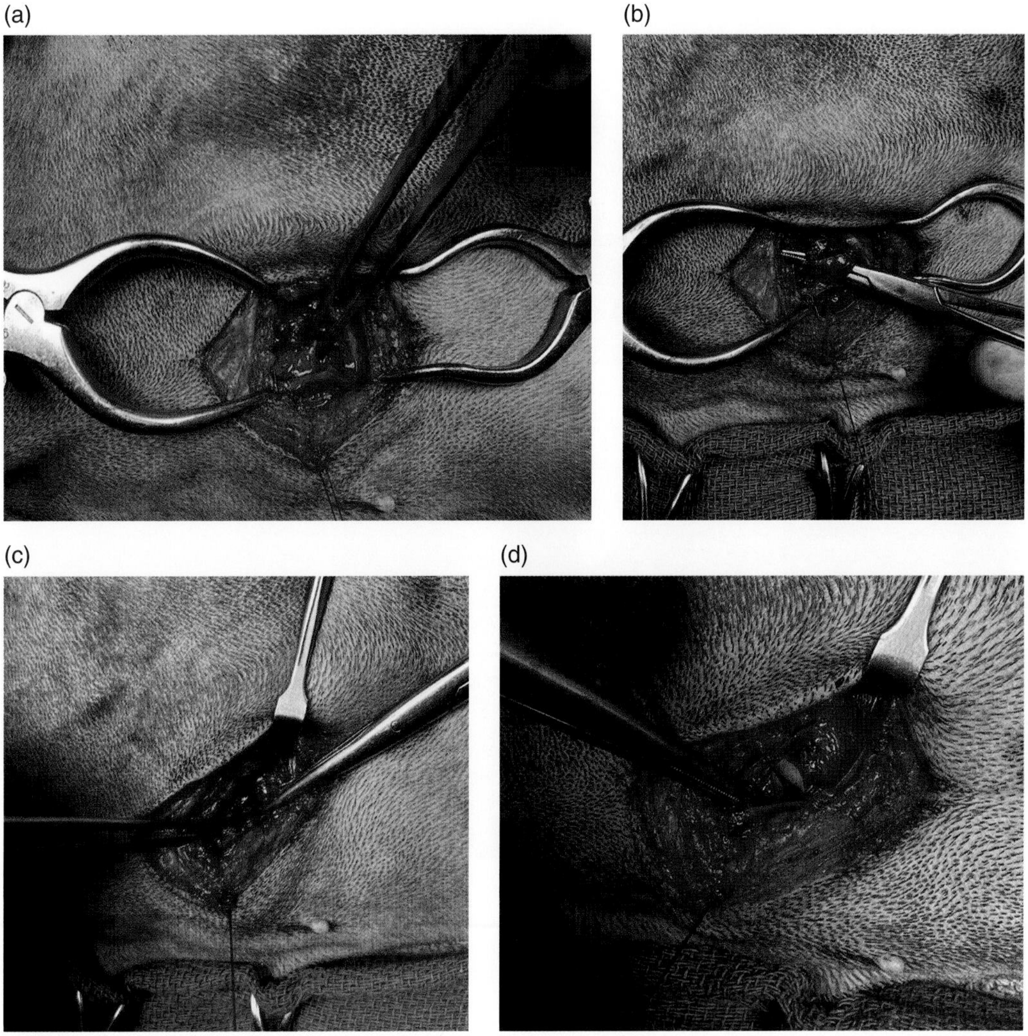

Figure 15.4 Dissection to the level of the cricoarytenoid joint during left unilateral cricoarytenoid lateralization on canine patient. Cranial is to the left and dorsal is to the top of the images. (a) Following incision of the membrane medial to the thyroid cartilage, the muscular process is again palpated and is being grasped by the DeBakey forceps here. (b) The CAD muscle, which may be barely present due to chronic atrophy or more robust as in this patient, should be undermined with curved mosquito hemostats and transected. It is recommended to leave a small tag of muscle attached to the muscular process to provide a handle for manipulation for the rest of the procedure. (c) Thumb forceps may then be used to lift the muscular process, and small curved Metzenbaum scissors are used to gradually incise into the joint capsule, which attaches the muscular process to the underlying cricoid cartilage (i.e., cricoarytenoid joint). (d) This view of the articular cartilages of both the muscular process and cricoid cartilage should be achieved prior to proceeding with the remainder of surgery. *Source:* © Kristin Coleman.

avoided. The mouth is suctioned prior to extubation. It is the author's preference that the patient be fasted for overnight following surgery and then offered 2–3 golfball-sized meatballs the following morning, while it is the editor's preference to perform a food trial with the same golfball-sized meatballs within hours after surgery and discharge the patient to avoid stress and excessive panting in hospital. Both are acceptable methods of postoperative management.

Reported postoperative complications include incisional complications, seroma or hematoma formation, persistent gagging/hacking, recurrence of respiratory signs (suture failure), laryngeal webbing, and aspiration pneumonia. Aspiration pneumonia is a life-long risk following surgery and has been reported in up to 21% of dogs.[9,13] Return of moderate to severe symptoms (suture failure or cartilage fracture is suspected) may require surgery to be performed on the contralateral side.[8] Overall, postoperative improvement occurs in up to 90% of cases.[14] The author recommends postoperative lifestyle changes, which include avoiding swimming, neck leads, high impact exercise, and hot and humid weather. Feeding smaller more frequent meals (3–4 times per day) is also recommended.

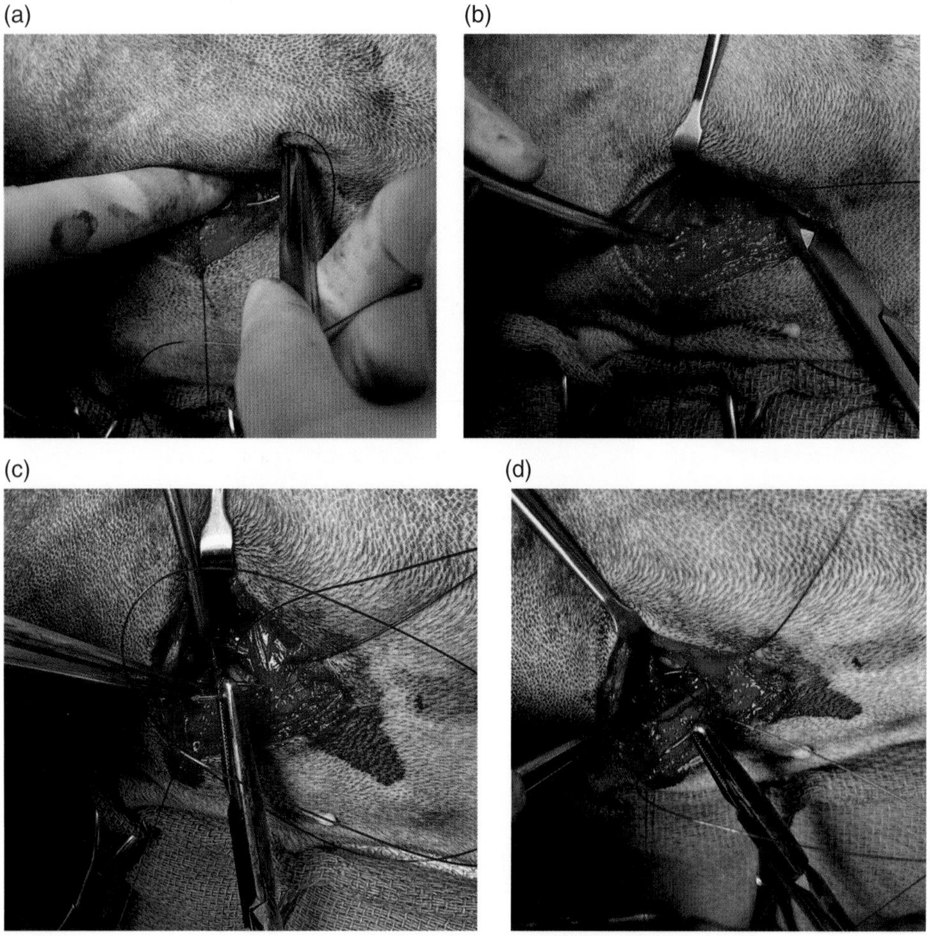

Figure 15.5 Passage of the suture during left unilateral cricoarytenoid lateralization on canine patient. Cranial is to the left and dorsal is to the top of the images. (a) Palpating the step from cricoid cartilage to trachea, the needle should be held in a way where the arc is parallel with the surface, which should reduce the risk of endotracheal tube penetration during passage of the needle around and through the cricoid cartilage. (b) Based on the article by Gauthier and Monnet,[11] the needle should pass around the caudodorsal aspect of the cricoid cartilage, then exit at the "1" or "2" sites near the caudal edge from where the muscular process was detached, and the needle in this image is exiting at the "1" site. (c) Once the suture has been passed around and through the cricoid cartilage, the surgeon should lift the suture and request that the anesthetist deflate the ET tube cuff and be able to shift the tube a few centimeters cranially and caudally, ensuring that the suture has not grasped the ET tube. (d) Once this is confirmed, the ET tube cuff is re-inflated, and the needle should be passed into the center of the muscular process. *Source:* © Kristin Coleman.

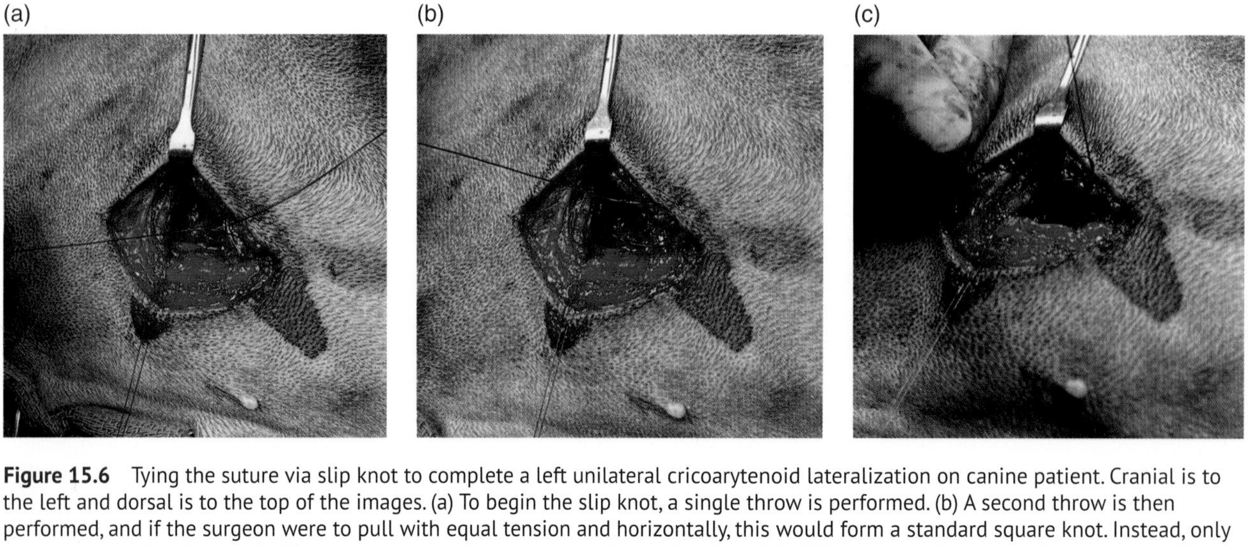

Figure 15.6 Tying the suture via slip knot to complete a left unilateral cricoarytenoid lateralization on canine patient. Cranial is to the left and dorsal is to the top of the images. (a) To begin the slip knot, a single throw is performed. (b) A second throw is then performed, and if the surgeon were to pull with equal tension and horizontally, this would form a standard square knot. Instead, only one strand has tension applied in order to control eventual formation of the knot. (c) A "D" should be formed by the suture, in which one strand has continuous tension applied and the other strand is slack until the desired point of adequate suture tightening, at which point both strands have equal and horizontal tension applied to "lock" the knot. Additional throws should then be applied. *Source:* © Kristin Coleman.

References

1 Monnet, E. and Tobias, K.M. (2012). Larynx. In: *Veterinary Surgery Small Animal* (ed. K.M. Tobias and S.A. Johnston), 1718–1733. WB Saunders.

2 Millard, R.P. and Tobias, K.M. (2009). Laryngeal paralysis in dogs. *Compend. Contin. Educ. Vet.* 31 (5): 212–219.

3 MacPhail, C.M. (2020). Laryngeal disease in dogs and cats: an update. *Vet. Clin. North Am. Small Anim. Pract.* 50 (2): 295–310. https://doi.org/10.1016/j.cvsm.2019.11.001.

4 Shelton, G.D. (2010). Acquired laryngeal paralysis in dogs: evidence accumulating for a generalized neuromuscular disease. *Vet. Surg.* 39 (2): 137–138.

5 Stanley, B.J., Hauptman, J.G., Fritz, M.C. et al. (2010). Esophageal dysfunction in dogs with idiopathic laryngeal paralysis: a controlled cohort study. *Vet. Surg.* 39 (2): 139–149.

6 Tobias, K.M., Jackson, A.M., and Harvey, R.C. (2004). Effects of doxapram HCl on laryngeal function of normal dogs and dogs with naturally occurring laryngeal paralysis. *Vet. Anaesth. Analg.* 31 (4): 258–263.

7 Miller, C.J., McKiernan, B.C., Pace, J. et al. (2002). The effects of doxapram hydrochloride (dopram-V) on laryngeal function in healthy dogs. *J. Vet. Intern. Med.* 16 (5): 524–528.

8 Monnet, E. (2016). Surgical treatment of laryngeal paralysis. *Vet. Clin. North Am. Small Anim. Pract.* 46 (4): 709–717. https://doi.org/10.1016/j.cvsm.2016.02.003.

9 MacPhail, C.M. and Monnet, E. (2001). Outcome of and postoperative complications in dogs undergoing surgical treatment of laryngeal paralysis: 140 cases (1985–1998). *J. Am. Vet. Med. Assoc.* 218 (12): 1949–1956.

10 von Pfeil, D.J.F., Edwards, M.R., and Dejardin, L.M. (2014). Less invasive unilateral arytenoid lateralization: a modified technique for treatment of idiopathic laryngeal paralysis in dogs: technique description and outcome. *Vet. Surg.* 43 (6): 704–711.

11 Gauthier, C.M. and Monnet, E. (2014). In vitro evaluation of anatomic landmarks for the placement of suture to achieve effective arytenoid cartilage abduction by means of unilateral cricoarytenoid lateralization in dogs. *Am. J. Vet. Res.* 75 (6): 602–606.

12 Bureau, S. and Monnet, E. (2002). Effects of suture tension and surgical approach during unilateral arytenoid lateralization on the rima glottidis in the canine larynx. *Vet. Surg.* 31 (6): 589–595.

13 Wilson, D. and Monnet, E. (2016). Risk factors for the development of aspiration pneumonia after unilateral arytenoid lateralization in dogs with laryngeal paralysis: 232 cases (1987–2012). *J. Vet. Med. Assoc.* 248 (2): 188–194.

14 Hammel, S.P., Hottinger, H.A., and Novo, R.E. (2006). Postoperative results of unilateral arytenoid lateralization for treatment of idiopathic laryngeal paralysis in dogs: 39 cases (1996–2002). *J. Am. Vet. Med. Assoc.* 228 (8): 1215–1220.

16

Peripheral Lymph Node Extirpation in the Dog and Cat

Arathi Vinayak

VCA West Coast Animal Emergency and Specialty Hospital, Fountain Valley, CA, USA

Key Points

- Common indications for lymph node extirpation are for lymphadenitis due to infection or inflammation, for staging and prognosis, and for improvement in prognosis in certain malignancies.
- Thorough knowledge of anatomy is required for atraumatic dissection to minimize complications. With appropriate tissue-handling, complication rate, and patient morbidity are very low.
- Knowledge of regions of afferents received by each node type will allow veterinarians to extirpate the node most likely affected by malignancy depending on location of the neoplastic process.
- Sentinel lymph nodes are the at-risk lymph nodes for metastasis from a primary tumor and may not necessarily be the nearest lymph node. In fact, nearly half of the time, the sentinel node differed from the nearest node in a recent study. Nodal mapping is required to identify these at-risk lymph nodes.

Introduction

The number of lymphocenters in dogs is relatively small with small groups and number of nodes in each group.[1] Shapes vary with some nodes being oval or round, bean-shaped, bilobed, elongated, etc. Most nodes have between 1 and 3 afferent lymphatics with upward of 50 efferents exiting a node that then combine to form three to five larger efferent lymphatics.[1] These efferent lymphatics then drain into either venous vasculature or directly into the thoracic duct. Lymphatic vessels transport lymph from organs and tissues, lipids from the intestines and liver, and fluid from local sites back into circulation.[2] The lymphatic system also functions to mount an immune response when it detects foreign materials and infectious agents from the skin, respiratory, and gastrointestinal systems. These foreign or infectious agents are presented to the nodes via afferent lymphatics,[2] which divide into branches within the cortex, then drain into the medulla of the node from where the efferent lymphatics exit the node. The nodal cortex is primarily comprised of B-lymphocytes arranged into follicles; the medulla consists of lymphocytes, macrophages, and plasma cells; and the paracortex between the cortex and medulla consists of T-lymphocytes.[2,3] The three regions work in tandem to present antigens and elicit a primary immune response.[2,3]

Nodal involvement is an integral part of staging a cancer patient. In addition to distant metastasis, locoregional nodal involvement is part of the World Health Organization TNM system.[4] The primary tumor extent is T, nodal (lymph node) extent is N, and M represents distant metastasis. Stage of the tumor affects prognosis and the treatment plan for the patient. Knowledge of cancer behavior, as well as knowledge of draining lymph nodes relative to site of the primary tumor, sheds light on whether nodal involvement is possible and how this affects prognosis, treatment plan, and patient survival. For example, mast cell tumors, oral melanoma, and anal sac adenocarcinomas are a few

Techniques in Small Animal Soft Tissue, Orthopedic, and Ophthalmic Surgery, First Edition. Edited by Kristin A. Coleman.

Companion website: www.wiley.com/go/coleman/surgeries

commonly encountered tumors that metastasize to regional lymph nodes. Nodal staging is accomplished by palpation, imaging, sentinel lymph node mapping, cytology, and histopathology.[1] Palpation alone has a sensitivity of 60% and specificity of 72% in predicting metastasis; thus, it should be used in conjunction with other modalities.[5] Cytology has a 66.6–100% sensitivity, 91.5–96% specificity, and 77.2% accuracy.[5,6] The correlation between cytology and histopathology is 90.9%.[7]

Cancer can alter lymphatic drainage, so lymph nodes other than the nearest draining regional lymph node may be affected. In fact, the sentinel lymph node differed from the regional lymph node in 52% of dogs in a recent study.[8] Identification of the at-risk lymph node can be accomplished using contrast lymphography followed by imaging, such as radiography or CT, lymphoscintigraphy using a radioactive tracer, or perioperative injection of a dye. This at-risk lymph node is the sentinel node, and identification of these nodes is called sentinel lymph node mapping. The sentinel node identification in and of itself does not mean the node is metastatic; it simply means that if cancer is going to spread via the lymphatic system, it would spread first to the sentinel lymph node. Extirpation of the lymph node with histopathology identifies whether a node is metastatic, and metastasis in the sentinel node is reported in 42–45% of the lymph nodes.[8,9]

Pre-operative Considerations/Indications

Lymphadenitis, inflammation, and subsequent enlargement of lymph nodes, most commonly due to infection, are indications for removal (i.e., lymphadenectomy or lymph node extirpation). Presurgical culture and antibiotics are indicated if bacterial infection has led to marked cellulitis around the surgery site and to decrease the odds of an incisional infection. A macerated tissue culture of nodal tissue at the time of surgery is also indicated to ensure that the antibiotics used have treated the infection. Another common reason for marked nodal enlargement is malignancy that may be identified on cytology. Removal of lymph nodes that are metastatic may be the part of treatment with improvement in prognosis for some cancers, such as canine mast cell tumors. Removal of regional lymph nodes is also indicated for highly malignant tumors like melanoma, after which the node can be thoroughly evaluated for malignancy to aid in staging, prognosis, and guidance for adjuvant therapy recommendations. Sentinel lymph node mapping as discussed above to help identify at-risk lymph nodes is becoming increasingly popular in veterinary medicine.

Commonly extirpated peripheral lymph nodes are mandibular, medial retropharyngeal, prescapular (i.e., superficial cervical), popliteal, and superficial inguinal lymph nodes. The axillary lymph node is also accessible for extirpation; however, thorough knowledge of anatomy in and around the brachial plexus is needed before undertaking removal.

Mandibular lymph nodes are readily palpable and are easy to approach surgically. Landmarks include the bifurcation of the external jugular vein into the linguofacial vein and external maxillary vein, but this palpable structure is not to be confused with the normally larger but similarly located mandibular salivary gland. The linguofacial vein divides the mandibular nodes into dorsal and ventral groups. Each group consists of one to two nodes, thus making a total of two to four nodes in the mandibular lymph node basin in most companion animals.[1] These nodes receive afferent drainage from the nose, lips, cheek, intermandibular region, zygomatic arch, gums, hard and soft palate, eyelids, various bones of the head, and muscles of the head and neck.[1]

The medial retropharyngeal lymph nodes serve as the lymphatic collection center of the head and receives efferent drainage from the lateral retropharyngeal, parotid, and mandibular lymph nodes. This lymph node tends to yield the most diagnostic information for potential metastatic spread of oral cancers.[10] This node is located caudomedial to the mandibular salivary gland, caudal to the digastricus muscle, ventral to the wing of the atlas and the longus colli muscle, medial to the mastoid aspects of the brachiocephalicus and sternocephalicus muscles, and dorsal to the thyroid cartilage of the larynx, and these structures serve as landmarks for locating this lymph node. Afferent drainage is from similar regions as the mandibular lymph nodes, in addition to drainage from the tonsils, pharynx, esophagus, thyroid, larynx, trachea, and ears.[1] There is sometimes but inconsistently a lateral retropharyngeal lymph node present.

Superficial cervical nodes are relatively deep lymph nodes in the neck located at the junction of the neck and shoulder. Most dogs have one to two nodes on each side. They are sandwiched between the supraspinatus muscles and the brachiocephalicus and omotransversarius muscles superficially, which serve as landmarks for localization in surgery. The bulk of the afferent drainage is received from the skin of the caudal part of the dorsal head region, pinna, parotid and neck areas, caudal half of the cranial neck region, forelimb digits, metacarpus, carpus and forearm, most of the lateral side of the upper shoulder, upper foreleg region, medial side of the humeral region, thoracic inlet, and cranial part of the ventral thorax.[1]

The axillary lymph node lies in the brachial plexus region at the level of the shoulder joint. There is usually only one axillary node in dogs, and this lymph node receives afferent drainage from nearly all bones of the forelimb and the cranial mammary glands. It also receives afferent drainage from the skin lying between the shoulder and the last rib on the lateral and ventral thoracic wall, lateral side of the shoulder, lateral brachium, olecranon, and nearly all muscles of the forelimb.[1]

Located on the caudal aspect of the stifle joint between the distal end of the biceps femoris and semitendinosus muscles encased in fatty tissue is the popliteal lymph node. Typically, this is only a single node in this location with rare occurrence of two nodes. Most of the afferents are received from the skin on the lateral aspect of the stifle joint and lower leg, metatarsus and digits, tibia, fibula, tarsal and metatarsal bones, phalanges, and muscles distal to the stifle joint.[1]

The superficial inguinal lymph nodes are located just medial to the fifth mammary nipple in dogs and fourth mammary nipple in cats (i.e., the most caudal nipples). The external pudendal artery and vein serve as landmarks where one to three nodes are typically present. Most of the afferent drainage is received from the ventral half of the abdomen caudal to the 13th rib, prepuce, penis and scrotum, vulva and clitoris, mammary glands, skin of the caudal pelvis, skin of the lateral and medial thighs, skin of the medial and cranial half of the lateral stifle, and the medial and cranial half of the lateral lower leg.[1]

Surgical Procedures

A) **Mandibular lymph node extirpation** (Figure 16.1): The patient is positioned in lateral recumbency with the affected lymph node side up. The most superficial of the many nodes in this nodal basin is palpable caudal to the angle of the mandible. The incision is made

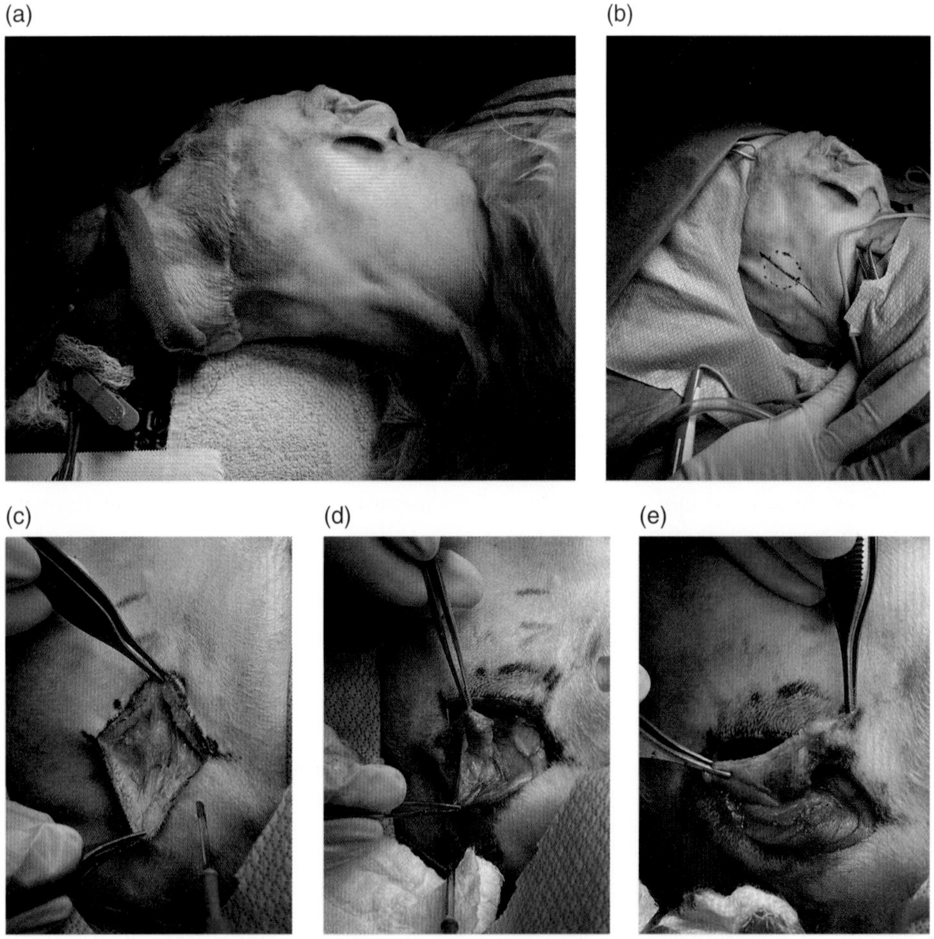

Figure 16.1 Left mandibular lymph node extirpation in a dog. (a) An area caudal to the angle of the mandible is shaved, exposing the external jugular vein and its bifurcation into the dorsally located maxillary vein and ventrally located linguofacial vein. (b) An incision is made dorsal to the linguofacial/facial vein over the most superficial of the mandibular lymph nodes that are palpable. (c) The incision is continued through the subcutaneous tissue and platysma muscle. (d) The node(s) dorsal to the linguofacial vein are dissected free, taking care to not damage the vein in close proximity. The vein is seen in the image near the bottom thumb forceps. (e) Nodes in the group ventral to the linguofacial vein are then dissected free. Closure is as described in Figure 16.2 for medial retropharyngeal lymph node extirpation that uses a similar approach.

just dorsal to the linguofacial vein separating these nodes into dorsal and ventral sections. The incision is continued through the subcutaneous tissues and platysma muscle. The mandibular lymph nodes are palpated and extirpated using thumb forceps, Allis tissue forceps, or a stay suture to hold the node while dissection is continued around to free it from the surrounding tissues. Any small blood vessels at the nodal hilus are cauterized as they are encountered. Closure consists of apposition of the platysma as the deep layer in a simple continuous pattern using a long-lasting synthetic monofilament absorbable suture (3-0 or 4-0), followed by subcutaneous tissues in a simple continuous pattern using a medium-lasting synthetic monofilament absorbable suture (3-0 or 4-0). The external skin is apposed with a pattern of the clinician's choice, and the author uses either a simple interrupted or interrupted cruciate pattern of nonabsorbable suture (3-0 or 4-0). The procedure is repeated on the contralateral side if warranted.

B) **Medial retropharyngeal lymph node extirpation** (Figure 16.2): The patient is positioned in lateral recumbency with the affected lymph node side up. Knowledge of anatomy is critical to prevent inadvertent dissection and damage to the common carotid artery, which is medial to the node, vagosympathetic trunk, hypoglossal nerve, recurrent laryngeal nerve, internal jugular vein, and the larynx. This node, grossly similar in appearance to the thyroid gland, must not be confused with the thyroid gland, which lies just caudal and dorsal to the thyroid cartilage and closer to midline. The initial approach is similar to mandibular lymph node extirpation, and this retropharyngeal lymph node is often extirpated in conjunction with mandibular nodes using a single approach. The skin, subcutaneous tissue, and platysma muscle are incised. Dissection is carried out medial to the mandibular salivary gland, and the salivary gland is gently elevated until the thyroid cartilage is palpable. Nodal dissection is carried out dorsal to the thyroid cartilage at a level just caudal to the mandibular salivary gland. Closure consists of apposition of the platysma as the deep layer in a simple continuous pattern using a long-lasting synthetic monofilament absorbable suture (3-0 or 4-0) and subcutaneous tissues in a simple continuous pattern. The external skin is apposed with a pattern of the clinician's choice, and the author uses either a simple interrupted or interrupted cruciate pattern of nonabsorbable suture (3-0 or 4-0). The procedure is repeated on the contralateral side if warranted.

C) **Superficial cervical (i.e., prescapular) lymph node extirpation** (Figure 16.3): The patient is positioned in lateral recumbency with the affected lymph node side up. The lymph node is palpable medial to (under) the omotransversarius muscle. A skin incision is made over the node, and the subcutaneous tissue is dissected to expose the omotransversarius muscle. Muscle fibers are bluntly separated along the fiber orientation, and the lymph node is bluntly dissected free. Any small blood vessels at the nodal hilus are cauterized, as they are encountered. The muscle fibers are apposed in a simple continuous pattern using a long-lasting synthetic monofilament absorbable suture (3-0 or 4-0), and closure is continued by apposing subcutaneous tissue in a simple continuous pattern. The external skin is apposed with a pattern of the clinician's choice, and the author uses either a simple interrupted or interrupted cruciate pattern of nonabsorbable suture (3-0 or 4-0).

D) **Axillary lymph node extirpation** (Figure 16.4): The patient is positioned in dorsal recumbency, and the ipsilateral forelimb with ventrolateral thoracic area is shaved, prepped, and draped in a standard hanging limb prep/drape. This lymph node is seldom palpable unless markedly enlarged. A skin incision is made over the axilla, and subcutaneous tissue is dissected to reveal the superficial pectoral muscle. These muscle fibers are bluntly separated to reveal the brachial plexus. With gentle digital exploration, the axillary artery pulse is palpated. The axillary vein runs along with this artery, and the axillary lymph node is adjacent to the axillary vein wall. Gentle blunt dissection is carried out until the lymph node is gently dissected away without damage to the artery, vein, and nerves of the brachial plexus. Closure is routine with apposition of the incised superficial pectoral muscle and subcutaneous tissues closed in separate layers in a simple continuous pattern using a long-lasting synthetic monofilament absorbable suture (e.g., 3-0 or 4-0 polydioxanone or polyglyconate). The external skin is apposed with a pattern of the clinician's choice, and the author uses either a simple interrupted or interrupted cruciate pattern of nonabsorbable suture (3-0 or 4-0).

E) **Popliteal lymph node extirpation** (Figure 16.5): The patient is positioned in lateral recumbency with the affected lymph node side up. The node is palpable in the popliteal fossa on the caudal aspect of the stifle. A small proximal to distal skin incision is made in this region, and subcutaneous tissue is dissected. Gentle dissection in the popliteal fat should yield a superficially located popliteal node, which has a small blood vessel requiring ligation and transection with care being taken to avoid the large underlying lateral saphenous vein. The lymph node is then dissected free. Closure consists of apposition of the subcutaneous tissues

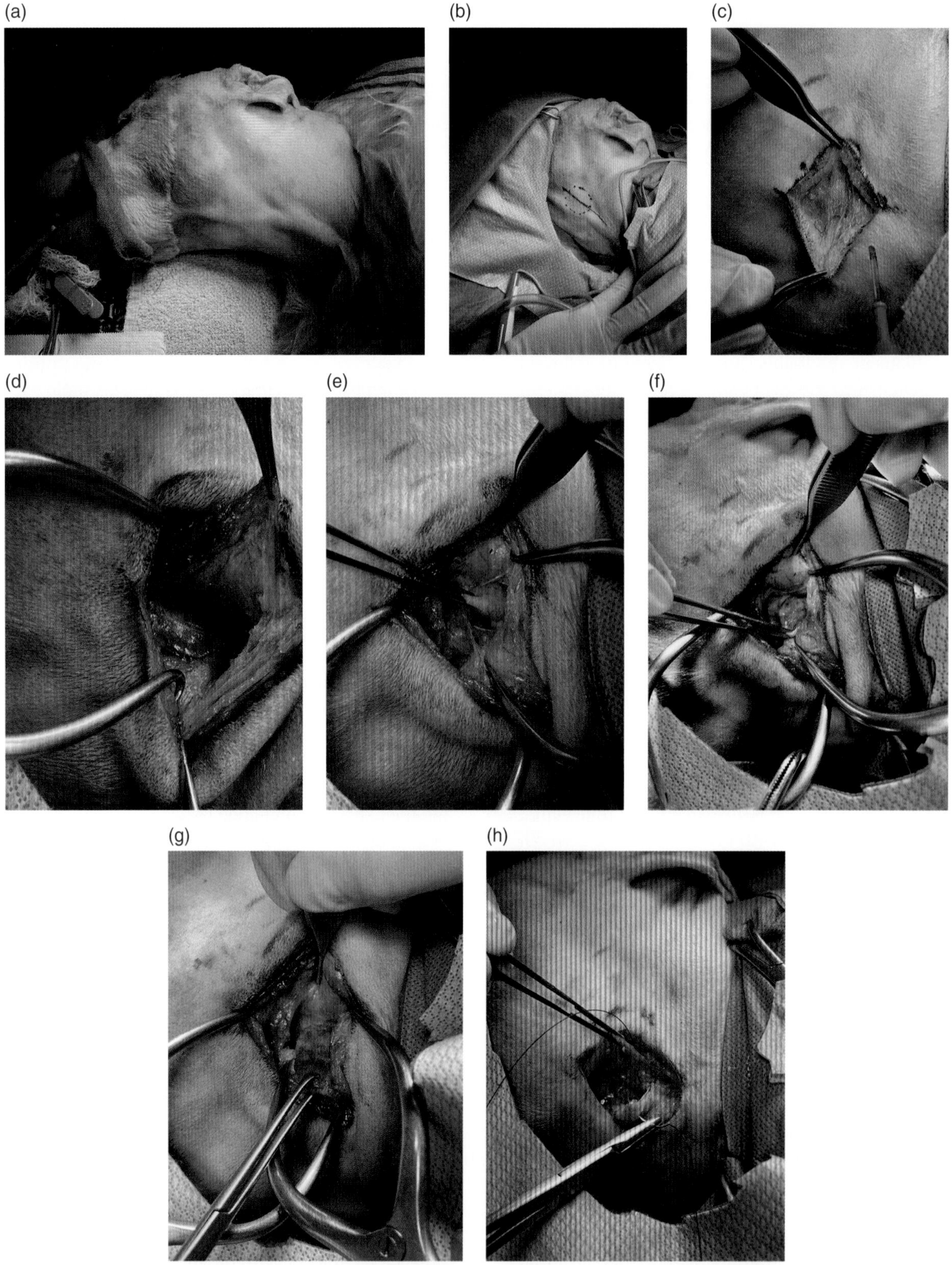

Figure 16.2 Left medial retropharyngeal lymph node extirpation in a dog. (a) An area caudal to the angle of the mandible is shaved, exposing the external jugular vein and its bifurcation into the dorsally located maxillary vein and ventrally located linguofacial vein. (b) An incision is made dorsal to the linguofacial/facial vein over the palpable mandibular salivary gland. (c) The incision is continued through the subcutaneous tissue and platysma muscle. (d) Dissection is carried medial to the mandibular salivary gland. (e) The medial retropharyngeal lymph node is identified just along the caudal edge of the mandibular salivary gland seen in the top thumb forceps with the DeBakey thumb forceps grasping the node. (f,g) The node is gently teased from surrounding fat, vasculature, and nerves, being careful to not damage the common carotid artery and vagosympathetic trunk medial to the node. This node is a flattened and long node that requires patient gentle dissection to free it in its entirety. (h) The deeper subcutaneous tissue and platysma are sutured as a single layer, followed by routine closure of the superficial subcutaneous tissue and external skin.

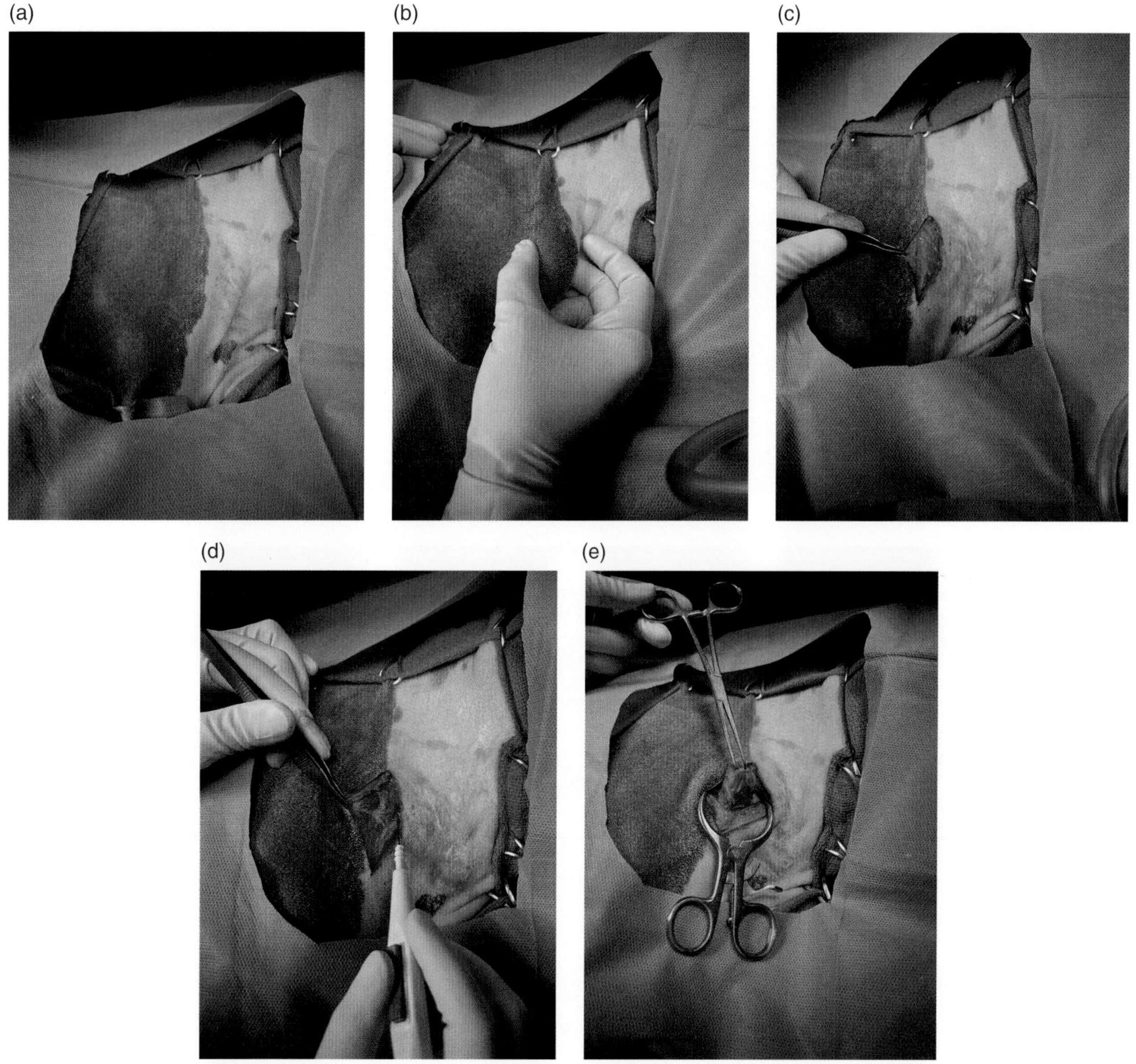

Figure 16.3 Right superficial cervical lymph node extirpation in a dog. (a) The patient is positioned in lateral recumbency with the affected lymph node side up. (b) The lymph node is palpable medial to (under) the omotransversarius muscle. (c) A skin incision is made over the node, and the subcutaneous tissue is dissected to expose the omotransversarius muscle. (d) Omotransversarius muscle fibers are bluntly separated along the fiber orientation until the node is visible. (e) The lymph node is bluntly dissected free. The muscle fibers and subcutaneous tissue are apposed in two layers using a simple continuous pattern using a long-lasting synthetic monofilament absorbable suture (3-0 or 4-0). External skin with simple interrupted or interrupted cruciate patterns using nonabsorbable suture (3-0 or 4-0). *Source:* © Kristin Coleman.

in a simple continuous pattern subcutaneous tissues using a medium-lasting synthetic monofilament absorbable suture (e.g., 3-0 or 4-0 poliglecaprone 25 or glycomer 631). The external skin is apposed with a pattern of the clinician's choice, and the author uses either a simple interrupted or interrupted cruciate pattern of nonabsorbable suture (3-0 or 4-0).

F) **Superficial inguinal lymph node extirpation** (Figure 16.6): The patient is positioned in dorsal recumbency. A skin incision is made medial and caudal to the last (most caudal) mammary nipple. Dissection is gentle and is carried out until the caudal superficial epigastric vessels are observed. One to two nodes may be found in this location and are bluntly dissected, taking

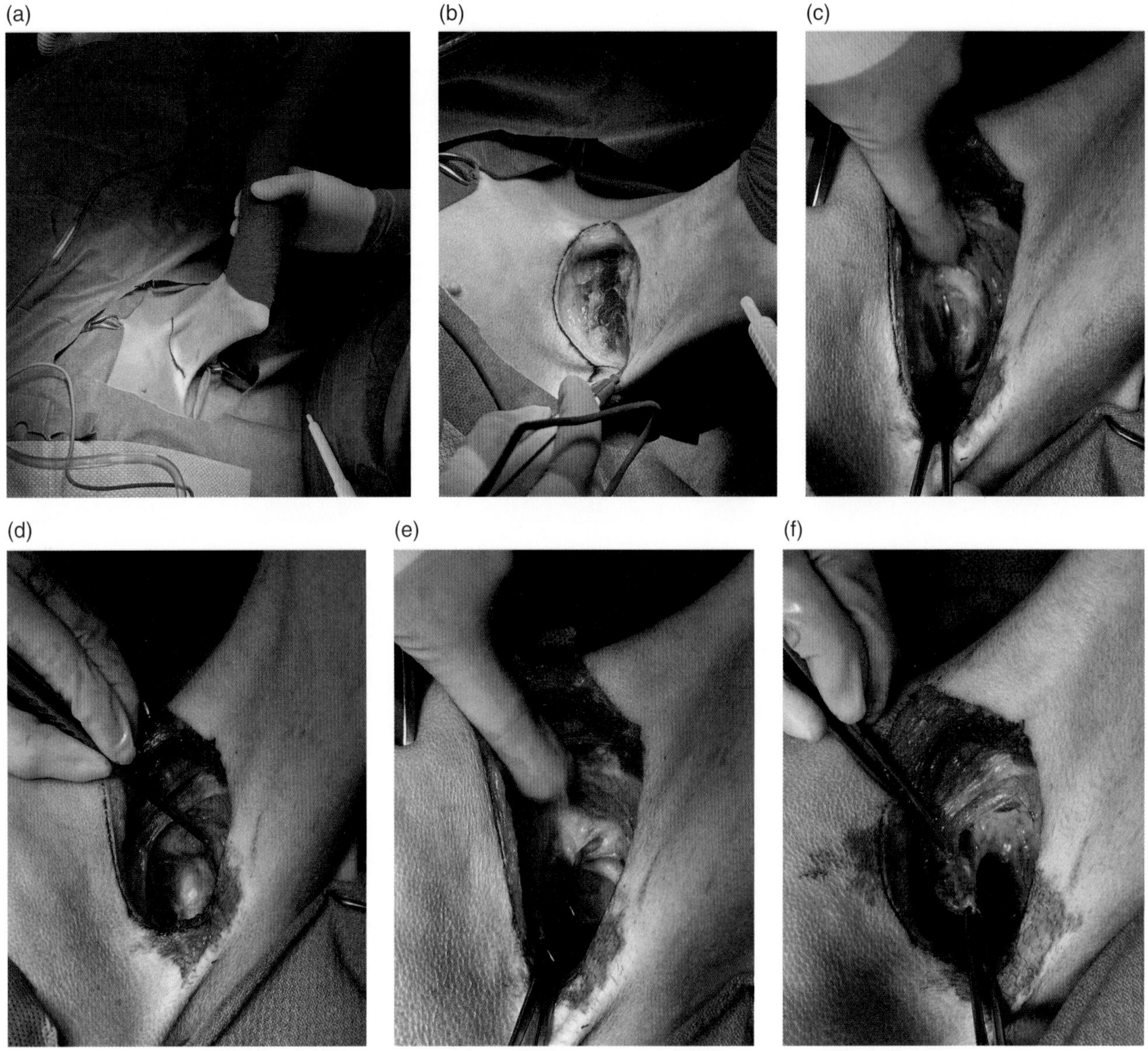

Figure 16.4 Left axillary lymph node extirpation in a dog. (a) The proposed incision is shown in the left axillary region in purple surgical marker. (b) The skin and subcutaneous tissues have been dissected to reveal the superficial pectoral muscle. (c) The axillary region is gently digitally palpated until the pulse of the axillary artery is identified. The tip of the right-angle forceps in the image points to the axillary artery. (d) Gentle palpation reveals the axillary node alongside the axillary artery and vein. The tip of the DeBakey thumb forceps points to the location of the node. (e) Gentle dissection of the fat around the node reveals the node. (f) Grasping the node with Allis tissue forceps to provide traction once the node is revealed aids in dissection, as long as care is taken to not grasp nerves or vasculature with the node! Closure of this area is very straightforward with closure of the incised superficial pectoral muscle, subcutaneous tissue, and skin in a standard three-layer closure.

care to not damage the caudal superficial epigastric vasculature nearby. Closure consists of apposition of the subcutaneous tissues in a simple continuous pattern. The external skin is apposed with a pattern of the clinician's choice, and the author uses either a simple interrupted or interrupted cruciate pattern of nonabsorbable suture (3-0 or 4-0).

Potential Complications

Like complications with any incision, infection, dehiscence, and seroma are potential complications. Thorough knowledge of the local anatomy is warranted prior to undertaking lymphadenectomy to prevent iatrogenic damage to vasculature and nerves. Unnecessary wide

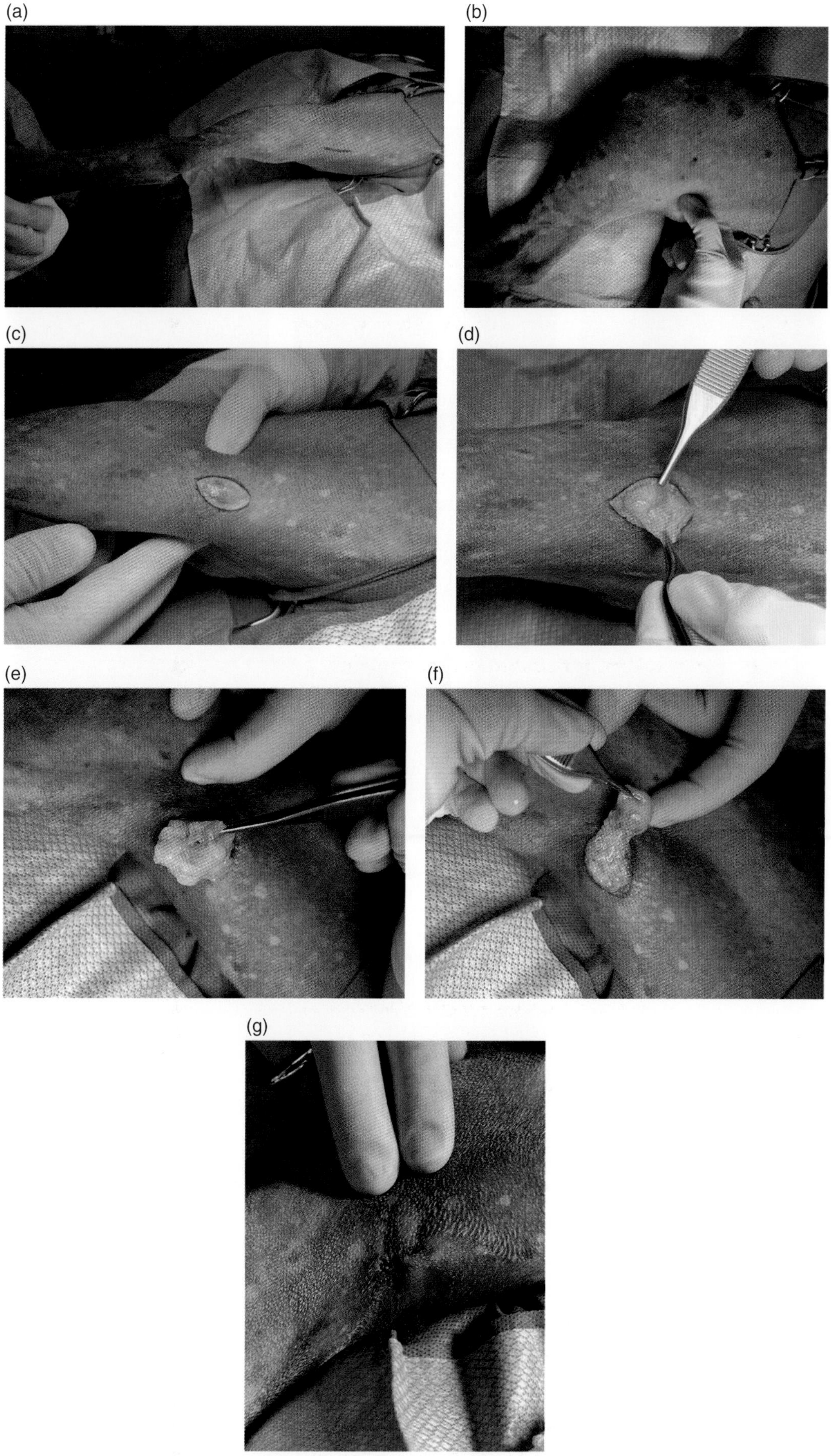

Figure 16.5 Left popliteal lymph node extirpation in a dog. (a) The caudal aspect of the left rear leg is shown. (b) The popliteal node is palpable in the popliteal fossa on the caudal aspect of the stifle. (c) An incision is made in the skin over the popliteal fossa. (d) The fat in the fossa is gently dissected. (e,f) The lymph node is found and gently extirpated from surrounding fat, and caution is taken to not damage the popliteal vasculature (lateral saphenous vein) just deep to the node. (g) Subcutaneous tissue and skin are closed routinely.

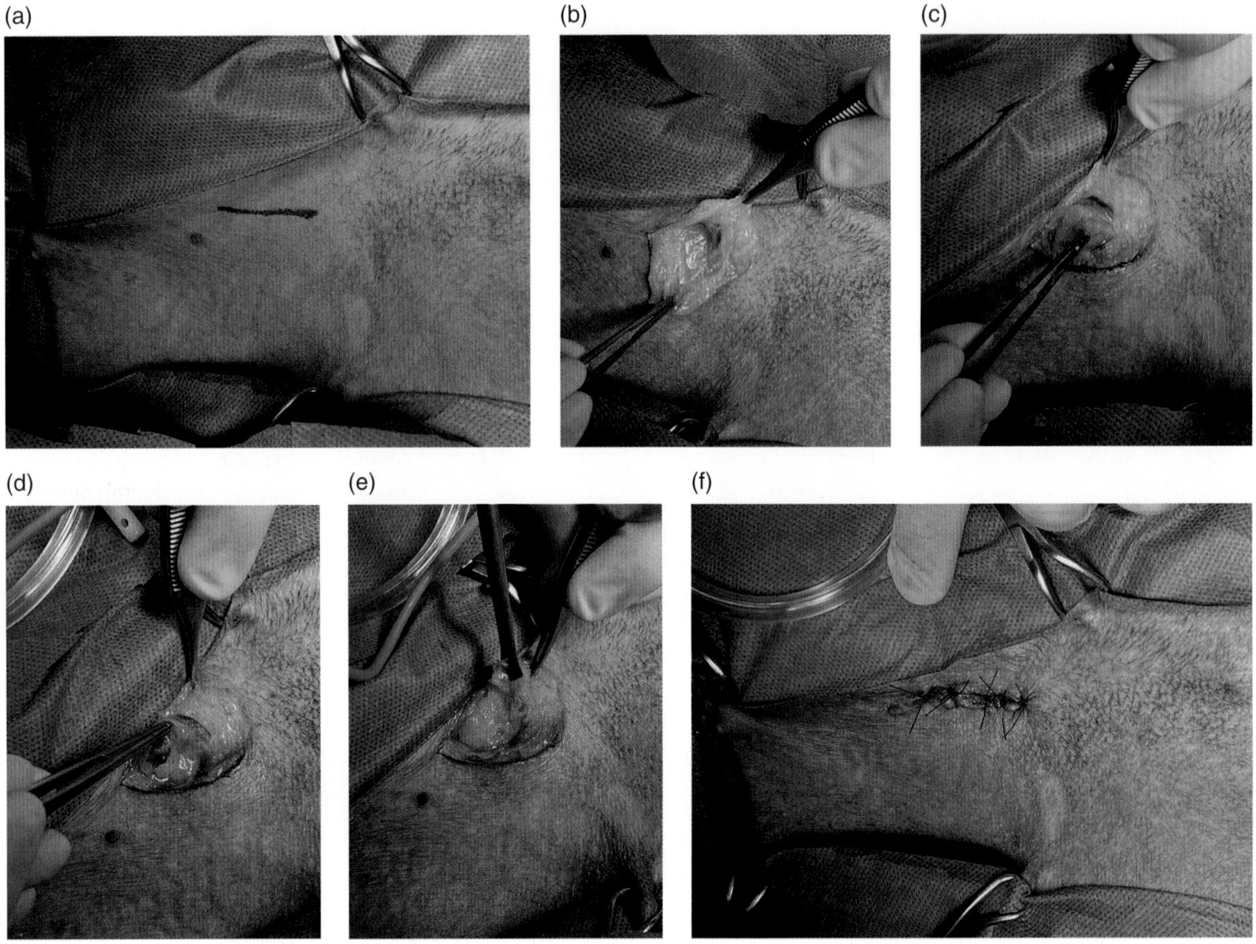

Figure 16.6 Right inguinal lymph node extirpation in a dog. (a) Cranial is to the left of the image and caudal is on the right of the image. The proposed incision is made just medial and caudal to the most caudal mammary nipple. (b) Blunt dissection is carried deeper until the caudal superficial epigastric artery and vein are encountered to serve as landmarks. (c) One to two nodes are generally present and are located near the vessels. The thumb forceps in the figure show nodal tissue visible in the inguinal fat. (d) A smaller node is dissected first. (e) A larger node is then dissected more caudally along the incision. (f) The site is then closed routinely.

dissection can help prevent dead space formation. Lymphedema, an accumulation of protein-rich fluid drained by lymphatics, can occur after lymphadenectomy but tends to be a self-limiting complication. The overall complication rate for lymphadenectomy is low and reported to be between 21.24% and 22%, of which 91.67% were self-limiting and minor.[8,9]

Postoperative Care

Pain medications +/− antibiotic therapy is recommended as with any surgical procedure. Infiltration of the surgery site with a local anesthetic can help with postoperative pain relief, especially with large nodal bed dissections. Warm compresses to the surgery site and proper activity restrictions for the patient can help minimize seroma formation.

Prognosis

Prognosis following lymphadenectomy depends on whether the procedure is considered for benign versus neoplastic disease. If benign, prognosis following lymphadenectomy could be good. No long-term negative effects have been documented in cats or dogs that have had one or more peripheral lymph nodes extirpated. If neoplastic, node positivity and stage of disease would offer a more guarded to potentially a poor prognosis depending on the malignancy.

References

1 Baum, H. (2021). *The Lymphatic System of the Dog* (ed. M. Mayer, L. Bettin, K. Bellamy, and I. Stamm).

2 van Nimwegen, S.A. and Kirpensteijn, J. (2018). Specific disorders of the skin and subcutaneous tissues. In: *Veterinary Surgery: Small Animal*, 2e, vol. 2 (ed. S.A. Johnston and K.M. Tobias), 1511–1514. Elsevier.

3 Samuelson, D.A. (2007). *Textbook of Veterinary Histology*. Saunders.

4 Owen, L.N. (1980). TNM classification of tumors in domestic animals. World Health Organization.

5 Langenbach, A., McManus, P.M., Hendrick, M.J. et al. (2001). Sensitivity and specificity of methods of assessing the regional lymph nodes for evidence of metastasis in dogs and cats with solid tumors. *J. Am. Vet. Med. Assoc.* 218 (9): 1424–1428. https://doi.org/10.2460/javma.2001.218.1424.

6 Ku, C.-K., Kass, P.H., and Christopher, M.M. (2017). Cytologic-histologic concordance in the diagnosis of neoplasia in canine and feline lymph nodes: a retrospective study of 367 cases. *Vet. Comp. Oncol.* 15 (4): 1206–1217. https://doi.org/10.1111/vco.12256.

7 Ghisleni, G., Roccabianca, P., Ceruti, R. et al. (2006). Correlation between fine-needle aspiration cytology and histopathology in the evaluation of cutaneous and subcutaneous masses from dogs and cats. *Vet. Clin. Pathol.* 35 (1): 24–30. https://doi.org/10.1111/j.1939-165X.2006.tb00084.x.

8 Chiti, L.E., Stefanello, D., Manfredi, M. et al. (2021). To map or not to map the cN0 neck: impact of sentinel lymph node biopsy in canine head and neck tumours. *Vet. Comp. Oncol.* 19 (4): 661–670. https://doi.org/10.1111/VCO.12697.

9 Chiti, L.E., Gariboldi, E.M., Ferrari, R. et al. (2023). Surgical complications following sentinel lymph node biopsy guided by γ-probe and methylene blue in 113 tumour-bearing dogs. *Vet. Comp. Oncol.* 21 (1): 62–72. https://doi.org/10.1111/VCO.12861.

10 Belz, G.T. and Heath, T.J. (1995). Lymph pathways of the medial retropharyngeal lymph node in dogs. *J. Anat.* 186 (Pt 3): 517–526. http://www.ncbi.nlm.nih.gov/pubmed/7559125.

17

Limb Amputation in Companion Animals: Thoracic and Pelvic Limb Amputations

Arathi Vinayak

VCA West Coast Animal Emergency and Specialty Hospital, Fountain Valley, CA, USA

Key Points

- Most animals return to normal activity within a month following amputation.
- There does not appear to be a difference in recovery between thoracic and pelvic limb amputations.
- Age and breed size do not appear to be negative prognostic indicators in amputees.
- Despite owner and veterinarian reservations against amputations, clients should be educated that owner satisfaction in both dogs and cats based on studies is high with most owners willing to consider amputation again if given a choice.
- A forequarter amputation for the thoracic limb and coxofemoral disarticulation for the pelvic limb have become the preferred options, as muscle atrophy post-amputation and disuse of the stump can lead to protrusion of bony prominences against the skin. Secondary irritation can result with potential need for revision surgery.
- Knowledge of anatomy and limited use of bipolar electrosurgery can help minimize intraoperative and postoperative morbidity.
- The overall complication rate is low in both dogs and cats with a relatively low infection rate.

Introduction

Thoracic and pelvic limb amputations are routinely performed procedures in small animal practice. The procedure is a salvage option when medical management or other limb-sparing surgical options fail to address the problem. It is also considered when the cost of treatment for the owner becomes prohibitive to save the limb. Careful orthopedic and neurologic evaluation of the animal should be performed to ensure compensation with the remaining three limbs occurs following amputation. Marked obesity and significant orthopedic and/or neurologic disease of the remaining limbs are contraindications for amputation of a limb.[1]

Despite how well veterinary amputees recover, there is still considerable reservation against the procedure from owners and some veterinarians. It is, thus, important to prepare the owner about amputation as an option and regarding surgical esthetics and recovery, as adequate owner preparation in advance of the procedure showed higher owner satisfaction with the procedure.[1] Concerns regarding the ability to compensate, concurrent osteoarthritis in remaining limbs/spine, compromise of other limbs due to compensation, change in attitude after surgery, postoperative pain, fear of anesthesia in an older pet, ability to resume normal activity, prognosis if cause of amputation is neoplasia, and thoracic limb versus pelvic limb are some of the more common owner concerns.[2,3]

The reality is that most dogs are reported to return to normal activity within one month following amputation.[1,4] In clinically normal dogs, the thoracic limbs each take on 30% of the body weight while the pelvic limbs each distribute 20% body weight.[5,6] This finding, however, does not appear to affect recovery from thoracic limb compared to pelvic limb amputation, as several studies show that there is no difference in owner perception of recovery.[1,3] Age and breed size have not been found to be factors impeding recovery.[1,3] Body weight did not appear to affect the time to reach best quality of life.[3] Objective data regarding adaptation have

Techniques in Small Animal Soft Tissue, Orthopedic, and Ophthalmic Surgery, First Edition. Edited by Kristin A. Coleman.

Companion website: www.wiley.com/go/coleman/surgeries

been evaluated using spatial kinematic and kinetic data in pelvic limb amputee dogs, and it was shown that this adaptation occurs from increased range of motion at the contralateral tarsal joint, thoracolumbar and cervicothoracic vertebral regions, and extension of the lumbosacral vertebrae.[6] A similar study evaluating adaptations for forelimb amputee dogs has shown that the ipsilateral pelvic limb served a dual thoracic and pelvic limb role during trotting.[7] In fact, a study evaluating adaptations has shown that the adaptation process began before the amputation was even performed, contributing to the rapid recovery seen in most pelvic limb amputees.[2] Magnetic resonance imaging evaluating the contralateral stifle in pelvic limb amputee dogs 120 days after amputation showed no cartilage damage or osteoarthritis.[2] Overall, 91% of dog amputee owners perceived no change in attitude, 88% reported complete to near complete return to life prior to amputation, 78% indicated that the recovery was better than they were expecting, and 86% of owners indicated they would elect amputation again if given a choice based on their experience.[3]

While kinetic and kinematic studies are hard to perform in cats, a client survey in a multi-institutional study of nearly all owners reported a good to excellent satisfaction with only 1.7% reporting fair satisfaction. In this same study, 84.7% of owners would elect for an amputation in another pet if needed based on their current experience.[8]

It is our responsibility as veterinarians to present objective information to owners regarding prognosis if amputation is being considered for malignancy. Bloodwork is indicated prior to amputation to determine general health status, and staging diagnostics are recommended as well if the procedure is being considered for neoplasia.

Indications

Indications for limb amputation include trauma, neoplasia, neurological dysfunctions confined to one limb, chronic osteomyelitis, limb deformities (congenital, malunion fractures), severe infection, and vascular disease (thromboembolism, arteriovenous fistulas).[9]

Pre-operative Considerations

Thorough knowledge of the intrinsic and extrinsic muscles of the limb is required prior to amputation, since only the extrinsic muscles need transection for successful amputation. Transection of the intrinsic muscles leads to surgical morbidity, longer anesthesia times, and increase in surgical blood loss. Maintaining hemostasis is paramount during the procedure. Anatomic location of large caliber blood vessels must be known such that these vessels can be isolated and ligated prior to transection. Smaller arteries and veins encountered should be addressed with electrocautery, hemoclips, or ligatures. While forelimb amputation can be performed distal to the scapula with a disarticulation at the level of the scapulohumeral joint leaving the scapula on the thoracic wall, there is no literature to support the procedure. Like a mid-femoral amputation, muscle atrophy from disuse that occurs over time can lead to protrusion of the bony remnants against the skin, leading to ulceration and sores over the sites. Thus, the amputation preference in veterinary medicine is a complete forequarter amputation for the thoracic limb and a coxofemoral disarticulation for the pelvic limb.

Multimodal analgesia should be considered in conjunction with opioids, *N*-methyl-D-aspartate (NMDA) receptor antagonists-antagonists, and anti-inflammatories with local blocking of the nerve sheaths with lidocaine or bupivacaine prior to transection, which should ideally be performed with a blade instead of scissors for the sharpest transection. Infiltration of the transected muscle with liposome-encapsulated bupivacaine available commercially should be considered at the time of surgical closure.

Surgical Procedure

Thoracic Limb Amputation (Forequarter Amputation)

Forequarter amputation is a procedure that disarticulates the scapula from the thoracic wall, removing the scapula with the limb (Figures 17.1 and 17.2). The entirety of the front leg to dorsal midline, cranial thorax, and thorax ventral to the front leg are clipped, and a rough prep is performed outside of the operating room. The patient is placed in lateral recumbency with the affected side up, and the leg is draped in using a standard hanging leg technique after a final surgical prep is performed in the operating room.

A teardrop skin incision is made along the spine of the scapula to the acromion and continued circumferentially around the limb ventrally. Subcutaneous tissue is dissected away, to reveal the omotransversarius muscle along the cranial and ventral aspect of the scapula and the trapezius cranial and dorsal to the scapula. The omotransversarius and trapezius (both cervical and thoracic portions) muscles are transected at the spine of the scapula where it is least vascular, and the entirety of these muscles are saved for closure. Distal to the omotransversarius and cranial to the scapula, the cleidobrachialis muscle is transected near its insertion onto the humeral crest, or if amputating for neoplasia, transected mid-belly. Cephalic and omobrachial veins encountered in this area are isolated and ligated with a suture ligature, hemoclip, or vessel-sealant device prior to transection.

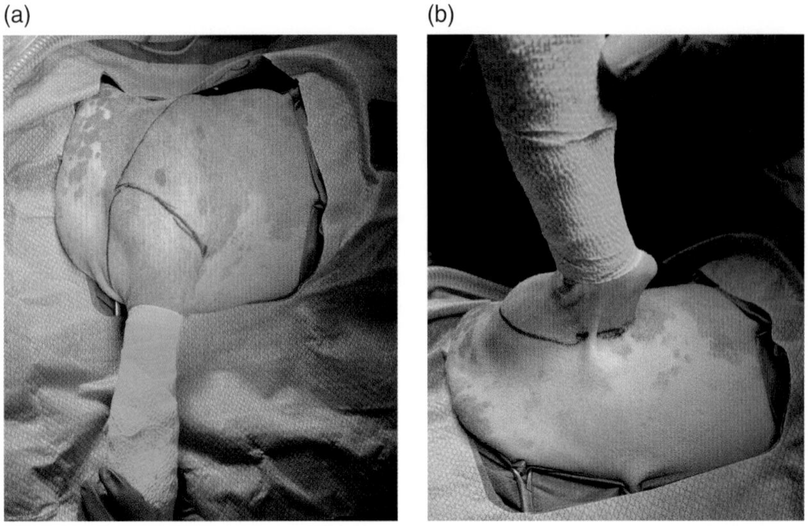

Figure 17.1 Proposed incision for forequarter amputation of the left thoracic limb in a 10-year-old spayed female mixed-breed dog. (a) Surgical markings in purple for proposed incisions indicate the dorsoventral line over the scapular spine to the acromion and continued circumferentially around the leg. (b) The ventromedial aspect of the leg showing continuation of the proposed circumferential incision.

The dorsal spine of the scapula is grasped with a towel clamp and lifted laterally to expose the rhomboideus muscle attaching to the dorsal border of the scapula, which is transected along the scapula to expose the serratus ventralis muscle, which is also transected along its scapular attachment. The subcutaneous dissection is carried along the caudal aspect of the scapula with monopolar electrosurgery, a Freer or other periosteal elevator, or curved Mayo scissors to expose the caudally located latissimus dorsi muscle. This muscle is then transected carefully and methodically to identify the thoracodorsal neurovascular bundle along the deep fibers of the latissimus. The thoracodorsal artery and vein can be quite sizable in large dogs and can be a source of hemorrhage during dissection if they are not identified and ligated, being mindful to separate the nerve to sharply transect instead of ligating with the artery and vein.

The scapula should now be fully mobilized from dorsal and lateral attachments, and lateral elevation of the scapular with the towel clamp should become easier. The brachial plexus consisting of the ventral nerve branches of C6, C7, C8, T1, and T2 are identified. Nerves are blocked with a local anesthetic closer to the thoracic wall and then transected. The axillary artery and vein are individually isolated and double-ligated before transection. This is preferentially done with a proximal encircling ligature (toward the patient) and a distal modified transfixation ligature (toward the cut vessel edge) of a long-term monofilament synthetic absorbable suture. Superficial and deep pectoral muscles are transected ventrally with any remaining subcutaneous attachments to free the leg completing the forequarter amputation, taking care to ensure the axillary lymph node is excised with the leg for nodal evaluation in the case of neoplasia. The axillary lymph node is located just caudal to the axillary vein and medial to the latissimus dorsi muscle.

During this dissection, the lateral thoracic artery will need to be ligated. Additionally, in the case of neoplasia, the regional prescapular lymph node is identified and dissected bluntly for removal for histopathology and is located along the cranial aspect of the incision deep to the brachiocephalicus muscle. Routine thorough lavaging is performed with sterile saline. Gloves and instruments are changed in the case of neoplasia and infection. Suture size is selected based on the size of the patient, and when suturing the transected muscles with long-lasting synthetic monofilament absorbable suture, the fascia surrounding the muscle is the holding layer; not the muscle belly itself. Closure after lavage is done with apposition of the serratus ventralis to itself ("serratus taco"), and the trapezius and omotransversarius are apposed to the latissimus dorsi dorsally. The pectoral muscles are apposed over the top of the ligated axillary artery and vein and brachial plexus to the previous muscle closure. This protects the plexus and the ribs with a layer of muscle. Subcutaneous tissue and skin are closed routinely.

Pelvic Limb Amputation

Mid-Femoral Amputation

The entirety of the affected pelvic limb, ventral and caudal abdomen adjacent to the leg to ventral midline, caudal to the ischiatic tuberosity, cranial to the mid-abdomen level, and dorsal hip and lumbar region just past dorsal midline are clipped, and a rough prep is performed outside of the operating room. The patient is positioned in lateral recumbency with the affected leg up, and the leg is draped using

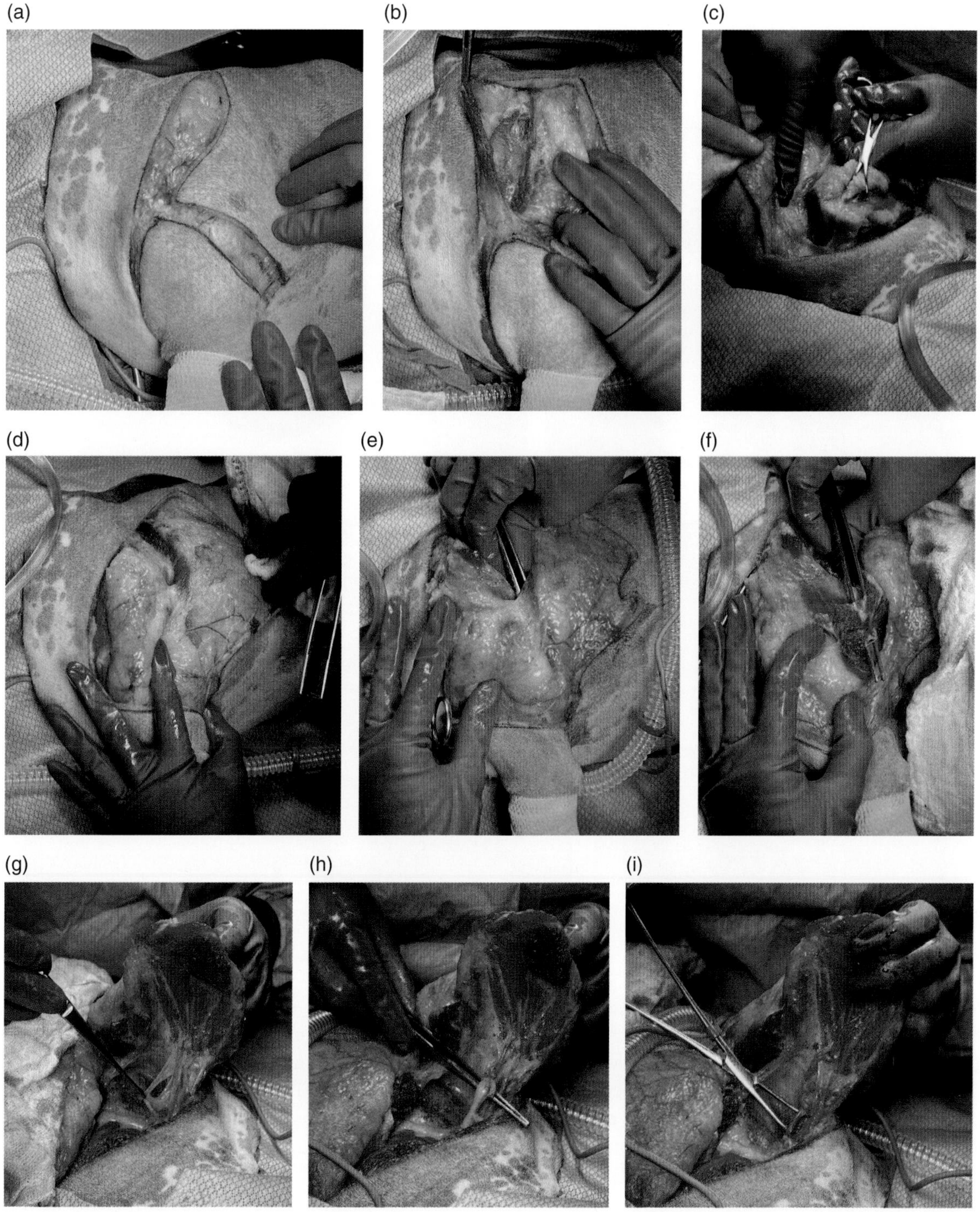

Figure 17.2 (a–f) Forequarter amputation of the left thoracic limb in a 10-year-old spayed female mixed-breed dog. (a) A skin incision has been made as described in Figure 17.1, exposing the subcutaneous tissue. (b) Subcutaneous tissue has been dissected away, and the omotransversarius muscle along the cranial aspect of the scapula grasped by the thumb forceps has been transected off the scapular spine. This transection is carried proximally to elevate the trapezius from its attachment to the spine of the scapula. (c) The dorsal spine of the scapula is lifted laterally with a towel clamp through the scapular spine to expose the rhomboideus muscle, which is transected to expose the serratus ventralis muscle, which is also then transected along its scapular attachment. (d) The subcutaneous dissection is carried along the caudal aspect of the scapula. (e) The latissimus dorsi muscle along the caudal aspect of the scapula is identified under the subcutaneous tissue. (f) The latissimus dorsi muscle is then transected, and the thoracodorsal neurovascular bundle is identified and ligated prior to transection. This neurovascular bundle is identified by the thumb forceps. (g–j) (g) The scapula is now fully mobilized from its dorsal attachments, and the brachial plexus is identified. Nerves are blocked with a local anesthetic closer to the thoracic wall and then transected. (h) Nerves in the process of transection. (i) The axillary artery (shown in the right-angle forceps) is dissected, double-ligated, and transected. (j) The axillary vein (shown in the right-angle forceps) is similarly dissected, double-ligated, and transected. (k–n) (k) Superficial and deep pectoral muscles are transected ventrally with any remaining subcutaneous attachments completing the forequarter amputation. (l) Prescapular lymph node is identified for removal in cases with neoplastic disease and is located along the cranial aspect of the incision deep to the omotransversarius muscle. (m) Closure after lavage is done with apposition of the serratus ventralis rolled to appose itself and the trapezius and omotransversarius muscles to the latissimus dorsi. Pectoral muscles are apposed over the top of the ligated axillary artery and vein and brachial plexus to the previous muscle closure. (n) Subcutaneous tissue and skin are closed routinely.

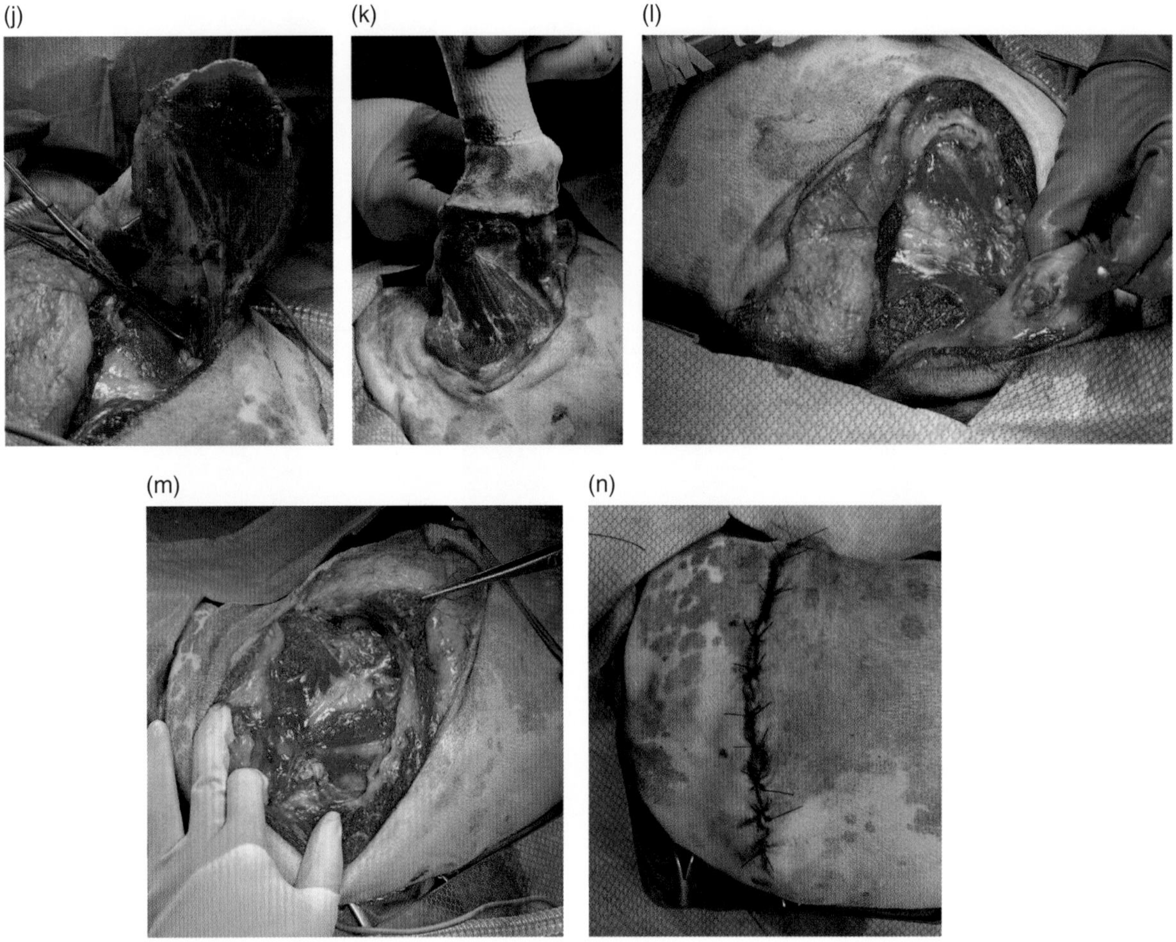

Figure 17.2 (Continued)

the standard hanging leg technique after a final surgical prep is performed.

The skin incision is planned at the distal third level of the femur or near the level of the stifle joint. Dissection is continued through the subcutaneous tissue to expose underlying muscles laterally, cranially, medially, and caudally. The cranial and caudal sartorius muscle bellies and the gracilis muscle are transected mid-belly. The femoral neurovascular bundle is identified cranial to the pectineus muscle. The femoral nerve is blocked with a local anesthetic and sharply transected. The femoral artery and vein are dissected individually and double-ligated prior to transection. It is preferred to perform a proximal encircling ligature (toward the patient) and a distal modified transfixation ligature (toward the cut vessel edge) of a long-term monofilament synthetic absorbable suture prior to transection of the vessels.

The pectineus muscle is located just caudal to the femoral neurovascular bundle and is transected close to the pubis. The quadriceps muscles are transected at the level of the proximal patella. Laterally, the biceps femoris muscle is transected to expose the sciatic nerve at the same level of excision as the quadriceps muscle. The nerve is infiltrated with a local anesthetic and sharply transected at the proximal third of the femur. The adductor, semimembranosus, and semitendinosus muscles and any remaining muscles are excised at the same level. The adductor and vastus medialis are elevated off the proximal femur to the site of the proposed osteotomy. Once the osteotomy has been performed, an ideally tension-free closure is performed with apposition of the deeper muscles first, followed by the superficial muscles, like the biceps and gracilis. Transected muscle bellies should be apposed by suturing the fascia overlying the muscle belly in an appositional or inverted interrupted pattern, such as with cruciate mattress. Subcutaneous and skin are closed routinely.

Coxofemoral Disarticulation

The entirety of the affected pelvic limb, ventral and caudal abdomen adjacent to the leg to ventral midline, caudal to the ischiatic tuberosity, cranial to the mid-abdomen level, and dorsal hip and lumbar region just past dorsal midline

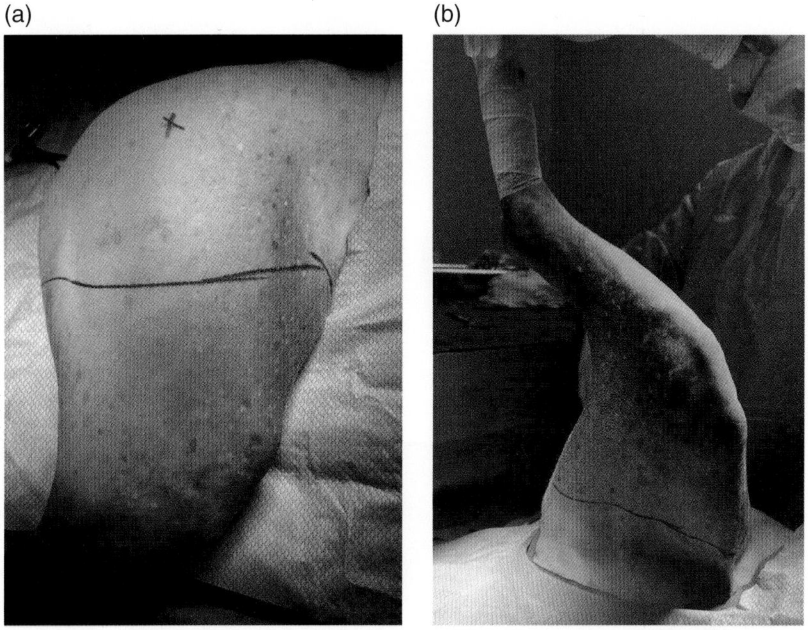

Figure 17.3 Proposed incision for a coxofemoral amputation of right rear limb in a 12-year-old castrated male mixed-breed dog. (a) Surgical markings in purple indicate proposed incision around the lateral aspect of the leg between the proximal one-third and mid-femoral level with an "X" on the greater trochanter. (b) The medial aspect of the thigh showing continuation of the proposed circumferential incision.

are clipped, and a rough prep is performed outside of the operating room (Figures 17.3 and 17.4). The patient is positioned in lateral recumbency with the affected leg up, and the leg is draped using the standard hanging leg technique after a final surgical prep is performed.

The skin incision is semicircular and centered at the mid- to proximal third femoral level. The incision is continued around the circumference of the leg at this level. Subcutaneous tissue is dissected along the medial thigh incision to expose the cranial and caudal bellies of the sartorius, pectineus, gracilis, and adductor muscles. The femoral artery, vein, and nerve are identified just cranial to the pectineus muscle and is often more accessible for dissection after careful transection of the pectineus muscle. The femoral nerve is blocked with a local anesthetic and sharply transected. The femoral artery and vein are dissected individually and double-ligated prior to transection. It is preferred to perform a proximal encircling ligature (toward the patient) and a distal modified transfixation ligature (toward the cut vessel edge) of a long-term monofilament synthetic absorbable suture prior to the transection of vessels. The medial muscles are then transected close to the coxofemoral joint. The semimembranosus and semitendinosus muscles are transected caudally. The sciatic nerve is identified, blocked with a local anesthetic, and sharply transected. The dissection of the subcutaneous tissues is continued laterally to expose the biceps femoris, abductor, and tensor fascia latae muscles that are then transected close to the hip joint and reflected dorsally to reveal the superficial, middle, and deep gluteal muscles, external rotators, and quadratus femoris, which are all transected near their attachments on the femur. The coxofemoral joint capsule is accessed via the medial aspect, and the ligament of the head of the femur is transected with a blade, curved Mayo scissors, or a Hat spoon to remove the leg. The site is lavaged and checked for any bleeding. Gloves and instruments are changed in the case of neoplasia and infection. Deeper muscles are apposed to minimize dead space and cover the hip socket. Superficial muscles, like the biceps femoris and gracilis, are then approximated, followed by routine closure of the subcutaneous tissue and skin. As noted previously, transected muscle bellies should be apposed by suturing the fascia overlying the muscle belly in an appositional or inverted interrupted pattern, such as with cruciate mattress, using a long-term monofilament absorbable suture.

Tips for amputations:

- Staying close to the extrinsic musculature insertion when transecting will result in less post-op pain, less intra-op bleeding, and presumably less potential seroma formation.
- Separately ligate large arteries and veins to reduce the risk of the rare complication: arteriovenous fistula.
- Clients should be prepared that the forelimb amputation skin incision is different for the shape and skin closure tensions for every dog, which may be "L-shaped," straight dorsoventral line, or even the traditional "upside-down T-shaped."
- To further reduce the risk of seroma formation, the muscle edges may be inverted when suturing together, as the lymphatic fluid may be a factor in post-op seroma formation.

(a) (b) (c) (d) (e) (f) (g) (h) (i)

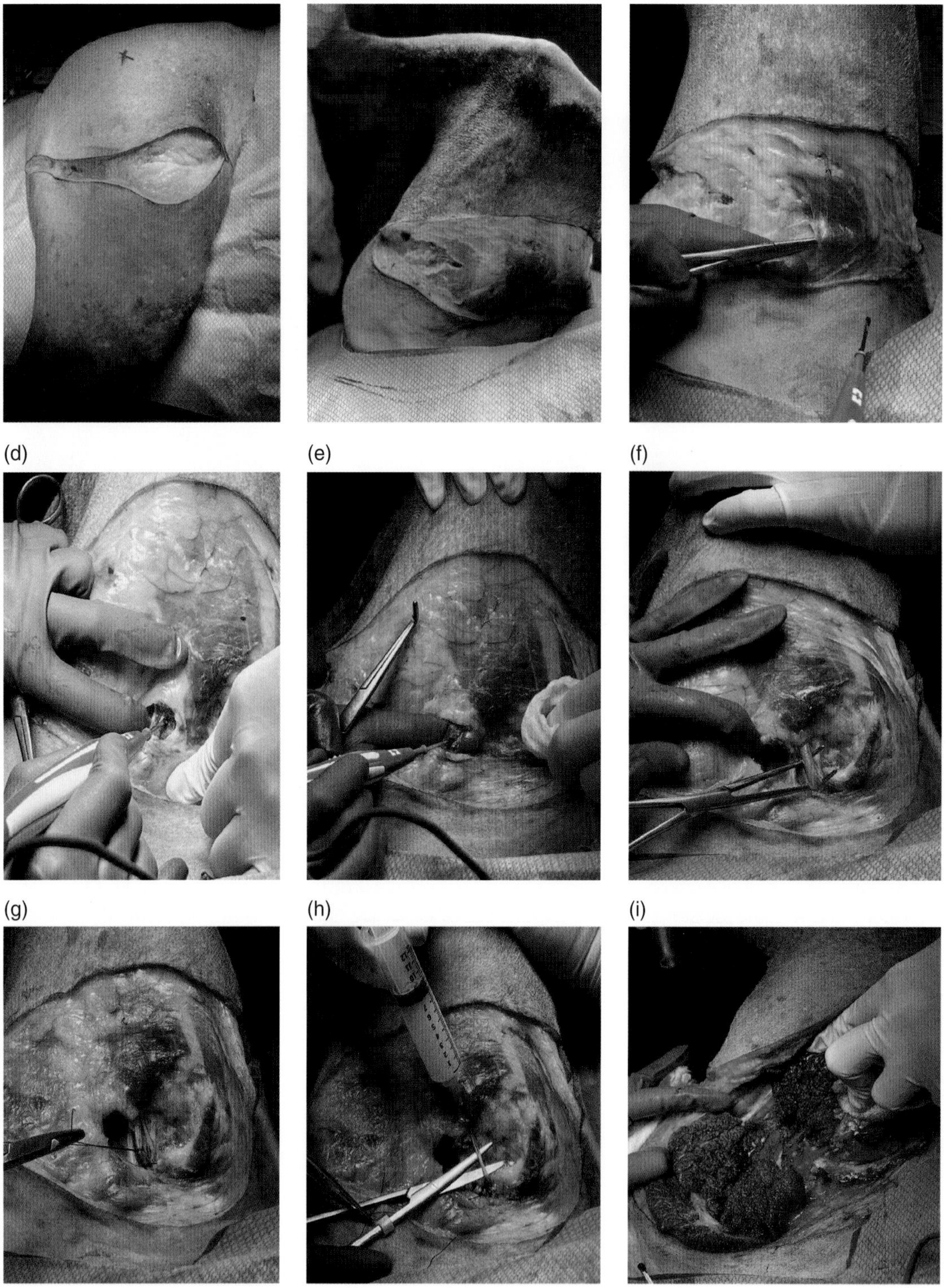

Figure 17.4 (a–f) Coxofemoral amputation of the right rear limb in a 12-year-old castrated male mixed-breed dog. (a) A skin incision has been made as described in Figure 17.3, exposing the subcutaneous tissue laterally. (b) The incision has been continued medially. (c) The caudal belly of the sartorius muscle is elevated and transected. (d,e) Careful transection of the pectineus muscle with either an instrument or finger placed deep to the muscle during transection to protect the surrounding structures. (f) The femoral neurovascular bundle is now exposed, and the vessels are dissected individually for ligation. The femoral artery is shown in the right-angle forceps. (g–l) (g) The femoral vessels are double-ligated proximally and distally with a modified transfixation ligature just distal to the encircling ligature proximally. (h) Infiltration of the femoral nerve with a local anesthetic prior to transection. A 25-gauge needle is used with the bevel facing up, as the anesthetic is injected into the nerve sheath toward the patient. (i) Transection of the medial thigh muscles. (j) Transection of the biceps femoris laterally. A tip is to place an instrument or finger deep to the muscle during transection due to the proximity of the sciatic nerve. (k) Transection of the semitendinosus muscle just caudal to the biceps femoris laterally. (l) Exposure of the sciatic nerve for infiltration and sharp transection, which is performed as proximally as possible to prevent excess nerve in the surgical site. (m–s) (m) Elevation of the biceps femoris to expose the gluteal muscles for transection. The right-angle forceps points to the greater trochanter, onto which the middle and deep gluteal muscles insert. (n) Elevation of the gluteal muscles for transection. (o) Exposure of the joint capsule of the coxofemoral joint medially once all muscle transections are completed. (p) Lateral traction on the limb allows exposure and transection of the ligament of the head of the femur, freeing the leg. (q) Appearance of the amputation site at the time of closure. (r) Closure of the musculature with apposition of the deeper muscles first, followed by the more superficial muscles. (s) Appearance of the amputation site after closure.

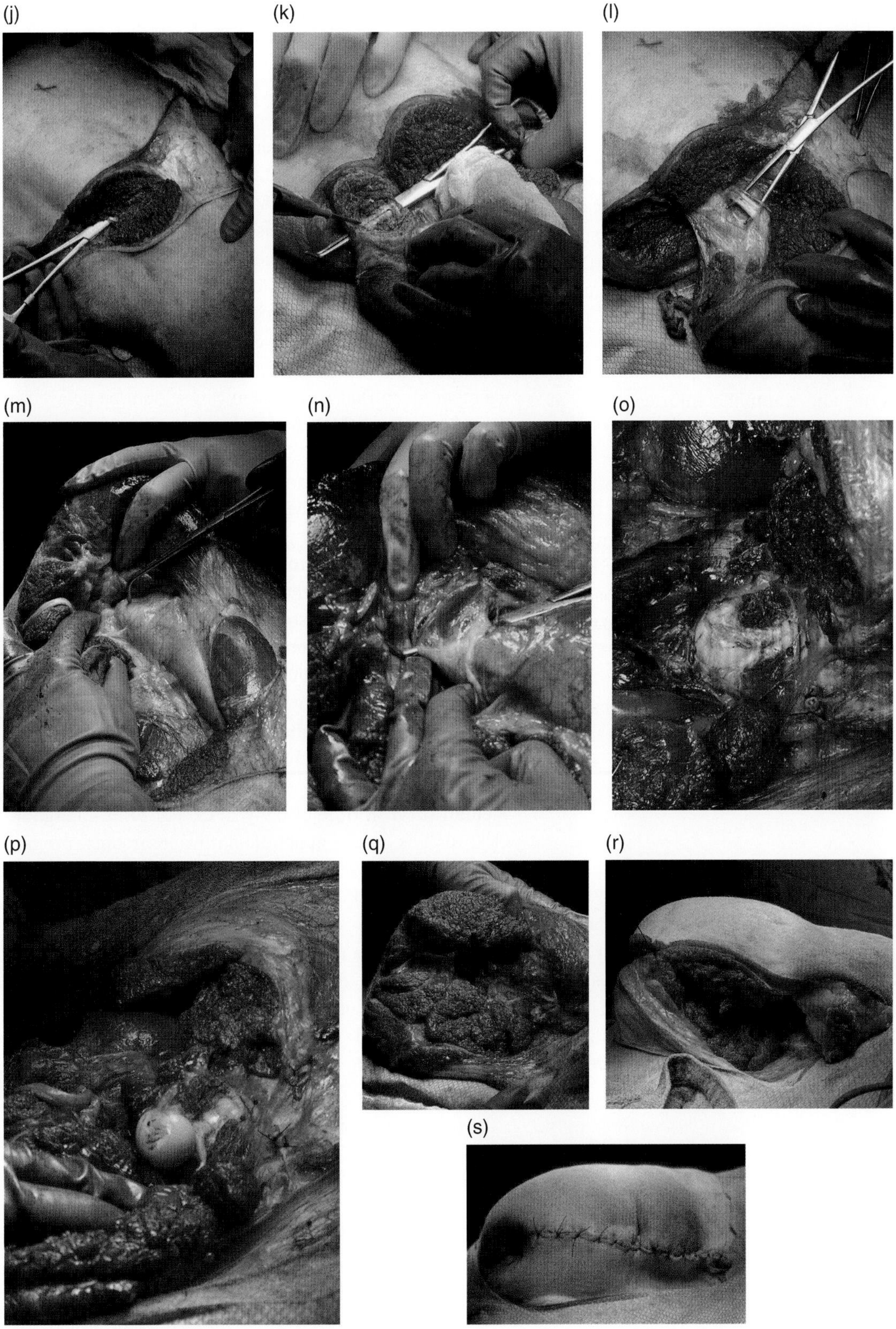

Figure 17.4 (Continued)

Potential Complications

Like with other surgical procedures, complications can include hemorrhage, inflammation, seroma, dehiscence, and infection. In one study of canine and feline amputees, the overall complications following amputation was low and included an infection/inflammation rate of 12.8% in dogs and 3.6% in cats with a reported major complication rate of only 1.5%.[10] More specifically in another study, in dogs, the incidence of surgery site infection was 12.5% for all amputations with a lower rate (10.9%) for clean procedures.[12] Factors that increased rate of infections included use of a bipolar sealing device for muscle transection, procedures classified as not clean, amputation for bacterial infection, and traumatic injuries.[11] Use of electrocautery or sharp dissection resulted in lower infection rates.[11]

In cats, postoperative complication rates are reported to be similar for thoracic and pelvic limb amputations. In one study, 57.6% (34 of 59) of cats had postoperative complications, of which only 5.1% was considered a major complication.[8] Minor complications included mild balance difficulty in 20.3% (12/59 cats), mild incisional pain in 23.7% (14/59 cats), mild depressed mentation in 6.8% (4/59 cats), and a combination of mild incisional pain and mild balance difficulty in 1.7% (1/59 cat). Major complications included severe balance difficulty in 3.4% (2/59 cats) and a combination of major decrease in appetite and severe balance difficulty in 1.7% (1/59 cat).[8]

Postoperative Care/Prognosis

Analgesia, injectable and/or oral, consisting of opioids, NMDA-receptor antagonists, and anti-inflammatories is provided depending on status of the liver and kidneys. Age has been associated with an increase in postoperative infection/inflammation rates in dogs following amputation.[10] Thus, postoperative antibiotics should be considered in geriatric amputees, trauma cases, and bacterial infections as the reason for amputation. Ice-packing for the first three days followed by warm-packing of the area for the next week can help prevent seroma formation. Body harnesses are helpful with patients that require assistance during the recovery period. Exercise restriction to slow walks is recommended for the first two weeks to prevent injury to the surgical site and seroma formation from over-activity. Rehabilitation with a licensed rehabilitation expert is a consideration in all amputees and especially the few that are having a difficult transition.

Increase in body condition scores and body weight at the time of surgery were negatively correlated to recovery after surgery, stressing the need for postoperative weight management given that amputation can seldom be delayed in an overweight patient for conditions such as trauma and neoplasia.[3]

Prognosis following amputation for non-neoplastic conditions can be guarded to good depending on etiology and patient status during the amputation. Prognosis for neoplasia can range from good to poor depending on tumor type on histopathology, stage of disease, grade for certain malignancies, soft tissue versus bone neoplasia, and bone versus joint neoplasia. For certain malignancies, such as canine appendicular low-grade chondrosarcoma (grade 1), amputation of the limb could prove to be curative in patients with a median survival time of 6 years as opposed to a grade 2 chondrosarcoma having a median survival time of 2.7 years and a grade 3 having a median survival time of 0.9 years.[12] For other malignancies, such as canine appendicular osteosarcoma, prognosis is poor even with amputation and chemotherapy[13] due to development of macroscopic pulmonary metastasis in 87.2% and a one-year survival rate of 14.3% in a recent study.[14] In a recent study of appendicular and scapular osteosarcoma in cats, the distant metastatic rate was 46.3% at the time of limb amputation and 41.9% after limb amputation, and the median survival time following amputation was 527 days.[14]

References

1 Kirpensteijn, J., van den Bos, R., and Endenburg, N. (1999). Adaptation of dogs to the amputation of a limb and their owners' satisfaction with the procedure. *Vet. Rec.* 144 (5): 115–118.

2 Galindo-Zamora, V., von Babo, V., Eberle, N. et al. (2016). Kinetic, kinematic, magnetic resonance and owner evaluation of dogs before and after the amputation of a hind limb. *BMC Vet. Res.* 12 (1): 20. https://pubmed.ncbi.nlm.nih.gov/26810893.

3 Dickerson, V.M., Coleman, K.D., Ogawa, M. et al. (2015). Outcomes of dogs undergoing limb amputation, owner satisfaction with limb amputation procedures, and owner perceptions regarding postsurgical adaptation: 64 cases (2005–2012). *J. Am. Vet. Med. Assoc.* 247 (7): 786–792.

4 Carberry, C.A. and Harvey, H.J. (1987). Owner satisfaction with limb amputation in dogs and cats. *J. Am. Anim. Hosp. Assoc.* 23: 227–232.

5 Budsberg, S.C., Verstraete, M.C., and Soutas-Little, R.W. (1987). Force plate analysis of the walking gait in healthy dogs. *Am. J. Vet. Res.* 48: 915–918.

6 Hogy, S.M., Worley, D.R., Jarvis, S.L. et al. (2013). Kinematic and kinetic analysis of dogs during trotting after amputation of a pelvic limb. *Am. J. Vet. Res.* 74 (9): 1164–1171.

7 Jarvis, S.L., Worley, D.R., Hogy, S.M. et al. (2013). Kinematic and kinetic analysis of dogs during trotting after amputation of a thoracic limb. *Am. J. Vet. Res.* 74 (9): 1155–1163.

8 Wagner, J.R., DeSandre-Robinson, D.M., Moore, G.E. et al. (2022). Complications and owner satisfaction associated with limb amputation in cats: 59 cases (2007–2017). *BMC Vet. Res.* 18 (1): 1–7.

9 Stone, E.A. (1985). Amputation. In: *Textbook of Small Animal Orthopaedics* (ed. C.D. Newton and D.M. Nunamaker), 577–588. New York: Lippincott Williams and Wilkins.

10 Raske, M., McClaran, J.K., and Mariano, A. (2015). Short-term wound complications and predictive variables for complication after limb amputation in dogs and cats. *J. Small Anim. Pract.* 56 (4): 247–252.

11 Farese, J.P., Kirpensteijn, J., Kik, M. et al. (2009). Biologic behavior and clinical outcome of 25 dogs with canine appendicular chondrosarcoma treated by amputation: a Veterinary Society of Surgical Oncology retrospective study. *Vet. Surg.* 38 (8): 914–919.

12 Billas, A.R., Grimes, J.A., Hollenbeck, D.L. et al. (2022). Incidence of and risk factors for surgical site infection following canine limb amputation. *Vet. Surg.* 51 (3): 418–425. https://pubmed.ncbi.nlm.nih.gov/35006627.

13 Guim, T.N., Bianchi, M.V., De Lorenzo, C. et al. (2020). Relationship between clinicopathological features and prognosis in appendicular osteosarcoma in dogs. *J. Comp. Pathol.* 180: 91–99.

14 Nakano, Y., Kagawa, Y., Shimoyama, Y. et al. (2022). Outcome of appendicular or scapular osteosarcoma treated by limb amputation in cats: 67 cases (1997–2018). *J. Am. Vet. Med. Assoc.* 260 (S1): S24–S28.

18

Summary of Skin Reconstruction Options

David Michael Tillson

Department of Clinical Sciences, Auburn University, Auburn, AL, USA

Key Points

- Mass excisions are one of the most common veterinary procedures.
- Simple excisions require a good surgical technique to consistently have a high-quality outcome for the patient.
- There are numerous techniques available for wound closure; typically, the least complicated procedure will have the greatest chance of success without postoperative complications.
- The use of various subcutaneous suture patterns will eliminate dead space, resist tensile forces trying to disrupt the incision, and help maintain wound apposition for better wound closure.
- Local skin flaps, such as advancement and rotational flaps, are useful for primary wound closure but require preoperative planning for successful execution. These flaps are limited in scope and may be insufficient for larger wounds.
- Axial pattern flaps offer a more advanced surgical option for single-stage wound closure of large wounds created by mass resection or other full-thick skin injuries. Accurate planning and dissection are essential for success.

Introduction

Basic Principles

Mass excision is one of the most common surgical procedures in veterinary medicine. On the surface, mass excision is simple to accomplish, but so many factors can turn a simple procedure into a complex headache, resulting in angry clients, uncomfortable patients, and increased personal stress. The steps for a mass excision are planning, preparation, incision, dissection and hemostasis, wound closure, and postoperative management. This chapter will focus on these steps and they are all essential for the effective surgical management of masses. Some mass removals will be simple and straightforward, while others require detailed thought for each of the steps outlined, as there may be multiple techniques for managing them. To start, a brief review of wound healing will be included in a chapter focused on wound creation and reconstruction.

Wound Healing

Wound healing is divided into an inflammatory phase, a proliferative phase, and a remodeling or maturation phase.[1,2] Each of these phases is characterized by some specific processes occurring during each phase of healing. It is clinically important to remember there are often multiple phases of wound healing occurring within a single wound simultaneously, as some areas of the wound progress faster than other areas. The ultimate goal of the surgeon when managing a wound is to promote effective healing while minimizing actions or conditions that would negatively impact wound healing.

The inflammatory phase occurs immediately after wounding occurs. There is trauma to vascular structures, resulting in vasoconstriction followed by vasodilation and clot formation that creates the fibrin meshwork for future cell migration. Leukocytes, monocytes, and neutrophils begin to move into the wound bed within 30–60 minutes

Techniques in Small Animal Soft Tissue, Orthopedic, and Ophthalmic Surgery, First Edition. Edited by Kristin A. Coleman.

Companion website: www.wiley.com/go/coleman/surgeries

after injury. The neutrophils release proteinases that begin to break down damaged tissue. Monocytes activate, becoming tissue macrophages, and continue the process of transforming the wound environment into one that will promote future healing. Monocytes can survive the lower oxygen environment of a fresh wound while phagocytizing bacteria and other contaminants release proteases that continue the process of tissue debridement. Surgical debridement of necrotic tissue and wound lavage can reduce the workload on the macrophages and promote wound healing during this phase. Classically, the inflammatory phase continues for three to five days; however, increased wound contamination can prolong this phase.

The proliferative phase starts as the inflammatory phase winds down, typically around four days after injury. Macrophage-released cytokines stimulate fibroplasia and angiogenesis, which is characteristic of this stage. The proliferative phase includes the processes of neovascularization, or angiogenesis, fibroplasia and deposition of collagen within the wound, the migration of epithelial cells over the wound surface, and wound contraction. Neovascularization begins in response to low oxygen tension within the wound bed, stimulating the release of angiogenic factors from tissue macrophages within the wound. These factors stimulate vascular ingrowth and the formation of the capillary loops associated with granulation tissue. This vascular ingrowth is critical since fibroplasia and collagen deposition are dependent on an oxygen-rich environment. Fibroblasts migrate along the fibronectin mesh left over from the wound clot and begin to secrete the fibronectin extracellular matrix followed by type III collagen. Type III collagen is eventually replaced by the more organized, stronger type I collagen; this process will continue into the maturation phase before it is completed. Epithelization starts along the wound edges within days of injury as the cells begin to proliferate and start moving over the surface of the wound. Epithelial cells undergo morphologic changes as they migrate into the wound, becoming larger in size and flatter, less plump than normal epithelial cells. While sutured wounds may have epithelial coverage in as few as two days, open or problematic wounds or those with necrotic tissues, foreign debris, or infection may result in the epithelialization process continuing into the maturation phase or later. This type of migrating epithelial surface is initially very thin and fragile. It is easily traumatized, which may lead to chronic problems with tissue injury, requiring wound revision or placement of a full-thickness skin flap or graft for optimal function.

If epithelialization has occurred but the collagen deposition within the wound bed is insufficient, the phenomenon of "pseudo-healing" may occur. Pseudo-healing is when the wound appears to be grossly healed, but due to minimal tissue strength, the wound easily reopens. Pseudo-healing is reported to be a substantial issue in cats[3] and can be encountered in dogs as well, especially those dogs with a history of chronic glucocorticoid steroid use.

Wound contraction occurs when the wound bed decreases in size as the contraction process moves the full-thickness skin surrounding a defect toward the center of the wound. This action decreases the distance epithelial cells must cover in the process of healing. This centripetal tissue movement begins during the proliferative phase as a result of the contraction of fibroblasts and myofibroblasts, and it typically continues into the maturation phase, moving at a rate of 0.5–0.75 mm per day and continuing for up to six weeks.[1,4] Wound contraction after that time should not be expected, and surgical intervention may be needed to achieve sturdy wound closure. Wound healing by contraction is very effective in dogs and cats when there is adequate skin available, such as wounds on the thorax or lateral flanks. Contraction results in a small scar with haired skin adjacent to the epithelial scar. However, if the opposing tension on the skin reaches an equilibrium with the contractile force generated within by the wound, the contraction process is halted. This typically results in a large open wound with an epithelial covering. This type of wound epithelialization creates a large area of hairless, depigmented skin covered by thin, fragile epithelial tissue. Thus, wound healing through contraction is typically better than simple wound epithelialization over a granulation tissue bed.

Contracture is the term applied when wound contraction results in impediment of function, typically with movement of limbs, due to excessive tissue contraction and subsequent scarring. This is commonly encountered with large wounds left to heal on their own or those that are near high-motion areas. In cases of severe contracture, surgical revision may be required to restore some of the normal function of the affected area.

The remodeling (maturation) phase can begin as early as 20 days after wounding and extend up to a year. During that time, the collagen deposition and resorption replaces type III collagen with the stronger, more organized type I collagen slowly increasing the wound tensile strength. Most wounds only achieve 70–80% of their original wound strength. At the same time, the proliferative capillary bed of granulation tissue gradually regresses toward the normal vascular arrangement. Chronic wounds may undergo a similar regression of the vascular bed, resulting in tissue that is incapable of supporting grafts or other efforts at getting the wound to heal. If further surgical intervention is planned, the wound should be freshened through the removal of the granulation bed then giving the wound four to seven days to establish a new bed of granulation tissue. With a new bed of granulation tissue, the wound is prepared for and supportive of primary wound closure or wound closure with flaps or grafts.

Planning

Mass excisions are often seen as uncomplicated surgical procedures, and while many of them are, even small or moderately-sized masses can be challenging to remove without complications. This is because factors, such as the biologic nature of the mass or mass location, may complicate the surgical procedure or the postoperative period. Non-surgical factors, such as patient health status, owner expectations, and budgetary restrictions, can also create complications for the patient, owner, and surgeon.

For small animal patients, location is one of the primary considerations when planning a mass resection and subsequent wound closure. Mass resections on the thoracic wall or abdominal flank offer substantial skin to permit primary wound closure. Distal limb masses have little extra skin for reconstruction and may require the use of flaps, grafts, or even open wound management to achieve wound healing. Furthermore, locations near joints must be able to withstand the constant tension on the wound from the animal's normal activities, even when an owner complies with efforts to restrict activity, and locations over pressure points, such as the elbows, sternum, or hip, must be able to heal despite constant pressure on the wound. The ability of the veterinarian to protect the surgical site can also be complicated by the location. Inguinal wounds, especially in the male dog, can be difficult to bandage. Limbs can be bandaged, but bandage management is time-consuming for the veterinarian and the client, and bandage-related complications are common and can have devastating results. Planning is essential to surgical success and can give the client realistic expectations about the postoperative path to wound healing.

"Surgical margin" is the term applied to how much tissue is removed along with the target mass. Some refer to margins as the "surgical dose" and try to determine the appropriate dose for each patient and for each tumor type.

Various descriptions can be found on surgical margins.[4] *Intralesional resection* is often referred to as "debulking," and there is typically gross disease or bits of the mass left behind after the resection of the target tissue. *Marginal resection* is a limited resection, and it may be the most misused surgical procedure. With the marginal resection, the mass is removed at the level of the pseudocapsule surrounding the mass. There is residual, microscopic disease remaining in the wound bed. As with the debulking procedure, this is likely to lead to the re-establishment of any aggressive mass in the same location. Ideally, a marginal resection is only used for benign masses or for tumors that will be subjected to other means of control, such as radiation or chemotherapy. If the biologic nature of the mass is unknown prior to excision, it is better to perform a wider resection.

A *wide resection* is a larger dose of surgery, and it is the recommended technique when removing malignant tumors or masses of unknown etiology. Typically, a "wide margin" involves resecting 2–3 cm of normal tissue surrounding the target mass and taking a deep margin, defined as removal of a fascial tissue plane beneath the target. A wide margin may still have local, residual neoplastic tissue, especially with spindle cell neoplasms that have branching projections radiating from the neoplasia.

A *radical resection* should result in no localized, residual neoplastic tissue remaining on the patient; however, to accomplish this, there is the loss of a substantial volume of normal, unaffected tissue. Examples of a radical resection would be an amputation or hemipelvectomy for a distal cutaneous sarcoma or a lung lobectomy for a peripheral lung nodule. The significant morbidity associated with performing a radical resection may dissuade owners from pursuing this option; however, it is often the recommended technique to effectively manage a malignant tumor. At the same time, the nature of a radical resection also requires the veterinarian to have definitively diagnosed the offending mass, to make sure other management options are not available, and to then present all options to the owner in order to meet the expectation of having obtained informed consent before surgery.

Any limitations on the effectiveness of a mass excision must be discussed with owners prior to surgery. When a patient has a mass of unknown etiology, which could require a radial resection, i.e., amputation, to obtain adequate margins, the author believes incisional biopsy or a marginal resection would be warranted prior to the radical surgery with the client's understanding that the more aggressive surgical procedure would be needed if the mass is deemed malignant.

The effectiveness of a surgical margin in managing a mass is based on the histopathologic description of the mass.[4] An *incomplete* margin is reported when the targeted tissue reaches the cut edge of the histopathological specimen. If the target tissue is less than 3 mm from the cut edge, the margin is noted to be *narrow*, while specimens with more than 3–5 mm of normal tissue between the target tissue and the cut edge are considered to have been *completely* resected. These descriptions take into consideration the potential for tissue shrinkage at resection and during specimen fixation, staining, and processing.[5,6] Based on the tissue diagnosis and the accompanying descriptions, the veterinarian needs to determine if the resection was effective or if additional surgery or other treatment methods are needed.

The above statement emphasizes the need for appropriate histopathologic evaluations of all resected masses. In the author's referral practice, the surgeons are frequently told that the original mass was "tossed in the trash" at the time of their first surgery and that no histopathologic diagnosis is available. While histopathology is an additional expense, it is an important diagnostic test and should be standard for any mass resection. One approach is to not break out the histopathologic submission as a separate charge, but rather include it as a part of the surgical fee. This way, the surgeon is less likely to be swayed by the client to not submit the mass for the sake of costs. Another method is to take advantage of state diagnostic laboratories that, while slower than commercial laboratories, often offer a bargain price for histopathologic evaluations.

A couple of final planning considerations are associated with a decision to remove multiple masses during a single procedure. The first is that this may require unique positioning and draping, or it might be determined that patient repositioning, along with re-prepping and re-draping, would be the most efficient and effective way to manage this. The operating room staff should be prepared for this step, and the surgeon will need to determine if they need to rescrub as well.

Next, whenever multiple masses are being resected during a single procedure, the surgeon must decide the order of attack. Ideally, any benign masses should be removed first. The progression should then be to those with a greater potential to be malignant. If the malignant mass must be resected first, there should be a change out of instruments, gloves, and any other materials that came into contact with the suspected malignant mass. This will reduce the potential for surgical transfer, or "seeding," of the secondary wounds with tumor cells from the primary tumor.

The third concern when removing multiple masses is the effect each resection will have on the adjacent resection sites (i.e., will the closure of one site impact the planned closure of the other sites?) (Figure 18.1). If the plan to close one surgical wound ends up using the loose skin that was also part of the plan to close the additional surgical wound, the surgeon will need to modify their plan on-the-fly. This situation can be challenging to anticipate but is an important consideration in surgical planning.

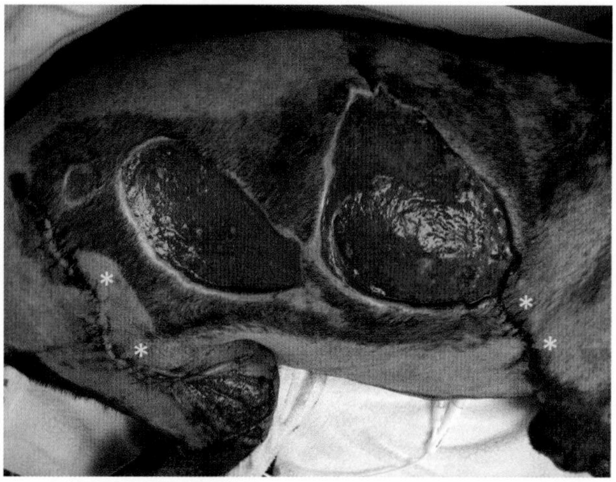

Figure 18.1 When planning to close multiple wounds or to resect multiple masses, the surgeon must consider the effect closing one wound will have on the availability of tissue and the surgical plan for closing any additional wounds. In some settings, combining multiple small resections into a single larger wound may allow for a more effective closure. In this image, the closure of the more difficult wounds on the right lateral hindlimb and right axillary areas (asterisks) utilized all the easily available tissue, requiring that the thorax and flank wounds to be managed in an open manner for an additional period of time.

Preparation

Surgical preparation for a mass excision begins with clipping of the patient's hair in the necessary surgical field. In the planning stage of the mass excision, the boundaries anticipated should be clearly defined for the technical staff that is preparing the patient. Hair removal needs to be sufficient to prevent pulling unprepped skin into the surgical field as skin is advanced for wound closure. It is also useful to secure the field drapes with extra towel clamps or skin staples to minimize this issue. Another technique would be to have additional drapes or sterile surgical towels to cover any unprepped skin pulled into the primary field during wound closure.

Once the surgical field has been clipped, the surgeon should review their surgical plan before moving to the OR. This may include using a marker to diagram the proposed procedure, including the primary incision and excision of the mass, the location, and the extent of any flap intended for primary closure. Diagramming out the proposed incision(s) with a sterile marker on the skin is useful and helps ensure the plan is appropriate and achievable.

Peri-operative planning also includes the potential need for wound drains, wound diffusion catheters for administration of analgesics, supportive bandaging, or limb immobilization. During the patient prep, the surgeon should anticipate and clip for any of these needs, as well as make sure that all appropriate materials are available in the OR.

Once the patient is moved into the OR, a final skin prep is performed with the antiseptic of choice. While the author's practice primarily uses chlorhexidine-based antiseptics, some prefer to use a final application of an iodine-based antiseptic, as the distinctive iodine color helps to confirm the surgical field is ready. Regardless of the product used, it is important to make sure there is no standing fluid on the field and that the surgical field is allowed to dry prior to surgical draping. Many practices use a surgical checklist, and this is the point in the procedure where the checklist is reviewed with the OR staff.[7] Once the checklist is completed, the surgeon can begin the procedure.

Incision

After the patient draping is completed and the surgical field established, the surgeon starts their incision. If the goal is a wide surgical margin, the proposed incision lines should be drawn out on the patient with a sterile surgical marker. Most of these markers come with a paper ruler, allowing the surgeon to accurately determine measured margins around the mass (Figure 18.2). Other surgeons use a graduated scalpel handle for measurements or a premeasured digit. Sutures, staples, or electrosurgery spots can be used to mark the patient's skin along the proposed margin. Once the margins have been marked, the surgeon determines the best shape for the complete skin incision. This is important since following the margins around a mass will typically result in a circular wound, which is a difficult shape to effectively close. There are a variety of shapes for a surgical wound that will both maintain the desired margins and allow for advantageous wound closure. Most surgeons will try to modify the circular wound into an elliptical or fusiform-shaped wound, although the use of flaps can force this plan to be modified. Ultimately, the final wound shape is influenced by skin tension lines, adjacent structures, or other wounds that may exist or be created.

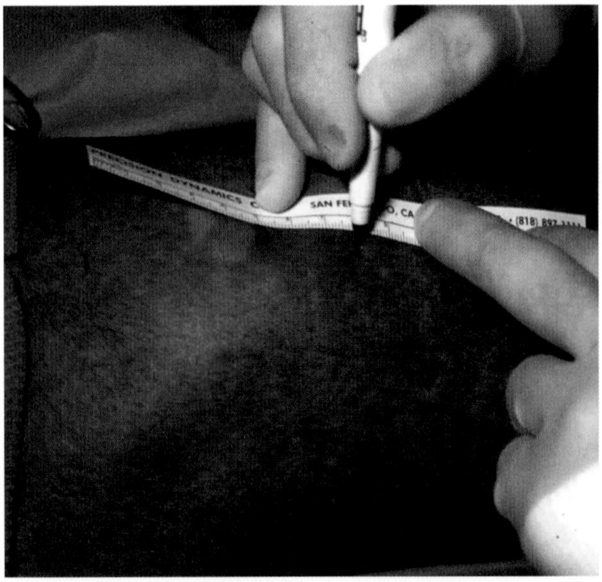

Figure 18.2 Once the surgical field is established, the surgeon should use a sterile marking pen to determine the margins for a mass resection. Using the sterile ruler supplied with many markers ensures that accurate margins are drawn prior to wound resection.

A variety of scalpel blades can be used for the skin incision associated with routine mass resection. The typical #10 blade is good for longer incisions, while the #15 blade is normally used for shorter incisions. The author has started to more frequently ask for a #11 blade for more precise incisions and for undermining tissues. Electrosurgical devices or CO_2 lasers can also be used for creation of the surgical incision; however, the author minimizes direct incision with either, preferring to use the scalpel through the epidermis and dermis and then switching to electrosurgery for continuing the incision. If either electrosurgery or CO_2 lasers are being used for primary incision, the surgeon should be comfortable with the guidelines for usage and wound closure.

When performing the incision for a mass resection, care is taken to have the scalpel blade maintain a perpendicular orientation to the skin surface. Failure to maintain this orientation results in beveling of the skin incision, especially as the incision curves around the mass. A beveled wound edge is more challenging to close, can result in gaping along the wound edge, and can shrink the intended surgical margin. Using the fingers of the non-dominant hand, tension can be placed across the proposed incision site. The fingers are moved as the scalpel advances, maintaining this tension, which encourages the easy separation of the wound edges during incision. As with all surgical incisions, the surgeon must carefully adjust the pressure on the blade to accommodate the skin thickness and the potential for injuring tissues beneath the incision. Once the initial incision has been created, modifications can be made as required for better visualization or improved wound closure. The final incisional adjustment may occur as the surgeon is adjusting the wound conformation for closure.

Dissection and Hemostasis

Gentle tissue handling is an essential component of wound reconstruction and closure. Aggressively grasping the edges of the wound or of flaps being developed can result in damage to the tissue and the associated vascular supply. While using thumb forceps, there is a natural tendency to grasp tissues tighter when struggling with them, this can result in excessive tissue trauma to the skin edge. Thumb forceps with worn, dulled, or no teeth actually cause the surgeon to increase the pressure on the tissues being held.

To minimize trauma to the wound edge, it is recommended that the surgeon takes care to avoid excessive skin manipulation with forceps. A method to minimize repetitive grasping of a skin edge is to use items that can be left in place in the wound edges for manipulation, such as stay sutures placed at the corners of flaps or the use of skin hooks, specialized skin forceps (e.g., LaLonde forceps), or

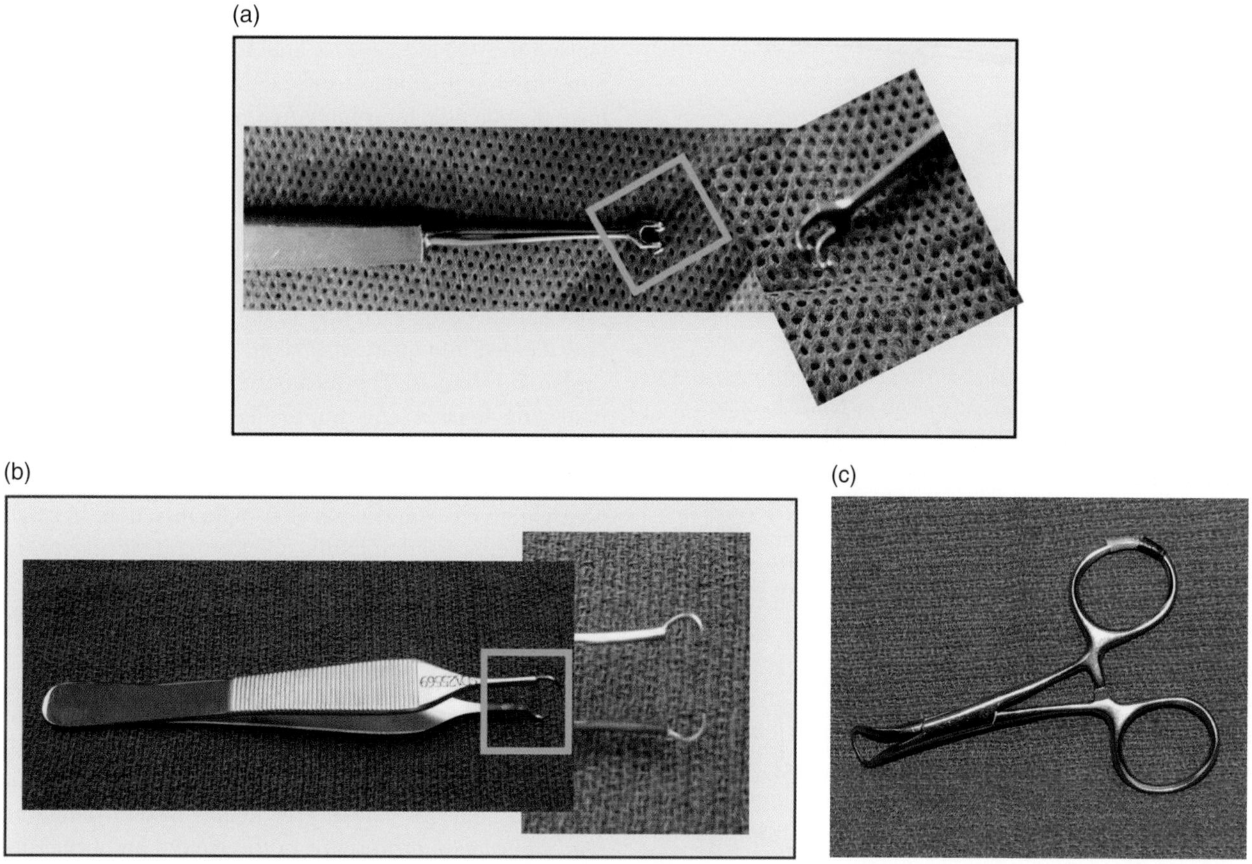

Figure 18.3 Instruments with sharp points often create less trauma to a wound edge than do normal tissue forceps. This is especially true if there is significant tension, as this causes the surgeon to exert significant force on tissue forceps to maintain a grip on the tissue. (a) Skin hooks. (b) LaLonde tissue forceps. These forceps have skin hooks rather than teeth and have a carbide insert to grasp the surgical needle. (c) Backhaus towel clamps are routinely used to hold tissue edges during dissection. Additionally, they can be used to hold tissues in apposition while trying to determine the best method of wound closure.

even penetrating towel clamps to manipulate tissue edges (Figure 18.3). Crushing clamps (e.g., Allis tissue forceps) or hemostatic forceps can be used to grasp the mass and any resected tissue surrounding it, but they should not be used on the incision edges.

Tissue dissection and undermining are essential skills for mass removal and subsequent wound closure. This can be accomplished using a sharp scalpel blade, Metzenbaum scissors, or electrosurgical instruments.[8,9] In the author's opinion, a combination of these instruments will probably provide the best results for effective dissection. Sharp dissection is effective and gives the best tactile feedback during dissection but can result in more hemorrhage from the transection of the numerous small vessels in the subcutaneous space than would be encountered with electrosurgery. Using electrosurgery will minimize capillary and small vessel hemorrhage, thus reducing the potential for hematoma formation; however, it does create carbon residue or char that remains behind. Excessive char, typically created by inappropriate electrosurgical or laser settings, increases inflammation and may negatively impact wound healing. Judicious use of the electrosurgical device at appropriate settings and generous lavage of the subcutaneous space will help reduce the remaining char prior to closure.

A principle of dissection that is underappreciated is the use of "traction-countertraction."[10] This simple technique enhances the precision of tissue dissection by using gentle tension to separate the various tissue planes more easily. The surgeon places tension on one side of an incision, while an assistant provides traction in the opposite direction (i.e., "countertraction"). This is the same principle being used when the non-dominant fingers are used during the initial skin incision. This traction-countertraction helps define tissue planes and keeps the surgeon from deviating in a manner that could compromise the development of tissue margins around a mass (Figure 18.4).

Hemostasis during dissection can often be managed exclusively by the use of electrosurgery, or it may be achieved by small vessels being crushed with hemostats or by large vessels being ligated by suture, clips, or bipolar vessel sealing devices. Most skin masses do not require exceptional techniques for hemostasis; electrosurgery and

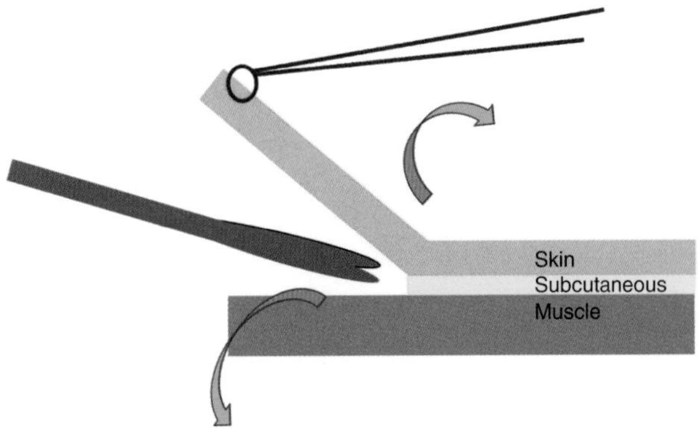

Figure 18.4 Using "traction and countertraction" allows for effective dissection of soft tissues and aids the surgeon in staying within the optimal tissue plane. This is accomplished by the surgeon gently placing tension on the tissues on their side of the surgical wound and having their assistant gently retract in the opposite direction. An experienced assistant will move with the surgeon, maintaining a 180° position to maintain effectiveness.

a fine, short-term absorbable monofilament suture will manage most situations. It is helpful, however, to employ caution during dissection. It is easier to identify and occlude a vessel before cutting it than it is to cut it and then struggle to find the bleeding end that retracted into the middle of the tissue dissection! It is also important to remember that most neoplastic masses will develop an increased blood supply through increased vessels leading to and from the mass (i.e., neovascularization). Be prepared for more hemorrhage than normal.

Wound Closure

Wound closure options range from simple to complex; however, the principles of wound healing are essentially the same no matter the method of closure. They include gentle tissue handling, effective dead space closure, tension-free wound closure, and accurate wound apposition. Striving to adhere to these principles should maximize the potential for trouble-free wound healing.[8–11]

The "rule of ½" is a suturing technique that helps create accurate wound apposition and decrease tension across the surgical wound during closure. The first suture is placed in the center of the incision, effectively dividing the length into halves. The next sutures are placed in the center of each half, dividing each half in half again; the incision is now divided into quarters. This process is repeated, until the wound is closed. This technique is especially helpful in managing tension and improving the spacing of skin sutures along the incision.

Undermining and advancement of the wound edges can be useful in closing wounds after mass resection. In small mass resections with minimal or wide margins, undermining the adjacent skin and subcutaneous tissue releases it and allows one wound edge to be moved toward the opposite wound edge. The principles of dissection given earlier in the chapter should be adhered to when undermining the wound edges. Once the skin has been freed sufficiently to permit wound edge apposition, additional dissection will simply create dead space for seroma or hematoma formation. Subcutaneous sutures (see details below) should be used to decrease dead space in the wound and bring the wound edges closer together for better apposition and a tension-free closure.

Relaxing/releasing incisions can be either small, punctuate incisions or a longer, full-thickness incision made through the skin adjacent to the wound closure.[8–10] With either, the aim is to release some of the tension across the wound by allowing a longitudinal incision, made perpendicular to the tension line but parallel to the long axis of the wound, to expand from a slit to a diamond (Figure 18.5),

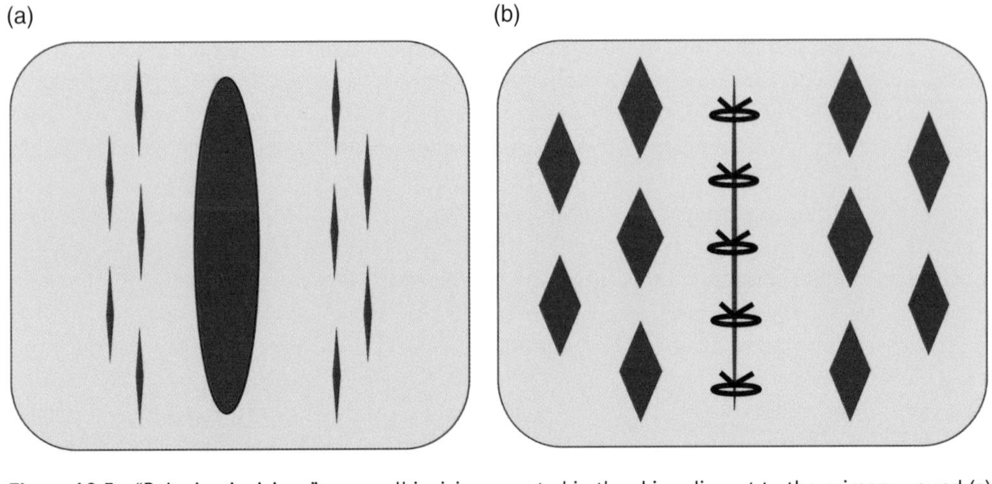

Figure 18.5 "Relaxing incisions" are small incisions created in the skin adjacent to the primary wound (a). When the primary wound is closed, the relaxing incisions expand (b) to allowing the apposition of the wound edges with minimal tension.

creating a small to moderate amount of release. When small, punctuate, relaxing incisions are used, they are made by cutting through the skin into the subcutaneous tissue with a #11 scalpel blade. The number of relaxing incisions will range from a few to a dozen or more incisions on either side of the wound. These small relaxing incisions are allowed to heal through secondary intention healing, so no additional surgery is required. Larger releasing incisions can run the length of the original wound. These incisions can also be allowed to heal by secondary intention, or, if the causes that inhibited primary closure of the original wound have been eliminated, primary closure can be considered.

Subcutaneous sutures are important for successful wound management, especially when skin advancement or reconstructive procedures are being performed. Different subcutaneous suture patterns can be used to accomplish different tasks during wound closure. The most basic suture pattern is a buried, simple interrupted subcutaneous suture. This suture type is generally placed to help decrease dead space through the apposition of subcutaneous fascia and adipose tissue. There is some benefit at reducing future tension when the overlying skin is subjected to motion in the awake animal.

Normally, the author uses a small, 3-0 to 5-0, short-term absorbable suture material for all the various subcutaneous patterns. Poliglecaprone 25 (Monocryl®; Ethicon, Somerville, NJ) is the author's "go-to" choice for subcutaneous sutures; however, sometimes, it is the multifilament, polyglactin 910 (Vicryl®; Ethicon, Somerville, NJ) suture that is chosen for its handling characteristics and knot security. Monocryl and Vicryl have a short duration in tissues, losing >50% of their tensile strength by 21 days and undergoing complete absorption by 120 and 70 days, respectively.[11] Only when there is a significant concern for delays in wound healing would a longer-lasting suture material be required for subcutaneous placement.

"Walking" sutures are another subcutaneous suture pattern that is used to advance a skin edge toward the opposite side for closure and to counteract tension within the wound.[8–10] The suture pattern is accomplished by pulling the skin edge back and exposing the underside. A suture bite is directed from within the incision outwards, taking a bite of the dermal layer in the process. The suture needle is pulled free and the next bite is taken in some sturdy subcutaneous tissue or deep fascia coming back toward the first bite (Figure 18.6). This allows the suture knot to be buried within the deep tissues. When the walking suture's dermal bite is placed several mm (5–10 mm) laterally to the fascial bite, the process of tightening the suture will pull the dermis toward the center of the wound. These steps are repeated in a methodical pattern to slowly advance the wound edge further and further toward the center of

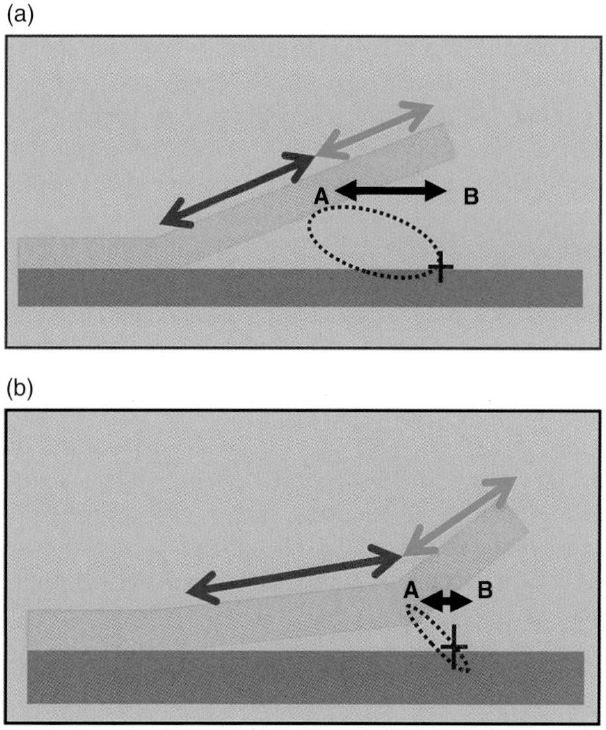

Figure 18.6 Walking sutures are used to advance tissues toward a central point and to assist in the closure of dead space. (a) When a walking suture is placed, the first bite is through the dermis (**A**), and the next bite is taken through the fascia (**B**). The fascial bite (**B**) is taken 5–10 mm ahead of the dermal bite (**A**) in the direction of skin advancement. (b) When the suture is tightened, the dermal bite (**A**) is drawn forward toward the fascial bite (**B**), advancing the skin edge. Multiple rows of walking sutures may be required to advance wound edges sufficiently to close the primary wound.

the wound. Correctly placed, walking sutures can advance a skin edge of a wound dramatically, ultimately allowing the skin edges to be in close application without excessive tension, while also reducing dead space in the wound bed. If the placement of the walking sutures tries to advance the tissues too aggressively or they are not anchored securely to fascia or in the dermis, suture pull-out will occur. If there is limited tissue available for a solid suture purchase, more sutures should be placed with each suture advancing the wound edge a shorter distance. This will accomplish the same objective.

Pulley sutures are another subcutaneous suture pattern that will help appose a wound while overcoming the tension within the wound.[12] A subcutaneous "pulley suture" involves taking a double pass with a suture needle on each side of the wound. Each suture bite must engage sturdy tissue, or pull-out is likely to occur. Specifically, the surgeon takes a deep to superficial bite on the near side, then takes a superficial to deep bite on the far side. At this point, it is the same as a buried knot. The difference with a modified pulley is that a second pass, running deep-to-superficial (near side) and superficial-to-deep (far side), is taken. It is important to pass the second bite immediately adjacent to or even in the same plane as the first suture passage. Spreading the bites apart seems to reduce some of the effectiveness of the pulley suture. Both the suture tag and the needle end should come through the middle of the suture pattern. The suture is slowly tightened until the degree of closure desired is achieved, and a knot is tied. The pulley suture can overcome significant tension within a wound bed and is especially helpful for wounds like unilateral or bilateral mastectomy. Multiple sutures should be placed until the skin edge has been advanced sufficiently to permit closure (Figure 18.7). Based on the needs of a particular closure, the pulley suture can be used in a similar manner to the walking suture, to help with the initial mobilization of the skin edges for closure. Pulley sutures and walking sutures can also be in open wounds to help prevent retraction of the wound edges during initial management.

Advancement and Rotational Flaps

Advancement, transposition, and rotational flaps are skin flaps that rely on the subdermal plexus of vessels for the survival of the overlying skin. It is this reliance that limits these flaps. As the flap is developed, the blood supply is severed on three sides, with only the vessels crossing the flap base onto the pedicle remaining. While it was once felt there was an ideal width-to-length ratio for a pedicle flap, it appears, within reason, that the survival of these flaps is based more on the characteristics of the subdermal plexus in the immediate area rather than the width of the base or the length of the flap.[8,13–15] The same flap, created in two different locations, may have different clinical outcomes.

The primary indication for the use of skin flaps during a mass resection is the potential for the flap to allow a more effective tension-free closure of the wound created during removal of the mass. This may be in the form of (1) bringing healthy skin into a compromised area, (2) releasing

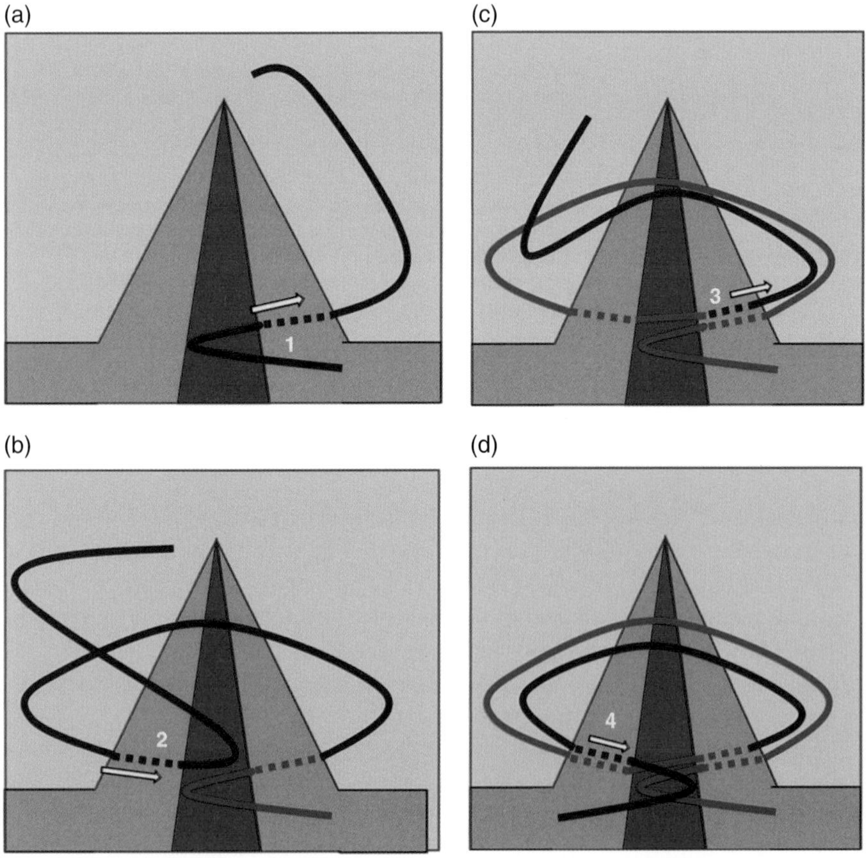

Figure 18.7 Pulley suture. Pulley sutures are typically used when the skin around the surgical wound is plentiful, but it will be under tension when apposed. The placement of several pulley sutures in a wound can bring the skin edges closer, neutralizing the distractive tension. Pulley sutures can also be combined with interrupted subcutaneous sutures or walking sutures for optimal results. (a) The first pass is deep to superficial to bury the knot on the near side. (b) A superficial to deep bite is taken on the far side. (c) The next pass is taken immediately beside (or even in the same plane as) the first bite. (d) The final pass is superficial to deep immediately beside (or in the same plane as) the second bite. It is important to keep the suture passes closely associated to maximize the benefits of the pulley suture.

excessive tension on the surgical wound, or (3) allowing closure of a difficult spot in a single session. Despite these advantages, the process of flap creation increases the amount of surgery a patient is receiving; therefore, flaps should be used only when necessary, relying on simpler closure techniques when appropriate.

Vascular Supply to the Skin

The skin has a rich vascular supply; however, this vascular support can be easily disrupted, impairing the health of the skin the surgeon is relying on to close the wound. The normal vascular supply to the skin begins with the direct (deep) cutaneous arteries.[11] These arteries supply specific zones within the skin and subcutaneous tissue and are the basis for axial pattern flaps. The direct cutaneous arteries give rise to a mid-level arterial supply to the skin that further branches into the small vessels or capillaries in the dermis. These form a meshwork of small, anastomosing "subdermal" vessels that support the overlying skin. The subdermal plexus can be damaged during manipulation, but the meshwork nature of these vessels and their inherent redundancy give the skin resilience. However, when a flap is elevated, this redundancy and resiliency are diminished; thus, adherence to the Halstedian principle of "gentle tissue handling" to protect the blood supply to a skin flap is essential to optimize healing. Many of the techniques for gentle tissue handling, discussed earlier in the chapter, become even more important when dealing with flaps.

When dealing with skin flaps, the "delayed phenomenon" is a technique used to enhance the vascular support of a planned subdermal plexus flap.[16] This is a two-step process that begins with elevation of the planned flap, including freeing of the skin from the underlying subcutaneous tissue, and then replacing the flap in its original location. The flap is sutured back in place and allowed to heal. This time stimulates the skin to reestablish a more robust subdermal plexus to support the overlying skin. In a few weeks, a second surgery is performed with resection of the target mass, and the flap previously elevated is again elevated, incising along the same lines as the previous surgery. The flap is then shifted to the recipient bed and sutured into place. Flap survival is expected to be improved with this technique. The primary disadvantage of the delayed transfer technique is the requirement for it being a two-stage process; requiring two separate surgical procedures before a mass can be resected and the wound closed.

Subdermal plexus flaps are what most veterinarians think of as skin flaps. These flaps are variations of advancement flaps, transposition, and rotational flaps. These flaps rely on the normal subdermal vascular plexus in the skin to support the flap.[14,15,17,18] For that reason, they need to be planned prior to development, and care must be taken during manipulation of the flaps to avoid injuring the subdermal plexus, as this will increase the potential for primary wound dehiscence. While there are numerous variations on subdermal plexus flaps, this discussion will focus on advancement flaps, such as the single-pedicle flap, the "H-plasty," the bipedicle flap, and the rotational flap.

Single-pedicle advancement flap is the most common flap for wound closure.[8,11,15,17–19] It involves the creation of a skin flap from the available skin immediately adjacent to the wound bed to be closed. The length of the flap is created by extending parallel incisions away from the wound bed that are 1–1.5x the length of the wound bed to be closed. It is important that the base of the flap is maintained at least the width of the original flap, although the author tends to widen the base slightly (Figure 18.8a). After the flap is elevated, the only remaining connection to the subdermal plexus is across the base of the flap, so keeping it as wide as possible should be beneficial. Advancement flaps tend to create "dog-ears" at the point where the flap slides onto the wound bed. Most of the time, these can be left in situ, and they will smooth out as the healing process continues; however, if resection of the dog-ears is attempted, it is essential that the process does not impinge on or diminish the base width of the advancement flap. Metzenbaum scissors or a scalpel blade is used to undermine the proposed flap, releasing it from any subcutaneous attachments, and the flap is advanced toward the far side of the wound bed. The author uses a combination of interrupted, subcutaneous, and walking sutures (Figure 18.8b) to advance the flap until it reaches the point of close apposition to the target edge in a relatively tension-free manner. This means the flap should maintain its position when it is released from external forces; if the flap retracts substantially, additional supporting sutures are needed to address the tension.

H-plasty advancement flaps are a modification of the single advancement flap.[8,14,16,17,19] This flap, also referred to as a double advancement flap, elevates two opposing subdermal advancement flaps, allowing the length of each flap to be more conservative than a single advancement flap would need to be. The shorter flaps are less likely to exceed the capacity of the subdermal plexus to support them once they are advanced. Once the flaps are elevated, they are advanced toward the middle of the defect, using a combination of subcutaneous, interrupted, and walking sutures to counteract any retraction. The flaps are advanced until they can be apposed without tension, and skin sutures are placed for final apposition of the first flap to the flap from the opposite side. Skin sutures are then continued along the incision lines created when the flap was raised. The final incision's appearance is a capital "H." The main advantage of the "H-plasty" is reducing the length of a

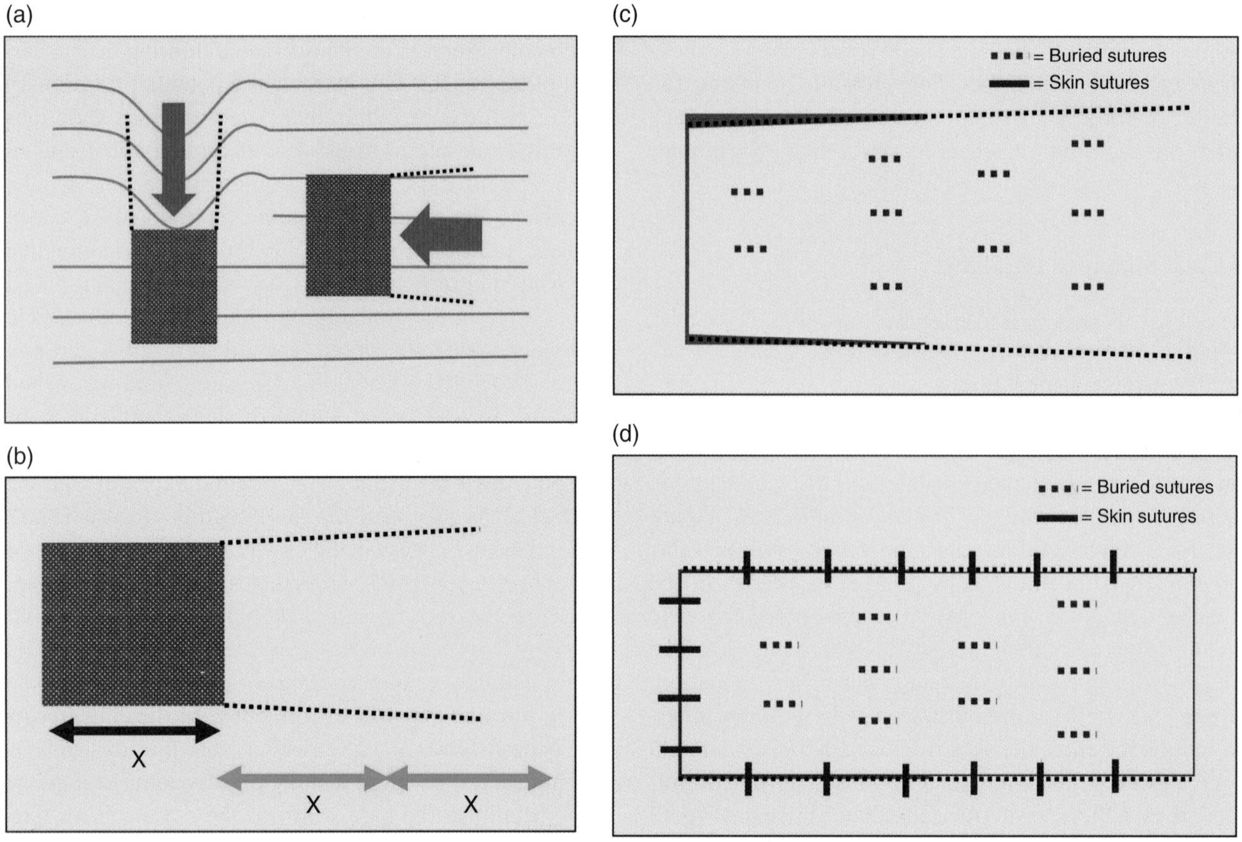

Figure 18.8 Single pedicle advancement flap. (a) During the planning stage, the surgeon must check tension lines of the skin (brown lines) to ensure there is sufficient skin available for the flap without excessive tension. (b) The flap is created by making parallel incisions that develop a flap at least 1–1.5x the length of the defect to be closed. (c) The flap is undermined and advanced using subcutaneous sutures to eliminate tension. The flap is stretched until it apposes the distant wound edge. (d) The wound edges are apposed to the flap edges for final closure. Additional wrinkles or "dog ears" created by the advancement of the flap can be cut off or allowed to remain.

single flap that would be required to close an incision by using two shorter flaps. In addition to improving the vascular support with a shorter flap, this technique should also reduce the tension on the final closure.

A *bipedicle advancement flap* uses an adjacent, releasing incision to create the flap. First, the length of the wound, as measured along the long axis, is determined.[8,15,17,19] The releasing incision is made parallel to this long axis at a distance that is ½ of the long axis length from the wound bed (Figure 18.9). The skin between the wound bed and the releasing incision is undermined, creating a skin flap anchored at each end. The bipedicle flap is then advanced laterally, over the wound bed and sutured in place, covering the exposed bed.

This process obviously creates a secondary wound to be closed. Ideally, the change in location of the defect will permit the definitive closure of the secondary wound. The ability to close this wound could be possible because the flap bed wound may not be constrained by the same factors that prevented closure of the primary wound and necessitated the bipedicle flap usage. These could be issues with wound tension or concerns about movement prompting use of the flap, which may not be the situation for the new location of the flap bed wound because of more availability of adjacent skin for closure or the use of the bipedicle flap could move the wound away from a high-motion zone. One final reason to consider the use of a bipedicle flap, even if the secondary wound cannot be immediately closed, would be the option of closing the primary wound that may be in a sensitive area, such as exposed bone or tendon, exposed major vessels, or an open wound over an orthopedic implant. In this situation, once the flap is moved and the primary wound is closed, the secondary wound can then managed.

Rotational flaps are most useful when the defect is triangular in shape.[8,14] In describing this type of flap, the defect can be thought of as a wedge, and the flap is created such that the clockwise (or counterclockwise) rotation of the flap will "close the wedge." To begin, the wound defect is debrided, and the wound edges freshened so the defect

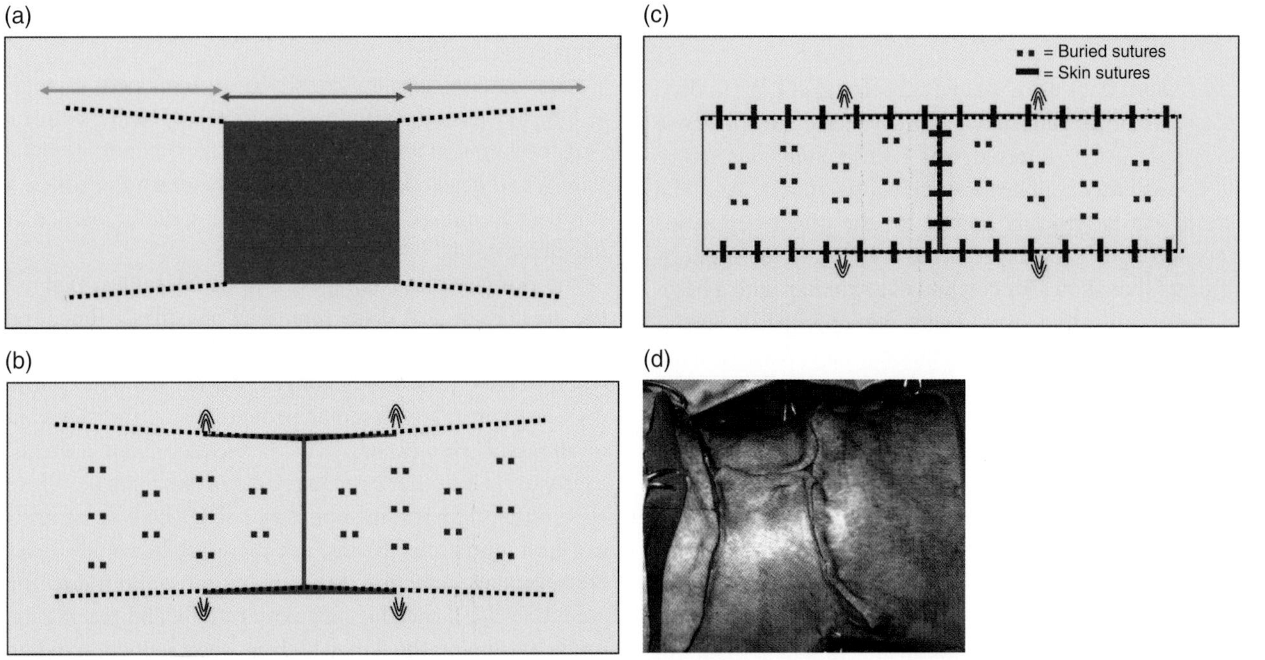

Figure 18.9 "H-plasty" advancement flap. (a) An advancement flap is outlined on opposite sides of a wound bed. Since two flaps are being elevated, the flaps are typically shorter than a single flap would be. (b) The flaps are undermined and advanced using subcutaneous sutures to eliminate tension. Each flap is advanced until they meet midway across the wound. (c) The flaps are apposed, and the edges are sutured to maintain apposition and positioning. (d) H-plasty advancement flap prior to placement of the skin sutures.

forms a roughly triangular shape. Using one of the long edges of the defect, a curving arc of the rotation is drawn beginning at the base of the triangle and creating a semicircular incision, which encompasses the wound defect at one end. The skin is undermined along the incision moving inward until the flap is freed. The flap is then pivoted into the defect, with the outer edge moving further than the inner edge, until the flap reaches the far side of the triangle and the defect is closed. Tension along the flap is controlled with subcutaneous sutures, as previously described, and the incisions are closed using an appositional suture pattern.

Transposition flaps are similar to advancement flaps, but they are developed at an angle to the recipient wound bed, generally between 45° and 90°.[8,14] One side of a transposition flap will be the edge of the wound defect to be closed. This is in contrast to the advancement flap, where it is the leading edge of the flap that is one of the wound edges. Because a transposition flap will be raised and then rotated into the wound bed, it is important to check skin tension on all sides of the wound to determine which side is optimal for flap development.

The transposition flap width is determined by the width of the wound bed. The length of a transposition flap is estimated by determining the distance from the far edge of the flap base and the farthest point away from the wound bed to the far side of the wound defect. The outline of the proposed flap is drawn adjacent to the wound, then the skin is incised and undermined. The flap can now be rotated into the wound bed, where it is secured with subcutaneous sutures. The flap edges are apposed with skin sutures, and the first portion is completed. Ideally, the open donor site from where the flap was elevated can be closed primarily to complete the procedure. As a subdermal plexus flap, transposition flaps need to have a substantial base to support the flap. Some surgeons consider the 90° rotational flap to be the most versatile.[8,14] When raising a transposition flap on a limb, the base of the flap must be the most proximal point with the flap extending distally down the leg. With increasing rotation, the flap is more likely to suffer flap necrosis and incisional dehiscence. Closure of the donor site, when a flap is raised on a limb, is more difficult due to the limited amount of loose skin on the limbs.

When moving the transposition flap into the recipient bed, the skin can bunch along the base of the flap. These areas, referred to as "dog-ears," tend to get larger the more the flap has to be rotated to fit into the recipient bed.[14] Surgical removal of dog-ears may create a more esthetically-pleasing wound closure; however, there is little reason to actually remove them. Furthermore, careless action while trying to remove dog-ears can impinge on the flap base, increasing the risk of flap necrosis.

Axial Pattern Flaps

Axial pattern flaps are a unique subset of skin flaps in dogs and cats. An axial pattern flap is predicated on the presence of a specific artery, referred to as a direct cutaneous artery, that consistently supplies a specific area of skin. An axial pattern flap is typically named for the direct cutaneous artery supporting the flap. It is the presence of the supporting artery that allows for creation of a skin flap with a base-to-length ratio that would not be appropriate for a subdermal advancement or rotational flap. With an axial pattern flap, the length and width of the flap is only limited by the circulatory distribution of its supporting artery. Axial pattern flaps are typically rectangular in shape but some of the flaps can be extended at a 90° angle at the end of the flap, creating an inverted "L" shape for rotation into the recipient wound bed.[20,21] The standard axial pattern flap is sometimes referred to as a "peninsula" flap. This term is applied since the standard axial pattern flap is a long strip of skin that maintains an attachment to the main body. This terminology differentiates the standard axial pattern flap from an "island" flap (to be discussed later). Table 18.1 summarizes the uses of and the surgical guidelines for elevating the caudal superficial epigastric flap (Figure 18.10), the thoracodorsal flap, the omocervical flap, the caudal auricular flap, the dorsal and ventral deep circumflex iliac flaps, and the related, flank fold flap.[20–23] Details for other axial pattern flaps can be found in detail elsewhere.[8,20,21]

The versatility of the axial pattern flap allows the surgeon to employ it for difficult areas to reach or challenges in wound closure. The most common usage is where the flap is raised, its base is maintained, and then the flap is rotated into a wound bed. This can be done with more chronic wounds after open wound management or with acute, surgical wounds. Care needs to be taken whenever the plan is to employ an axial pattern flap for closure of a traumatic wound. There is a risk that the traumatic episode could have damaged the direct cutaneous artery that supports the flap, rendering the axial pattern flap into a simple rotational flap. In this circumstance, there is likely to be significant necrosis of the flap and wound dehiscence.

The advantages of axial pattern flaps include the ability to combine the initial mass removal with closure using an axial pattern flap, providing a single-stage resection and closure of a surgical wound. This flexibility to provide a primary closure reduces the need for open wound management and the need for additional surgery, resulting in less cost and hospitalization time for the patient and client. Axial pattern flaps also offer the potential for primary closure of large wounds in a manner that minimizes tension across the site.

Axial pattern flaps are consistent in their performance, as long as the surgeon follows the reported borders during flap development and is careful with tissue handling of the flap. When developed correctly, axial pattern flaps have a survivability rate of 85–100%, depending on the particular flap being used.[20]

The primary disadvantages of an axial pattern flap are the greater surgical dose, increased anesthesia time, and costs required to elevate and secure the flap in the recipient wound bed. Other disadvantages include the potential to disrupt the primary vascular pedicle during the elevation of the axial pattern flap with subsequent flap necrosis. Injury to the vascular pedicle results in two large defects to close rather than just the one, original defect. Flap necrosis can have numerous causes, but the most common causes are secondary infection, the surgeon failing to follow the guidelines for a specific axial pattern flap, and placing too much tension on the flap, which causes a reduction in flap perfusion. Appropriate perioperative antibiotic administration and judicious postoperative antimicrobial therapy can help prevent or treat bacterial infections associated with the flap. Early intervention to reduce tension, correct vascular pedicle occlusions, or relieve excessive fluid accumulations under the flap may help with salvaging a compromised flap. A closed suction drain is often placed at the time of flap development and suturing into the recipient bed, which will reduce the fluid build-up beneath the flap. Additional therapies, such as hyperbaric oxygen and negative-pressure wound therapy, have shown to have some benefits in human medicine, but the role and the benefit of these modalities in veterinary medicine remain unclear.[20]

Preoperative planning is essential for successful outcomes with axial pattern flaps. The anticipated origin of the direct cutaneous vessels should be carefully marked, followed by diagramming the borders of the proposed flap. The flap length must be measured to ensure it will be sufficient for the wound to be closed. This can be accomplished by using a 4×4 gauze, or similar non-stretchy material, to represent the flap, anchoring it to the proposed flap base then rotating the gauze into the recipient wound bed. If the gauze bunches too much or is insufficient in length, changes need to be made to the plan. This could consist of (1) using a different axial flap, if available, (2) altering the length of the proposed flap within acceptable parameters, or (3) by determining a different closure technique may offer a better outcome compared to the planned axial pattern flap.

Table 18.1 Common axial pattern flaps.

Name	Borders	Uses
Caudal superficial epigastric flap		
This flap is based on the caudal superficial epigastric vessel. This vessel arises from the external pudendal artery as it exits the inguinal ring and runs cranially.	Base: Between the last mammary gland and the inguinal ring. Central axis: The nipple line of the mammary chain. Medial border: The ventral midline. Lateral border: A parallel incision equidistance to the distance between the central axis and the ventral midline. Cranial border: The flap can run cranially to the third or even extended to the second mammary gland in the dog and cat (i.e., glands 2–5 in the dog, glands 2–4 in the cat).	Can be stretched up to the dorsum in the flank area, rotated down the proximal portion of the rear leg to the stifle, or shifted anywhere within 180° of the base of the flap, including the perineal region. Dissection should be deep to the mammary tissue. Require a bridging incision to rotate into wound beds.
Caudal auricular flap		
Based on the caudal auricular artery.	Base: Centered over the lateral wing of the atlas. Cranial/Caudal incisions: Parallel incisions running caudally to the edge of the scapula. Flap width: The width of the flap can vary but is typically 1/3–1/2 of the distance from the dorsal cervical midline to the ventral cervical midline. Flap length: The edge of the scapula.	Wounds on the head (dorsal), neck, fascial area, and the ear.
Thoracodorsal flap		
Based on a cutaneous branch of the thoracodorsal artery. Creation of an "inverted-L" shape is possible with this flap.	Base: Caudal depression of the shoulder (with the vessel just caudal to the acromion) Central axis: Runs along the caudal border of the scapula Cranial: From the acromion running dorsally along the spine of the scapula. Caudal: Parallel to the cranial incision, equidistance from the central axis to the scapular spine (cranial incision) Flap length: Can run dorsally to the dorsal midline or to the contralateral dorsal scapula; a "L-shaped" flap can be raised along the dorsum with the short leg moving caudally	Shoulder, axilla, thoracic wall, upper arm, and forearm in cats and certain dog breeds. Flap is raised deep to the cutaneous trunci muscle; the thoracodorsal artery is vulnerable to injury. This flap can extend to the dorsal midline and even beyond, although the further over the dorsal it extends, the greater the risk for distal flap necrosis.
Deep circumflex iliac flap – dorsal branch		
Based on the dorsal branch of the deep circumflex iliac artery.	Base: The artery exits the flank area just below the wing of the ilium. It branches into a ventral and dorsal branch. The central axis runs from the base dorsally along the cranial edge of the ilium. Caudal: The caudal incision runs from the base dorsally between the cranial edge of the ilium and the greater trochanter. Cranial: A parallel incision equidistance to the measured distance between the central axis and the caudal border (over the ilium). Flap length: Can extend to the dorsal spine and over the dorsum to the flank fold on the opposite side.	Used for lesions in the ipsilateral flank, pelvic, lumbar, and defects of the greater trochanter and lateromedial thigh.

(Continued)

Table 18.1 (Continued)

Name	Borders	Uses
Deep circumflex iliac flap – ventral branch		
Based on the ventral branch of the deep circumflex iliac artery.	Base: The artery exits the flank area just below the wing of the ilium. It branches into a ventral and dorsal branch. The central axis, for the ventral branch, runs ventrally toward the flank fold. Caudal: The caudal incision runs from the base ventrally from a point midway between the cranial ilium and the greater trochanter. This incision runs parallel to the shaft of the femur. Cranial: A parallel incision equidistance to the distance measured between the central axis and the caudal incision (parallel to femur). Flap length: Can extend ventrally to the level of the patella.	Can be used as a rotational flap or as an island flap. As a peninsula flap, it can rotate cranially or caudally to reach the lateral abdominal wall, flank, and lateromedial thigh; as an island flap, it can be rotated to reach lesions associated with the sacral and lateral pelvic injuries. This flap is reportedly more versatile than the flap based on the dorsal branch.
Flank fold flap (rear)		
Based off the ventral branch of the deep circumflex iliac artery, this flap is based on the loose skin at the front of the thigh between the body wall and the stifle, associated with the flank area.	Base: The proximal area of the flank fold. Flap: The flap is raised by grasping the loose skin of the flank skin fold and starting the incision distally. The incision is extended dorsally into the flank exposing the proximal thigh. This incision frees the flap flank fold but must be created to permit a tension-free closure over the cranial portion of the thigh. The flap can be rotated ventrally to close wounds in the inguinal area with a bridging incision.	This flap is useful for ventral abdominal and inguinal wounds. It is especially useful when injury or trauma may have rendered the caudal superficial epigastric flap unreliable.
Omocervical flap		
The omocervical artery emerges cranial to the scapula and gives off the superficial cervical branch that supports this flap. Creation of an "inverted-L" shape is possible with this flap.	Base: Level of the superficial scapular lymph node with the central axis of the flap running parallel to the cranial edge of the scapula. Caudal border: An incision along the scapular spine. Cranial border: A parallel incision equidistance to the measured distance between the central axis and the caudal border (scapular spine). Flap length: The location of the dorsal connecting incision is determined by the desired length of the flap. This flap is reportedly supported as far as the scapulohumeral joint on the opposite side.	Can be used for defects of the head, neck, face, ear, shoulder, and axilla.

Adapted from Fossum, Wardlaw and Lanz, and Pavletic.[8,20–22]

If the recipient wound bed exists due to a traumatic wound, it will need to be managed until there is a healthy bed of granulation tissue. Once this is the case, a tissue culture should be obtained and the wound bed should be covered with a topical antimicrobial cream for 24–48 hours before the final procedure, and then it should be sterilely bandaged. Once in surgery, the wound edges are freshened, and efforts made to reduce the biofilm on the granulation tissue surface before transferring the axial pattern flap to the recipient bed.

For standard axial pattern flaps, the attached base of the flap can rotate no more than 180° without risking compression of the vascular pedicle. Careful dissection of fat and subcutaneous tissue surrounding the vascular pedicle

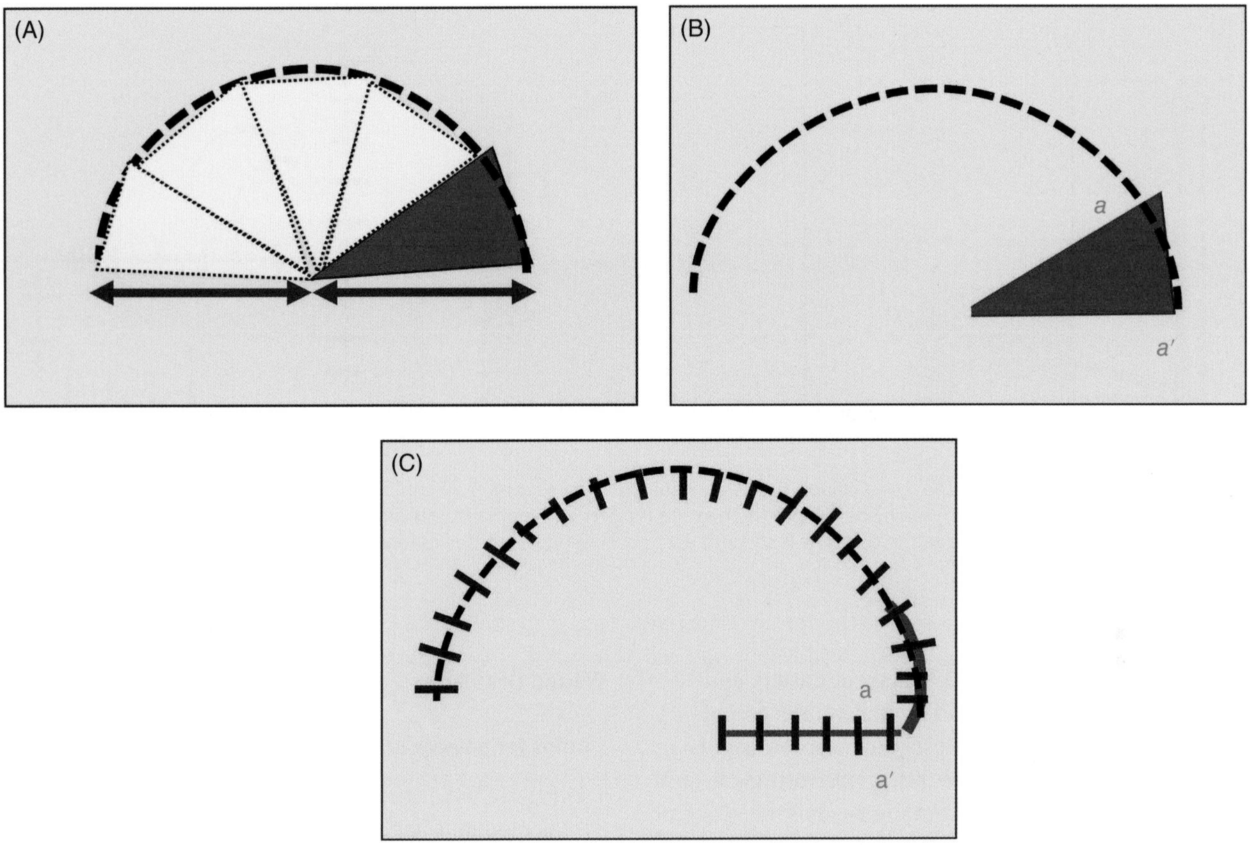

Figure 18.10 The rotational flap is useful for closing triangular defects or defects that can be debrided to a triangular shape. (A) Flap shape and size are estimated by taking the wound bed and using the size to create an arc that pivots around the narrow point for 180°. (B) The line of the arc is incised, and the skin is elevated from the subcutaneous layer. The leading edge of the flap (a) is to be advanced to the far edge of the defect (*a*′). (C) The flap is advanced (point *a* meets *a*′) and secured in place with subcutaneous sutures and skin sutures.

can reduce the pressure exerted against the pedicle when rotating the flap but this action increases the risk of iatrogenic damage to the vascular pedicle.

Vascular compromise associated with flap rotation is typically from compression of the vein draining the flap, since veins are low pressure, thin-walled, and easily compressible. The result of venous outflow obstruction is mild to severe venous congestion of the flap, leading to flap necrosis. This can be treated by surgical means to relieve venous congestion (e.g., flap revision), flap drainage through the use of punctuate incisions to allow congested blood to escape into a bandage, or application of medicinal leeches (hirudotherapy).[24,25] The more aggressive the axial pattern flap is rotated, the greater the risk of compromising the artery causing ischemic flap necrosis. To minimize this complication, an axial pattern peninsular flap that needs to have greater than 120° rotation can be converted to an axial pattern "island" flap allowing up to 180° of flap rotation (Figure 18.11).

To create an axial pattern island flap,[20,21] the surgeon first develops a standard axial pattern flap. After elevating the flap, the surgeon carefully severs the skin attachment at the flap's base. With the base severed, the flap is now simply an island of skin that is only anchored by the vascular pedicle. This island of skin can be elevated and rotated up to 180° with less risk of twisting or compressing the vascular supply, potentially causing vascular compromise and flap necrosis. There is, however, an increased risk of surgically damaging the vascular pedicle of the supporting artery and vein during the dissection required to create the island flap.

Finally, surgeons who are comfortable with microsurgical techniques may use an axial pattern flap as the donor flap for a free vascular graft. The consistent blood supply means the flap can be raised from the donor site, and the pedicle vessels are dissected clear and transected. The surgeon may now free up the newly created graft, which is transferred to a new location. Once the microvascular

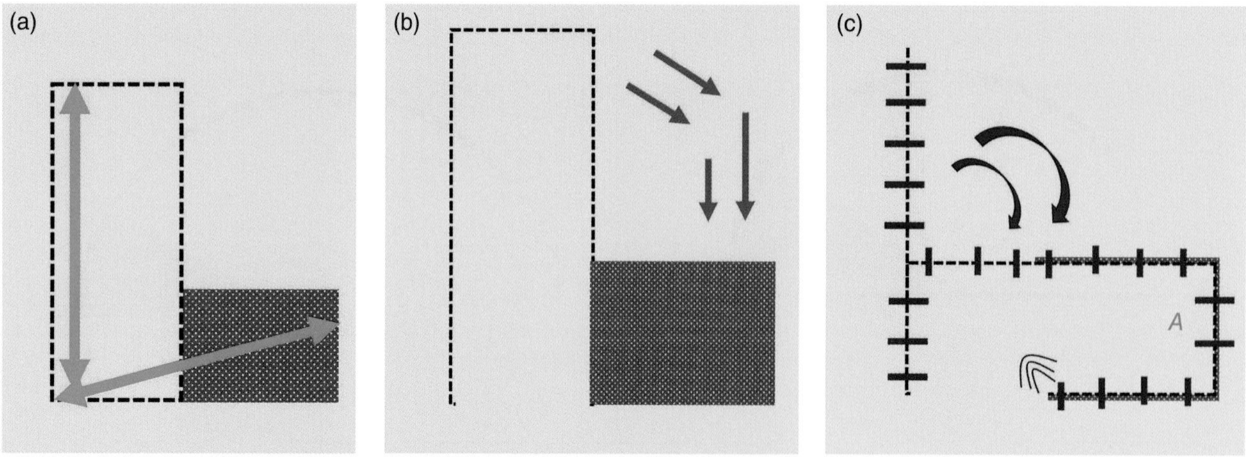

Figure 18.11 (a) The length of the transposition flap is determined by measuring from the far corner of the flap base to the distant edge of the defect (green arrows). (b) The borders of the flap are incised, and the flap is elevated in preparation for rotation into the defect. (c) Once the flap is placed in the defect, it is secured with subcutaneous sutures followed by skin sutures. The donor site is closed primarily.

anastomosis between the direct cutaneous artery and vein of the graft and a recipient artery and vein is completed, the newly re-vascularized graft should have consistent survival in its new location. Details of microsurgical graft transfers have been reported but are beyond the scope of this chapter.[26]

When the wound bed that needs the axial pattern flap is not immediately adjacent to the base of the axial pattern flap, a "bridging incision" will be needed to move the flap into the correct position. The bridging incision is created by incising the skin and subcutaneous tissue between the base of the axial pattern flap and the recipient wound bed, permitting the flap to contact the edges of the bridging incision as it travels to the wound bed. The location of the incision should accommodate any anticipated tension or stresses from movement. Hemostasis is established but care must be taken to not compromise the primary blood supply to the newly raised flap.

Once the flap is rotated into the recipient wound bed, it is secured in place. Some surgeons simply secure the flap in place with skin sutures (or staples) after placing an active or a passive drain in the recipient wound bed underneath the flap. The author prefers to use a combination of buried, simple interrupted sutures and walking sutures to decrease dead space under the graft and help dissipate any tensile forces on the flap, while the editor prefers to place a closed suction drain and not place walking sutures, which could increase the risk of flap vascular compromise if sutures grab any of the small vessels. Care must be taken to not damage or occlude the direct cutaneous artery when placing these sutures, or distal graft necrosis is likely to be the result.

Wound Drainage

Rules for passive drainage:

1) Passive drains need only have a single exit site with a single suture applied. The dorsal aspect may be secured by a skin suture passed into the wound bed, passed in a mattress pattern through an uncut end of the drain, and passed back through the skin where it is tied. Leave these suture tags long for easy identification. A dorsal suture is not essential for securing of the drain.
2) The exit site needs to be large enough to not impinge on the drain. This will inhibit drainage.
3) Passive drains act by capillary action, so fenestration is not needed.
4) Drains are a two-way path. Bacteria can move up the drain into the wound in less than 48 hours, so whatever the drain touches can shortly be in the wound.
5) The exposed end of the drain should remain covered with an adsorptive dressing and protective covering.
6) Drains should be removed as soon as practical.

The use of passive or active wound drains after mass resection is at the discretion of the attending surgeon. The author acknowledges a hesitancy to use drains, preferring to rely heavily on sutures to minimize dead space and gentle pressure wraps; however, if a drain is going to be placed, it is essential to manage it appropriately. Passive drains (e.g., Penrose drains) must be placed so that gravity can encourage drainage. Ideally, the drain should be placed before closure, but care is needed to ensure the drain is not incorporated into any sutures during wound closure.

Active wound drains can be used for wound beds under flaps or large wounds, such as amputations. A Jackson-Pratt-type drain with an external vacuum source or a butterfly catheter with a vacutainer is an example of active wound/closed suction drains. The incorporation of a vacuum source (i.e., the collapsible "grenade") helps to overcome situations where gravity drainage is not able to accommodate the needs of the wound. Benefits of active suction drains include decreased risk of ascending infection as compared to passive drains, no need to cover the exit site, and no requirement for the exit site to be in a gravity-dependent location.

Active drains also require that the wound be closed completely, creating an air-tight pocket around the drain. Wound dehiscence or incomplete closure renders a limited vacuum-source drain, like the Jackson-Pratt, ineffective. In situations where the wound is not able to be effectively sealed at closure, options such as placing an air-tight wound cover (e.g., Ioban™), changing to passive drainage, using open wound management (open wounds drain surprising well!), or resorting to negative pressure wound therapy should be considered.

Potential Complications?

The major complications associated with mass resection and wound closure include incisional dehiscence, wound infection, seroma formation, and flap necrosis (partial versus full). The other significant complication is not getting effective surgical margins on the mass being removed. This failure subjects the pets to additional surgery, and their owners to increased costs and anxiety. This is minimized by planning for appropriate margins prior to the initial surgery and by having frank discussions with the owner when they want lower doses of surgery than what might be ideal.

Incisional dehiscence is always a potential complication; however, it is the goal of the advanced planning efforts to minimize tension across incisions and to select the best procedure to minimize this risk. Using the various layers of subcutaneous sutures, adding an intradermal or skin suture pattern, and accurate skin apposition are essential for reducing this complication. Emphasizing good follow-up care is also important. Wound infection can be minimized with the use of good surgical technique, intravenous administration of peri-operative antibiotics, gentle tissue handling, and good wound management, including covering all incisions, effective analgesia, oral antibiotics if indicated, and early discharge from hospital. Ensuring that the patient is prevented from self-mutilation with a hard cone collar of adequate length is also important.

Flap necrosis (Figure 18.12) is one of the most frustrating complications after reconstructive procedures. Again, the

(a)

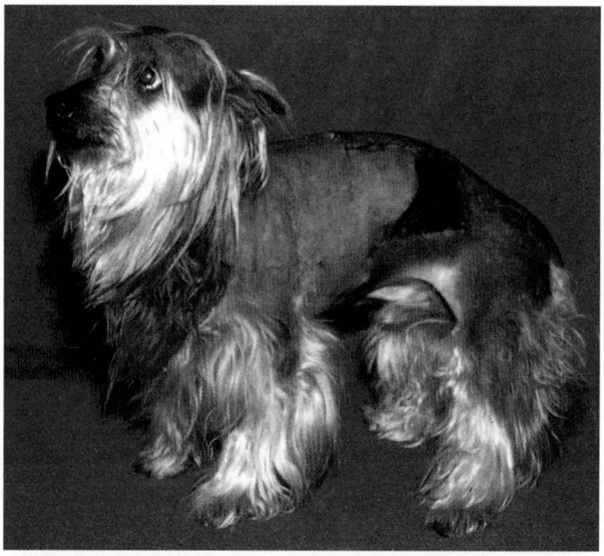

(b)

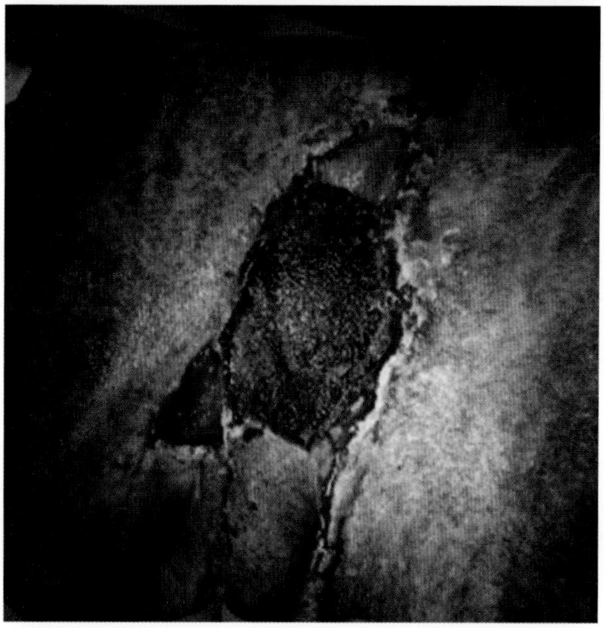

Figure 18.12 Flap necrosis. (a) Advancement flap necrosis was seen with this advancement flap about three to four days after surgical resection of a cutaneous lymphoma lesion. (b) A caudal superficial epigastric flap was elevated after resection of a large cutaneous Pythiosis lesion. The wound location was ideal for this axial pattern flap; however, five days after surgery, a Penrose drain was placed for a suspected seroma. A few days later, flap necrosis was apparent. The Penrose drain was reported to have exited at the level of the tissue demarcation, suggesting it damaged the supporting vessels during placement. Due to the location and the significant volume of tissue resected with the original lesion, this wound had to be managed with debridement, partial wound closure, and as an open wound for another six weeks prior to delayed primary closure.

planning process before surgery is aimed at reducing this potential, but it is always a possible outcome. Flap necrosis can be caused by surgical failures (e.g., transecting or otherwise damaging the direct cutaneous artery and roughly handling the flap), by compromising the flap blood supply (e.g., applying bandages and applying cold compresses), by self-inflected trauma, by wound infection and subsequent dehiscence, or by poor postoperative management. If a flap has developed necrosis, it will need to be debrided and managed as an open wound until the wound bed is healthy. Some wounds may only have a partial failure, and the remaining wound may be closed by wound contraction with open wound management and no additional surgery required.

Otherwise, once the wound bed is ready, another attempt at surgical closure can be considered. This second attempt at wound closure will be more challenging, especially if the attempt is made too soon after the initial closure. This is because the skin and subcutaneous tissue surrounding the open wound may not have rebuilt the reserves or have the ability to stretch via mechanical creep in the edges needed for closure, whether that is through the creation of alternative flaps or through attempts at primary closure. For many patients, waiting a few weeks will not only give a greater chance of being successful, but it might also reduce the wound size, making subsequent closure easier. Patience, on the part of the surgeon and the owners, will be essential. Intervening too early will likely result in a poor outcome a second time as well.

Postoperative Management

Incision care is particularly important after mass resection and reconstructive procedures. Opinions vary about the necessity of covering surgical incisions; however, it is generally accepted that the incision must be protected from licking, chewing, or other patient self-mutilation activities. Employing an Elizabethan collar, a surgical shirt, or routine bandaging to cover the surgical site(s) is the basic expectation for after-care. All coverings must be managed carefully to ensure the wound covering is not rubbing against that incision, which could create pressure points or harbor excessive moisture that can impair wound healing, cause wound irritation, and ultimately, lead to wound dehiscence. Whatever dressing is used, it must be checked frequently and changed on a regular basis for the first several days.

Suture removal for a healthy patient can be removed in 10–14 days. Patients with medical conditions or that are receiving treatments that may negatively impact healing may need to have their sutures left in place for a longer period (up to 21 days). When an intradermal suture line is placed in addition to skin sutures, the skin sutures can be removed earlier (7–10 days), allowing the intradermal sutures to maintain wound apposition. The author routinely removes half or all of a patient's skin staples at 7–10 days as well, depending on the spacing of the staples.

While a wound can undergo dehiscence at any time, most surgically closed wounds will dehisce between days 3 and 5 as the inflammatory phase is transitioning into the proliferative phase of wound healing. The typical approach, rechecking the wound at the time of suture removal, is often much too late to allow for early intervention if any wound complications have arisen. If there is concern about the integrity of a postoperative wound, it should be repeatedly evaluated during the two- to six-day period after surgical closure.

A supportive bandage, such as a modified Robert-Jones bandage, can be applied when appropriate; however, if rigid stabilization of a wound is required, more aggressive bandaging, using either a pre-made spoon splint or a custom splint made with fiberglass-casting tape, can be incorporated in the modified Robert-Jones bandage. In a few situations, the author has used a temporary, trans-articular, external fixator to protect a vulnerable flap. The primary advantage of this technique is that the rigid stabilization is maintained even if the bandage becomes displaced during bandage changes. The disadvantage is the time and expense of the fixator placement and the need to have a second anesthetic event for pin removal.

Exercise restriction should be expected after mass resection and wound reconstruction. The severity and duration of exercise restriction is influenced by the size and complexity of the wound closure, the tension on the incision, and the wound location. Wounds with minimal tension across the site or those that are along the ventral midline or on the chest wall are subjected to minimal disruptive forces. These wounds may only require a light wrap or shirt to protect them during healing. Other wounds, such as those in a high-motion location and or those closed under tension, should have more restrictive exercise restriction. Each wound and each patient should be evaluated individually for the best postoperative plan that will get the best client compliance and the optimal healing for the patient.

Every owner should also receive clear instructions for incision monitoring. In addition to twice daily checks, the author recommends warm, moist compresses over the surgical site. This gets the owner to indirectly monitor the incision for the 5–10 minutes that the compress is being applied. Discharge instructions should also include "trigger points" or "signposts" the owners can use for monitoring the incision, with the instruction to return for an incision recheck if any of these points are encountered. These can include increasing redness, a bruised appearance around the wound that appears more pronounced or is spreading, purulent wound discharge or persistent serous discharge, hemorrhage, pain on gentle palpation of the incision, or significant swelling of the surgical site. The presence of one or more of these findings when combined with general health parameters like decreased appetite, alertness, and/or normal interest in interactions with family members is useful to detect early problems and prevent them from becoming more serious complications.

References

1 Pavletic, M.M. (2010). Basic principles of wound healing. In: *Atlas of Small Animal Wound Management and Reconstructive Surgery*, 17–30. Ames, IA: Wiley-Blackwell.

2 Hunt, G.B. and Cornell, K. (2018). Wound healing. In: *Veterinary Surgery-Small Animal*, 2e (ed. S.A. Johnson and K.S. Tobias), 132–147. Elsevier.

3 Bohling, M.W., Henderson, R.A., Swaim, S.T. et al. (2004). Cutaneous wound healing in the cat: a macroscopic description and comparison of cutaneous wound healing in the dog. *Vet. Surg.* 33: 579–587. https://doi.org/10.1111/j.1532-950X.2004.04081.x.

4 van Nimwegen, S.A. and Kirpensteijn, J. (2018). Specific disorders of the skin and subcutaneous tissues. In: *Veterinary Surgery-Small Animal*, 2e (ed. S.A. Johnson and K.S. Tobias), 1508–1550. Elsevier.

5 Risselada, M., Mathews, K.G., and Griffith, E. (2016). The effect of specimen preparation on post-excision and post-fixation dimensions, translation, and distortion of canine cadaver skin-muscle-fascia specimens. *Vet. Surg.* 45: 563–570. https://doi.org/10.1111/vsu.12481.

6 Terry, J.L., Milovancev, M., Nemanic, S., and Löhr, C.V. (2017). Quantification of surgical margin length changes after excision of feline injection site sarcomas—a pilot study. *Vet. Surg.* 46: 189–196. https://doi.org/10.1111/vsu.12602.

7 Thieman-Mankin KM, Jeffery ND, Kerwin SC. (2021). The impact of a surgical checklist on surgical outcomes in an academic institution. *Vet. Surg.* 50(4):848–857. https://doi.org/10.1111/vsu.13629.

8 MacPhail, C. and Fossum, T.W. (2018). Surgery of integumentary system. In: *Small Animal Surgery*, 5e (ed. T.M. Fossum), 512–539. Mosby.

9 Stanley, B.J. (2018). Tension relieving techniques. In: *Veterinary Surgery-Small Animal*, 2e (ed. S.A. Johnson and K.S. Tobias), 1422–1445. Elsevier.

10 Swaim, S.A. and Henderson, R.H. (1997). Management of skin tension. In: *Small Animal Wound Management*, 143–190. Baltimore: William & Wilkins.

11 Tobias, K.M. (2017). Lumpectomy and primary closure. In: *Manual of Small Animal Soft Tissue Surgery*, 2e, 15–24. Wiley.

12 Schmiedt, C.W. (2018). Suture material, tissue staples, ligation devices and closure methods. In: *Veterinary Surgery-Small Animal*, 2e (ed. S.A. Johnson and K.S. Tobias), 1210–1225. Elsevier.

13 Austin, BR, Henderson RA. (2006). Buried tension sutures: force-tension comparisons of pulley, double butterfly, mattress, and simple interrupted suture patterns. *Vet. Surg.* 35: 43–48. https://doi.org/10.1111/j.1532-950X.2005.00110.x.

14 Pavletic, M.M. (2010). Local flaps. In: *Atlas of Small Animal Wound Management and Reconstructive Surgery*, 307–336. Ames, IA: Wiley-Blackwell.

15 Hunt, G.B. (2018). Local or subdermal flaps. In: *Veterinary Surgery-Small Animal*, 2e (ed. S.A. Johnson and K.S. Tobias), 1446–1456. Elsevier.

16 Pavletic, M.M. (2010). Distant flap techniques. In: *Atlas of Small Animal Wound Management and Reconstructive Surgery*, 337–343. Ames, IA: Wiley-Blackwell.

17 Pavletic, M.M. (1990). Skin flaps in reconstructive surgery. *Vet. Clin. North Am. Small Anim. Pract.* 20 (1): 81–103. https://doi.org/10.1016/s0195-5616(90)50005-4.

18 Swaim, S.A. and Henderson, R.H. (1997). Various shaped wounds. In: *Small Animal Wound Management*, 235–274. Baltimore: William & Wilkins.

19 Tobias, K.M. (2017). Basic flaps. In: *Manual of Small Animal Soft Tissue Surgery*, 2e, 25–33. Wiley.

20 Wardlaw, J.L. and Lanz, O.I. (2018). Axial pattern and myocutaneous flaps. In: *Veterinary Surgery-Small Animal*, 2e (ed. S.A. Johnson and K.S. Tobias), 1457–1473. Elsevier.

21 Pavletic, M.M. (2010). Axial pattern skin flaps. In: *Atlas of Small Animal Wound Management and Reconstructive Surgery*, 357–402. Ames, IA: Wiley-Blackwell.

22 Pavletic, M.M. (1981). Canine axial pattern flaps, using the omocervical, thoracodorsal, and deep circumflex iliac direct cutaneous arteries. *Am. J. Vet. Res.* 42 (3): 391–406.

23 Hunt, G.B., Tisdall, P.L., Liptak, J.M. et al. (2001). Skin-fold advancement flaps for closing large proximal limb and trunk defects in dogs and cats. *Vet. Surg.* 30 (5): 440–448. https://doi.org/10.1053/jvet.2001.25868.

24 Sobczak, N. and Kantyka, M. (2014). Hirudotherapy in veterinary medicine. *Ann. Parasitol.* 60 (2): 89–92.

25 Kermanian, C.S., Buote, N.J., and Bergman, P.J. (2022). Medicinal leech therapy in veterinary medicine: a retrospective study. *J. Am. Anim. Hosp. Assoc.* 58 (6): 303–308. https://doi.org/10.5326/JAAHA-MS-7146.

26 Valery, F. and Scharf, V.F. (2017). Free grafts and microvascular anastomoses. *Vet. Clin. North Am. Small Anim. Pract.* 47 (6): 1249–1262. https://doi.org/10.1016/j.cvsm.2017.06.009.

19

Digit Amputation

David Michael Tillson

Department of Clinical Sciences, Auburn University, Auburn, AL, USA

Key Points

- Local or regional anesthetic protocols are effective adjuncts to general anesthesia.
- The incision for a digital amputation should be planned to allow for adequate exposure, appropriate tissue margins, and tension-free closure.
- Creation and maintenance of a "bloodless surgical field" will aid the surgical procedure.
- Minor wound dehiscence is a common sequela from self-trauma, weight-bearing, or excessive tension across the surgical site.
- Patient bandaging is important for protect and support; however, bandage complications can be severe if the bandage is too tight or not maintained.

Introduction/Anatomy

Dogs have five digits on the foreleg and four to five digits on the rear leg. The first digit, the "dewclaw," is not weight-bearing and is the digit typically absent on the rear leg. Digits 3 and 4 are referred to as "weight-bearing" digits, while 2 and 5 play a lesser role.[1] Thus, amputation of either digits 2 or 5 should result in minimal clinical impairment.

Each digit consists of three small bones: proximal, middle, and distal phalanges. These bones are also referred to as P1, P2, and P3, respectively. The proximal phalanx of each digit articulates with the metacarpal or metatarsal bones. Each digit has a sesamoid bone over the P1–P2 and the P2–P3 joints on the dorsal surface and paired sesamoid bones on the ventral aspect at the P1–P2 joint. Fractures of the sesamoid bones can occur and are typically treated by removal of the sesamoid fragments. Most surgeons will remove the sesamoids when performing a partial digital amputation.

The vascular supply to the digit is primarily from the dorsal and palmar/plantar digital arteries and their branches that supply each digit along with the corresponding veins. Tendinous insertions of the common digital extensor (digits 1–5) and the lateral digital extensor (digits 3–5) attach to the dorsal aspect of the digits while the superficial and deep digital flexors attach on the palmar/plantar aspect of the paw.[2] The skin over the proximal portion of the proximal phalanges is fused and then separates to cover each individual digit near the end of the proximal phalanges.

As noted previously, the first digit (i.e., dewclaw) is seldom an issue regarding locomotion or lameness. It is still common to see dewclaws being removed for cosmetic or functional reasons, especially when they are very loosely attached and there is concern about trauma. Digits 2 and 5 are the outside digits and are considered to not be weight-bearing. Therefore, amputation of one of these digits is seldom associated with significant gait changes or lameness.

Techniques in Small Animal Soft Tissue, Orthopedic, and Ophthalmic Surgery, First Edition. Edited by Kristin A. Coleman.

Companion website: www.wiley.com/go/coleman/surgeries

When amputating digit 3 or 4, there can be changes to the animal's gait due to the weight-bearing nature of these digits. The clinical significance of amputation of the central digits has not been sufficiently documented and may only be significant in working or racing animals. It is generally accepted that more distally located amputations, or partial amputation, will have a more limited clinical impact on the patient.

Indications

Indications for a digital amputation include traumatic injury, osseous or soft tissue infection, and neoplastic conditions are the most common reasons for digital amputation.[2,4] In some situations, owners may request a digital amputation(s) for cosmetic or behavior reasons. Iatrogenic injuries, such as the application of an excessively tight bandage, can also prompt the need for a digital amputation. Traumatic injury can result in dislocation of the digits, phalangeal fractures, or loss of the nail, resulting in a painful toe. Some dogs will further exacerbate the situation by inflicting self-trauma to the damaged digit. In some situations, digit amputation is used to create tissue for wound or surgical site closure, such as managing significant foot pad injuries by generating digital pad tissues used in reconstructive procedures. Infectious conditions, such as suspected or documented osteomyelitis, soft tissue infections from bacterial or fungal sources, or the chronic presence of foreign material adjacent to a digit, may prompt amputation. In these cases, it is important to get deep tissue samples for bacterial or fungal culture and to have histopathological evaluation of the digit performed.

Several neoplastic conditions can originate on the digits. While osteosarcoma of a digit is reported, neoplasms associated with the soft tissues are more frequently encountered. In the dog, the most common digital tumors include squamous cell carcinoma (SCC), melanoma, soft tissue sarcomas, and mast cell tumors; however, numerous other tumor types have been reported to affect the digit.[3–8] A recent report of 2912 digital amputations from dogs found that 52% of submissions were for suspected neoplasm and 80% of these were malignant tumors.[6] The most common diagnosis in dogs was SCC, accounting for 63% of diagnosed malignancies, with melanoma, soft tissue sarcomas, and mast cell tumors accounting for another 27%. Tumors originating from the subungual epithelium (nail bed) are thought to have a more aggressive metastatic pattern, and dogs with darker coats, as well as Schnauzers and Poodles, have been suggested to be at higher risk of digital SCC.[7,8] In cats, SCC and fibrosarcoma are the most commonly reported neoplastic conditions. There is a unique condition, "feline lung-digit syndrome," in which cats may present with a lameness caused by a metastatic lesion from a bronchogenic carcinoma,[9,10] although metastasis to other sites has also been documented.[11] Since most of the cases reported did not have a prior diagnosis of lung cancer, thoracic radiographs should be obtained in cats with digital lesions.

Techniques

In the descriptions below, the terminology used is for amputation of a digit on the foreleg; however, the techniques are applicable to both the front and rear legs.

Surgical preparation of the paw is important and can be time-consuming. Hair is carefully clipped from the carpus distally toward the digits, including the interdigital spaces and between the digital pads. Once clipped, the paw can be prepared using a standard surgical preparation with chlorhexidine or povidone-iodine. Some prefer to soak the paw in an aseptic solution; however, gentle mechanical cleansing to remove dirt and debris is still required. For the final surgical prep, it is common to hang the leg, allowing prep solution to run away from the surgical site. This solution should be blotted up prior to release of the limb. The hanging leg positioning also facilitates application of a sterile wrap over the end of the limb (Figure 19.1).

Establishing a "bloodless" surgical field is useful when doing a digital amputation. Typically, this is accomplished by placing a tourniquet on the limb, and this can be accomplished using a standard tourniquet, a pneumatic cuff, or a sterile Penrose drain placed proximal to the surgical site.

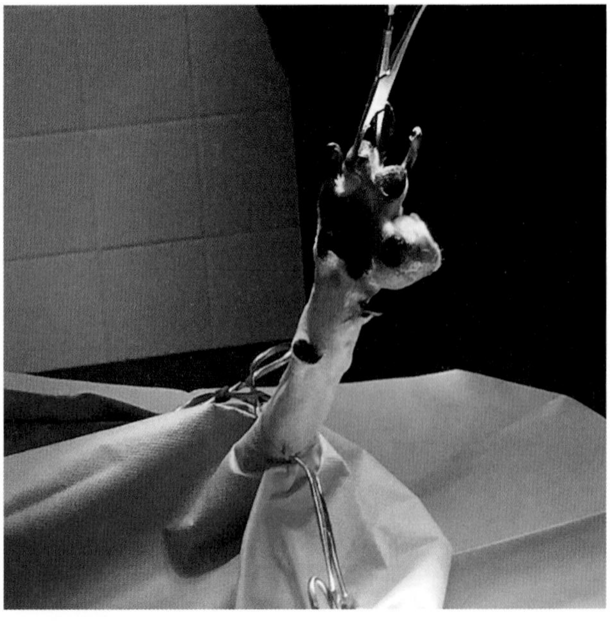

Figure 19.1 After clipping and an initial preparation, the patient is moved to the operating room. A "hanging leg" prep was used and the field draped. Once the drapes are in place, a tourniquet or an Esmarch bandage can be placed before releasing the leg.

Application after the leg has been in the hanging leg position for a few minutes will allow gravity to help drain blood from the distal limb. Another useful option is to use a modification of the Esmarch bandage. This type of bandage is both a tourniquet and a method to exsanguinate the distal limb. While a true Esmarch bandage is based on a latex wrap, an elastic bandage material, such as sterile Vetrap™ (3M™ Animal Care Products, St. Paul, Minnesota), can be used. When applying the Esmarch, start at the toes, firmly wrap the bandage material around the leg from distal to proximal, forcing blood out of the distal limb. When the wrap is completed, it should extend 2–4 in. beyond the top of the planned incision. The surgeon can now incise through the bandage material, removing the distal portion for access while the proximal portion maintains tourniquet-like pressure, minimizing blood in the surgical field. As when using a tourniquet, the surgeon needs to be mindful of how long the Esmarch bandage has been in place, and they must ensure the entire bandage is removed after the procedure and not incorporated into the postoperative bandage.

Tourniquet use should be monitored closely and kept in place for the least amount of time possible, which may be facilitated by the circulating nurse or anesthesia personnel charting the time of application and removal. Most sources suggest that application times of less than 60 minutes will result in minimal issue; however, earlier release might be better. Many animals have increased postoperative swelling after tourniquet use, so it is recommended to support the paw with a supportive, compression bandage (modified Robert Jones) and avoid casts and rigid splints for 24–48 hours after surgery.[1]

Regional anesthesia is appropriate for a digital amputation. A ring block with an injectable local anesthetic, such as lidocaine or bupivacaine, is a simple technique for adjunctive anesthesia and can be placed at the level of metacarpal/metatarsal bones or immediately above the target digit. Regional limb infusion can also be used for more extensive anesthesia. Details of these techniques are available elsewhere.[3,12]

Complete Digital Amputation (P1–P3) (i.e., Metacarpo- or Metatarsophalangeal Joint Amputation)

Before the initial skin incision is made, the desired joint space for the amputation is determined. A 25-gauge hypodermic needle can be used to locate the joint space at the proximal aspect of the amputation. The needle is walked along the dorsal surface of the digit until it drops into the desired joint space. The space can be marked with a sterile marking pen, or the needle can be left in the joint space during creation of the initial incision. The skin incision can be made with a blade, electrosurgical device, a CO_2 laser, or a combination of these methods. The mechanism of incision is up to the surgeon, but the improved hemostasis associated with laser and electrosurgical device incisions may offset the slight increase in time expected for wound-healing.

The classic incision for a complete digital amputation is an "inverted Y" incision (Figure 19.2). For the second and fifth digits, this incision can be made on the lateral aspect of the digit. For digits 3 and 4, the "Y" incision is typically

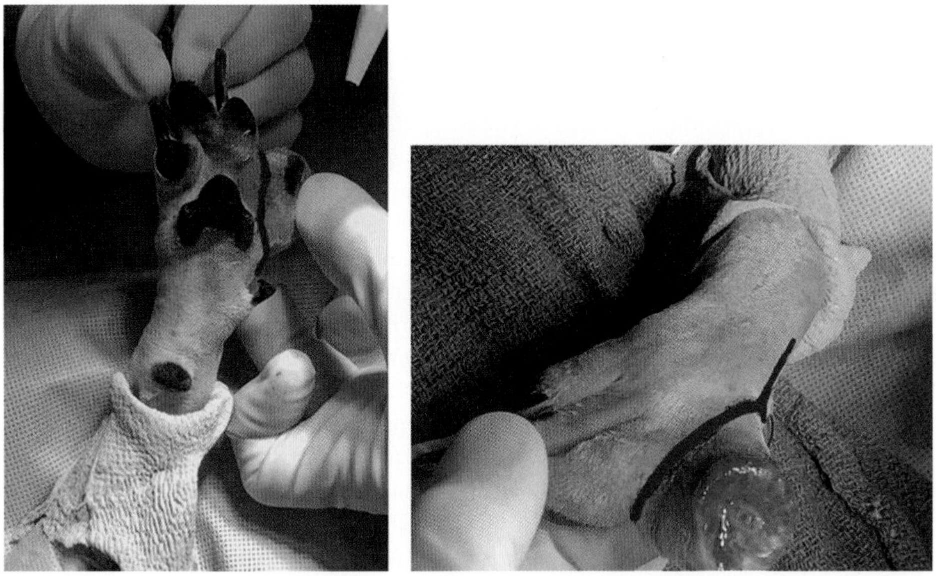

Figure 19.2 After the sterile surgical filed is established, a marking pen can be utilized to clarify surgical boundaries. The lateral digit can use a modified Y incision where the two arms meet distally to create an elliptical or teardrop incision. Note the brown bandage material proximally. It is sterile elastic bandage that was placed as an Esmarch-type bandage. It was opened distally to allow access to the incision site and reflected proximally to act as a tourniquet.

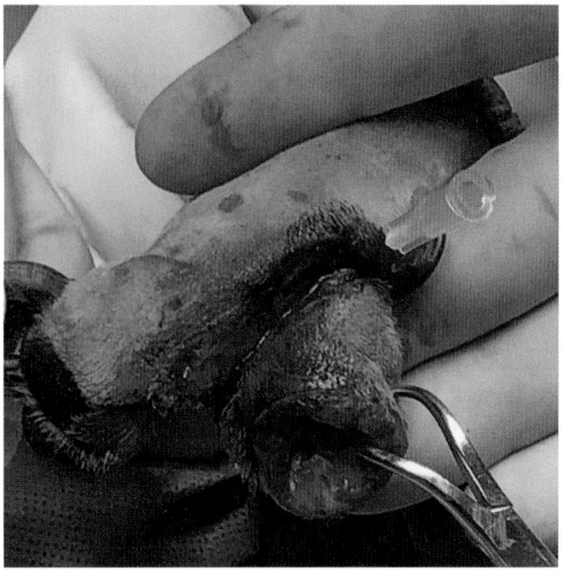

Figure 19.3 The initial incision had been made. Note the effective hemostasis provided by the Esmarch bandage. A hypodermic needle has been used to identify the joint space for the amputation.

created on the dorsal surface of the paw. The base of the V of the "Y" incision is stopped just proximal to the anticipated joint space for the amputation (e.g., the first metacarpophalangeal joint space if amputating digit 1). The branches of the Y are extended distally down the sides, encircling the digit like a teardrop. The skin can be retracted proximally to expose the tendons and vascular structures underneath, and the desired joint space for amputation is again located (Figure 19.3). Using a #11 scalpel blade, the joint space is opened by transecting the overlying tendons and incising the joint capsule. Having a clamp on the toe of the target digit will improve the manipulation of the toe, allowing the surgeon to gently rotate the phalanges during the dissection.

Once the joint space has been transected, any remaining soft tissues are freed from the digit. It is a good idea to carefully examine the wound bed to locate the transected blood vessels. Since a tourniquet is in place, there shouldn't be significant hemorrhage at this point, but failure to occlude these vessels will result in substantial hemorrhage once the tourniquet is released.

For full or partial digital amputations, exposed sesamoid bones are dissected free from the wound before closure. The cartilage covering the distal end of the remaining bone is removed until bleeding bone is exposed. A bone rongeur can easily accomplish this task, although others may prefer to use a bone saw or bone cutter for this task, especially in larger patients. Any jagged edges are smoothed out and after amputation of the second or fifth digit, the distal end of the corresponding metacarpal bone is contoured at an

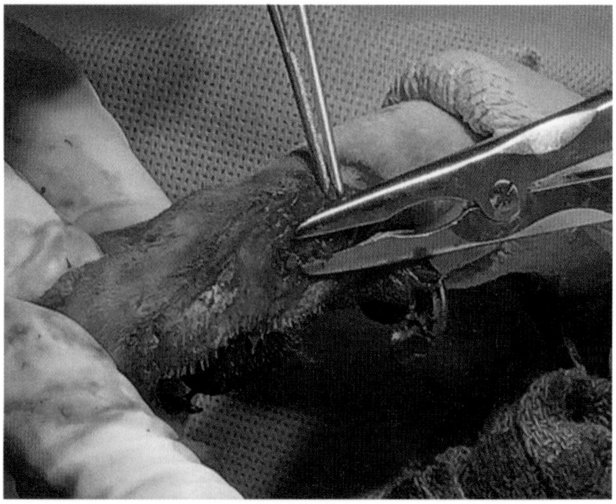

Figure 19.4 After amputation is complete, bone rongeurs are used to remove the cartilage and smooth the edges of the remaining bone.

angle to eliminate protruding edges, which can create pressure points under the skin after amputation (Figure 19.4). Such sculpting will both make incision closure easier and improve the appearance of the amputation site.

Prior to wound closure, the tourniquet is relaxed allowing for reperfusion of the distal limb. This exposes any significant bleeding prior to closure and shortens the duration of tourniquet application. If there is hemorrhage, this is controlled using direct pressure, pinpoint cautery, or vessel ligation for larger blood vessels. In cases of substantial hemorrhage, it might be appropriate to reapply the tourniquet until the hemorrhage can be controlled. Alternatively, the wound closure could be completed before releasing the tourniquet, but this can result in unexpected significant hemorrhage from the incision, necessitating reopening the incision or the need for a pressure bandage after surgery. Experience has shown that the presence of a large hematoma after such an event can be detrimental to trouble-free wound-healing after digital surgery.

While it can be tempting to simply close the amputation incision with a few skin sutures, the addition of some supportive deep sutures helps prevent incisional complications. Prior to suture placement, the wound edges can be trimmed to remove damaged tissues and to conform the surgical wound to an appropriate shape to closure. Any trimming should be judicious to avoid creating additional tension on the final wound closure. For wound closure, two to five deep sutures, using a fine (3–0 → 5–0) monofilament absorbable suture material, are placed to help pull soft tissues over the end of the bone, to counteract tension across the incision and to improve skin apposition. A buried, interrupted suture pattern is used, and the suture tags are cut short. It may be useful to preplace these sutures, as placement will get more

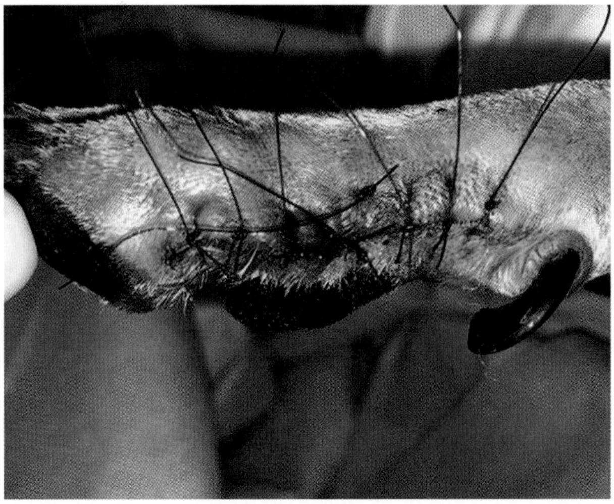

Figure 19.5 Immediate appearance after surgery and prior to bandaging. The incision is apposed with simple interrupted sutures. The Esmarch bandage has been removed, and no hemorrhage is noted through the incision.

challenging as the wound is closed. Final skin apposition is accomplished with appropriately sized (2-0 → 4-0), monofilament non-absorbable sutures in an interrupted pattern (Figure 19.5). In patients where suture removal would be challenging, an absorbable suture can be used in the skin; however, it is not the author's general preference.

First Digit (Dewclaw) Amputation

When considering amputation of a dewclaw in an adult dog, several factors should be considered. First, most dogs have front dewclaws, but dewclaws can be found on both the front and rear legs in many dogs. There are several breeds in which the presence of rear dewclaws is considered to be "standard" for the breed, and these typically include the larger mountain breeds (e.g., Great Pyrenees, Anatolian shepherds). There are other breeds that actually have a double dewclaw (e.g., Icelandic sheepdog, Briard) on the rear. Otherwise, the rear dewclaws are often absent or vestigial in dogs. Second, the attachment of dewclaws vary greatly, with some being as strongly attached to the paws as any other digit and others will have only soft tissue attachments to the underlying paw. Owners also have various degrees of attachment to their pet's dewclaws. While removal is not required, owners do need to be counseled about appropriate nail trimming, as dewclaws can easily overgrow, curling into the pad or surrounding soft tissues.

If a dewclaw is amputated in an adult dog, they typically require less extensive preparation, as the local area can be clipped and prepped without involving the other digits. Furthermore, while using a tourniquet with the procedure is still helpful, it is less essential than with the full-digit amputation.

With the patient positioned laterally, the dewclaw is exposed, prepped, and draped. An elliptical incision works well for dewclaw amputation, taking care not to be too wide at the midpoint, as this will create more tension on the incisional closure. The initial incision is shallow to prevent prematurely incising the dorsal common and axial palmar artery and vein at the proximal aspect of the incision. Dissection at the proximal aspect of the incision will allow identification of these vessels, permitting ligation or cauterization before transection, making the procedure much easier and less bloody. The elliptical incision can then be deepened, and any soft tissue or tendinous attachments transected. Abaxial tension on the dewclaw will assist during the soft tissue dissection. A 25-gauge needle can be used to determine the desired joint space for amputation, which may be either the complete digit or between P1 and P3 (since many dewclaws lack a middle phalanx). The tendons and joint capsule are transected, and the distal phalanges removed. If there is an exposed end to P1, removal of the cartilage and sculpting of the end of the bone are recommended. In patients where the dewclaw has minimal osseous attachment, this step may not be required. While a P3 disarticulation technique would result in the removal of the offending nail from a dewclaw, the continued presence of P1 or P2 underneath the skin can be unsightly, as well as a source of irritation to the patient. Managing any hemorrhage and the subsequent wound closure is as described above.

Distal Phalangeal Amputation

When amputating the distal digit (P3) alone, the digital pad should be retained. After clipping and preparation, the toenail of the offending digit is grasped with a clamp and the joint space located. This can be done with a needle as described above or with the spine of the scalpel blade as it sinks into a noticeable gap between P2 and P3. A #11 blade works well for this, although some surgeons prefer the curved shape of a #12 blade for this type of dissection. The skin overlying P3 can be pushed proximally, and the incision is made on the dorsal aspect over the joint space incising down into the joint.

In the cat, a P3 amputation is more nuanced, as the proximal end of the feline P3 forms a small ledge that slides under the dorsal protrusion of P2. This difference results in a need to gently manipulate P3 around the scalpel blade, working it into the joint space as it transects the collateral ligament of the joint. In the dog, the scalpel blade can be worked into the joint space. A twisting motion of the scalpel will sever several small collateral ligaments between P2 and P3, allowing the joint space to be further exposed. Rotating the clamp on the toenail downward will open the joint angle, making the final dissection of P3 easier.

In both species, care must be taken as the soft tissue dissection continues around the palmar or plantar aspect of P3, since the scalpel blade can travel downward unexpectedly when transecting the deep flexor tendon, which could cut through a significant portion of the digital pad. Finally, after the deep digital flexor tendon is transected, the remaining soft tissue attachments are freed.

Due to the small incision associated with a P3 amputation, wound closure typically only involves the placement of a few skin sutures, although the use of buried subcutaneous sutures, as previously described, may be warranted in larger animals.

Sequelae and Complications

Normal sequelae to a digital amputation include tissue swelling, edema, and postoperative pain. Swelling can be mitigated by gentle tissue-handling during surgery and limiting the duration of tourniquet application. Gentle compression and aggressive tissue cooling after surgery may be beneficial. Pain can be effectively managed with local or regional anesthetics, non-steroidal anti-inflammatory medications, and other analgesics, such as opioids or gabapentin, as required.

Complications after digital amputation include hemorrhage, incision dehiscence, lameness, or surgical site infection (SSI) (Figure 19.6). A review of 33 cases identified a short-term complication rate of almost 40% after digital amputation, exclusive of short-term lameness. Incisional dehiscence was the most common complication, and complications were significantly more likely to occur with rear digit amputations.[13] The same report noted that while 25% of dogs had long-term issues with lameness, outcomes for amputations involving the central, weight-bearing digits (digits 3 and 4) compared favorably to those involving the outer digits (2 and 5).[13] Careful attention to hemostasis during the procedure should limit the potential for hemorrhage and hematoma formation, since this can be a significant complication and contribute to patient discomfort and to potential wound dehiscence and/or SSI. Managing the tension of the surgical closure, providing a supportive bandage in the postoperative period, and reducing the risk of SSI, will help prevent wound dehiscence. Careful management of the surgical site, such as keeping the site free of blood and serum accumulations, minimizing the moist environment with appropriate bandaging, and application of topical antimicrobial medications when appropriate, will minimize the risk of SSI.

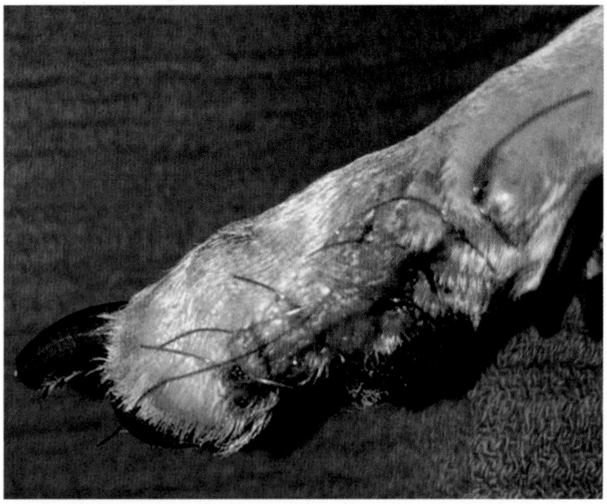

Figure 19.6 Incision appearance five days after amputation. There is slight gapping of the surgical incision, but overall, healing appears to be progressing. The dog is using the foot when not bandaged. Final diagnosis was a soft tissue sarcoma with clean surgical margins.

Postoperative Management

Once surgery is complete, any blood is removed from the surgical field with saline, and the area is completely dried. Use of a light layer of antibiotic ointment along the incision line and covering the surgical site with a non-adherent dressing are at the discretion of the surgeon. Tape stirrups are placed, and the foot is wrapped with an absorbent layer and covered with a protective bandage layer. For most bandages, the distal end of two central toes should be exposed, which will allow owners to check for dangerous swelling with spreading of the two central toes, indicative of the bandage compromising blood flow to the foot.

The use of bandages after a dewclaw or digit amputation must be done with care. Careful attention to the need for hemostasis during the surgical procedure should eliminate the need for a pressure bandage over the surgical site and should decrease the development of hematomas under the bandage. While lightly compression bandages can be applied, pressure bandages should be avoided or limited to a brief period (30–60 minutes) of application, after which a protective bandage is placed. Severe complications, including wound dehiscence, local skin or digital pad sloughing, and even amputation of other digits or the entire limb, have been seen as a result of poorly applied and maintained bandages.

Any bandage over a digital amputation should be changed daily for the first several days until the clinician is comfortable there is routine wound-healing. Once any swelling has resolved and healing appears to normal, the mildly compressive bandage can be changed to a bandage or some other cover, such as a bootie or sock, to provide coverage of the surgical site. Alternatively, the time between bandage changes can be increased. Owners should be instructed to check for swelling of the foot several times a day by inserting a finger into the space between exposed toes or monitoring the orientation of the exposed toenails, which spread apart if there is significant swelling under the bandage. The owners must be reminded to cover the bandage when in moist environments (outside), to remove that protective cover when returned to the indoors, and to have the bandage changed if it becomes wet or excessively soiled or if the pet seems to be excessively irritated by the bandage. Use of an Elizabethan collar is appropriate while the sutures are in place. Typically, suture removal is 10–14 days after surgery.

Activity is limited while the bandage and sutures are in place. Bandages should be covered with a waterproof cover when taken outside, and the covering should be removed when returning inside.

References

1 DeCamp, C.E., Johnston, S.A., Déjardin, L.M., and Schaefer, S.L. (2016). Fractures and other orthopedic conditions of the carpus, metacarpus and phalanges. In: *Brinker, Piermattei and Flo's Handbook of Small Animal Orthopedics and Fracture Repair*, 5e, 430–432. Elsevier.

2 Done, S.H., Goody, P.C., Evans, S.A. et al. (1996). *Color Atlas of Veterinary Anatomy (Dog and Cat)*, vol. 3. Edinburg: Mosby.

3 Kapatkin, A.S., Garcia-Nolen, T., and Hayashi, T. Carpus, metacarpus and digits. In: *In: Veterinary Surgery-Small Animal*, 2e (ed. S.A. Johnson and K.S. Tobias), 936–937. Elsevier.

4 MacPhail, C. and Fossum, T.W. (2018). Surgery of the integumentary system. In: *Small Animal Surgery*, 5e (ed. T.W. Fossum), 255–262. Mosby.

5 Henry, C.J., Brewer, W.G. Jr., Whitley, E.M. et al. (2005). Canine digital tumors: a veterinary cooperative oncology group retrospective study of 64 dogs. *J. Vet. Intern Med.* 19 (5): 720–724. https://doi.org/10.1892/0891-6640(2005)19[720:cdtavc]2.0.co;2.

6 Grassinger, J.M., Floren, A., Müller, T. et al. (2021). Digital lesions in dogs: a statistical breed analysis of 2912 cases. *Vet. Sci.* 8 (7): 136. https://doi.org/10.3390/vetsci8070136.

7 Marconato, L., Murgia, D., Finotello, R. et al. (2021). Clinical features and outcome of 79 dogs with digital squamous cell carcinoma undergoing treatment: a SIONCOV observational study. *Front. Vet. Sci.* 8: 645982. https://doi.org/10.3389/fvets.2021.645982.

8 Marino, D.J., Matthiesen, D.T., Stefanacci, J.D. et al. (1995). Evaluation of dogs with digit masses: 117 cases (1981-1991). *J. Am. Vet. Med. Assoc.* 207: 726–728.

9 Gottfried, S.D., Popovitch, C.A., Goldschmidt, M.H. et al. (2000). Metastatic digital carcinoma in the cat: a retrospective study of 36 cats (1992-1998). *J. Am. Anim. Hosp. Assoc.* 36 (6): 501–509. https://doi.org/10.5326/15473317-36-6-501.

10 van der Linde-Sipman, J.S. and van den Ingh, T.S. (2000). Primary and metastatic carcinomas in the digits of cats. *Vet. Q.* 22 (3): 141–145. https://doi.org/10.1080/01652176.2000.9695043.

11 Thrift, E., Greenwell, C., Turner, A.-L. et al. (2017). Metastatic pulmonary carcinomas in cats ('feline lung–digit syndrome'): further variations on a theme. *J. Feline Med. Surg. Open Rep.* 3 (1): 2055116917691069. https://doi.org/10.1177/2055116917691069.

12 Grubb, T. and Lobprise, H. (2020). Local and regional anaesthesia in dogs and cats: descriptions of specific local and regional techniques (part 2). *Vet. Med. Sci.* 6: 218–234.

13 Kaufman, K.L. and Mann, F.A. (2013). Short- and long-term outcomes after digit amputation in dogs: 33 cases (1999-2011). *J. Am. Vet. Med. Assoc.* 242 (9): 1249–1254. https://doi.org/10.2460/javma.242.9.1249.

20

The Art of the Abdominal Explore

Heidi Hottinger

Gulf Coast Veterinary Specialists, Houston, TX, USA

Key Points

- A proper abdominal explore requires an adequate incision length and good retraction.
- Use a repeatable, systematic approach every time.
- Complete the full exploratory exam before focusing on abnormalities (with a few exceptions).
- Perform a complete exploratory exam every time to help recognize normal vs. abnormal and to prevent missed lesions.

Instruments and Equipment

A proper exploratory laparotomy requires appropriate surgical instruments and equipment. Important instruments and equipment that make an abdominal surgery most efficient include four-pack of sterile Huck towels or sticky drapes for adequate quarter-draping, Backhaus towel clamps (minimum 8), patient and table drape, laparotomy sponges, a variety of hemostats (e.g., mosquito, Kelly, and Rochester-Carmalt), sterile bowl for warm saline lavage, curved Mayo scissors, curved Metzenbaum scissors, needle-holders, suture-cutting scissors, and a variety of thumb forceps (e.g., Brown-Adson or Adson with teeth for closure and DeBakey or Semken forceps for handling delicate tissues). Proper suction tips to remove peritoneal fluid or lavage are also beneficial when working in the abdominal cavity. A Poole suction tip is very helpful in the abdomen and will allow fluid to be removed without suction attachment and trauma to abdominal organs. If a Poole suction tip is not available, a laparotomy sponge can be wrapped around a standard suction tip to dissipate the force of suction present at the tip and prevent tissue trauma. Abdominal retractors are also important for proper visualization and exposure. Balfour retractors are recommended for abdominal wall retraction and can be purchased in a variety of sizes. The clinician may wish to start with a single Balfour retractor, in which case a large size (10″ spread) would be recommended. This size can be used in medium- and large-size dogs. For cats and small dogs, a small or medium Balfour retractor can be used, or a pair of Gelpi retractors with 7″ arms can be placed at either end of the incision. Other types of retractors that may be used if Balfours are not readily available include Weitlaner or Williams retractors.

Proper Abdominal Incision

A proper abdominal explore requires that you fully open the abdomen. This does not mean a slightly extended spay incision, and it does not mean stopping in front of the prepuce; it means the abdomen should be opened from xiphoid to pubis. An adequate cranial extent of the incision is necessary to properly examine the liver and stomach, and it is also crucial to performing surgical procedures on those structures. An adequate caudal extension of the

Techniques in Small Animal Soft Tissue, Orthopedic, and Ophthalmic Surgery, First Edition. Edited by Kristin A. Coleman.

Companion website: www.wiley.com/go/coleman/surgeries

incision is equally important to open the abdominal space enough to work cranially and properly evaluate and work on the urinary bladder and prostate. When doing surgery on the urinary bladder, and especially when needing to evaluate the prostate, the midline incision must extend to the pubis for proper access and visualization.

To create an abdominal incision of the appropriate length, the patient must be properly prepared for surgery. A surgical clip and scrub should begin 1–2 inches cranial to the xiphoid and 1–2 inches past the pubic brim. The lateral patient prep should be lateral to the mammary chains. In male dogs, the prepuce must also be clipped and then lavaged with a dilute iodine solution. If the prepuce is not to be included in the surgical field, it can be clamped to the left side (or the opposite side from where the clinician is standing) with a towel clamp, being sure to engage just the skin of the prepuce and not the penis, so the abdominal incision can be continued to the right (or left) side of the prepuce. Four quarter-draping should be utilized with sterile Huck towels or sticky drapes secured with towel clamps. The quarter drapes should be placed just medial or lateral to the nipples of the mammary chain, proximal to the xiphoid cranially, and to the level of the pubis caudally. A large fluid impervious surgical drape is then placed, which covers the patient and instrument table. A fenestration is then cut in the drape to expose the proposed incision site. If spillage of free abdominal fluid is anticipated, an Ioban™ or similar adhesive drape may be adhered to the ventral abdomen over the exposed skin and patient drape immediately prior to incision. This will help the patient stay dry and may help maintain the patient's temperature. Once the patient is properly prepped, a sponge and instrument count should be completed and recorded. These counts can be included as components of a surgical checklist, which is now utilized by many hospitals. The benefits of surgical checklists have been well documented,[1] and numerous examples of veterinary-specific lists are available online.

When making the incision, the skin should be incised, followed by a direct incision through the subcutaneous tissues to the linea alba (i.e., aponeurosis of the rectus abdominis muscles or external rectus sheath). Do not remove the subcutaneous tissue in search of the linea, as this creates dead space that can lead to seromas and surgical site infections. Judicious undermining can be utilized as needed to ensure that the external rectus sheath is easily visualized for purposes of incision closure. To help identify the midline/linea, approach the umbilicus, which is usually easy to identify (Figure 20.1). Tent the body wall with thumb forceps at the umbilicus and use a #10 or #15 scalpel blade with the sharp blade facing away from the abdomen to make a stab incision at the umbilicus. A #11 blade can also be used but requires more caution and precision to prevent

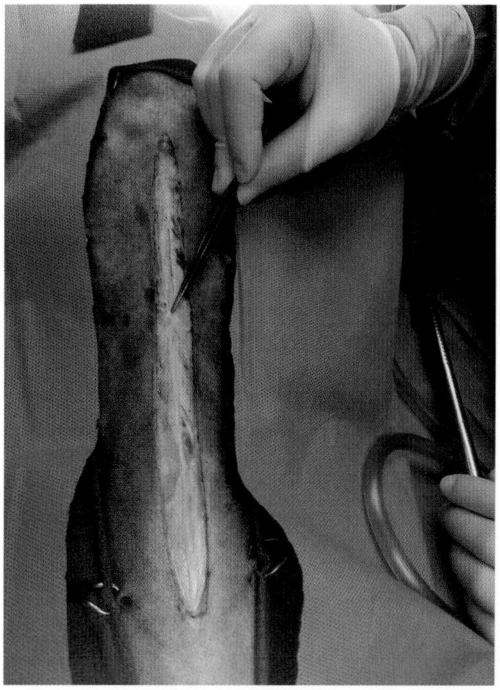

Figure 20.1 Location of the umbilicus to establish midline of the incision. Note that the quarter-draping is just outside of the nipple line. Cranial is to the bottom of the image. *Source:* © Heidi Hottinger.

the sharp tip from impaling organs next to the body wall. Mayo scissors, or the technique of your choosing, can then be used to extend the incision in both directions (Figure 20.2). Prior to extending the incision, be sure to see or feel the internal side of the linea, which may be done easily by sweeping the finger in advance of sharp transection on the linea alba. This "digital sweeping" is performed to avoid damage to abdominal viscera that may be close to, or adherent to, the body wall. The falciform ligament should be removed next. Removal of the falciform ligament allows for better inspection of the viscera, facilitates easier closure of the abdomen, and prevents postoperative steatitis from trauma to the adipose tissue during the procedure. It can be excised with electrosurgery, scissors, or blunt traction with hemostats from its attachments to the midline of the body wall. There will be a blood vessel at the level of the xiphoid process and one or two small blood vessels laterally that may require ligation. The incision should extend to, but not cranial to, the xiphoid process due to the close proximity of the diaphragm and risk of iatrogenic pneumothorax if the diaphragm is punctured. Should the diaphragm be accidentally opened, management is easily accomplished. The clinician should first request manual ventilation of the patient, and then ask for suture material to close the defect. The defect can be closed in a continuous pattern with long-term monofilament absorbable suture, and then free air within the thorax can be removed with a syringe and needle. The

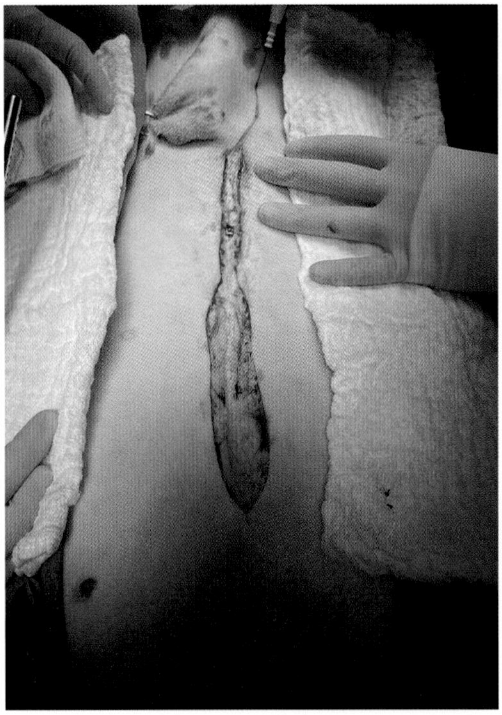

Figure 20.2 An approach to the abdomen for an explore should extend from the xiphoid process to the pubis. In a male dog, a right-handed surgeon standing on the patient's right side will incise to the right of the prepuce, which is clamped to the opposite side of the sterile field. Cranial is to the bottom of the image. *Source:* © Kristin Coleman.

patient can then be gradually weaned from manual ventilation to ensure they are appropriately oxygenating without assistance.

Proper Retraction

Once the abdomen is open, the incision needs to be retracted open to improve visualization and working space. An appropriate abdominal incision without proper retraction (Figure 20.3a) limits visualization significantly. Following proper retraction (Figure 20.3b), the liver and stomach in the cranial abdomen, as well as a large left renal cyst, can now be easily visualized and accessed. Moistened laparotomy sponges should be placed along the exposed subcutaneous tissues prior to placing the abdominal retractors. The laparotomy sponges will help to prevent direct contact of abdominal viscera with exposed skin, and they will also prevent desiccation and contamination of the subcutaneous tissues, both of which can contribute to postoperative incisional infections. Once the laparotomy sponges are in place, abdominal retractors can be placed and expanded (Balfour retractors are advised, but Gelpi, Weitlaner, or Williams retractors placed at either end of the incision can be used in cats and small dogs).

The Systematic Exploratory Laparotomy

Once the abdomen is properly opened and retractors are in place, the abdominal explore can begin. It is very important to develop a systematic approach that is followed every time. This ensures all structures are evaluated without getting distracted by an abnormal finding. Once abnormal findings are noted, it becomes very easy to focus on the abnormality and forget to perform the rest of the exploratory. Resist this temptation and complete the explore before beginning any projects or procedures. There are a few times when you may wish to ignore this guideline, such as when an active source of hemorrhage is present, or a gastric dilatation-volvulus (GDV) needs to be decompressed for the viability of the stomach and to allow room for an adequate explore. Similarly, an extremely large mass may prevent appropriate exploratory surgery until it has been removed. Aside from these exceptions, the full exploratory should be completed, then abnormalities can biopsied or definitively managed.

For a systematic approach, the abdomen can be divided into five regions, with each region evaluated in an orderly fashion. These five regions are the cranial abdomen, the right and left gutters, the caudal abdomen/pelvic region, and the central abdomen.

1) The **cranial abdomen** contains the liver, gall bladder and common bile duct, stomach (dorsal and ventral surfaces), left pancreatic limb, hepatic lymph nodes, and the diaphragm. The liver has six liver lobes: the left lateral, left medial, quadrate, right medial, right lateral, and caudate lobe, which is divided into the caudate process, which cups the right kidney, and the papillary process, which sits in the lesser curvature of the stomach. All lobes should be inspected visually on each surface, noting color, size, texture, and presence of nodules or other abnormalities. The gall bladder sits between the quadrate and right medial liver lobes and should be gently expressed using flattened fingers with slow, steady pressure. The gall bladder empties via the common bile duct into the proximal duodenum through a very small opening at the sphincter of Oddi, so vigorous attempts at expression can result in tearing or crushing of surrounding hepatic parenchyma or even rupture of the gall bladder itself. If expression of the gall bladder is unsuccessful, the common bile duct should be closely inspected for the presence of dilation or pieces of inspissated bile or stones within the lumen that could be causing obstruction. The stomach should be palpated for foreign objects, masses, wall thickness, or visual abnormalities, such as focal inflammation that may indicate an ulcer. The ventral wall of the stomach is readily visible, but to evaluate the dorsal wall of the stomach and

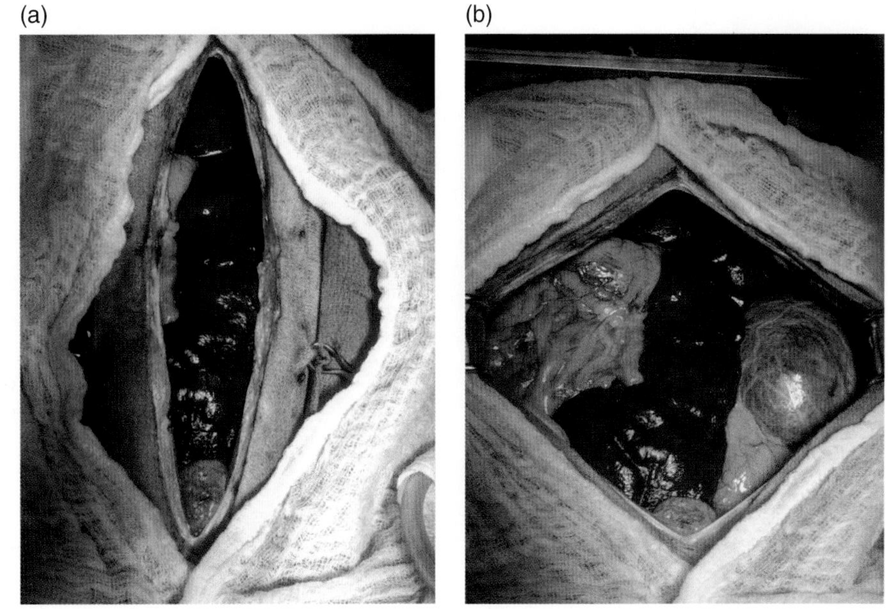

Figure 20.3 (a) Appropriate length abdominal incision prior to placement of retractor. (b) Placement of Balfour retractor allows visualization of organs not well-visualized prior to proper retraction, including liver, stomach, and a large left renal cyst. Cranial is to the top of both images. *Source:* © Heidi Hottinger.

the left limb of the pancreas, the omental bursa must be opened by following the omentum to its furthest extent where vessels are smaller, and tearing an opening in the tissue. (Tip: the omentum is the "belly's band-aid" and does not need to be sutured closed.) Once inside the bursa (Figure 20.4), the dorsal wall of the stomach, left limb of the pancreas, and hepatic lymph nodes can all be evaluated. The hepatic lymph nodes will border the epiploic foramen along the portal vein. These are important lymph nodes to evaluate for possible metastatic disease, especially when masses are present in the liver, spleen, and pancreas. The left limb of the pancreas runs parallel to the greater curvature of the stomach in the dorsal leaf of the omentum and should be visually inspected for nodules, masses, and fibrosis. Very gentle palpation of the pancreas is acceptable and will help to identify small, firm nodules and fibrosis. The diaphragm should also be evaluated in the cranial abdomen. It is best visualized by gently retracting the liver lobes caudally, and then inspecting for inflammatory fibrin debris, or nodules (which could indicate carcinomatosis from an abdominal tumor) on the surface of the diaphragm. Fluid within the chest cavity can usually be seen through the diaphragm's central tendon as well.

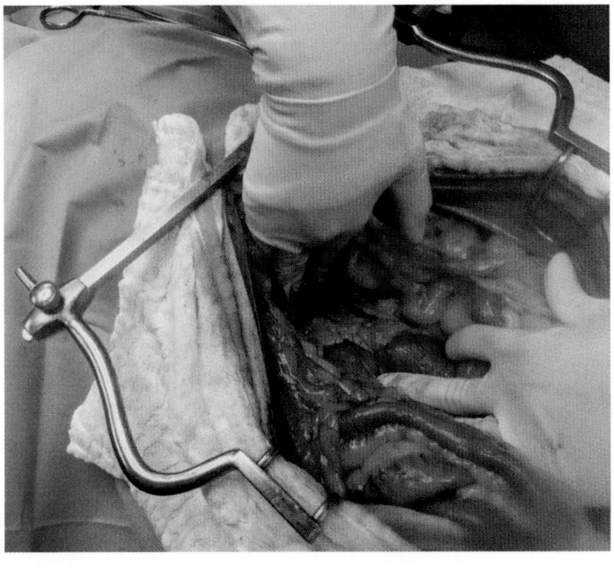

Figure 20.4 Omental bursa. Cranial is to the left of the image. *Source:* © Heidi Hottinger.

2) The **left gutter** contains the spleen, left adrenal gland, left kidney and ureter, ovary and uterine horn in an unspayed female, or ovarian pedicle remnant in a spayed female. The spleen should be lifted from the abdomen and evaluated along its entire length on both the parietal and visceral surfaces, and hilar vessels should be palpated for pulses. Proper orientation of the spleen should also be noted, with the head of the spleen in the left craniodorsal quadrant more closely tethered to the greater curvature of the stomach by the short gastric vessels, and the tail of the spleen being more freely movable and typically located ventrally across the center of the abdominal contents. This orientation is important to become familiar with in order for splenic torsions to be recognized. The spleen can then be set to the side, even outside of the abdomen, to allow for better visualization of the remaining left gutter structures. The descending colon is the natural internal retractor for viewing these structures (Figures 20.5 and 20.6). The colon can be differentiated from the jejunum by its slightly larger size, linear striations that allow for distention, and often a slight green or gray color to the

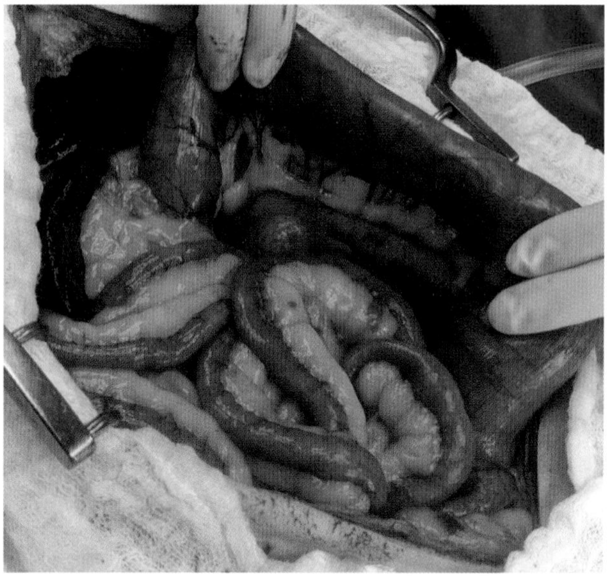

Figure 20.5 Colon and mesocolon as internal retractors for the left gutter. Cranial is to the top left of the image. *Source:* © Heidi Hottinger.

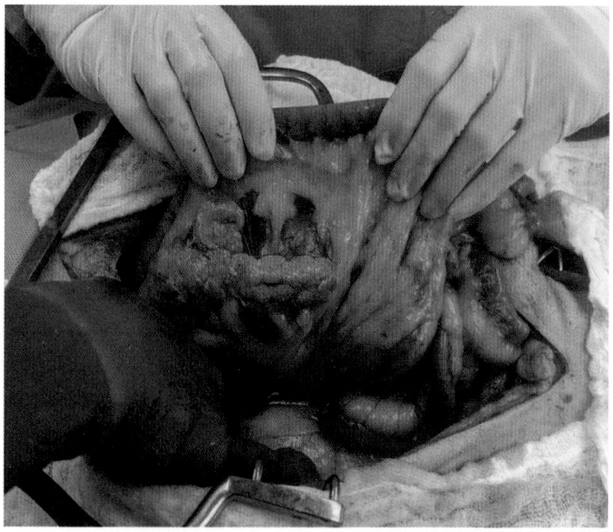

Figure 20.7 Duodenum and mesoduodenum as internal retractors for the right gutter. Note the left limb of the pancreas parallel to the duodenum. Cranial is to the left of the image. *Source:* © Heidi Hottinger.

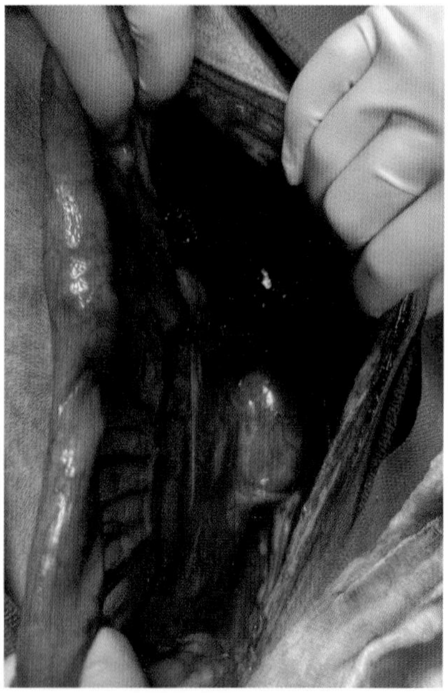

Figure 20.6 The left gutter contents are investigated with medial retraction of the descending colon. Cranial is at the top of the image. *Source:* © Kristin Coleman.

tissue (Figure 20.5). The colon and mesocolon can be evaluated at this time, as well as colonic lymph nodes that reside along the colonic vessels in the mesocolon. The colon and mesocolon can be used to retract the intestinal viscera medially and allow for evaluation of the left adrenal gland, which sits cranial to the kidney near the caudal vena cava, the left kidney and ureter, and the ovary and uterus. If the patient was previously spayed, an omental adhesion to the location of the ovarian pedicle may prevent proper visualization of the area and can be ligated with cautery or suture if needed.

3) The **right gutter** contains the same structures as the left, except for the spleen. The natural retractor on the right is the duodenum, which can be recognized by the closely associated right limb of the pancreas. Evaluation of the right gutter is also a perfect time to evaluate the duodenum and right pancreatic limb on the mesenteric aspect. The portal vein can also be seen running in the mesoduodenum. Using the duodenum and mesoduodenum to retract the intestinal viscera medially (Figures 20.7 and 20.8), the adrenal gland on the right side is found on the dorsal surface of the vena cava and often requires visualization and palpation through the wall of the cava (Figure 20.9). The right kidney sits further cranial than the left and is usually less mobile. There may again be an omental adhesion to the ovarian pedicle location in spayed females, which can be released by ligation as needed (Figure 20.8).
4) The **caudal abdomen/pelvic region** contains the urinary bladder and sublumbar lymph nodes. The sublumbar lymph nodes can be palpated along either side of the terminal aorta if they are enlarged but are not typically visible or even palpable in a normal state (Figure 20.10). The prostate should be palpated in males (Figure 20.11), and the uterine body, which will sit dorsal to the bladder, should be evaluated in females. The bladder has three ligaments that support it, which should also be examined so that familiarity develops. The ventral ligament is a reflection of the peritoneum and can be transected to allow better access to the bladder and identification of the ventral aspect if needed. The left and

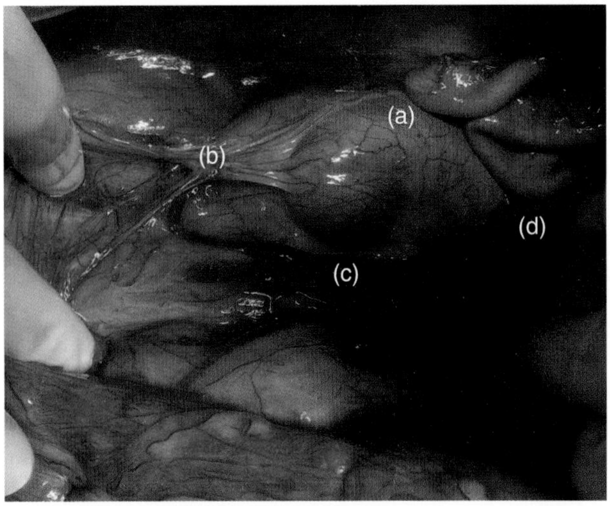

Figure 20.8 Contents of the right gutter with medial retraction of the descending duodenum. Cranial is to the right of the image. (a) Right kidney. (b) Scar from right ovariectomy. (c) Caudal vena cava. (d) Caudate process of caudate liver lobe. *Source:* © Kristin Coleman.

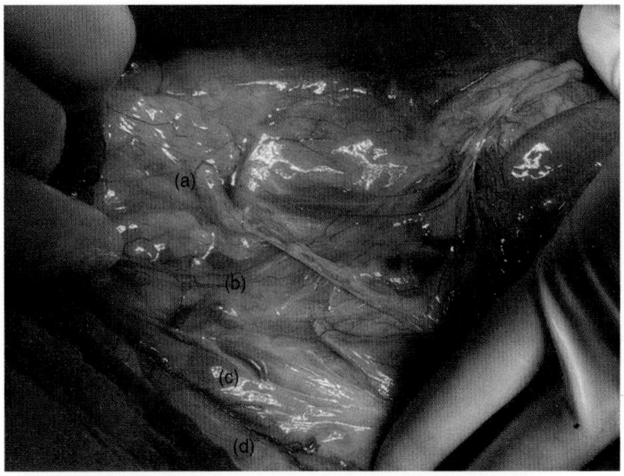

Figure 20.10 Examining the caudal abdominal contents on the dorsal aspect, caudal is to the left of the image and cranial is to the right of the image. (a) If any of the sublumbar lymph nodes are enlarged, they should be palpable in this region where the aorta bifurcates. (b) Ureter. (c) Colonic lymph node. (d) Descending colon. *Source:* © Kristin Coleman.

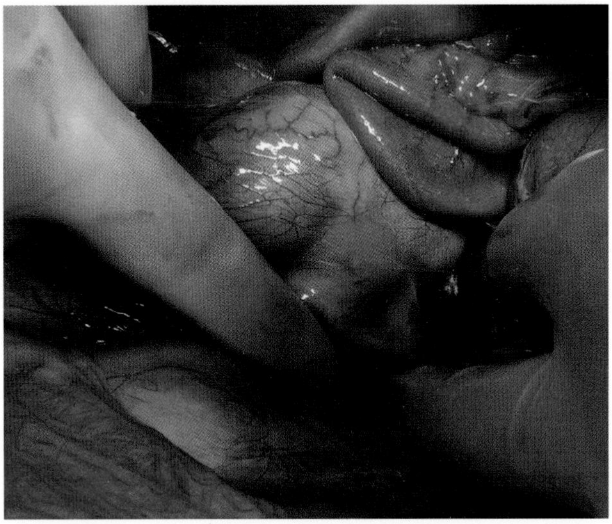

Figure 20.9 The right adrenal gland is often not visible during an abdominal exploratory and is instead palpated dorsal to the caudal vena cava. Cranial is to the right of the image. *Source:* © Kristin Coleman.

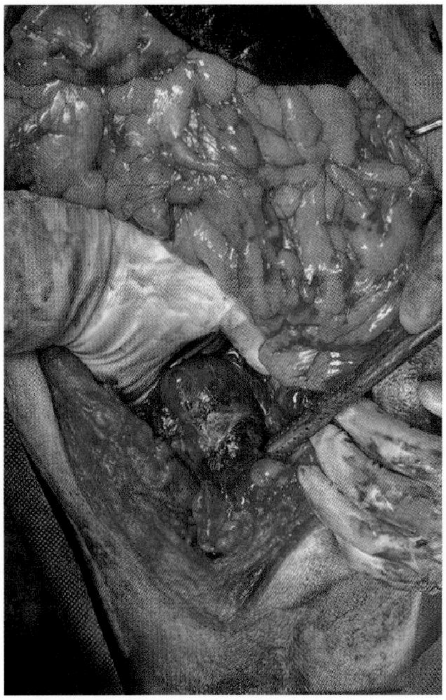

Figure 20.11 An incidental finding of an enlarged, friable, hemorrhagic prostate in an 8-year-old castrated male Boxer; cranial is at the top of the image and caudal is at the bottom of the image. If any abnormalities are discovered during the abdominal explore, they should be documented and potentially sampled. This prostate was biopsied and diagnosed as hemangiosarcoma. *Source:* © Kristin Coleman.

right lateral ligaments should NOT be cut, as they contain the ureters, hypogastric nerves, and primary vascular supply to the bladder. Spayed females may again have an omental adhesion to the uterine stump, which can be broken down bluntly or ligated with cautery or suture.

5) The **central abdomen** contains the omentum, intestines, and mesenteric lymph nodes. The omentum should have been lifted away from the intestines and shifted cranially when the omental bursa was entered. An understanding of the normal anatomical location of each section of the intestines and how each section relates to one another is important for proper evaluation and for ensuring proper replacement at the completion of the exploratory. At the point of the pylorus, the descending duodenum begins at the cranial duodenal flexure and travels down the right side of the abdomen, crosses the caudal abdomen as the caudal

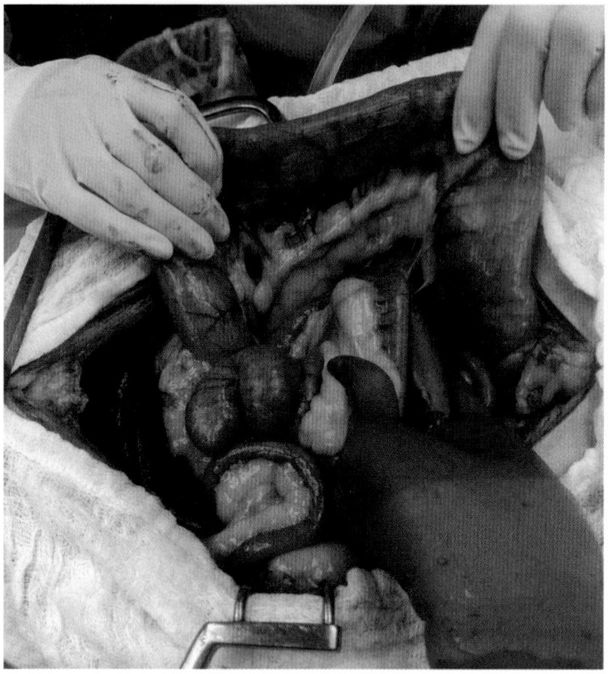

Figure 20.12 Caudal duodenal flexure attached to the mesocolon via the duodenocolic ligament. Cranial is to the left of the image. *Source:* © Heidi Hottinger.

duodenal flexure, and attaches to the mesocolon on the left via the duodenocolic ligament. The combined structure of the duodenum/mesoduodenum and the colon/mesocolon creates a chalice or cup effect that holds the remaining small intestines. The small intestines should be evaluated along their entire length, being sure to start at one end and progress to the other. The clinician can start at the caudal duodenal flexure on the left, where it is attached to the mesocolon (Figure 20.12) and then progress to the ileum and cecum or vice versa, but always start on one end and progress to the other; not in the middle. When "running the bowel" (i.e., evaluating all small intestines), execute Halstead's principle of *gentle tissue-handling*, which may involve using the sides of your fingers and not the fingertips when palpating. The mesenteric lymph nodes sit at the root of the mesentery and should be palpated. Keep in mind that the mesenteric lymph nodes can be carefully biopsied with a wedge incision, but they CANNOT be safely removed if they are enlarged. Removal of the mesenteric lymph nodes can result in irreparable damage to the mesenteric vessels, which will result in death of the small intestines: a condition incompatible with life. Once the intestines have been evaluated along their entire length for masses, foreign objects, wall thickness, etc., they should be returned to their proper location in the "chalice" and the omentum draped back over them.

Proper Abdominal Closure

Prior to closing the abdomen, sponge and instrument counts should be performed to ensure there are no retained surgical items. The sponge and instrument counts should be recorded and included in the surgical checklist. A retained gauze item results in the formation of a gossypiboma that can become debilitating or even life-threatening (Figure 20.13) and requires additional surgery for the patient.

Proper closure of the long abdominal incision created for an appropriate exploratory can seem a bit daunting. However, closure of such a long incision can be rapid and secure by using a simple continuous suture pattern, although a simple interrupted closure pattern is certainly appropriate as well. Simple continuous abdominal wall closure can be very strong when performed properly, is much faster than an interrupted closure, and places less foreign material and knots in the incision.[2–4] To ensure a strong closure, the external rectus sheath must be engaged with every suture bite. This is especially important in male dogs, where the preputial ligament can be confused with the linea alba.

The continuous suture line is dependent on secure knots at both ends of the closure. Therefore, techniques to stress-protect the knots and to ensure secure knots are very important. The first recommended technique is to start and end the suture line off the incision. Starting before and ending after the incision allows the knots to be placed in a very low tension, stress-protected position. Care should be taken to avoid ending and starting a continuous closure line in the middle of an incision, as this will place knots in the highest tension location of the incision. An additional technique to stress-protect the knot is to start with a cruciate mattress pattern stitch before tying the knot. The cruciate mattress pattern has an inherent holding capability of its own (note tissue drag when pulling the suture through), which adds a small amount of protection to the knot. When tying the knot at either end of a simple continuous line, at least five to six throws should be used on each knot, and each throw should be snugged securely.[5] Suture bites should be 4–6 mm apart and should engage 4–6 mm of tissue on each side of the body wall. If the incision is on midline, suture bites should engage full thickness body wall, which will include the external rectus sheath, internal rectus sheath, and peritoneal lining as they converge to create the linea alba. For paramedian incisions, the suture bites should only include the external rectus sheath, not the underlying muscle or peritoneum (Figure 20.14). Muscle becomes inflamed and painful when strangulated in suture, and the peritoneum has no substantial holding strength to add to the incision and does not need to be apposed for proper healing.

Suture selection is typically recommended to be a monofilament, long-term absorbable material that retains

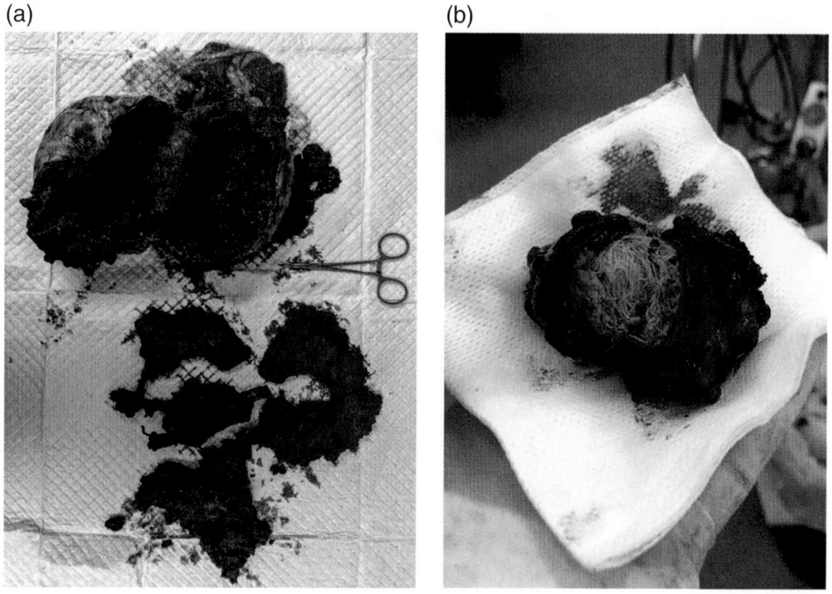

Figure 20.13 Gossypibomas.
(a) *Source:* © Heidi Hottinger; (b) *Source:* Kristin Coleman.

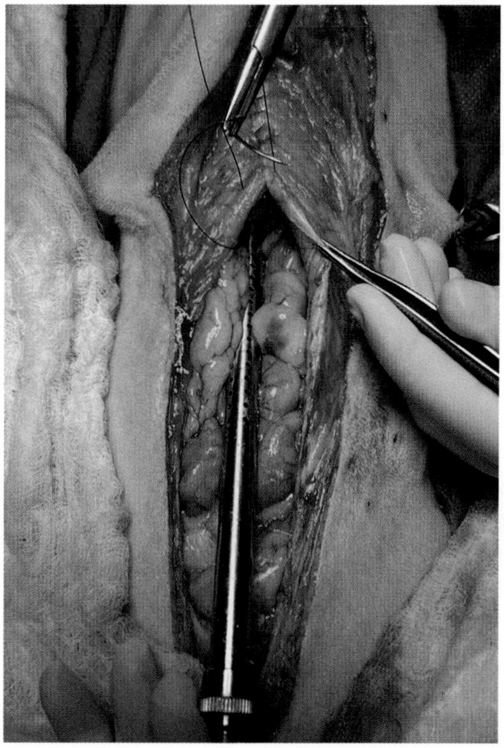

Figure 20.14 When closing the body wall (holding layer: external rectus sheath), be careful to not grab any of the abdominal contents with each pass of the needle. The risk of this can be mitigated by putting an object, such as the Poole suction tip, just beneath the body wall to push away the abdominal contents. Cranial is to the bottom of the image. *Source:* © Kristin Coleman.

approximately 50% of its tensile strength at four weeks. Non-absorbable and braided materials can be associated with a higher rate of incisional infections or suture sinus draining tracts,[6] but they can still be used successfully if used carefully. Suture size will typically be 0-gauge for large dogs, 2-0 for medium dogs, and 3-0 for cats and small dogs. Once the linea is closed, there are a few tips for closing the remaining incision that can be useful as well. In male dogs, the preputial muscle fibers and ligament should be apposed to close dead space and allow proper alignment of the prepuce, preventing urine-soiling of the front legs postoperatively. Closure of the subcutaneous fatty tissue is surgeon preference. Some surgeons prefer not to close this layer and move directly to the intradermal closure, while others prefer to close this layer to help minimize tissue dead space. The subcutaneous tissue does not provide substantial holding strength to the incision, so small gauge suture is recommended to limit inflammation and foreign material within the incision. The skin can be closed in a simple interrupted or continuous pattern, using monofilament absorbable or non-absorbable suture, or skin staples can be used.

Documentation

The importance of a surgical checklist was previously discussed and should be part of the documentation in the patient record. A surgical report should be created immediately following surgery so details are not forgotten. A complete surgical report should include all abnormal findings and measurements of any masses noted (Figure 20.15), as well as notation of structures that were within normal limits, as this verifies all structures were evaluated. If a mass or abnormality is sampled (e.g., biopsy, aspirate, culture), this should be recorded. Similarly, structures not able to be evaluated should also be noted. All procedures performed should also be included in the report, as well as suture types and sizes for ligations and closure.

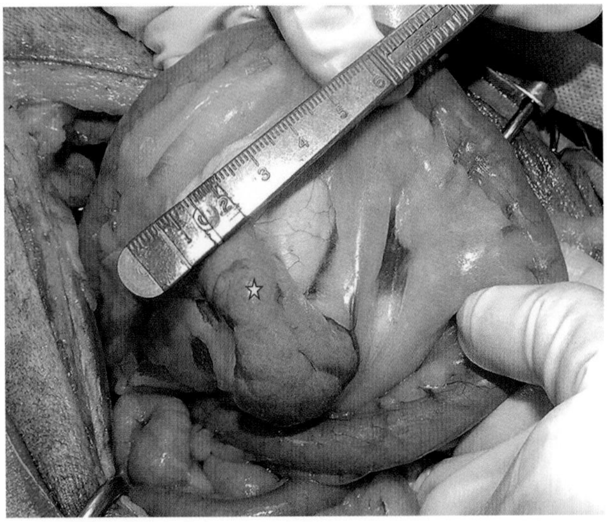

Figure 20.15 Mass within the left limb of pancreas (denoted by a yellow star) of a middle-aged dog. A thorough systematic investigation of all abdominal contents is key to recognizing abnormalities, and measurement of any masses before aspiration or removal could aid in prognostication of certain neoplasias. *Source:* © Kristin Coleman.

Conclusion

A proper abdominal exploratory requires recognition of normal to be able to identify abnormal, and documentation is key to recording all findings in the abdomen of a patient and to remembering to check all aspects of the peritoneal cavity. The only way to recognize normal is to do a thorough exploratory surgery every time and to carefully look at and palpate every structure in every patient. Doing quick exploratory surgeries and taking shortcuts will not allow for development of the experience required to recognize subtle changes or the judgment to know whether changes are significant. With experience, a complete and thorough abdominal exploratory can be performed in less than five minutes. Every laparotomy procedure offers the opportunity to observe normal structure, color, consistency, and position of structures to help gain the experience required for a confident and thorough exploratory. Using a consistent technique in every patient will also help to prevent missing a second foreign body, an incidental tumor, or a metastatic lesion.

References

1. Boston, S. (2015). The use of surgical checklists in veterinary surgery. WSAVA 2015 Congress – VIN.
2. Kummeling, A. and van Sluijs, F.J. (1998). Closure of the rectus sheath with a continuous looped suture and the skin with staples in dogs: speed, safety, and costs compared to closure of the rectus sheath with interrupted sutures and the skin with a continuous subdermal suture. *Vet. Q.* 20 (4): 126–130.
3. Crowe, D.T. (1978). Closure of abdominal incisions using a continuous polypropylene suture: clinical experience in 550 dogs and cats. *Vet. Surg.* 7 (3): 74–77.
4. Bula, E., Upchurch, D.A., Wang, Y. et al. (2018). Comparison of tensile strength and time to closure between an intermittent Aberdeen suture pattern and conventional methods of closure for the body wall of dogs. *Am. J. Vet. Res.* 79 (1): 115–123.
5. Marturello, D.M., McFadden, M.S., Bennett, R.A. et al. (2014). Knot security and tensile strength of suture materials. *Vet. Surg.* 43 (1): 73–79.
6. Markel, D.C., Bergum, C., Wu, B. et al. (2019). Does suture type influence bacterial retention and biofilm formation after irrigation in a mouse model? *Clin. Orthop. Relat. Res.* 477 (1): 116–126.

21

Gastropexy

Kristin A. Coleman

Gulf Coast Veterinary Specialists, Houston, TX, USA

Key Points

- Gastropexy is an essential surgery to learn for both emergent intervention with a gastric dilatation-volvulus (GDV) and prophylactically when in the abdominal cavity for other procedures in at-risk breeds of dogs.
- If not performing pediatric spays and neuters (under six to eight months of age), a gastropexy may ideally be done concurrently at the time of sterilization in at-risk breeds of dogs.
- The length, location, and orientation of gastropexy all contribute to a successful surgery with a low risk of side effects.
- There are many ways to perform a right-sided gastropexy for the treatment or prevention of GDV; it is advised to choose one method with which to become comfortable to ensure consistent outcomes.

Introduction

A gastropexy is the creation of a permanent adhesion between the stomach and the peritoneal wall, and it may be performed as a right-sided or left-sided procedure. A right-sided gastropexy is primarily performed to prevent either the life-threatening occurrence or recurrence of a gastric dilatation-volvulus (GDV). A left-sided gastropexy is most commonly performed as part of the treatment for hiatal hernias. The focus of this chapter will be on the right-sided gastropexy in dogs.

Gastric volvulus was first described in humans by Berti in 1866 and in dogs by Funkquist and Garmer in 1967,[1] who referred to the disorder as "gastric torsion." It is defined as a rotation (commonly, in a clockwise direction) of all, or part, of the stomach either along the longitudinal or transverse axis that prevents evacuation of the luminal gastric contents into the esophagus or small intestines.[1–11] Technically, a torsion is twisting of bowel on its longitudinal axis and volvulus is rotation of bowel on its mesenteric axis, so gastric dilatation and *volvulus* is the correct phrasing. To facilitate emptying of the stomach after a GDV, pyloroplastic surgery was first attempted as a means to prevent recurrence,[12] but this was unsuccessful to treat this deadly "disease of domestication."[13]

Gastropexy following gastric repositioning after GDV was first described in 1979 as a way of successfully preventing recurrence of GDV, which is known to have a recurrence rate of up to 86% if the volvulus simply resolves after the first episode or is manually repositioned into normal anatomic location. One of the first successful gastropexy techniques was described by suturing the fundus to the diaphragm using silk suture (fundupexy) as a "relapse-preventing procedure of gastric torsion" by Funkquist et al.[14,15] This was a staged procedure performed approximately five days after the onset and surgical de-torsion of the stomach. The gastropexy procedure has continued to evolve and improve with many technical variations over the years, including performing the surgery on a prophylactic basis in at-risk breeds of dogs. With every passing year, there are more gastropexy techniques from which to choose to give more options to surgeons while attempting to improve efficiency and reduce potential complications associated with the surgery.

With the gastropexy being a life-saving surgery that every surgeon and general practitioner should know how to

Techniques in Small Animal Soft Tissue, Orthopedic, and Ophthalmic Surgery, First Edition. Edited by Kristin A. Coleman.

Companion website: www.wiley.com/go/coleman/surgeries

perform in order to both treat and prevent a GDV,[16,17] several variations have been described and continue to be altered as new ideas arise for making a gastropexy less invasive and/or more efficient than the original procedure. Every veterinarian performing gastropexy should be comfortable with one type of right-sided gastropexy, and it is not necessary to know how to do all of the varieties. Knowing one technique to grow comfortable with over time and with practice will allow an anatomically correct gastropexy to be done, which reduces both the risk of GDV and the iatrogenic complication of a partial pyloric outflow obstruction.[18] Some of the open gastropexy techniques that are recommended and proven to be successful at preventing a GDV include incisional,[19,20] belt-loop,[21] circumcostal,[22–25] and tube gastropexy.[26,27] Minimally invasive gastropexy techniques include grid,[28] laparoscopic-assisted,[29–31] total laparoscopic,[32–41] and endoscopic-assisted.[42,43]

Incisional Gastropexy

One of the earliest described and still one of the most commonly performed gastropexy techniques is the incisional gastropexy, which was described by MacCoy et al. in 1982.[19] This procedure was performed by suturing the serosamuscular layers of the stomach wall to the internal intercostal musculature between the 11th and 12th ribs on the right side and approximately 1/3 of the distance from ventral midline to the dorsal aspect of the patient, which presumably allows the stomach to be in an anatomically normal position. To promote avoidance of the diaphragm and possible iatrogenic pneumothorax, an *ideal position* for the body wall incision is now caudal to the last rib with suturing of the transversus abdominis, as opposed to the intercostal musculature. The recurrence rate of GDV after gastropexy varies greatly, and, in most of the literature, an incisional gastropexy has a 0–5% recurrence rate.

Due to the relative ease, rapidity, effectiveness, and low recurrence rate associated with the incisional gastropexy, this is the technique that is recommended and is described below. As with all gastropexies, ~4 cm incisions in both the right abdominal wall and seromuscular layer of the pyloric antrum are recommended, both because of approximately 47% contraction of the incision with healing and remodeling over time[44,45] and because of a 4 cm incision having a higher load to failure compared to a 2 cm incision in a cadaveric study.[46] There have been many varieties of incisional gastropexy described using several materials for apposition, including suture (both barbed[47,48] and smooth), staples,[49,50] and others, in addition to using one or two suture lines. Although one suture line was recently shown in a cadaveric biomechanical study to have a similar load to failure as two suture lines for incisional gastropexy,[46] the traditional use of two suture lines will be described in this chapter.

This technique may be performed either solo[51] or with the help of an assistant, and since some veterinarians are alone when performing this surgery on an emergency basis, both techniques will be described in detail.

Belt-Loop Gastropexy

A belt-loop gastropexy is a technique described by Whitney et al. in 1989[21] and is a method that involves a U-shaped flap from the seromuscular layer of the pyloric antrum (incorporating a branch from the right gastroepiploic artery and vein at the base) that is passed through a muscular tunnel (under a segment of transversus abdominis muscle on the right lateral body wall caudal to the last rib) then sutured back to the pyloric antrum. Although slightly stronger than an incisional gastropexy adhesion, which are both believed to be supraphysiologic in their strength, this technique is more time-consuming and more difficult for a novice surgeon to perform.[52] A modified belt-loop gastropexy utilizing an antral fold instead of an antral flap was recently described,[53] which, based on the results of the study, prevents recurrence of GDV in dogs.

Circumcostal Gastropexy

A circumcostal gastropexy, which is technically the strongest of the gastropexy options, is a technique described by Fallah et al. in 1982.[22] This technique involves the creation of a flap from the seromuscular layer of the pyloric antrum that is passed around a rib through a tunnel under the 11th or 12th ribs at the level of the costochondral junction and then sutured back to the pyloric antrum. Potential complications include pneumothorax, rib fracture, and a 3.3–9% recurrence rate of GDV.[24,54–58]

Laparoscopic-Assisted and Total Laparoscopic Gastropexy

The first laparoscopic-assisted gastropexy was described by Rawlings et al. in 2001,[29] and this development, along with the increasing interest in and availability of laparoscopy, led to total laparoscopic gastropexy techniques. These minimally invasive procedures allow for a faster return to normal activity, have smaller incisions, and result in decreased post-operative pain; however, compared to the incisional gastropexy, these require advanced minimally invasive surgery (MIS) training and expensive laparoscopic equipment. Description of each type of laparoscopic gastropexy is beyond the scope of this chapter, and for those who prefer minimally invasive options for this procedure, particularly for prophylactic purposes, other textbooks are available.

Those gastropexy techniques that are described, but are not recommended, by the author include incorporating, gastrocolopexy, and fundic.

Incorporating Gastropexy

An incorporating, or ventral midline, gastropexy is a technique described by Meyer-Lindenberg et al. in 1993,[59] in which the pyloric antrum is incorporated into the cranial aspect of the linea alba closure when suturing the abdominal wall to close at the end of a celiotomy.[59,60] The seromuscular layer of the ventral pyloric antrum is incorporated into the cranial linea alba for approximately 5 cm using a continuous suture pattern of absorbable suture material without incision into the gastric wall. Proponents of this technique claim that it is a simple and fast way to reduce the risk of a GDV by saving time with suturing, but the critics have concerns regarding gastric penetration that may occur upon peritoneal cavity entry during subsequent midline celiotomies,[8,45,59] in addition to gastric malpositioning.[18] In a recent retrospective study looking at over 200 dogs undergoing an incorporating gastropexy, a unique complication with this technique is diffuse bleeding into the subcutaneous tissues or the possible need to re-perform the gastropexy if the surgeon accidentally incises the site of gastric adherence to the cranial linea alba.[60]

To avoid this potential complication, the authors of the study suggested not incising the linea alba along the cranial aspect during subsequent celiotomies unless the surgeon specifically needs access to the diaphragm, stomach, or liver. In the author's opinion, this is not an appropriate recommendation, since thorough abdominal exploratory surgeries should aim to evaluate every aspect of the peritoneal cavity, which includes palpating and visualizing all lobes of the liver, gallbladder, and biliary tree (see Chapter 20 for more details). With many other gastropexy techniques available that are also quick to perform once proficient, this technique is not recommended.

Gastrocolopexy

Gastrocolopexy is a technique described by Christie and Smith in 1976[61] that involves serosal scarification followed by suturing of the seromuscular layers of the gastric greater curvature to the transverse colon. Unlike some of the other gastropexies, a gastrocolopexy had an increased risk of recurrence with time (9% after 365 days compared to 20% after 457 and 530 days).[55] With this in mind and other techniques associated with lower recurrence rates, this technique is also not recommended.

Indications/Pre-op Considerations

There are several studies describing risk factors for a dog, such as breed, age, gender, temperament, dietary aspects (e.g., only fed once daily with a large amount of food, eating from a raised bowl, rapidly eating), concurrent disease, and management, that predispose certain dogs to developing a GDV.[62–70] These factors should be known in order to guide veterinarians into recommending prophylactic gastropexy for the at-risk individuals, which may be easiest to perform at the time of sterilization or any other surgery requiring entry into the abdominal cavity.

A higher risk of developing GDV, compared to the general canine population, is associated with a large chest depth-to-width ratio, increasing age, having a first-degree relative with a history of GDV, gastrointestinal disease, and being an at-risk breed.[62–66,69,70] Stressful events may predispose dogs to GDV, as well as an anxious disposition. The lifetime risk of developing GDV in large and giant breeds of dogs is 6%, and the Great Dane has a 42% risk of developing GDV in the course of its life, which highlights the importance of prophylactic gastropexies in most large and giant breeds of dogs.[63,64,68]

Splenectomy – To Pexy or Not to Pexy?

Splenectomy may or may not predispose a dog to developing GDV,[71–75] but the general recommendation is to perform a gastropexy when in the abdominal cavity of patients with risk factors, such as breed, conformation, temperament, or a history of gastrointestinal disease; a gastropexy is a quick additional procedure to perform if already in the peritoneal cavity with minimal potential for unwanted long-term effects. One theory as to why GDV may follow splenectomy is that stretching and disruption of gastric ligaments (e.g., gastrosplenic ligament when removing head of spleen) increases stomach mobility.[76,77] Some studies[72,73,75] found no evidence that splenectomy was associated with an increased incidence of subsequent GDV, while other authors have recommended prophylactic gastropexy at the time of splenectomy for splenic torsion,[74,78] splenic neoplasia,[76] and other causes of splenomegaly.[11,77,79] In summary, because both splenic disease and GDV are more prevalent in large breed, deep-chested dogs, the author recommends prophylactic gastropexy if already in the abdomen and performing a splenectomy in at-risk breeds or those with other risk factors.

Surgical Procedure

Once a gastropexy is planned, standard IV catheter placement, induction for anesthesia, and preparation for abdominal exploratory are performed (see Chapter 1 for details). If no source of infection is found (at which point another type of antibiotic may be indicated), cefazolin (22 mg/kg IV) should be given slowly every 90 minutes peri-operatively, beginning 30–60 minutes prior to creation of the incision.

The details of GDV management are beyond the scope of this chapter, so the following discussion will revolve around prophylactic gastropexy.

The patient is positioned in dorsal recumbency, and the ventral abdomen and caudal thorax are clipped, prepped in standard aseptic fashion, and draped to allow for celiotomy. Celiotomy is performed on ventral midline extending from the xiphoid process to at least caudal to the umbilicus, and the falciform ligament is removed with either sharp transection or monopolar electrosurgery to allow for improved visualization of the peritoneal cavity and to provide easier identification of the external rectus sheath edge during closure. While Balfour retractors need to be placed for most procedures in the peritoneal cavity, especially for abdominal exploration, the retractors should be removed when the gastropexy is being performed in order to minimize distortion of the spatial relationship between the body wall and the stomach.

TIPS: While this surgery may be performed alone or with the help of an assistant, the location, length, and depth of the gastropexy are always the same:

- **Location**: pyloric antrum (between the body and pylorus, halfway between the vasculature of the greater and lesser curvatures to reduce risk of bleeding) is sutured to the right transversus abdominis muscle (caudal to the 13th rib, ~2 cm caudal to the diaphragm to reduce risk of iatrogenic pneumothorax, at least 2 cm lateral to the rectus abdominus muscle [~6 cm from ventral midline] to position the site dorsal enough to be anatomically appropriate). Prior to definitive gastropexy, the planned gastric incision site should be approximated to the planned body wall incision site to ensure that there is no excessive tension placed on the remainder of the stomach.
- **Length**: 3–5 cm.
- **Depth**: through the seromuscular layer of the stomach, incising through the transversus abdominis muscle (or at least the fascia and some of the muscle).
- Suture bite size (e.g., distance of suture bites from cut edge): ~3 mm.

One-Person Technique

TIP: If this technique is pursued, it is recommended to aseptically prepare the patient to include dorsally past the flank folds and continue about 10 cm cranial to the xiphoid process. This will allow for proper retraction with the towel clamps.

The surgeon should stand on the right side of the patient, and no assistant is needed with this procedure. With four fingers of both hands on the peritoneal surface of the right body wall and thumbs of both hands on the skin along the palpable costal arch, the right ventral body wall is folded over the ribs of the costal arch, which are pushed in toward the abdomen and ventrally using the thumbs to essentially evert the peritoneum. This results in the pronounced palpable ribs just beneath the peritoneal surface of the transversus abdominis muscle. Two Backhaus towel clamps are placed around the costal arch ~5 cm apart, ensuring that the cranial most clamp is at least 2 cm caudal to the white line costal origin of the diaphragm (Figure 21.1a–c). Once these towel clamps are in place, they are pulled laterally and dorsally to further push the costal arch into a ventral position, and the rings are secured to the patient's sterile lateral body wall skin using an additional towel clamp (Figure 21.2).

To create an incision into the pyloric antrum, a 3–5 cm longitudinal incision is made into the ventral aspect of the pyloric antrum halfway between the greater and lesser curvatures, which may be accomplished in two ways. The preferred method by the author is to pinch the stomach with the non-dominant hand as if assessing for a gastric slip, and when the seromuscular layer is isolated after slipping away of the mucosal–submucosal layer, Mayo tissue scissors are used to cut the pinched seromuscular layer. The submucosa is then exposed, and the Mayo scissors may be used to extend the longitudinal incision both orad and aborad, ensuring that the incision remains halfway between the greater and lesser curvatures of the stomach and their associated vasculature. The alternative method is to use a #15 blade to incise through the seromuscular layer of the pyloric antrum, and once appropriate depth is achieved, Mayo scissors may be used to extend the incision orad and aborad, similarly as described above. The gastric incision may then be manipulated to the transversus abdominis muscle isolated between the towel clamps to match incision length (Figure 21.2).

A scalpel blade (#10, #11, or #15 preferred) is then used to incise the transversus abdominis muscle between the two towel clamps along the ventral-most edge of the costal arch with resistance being met by the ribs of the costal arch, and the muscle should fall away on either side to reveal the white portion of the costal arch deep to the muscle. This incision should be at least 2 cm lateral to the approximate lateral aspect of the rectus abdominis musculature, which prevents the gastropexy from being too far ventral. Minimal self-limiting hemorrhage may be encountered (Figure 21.3). Ensure adequate length of this incision prior to suturing.

The suturing may proceed with one or two packs of long-lasting synthetic monofilament absorbable suture

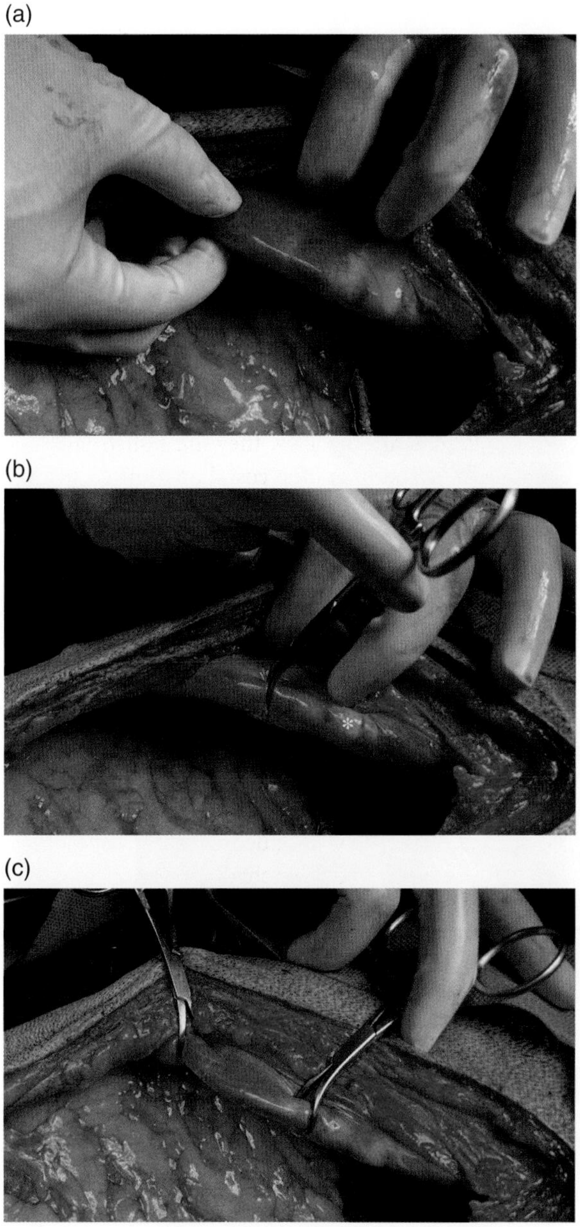

Figure 21.1 One-person incisional gastropexy technique: placement of towel clamps. Cranial is to the right in this image with the patient in dorsal recumbency. (a) With fingers folding the abdominal wall and peritoneum and thumbs pushing the costal arch ventrally and medially, the costal arch is palpable with overlying transversus abdominis musculature. (b) While holding the costal arch with one hand, the first towel clamp is placed on the cranial aspect to grasp the 12th rib about 2 cm caudal to the white line of the diaphragmatic costal attachment (denoted by a yellow *). (c) The second towel clamp is around the costal arch rib (~12th rib) approximately 5 cm caudal to the first, which will allow for a 4–5 cm transversus abdominis incision for the gastropexy. *Source:* © Kristin Coleman.

(e.g., polyglyconate or polydioxanone), usually 2-0 in size for most large breed dogs and 0 for giant breed dogs. If two suture lines are chosen, each simple continuous suture line is initiated with one corner apposing the cranial transversus incision and the aborad antral incision and the other corner apposing the caudal transversus incision and orad antral incision (Figures 21.4 and 21.5). A Kelly hemostat may be used to clamp the end of the suture tag left long from each corner's simple continuous suture lines, which may be used for tying the knot of the opposite strand's line. Suturing of the simple continuous suture line proceeds with the dorsal aspect first to appose the antral muscular flap (the edge closer to the greater curvature) to the transversus cut edge (the dorsal edge), and this simple continuous line terminates by tying a knot using the suture tag of the opposite corner's simple continuous suture line (Figure 21.5). Once this is done, hemostasis is confirmed, the area is locally lavaged, and standard celiotomy closure may commence.

Two-Person Technique

The surgeon should stand on the left side of the patient to better visualize the right lateral body wall while suturing, and the assistant should stand on the right side of the patient. The assistant will place two Backhaus towel clamps on the right body wall (not to include the skin) in order to provide ventral traction via lifting of the clamps when needed (Figure 21.6).

A 3–5 cm longitudinal incision is made into the ventral aspect of the pyloric antrum halfway between the greater and lesser curvatures, which may be accomplished in two ways. The preferred method by the author is to pinch the stomach with the non-dominant hand as if assessing for a gastric slip, and when the seromuscular layer is isolated after slipping away of the mucosal–submucosal layer, Mayo tissue scissors are used to cut the pinched seromuscular layer. The submucosa is then exposed, and the Mayo scissors may be used to extend the longitudinal incision both orad and aborad, ensuring that the incision remains halfway between the greater and lesser curvatures of the stomach and their associated vasculature. The alternative method is to use a #15 blade to incise through the serosa and muscular layers (grossly seem to palpate as one seromuscular layer) of the pyloric antrum, and once appropriate depth is achieved, Mayo scissors may be used to extend the incision orad and aborad, similarly as described above (Figure 21.7).

The stomach is gently lifted ventrally toward the right lateral transversus abdominis to assess where the stomach may naturally appose, ensuring that the "kissing mark" of blood of the gastric incision onto the body wall is at least 2 cm caudal to the white line denoting the costal origin of the diaphragm. Along this mark, a 3–5 cm incision is made with a scalpel blade through the transversus abdominis muscle from ventral to dorsal (Figure 21.8). This incision should be at least 2 cm lateral to the approximate lateral

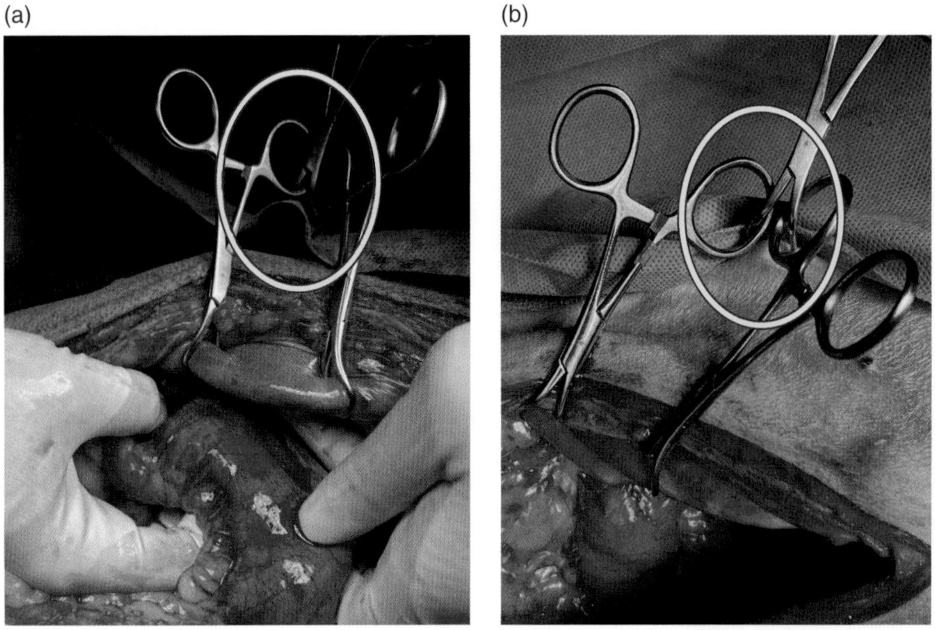

Figure 21.2 One-person incisional gastropexy technique: stabilization of the towel clamps. Cranial is to the right in this image with the patient in dorsal recumbency. A third towel clamp is passed around a ring from each of the previously placed towel clamps then secured to the patient's right dorsolateral body wall (denoted with a yellow circle), which is why additional clipping and prepping is necessary on the patient's right side if this procedure is anticipated. In this image, the gastric incision is being elevated to the proposed site of the transversus abdominis incision to both match length and ensure proper positioning. *Source:* © Kristin Coleman.

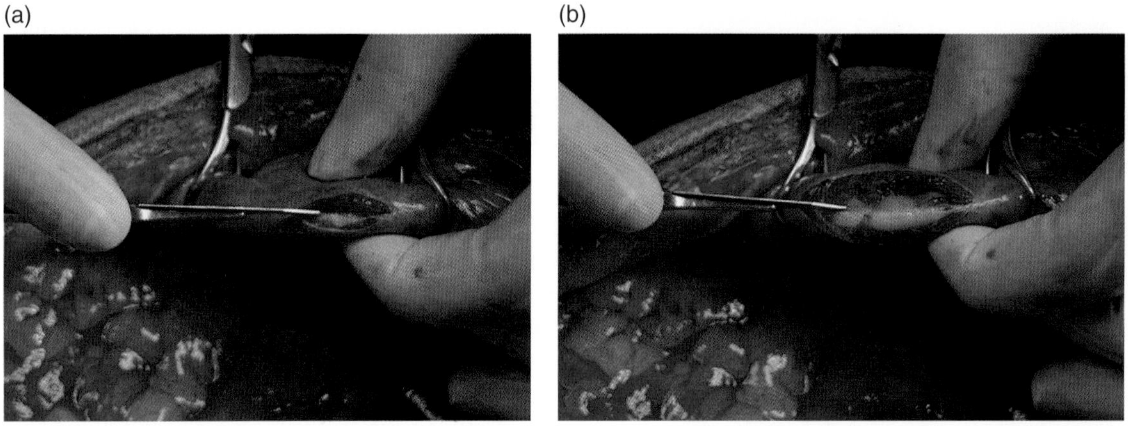

Figure 21.3 One-person incisional gastropexy technique: creating the transversus abdominis mm incision. Cranial is to the right in this image with the patient in dorsal recumbency. A #15 scalpel blade is used to incise through the transversus abdominis muscle over the costal arch for a length of ~4 cm to create two muscular flaps for suturing. *Source:* © Kristin Coleman.

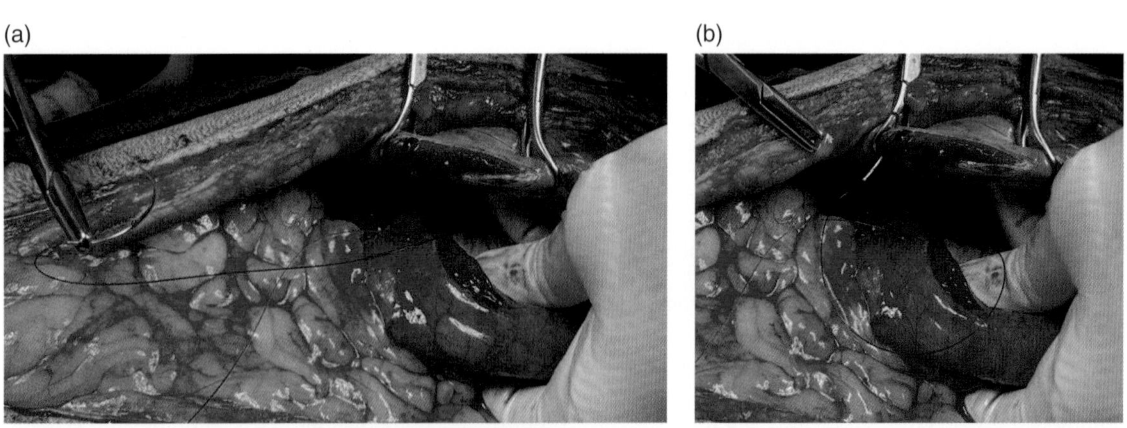

Figure 21.4 One-person incisional gastropexy technique: beginning the suture lines. Cranial is to the right in this image with the patient in dorsal recumbency. (a) The first simple continuous suture line of 2-0 polydioxanone is initiated by passing through the seromuscular apex of the gastric incision, then (b) the suture is passed through the matching incision of the transversus abdominis muscle. To have proper orientation and maintain normal gastric anatomy within the abdominal cavity, the orad aspect of the gastric incision is typically sutured to the caudal aspect of the transversus incision, and the aborad aspect of the stomach (with the pylorus) faces cranially to then flow naturally into the descending duodenum at the level of the cranial duodenal flexure. *Source:* © Kristin Coleman.

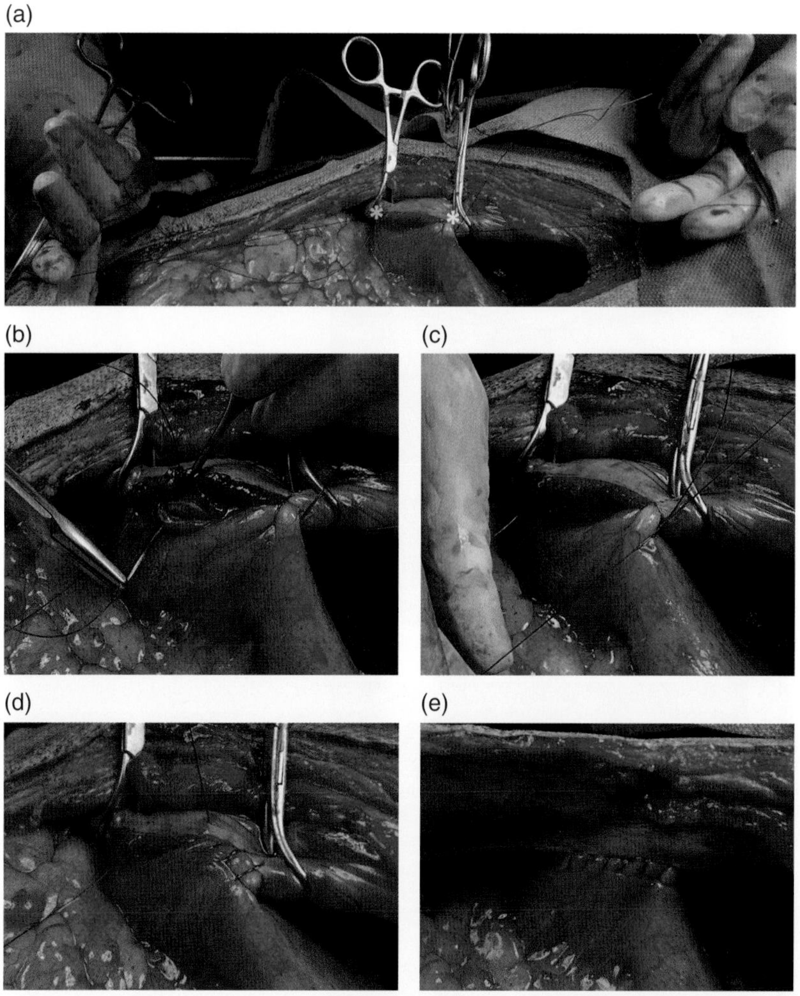

Figure 21.5 One-person incisional gastropexy technique: suturing the gastropexy with two lines. Cranial is to the right in this image with the patient in dorsal recumbency. (a) A simple continuous suture line of 2-0 polydioxanone is initiated on both sides of the gastropexy to join the corners of the gastric and right body wall incisions: orad gastric to caudal transversus abdominis mm (denoted with cyan *), aborad gastric to cranial transversus abdominis mm (denoted with a yellow *). Note how each simple continuous suture line's suture tag is left long and is clamped on the end with a hemostat, which allows for the opposite strand to end its line by suturing to the other's suture tag. (b) The first simple continuous line of suture should be the line that is most difficult to see the dorsal muscular flap of the transversus abdominis incision and the gastric seromuscular flap closest to the greater curvature. In this image, the needle is passing through the gastric seromuscular flap. (c) The first simple continuous suture line is ended by tying to the suture tag of the cranial strand. (d) The second simple continuous suture line apposes the ventral muscular flap of the transversus abdominis incision to the gastric seromuscular flap closest to the lesser curvature. (e) Completed gastropexy. While no studies have been done to investigate the number of suture bites required per simple continuous line, the author recommends four to seven bites per side. *Source:* © Kristin Coleman.

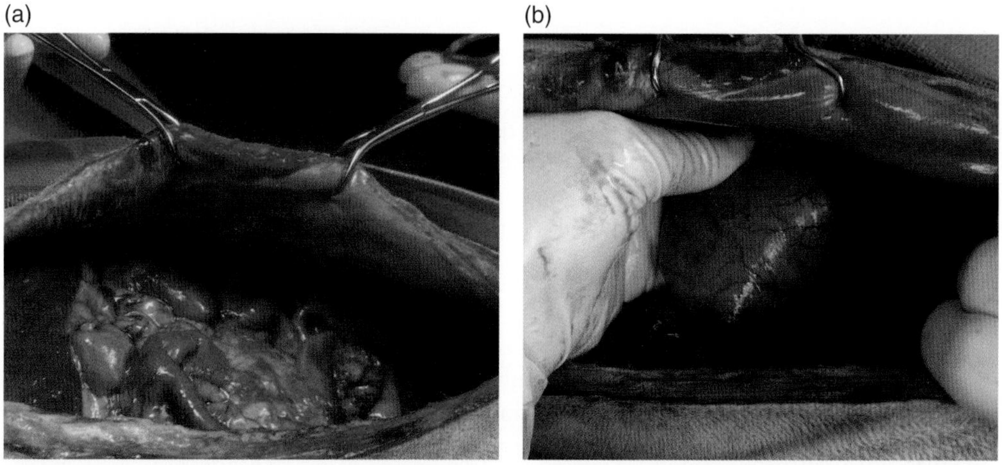

Figure 21.6 Two-person incisional gastropexy technique: placement of towel clamps. Cranial is to the right in this image with the patient in dorsal recumbency. (a) Two Backhaus towel clamps are placed in the right ventral body wall near the level of the gastropexy. Do not include the skin. With the surgeon on the patient's left side and the assistant on the right side, the assistant is able to lift the patient's right side to allow easier suturing for the surgeon. (b) The stomach may be elevated to assess the level of antral and transversus abdominis gastropexy sites. *Source:* © Kristin Coleman.

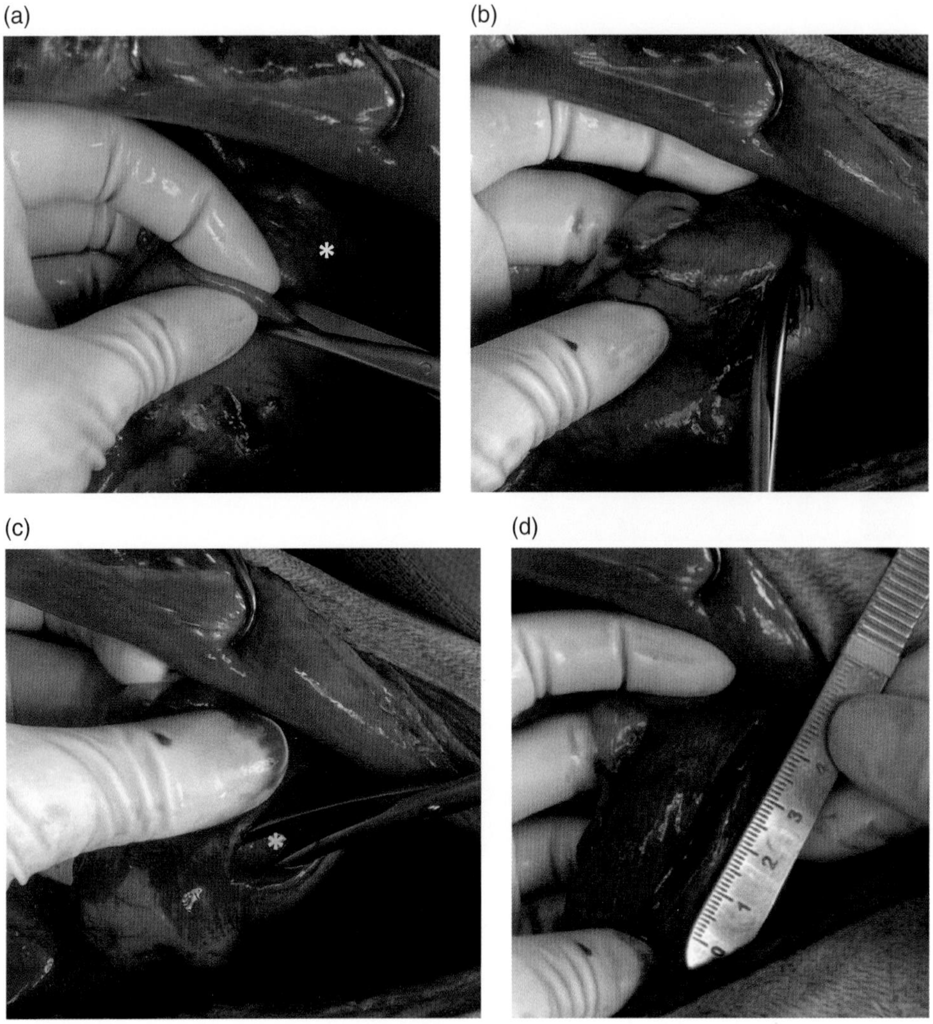

Figure 21.7 Two-person incisional gastropexy technique: creating the gastric incision. Cranial is to the right in this image with the patient in dorsal recumbency. (a) Midway between the lesser and greater curvatures of the pyloric antrum (muscular pyloric sphincter is denoted with a yellow *), the stomach wall is pinched with the non-dominant hand orad to aborad to isolate the seromuscular layers. Mayo scissors are used to incise the pinched tissue, which allows for exposure of the submucosal layer. (b) The gastric incision is continued along the longitudinal axis of the pyloric antrum until adequate length (~4 cm) is obtained. (c) Adequate depth of the gastric incision (through the seromuscular layers) should be confirmed with visualization of the submucosal tissue (denoted by cyan *). (d) A gastric incisional length of 4 cm is confirmed. *Source:* © Kristin Coleman.

aspect of the rectus abdominis musculature, which prevents the gastropexy site from being too far ventral.

The suturing should proceed with two packs of long-lasting synthetic monofilament absorbable suture (e.g., polyglyconate or polydioxanone), usually 2-0 in size for most large breed dogs and 0 for giant breed dogs. With two edges to each incision, two simple continuous suture lines are used to appose the stomach to the body wall from dorsal (aborad aspect of pyloric antrum) to ventral (orad aspect of pyloric antrum). Especially at the initiation of the two separate suture lines with the aborad gastric flaps being apposed to the dorsal transversus abdominis mm flaps, it is helpful for the assistant to elevate the body wall by lifting the towel clamps. A minimum of four to seven suture bites per simple continuous line is recommended prior to ending the pattern (Figure 21.9).

TIP: Take two bites per suture line at a time to gradually appose the two tissues without losing visualization.

Once this is done, hemostasis is confirmed, the area is locally lavaged, and standard celiotomy closure may commence.

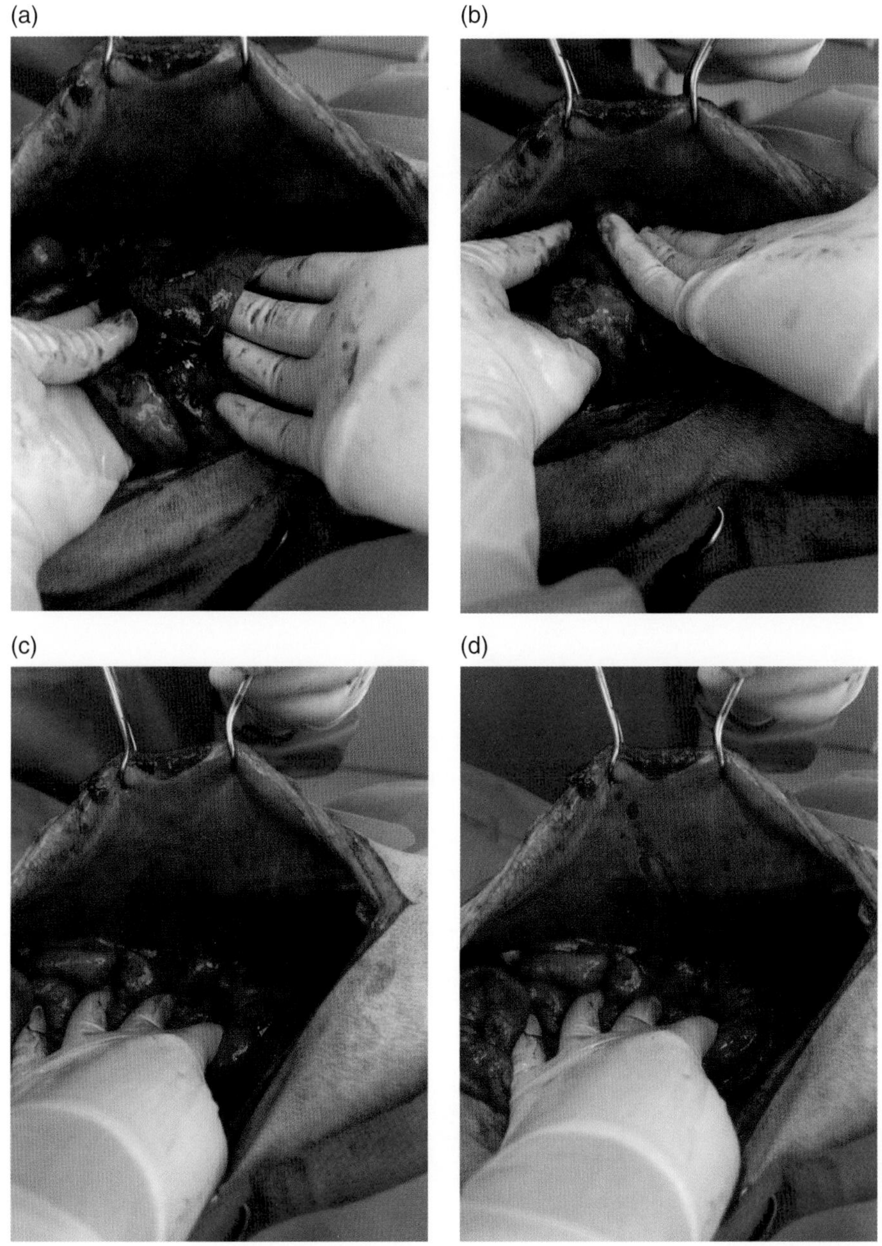

Figure 21.8 Two-person incisional gastropexy technique: creating the transversus abdominis mm incision. Cranial is to the right in this image with the patient in dorsal recumbency. (a) Placing one hand into the lesser curvature/angular incisure of the stomach allows the pyloric antrum to be gently lifted to the right ventrolateral body wall to assess for normal anatomic apposition for the gastropexy site. This particular patient had a gastrotomy performed in the body of the stomach immediately prior to performing this prophylactic gastropexy. (b) The antrum is pressed against the proposed transversus incision, which should be with minimal to no tension and at least 2 cm caudal to the white line of the diaphragmatic costal origin. (c) The "kissing mark" left by the antral incision, which is a guide for then incising the transversus abdominis mm. (d) A ~4 cm incision is made in the area of the "kissing mark" and has a trajectory that is slightly craniodorsal to caudoventral. *Source:* © Kristin Coleman.

Potential Complications

The normal risk of post-operative complications after any body cavity incision exists similarly after a gastropexy, including bleeding, infection, dehiscence, suture reaction, seroma, aspiration pneumonia, and gastrointestinal ileus. Intra-operatively, the risk of pneumothorax may be avoided by remaining caudal to the visible white line delineation laterally between the diaphragm and transversus abdominis musculature. Absorbable suture is recommended over non-absorbable suture due to the risk of fistula formation with non-absorbable materials. Post-operatively, the risk

(a) (b)

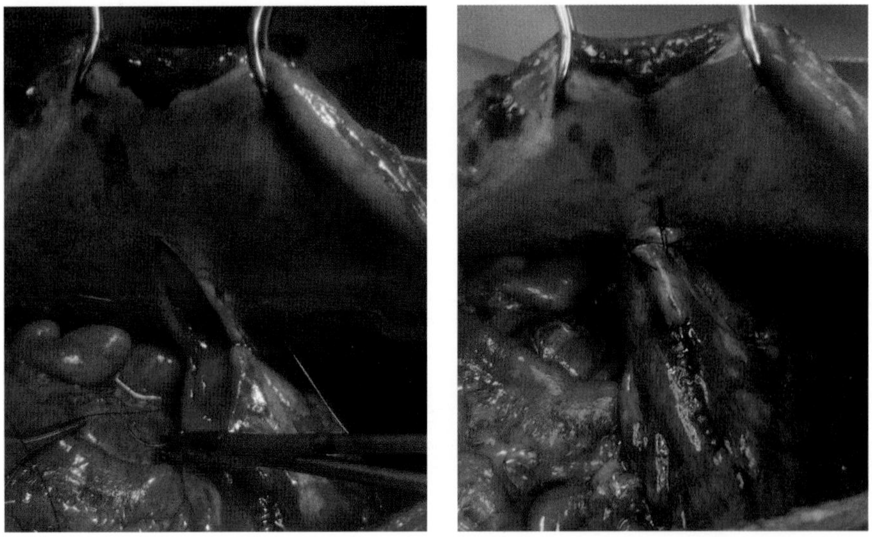

Figure 21.9 Two-person incisional gastropexy technique: suturing the gastropexy with two lines. Cranial is to the right in this image with the patient in dorsal recumbency. (a) Two simple continuous suture lines of 2-0 polydioxanone are initiated on the cranial and caudal aspects of the site to appose the two gastric seromuscular flaps to the transversus abdominis mm flaps. Two suture bites are taken per side to gradually complete the two lines simultaneously. (b) The two simple continuous lines may either be terminated separately or by suturing them together. *Source:* © Kristin Coleman.

for gastric dilatation is still possible, so advising owners to feed more than one meal per day to their dogs is recommended. Another potential complication is that of gastric malpositioning (if too acute of an angle is created with the gastropexy) leading to chronic intermittent vomiting secondary to partial gastric outflow tract obstruction,[18] which can be avoided by ensuring proper anatomic placement of the stomach to the right lateral body wall.

According to one study evaluating incorporating gastropexy, there was a 9.4% risk of wound-healing complications (mild seroma, swelling or purulent discharge, dehiscence) and a 3.4% risk of intra-abdominal hematoma or diffuse bleeding in the subcutaneous fatty tissue associated with that type of gastropexy.[60] While extremely rare if proper technique is followed, recurrence has been reported in a Rottweiler, who experienced a second 180° clockwise GDV approximately four months after the initial gastropexy for treating a GDV.[80] The recurrence was thought to be due to stretching of the adhesion at the gastropexy site, and, although rare, a GDV recurrence rate of 0–5% is documented for those dogs that had incisional gastropexy performed for treatment of a GDV.[10,81] Another rare but documented sequela to gastropexy is development of a soft tissue sarcoma at the gastropexy site.[82] In a case report of an eight-year-old spayed female Doberman Pinscher, a grade III soft tissue sarcoma was excised from the laparoscopic-assisted gastropexy site that was performed three years prior to tumor discovery, which the authors hypothesized may have been associated with inflammation and the process of scar formation that would occur secondary to any incision or surgical site.[82] On a positive note, prophylactic gastropexy does not seem to affect gastric motility or gastrointestinal transit time in dogs.[83,84]

Post-op Care/Prognosis

Depending on the gastropexy technique chosen, the other procedures performed in the same anesthetic event, the anesthetic protocol with possible incisional nerve block, the availability of overnight monitoring and care, and the potential co-morbidities present in the patients, these patients may either be discharged from the hospital within a few hours post-operatively or be kept overnight for observation and gradual transition from injectable to oral medications. The author recommends placement of a nasogastric tube intra-operatively after removal of the orogastric tube (if performing gastropexy to treat GDV); benefits include continuous decompression of the stomach, monitoring the color, quality, and volume of gastric contents in cases of questionable gastric viability, and trickle-feeding a liquid diet if prolonged anorexia (typically considered >12 hours post-operatively) is noted.

The at-home post-op care instructions for clients should include administration of pain medications (gabapentin 10 mg/kg by mouth every 8–12 hours +/− NSAID if no contraindications exist and if gastropexy performed for prophylaxis), applying compresses to the surgical site, application of a hard cone collar and/or T-shirt, and confinement to a crate, pen, or small room with no running, jumping, or playing for two weeks after surgery. Unless the patient had a pre-existing dermatitis, other source of infection, or suspicion for an aspiration event, no post-operative antibiotics need to be dispensed. Exceptions would include if gastric rupture was present at the time of exploratory celiotomy due to gastric necrosis, in which case broad-spectrum antibiotics should be administered until culture results are finalized. Even if a minimally invasive gastropexy technique is pursued and there is technically "faster return to normal activity" with these gastropexies, confinement and limiting activity to short (~5 minute duration) leashed walks only is still recommended for two weeks post-operatively.

Prognosis is excellent after gastropexy, especially when performed prophylactically in at-risk breeds of dogs. While certain types of gastropexy are associated with high recurrence rates of GDV after surgery (e.g., gastrocolopexy),[80] the incisional gastropexy as described here technically has very low recurrence rate but could still result in the patient developing gastric dilatation requiring hospitalization in the future.[85]

References

1 Funkquist, B. and Garmer, L. (1967). Pathogenetic and therapeutic aspects of torsion of the canine stomach. *J. Small Anim. Pract.* 8 (9): 523–532.

2 Ellison, G.W. (1993). Gastric dilatation volvulus. Surgical prevention. *Vet. Clin. North Am. Small Anim. Pract.* 23: 513–530.

3 Burrows, C.F. and Ignaszewski, L.A. (1990). Canine gastric dilatation-volvulus. *J. Small Anim. Pract.* 31 (10): 495–501.

4 Andrews, A.H. (1970). A study of ten cases of gastric torsion in the bloodhound. *Vet. Rec.* 86: 689–693.

5 Hosgood, G. (1994). Gastric dilatation-volvulus in dogs. *J. Am. Vet. Med. Assoc.* 204 (11): 1742–1747.

6 Rosselli, D. (2022). Updated information on gastric dilatation and volvulus and gastropexy in dogs. *Vet. Clin. North Am. Small Anim. Pract.* 52 (2): 317–337.

7 Brockman, D.J., Washabau, R.J., and Drobatz, K.J. (1995). Canine gastric dilatation/volvulus syndrome in a veterinary critical care unit: 295 cases (1986-1992). *J. Am. Vet. Med. Assoc.* 207 (4): 460–464.

8 Broom, C.J. and Walsh, V.P. (2003). Gastric dilatation volvulus in dogs. *N. Zeal. Vet. J.* 51: 275–283.

9 Muir, W.M. (1982). Gastric dilatation-volvulus in the dog, with emphasis on cardiac arrhythmias. *J. Am. Vet. Med. Assoc.* 180: 739–742.

10 Glickman, L.T., Lantz, G.C., Schellenberg, D.B. et al. (1998). A prospective study of the survival and recurrence following the acute gastric dilatation-volvulus syndrome in 136 dogs. *J. Am. Anim. Hosp. Assoc.* 34: 253–259.

11 Monnet, E. (2003). Gastric dilatation-volvulus syndrome in dogs. *Vet. Clin. North Am. Small Anim. Pract.* 33: 987–1005.

12 Wingfield, W.E. (1976). Pathophysiology associated with GDV in the dog. *J. Am. Anim. Hosp. Assoc.* 12: 136–141.

13 Lyman, D. (1981). Gastric dilatation-volvulus in the dog. *Iowa State Vet.* 3: 112–115.

14 Frendin, J. and Funkquist, B. (1990). Fundic gastropexy for prevention of recurrence of gastric volvulus. *J. Small Anim. Pract.* 31 (2): 78–82.

15 Funkquist, B. (1979). Gastric torsion in the dog III. Fundic gastropexy as a relapse-preventing procedure. *J. Small Anim. Pract.* 20: 103–109.

16 Eggertsdóttir, A.V. and Moe, L. (1995). A retrospective study of conservative treatment of gastric dilatation-volvulus in the dog. *Acta Vet. Scand.* 36: 175–184.

17 Ward, M.P., Patronek, G.J., and Glickman, L.T. (2003). Benefits of prophylactic gastropexy for dogs at risk of gastric dilatation-volvulus. *Prev. Vet. Med.* 60: 319–329.

18 Sutton, J.S., Steffey, M.A., Bonadio, C.M. et al. (2015). Gastric malpositioning and chronic, intermittent vomiting following prophylactic gastropexy in a 20-month-old great Dane dog. *Can. Vet. J.* 56 (10): 1053–1056.

19 MacCoy, D.M., Sykes, G.P., Hoffer, R.E. et al. (1982). A gastropexy technique for permanent fixation of the pyloric antrum. *J. Am. Anim. Hosp. Assoc.* 18: 763–768.

20 Benitez, M.E., Schmiedt, C.W., Radlinsky, M.G. et al. (2013). Efficacy of incisional gastropexy for prevention of GDV in dogs. *J. Am. Anim. Hosp. Assoc.* 49 (3): 185–189.

21 Whitney, W.O., Scavelli, T.D., Matthiesen, D.T. et al. (1989). Belt-loop gastropexy: technique and surgical results in 20 dogs. *J. Am. Anim. Hosp. Assoc.* 1989; 25: 75–83.

22 Fallah, A.M., Lumb, W.M., Nelson, A.W. et al. (1982). Circumcostal gastropexy in the dog: a preliminary study. *Vet. Surg.* 11: 19–22.

23 Leib, M.S., Konde, L.J., Wingfield, W.E. et al. (1985). Circumcostal gastropexy for preventing recurrence of gastric dilatation-volvulus in the dog: an evaluation of 30 cases. *J. Am. Vet. Med. Assoc.* 187 (3): 245–248.

24 Woolfson, J.M. and Kostolich, M. (1986). Circumcostal gastropexy: clinical use of the technique in 34 dogs with gastric dilatation-volvulus. *J. Am. Anim. Hosp. Assoc.* 22: 825–830.

25 Pope, E.R. and Jones, B.D. (1999). Clinical evaluation of a modified circumcostal gastropexy in dogs. *J. Am. Vet. Med. Assoc.* 215: 952–955.

26 Parks, J. (1979). Surgical management of gastric torsion. *Vet. Clin. North Am. Small Anim. Pract.* 9: 259–267.

27 Belch, A., Rubinos, C., Barnes, D.C. et al. (2017). Modified tube gastropexy using a mushroom-tipped silicone catheter for management of gastric dilatation-volvulus in dogs. *J. Small Anim. Pract.* 58 (2): 79–88.

28 Steelman-Szymeczek, S.M., Stebbins, M.E., and Hardie, E.M. (2003). Clinical evaluation of a right-sided prophylactic gastropexy via a grid approach. *J. Am. Anim. Hosp. Assoc.* 39: 397–402.

29 Rawlings, C.A., Foutz, T.L., Mahaffey, M.B. et al. (2001). A rapid and strong laparoscopic-assisted gastropexy in dogs. *Am. J. Vet. Res.* 62: 871–875.

30 Rawlings, C.A. (2002). Laparoscopic-assisted gastropexy. *J. Am. Anim. Hosp. Assoc.* 38: 15–19.

31 Rawlings, C.A., Mahaffey, M.B., Bement, S. et al. (2002). Prospective evaluation of laparoscopic-assisted gastropexy in dogs susceptible to gastric dilatation. *J. Am. Vet. Med. Assoc.* 221: 1576–1581.

32 Runge, J.J., Mayhew, P., and Rawlings, C.A. (2009). Surgical views: laparoscopic-assisted and laparoscopic prophylactic gastropexy: indications and techniques. *Compend. Contin. Educ. Vet.* 31: 58–65.

33 Mayhew, P.D. and Brown, D.C. (2009). Prospective evaluation of two intracorporeally sutured prophylactic laparoscopic gastropexy techniques compared with laparoscopic-assisted gastropexy in dogs. *Vet. Surg.* 38: 738–746.

34 Hardie, R.J., Flanders, J.A., Schmidt, P. et al. (1996). Biomechanical and histological evaluation of a laparoscopic stapled gastropexy technique in dogs. *Vet. Surg.* 25 (2): 127–133.

35 Giaconella, V., Grillo, R., Giaconella, R. et al. (2021). Outcomes and complications in a case series of 39 total laparoscopic prophylactic gastropexies using a modified technique. *Animals* 11 (2): 255.

36 Takacs, J.D., Singh, A., Case, J.B. et al. (2017). Total laparoscopic gastropexy using 1 simple continuous barbed suture line in 63 dogs. *Vet. Surg.* 46 (2): 233–241.

37 Deroy, C., Hahn, H., Bismuth, C. et al. (2019). Simplified minimally invasive surgical approach for prophylactic gastropexy in 21 cases. *J. Am. Anim. Hosp. Assoc.* 55 (3): 152–159.

38 Coleman, K.A., Adams, S., Smeak, D.D. et al. (2016). Laparoscopic gastropexy using knotless unidirectional suture and an articulated endoscopic suturing device: seven cases. *Vet. Surg.* 45 (S1): O95–O101.

39 Coleman, K.A. and Monnet, E. (2017). Comparison of laparoscopic gastropexy performed via intracorporeal suturing with knotless unidirectional barbed suture using a needle driver versus a roticulated endoscopic suturing device: 30 cases. *Vet. Surg.* 46 (7): 1002–1007.

40 Spah, C.E., Elkins, A.D., Wehrenberg, A. et al. (2013). Evaluation of two novel self-anchoring barbed sutures in a prophylactic laparoscopic gastropexy compared with intracorporeal tied knots. *Vet. Surg.* 42: 932–942.

41 Lacitignola, L., Crovace, A.M., Fracassi, L. et al. (2021). Comparison of total laparoscopic gastropexy with the Ethicon Securestrap fixation device versus knotless barbed suture in dogs. *Vet. Rec.* 188 (7): e113.

42 Dujowich, M. and Reimer, S.B. (2008). Evaluation of an endoscopically assisted gastropexy technique in dogs. *Am. J. Vet. Res.* 69: 537–541.

43 Dujowich, M., Keller, M.E., and Reimer, S.B. (2010). Evaluation of short- and long-term complications after endoscopically assisted gastropexy in dogs. *J. Am. Vet. Med. Assoc.* 236: 177–182.

44 Wacker, C.A., Weber, U.T., Tanno, F. et al. (1998). Ultrasonographic evaluation of adhesions induced by incisional gastropexy in 16 dogs. *J. Small Anim. Pract.* 39 (8): 379–384.

45 Tanno, F., Weber, U., Wacker, C. et al. (1998). Ultrasonographic comparison of adhesions induced by two different methods of gastropexy in the dog. *J. Small Anim. Pract.* 39: 432–436.

46 Webb, R.J. and Monnet, E. (2019). Influence of length of incision and number of suture lines on the biomechanical properties of incisional gastropexy. *Vet. Surg.* 48 (6): 933–937.

47 Arbaugh, M., Case, J.B., and Monnet, E. (2013). Biomechanical comparison of glycomer 631 and glycomer 631 knotless for use in canine incisional gastropexy. *Vet. Surg.* 42 (2): 205–209.

48 Imhoff, D.J., Cohen, A., and Monnet, E. (2015). Biomechanical analysis of laparoscopic incisional gastropexy with intracorporeal suturing using knotless polyglyconate. *Vet. Surg.* 44 (Suppl 1): 39–43.

49 Belandria, G.A., Pavletic, M.M., Boulay, J.P. et al. (2009). Gastropexy with an automatic stapling instrument for the treatment of gastric dilatation and volvulus in 20 dogs. *Can. Vet. J.* 50: 733–740.

50 Coolman, B.R., Manfra Marretta, S., Pijanowski, G.J. et al. (1999). Evaluation of a skin stapler for belt-loop gastropexy in dogs. *J. Am. Anim. Hosp. Assoc.* 35 (5): 440–444.

51 Touru, S.H. and Smeak, D.D. (2005). A practical right-sided incisional gastropexy technique for treatment or prevention of gastric dilatation volvulus. *Suomen Elainlaakarilehti* 111 (3): 123–128.

52 Wilson, E.R., Henderson, R.A., Montgomery, R.D. et al. (1996). A comparison of laparoscopic and belt-loop gastropexy in dogs. *Vet. Surg.* 25 (3): 221–227.

53 Formaggini, L. and Degna, M.T. (2018). A prospective evaluation of a modified belt-loop gastropexy in 100 dogs with gastric dilatation-volvulus. *J. Am. Anim. Hosp. Assoc.* 54 (5): 239–245.

54 Degna, M.T., Formaggini, L., Fondati, A. et al. (2001). Using a modified gastropexy technique to prevent recurrence of gastric dilatation-volvulus in dogs. *Vet. Med.* 96 (1): 39–50.

55 Eggertsdóttir, A.V., Stigen, Ø., Lønaas, L. et al. (2001). Comparison of the recurrence rate of gastric dilatation with or without volvulus in dogs after circumcostal gastropexy versus gastrocolopexy. *Vet. Surg.* 30 (6): 546–551.

56 Eggertsdóttir, A.V., Stigen, Ø., Lønaas, L. et al. (1996). Comparison of two surgical treatments of gastric dilatation-volvulus in dogs. *Acta Vet. Scand.* 37: 415–426.

57 Eggertsdóttir, A.V., Langeland, M., and Fuglem, B. (2008). Long-term outcome in dogs after circumcostal gastropexy or gastrocolopexy for gastric dilatation with or without volvulus. *Vet. Surg.* 37: 809–810.

58 Hall, J.A., Willer, R.L., Seim, H.B. III et al. (1992). Gastric emptying of nondigestible radiopaque markers after circumcostal gastropexy in clinically normal dogs and dogs with gastric dilatation-volvulus. *Am. J. Vet. Res.* 53: 1961–1965.

59 Meyer-Lindenberg, A., Harder, A., Fehr, M. et al. (1993). Treatment of gastric dilatation-volvulus and a rapid method for prevention of relapse in dogs: 134 cases (1988-1991). *J. Am. Vet. Med. Assoc.* 203 (9): 1303–1307.

60 Ullmann, B., Seehaus, N., Hungerbuhler, S. et al. (2016). Gastric dilatation volvulus: a retrospective study of 203 dogs with ventral midline gastropexy. *J. Small Anim. Pract.* 57: 18–22.

61 Christie, T.R. and Smith, C.W. (1976). Gastrocolopexy for prevention of recurrent gastric volvulus. *J. Am. Anim. Hosp. Assoc.* 12: 173–176.

62 Raghavan, M., Glickman, N., McCabe, G. et al. (2004). Diet-related risk factors for gastric dilatation-volvulus in dogs of high-risk breeds. *J. Am. Anim. Hosp. Assoc.* 40 (3): 192–203.

63 Glickman, L.T., Glickman, N.W., Schellenberg, D.B. et al. (2000). Non-dietary risk factors for gastric dilatation-volvulus in large and giant breed dogs. *J. Am. Vet. Med. Assoc.* 217: 1492–1499.

64 Glickman, L.T., Glickman, N.W., Schellenberg, D.B. et al. (1997). Multiple risk factors for the gastric dilatation-volvulus syndrome in dogs: a practitioner/owner case-control study. *J. Am. Anim. Hosp. Assoc.* 33: 197–204.

65 Schellenberg, D., Yi, Q., Glickman, N.W. et al. (1998). Influence of thoracic conformation and genetics on the risk of gastric dilatation-volvulus in Irish setters. *J. Am. Anim. Hosp. Assoc.* 34 (1): 64–73.

66 de Battisti, A., Toscano, M.J., and Formaggini, L. (2012). Gastric foreign body as a risk factor for gastric dilatation and volvulus in dogs. *J. Am. Vet. Med. Assoc.* 241 (9): 1190–1193.

67 Theyse, L.F.H., van de Brom, W.E., and van Sluijs, F.J. (1998). Small size of food particles and age as risk factors for gastric dilatation volvulus in great danes. *Vet. Rec.* 143 (2): 48–50.

68 Glickman, L.T., Glickman, N.W., Perez, C.M. et al. (1994). Analysis of risk factors for gastric dilatation and dilatation-volvulus in dogs. *J. Am. Vet. Med. Assoc.* 204: 1465–1471.

69 Braun, L., Lester, S., Kuzma, A.B. et al. (1996). Gastric dilatation-volvulus in the dog with histological evidence of preexisting inflammatory bowel disease: a retrospective study of 23 cases. *J. Am. Anim. Hosp. Assoc.* 32 (4): 287–290.

70 Evans, K.M. and Adams, V.J. (2010). Mortality and morbidity due to gastric dilatation-volvulus syndrome in pedigree dogs in the UK. *J. Small Anim. Pract.* 51 (7): 376–381.

71 Sartor, A.J., Bentley, A.M., and Brown, D.C. (2013). Association between previous splenectomy and gastric dilatation-volvulus in dogs: 453 cases (2004-2009). *J. Am. Vet. Med. Assoc.* 242 (10): 1381–1384.

72 Grange, A.M., Clough, W., and Casale, S.A. (2012). Evaluation of splenectomy as a risk factor for gastric dilatation-volvulus. *J. Am. Vet. Med. Assoc.* 241: 461–466.

73 Goldhammer, M.A., Haining, H., Milne, E.M. et al. (2010). Assessment of the incidence of GDV following splenectomy in dogs. *J. Small Anim. Pract.* 51: 23–28.

74 Millis, D.L., Nemzek, J., Riggs, C. et al. (1995). Gastric dilatation-volvulus after splenic torsion in two dogs. *J. Am. Vet. Med. Assoc.* 207: 314–315.

75 Maki, L.C., Males, K.N., Byrnes, M.J. et al. (2017). Incidence of gastric dilatation-volvulus following a splenectomy in 238 dogs. *Can. Vet. J.* 58 (12): 1275–1280.

76 Marconato, L. (2006). Gastric dilatation-volvulus as complication after surgical removal of a splenic haemangiosarcoma in a dog. *J. Vet. Med. A Physiol. Pathol. Clin. Med.* 53 (7): 371–374.

77 Tillson, D.M. (2003). Spleen. In: *Textbook of Small Animal Surgery*, 1e (ed. D. Slatter), 1058. Philadelphia, PA: Saunders.

78 Neath, P.J., Brockman, D.J., and Saunders, H.M. (1997). Retrospective analysis of 19 cases of isolated torsion of the splenic pedicle in dogs. *J. Small Anim. Pract.* 38 (9): 387–392.

79 Rasmussen, L. (2003). Stomach. In: *Textbook of Small Animal Surgery*, 3e (ed. D. Slatter), 592–643. Philadelphia, PA: Saunders.

80 Hammell, S.P. and Novo, R.E. (2006). Recurrence of gastric dilatation-volvulus after incisional gastropexy in a Rottweiler. *J. Am. Anim. Hosp. Assoc.* 42 (2): 147–150.

81 Przywara, J.F., Abel, S.B., Peacock, J.T. et al. (2014). Occurrence and recurrence of gastric dilatation with or without volvulus after incisional gastropexy. *Can. Vet. J.* 55 (10): 981–984.

82 Allegrini, G., Linden, A.Z., Singh, A. et al. (2021). Soft tissue sarcoma at the site of a previous laparoscopic-assisted gastropexy in a dog. *Can. Vet. J.* 62 (2): 173–178.

83 Coleman, K.A., Boscan, P., Ferguson, L. et al. (2019). Evaluation of gastric motility in nine dogs before and after prophylactic laparoscopic gastropexy: a pilot study. *Aust. Vet. J.* 97 (7): 225–230.

84 Balsa, I.M., Culp, W.T.N., Drobatz, K.J. et al. (2017). Effect of laparoscopic-assisted gastropexy on gastrointestinal transit time in dogs. *J. Vet. Intern. Med.* 31: 1680–1685.

85 Jennings, P.B. Jr., Mathey, W.S., and Ehler, W.J. (1992). Intermittent gastric dilatation after gastropexy in a dog. *J. Am. Vet. Med. Assoc.* 200: 1707–1708.

22

Gastrointestinal Procedures

Penny J. Regier

Department of Clinical Sciences, University of Florida, Gainesville, FL, USA

Key Points

- The most common indication for gastrointestinal (GI) surgery in dogs is a foreign body (FB) obstruction, which accounts for approximately 80% of all mechanical GI obstructions in dogs.
- Other indications for intestinal surgery include intestinal biopsies, neoplasia, intussusceptions, and penetrating trauma.
- Dehiscence is a potentially life-threatening complication of GI surgery and requires surgical intervention with anastomotic dehiscence rates reported to be as high as 28%.
- These surgical procedures are commonly performed in veterinary medicine, and an understanding of normal intestinal healing, suturing, and stapling techniques, and consequences of impaired intestinal healing resulting in dehiscence is critical for the veterinary surgeon.

Introduction

Gastrointestinal (GI) surgery is commonly performed in veterinary medicine for numerous indications. However, small intestinal foreign bodies (FBs) are one of the leading causes of exploratory abdominal surgery in dogs, often resulting in either a gastrotomy or an enterotomy. When devitalized intestine is identified in surgery, patients may require resection of the necrotic intestine and anastomosis of the remaining healthy intestine. An understanding of how to assess tissue viability and knowing when to resect devitalized tissue is imperative for surgical success. Other indications for intestinal surgery include intestinal biopsies, neoplasia, intussusceptions, hernia repair, and penetrating trauma.[3,6] Dehiscence is a potentially life-threatening complication of GI surgery, resulting in septic peritonitis (SP) and requiring surgical intervention. An understanding of indications for surgery, normal intestinal healing, suturing and stapling techniques, potential complications, consequences of dehiscence, and post-operative care are critical for the veterinary surgeon and positive surgical outcomes.

Indications and Preoperative Considerations

Clinical Signs/Physical Exam

Surgical management of GI FBs varies depending on the type and location of the FB. Sharp FBs, such as straight pins, safety pins, bones, nails, or glass, will usually pass through the GI tract without creating intestinal perforation. Rubber balls, cellophane, or corncobs tend to pass slower or not at all and are more likely to cause complete mechanical obstruction requiring emergency laparotomy.

Gastric FBs can be seen in any age animal but are most common in puppies or kittens because of their indiscriminate eating habits. Common gastric FBs seen in dogs include bones, balls, corn cobs, rope toys, and cellophane

Techniques in Small Animal Soft Tissue, Orthopedic, and Ophthalmic Surgery, First Edition. Edited by Kristin A. Coleman.

Companion website: www.wiley.com/go/coleman/surgeries

wrappers. Linear FBs, such as yarn, tinsel, or string, are more common in cats.

Clinical signs associated with gastric FBs are highly variable. If the structure moves freely about the gastric lumen, sporadic vomiting, inappetence, or weight loss is commonly reported. Occasionally animals are completely asymptomatic. However, if the FB lodges in the pylorus, acute profuse projectile vomiting results and rapid dehydration is often noted. Gastric fluids rich in K^+, Na^+, H^+, and Cl^- are lost, sometimes resulting in a hypokalemic hypochloremic metabolic alkalosis.

Animals may be categorized as having either an incomplete (partial) or complete obstruction. Patients with incomplete obstructions caused by intraluminal linear FBs or neoplasia usually present with sporadic vomiting, anorexia, and weight loss, which often progresses in severity over days or weeks. Conversely, complete obstructions caused by FBs, strangulated intestines, acute intussusceptions, or intestinal volvulus usually cause acute bowel distention and more severe clinical signs than in those with partial obstructions. The presence and character of feces is sometimes important in establishing the type of obstruction. Scant stools often indicate an incomplete obstruction is present. Blood or melena may indicate intestinal strangulation, ulceration, neoplasia, or parasitism. Diarrhea, tenesmus, and/or scant amounts of blood-stained feces are also often seen in patients with intussusception.

Animals may also be categorized as having high (proximal) versus low (distal) obstruction. With proximal (pylorus or duodenum) and complete obstructions, vomiting is often projectile, and the patient has more acute and severe clinical signs with rapid electrolyte changes and dehydration. Duodenal obstruction prevents large quantities of salivary, gastric, pancreatic, or duodenal secretions from contacting the jejunal and ileal mucosal surfaces for reabsorption, resulting in rapid dehydration. The major cause of mortality from upper small intestinal obstruction is severe hypovolemia and electrolyte disturbances. With distal jejunum, ileum, ileocecal junction, and incomplete intestinal obstruction, clinical signs may be more chronic and vague with intermittent anorexia, lethargy, diarrhea, and occasional vomiting. More than half of all the fluids and electrolytes are added in the stomach and duodenum, and the majority of these are reabsorbed by the jejunum and ileum. Obstruction of the distal small intestine spares most of this absorptive surface. Signs with distal obstructions are associated with maldigestion and malabsorption of nutrients.

Animals may also be categorized as having a simple mechanical versus a strangulated (ischemic) obstruction. Distinguishing between simple mechanical and strangulated (ischemic) bowel obstruction is critical because the latter condition requires early and rapid surgical intervention. Mechanical obstructions can be luminal (FBs), intramural (neoplasia), or extramural (adhesions). With simple mechanical luminal obstruction, blood flow to the distended bowel is not completely obliterated, but increased bowel wall tension may cause both histological and physiologic changes. Strangulated obstruction may occur from intraluminal obstruction with local pressure necrosis. More commonly, strangulation obstruction occurs secondarily to mesenteric vascular disruption caused by intestinal volvulus, intussusception, or a strangulated hernia.

Diagnostics

Most importantly, the clinician should consider history and physical exam findings when considering whether a patient needs emergent surgery or not. Abdominal palpation is of utmost importance to evaluate for pain and tenderness in the abdomen. In some cases, foreign material may be palpated on examination. A rectal exam should also be included as part of a thorough physical exam.

Diagnosis of gastric FBs is often made based on plain abdominal radiographs. Focal gas dilation of the small intestines is consistent with intestinal FB obstruction with an 80% greater chance of obstruction if the maximal SI diameter is >2x compared to the height of L5 at the mid-centrum in dogs.[11,12] In cats, similar ratio measurements are taken with maximum small intestinal diameters compared to the height of the cranial end plate of the second lumber vertebra (L2) on a lateral view radiograph, and cats with ratios <2.0 are more likely to have non-obstructed intestines.[13] In cats, the maximal small intestinal diameters should not exceed 12 mm.

Metal objects are easily identifiable, and objects such as bones, racket balls, or corn cobs often can be seen without contrast studies. Radiolucent objects causing an obstruction may be more challenging to diagnose. In these cases, barium sulfate may be administered to help delineate the object. Caution should be taken with barium administration, as it should not be used if a GI perforation is suspected or when there is concern for aspiration pneumonia with continuous regurgitation. If free gas is visualized in the abdomen on radiographs, this is an indication of a possible GI perforation, and an abdominal explore is recommended. Linear FBs pass down into the small intestine resulting in "pleating" of the small bowel, although the proximal anchor point is usually located in the stomach (dogs > cats) or under the tongue (cats > dogs).[14–16] This often appears in the right cranial quadrant of the abdomen in the ventral–dorsal (VD) radiograph or cranioventral portion of the abdomen in the lateral view.

Ultrasonography is another diagnostic tool often used to help diagnose GI FBs and is preferred over radiographs by some clinicians. An advantage of ultrasound is that if free fluid is present in the abdomen, the fluid may be aspirated via ultrasound guidance to assess for SP. With the use of radiographs and ultrasound, barium is not commonly used. In recent years, endoscopes have become invaluable in diagnosing gastric FBs, ulcerations, or neoplasms, which were not apparent radiographically.

Treatment Options

In some cases, medical or conservative management may be pursued. This is only an option if the material is small enough to pass through the GI tract or if there is an acute presentation. Rehydration with high rates of IV fluids is a key component of medical management and may help to move the obstruction through the GI tract once the bowel is rehydrated. Prokinetics, such as cisapride or metoclopramide, are contraindicated for use with GI FB obstructions, as these medications will increase the likelihood of GI perforation. Abdominal radiographs are repeated every 8–12 hours to monitor for movement of the foreign material and monitor for progressive gas distention in the bowel. If the patient has progressive vomiting or becomes more painful on abdominal palpation during this time, surgery should be recommended. A potential concern, which owners should be aware of with medical management, is that the foreign material may continue to stay lodged in place, and the bowel may perforate from continued pressure necrosis. Medical management is contraindicated in the case of linear FB obstructions and SP.

Endoscopic FB removal is also an option for gastric FBs in the case of smaller FBs or less numerous FBs. Endoscopes are frequently invaluable for removing FBs, such as silk stockings or rags, which may be easily grasped with forceps. Endoscopy is not ideal with numerous FBs, larger FBs, or FBs that may be linear or lodged in part of the small intestines. Rubber balls or bones cannot usually be removed with endoscopy.

Careful client consultation is important when managing gastric FBs. Surprisingly, sharp FBs, such as nails, straight pins, and bones, will usually pass spontaneously through the entire intestinal tract without causing perforation. The animal should be fed a high-fiber diet and carefully monitored for the onset of vomiting, abdominal tenderness, or fever. Radiographs should be repeated daily to ensure that aboral passage is occurring. Complete passage usually takes three to four days. With larger FBs, the owner must be made aware that at any time, complete intestinal obstruction may occur that necessitating surgery.

If the FB has a relatively smooth surface and appears as though it is too large to pass distally, induction of vomiting may be considered. Dogs may be induced to vomit with apomorphine or cats with xylazine. Induced vomiting for attempted gastric evacuation of a sharp FB should be approached with great caution because of the danger of the FB lodging in the esophagus. For this reason, some veterinarians will feed cotton prior to inducing emesis. The author's preference is to not induce vomiting with foreign material due to the concern for the material lodging in the esophagus.

The treatment most commonly used for recovering gastric FBs if spontaneous passage does not occur is gastrotomy. With linear FBs like strings or abrasive FBs like corn cobs, exploration and gastrotomy should be recommended immediately because they rarely pass without causing obstruction or perforation. The prognosis with a gastric FB is considered very good if there is no evidence of perforation.

Preoperative Considerations

The patient should be optimized for anesthesia and surgery. Prolonged stabilization may be limited if in an emergency setting. Ideally, the patient would be physiologically stable and would be rehydrated, and any acid-base or electrolyte abnormalities would be addressed prior to surgery. A minimum database with a complete blood cell count and diagnostic panel should be performed, along with a urinalysis and coagulation panel depending on the patient. A venous blood gas may also be performed to evaluate for electrolytes and lactate. Electrolyte loss is dependent upon the level of obstruction. With obstructions proximally, gastric fluids rich in potassium (K^+), sodium (Na^+), hydrogen (H^-), and chloride (Cl^-) ions are vomited, and a hypochloremic, hypokalemic, hyponatremic metabolic alkalosis with dehydration may result. Obstructions distal to the bile and pancreatic ducts result in loss of highly alkaline (HCO_3) duodenal, pancreatic, and biliary secretions, and metabolic acidosis usually results from loss of these bicarbonate-rich duodenal contents.

Prophylactic Antimicrobial Use

Prophylactic antibiotics are indicated to reduce the incidence of surgical site infections (SSIs) and are indicated in surgeries with prolonged surgery and anesthesia time and with a risk of contamination, among other factors. In the absence of GI perforation or SP, GI surgery is considered a clean-contaminated procedure with the risk of an SSI of less than 5%. The GI tract contains both Gram-positive (>upper GI) and Gram-negative (>lower GI) organisms. In these cases, the author prefers the use of cefoxitin, a second-generation cephalosporin that covers more anaerobes and Gram-negative bacteria found in the GI tract, in addition to Gram-positive bacteria.

Timing of antimicrobial administration is one of the most important factors when evaluating perioperative antimicrobial prophylaxis. Cephalosporins are time-dependent and well-tolerated, achieve targeted serum and tissue concentrations, are broad-spectrum, have a low incidence of adverse effects, are low cost, and are the preferred prophylactic antimicrobial for most surgical procedures. Dosing regimen should ensure adequate bactericidal drug concentrations are achieved and maintained at the site of invasion before potential contamination and until shortly after completion of surgery. Cefoxitin, similar to cefazolin, should be given at 22 mg/kg IV at induction of general anesthesia (complete administration 30–60 minutes before incision) and repeated every 90 minutes throughout the surgery or up to 12 hours after surgery.

Extended postoperative antibiotics are not indicated unless there is gross GI spillage or the presence of SP causing the surgery to be contaminated, in which case a more broad-spectrum antibiotic, like ampicillin sulbactam (Unasyn), would be preferred with ultimate selection based on culture/susceptibility results.[17] Postoperative antibiotics are not indicated in cases without contamination or SP, as extended use of antibiotics does not prevent infection, and it also contributes to increased antimicrobial resistance.[18] In addition, extended antibiotic use may mask clinical signs of dehiscence, which may delay treatment of SP and cause a more guarded prognosis.

Surgical Procedures

Stomach

The stomach is divided into four parts: the cardia, fundus, body, and pyloric portions. The cardia is located on the left side where the esophagus joins the stomach. The point where the intraabdominal esophagus blends into the stomach on the left side is termed the cardia. The fundus is an expansive sac that is located dorsal and to the left of the cardia. The body of the stomach is the largest part of the stomach and is set between the fundus and the pylorus, which is located on the right side and joins the stomach to the duodenum and is made up of the antrum and pyloric muscular sphincter. The greater curvature of the stomach is convex and is located on the more caudal aspect of the stomach, whereas the lesser curvature is concave and located at the more cranial aspect of the stomach between the dorsal and ventral aspects. Both the greater and lesser curvatures are where the greater and lesser omentum attach.

The celiac artery is a direct branch from the aorta and supplies the arterial blood flow to the stomach. From the celiac artery, there are three branches (splenic, hepatic, and left gastric arteries), each of which provides blood flow to the stomach. The stomach has an excellent redundant blood supply and subsequently great healing. The portal vein provides venous drainage of the stomach via the splenic vein and gastroduodenal vein.

The GI tract is made up of four layers, listed from the internal surface to the external, and consists of the mucosa, submucosa, muscularis, and serosa. The submucosa is the critical holding layer of the GI tract when performing GI surgery.

Gastrotomy Techniques

For any GI surgery, a full abdominal explore should be performed to evaluate the entire GI tract and abdomen, which entails a ventral midline abdominal incision that extends from the xiphoid and caudal to the umbilicus (Figure 22.1). A Balfour retractor (Figure 22.1) may be used as a self-retraining retractor to aid in visualization within the abdomen after the falciform ligament has been removed (Video 22.1). It is important to minimize the risk and consequences of gastric content spillage, and there are a number of important steps to aid in this process. First, separate clean instruments from clean-contaminated instruments. The same instruments used to create the gastrotomy or handle the tissue while the lumen is open should not be used to close the abdomen. Either using clean instruments separated before the procedure or using a new "closing" pack that is opened at the end of the procedure is ideal to reduce contamination. Second, place stay sutures in the stomach to elevate the stomach and

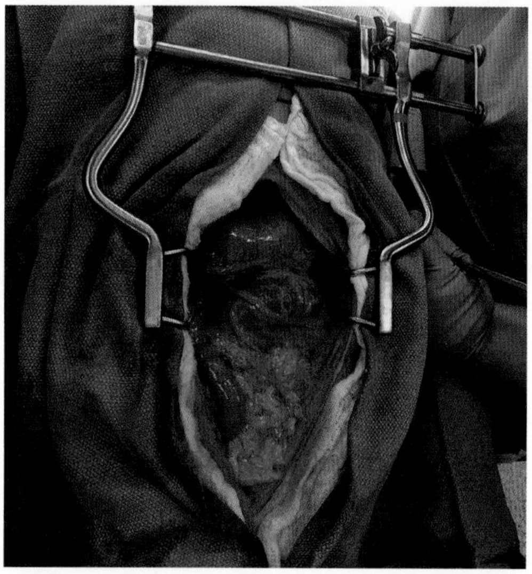

Figure 22.1 Balfour retractor placed after the falciform ligament is removed and prior to an abdominal explore to improve visualization. Top of the image is cranial and bottom of the image is caudal. *Source:* © Penny Regier.

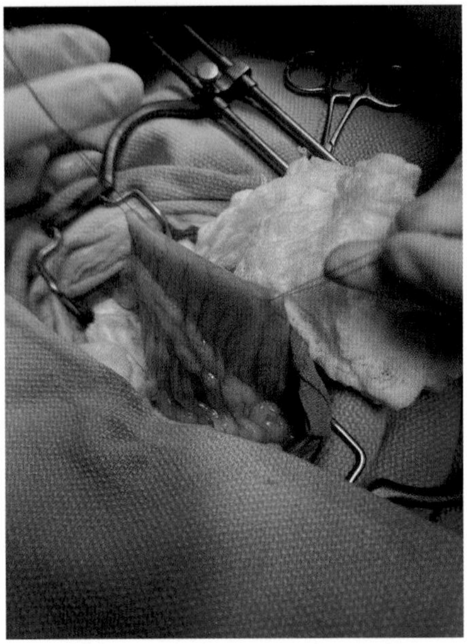

Figure 22.2 Image of pre-placed stay sutures prior to initial gastrotomy incision. Moist laparotomy sponges are placed both cranial and caudal to the stomach to prevent any contamination into the abdomen. A green towel is placed caudally on top of the laparotomy sponge to place any foreign material removed from the stomach and place dirty instruments used during the gastrotomy and foreign body removal. *Source:* © Penny Regier.

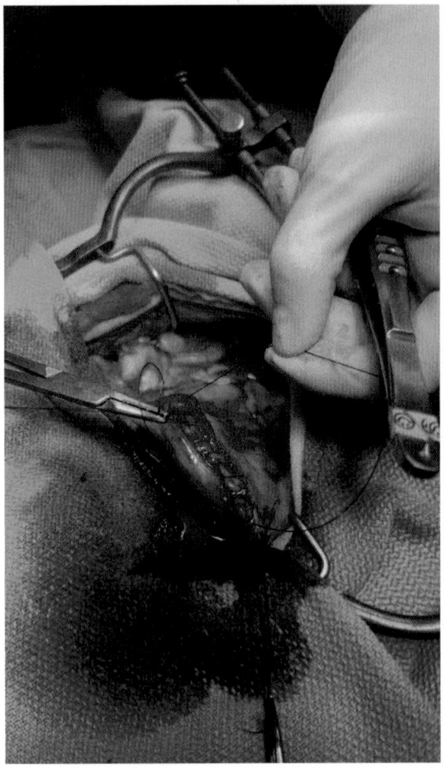

Figure 22.3 Image of gastrotomy while placing final bite of the first layer simple continuous appositional pattern. *Source:* © Penny Regier.

avoid spillage (Figure 22.2, Video 22.2). This entails taking large, full-thickness bites using 2-0 or 3-0 monofilament suture on a taper needle between the lesser and greater curvatures of the stomach on either side of where the intended gastrotomy site will be and elevating the stomach with hemostatic forceps holding the stay sutures. Third, thoroughly pack off the abdomen around the proposed surgical site with moist laparotomy sponges for inadvertent leakage (Figure 22.2) and have suction ready and available with a Poole tip. Lastly, remove contaminated instruments from the surgical field, change surgical gloves when closing, and lavage the abdomen with warm sterile saline. Abdominal lavage should occur with warm sterile saline (98.6–102.2 °F), which will not only aid in removing potential contaminates, but also warm the patient.

The gastrotomy incision should be made on the ventral aspect of the stomach and equidistant between the greater and lesser curvatures in a region with minimal vasculature. The size and exact location of the incision is dependent on the size and location of the foreign material. After the stomach has been packed off and stay sutures elevated and suction prepared, a stab incision is made into the stomach with a #11 blade and extended to the desired length with Metzenbaum scissors (Video 22.3). The area should be packed off with moist laparotomy sponges, and the author places a green towel just caudal to the stomach, so the foreign material can be placed on the towel once removed, along with the dirty instruments to be removed from the surgical field (Video 22.4). There are several techniques to close the stomach after a gastrotomy is performed. Closure may be performed with a single-layer appositional pattern making sure to engage the submucosa, the holding layer, in the closure. The author prefers a double-layer closure with the first layer (Figure 22.3, Video 22.5) being appositional and engaging both the mucosa and submucosa (inner layers of the stomach), and the second layer (Figure 22.4, Video 22.6) being an inverting pattern and engaging the muscularis and serosa (outer two layers of the stomach). Inverting patterns consist of the Cushing (author's preference), Connell, and Lembert patterns. Recommended suture material is a monofilament, synthetic absorbable suture, such as polydioxanone (PDS®; PDS II, Johnson & Johnson Medical, New Brunswick, NJ), glycomer 631 (Biosyn) (Biosyn™, Medtronic, Minneapolis, MN), or poliglecaprone 25 (Monocryl) (Monocryl®, Johnson & Johnson Medical, New Brunswick, NJ) on a taper-point needle. The author prefers 3-0 suture for the stomach unless the patient is a small/toy breed dog or cat, in which case 4-0 suture may be preferred pending stomach thickness. Stapling equipment, such as the thoracoabdominal (TA) (TA™ Single Use Reloadable Staplers, Medtronic, Minneapolis, MN) stapler or gastrointestinal anastomosis (GIA) (GIA™

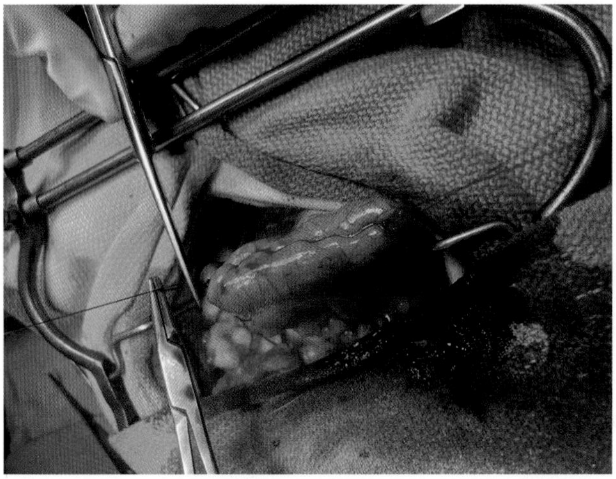

Figure 22.4 Image of gastrotomy after second layer inverting Cushing pattern was performed. Stay sutures intact on either side of the gastrotomy site. *Source:* © Penny Regier.

Single Use Reloadable Staplers, Medtronic, Minneapolis, MN) stapler may be used with partial gastrectomies, which may be indicated with a GDV, and gastric necrosis and will be discussed later with intestinal R&A.

Small Intestine

The small intestine begins with the duodenum, which makes up approximately 10% of the total small intestinal length, begins at the pylorus, and runs caudally in a dorsolateral direction to the right of the midline as the descending duodenum. The mesoduodenum becomes shorter, and at the level of the fifth lumbar vertebra, the duodenum turns medially (caudal duodenal flexure) to the left of the midline in close proximity to the root of the mesentery. The ascending duodenum is closely adhered to the mesocolon by the triangle-shaped duodenocolic ligament. Immediately cranial and to the left of the mesenteric root, the transition to jejunum begins. Unlike the relatively fixed duodenum with its short mesoduodenum and duodenocolic ligament, the jejunum and ileum are loosely coiled and freely moveable because they are suspended from a long mesentery. The jejunum comprises the bulk of the small intestine. A gross division between the jejunum and ileum is difficult to determine, but the terminal contracted portion of the ileum is characterized by prominent antimesenteric vessels. The ileum is attached to the cecum by the ileocecal fold and lies principally to the right of the midline.

The duodenum is supplied by the cranial pancreaticoduodenal off the celiac artery and the caudal pancreaticoduodenal off the cranial mesenteric artery. The jejunum is supplied by several jejunal arteries, which arise from the cranial mesenteric. The ileum is supplied by the ileocolic artery which arises from the cranial mesenteric, both on its mesenteric and antimesenteric surface. The four tissue layers of the intestine from external to internal include serosa, muscularis, submucosa, and mucosa. The muscular coat consists of a relatively thick outer longitudinal layer and a thinner inner circular layer. At the junction of the small and large intestine, this circular muscular layer is grossly thickened becoming the ileocolic sphincter. The submucosa contains the main vascular supply to the bowel wall, known as the submucosal plexus. It is also rich in collagen and is the layer of ***greatest suture-holding capacity***.

Enterotomy Techniques

Similar to a gastrotomy, a full ventral midline abdominal incision should be created with the falciform ligament removed, and a full abdominal explore should be performed (Figure 22.1). The entire GI tract should be explored and palpated for irregularities and foreign material prior to any surgical procedure. Once the foreign material is located, the segment of intestines should be assessed. If the foreign material is located in the duodenum, the author recommends attempting to milk the foreign material orad to the stomach to perform a gastrotomy. If the material cannot be milked to the stomach, the surgeon may attempt to milk the foreign material to the jejunum to perform an enterotomy, or perhaps milk to the colon where it will eventually be defecated. If the material is unable to be milked in either direction or excess trauma is being caused to the tissue from manipulation, a duodenotomy should be performed. Foreign material located in the colon should be able to pass on its own, and a colotomy is not recommended. Once the surgeon has determined where the surgical procedure will occur, the segment of intestine should be packed off with moist laparotomy sponges to prevent contamination.

If the distended segment of intestine is viable, an enterotomy is made. If the tissue has questionable viability, the GI obstruction should first be removed and the intestine assessed for viability prior to determining if a resection needs to be performed. After milking intestinal contents 10 cm to either side of the FB and packing the intestine off from the abdominal cavity with moist laparotomy sponges, the selected bowel is held by the assistant's fingers or with atraumatic Doyen intestinal forceps. A longitudinal incision is made in the antimesenteric border of the intestine in the viable tissue immediately distal or aborad to the FB. The incision is recommended in this distal location because the tissue is healthy and has not been traumatized by the FB passage, which is ideal for healing. The FB is gently delivered through the enterotomy incision, taking care not to tear the incisional margins.

Closure of the enterotomy incision is usually made in a longitudinal fashion. A variety of closure patterns are acceptable. Simple interrupted (Figure 22.5a) or simple continuous (Figure 22.5b) appositional patterns have sutures placed ~3 mm apart and ~3 mm from the cut edge, taking care to incorporate all layers of the intestinal wall. A modified Gambee pattern incorporates the serosa, muscularis, and submucosa but excludes the mucosa and is helpful in reducing mucosal eversion. If a simple continuous layer is performed, it is important to evaluate tension on the line and ensure the tissues are well-apposed prior to tying the end knot (Video 22.7). As each loop is placed for a simple continuous line, a curved mosquito hemostat or the curved needle may be used to gently place each loop and invert any mucosa that may be everting from the enterotomy site (Figure 22.6, Video 22.8a–c). Single-layer enterotomy closures are used because double-layer closures may cause excessive compromise of the lumen diameter. Recommended suture material is a monofilament, synthetic absorbable suture, such as polydioxanone (PDS; PDS II, Johnson & Johnson Medical, New Brunswick, NJ), glycomer 631 (Biosyn) (Biosyn, Medtronic, Minneapolis, MN), or poliglecaprone 25 (Monocryl) (Monocryl, Johnson & Johnson Medical, New Brunswick, NJ) on a taper-point needle with 3-0, 4-0, or 5-0 suture. Chromic surgical gut breaks down rapidly in the stomach because of the acidic environment. Also, surgical gut is not a good choice of suture for use in the colon because of that tissue's slow

(a) (b)

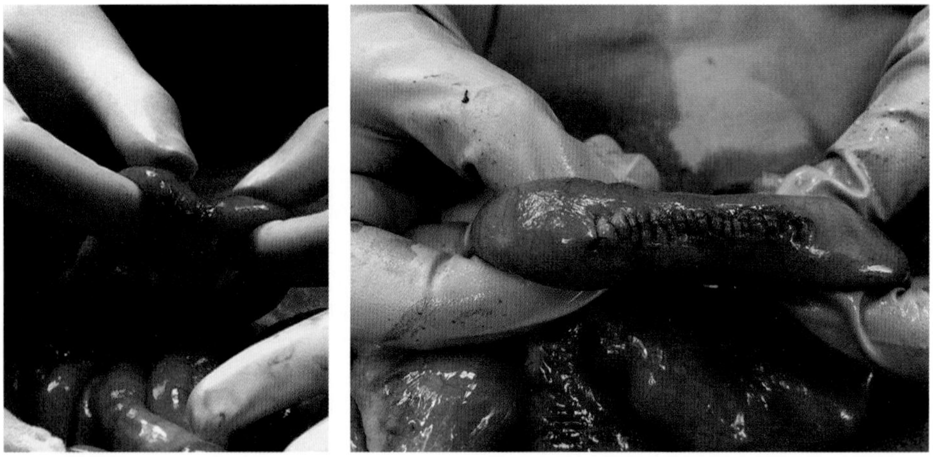

Figure 22.5 Enterotomy closure in the jejunum with a simple interrupted suture pattern (a) and simple continuous pattern (b) with suture bites taken approximately 3 mm from each other and 3 mm from the cut edge of the incision. *Source:* © Penny Regier.

(a) (b)

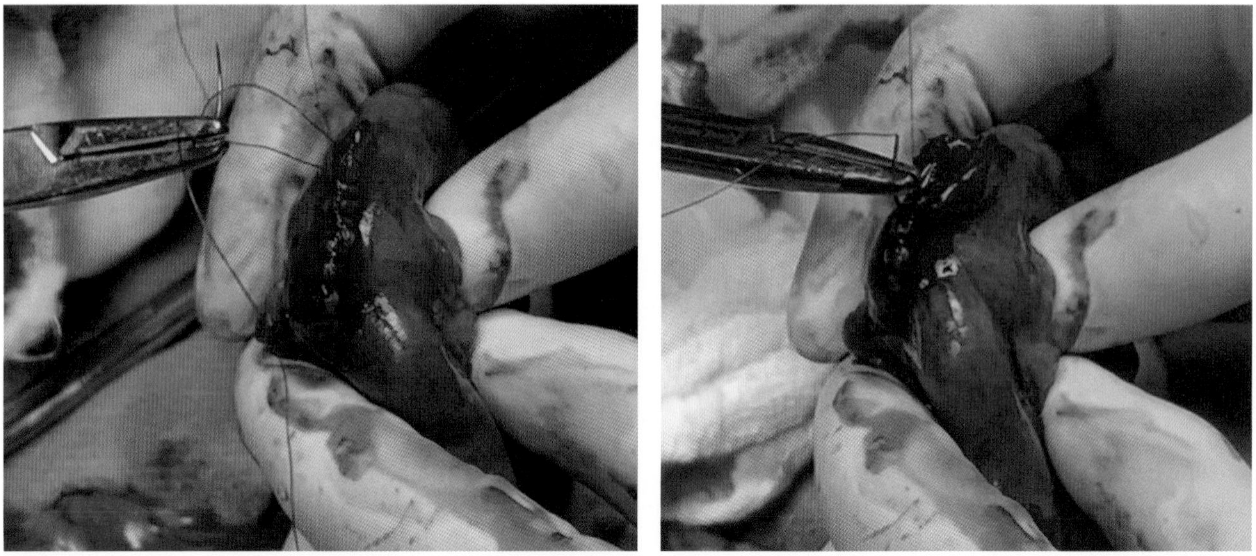

Figure 22.6 (a) Image of taper point needle at end of the suture line being used to gently hook under the suture loop to place loop from simple continuous in the precise location. (b) Image of the same taper point needle being used to place the suture loop over the enterotomy incision and simultaneously using the point of that needle to invert any mucosa everting from the closure. *Source:* © Penny Regier.

healing properties and the presence of collagenase, which may speed tensile strength loss of the suture. Prior to closure of the abdomen, the enterotomy site should be draped in omentum to aid in healing. The greater omentum may simply be draped over top of the surgery site (author's preference) (Video 22.9a) or it may be tacked down over the surgery site with a few simple interrupted sutures (Video 22.9b).

Linear FBs caused by such items as fishing line, sewing yarn, or rope toys present a difficult surgical problem. The trailing end of string FBs often catches over the base of the tongue or in the stomach and acts as an anchor. Intestinal peristalsis moves the FB aborally resulting in bowel plication (Figure 22.7). The string often embeds itself in the mesenteric mucosa and can cause necrosis of the tissue and potentially cut through the wall on the mesenteric border, resulting in peritonitis (Figure 22.8). Linear FBs should be managed by initially identifying and releasing the anchor point. If wrapped around the tongue, the FB should be released prior to laparotomy. More commonly, a gastrotomy is necessary to free the foreign material from its gastropyloric anchor. Multiple enterotomies are then usually required to facilitate the complete removal of the FB. If too few enterotomies are made with too much traction placed on the string, the mesenteric border may be perforated in an area that is difficult to explore and suture. Occasionally, the string has cut through at several locations, and peritonitis is evident. Sometimes, in long-standing cases, fibrosis has occurred around the FB so that even after its removal, the bowel retains its pleated conformation. In these cases, intestinal R&A may be necessary. Alternatively, the string can be removed by attaching it to a red rubber catheter and pushing it aborally to disengage it from the bowel wall. If successful, the string can sometimes be removed with a single enterotomy (Figure 22.9, Video 22.10a,b).

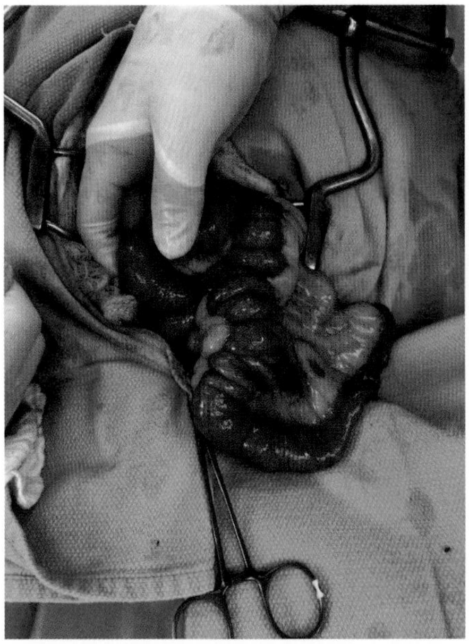

Figure 22.7 Image of a linear foreign body causing plication of the small intestines. *Source:* © Penny Regier.

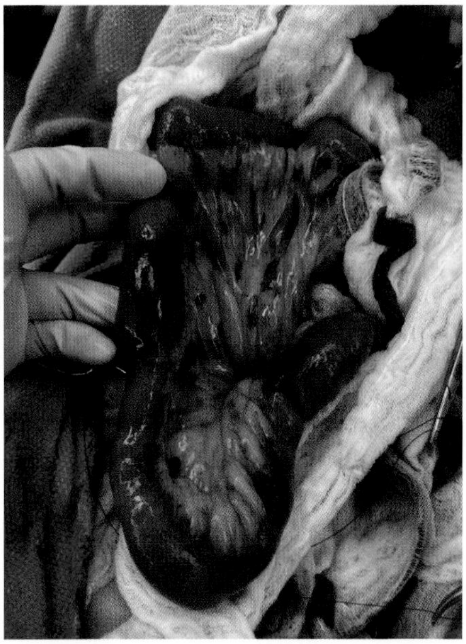

Figure 22.8 Image of necrotic bowel along mesenteric border from previous linear foreign body plication causing necrosis. *Source:* © Penny Regier.

Assessing Tissue Viability

With complete obstruction, intestinal distention is often severe, and the distended loops of bowel take on a cyanotic appearance. Intestinal viability is best evaluated after (1) decompression of dilated loops of intestine and (2) removal of the FB. If intestinal wall ischemia and necrosis (Figure 22.10) are present, then R&A is performed immediately. However, in most cases of simple

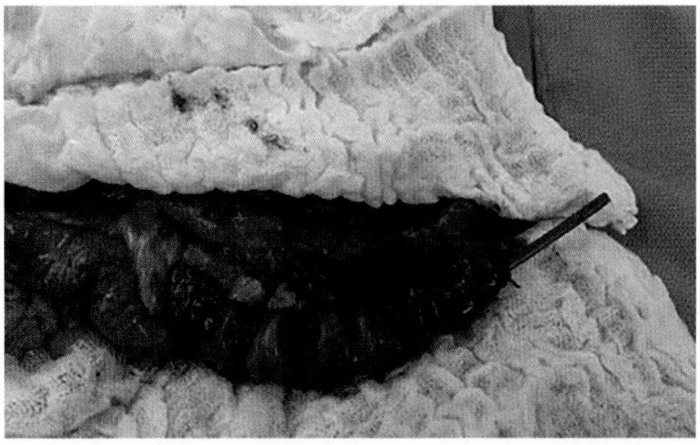

Figure 22.9 Image of red rubber catheter technique being used to remove linear foreign body embedded in the intestinal mucosa through a single enterotomy. *Source:* © Penny Regier.

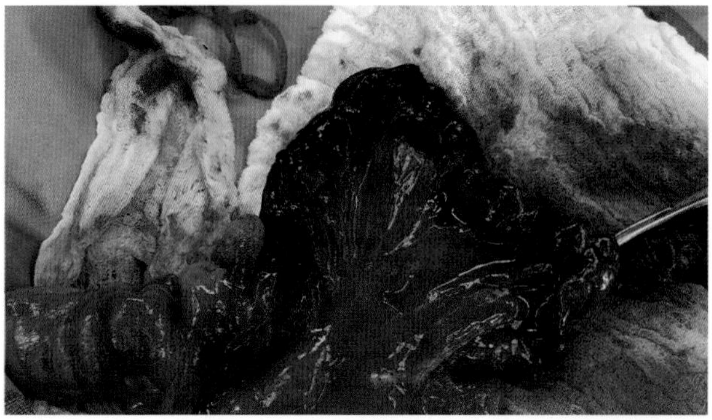

Figure 22.10 Image of necrotic bowel after manual reduction of an intussusception. *Source:* © Penny Regier.

non-strangulated obstruction, bowel viability is maintained, and the visual appearance of dark distended loops of bowel improves rapidly after removal of the obstruction.

Standard clinical subjective criteria for establishing intestinal viability are color (palor) (Figure 22.10), arterial pulsations (Video 22.11), thickness (palpation), and the presence of peristalsis, the four Ps. Of these parameters, experimental data has shown peristalsis to be the best and most dependable determinant of viability, although depending on the severity and chronicity of the obstruction, the intestines may have severe ileus. The "pinch test" should be performed on questionable bowel to determine if smooth muscle contraction and peristalsis can be initiated.

Intestinal Resection and Anastomosis

Intestinal R&A is a common procedure performed in small animal surgery in order to remove non-viable or diseased intestines with a reported incidence of dehiscence between 3% and 28%.[7–10] Currently, anastomoses in small animals are commonly performed with either a traditional hand-sewn technique or surgical stapling device.

When the bowel is devitalized, R&A is necessary. The mesenteric vessels to the affected bowel are isolated and ligated between ligatures (Video 22.12). The arcuate vessels located along the mesenteric boundary are then ligated. Alternatively, a small handheld vessel sealing device that both cauterizes and cuts is an option and decreases surgical time (Video 22.12). At least 1.5 cm of viable tissue is included in the proximal and distal boundaries of the devitalized tissue to be removed. Intestinal contents are milked proximally and distally and held by an assistant's fingers or with Doyen intestinal forceps to reduce the risk of spillage and contamination. Carmalt or other crushing clamps are placed in the area of intestine to be resected at an ~45° angle away from the long axis of the intestine (if lumen size needs to be increased at one end) or placed straight across the intestines (if there is no need to increase lumen size) (Figure 22.11a). A scalpel blade is used to excise the bowel along the outside of the crushing clamp (Video 22.13). The mesentery is then transected, and the excised bowel is removed from the surgical field. Up to 80% resection of the small intestine is consistent with quality of life. Resections greater than 75–80% may result in weight loss, cachexia, hypoproteinemia, and chronic diarrhca from short bowel syndrome.[19–21] The author also recommends avoiding resection of the ileocecocolic junction if possible, as resection will result in long-term diarrhea.

Differences in luminal diameter sometimes make end-to-end anastomosis difficult. The lumen diameter of the smaller segment can be enlarged by (1) cutting the tissue back at a more acute angle as discussed above, (2) making

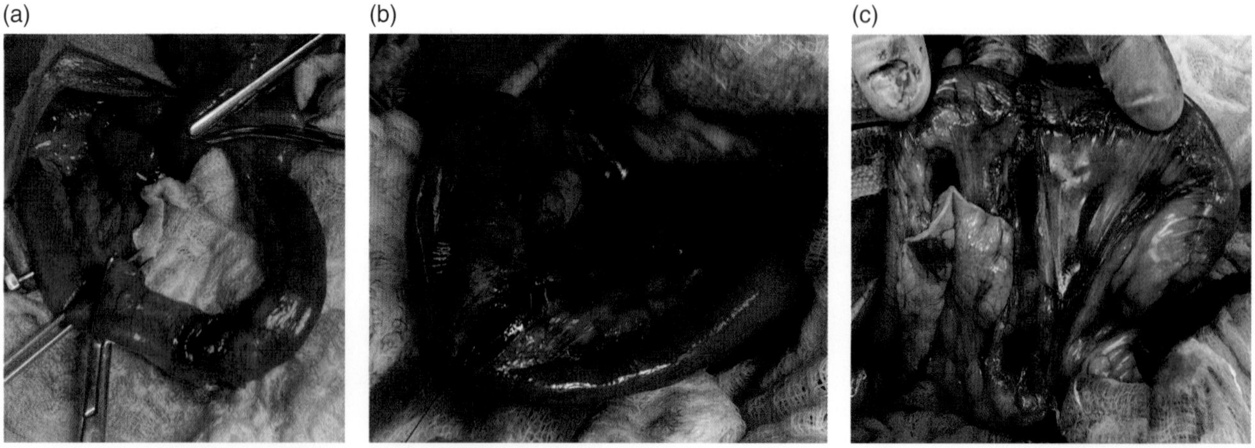

Figure 22.11 Intestinal handsewn resection and anastomosis. (a) Resection of small intestinal lesion with the mesentery removed from the mesenteric border of the segment of bowel being resected. Carmalt forceps are placed on the segment of bowel being excised and Doyen forceps are placed on the segment of bowel being anastomosed. (b) Handsewn anastomosis with two simple continuous suture patterns with one strand of 4-0 Biosyn (or other short-term absorbable monofilament) suture placed on the mesenteric border and a second strand of the suture placed on the antimesenteric border. (c) Final image of a simple continuous handsewn anastomosis with two strands of suture and prior to closure of the mesenteric rent. *Source:* © Penny Regier.

a longitudinal incision along the antimesenteric border creating a spatulated opening, or (3) "fudging" the suture placement and placing the sutures farther apart on the larger lumen side and closer together on the smaller lumen size for cases of mild lumen disparity.

A variety of suture patterns have been used successfully for end-to-end intestinal anastomosis in the small animal patient; currently, approximating patterns are recommended. Properly performed approximating patterns (1) create an increased lumen diameter when compared to everting or inverting patterns, (2) give rapid and precise primary intestinal healing, and (3) minimize the potential for postoperative adhesion formation. Everting anastomosis is not recommended due to narrowing and stenosis of the lumen, as well as delayed mucosal healing, prolonged inflammatory response, and increased adhesion formation. Inverting anastomoses have the advantage of a more leak-resistant serosa approximation but decreases the lumen diameter. Inflammation is more severe and the healing time of inverting patterns is delayed when compared to approximating techniques. Despite these disadvantages, inverting techniques may be considered for use in colonic R&A where the high bacterial content of feces makes leakage of the anastomosis extremely dangerous.

Simple interrupted approximating and simple continuous techniques are the most commonly used techniques for approximating end-to-end anastomosis. Eversion of mucosa from the bowel edge can be overcome by incising the mucosa with Metzenbaum scissors or by using a modified Gambee suture pattern. Regardless of the suture technique used, it is critical to secure the submucosa, which is the layer of greatest strength. The author recommends using a simple interrupted or simple continuous approximating anastomosis for handsewn R&A's.

Simple interrupted and continuous patterns can be performed by taking bites through all layers of the intestinal wall, approximately 3 mm from the tissue edge and 3 mm apart, with extraluminal knots. By engaging slightly more serosa than mucosa, the everted mucosal edge is forced back into the lumen using either a curved mosquito hemostat or the end of a curved needle. To place a modified Gambee suture, the needle is inserted through the serosa 3 mm from the edge of the incision and is passed through the muscularis and submucosa. Resistance is felt as the needle penetrates the collagen-dense submucosa. The needle is then directed toward the cut surface, so as to emerge at the junction of the submucosa and mucosa and pulled through. The needle is inserted into the second intestinal end at the mucosa–submucosa junction and passed through the submucosa, muscularis, and serosa in an arc to exit 3 mm from the cut surface. The suture is pulled just taut enough to appose tissues; if the suture is pulled too tightly, it will cut through the muscularis. The modified Gambee pattern works well to provide adequate submucosal apposition while inverting the mucosa. The Gambee suture depends on correct identification and inclusion of submucosa in each bite; inexperienced surgeons may be more likely to miss the submucosa, resulting in suboptimal leak pressures. A simple full-thickness closure pattern is therefore the preferred choice for enteric closure among novice and infrequent surgeons. The amount of force applied to the knot is decided by the surgeon and is based on surgeon experience, stretch of the suture, and deformation of tissue. The rule of thumb is that tissues should be well-apposed without being crushed. Poor apposition results in healing by second intention, which is not ideal, but overcompensation by crushing tissues between the sutures inhibits angiogenesis and impedes healing as well.

Simple interrupted – The anastomosis (Figure 22.12, Video 22.14a–c) begins at the mesenteric border with one to three interrupted sutures, because the presence of fat in this area makes suture placement most difficult and leakage is most likely to occur. A second suture is placed on the antimesenteric border with the third and fourth sutures placed at the 90° quadrants, respectively. Several more sutures are placed between each of the four quadrant sutures at ~3 mm intervals.

Simple continuous – The anastomosis consists of two separate lines of suture (Figure 22.11b,c). The first suture strand is placed beginning at the mesenteric border because the presence of fat in this area makes suture placement most difficult and leakage is most likely to occur, and the suture tag after tying the knot is held with a hemostat to provide a tag to which the other strand will be tied. A second suture strand is placed on the antimesenteric border. Each suture strand completes half the anastomosis with a simple continuous pattern to meet the other line of suture. These suture strands may be tied separately or may be tied to the suture tag of the opposite line. Often, the author will place an additional two simple interrupted sutures at the mesenteric border.

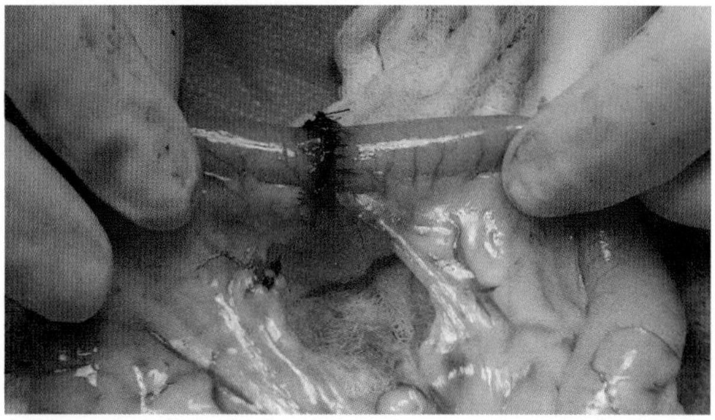

Figure 22.12 Handsewn resection and anastomosis with simple interrupted sutures prior to closure of the mesentery. *Source:* © Penny Regier.

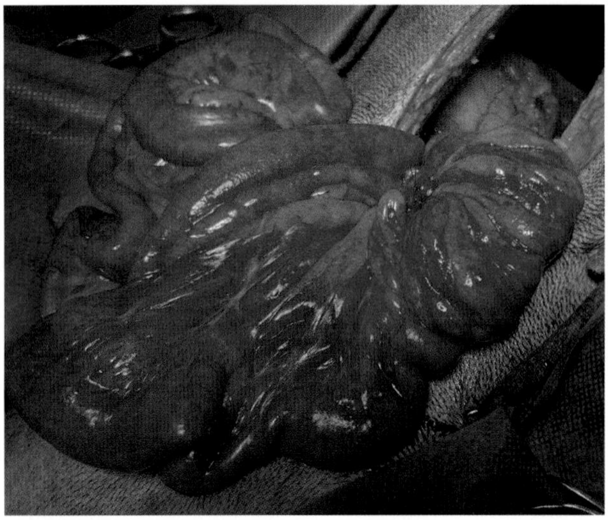

Figure 22.13 Omental wrap placed and tacked down over a FEESA site. *Source:* © Penny Regier.

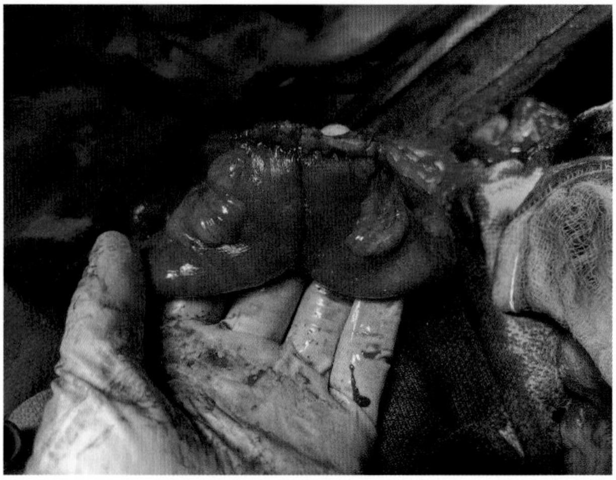

Figure 22.14 Functional end-to-end stapled anastomosis (FEESA). Image of FEESA created with a GIA™ stapler for the vertical staple line and a TA™ stapler for the transverse staple line. *Source:* © Penny Regier.

Recommended suture material is a monofilament, synthetic absorbable suture such as polydioxanone (PDS; PDS II, Johnson & Johnson Medical, New Brunswick, NJ), glycomer 631 (Biosyn) (Biosyn, Medtronic, Minneapolis, MN), or poliglecaprone 25 (Monocryl) (Monocryl, Johnson & Johnson Medical, New Brunswick, NJ) on a taper-point needle with 3-0 or 4-0 suture. After the anastomosis has been completed, the mesenteric defect (Figure 22.11c) is closed with a simple continuous pattern taking care not to include the mesenteric vessels within the sutures. The anastomosis is then covered with a pedicle of greater omentum (Figure 22.13). The omentum with its abundant vascular and lymphatic supply is critical to the successful healing of the intestinal wounds, especially in patients with peritonitis.[22–24] A serosal patch[25] can also be created by suturing an adjacent, healthy intestinal loop over the defect or suture line with simple continuous or interrupted sutures. Serosal patches are not commonly performed, and care should be taken to not create a tight hairpin turn with the intestinal loops, which may create a future site for obstruction.

Stapling Techniques

In addition to a handsewn end-to-end anastomosis, the most commonly used stapling technique used to perform an anastomosis is a functional end-to-end stapled anastomosis (FEESA) using a linear cutting GIA™ stapler for the vertical staple line and a TA™ stapler for the transverse staple line (Figure 22.14). Modifications to this technique, including the use of a GIA™ stapler for the transverse staple line,[26] which obviates the need to utilize more than one stapler type, or oversewing of the TA™ staple line with suture, which facilitates inversion of the everted TA™ staple line, have been described.[27–30] Each limb of the GIA™ stapler is placed within the lumen of the intestines both orally and aborally, and the antimesenteric borders are pressed together (Figure 22.15a, Video 22.15). The linear cutting GIA™ is then used to simultaneously staple and cut, creating three rows of staples on either side of the newly created lumen (Figure 22.15b). Next, the linear staple lines should be offset,[31] and either the GIA™ (three rows of staples) or a TA™ (two rows of staples) stapler can be used to seal off the remaining opening and create the transverse staple line (Figure 22.16). Placement of a crotch suture (Figure 22.17, Video 22.16a,b) is recommended to control tension and prevent separation of apposed jejunal limbs to increase leakage pressures or reduce tension.[32,33] The TA™ staple line has been identified as the most common site of dehiscence or leakage, so reinforcement of the transverse staple line with an oversewn pattern (Figures 22.18 and 22.19, Video 22.17) may be warranted. Also, as with any surgical procedure in the GI tract, an omental wrap is recommended over the R&A site to aid in healing (Video 22.18). Recent studies have shown a decreased rate of dehiscence with oversewn FEESAs compared to non-oversewn,[27] as well as increased leak pressures when using an inverting Cushing pattern.[28–30]

Staple size selection – The staples utilized by the GIA™ and TA™ stapler are color-coded based on staple size. The use of intestinal stapling is limited in application due to fixed staple heights. Too small of a staple size may result in compression of the microvasculature in the intestinal wall or failure to engage the submucosa, whereas too large of a staple may fail to create leak-resistant apposition of the intestinal ends. These limitations must be considered when utilizing surgical staples in addition to their purported benefits of reduced

(a) (b)

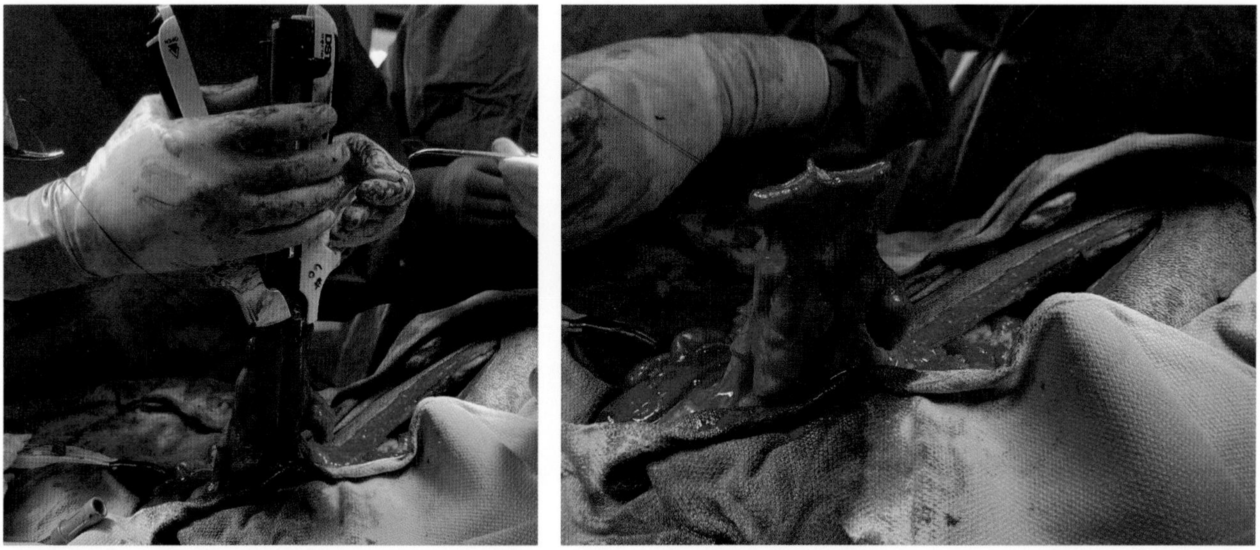

Figure 22.15 (a) GIA™ stapler limb placed at each end of the small intestine loops with the antimesenteric border serosa placed between the two limbs of the stapler and the mesenteric border facing outward. (b) Vertical staple line created by GIA™ stapler for FEESA. *Source:* © Penny Regier.

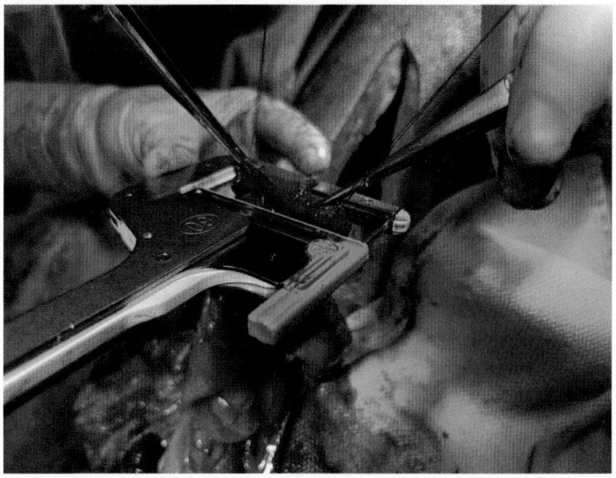

Figure 22.16 TA™ stapler with green cartridge being used to seal transverse staple line of FEESA. DeBakey forceps being used to offset the vertical staple line prior to closure of the TA™ staple device. *Source:* © Penny Regier.

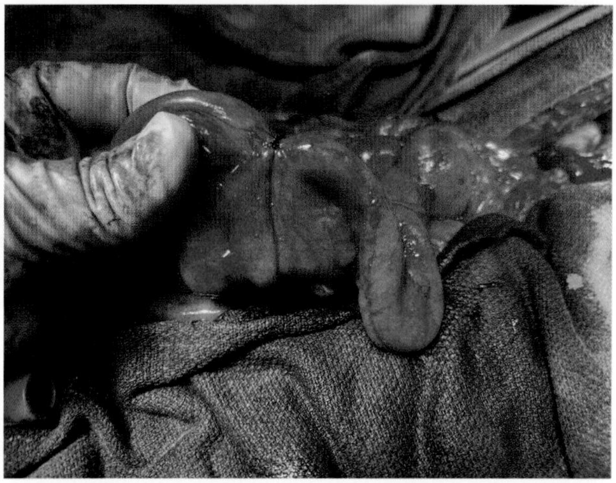

Figure 22.17 Two interrupted sutures placed at the crotch of FEESA to help relieve tension at the anastomosis site. *Source:* © Penny Regier.

surgical time, ability to address lumen disparity, decreased need for tissue handling, and ease of use for the novice surgeon.[7,29,34–36] The surgical stapling devices (TA™ and GIA™) and staple sizes presently used in small animals for FEESAs have been adopted from human medicine. Guidelines for their use in veterinary medicine were directly translated from man without formal investigation into differences in intestinal thickness, vascularity, and surgical indications in our small animal patients. For this reason, blue staple cartridges, with a closed staple height of 1.5 mm, were historically used in veterinary medicine, with reservation of the larger green staples (closed staple height of 2.0 mm) for gastric surgery. It has recently been reported that canine small intestinal thickness ranges between 2.06 and 3.13 mm in healthy dogs, which is thicker than human intestines (mean mural thickness of 1.5 mm), indicating that green staple cartridges with a closed staple height of 2.0 mm may be indicated.[29] The author routinely uses green staple cartridges when performing FEESA in small animal patients.

Handsewn Versus Stapled Anastomosis

Surgeon preference, equipment availability, patient intestinal size, and location of the intestinal resection

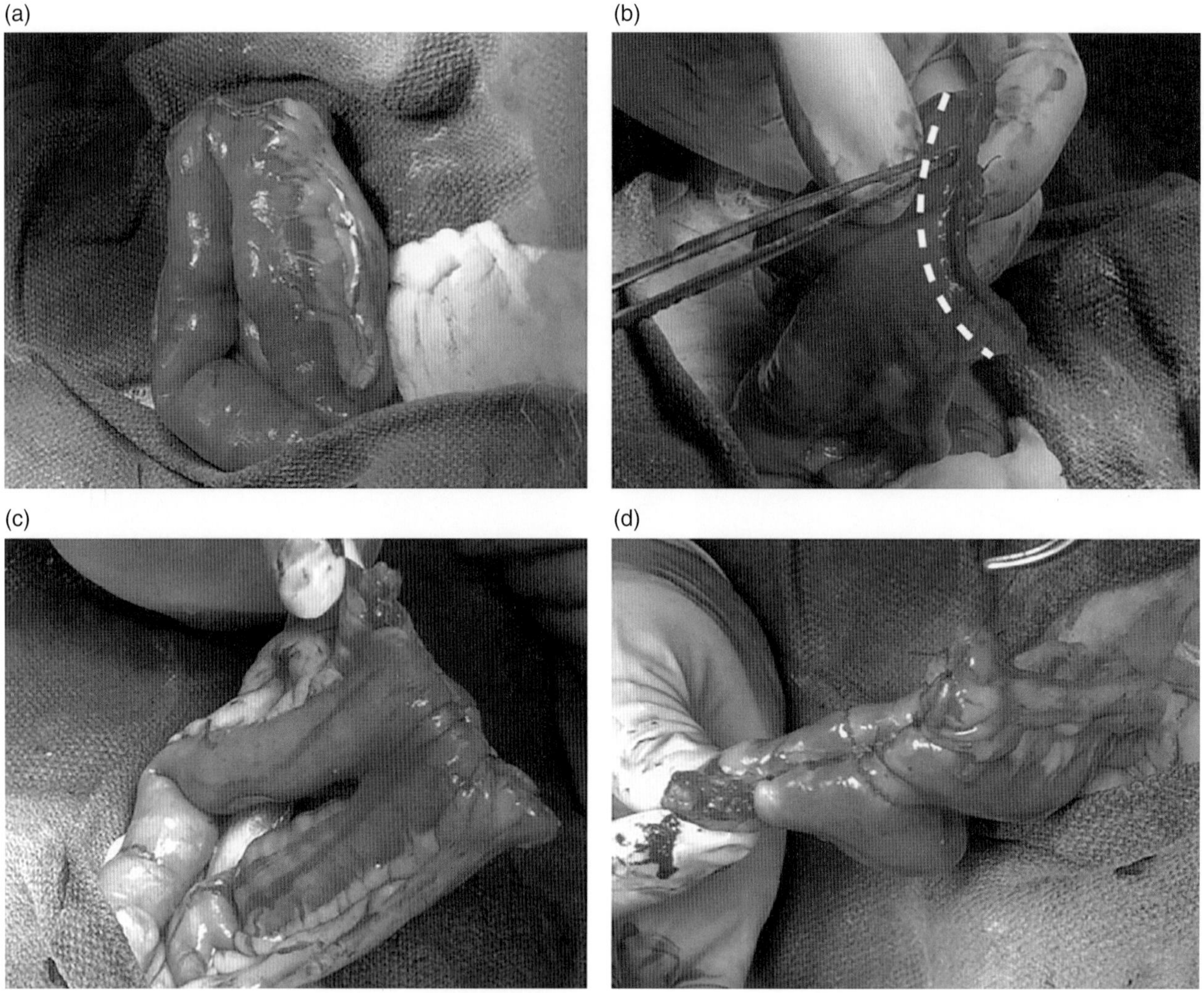

Figure 22.18 Oversewing a FEESA. After completion of the stapled anastomosis (a), the transverse staple line was oversewn along the white dashed line (b) to invert the transverse staple line (c,d). *Source:* © Penny Regier.

often dictate whether a handsewn anastomosis or stapled anastomosis is performed. Studies have shown that both handsewn and FEESA have similar dehiscence rates[7] and similar leak pressures.[29] Stapled anastomoses or FEESAs have been shown to have faster surgical times[7,29] when compared to handsewn anastomoses, and they may be preferred to address luminal disparity.[35,36] Most recently, FEESAs have been shown to have decreased dehiscence rates in the face of preoperative SP.[37,38] Literature in human medicine has shown that handsewn anastomoses have decreased dehiscence rates when compared to stapled anastomoses in trauma patients, which is likely attributed to intestinal edema and fixed staple heights.[39,40] Therefore, the author recommends considering factors such as preoperative SP, intestinal wall edema, patient stability, and other intraoperative factors when deciding whether to perform a handsewn or stapled anastomosis.

Gastrointestinal Biopsies

When full-thickness intestinal biopsy samples are needed for histopathologic evaluation, an elliptical incision is made in the antimesenteric border of the bowel. With a longitudinal incision with a longitudinal closure, there is no tension on the suture line, but it may reduce the lumen diameter. With a longitudinal incision with a transverse closure, there is more tension on the suture line than with other techniques, but it maintains lumen diameter. With the transverse biopsy technique, a full-thickness wedge of tissue (~3–4 mm × 1–2 mm) is removed by incising transversely with a #11 or #15 scalpel blade. The defect is closed with interrupted sutures. This permits removal of a small wedge of tissue without damage by thumb forceps, and the transverse orientation prevents bowel stenosis. The author's preference is to do a punch biopsy technique (Figure 22.20a, Video 22.19) using either a 4- or 6-mm skin punch biopsy instrument depending on the size of the bowel and a sterile

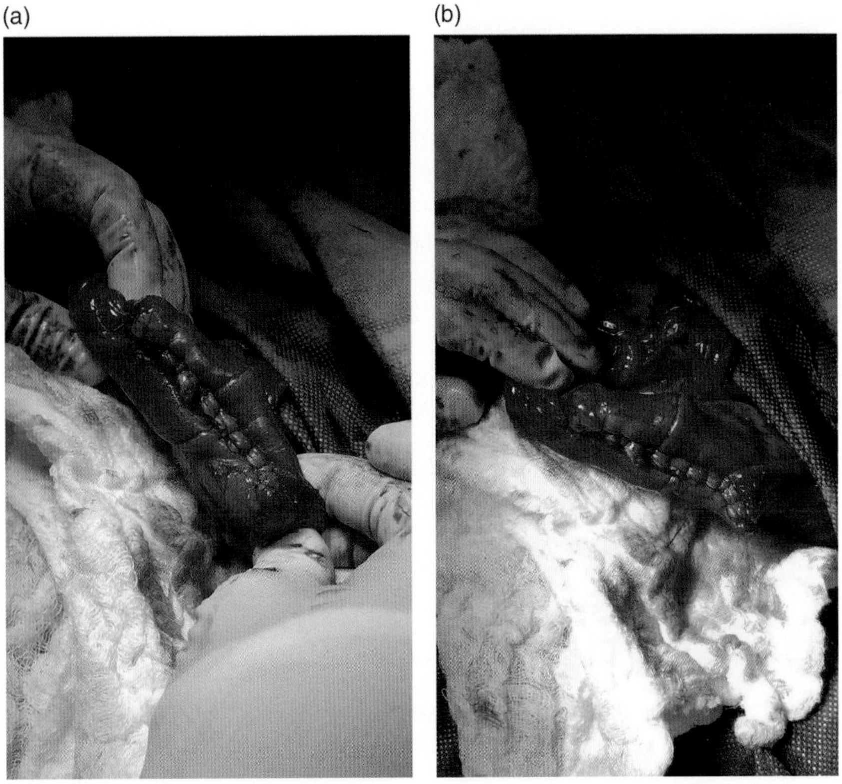

Figure 22.19 (a, b) Images of oversewn FEESA with a Cushing pattern over the transverse staple line to reduce the risk of postoperative dehiscence.
Source: © Penny Regier.

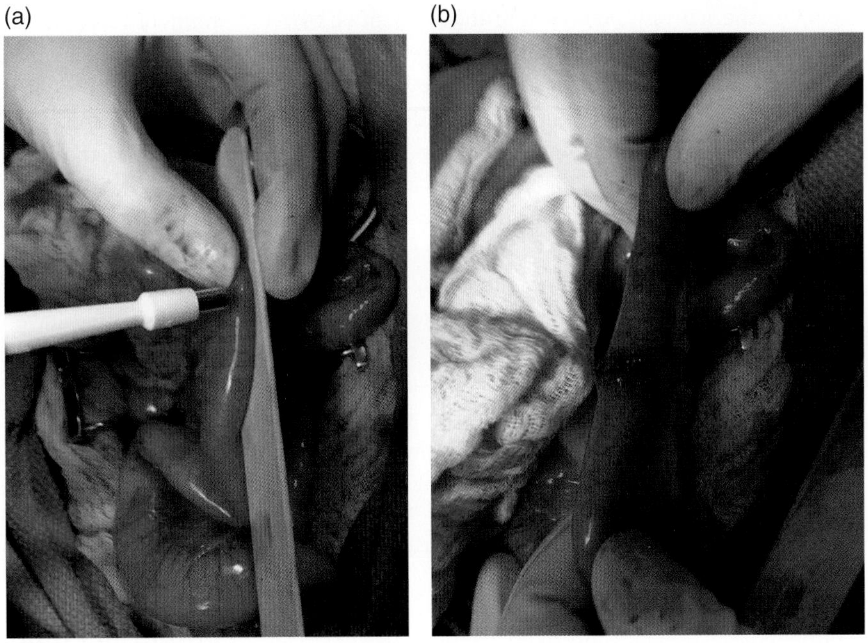

Figure 22.20 (a) GI punch biopsy technique using a sterile tongue depressor and a 4 mm punch to take a full-thickness biopsy on the antimesenteric border of the small intestine. (b) GI punch biopsy site closure with 4-0 Biosyn™ using a simple interrupted pattern.
Source: © Penny Regier.

wooden tongue depressor. With this technique, the surgeon places the antimesenteric border of the bowel against the tongue depressor and pushes the punch biopsy instrument down full thickness into the antimesenteric margin. The punch biopsy site is then closed transversely with simple interrupted sutures (Figure 22.20b). The surgeon should inspect each biopsy sample to ensure that all intestinal layers are represented, particularly mucosa.

Leak Testing

The intraoperative leak test is often recommended to assess security of enteric suture lines, identify imperfections in closure technique, and prevent postoperative leakage.[41] One method to perform a leak test is to simply milk the intestinal contents to the suture line and observe for leakage at the surgery site. This may be challenging if the bowel

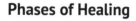

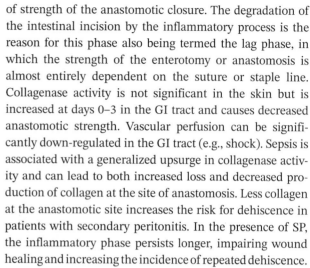

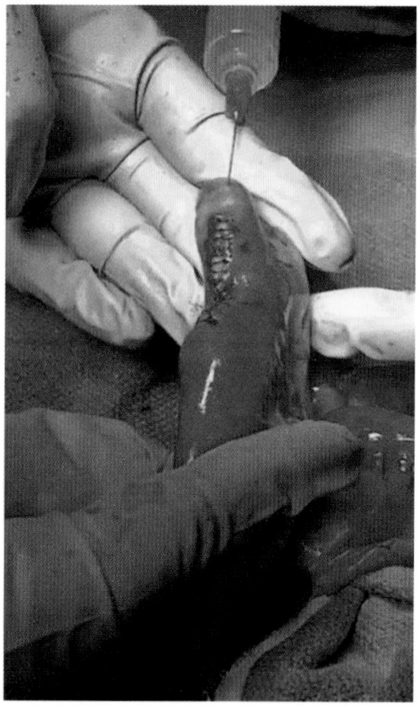

Figure 22.21 Image of leak testing being performed to assess enterotomy closure and evaluate surgical site for signs of leakage. *Source:* © Penny Regier.

is empty. Alternatively, both ends of the segment of bowel may be occluded with either digital pressure or Doyen forceps and saline injected into the lumen of bowel with a needle attached to a syringe (Figure 22.21, Video 22.20). The segment can be gently manipulated while observing the incision line for any leaks. All anastomoses can be made to leak with sufficient pressure. Traditionally, the leak test should be performed with a 22–25 gauge needle and 12 cc syringe holding an approximately 10 cm loop of bowel with Doyen forceps or fingers and injecting approximately 10 mL of water, known as the "rule of 10s." It is important to remember, however, that all incisions will leak with enough force. Alternatively, a curved hemostat can also be used to gently probe along the incision line and evaluate for defects (Video 22.21), which is the author's preference.[42]

Phases of Healing

Full-thickness wound healing in the GI tract begins with an inflammatory phase (lag phase), similar to that of cutaneous wound healing, and occurs at days 0–3. Neutrophils (first 24 hours) and macrophages (>48 hours) are predominant, and the wound is held together by sutures. Almost all leakages occur during this time. Strength of the anastomoses throughout the GI tract decreases significantly in the first 48 hours after surgery. Collagen breakdown secondary to collagenase activity within the wound occurs in the first one to two days of the healing process and results in net loss of strength of the anastomotic closure. The degradation of the intestinal incision by the inflammatory process is the reason for this phase also being termed the lag phase, in which the strength of the enterotomy or anastomosis is almost entirely dependent on the suture or staple line. Collagenase activity is not significant in the skin but is increased at days 0–3 in the GI tract and causes decreased anastomotic strength. Vascular perfusion can be significantly down-regulated in the GI tract (e.g., shock). Sepsis is associated with a generalized upsurge in collagenase activity and can lead to both increased loss and decreased production of collagen at the site of anastomosis. Less collagen at the anastomotic site increases the risk for dehiscence in patients with secondary peritonitis. In the presence of SP, the inflammatory phase persists longer, impairing wound healing and increasing the incidence of repeated dehiscence.

The inflammatory response begins to subside and cellular proliferation characteristic of the proliferative phase becomes the predominant process for up to two weeks postoperatively. During this phase, there is a rapid increase in anastomotic strength characterized by fibroblast proliferation, angiogenesis, contraction, and epithelialization. During this time, the suture or staple line reinforcement is less important. For this reason, if absorbable sutures or staples are to be used, the suture should possess adequate tensile strength for a minimum of two to three weeks, as in polydioxanone (PDS; PDS II, Johnson & Johnson Medical, New Brunswick, NJ), glycomer 631 (Biosyn) (Biosyn, Medtronic, Minneapolis, MN), or poliglecaprone 25 (Monocryl) (Monocryl, Johnson & Johnson Medical, New Brunswick, NJ), which maintain 80% and 50% tensile strength at two weeks, respectively. The final phase of healing, the maturation phase, can persist for up to six months postoperatively and is responsible for strengthening of the wound and providing a robust physical barrier.

Factors that have an effect on intestinal wound healing consist of the etiology of obstruction (FBs cause more intestinal leakages than neoplasia), failure to adequately identify ischemic tissue, improper suturing or stapling, sepsis, malnutrition, and antineoplastic therapy. Sepsis mortality is reported in up to 50–70% of cases; sepsis reduces the effect of omentum, increases collagenase at wound site, and causes protein loss and a catabolic state.[43,44]

Potential Complications

Dehiscence is a potentially life-threatening complication of GI surgery that leads to SP and requires surgical intervention. R&A, necessitated due to an intestinal FB obstruction, is associated with a high rate of postoperative dehiscence reported upwards of 28% with mortality rates over 85%. In comparison, when not associated with FB obstruction, the dehiscence rates following an enterotomy or R&A have been reported to be 0–12% with postoperative mortality rates of 0–7%.[4,6,8–10,26,31,37,38,45–51] It is believed that the increased morbidity and mortality associated with surgery for FB obstructions is due to our inability to reliably assess the viability of traumatized intestine intraoperatively or due to compromise of the vascular supply to the anastomotic edges by our presently employed anastomosis techniques. Dehiscence may be due not only to preoperative risk factors (i.e., preoperative SP, hypoalbuminemia, and surgical indication) but also to intraoperative risk factors (i.e., surgical technique, hypotension, and anastomotic reinforcement), patient-dependent risk factors (i.e., pre-existing systemic disease and medications), and intestine-dependent risk factors (i.e., vascularity, pre-existing inflammatory or neoplastic disease, and compliance to distension).[4,8–10]

SP is a challenging condition that requires rapid diagnosis and therapeutic intervention to maximize the chance of a successful outcome. The condition is most commonly secondary to compromise or rupture of a hollow viscera, and in dogs, it is frequently associated with GI FBs, neoplasia, and administration of medications such as nonsteroidal anti-inflammatory drugs. The peritoneal cavity has a very large surface area and is highly absorptive. Consequently, many deleterious substances, such as endotoxins and free radicals, are readily and efficiently absorbed into the systemic circulation. The result of which is disruption of normal physiologic processes, organ dysfunction/failure, and ultimately death in many cases. There are two major requirements of the veterinarian who is treating a patient with SP: (1) rapid resuscitation and appropriate antimicrobial administration and (2) rapid decontamination and source control. Unfortunately, despite aggressive and accurate intervention, SP is associated with a guarded prognosis.

SP after small intestinal surgery is most commonly associated with dehiscence of anastomotic or enterotomy sites, which is reported to occur in 7–16% of patients.[7–10,26,37,38,52,53] The reported incidence of dehiscence after full-thickness small intestinal biopsy is up to 12%, which is similar to enterotomy and anastomosis.[54,55] Hypoalbuminemia, hypotension, use of blood products, longer length of bowel resected, and delayed enteral feeding postoperatively are all likely important predictors of leakage for anastomoses or enterotomies with the role of intestinal FBs being a possibility as well. Also, the presence of preoperative SP is well-described as an important risk factor for GI leakage and ongoing sepsis with increased mortality.

Ileus is a common complication after surgery and is not only due to obstruction of the GI tract but also caused by manipulation of the GI tract, long operative time, and extensive resection. Ileus can cause postoperative clinical signs such as abdominal pain, regurgitation, vomiting, or abdominal distention from fluid and gas accumulation.

Other potential complications with GI surgery include pancreatitis, hypoalbuminemia, and aspiration pneumonia. Also, important complications to note would include SSIs (Figure 22.22), adhesions (Figure 22.23) that may cause extraluminal narrowing of the GI tract and subsequent obstruction, and short bowel syndrome if over ~75% of the small intestine are removed, especially the distal small intestine or ileocecal junction.

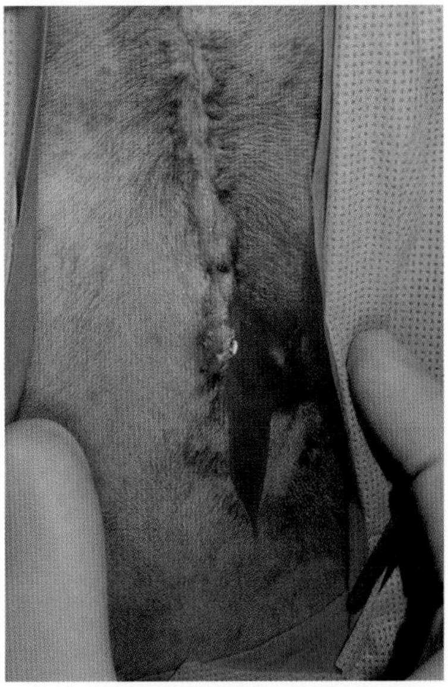

Figure 22.22 Surgical site infection noted with purulent material from the incision and treated with open wound management and oral antibiotics. *Source:* © Penny Regier.

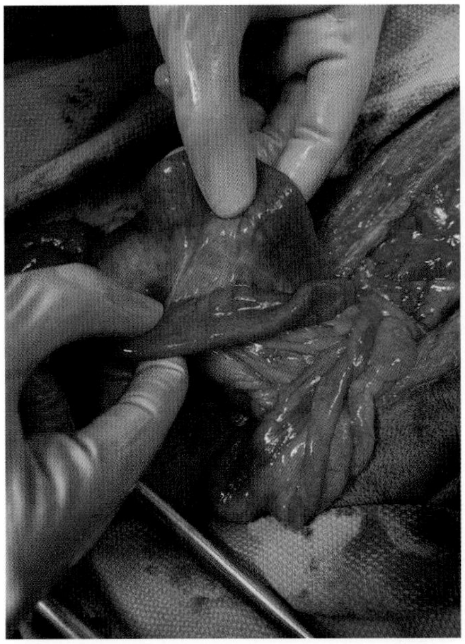

Figure 22.23 Jejunal adhesions noted intraoperatively during an abdominal explore for a GI foreign body obstruction. *Source:* © Penny Regier.

Postoperative Care and Prognosis

Enteral nutrition is vital for GI health and healing. Feeding may begin 6–12 hours after surgery once the patient is fully recovered from anesthesia and able to eat on its own.

Nasoesophageal (NE) feeding may be considered for animals that are too debilitated to undergo anesthesia for placement of other types of feeding tubes or may need short-term nutritional support. NE tubes are easy to place and well-tolerated by most animals. The author prefers placement of nasogastric (NG) tubes (Figure 22.24) intraoperatively to potentially reduce the risk for tube malpositioning and to enable gastric decompression. The surgeon can palpate placement in the stomach during surgery and avoid taking postoperative radiographs to confirm placement. NG tubes can feed a continuous rate infusion (CRI) of liquid diet, often started at 1/3 RER then increased daily if tolerated. Aspiration of the NG tube every four to six hours can determine if gastric stasis is present and can help reduce the risk of regurgitation and pneumonia. These tubes are generally used for less than one week but can be maintained for several weeks if necessary. They allow access for early feeding of the patient to help with GI healing. In several reports and in the author's experience, placement of NG tubes across the lower esophageal sphincter may increase the risk for regurgitation and gastroesophageal and reflux esophagitis, in which case the tube should be removed. NE and NG tube feeding is contraindicated for animals with an abnormal gag reflex, esophageal dysfunction, coma, or other condition that increases the risk for aspiration. It is also contraindicated in animals with persistent vomiting. A disadvantage of NE tubes is the small internal diameter, which necessitates the use of commercial liquid diets rather than blenderized pet foods. Also, some animals are reluctant to eat voluntarily while the tube is in place, making it difficult to determine when the tube feeding can be discontinued.

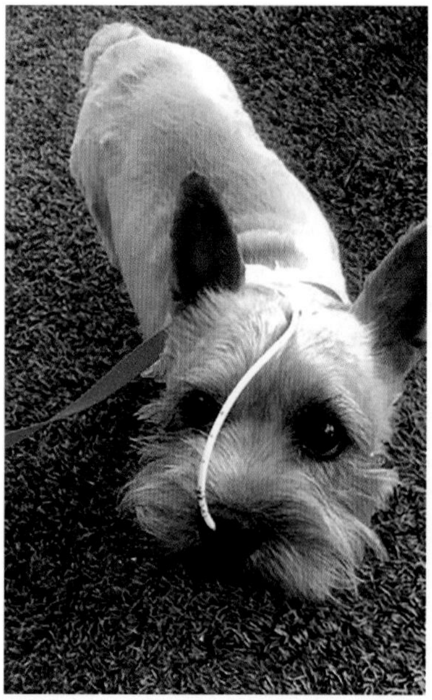

Figure 22.24 NG tube placed in a patient intraoperatively to aid in gastric decompression and enteral nutrition postoperatively. *Source:* © Penny Regier.

Intravenous fluid administration is important for preoperative treatment of hypovolemia secondary to intestinal obstruction and ileus, and it consists of a balanced electrolyte solution for correction of severe acid-base and electrolyte abnormalities. Fluid therapy is not only important preoperatively, but it is also important both during and after a GI surgical procedure, which may correct any deficits that may still be present at the start of surgery and to replace intraoperative fluid losses that occur from surgical handling during dissection and from expected evaporative loss. The type of solution used depends on serum electrolyte values with crystalloid solutions being the most commonly used solution. Additional potassium supplementation ($\leq$0.5 mEq/kg/h) should also be considered in these cases to address preoperative hypokalemia. After surgery, both hydration status and electrolyte values should be reassessed frequently and alterations made based on these assessments.

Gastroprotectants are among the most commonly used drugs in veterinary medicine because the GI tract can be injured secondary to a wide variety of diseases, which leads to their common use after surgery on the GI tract. These drugs include histamine (H2)-receptor antagonists, proton pump inhibitors (PPIs), sucralfate, misoprostol, antacids, and bismuth subsalicylate. Many of these drugs have been developed to decrease intraluminal acidity and/or promote mucosal protective defense mechanisms. PPIs, such as omeprazole and pantoprazole, inhibit gastric acid secretion and are commonly used after GI surgery with pantoprazole being the IV formulation. Famotidine is another commonly used gastroprotectant and is an H_2-antagonist that decreases HCl secretion.

Prokinetic drugs (i.e., metoclopramide or cisapride) may be indicated to treat postoperative ileus. Metoclopramide increases duodenal and jejunal peristalsis, increases gastric contractions, and is a commonly used prokinetic drug. Cisapride has become increasingly popular for treatment of ileus in veterinary medicine mainly due to its ability to support motility of the entire GI tract. In cases with severe ileus noted at the time of surgery, prokinetics may be initiated as part of the immediate postoperative plan. In cases that are perhaps more acute or peristalsis is noted intraoperatively, the surgeon may elect to withhold prokinetics immediately postoperatively and instead elect to monitor the patient for regurgitation or other signs of ileus prior to initiating.

Anti-emetic medications, including ondansetron (Zofran) or maropitant citrate (Cerenia), should also be considered to help address nausea that may be in part due to the GI FB obstruction and/or general anesthesia. Maropitant also has mild anti-inflammatory, pain relieving, and anti-anxiety effects, which may be beneficial as well.

Pain management is a very important aspect of postoperative management. Typically, pain management is initiated with IV pain medications until the patient is eating and can be transitioned to oral pain medications to go home. Common pain medications include opioids, such as methadone and fentanyl. Caution should be taken with hydromorphone in patients undergoing GI surgery, as vomiting could be a potential side effect. Another important caution to consider is that opioids may exacerbate ileus, and in patients that already have severe ileus due to their GI obstruction, opioids may not be an ideal choice. Ketamine is another great choice either alone or in combination with opioids to help with pain relief. The author does not recommend use of non-steroidal anti-inflammatory drugs (NSAIDS) in these patients as NSAIDS can delay healing. An epidural or transversus abdominis plane (TAP) block preoperatively with bupivacaine may also be used to aid in pain management and reduce the need for IV pain medications. Oral pain medications, such as gabapentin or buprenorphine, may be initiated once the patient is eating and may be sent home with the patient.

To access the videos for this chapter, please go to

www.wiley.com/go/coleman/surgeries

VIDEO 22.1 Falciform ligament excision prior to placement of the Balfour retractor. *Source:* © Penny Regier.

VIDEO 22.2 Video demonstrating placement of stay sutures in the ventral aspect of the stomach between the greater and lesser curvatures and prior to gastrotomy incision. *Source:* © Penny Regier.

VIDEO 22.3 Video demonstrating creation of a gastrotomy incision with a #11 blade and extended with Metzenbaum scissors. *Source:* © Penny Regier.

VIDEO 22.4 Video demonstrating the stomach packed off with moist laparotomy sponges both cranially and caudally to prevent contamination. The foreign material is removed with a Carmalt forcep onto a green towel placed over the laparotomy sponges, and the foreign material is placed on the towel with the contaminated instruments and removed from the surgical field. *Source:* © Penny Regier.

VIDEO 22.5 Video demonstrating start of the gastrotomy closure with a two-layer closure. The first layer closure involves the mucosa and submucosa and is performed with a simple continuous appositional pattern taking full-thickness bites. The first and last bites are taken before the incision into the stomach and past the gastrotomy incision. The taper point needle at the end of the suture line is used to gently place the loop of suture and invert any everting mucosa. The extraluminal knots should not overly the incision. *Source:* © Penny Regier.

VIDEO 22.6 Video demonstrating gastrotomy closure with a two-layer closure. The second layer closure involves the muscularis and serosa and is performed with an inverting Cushing pattern. *Source:* © Penny Regier.

VIDEO 22.7 Video demonstrating how to evaluate tension on the line and ensure the tissues are well-apposed prior to tying the extraluminal end knot for the enterotomy closure. *Source:* © Penny Regier.

VIDEO 22.8 (a–c) Videos demonstrating how to perform an enterotomy closure with a single layer simple continuous pattern. Each bite is taken deliberately on each side of the incision ~3 mm from each other and 3 mm apart along the incision. A curved hemostat is used to gently place each loop of suture and invert any everting mucosa. *Source:* © Penny Regier.

VIDEO 22.9 (a) An omental wrap is placed over the enterotomy site after abdominal lavage and prior to closure of the abdomen. (b) An omental wrap is placed over the enterotomy site with simple interrupted tacking sutures to hold the wrap in place and take care not to incorporate any of the mesenteric blood supply to the intestines. *Source:* © Penny Regier.

VIDEO 22.10 (a,b) Red Rubber Catheter (RRC) Technique. Video demonstrating how to perform the RRC technique to remove linear foreign material causing plication of the bowel through a single enterotomy. *Source:* © Penny Regier.

VIDEO 22.11 Arterial pulses noted in the jejunal arteries demonstrating tissue viability. *Source:* © Penny Regier.
VIDEO 22.12 Video demonstrating mesenteric artery ligation with both suture ligatures and using a vessel-sealing device for an intestinal resection and anastomosis. *Source:* © Penny Regier.
VIDEO 22.13 Video demonstrating placement of the Carmalt forceps and Doyen forceps at both the orad and aborad regions of intestinal resection and subsequent excision of the tissue with a #11 blade between the Carmalt and Doyen forceps. *Source:* © Penny Regier.
VIDEO 22.14 (a–c) Handsewn intestinal R&A. Video demonstrating simple interrupted suture placement for a hand-sewn intestinal R&A starting at the mesenteric border, followed by the antimesenteric border, then placed in between these two starting points until the anastomosis is complete with simple interrupted sutures spaced ~3 mm apart. *Source:* © Penny Regier.
VIDEO 22.15 Video showing each limb of the GIA stapler placed within the lumen of the intestines both orally and aborally, and the antimesenteric borders pressed together prior to deploying the linear stapling device. *Source:* © Penny Regier.
VIDEO 22.16 (a,b) Placement of simple interrupted crotch suture for a FEESA to help relieve tension at the site. *Source:* © Penny Regier.
VIDEO 22.17 Suture oversew of the transverse staple line of a FEESA using an inverting Cushing pattern. *Source:* © Penny Regier.
VIDEO 22.18 Omental wrap placed around a FEESA site prior to closing the mesenteric rent. *Source:* © Penny Regier.
VIDEO 22.19 GI punch biopsy technique using a 4 mm punch biopsy at the antimesenteric border of the intestines pressed against a sterile tongue depressor. *Source:* © Penny Regier.
VIDEO 22.20 Leak testing performed of an enterotomy site with a 25-gauge needle attached to a 12 cc syringe and injecting ~10 mL of saline into an ~10 cm segment of bowel. *Source:* © Penny Regier.
VIDEO 22.21 GI probing performed with a curved hemostat to identify regions along the enterotomy site that may need reinforcement with an additional simple interrupted suture. *Source:* © Penny Regier.

References

1 Ciasca, T.C., David, F.H., and Lamb, C.R. (2013). Does measurement of small intestinal diameter increase diagnostic accuracy of radiography in dogs with suspected intestinal obstruction? *Vet. Radiol. Ultrasound* 54: 207–211.

2 Sharma, A., Thompson, M.S., Scrivani, P.V. et al. (2011). Comparison of radiography and ultrasonography for diagnosing small-intestinal mechanical obstruction in vomiting dogs. *Vet. Radiol. Ultrasound* 52: 248–255.

3 Giuffrida, M.A. and Brown, D.C. (2012). Small intestine. In: *Veterinary Surgery: Small Animal* (ed. K.M. Tobias and S.A. Johnston), 1732–1760. St. Louis, MO: Saunders.

4 Grimes, J.A., Schmiedt, C.W., Cornell, K.K. et al. (2011). Identification of risk factors for septic peritonitis and failure to survive following gastrointestinal surgery in dogs. *J. Am. Vet. Med. Assoc.* 238: 486–494.

5 Ellison, G.W. (2010). Intestinal obstruction. In: *Mechanisms of Disease in Small Animal Surgery* (ed. M.J. Bojrab and E. Monnet), 183–187. Jackson, WY: Teton NewMedia.

6 Coolman, B.R., Ehrhart, N., Pijanowski, G. et al. (2000). Comparison of skin staples with sutures for anastomosis of the small intestine in dogs. *Vet. Surg.* 29: 293–302.

7 Fossum, T.W. (2012). Surgery of the digestive system. In: *Small Animal Surgery*, 4e (ed. T.W. Fossum), 497–552. St. Louis, MO: Mosby.

8 Duell, J.R., Thieman Mankin, K.M., and Rochat, M.C. (2016). Frequency of dehiscence in hand-sutured and stapled intestinal anastomoses in dogs. *Vet. Surg.* 45: 100–103.

9 Snowdon, K.A., Smeak, D.D., and Chiang, S. (2016). Risk factors for dehiscence of stapled functional end-to-end intestinal anastomoses in dogs: 53 cases (2001-2012). *Vet. Surg.* 45: 91–99.

10 Ralphs, S.C., Jessen, C.R., and Lipowitz, A.J. (2003). Risk factors for leakage following intestinal anastomosis in dogs and cats. *J. Am. Vet. Med. Assoc.* 223: 73–77.

11 Allen, D.A., Smeak, D.D., and Schertel, E.R. (1992). Prevalence of small intestinal dehiscence and associated clinical factors: a retrospective study of 121 dogs. *J. Am. Anim. Hosp. Assoc.* 28: 70–76.

12 Finck, C., D'Anjou, M.A., Alexander, K. et al. (2014). Radiographic diagnosis of mechanical obstruction in dogs based on relative small intestinal external diameters. *Vet. Radiol. Ultrasound* 55 (5): 472–479.

13 Graham, J.P., Lord, P.F., and Harrison, J.M. (1998). Quantitative estimation of intestinal dilation as a

predictor of obstruction in the dog. *J. Small Anim. Pract.* 39 (11): 521–524.

14 Adams, W.M., Sisterman, L.A., Klauer, J.M. et al. (2010). Association of intestinal disorders in cats with findings of abdominal radiography. *J. Am. Vet. Med. Assoc.* 236 (8): 880–886.

15 Evans, K.L., Smeak, D.D., and Biller, D.S. (1994). Gastrointestinal linear foreign bodies in 32 dogs: a retrospective evaluation and feline comparison. *J. Am. Anim. Hosp. Assoc.* 30 (5): 445–450.

16 Evans, K.L., Smeak, D.D., and Biller, D.S. (1992). Gastrointestinal linear foreign bodies in 32 dogs: retrospective clinical and prognostic evaluation. *Vet. Surg.* 21 (5): 388.

17 Felts, J.F., Fox, P.R., and Burk, R. (1984). Thread and sewing needles as gastrointestinal foreign bodies in the cat: a review of 64 cases. *J. Am. Vet. Med. Assoc.* 184 (1): 56–59.

18 Dickinson, A.E., Summers, J.F., Wignal, J. et al. (2014). Impact of appropriate empirical antimicrobial therapy on outcome of dogs with septic peritonitis. *J. Vet. Emerg. Crit. Care* 25 (1): 152–159.

19 Song, F. and Glenny, A.M. (1998). Antimicrobial prophylaxis in colorectal surgery: a systematic review of randomized controlled trials [erratum appears in Br J Surg 86(2):280, 1999]. *Br. J. Surg.* 85 (9): 1232–1241.

20 Gorman, S.C., Freeman, L.M., Mitchell, S.L. et al. (2006). Extensive small bowel resection in dogs and cats: 20 cases (1998-2004). *J. Am. Vet. Med. Assoc.* 228 (3): 403–407.

21 Orsher, R. and Rosin, E. (1993). Small intestines. In: *Textbook of Small Animal Surgery* (ed. D. Slatter), 593–712. Philadelphia, PA: Saunders.

22 Yanoff, S.R., Willard, M.D., Boothe, H.W. et al. (1992). Short-bowel syndrome in four dogs. *Vet. Surg.* 21 (3): 217–222.

23 McLachlin, A. and Denton, D. (1973). Omental protection of intestinal anastomosis. *Am. J. Surg.* 125: 134–140.

24 Katsikas, D., Sechas, M., Antypas, G. et al. (1977). Beneficial effect of omental wrapping of unsafe intestinal anastomoses. An experimental study in dogs. *Int. Surg.* 62 (8): 435–437.

25 Hosgood, G. (1990). The omentum-the forgotten organ: physiology and potential surgical applications in dogs and cats. *Compend. Contin. Educ. Pract. Vet.* 12 (1): 45–51.

26 Hansen, L.A. and Monnet, E. (2013). Evaluation of serosal patch supplementation of surgical anastomoses in intestinal segments from canine cadavers. *Am. J. Vet. Res.* 74: 1138–1141.

27 White, R.N. (2008). Modified functional end-to-end stapled intestinal anastomosis: technique and clinical results in 15 dogs. *J. Small Anim. Pract.* 49: 274–281.

28 Sumner, S.M., Regier, P.J., Case, J.B. et al. (2019). Evaluation of suture reinforcement for stapled intestinal anastomoses: 77 dogs (2008–2018). *Vet. Surg.* 48: 1188–1193.

29 Duffy, D.J., Chang, Y., and Moore, G.E. (2020). Influence of oversewing the transverse staple line during functional end-to-end stapled intestinal anastomoses in dogs. *Vet. Surg.* 49 (6): 1221–1229.

30 Mullen, K.M., Regier, P.J., Waln, M. et al. (2020). Gastrointestinal thickness, duration, and leak pressure of six intestinal anastomoses in dogs. *Vet. Surg.* 49 (7): 1315–1325.

31 Fealey, M.J., Regier, P.J., Steadman, B.C. et al. (2020). Initial leak pressures of four anastomosis techniques in cooled cadaveric canine jejunum. *Vet. Surg.* 49: 1–7.

32 Hansen, L.A. and Smeak, D.D. (2015). In vitro comparison of leakage pressure and leakage location for various staple line offset configurations in functional end-to-end stapled small intestinal anastomoses of canine tissues. *Am. J. Vet. Res.* 76: 644–648.

33 Ravitch, M.M. and Steichen, F.M. (1972). Technics of staple suturing in the gastrointestinal tract. *Ann. Surg.* 175: 815–837.

34 Duffy, D.J., Chang, Y., and Moore, G.E. (2022). Influence of crotch suture augmentation on leakage pressure and leakage location during functional end-to-end stapled anastomoses in dogs. *Vet. Surg.* 51 (4): 697–504.

35 Jardel, N., Hidalgo, A., Leperlier, D. et al. (2011). One stage functional end-to-end stapled intestinal anastomosis and resection performed by nonexpert surgeons for the treatment of small intestinal obstruction in 30 dogs. *Vet. Surg.* 40: 216–222.

36 Tobias, K.M. (2007). Surgical stapling devices in veterinary medicine: a review. *Vet. Surg.* 36: 341–349.

37 Ballantyne, G.H., Burke, J.B., Rogers, G. et al. (1985). Accelerated wound healing with stapled enteric suture lines: an experimental study comparing traditional sewing techniques and a stapling device. *Ann. Surg.* 201: 360–364.

38 Davis, D.J., Demianiuk, R.M., Musser, J. et al. (2018). Influence of preoperative septic peritonitis and anastomotic technique on the dehiscence of enterectomy sites in dogs: a retrospective review of 210 anastomoses. *Vet. Surg.* 47: 125–129.

39 DePompeo, C.M., Bond, L., George, Y.E. et al. (2018). Intra-abdominal complications following intestinal anastomoses by suture and staple techniques in dogs. *J. Am. Vet. Med. Assoc.* 253: 437–443.

40 Farrah, J.P., Lauer, C.W., Bray, M.S. et al. (2013). Stapled versus hand-sewn anastomoses in emergency general surgery: a retrospective review of outcomes in a unique patient population. *J. Trauma Acute Care Surg.* 74: 1187–1192.

41 Brundage, S.I., Jurkovich, G.J., Hoyt, D.B. et al. (2001). Stapled versus sutured gastrointestinal anastomoses in the trauma patient: a multicenter trial. *J. Trauma* 51 (6): 1054–1061.

42 Mullen, K.M., Regier, P.J., Fox-Alvarez, W.A. et al. (2021). Evaluation of intraoperative leak testing of small intestinal anastomoses performed by hand-sewn and stapled techniques in dogs: 13 cases (2008-2019). *J. Am. Vet. Med. Assoc.* 258 (9): 991–998.

43 Culbertson, T.F., Smeak, D.D., Pogue, J.M. et al. (2021). Intraoperative surgeon probe inspection compared to leak testing for detecting gaps in canine jejunal continuous anastomoses: a cadaveric study. *Vet. Surg.* 50 (7): 1472–1482.

44 Culp, W.T. and Holt, D.E. (2010). Septic peritonitis. *Compend. Contin. Educ. Vet.* 32: E1–E14.

45 Bellah, J.R. (2010). Peritonitis. In: *Mechanisms of Disease in Small Animal Surgery* (ed. M.J. Bojrab and E. Monnet), 84–90. Jackson, WY: Teton NewMedia.

46 Bennett, R.R. and Zydeck, F.A. (1970). A comparison of single layer suture patterns for intestinal anastomosis. *J. Am. Vet. Med. Assoc.* 157: 2075–2080.

47 Bone, D.L., Duckett, K.E., Patton, C.S. et al. (1983). Evaluation of anastomoses of small intestine in dogs: crushing versus noncrushing suturing techniques. *Am. J. Vet. Res.* 44: 2043–2048.

48 Rosenbaum, J.M., Coolman, B.R., Davidson, B.L. et al. (2016). The use of disposable skin staples for intestinal resection and anastomosis in 63 dogs: 2000 to 2014. *J. Small Anim. Pract.* 57: 631–636.

49 Weisman, D.L., Smeak, D.D., Birchard, S.J. et al. (1999). Comparison of a continuous suture pattern with a simple interrupted pattern for enteric closure in dogs and cats: 83 cases (1991-1997). *J. Am. Vet. Med. Assoc.* 214: 1507–1510.

50 Kieves, N.R., Krebs, A.I., and Zellner, E.M. (2018). A comparison of ex vivo leak pressures for four enterotomy closures in a canine model. *J. Am. Anim. Hosp. Assoc.* 54: 71–76.

51 Strelchik, A., Coleman, M.C., Scharf, V.F. et al. (2019). Intestinal incisional dehiscence rate following enterotomy for foreign body removal in 247 dogs. *J. Am. Vet. Med. Assoc.* 255: 695–699.

52 Wylie, K.B. and Hosgood, G. (1994). Mortality and morbidity of small and large intestinal surgery in dogs and cats: 74 cases (1980-1992). *J. Am. Anim. Hosp. Assoc.* 30: 469–474.

53 Hosgood, G. and Salisburg, S.K. (1988). Generalized peritonitis in dogs: 50 cases (1975-1986). *J. Am. Vet. Med. Assoc.* 193: 1448–1450.

54 Shales, C.J., Warren, J., Anderson, D.M. et al. (2005). Complications following full-thickness small intestinal biopsy in 66 dogs: a retrospective study. *J. Small Anim. Pract.* 46: 317–321.

55 Harvey, H.J. (1990). Complications of small intestinal biopsy in hypoalbuminemic dogs. *Vet. Surg.* 19: 289–292.

23

Splenectomy

Pamela Schwartz

Schwarzman Animal Medical Center, New York, NY, USA

Key Points
• Knowledge of the splenic and regional anatomy is imperative when performing splenectomy in order to avoid ligating the splenic vessels proximal to the pancreatic branches, causing iatrogenic compromise to the pancreas. • An online decision support calculator and a hemangiosarcoma likelihood prediction (HeLP) score were developed to help determine the risk of malignancy and risk of hemangiosarcoma (HSA), respectively. • Splenectomy can be performed through an open laparotomy or via minimally invasive techniques, the choice of which may be dictated by the size of the mass in relation to the patient. • Conventional techniques for splenectomy have largely been replaced with the use of a bipolar vessel sealing device (BVSD). • The overall prognosis associated with HSA is extremely poor with median survival times of 19–86 days with surgery alone. Referral to an oncologist is always recommended with the diagnosis of malignant splenic disease.

Anatomy

Knowledge of the splenic and regional anatomy is paramount prior to performing splenectomy. The spleen is a dynamic organ typically residing in the left cranial quadrant of the abdomen. The dorsal extremity (head) is less mobile, as it is tethered to the greater curvature of the stomach by the gastrosplenic ligament, in which the short gastric vessels are located. The larger ventral extremity (tail) is more mobile and generally resides across the ventral midline caudal to the ribs. The concave visceral surface of the spleen gives way to the attachments of nerves, vessels, and omentum.[1–3] The surgical approach to the spleen is simplified due to its peripheral location within the abdomen, moderately long vascular pedicle, and mostly loose mesenteric attachment.[4]

The main blood supply to the spleen is from the splenic branch of the celiac artery. The splenic artery generally gives off three to five primary branches as it courses in the greater omentum toward the spleen. The first branch is to the pancreas and is the main supply to the left limb of the pancreas. The two remaining branches run toward the spleen where they spread into several vessels supplying the splenic parenchyma. The dorsal branch continues toward the head of the spleen supplying the cranial parenchyma before coursing through the gastrosplenic ligament to supply the short gastric vessels, which provide blood to the fundus of the stomach. The caudal branch of the splenic artery is the left gastroepiploic artery, which supplies several branches to the caudal portion of the spleen, including the main splenic arteries (usually 2) and omental branch of the splenic artery, before turning back to the supply greater curvature of the stomach (Figure 23.1). The splenic vein drains the many hilar veins into the gastrosplenic vein prior to entering the portal vein.[1–3]

Pathology

Splenectomy is indicated in cases of torsion, trauma, diffuse infiltrative disease, splenomegaly, and solitary or multiple splenic masses caused by both neoplastic and

Techniques in Small Animal Soft Tissue, Orthopedic, and Ophthalmic Surgery, First Edition. Edited by Kristin A. Coleman.

Companion website: www.wiley.com/go/coleman/surgeries

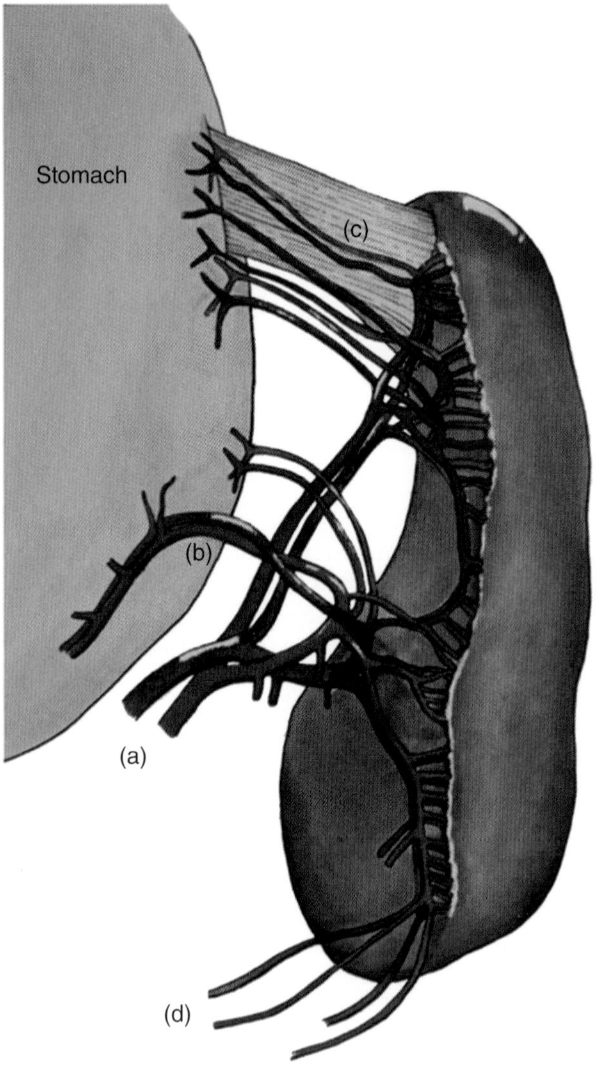

Figure 23.1 Diagram showing the splenic arterial supply. (a) Splenic artery and vein, (b) left gastroepiploic vessels, (c) short gastric vessels, and (d) branches to the greater omentum. Original artwork by Taylor Bergrud.

non-neoplastic causes (hematoma, nodular hyperplasia). Less frequently, splenectomy is performed as a treatment for immune-mediated disorders or splenic abscessation.[1,2,4] Splenic disorders are common in middle-aged to older dogs with clinical signs ranging from absent (incidentally found on palpation or with imaging) or vague signs to life-threatening (hemoperitoneum).[5]

The most common causes of splenic disease in dogs are hemangiosarcoma (HSA), extramedullary hematopoiesis, multicentric lymphoma, hematoma or nodular hyperplasia, and congestion.[4–7] The most common reasons for splenectomy in cats are mast cell tumors (53%) followed by HSA (21%) and lymphoma (11%).[8] HSA is the most common malignant splenic mass neoplasia in dogs.[7,9] Historically, the double two-thirds rule regarding HSA was relied on for all splenic masses (approximately two-thirds of dogs with splenic masses will have a malignant tumor, with two-thirds of those malignancies being HSA), although this appears to apply more closely to dogs with hemoperitoneum. A systematic review questioning the validity of the double two-thirds rule with non-traumatic hemoperitoneum found an even higher percentage of malignancy at 73%, with 87.3% of the malignant masses being HSA.[10] Another recent study documents a higher number of benign splenic tumors (37.5%) in dogs with hemoperitoneum associated with splenic rupture than previously reported.[11] Dogs that have splenic masses or nodules without associated hemoperitoneum more commonly have benign (70.5–72.7%) than malignant (27–29.5%) lesions.[12,13] Preoperative coagulation profiles should be performed, especially in cases of non-traumatic hemoperitoneum.[3]

Discrepancies in the literature make it difficult to interpret possible outcomes, and decisions should not be made based solely on the clinical presentation. Because the decision to proceed with surgery or not can be difficult, especially in the face of hemoperitoneum requiring emergent treatment, clinical decision tools based on initial assessments have been developed to help predict the risk of HSA. An online decision support calculator was developed to aid in the preoperative discrimination of benign from malignant splenic tumors on the basis of preoperative variables. The clinical variables used to estimate the probability of malignancy include serum total protein concentration, presence of (versus absence of) ≥ 2 nucleated red blood cells/100 white blood cells and ultrasound assessment of the following: splenic mass size, number of liver nodules, presence of multiple splenic masses/nodules, moderate to marked splenic mass inhomogeneity, marked to moderate abdominal effusion, and mesenteric, omental, or peritoneal nodules. Although this model has an accurate level to assist in clinical decision-making, the calculator should always be considered supplementary to the full clinical presentation.[7] A hemangiosarcoma likelihood prediction (HeLP) score was also developed for dogs with hemoperitoneum, which can facilitate identification of dogs at low ($\leq 40\%$) or high ($>55\%$) risk for HSA based on body weight, total plasma protein, platelet count, and thoracic radiographs. This score may help owners move forward with surgical treatment in dogs with lower risk; however, the decision to euthanize should not be made solely on a higher HeLP score. It is also important to note that a lower risk (non-HSA diagnosis) does not signify diagnosis of a benign disease, as alternate neoplasms (hepatocellular carcinoma, hepatoma, histiocytic sarcoma) were also included.[14]

Diagnostic Imaging Techniques

Abdominal masses are often initially diagnosed radiographically; however, there are many factors that can make definitive location of a mass within the spleen difficult (Figure 23.2). Either thoracic radiographs or thoracic CT should be performed in animals with splenic masses to screen for pulmonary or thoracic neoplasia or metastatic spread, especially to the right auricle or right atrium.[1] Brief echocardiogram may also be performed to evaluate for cardiac metastasis.

Ultrasonography is recommended to provide information regarding the location of a primary mass, evidence of metastasis if present, and surgical planning. Abdominal ultrasound (AUS) has a high sensitivity for detection of splenic masses (87.4%); however, benign and malignant lesions can be indistinguishable prior to pathologic evaluation.[10,15] Ultrasound is an excellent screening tool, but there are differences recognized between AUS and gross findings. In one study evaluating dogs with nontraumatic hemoperitoneum, differences were identified between AUS and gross findings in 54% of dogs.[15] It is important for clients to know that although obvious metastasis is not noted on AUS, it can still be present at the time of surgery. AUS does not accurately detect diffuse peritoneal or omental nodular metastasis in dogs in which it is identified grossly.[11,15] However, when diffuse omental or peritoneal nodular metastasis is evident on AUS, a neoplastic process is most likely supported. The correlation between the sizes of splenic masses detected on ultrasound in relationship to malignant or benign disease is also variable.[13,16] Ultrasound is often performed initially due to its wide availability and noninvasive nature.

Computed tomography (CT) is becoming more commonplace in veterinary medicine and has greatly improved the accuracy of imaging diagnosis.[13] One study evaluating the presurgical assessment of CT in dogs with splenic masses showed that precontrast lesion attenuation was

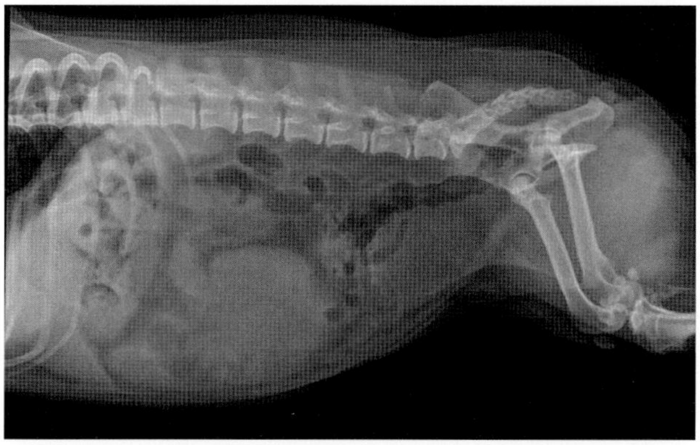

Figure 23.2 Left lateral radiograph of a dog with a suspected splenic tumor. The origin of the tumor was confirmed via ultrasound prior to splenectomy.

significantly different between malignant and benign tumors. The mean precontrast lesion attenuation of malignant tumors was 40.3 Hounsfield units (HU) compared to 52.8 HU for benign tumors, with most malignant tumors having attenuation lower than 50 HU.[13] A previous study noted significantly lower attenuation values on both pre- and post-contrast images; however, a postcontrast threshold value of 55 HU was the best at determining malignant from benign masses (<55 HU being malignant).[17] Another study evaluating dual-phase CT exhibited variable CT features, which do not corroborate with the previous studies.[18] A more recent study classifies focal splenic lesions based on their CT features, with a very high accuracy for sarcomas and a moderate accuracy for benign lesions and nodular hyperplasia, while round cell tumors could not be classified.[19] Investigation of triple-phase helical CT in dogs with solid splenic masses found that the enhanced volumetric ratio of HSA was significantly lower than that of hematoma and nodular hyperplasia in all phases; however, it was not possible to differentiate undifferentiated sarcomas with nodular hyperplasia or hematoma.[20]

While initial examination of CT to detect differences between malignant and benign disease is promising, disadvantages of utilizing CT for surgical decision-making are that it is limited to non-emergent cases, and cost may be preventive for some. Although CT shows significant promise to aid in identification of tumor features, it should not be the sole modality when considering splenectomy (Figure 23.3).

Magnetic resonance imaging (MRI) provides soft tissue contrast superior to that of ultrasound or CT; however, there has been very little investigation regarding the use of MRI for focal splenic lesions.[21,22] In a study of MRI results for focal splenic and hepatic lesions in dogs, the overall accuracy in differentiating malignant from benign tumors was 94.3%, although only eight of the cases included were of splenic origin.[21] While MRI is more readily available than previously, it is likely restricted to specialty facilities and limited by cost and duration of time required under anesthesia.

The decision for clients to move forward with surgery can be difficult since the prognosis varies significantly depending on the histopathologic diagnosis, which is usually not known prior to surgery. Owners should be counseled on all possible prognoses, cost, and aftercare to allow them to make the most informed decision given the work-up provided.

Surgical Techniques

Complete splenectomy is the most performed and recommended surgical treatment of suspected neoplasia, diffuse infiltrative disease, torsion, and most focal and/or generalized splenic enlargement. The spleen can be approached as an open abdominal procedure or with

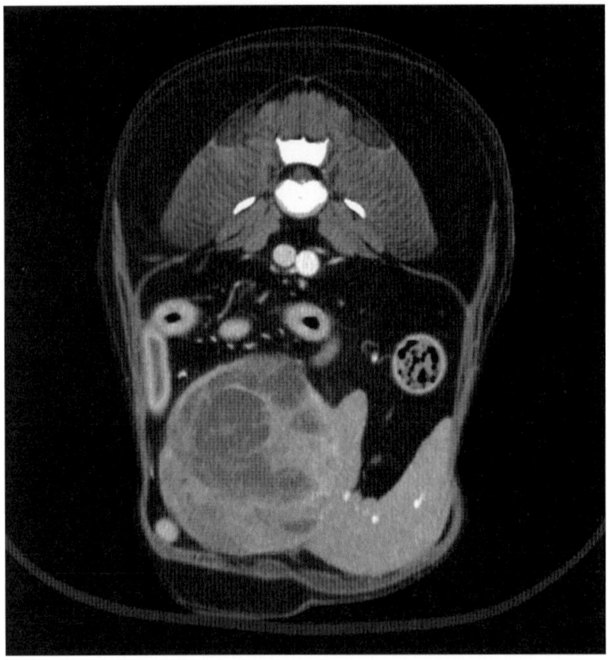

Figure 23.3 Axial CT image of a large (11.4 × 9.0 × 9.1 cm) heterogeneously contrast-enhancing mass expanding from the tail of the spleen. Histopathology was consistent with splenic nodular lymphoid hyperplasia and extramedullary hematopoiesis with infarction and hematoma formation.

laparoscopic assistance. Prior to surgery, patients with shock and coagulative dysfunction should be stabilized using appropriate supportive treatment and blood products.

Performing splenectomy as close to the hilus of the spleen as possible avoids ligating the splenic vessels proximal to the pancreatic branches, which could damage the pancreatic blood supply. The vessels are ligated as they terminate into the spleen. Conventional techniques for splenectomy include suture ligation or stapling devices. These have largely been replaced with the use of a bipolar vessel sealing device (BVSD), which is an electrosurgical instrument that can be utilized in both open and laparoscopic procedures. The BVSD applies direct pressure and bipolar energy to the tissue, causing vessel sealing by fusing the collagen and elastic fibers within the blood vessel walls. BVSDs have been shown to achieve sufficient and safe hemostasis during hilar splenectomy as well as shorten the surgical and anesthetic time.[23–26] There are several different commercial BVSDs available for veterinary use, such as the LigaSure™,[i] the EnSeal®,[ii] and the Harmonic device system.[iii,27] Each BVSD device will be slightly different depending on the system, but noted advantages include monopolar, bipolar, and vessel sealing capabilities within a single system (LigaSure™), variable handpieces, the ability to seal vessels of ≤7 mm diameter (LigaSure™ and EnSeal®), and the ability to reuse the handpieces for a limited number of times[28,29]

(a)

(b)

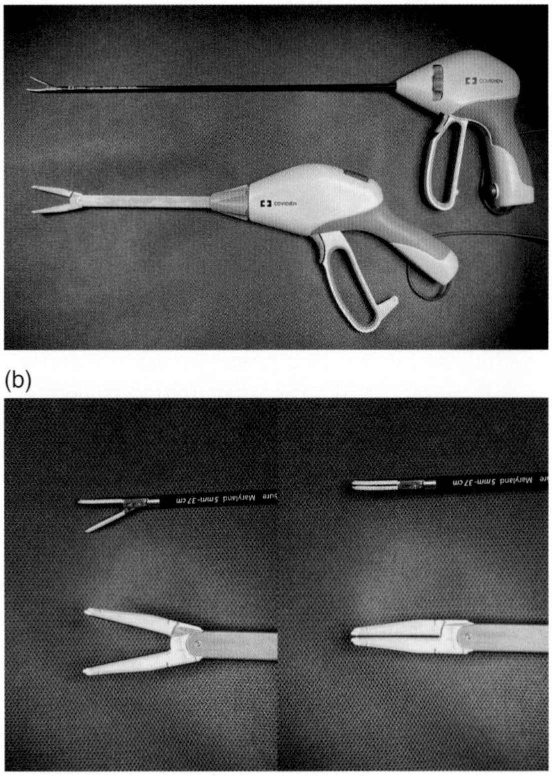

Figure 23.4 (a) LigaSure™ handpieces for laparoscopic use (top) and open laparotomy (bottom), although either can be used in both open and MIS cases. There are also a variety of other LigaSure™ handpieces not pictured. (b) The Maryland and Impact handpieces with jaws opened and closed. The seal length is 20 mm for the Maryland handpiece (top) versus 36 mm for the Impact (bottom).

(Figure 23.4a,b). Additional benefits include the ease of use and the lack of suture material needed.

Open laparotomy is often required due to the large size of a splenic mass in relation to the size of the patient and in cases of hemoperitoneum or splenic torsion. The presence of adhesions associated with larger masses may also limit minimally invasive procedures (Figure 23.5).

Historically, individual suture ligation of all short terminal branches at the hilus of the spleen was performed, preserving the left gastroepiploic artery and short gastric arteries. If the integrity of the blood supply to the stomach is not compromised (e.g., during gastric dilatation and volvulus if the short gastric arteries are torn), these vessels are not required to be preserved. Since the individual ligation technique is not necessary and is time-consuming, a modified en masse ligation technique has been described that only involves four ligatures of the short gastric arteries, dorsal branch of the splenic artery, main splenic artery, and omental branch of the splenic artery.[30] Complete splenectomy can be performed using sutures, staplers, or BVSDs. The Ligate and Divide stapler (LDS) places two U-shaped staples around a vessel and divides between the

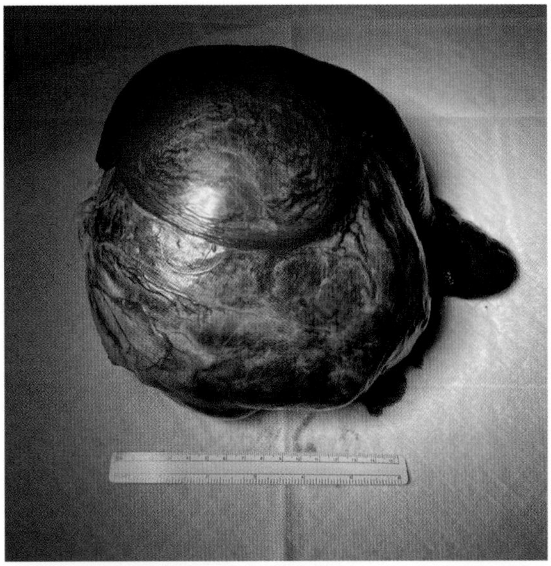

Figure 23.5 Note that large size of the splenic mass (>15 cm), which makes an open laparotomy approach to complete splenectomy more feasible than laparoscopic splenectomy. *Source:* © Pamela Schwartz.

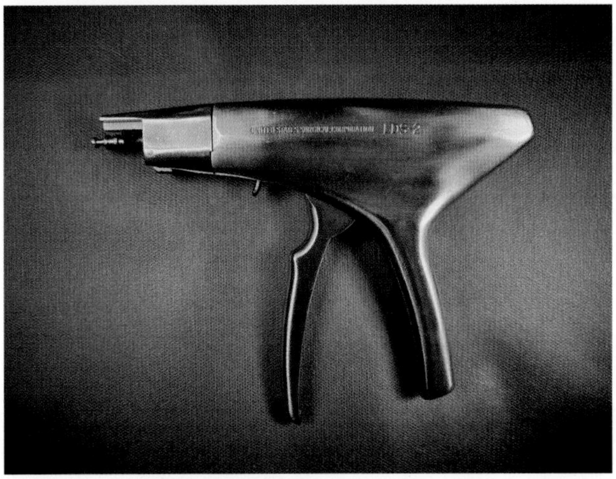

Figure 23.6 The Ligate and Divide Stapler handpiece, which can save time compared to hand sutures during hilar splenectomy. A disposable cartridge of staples is attached to the handpiece, which can be re-sterilized for multiple uses. There are single-use handles and cartridges available as well as power LDS staplers.

two (Figure 23.6). The LDSs can save a considerable amount of time for procedures that require multiple vessel ligation, such as the hilar ligation technique for splenectomy.[31]

Open Laparotomy with Suture Hilar Ligation Technique

This technique is reported as described by Fox-Alvarez and Case.[2] The patient is placed in dorsal recumbency, and the entire abdomen aseptically prepped. A ventral midline abdominal laparotomy is made starting caudal to the level of the xiphoid and extending as far caudally as necessary for full abdominal exploration and complete splenectomy. Removal of the falciform fat, using electrocautery or suture, and placement of the Balfour retractor improve visualization (Figure 23.7). If hemoperitoneum is present, the fluid should be suctioned to aid in visualization. The spleen is exteriorized and isolated from the remainder of the abdomen, which can conveniently stem active hemorrhage with the weight of the spleen compressing the splenic vessels against the patient's own body wall. In the author's experience, removal of Balfour retractors or loosening them allows improved exteriorization of the spleen against the patient's own body without the need for an assistant to retract the spleen. Any omental adhesions to the spleen are ligated with electrocautery, hemoclips, or suture. The spleen is positioned for visualization of the hilar vessels. Isolate each hilar vessel using hemostatic forceps to bluntly dissect a window through the fat surrounding the vessel for introduction of suture material. Circumferentially double-ligate using 3-0 absorbable, monofilament suture material. Prior to transection of the vessel, place a hemostatic forcep on the pedicle close to the spleen to prevent bleeding. Repeat this step for all the vessels along the splenic hilus until splenectomy is complete (Figure 23.8a–f). Blood pressure should be adequately maintained prior to the abdomen being assessed for hemostasis. The abdomen is lavaged with warm, sterile saline and subsequently suctioned of any remaining fluid prior to routine closure of the abdominal cavity.

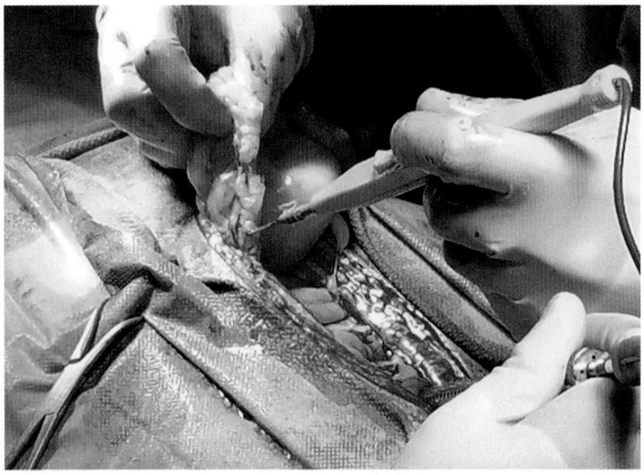

Figure 23.7 Cranial is to the left of the photo. Removal of the falciform fat is shown using monopolar electrocautery. This improves visualization during abdominal exploratory and splenectomy. *Source:* Reproduced with permission from Case and Fox-Alvarez et al.[2]/VetMedux.

Open Laparotomy with En Masse Ligation Technique

This technique is reported as described by Smeak.[30] The patient is placed in dorsal recumbency, and the entire abdomen aseptically prepped. A ventral midline abdominal

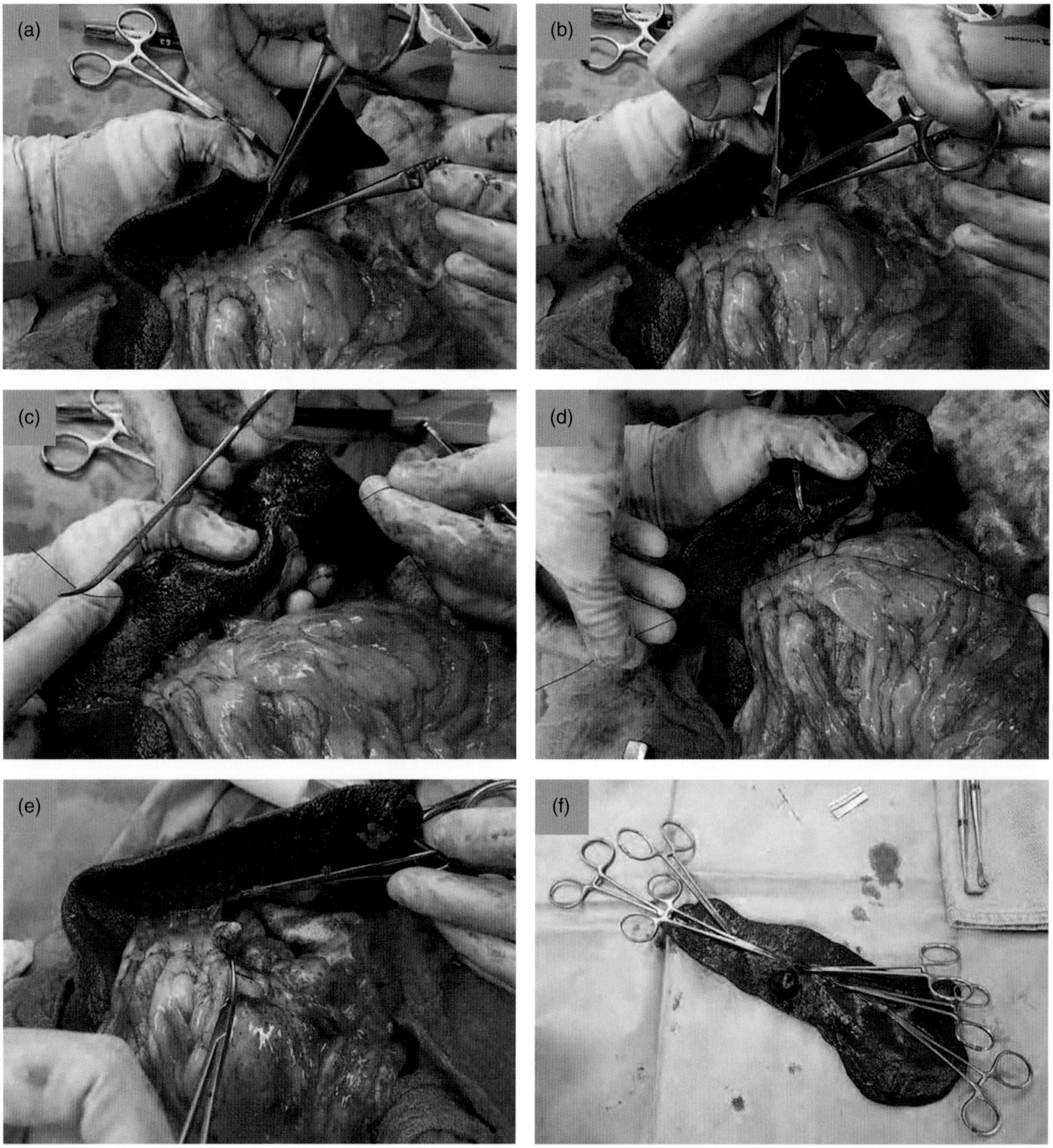

Figure 23.8 Hilar ligation technique for splenectomy. (a,b) The spleen is positioned for visualization of the hilar vessels. Each hilar vessel is isolated using hemostatic forceps to bluntly dissect a window through the fat surrounding the vessel for introduction of suture material. (c–e) Circumferentially double-ligate each vessel using 3-0 absorbable, monofilament suture material. Prior to transection of the vessel, place a hemostatic forcep on the pedicle closest to the spleen to prevent bleeding. (f) Repeat this step for all the vessels along the splenic hilus until splenectomy is complete. *Source:* Reproduced with permission from Case and Fox-Alvarez et al.[2]/VetMedux.

laparotomy is made starting caudal to the level of the xiphoid and extending as far caudally as necessary for full abdominal exploration and complete splenectomy. Removal of the falciform fat, using electrocautery or suture, and placement of the Balfour retractor improve visualization (Figure 23.7). If hemoperitoneum is present, the fluid should be suctioned to aid in visualization. Any omental adhesions to the spleen are ligated with electrocautery, hemoclips, or suture. The fundus of the stomach is exteriorized to expose the short gastric vessels tethered dorsally to the head of the spleen. Manually dissect a hole bluntly through an avascular area of the gastrosplenic ligament (Figure 23.9a). Cross-clamp and incise the short gastric vessels, which will release the head of the spleen. Ensure that the stomach wall is not inadvertently incorporated into the clamped pedicles (Figure 23.9b). When preserving the stomach vasculature is deemed necessary, open the gastrosplenic ligament in an avascular region. Locate the junction of the splenic artery and left gastroepiploic vessel and stay distal (toward the spleen) to this during isolation of the final three pedicles (Figure 23.10a). The three final pedicles are isolated with the index finger and cross-clamped: dorsal artery branch, main splenic artery, and caudal or omental branch. Use caution to preserve the left gastric epiploic artery, which is in close association with the dorsal branch (Figure 23.10b,c). The spleen, with associated forceps attached to the pedicles, is removed (Figure 23.11). Securely double-ligate the remaining pedicles within the crushed area of the previously placed forceps or ligate with a single friction knot, such as a strangle knot (Figure 23.12). Other procedures can be performed as required (i.e., biopsy of liver nodules). Blood pressure should be adequately maintained prior to the abdomen being assessed for hemostasis. The abdomen is lavaged with warm, sterile saline and subsequently suctioned of any remaining fluid prior to routine closure of the abdominal cavity.

Open Laparotomy with LigaSure Hilar Ligation Technique

The patient is placed in dorsal recumbency, and the entire abdomen aseptically prepped. A ventral midline abdominal laparotomy is made starting caudal to the level of the xiphoid and extending as far caudally as necessary for full abdominal exploration and complete splenectomy (Figure 23.13). Removal of the falciform fat, using electrocautery or suture, and placement of the Balfour retractor improve visualization (Figure 23.7). If hemoperitoneum is present, the fluid should be suctioned to aid in visualization. The spleen is exteriorized and isolated from the remainder of the abdomen, which can conveniently stem active hemorrhage with the weight of the spleen compressing the splenic vessels against the patient's own body wall (Figure 23.14). All vessels are sealed using a BVSD as close to the hilus as possible. Although commencing at the tail of the spleen is often more straightforward, since it

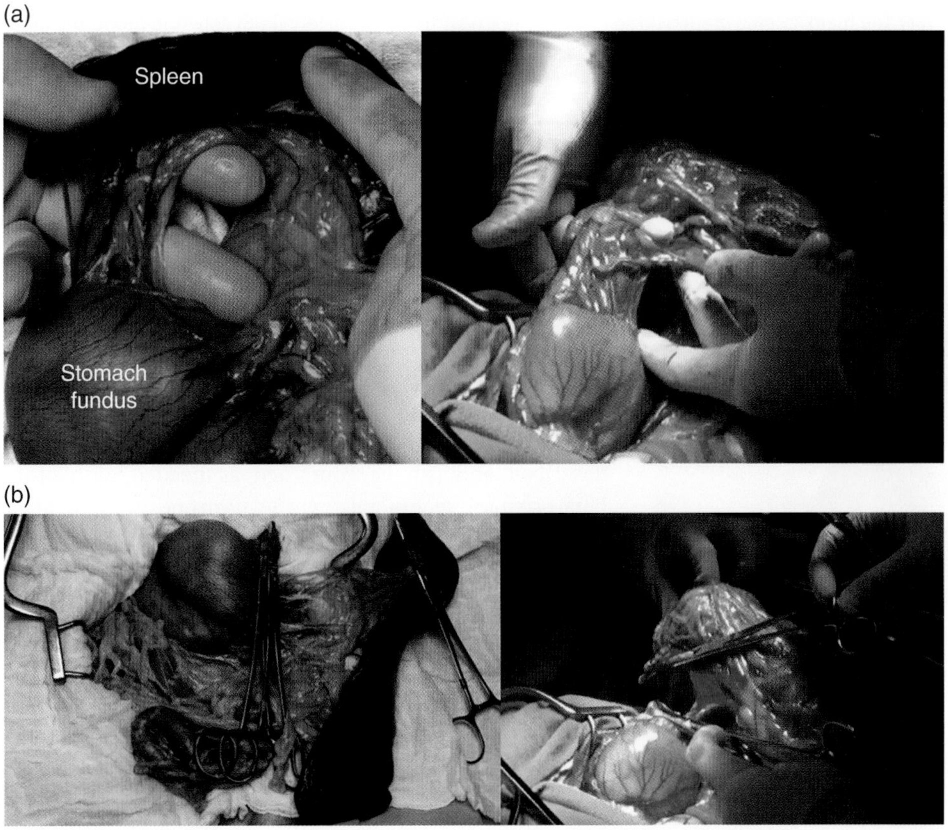

Figure 23.9 En masse four-ligature technique for splenectomy. (a) From a cranial to caudal direction, loop an index finger around the tethering vessel group and bluntly dissect a hole through an avascular region of the gastrosplenic ligament. (b) Cross-clamp and incise the short gastric vessels. The photos on the left are from a dog cadaver and the photos on the right are taken intraoperatively. *Source:* Reproduced with permission from Smeak[30] and Sarah Marvel.

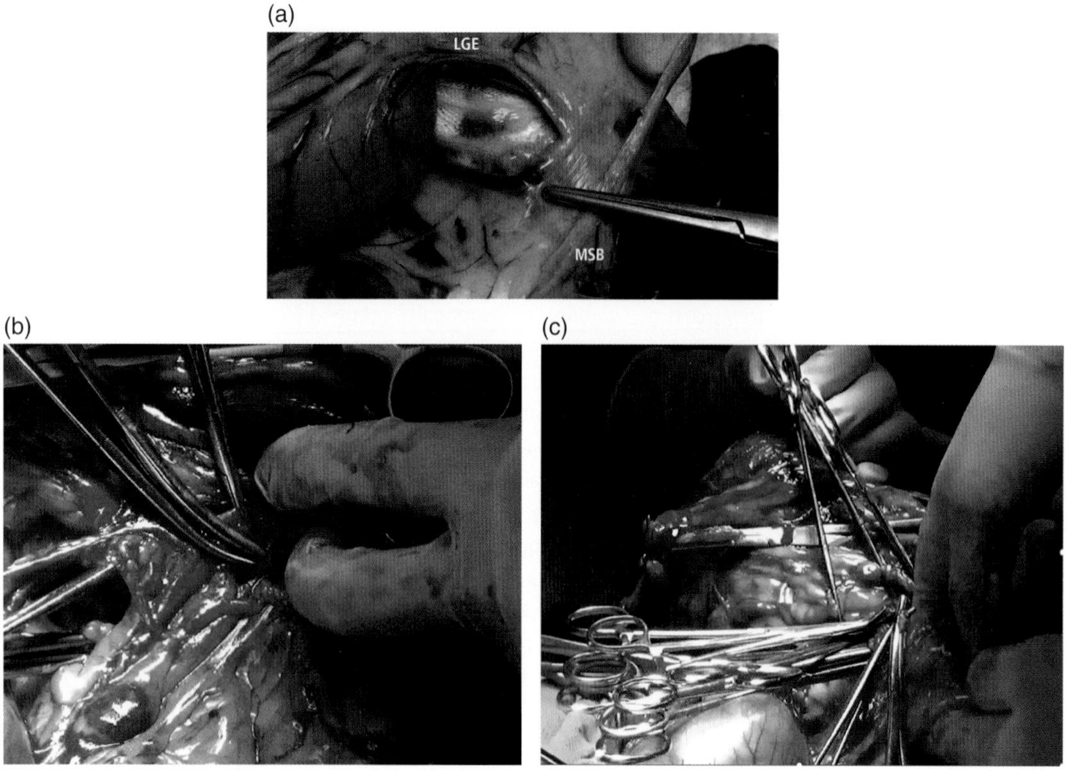

Figure 23.10 (a) In this figure, the splenic pedicle is viewed through a rent in the omentum in a dog cadaver. The forceps point to the junction of the main splenic artery, the main splenic branch (MSB), and the left gastroepiploic artery (LGE) coursing along the greater curvature of the stomach. (b) This figure depicts the pedicles cross-clamped distal to the LGE intraoperatively. (c) The caudal branch is isolated manually in preparation for cross-clamping. *Source:* Reproduced with permission from Smeak[30] and Sarah Marvel.

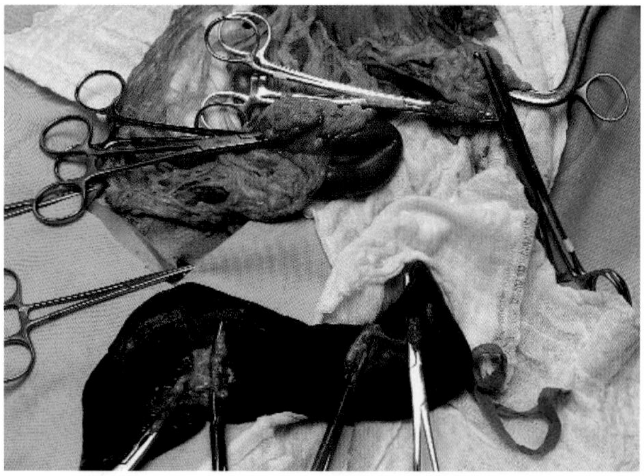

Figure 23.11 The spleen with associated forceps attached to the pedicles is removed and submitted for histopathology. *Source:* Reproduced with permission from Smeak.[30]

is more mobile than the head, adhesions may impair visualization or cause tethering of the tail of the spleen, rendering it more immobile than normal. Ligation can start at the head or tail of the spleen, and adhesions are likewise sealed and transected with a BVSD until complete splenectomy is achieved. Other procedures can be performed as required (i.e., biopsy of liver nodules). Blood pressure should be adequately maintained prior to the abdomen being assessed for hemostasis. The abdomen is lavaged with warm, sterile saline and subsequently suctioned of any remaining fluid prior to routine closure of the abdominal cavity.

Laparoscopic Splenectomy

Multiport total laparoscopic splenectomy has been described and can be combined as needed with other laparoscopic techniques (i.e., gastropexy and liver biopsy).[28,32,33] The size of the spleen and/or splenic mass obviates the need to extend one of the port sites in order to exteriorize and remove the spleen. Single incision laparoscopic surgery (SILS) is a growing technique that reduces the need for multiple laparoscopic ports. The SILS splenectomy is a safe and feasible option and can be used as an alternative approach to multiport laparoscopic surgery for dogs undergoing elective splenectomy. The advantages of SILS splenectomy are significantly faster operative time and smaller surgical scars without additional complications.[34] The disadvantage of splenectomy performed intracorporeally is the advanced training required in minimally invasive surgical techniques.

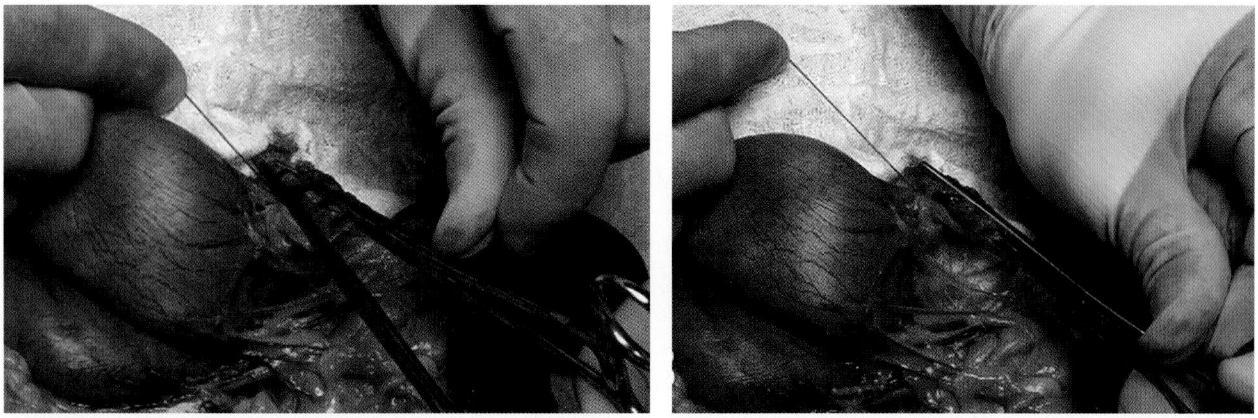

Figure 23.12 A ligature is shown encircling the short gastric artery pedicle just below the first forcep. Once ligation is complete via the three-clamp technique, the pedicles should be inspected for hemorrhage, and additional sutures placed as needed. A tip is to learn a reliable friction knot, which may be used as a single ligature (compared to the standard circumferential/transfixation combination) for a faster splenectomy. *Source:* Reproduced with permission from Smeak.[30]

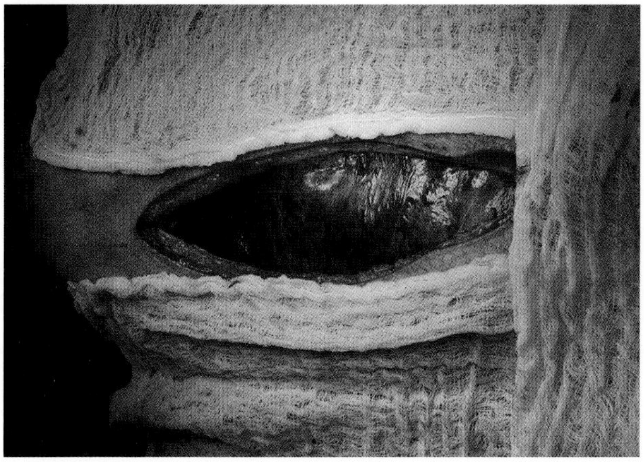

Figure 23.13 Cranial is to the left of the photo. The laparotomy commences at the level of the xiphoid and extends as far caudally as needed to exteriorize the spleen, which can be visualized upon entrance to the abdominal cavity due to the size of the mass (>15 cm). This particular incision will likely be extended further caudally to facilitate splenic mass exteriorization. *Source:* © Pamela Schwartz.

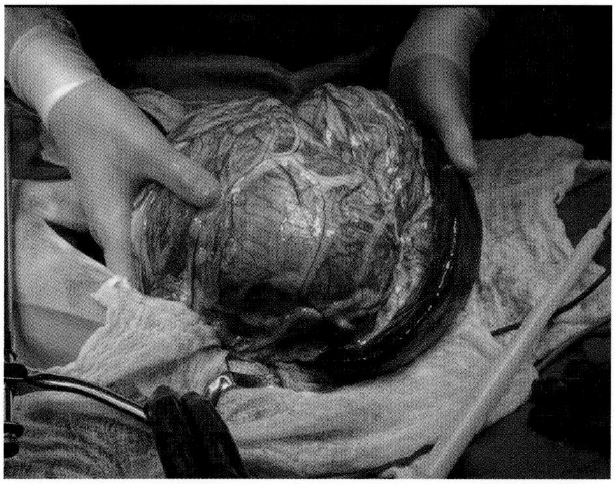

Figure 23.14 Cranial is to the left of the photo. Note the large size of the splenic mass (>15 cm). The spleen and associated mass are exteriorized from the abdomen prior to splenectomy. *Source:* © Pamela Schwartz.

Traditionally, splenic torsion and medium- to large-sized splenic masses have been considered a contraindication to laparoscopic splenectomy. A laparoscopic-assisted splenectomy (LAS) technique has been developed to accommodate medium to larger masses. One study documents LAS is possible in dogs with medium to large splenic masses, with the largest mass being 14.5 cm in diameter. The median minilaparotomy incision in this study was 7.5 cm, which is considerably shorter than that of a standard open laparotomy incision for medium- to large-breed dogs[35] (Figure 23.15). Another study documents LAS is possible in dogs with masses up to 15 cm in diameter.[36] Owners should be aware of the potential need for conversion to full laparotomy in cases of hemoperitoneum not recognized prior to surgery,

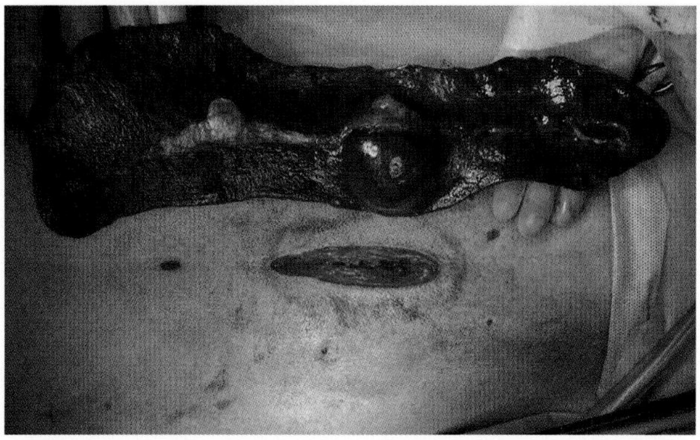

Figure 23.15 Note the size of the minilaparotomy incision in comparison to the size of the spleen and splenic mass. The 2 mm incision cranial to the minilaparotomy incision was placed for intracorporeal gastropexy prior to LAS. *Source:* © Pamela Schwartz.

adhesions that may prevent mobilization of the spleen, or hemorrhage that cannot be controlled with LAS alone.[36]

Total Laparoscopic Splenectomy Technique

This technique is reported as described by Shaver et al.[33] The patient is positioned in either dorsal or right lateral recumbency with the entire abdomen shaved and aseptically prepped. Initial port placement is established with three or four ports using a modified Hasson technique. Pneumoperitoneum is established using carbon dioxide (CO_2) insufflation, maintaining an intra-abdominal pressure of 8–12 mmHg. A camera is introduced, and the abdomen is inspected for any abnormalities. The spleen is elevated with the use of a blunt probe or a fan retractor. The table can be tilted to aid in visualization; rotating toward left lateral improves the visual field of the splenic vessels and surrounding structures, while rotation to right lateral facilitates dissection of the vessels at the dorsal extremity of the spleen and gastrosplenic ligament. Complete intracorporeal splenectomy at the hilus is performed using a BVSD, starting at the tail of the spleen and progressing toward the head. The location of the camera and instruments can be changed as needed throughout the procedure to aid in visualization. The spleen is exteriorized through enlargement of a paracostal or midline port. Routine closure of the ports and extended incision are performed. When indicated, the editor prefers total laparoscopic splenectomy utilizing a SILS™ Port in an infraumbilical position on midline (~3 cm incision) and a LigaSure™ Atlas (10 mm handpiece). Once the hilar vasculature is ligated and transected, the SILS™ Port is removed and replaced with a wound retractor, which facilitates gentle exteriorization of the entire spleen.

Laparoscopic-Assisted Splenectomy Technique

The patient is positioned in dorsal recumbency with the entire abdomen shaved and aseptically prepped. A 3 cm skin incision is made caudal to the umbilicus and continued through the subcutaneous tissue until the linea alba is approached. The incision can be adjusted cranially or caudally if needed, based on the patient's conformation and concern for ability to retract the spleen at the terminal portion of the splenectomy. The linea alba is incised, and a SILS™ Port[iv] is inserted through the fascial incision. The lubricated port can be inserted by folding it and placing 1–2 curved Carmalt hemostats at the base and directing it into the abdomen. Alternatively, the linea alba can be tented with rat-toothed forceps while manually directing the port into the abdomen (Figure 23.16). Making the abdominal incision too long will prevent an adequate seal between the incision and the SILS™ Port, and pneumoperitoneum will be more difficult to maintain. Three lubricated laparoscopic 5-mm cannulas are introduced through the access channels (Figure 23.17). Pneumoperitoneum is

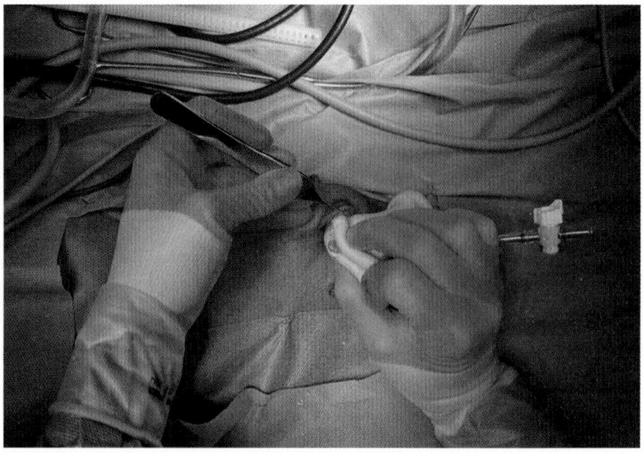

Figure 23.16 Placement of the SILS™ Port by tenting the linea alba with rat toothed forceps while manually directing the port into the abdomen. *Source:* © Pamela Schwartz.

established using CO_2, maintaining an intra-abdominal pressure of 8–12 mmHg. A camera is introduced, and the abdomen is inspected for any abnormalities. Following abdominal exploration, laparoscopic staging, and any additional procedures (e.g., liver biopsy and gastropexy), the camera, instruments, and SILS™ Port are removed.

The incision is extended into a minilaparotomy, which will vary in size depending on the size of the spleen[35] (Figure 23.15). A wound retraction device[v] may be inserted if preferred (Figure 23.18). For placement of the wound retractor device, the inner flexible ring is inserted through the abdominal incision, and the outer ring is then rolled toward the body until it results in taut circumferential retraction.[35] The tail of the spleen is grasped manually or with a dry gauze sponge or laparotomy pad, and the spleen is partially exteriorized through the wound retractor or minilaparotomy incision. A BVSD is used progressively toward the head of the spleen, while continually exteriorizing the spleen to seal the splenic hilar vessels and any omental adhesions (Figure 23.19).[35] Once splenectomy is complete and hemostasis confirmed, if used, the wound retractor is removed by simultaneously retracting the outer ring away from the body wall and compressing the inner ring, and the abdomen is routinely closed.

Postoperative Complications

Reported postoperative complications following splenectomy include hemorrhage, vascular compromise to the pancreas, systemic thrombosis, disseminated intravascular coagulation (DIC), cardiac arrhythmias, and gastric dilatation-volvulus (GDV).[1,37–39] The perioperative mortality rate after splenectomy in dogs varies from 5% to 33%.[11,38,40]

Intraoperative hemorrhage is most commonly from metastatic lesions.[38] The use of BVSDs significantly reduces

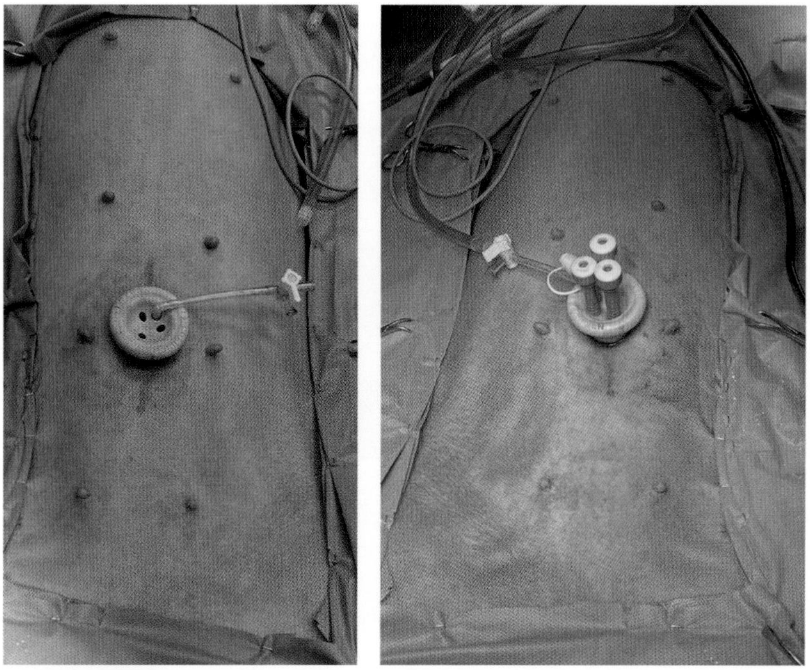

Figure 23.17 Cranial is to the top of the photo. The SILS™ Port is positioned within the abdominal cavity, and the laparoscopic cannulas are introduced through the channels. The insufflation tubing is attached. *Source:* © Daniel Spector.

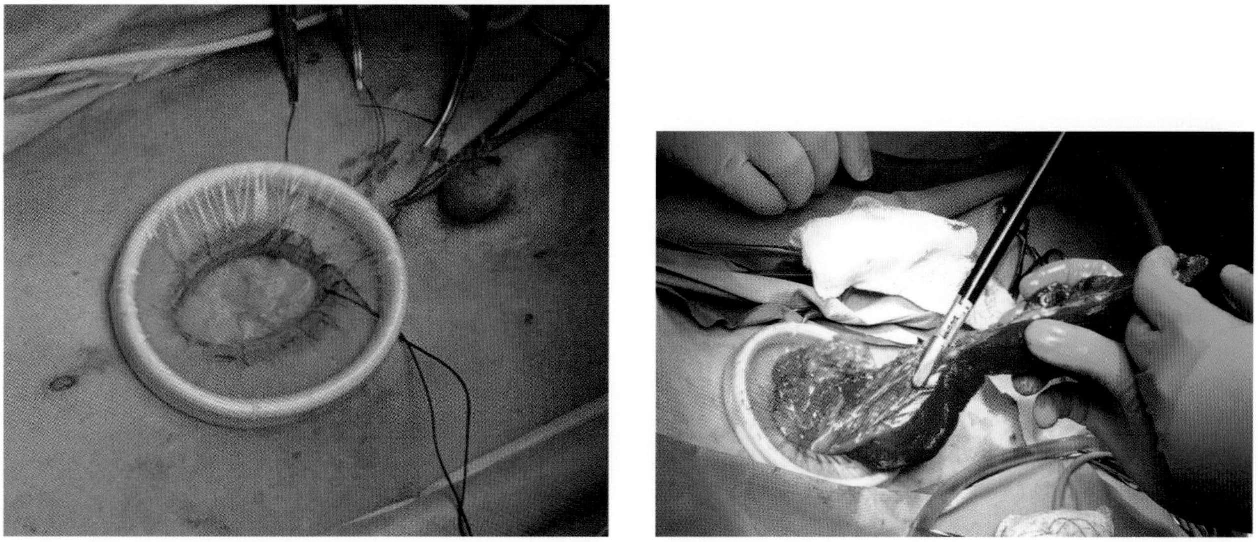

Figure 23.18 Following laparoscopic abdominal explore, the SILS™ Port is removed and replaced with a wound retraction device depicted in the top photo. Stay sutures are noted caudally that were previously placed on the body wall to facilitate port placement (Hasson technique). In the bottom image, a BVSD is used progressively toward the head of the spleen at the hilus, while continually exteriorizing the spleen. *Source:* © Pamela Schwartz.

intra- and post-operative blood loss.[25] Serial postoperative monitoring of hematocrit is recommended to monitor for hemorrhage from inadequately ligated vessels or vessels that were not obviously identified at the time of surgery due to intraoperative hypotension.

Vascular compromise to the pancreas can be iatrogenic in nature or secondary to another disease process, such as splenic torsion. Splenic torsion can either directly compromise the pancreatic branches or predispose the vasculature to thrombosis.[1,41] In dogs with splenic masses, hemorrhagic and thrombotic tendencies can occur separately or happen together within the same patient developing at different time points. Venous thrombosis can consume platelets and coagulation factors, leading to hemorrhagic tendencies.[38] One study documented that hypercoagulability was common during the first two weeks after splenectomy in dogs with splenic masses.[40] Thrombotic syndromes and coagulopathies combined were the most common cause of death

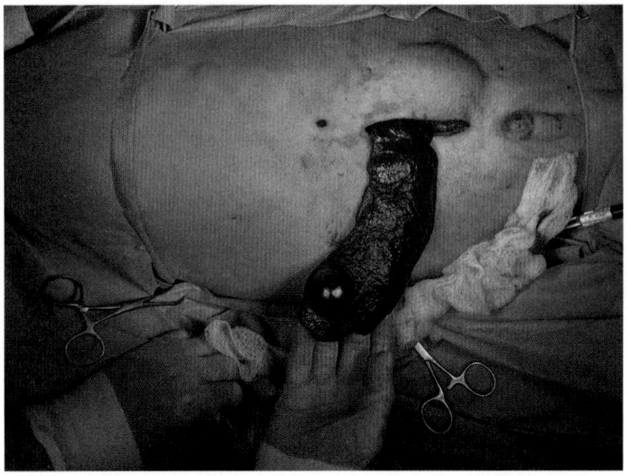

Figure 23.19 Minilaparotomy without a wound retractor device. The spleen is progressively exteriorized throughout LAS. *Source:* © Pamela Schwartz.

in one study.[38] Causes of venous thrombosis after splenectomy are not completely understood, although there are numerous potential risk factors for thrombosis. Large splenic masses may promote stasis of intra-abdominal blood flow, and manipulation of the splenic vasculature during splenectomy may contribute to portal system thrombosis. Portal system thrombosis is commonly accompanied by thrombocytopenia, elevated liver enzymes, and hypoalbuminemia, which are not uncommon in dogs presenting in hypovolemic shock.[38,42] Dogs with HSA appear to have a higher risk of DIC compared to other types of neoplasia. It is important to recognize DIC early and initiate treatment promptly due to its high mortality rate.[42]

Ventricular arrhythmias may develop in dogs with splenic masses due to anesthetic agents, thromboembolic events of the myocardium, and/or compromised venous return to the heart from compression of the vena cava or intra-abdominal hemorrhage. Continuous electrocardiogram (ECG) monitoring is recommended perioperatively to allow for immediate recognition and treatment of arrhythmias if they appear, as some types may be life-threatening by increasing susceptibility to cardiac arrest.[38] It is important to monitor continuous ECG postoperatively, even in the absence of pre- or intra-operative arrhythmias, as studies show the majority of arrhythmias develop in the postoperative period.[11,43] The need for transfusion or development of arrhythmias in the face of hemoperitoneum leads to longer hospitalization but can still carry a favorable perioperative outcome.[11] This is likely due to advancements in critical care of unstable patients. Dogs undergoing transfusion more commonly have hemoperitoneum, malignancy, and a higher odds of poor long-term outcomes compared with dogs that did not undergo transfusion.[44]

There is conflicting evidence in the literature regarding splenectomy as a risk factor for GVD, with some studies showing no risk and other studies showing an increased risk for GDV with a history of splenectomy.[37,45–47] It is possible that dogs with splenic neoplasia may skew the incidence of postoperative GDV, as this population may not survive long enough to subsequently experience GDV. It is also noted that both splenic disease and GDV are more prevalent in older, larger, deep-chested dogs.[11,45] Of the postoperative complications, GDV can be preventable by performing a prophylactic gastropexy (see Chapter 21) at the time of splenectomy. The author typically recommends prophylactic gastropexy (laparoscopically or open) in at-risk breeds of dogs or those with other risk factors at the time of splenectomy (Figure 23.15).

Prognosis

The overall prognosis for benign disease, such as splenic hematoma, is excellent, although a small proportion of these cases (11%) may have an undiagnosed malignant component presenting with metastatic disease at the time of death.[48] It is possible that these cases are misdiagnosed as benign, or there may be a different primary tumor than HSA in the spleen or elsewhere that is not initially detected. It is also possible that advancements in histopathologic characterization and immunohistochemical staining will make misdiagnosis less likely, but studies are warranted to support this theory. As most patients are older, the author recommends follow-up AUS even in benign cases, to monitor any comorbidities and for potential future metastasis.

The overall prognosis associated with splenectomy for treatment of splenic HSA is extremely poor with median survival times of 19–86 days with surgery alone.[9] Splenectomy with adjuvant treatment significantly extends medial survival to 117–273 days,[9,39] and with immunotherapy emerging in the oncologic world as an adjuvant option following surgery, referral to an oncologist is always recommended with a cancer diagnosis. Surgery is still the best option for HSA as a palliative treatment.

Yunnan Baiyao is a Chinese herbal remedy utilized for anti-inflammatory, hemostatic, wound-healing, and pain-relieving properties.[49,50] Yunnan Baiyao has been anecdotally reported to prolong survival times and control bleeding in dogs with HSA.[49] One study documents Yunnan Baiyao's ability to induce apoptosis in canine HSA cells.[49] Although further investigation in the treatment of HSA in dogs is warranted, Yunnan Baiyo appears to be safe in dogs. Since few patients survive beyond six months, its use should be considered. The author typically uses Yunnan Baiyo in cases of hemoperitoneum or when there is concern that additional sites may bleed and cannot be surgically controlled, such as with liver metastasis.

Much less is known regarding treatment and prognosis for splenic disease in cats, as it is much rarer compared to dogs. The prognosis for cats undergoing splenectomy is variable depending on the underlying cause, with median survival times as low as 132 days in cats with mast cell tumors and 197 days in cats with HSA.[8]

Notes

i LigaSure; Covidien/Medtronic; Mansfield, Massachusetts.
ii SurgRx EnSeal; Ethicon; Cincinnati, OH.
iii Harmonic system; Ethicon; Cincinnati, OH.
iv SILS Port; Covidien/Medtronic; Mansfield, Massachusetts.
v Alexis Wound Retractor; Applied Medical Resources Corp, Rancho Santa Margarita, California.

References

1 Richter, M.C. (2012). Spleen. In: *Veterinary Surgery: Small Animal* (ed. K.M. Tobias and S.A. Johnston), 1341–1352. Elsevier.
2 Case, J.B. and Fox-Alvarez, W.A. (2018). Splenectomy: hilar ligation technique. *Clinicians Brief* (April), 73–90, issued March 2018.
3 Fossum, T.W., Hedlund, C.S., Hulse, D.A. et al. (2019). *Small Animal Surgery E-Book*, 5e, 631–648.
4 Spangler, W.L. and Kass, P.H. (1997). Pathologic factors affecting postsplenectomy survival in dogs. *J. Vet. Intern. Med.* 11 (3): 166–171.
5 Sullivant, A. and Archer, T. (2018). Top 5 causes of splenomegaly in dogs. *Clinicians Brief* (April), 81–85, issued March 2018.
6 Corbin, E.E., Cavanaugh, R.P., Schwartz, P. et al. (2017). Splenomegaly in small-breed dogs: 45 cases (2005-2011). *J. Am. Vet. Med. Assoc.* 250 (10): 1148–1154.
7 Burgess, K.E., Price, L.L., King, R. et al. (2021). Development and validation of a multivariable model and online decision-support calculator to aid in preoperative discrimination of benign from malignant splenic masses in dogs. *J. Am. Vet. Med. Assoc.* 258 (12): 1362–1371.
8 Gordon, S.S., McClaran, J.K., Bergman, P.J. et al. (2010). Outcome following splenectomy in cats. *J. Feline Med. Surg.* 12 (4): 256–261.
9 Thamm, D.H. (2013). Miscellaneous tumors. In: *Withrow & MacEwen's Small Animal Clinical Oncology* (ed. D.M. Vail, S.J. Withrow, and R.L. Page), 697–688. St. Louis, MO: Elsevier.
10 Schick, A.R. and Grimes, J.A. (2022). Evaluation of the validity of the double two-thirds rule for diagnosing hemangiosarcoma in dogs with nontraumatic hemoperitoneum due to a ruptured splenic mass: a systematic review. *J. Am. Vet. Med. Assoc.* 261 (1): 69–73.
11 Stewart, S.D., Ehrhart, E.J., Davies, R. et al. (2020). Prospective observational study of dogs with splenic mass rupture suggests potentially lower risk of malignancy and more favourable perioperative outcomes. *Vet. Comp. Oncol.* 18 (4): 811–817.
12 Cleveland, M.J. and Casale, S. (2016). Incidence of malignancy and outcomes for dogs undergoing splenectomy for incidentally detected nonruptured splenic nodules or masses: 105 cases (2009-2013). *J. Am. Vet. Med. Assoc.* 248 (11): 1267–1273.
13 Lee, M., Park, J., Choi, H. et al. (2018). Presurgical assessment of splenic tumors in dogs: a retrospective study of 57 cases (2012-2017). *J. Vet. Sci.* 19 (6): 827–834.
14 Schick, A.R., Hayes, G.M., Singh, A. et al. (2019). Development and validation of a hemangiosarcoma likelihood prediction model in dogs presenting with spontaneous hemoabdomen: the HeLP score. *J. Vet. Emerg. Crit. Care* 29 (3): 239–245.
15 Cudney, S.E., Wayne, A.S., and Rozanski, E.A. (2021). Diagnostic utility of abdominal ultrasonography for evaluation of dogs with nontraumatic hemoabdomen: 94 cases (2014–2017). *J. Am. Vet. Med. Assoc.* 258 (3): 290–294.
16 Mallinckrodt, M.J. and Gottfried, S.D. (2011). Mass-to-splenic volume ratio and splenic weight as a percentage of body weight in dogs with malignant and benign splenic masses: 65 cases (2007-2008). *J. Am. Vet. Med. Assoc.* 239 (10): 1325–1327.
17 Fife, W.D., Samii, V.F., Drost, W.T. et al. (2004). Comparison between malignant and nonmalignant splenic masses in dogs using contrast-enhanced computed tomography. *Vet. Radiol. Ultrasound* 45 (4): 289–297.
18 Jones, I.D., Lamb, C.R., Drees, R. et al. (2016). Associations between dual-phase computed tomography features and histopathologic diagnoses in 52 dogs with hepatic or splenic masses. *Vet. Radiol. Ultrasound* 57 (2): 144–153.
19 Burti, S., Zotti, A., Bonsembiante, F. et al. (2022). A machine learning-based approach for classification of focal splenic lesions based on their CT features. *Front. Vet. Sci.* 9: 872618.
20 Kutara, K., Seki, M., Ishigaki, K. et al. (2017). Triple-phase helical computed tomography in dogs with solid splenic masses. *J. Vet. Med. Sci.* 79 (11): 1870–1877.
21 Clifford, C.A., Pretorius, E.S., Weisse, C. et al. (2004). Magnetic resonance imaging of focal splenic and hepatic lesions in the dog. *J. Vet. Intern. Med.* 18 (3): 330–338.

22 Martin, D.R. and Semelka, R.C. (2001). Imaging of benign and malignant focal liver lesions. *Magn. Reson. Imaging Clin. North Am.* 9 (4): 785–802, vi–vii.

23 Royals, S.R., Ellison, G.W., Adin, C.A. et al. (2005). Use of an ultrasonically activated scalpel for splenectomy in 10 dogs with naturally occurring splenic disease. *Vet. Surg.* 34 (2): 174–178.

24 Sirochman, A.L., Milovancev, M., Townsend, K. et al. (2020). Influence of use of a bipolar vessel sealing device on short-term postoperative mortality after splenectomy: 203 dogs (2005-2018). *Vet. Surg.* 49 (2): 291–303.

25 Monarski, C.J., Jaffe, M.H., and Kass, P.H. (2014). Decreased surgical time with a vessel sealing device versus a surgical stapler in performance of canine splenectomy. *J. Am. Anim. Hosp. Assoc.* 50 (1): 42–45.

26 Rivier, P. and Monnet, E. (2011). Use of a vessel sealant device for splenectomy in dogs. *Vet. Surg.* 40 (1): 102–105.

27 Sackman, J.E. (2012). Surgical modalities: laser, radiofrequency, ultrasonic, and electrosurgery. In: *Veterinary Surgery: Small Animal* (ed. K.M. Tobias and S.A. Johnston), 180–186. Elsevier.

28 Collard, F., Nadeau, M.E., and Carmel, E.N. (2010). Laparoscopic splenectomy for treatment of splenic hemangiosarcoma in a dog. *Vet. Surg.* 39 (7): 870–872.

29 Kuvaldina, A., Hayes, G., Sumner, J. et al. (2018). Influence of multiple reuse and resterilization cycles on the performance of a bipolar vessel sealing device (LigaSure) intended for single use. *Vet. Surg.* 47 (7): 951–957.

30 Smeak, D.D. (2008). Total splenectomy. *Clinicians Brief* (September), 13–17, issued August 2008.

31 Liscomb, V. (2012). Surgical staplers: toy or tool? *Compan. Anim. Pract.* 34: 472–479.

32 Ezzeldein, S.A., Elgaml, S.A., Elseddawy, N.M. et al. (2022). Assisted laparoscopic splenectomy: current concept for treatment of splenic hemangiosarcoma in dogs. *Iran. J. Vet. Res.* 23 (1): 46–52.

33 Shaver, S.L., Mayhew, P.D., Steffey, M.A. et al. (2015). Short-term outcome of multiple port laparoscopic splenectomy in 10 dogs. *Vet. Surg.* 44 (Suppl. 1): 71–75.

34 Khalaj, A., Bakhtiari, J., and Niasari-Naslaji, A. (2012). Comparison between single and three portal laparoscopic splenectomy in dogs. *BMC Vet. Res.* 8: 161.

35 Wright, T., Singh, A., Mayhew, P.D. et al. (2016). Laparoscopic-assisted splenectomy in dogs: 18 cases (2012-2014). *J. Am. Vet. Med. Assoc.* 248 (8): 916–922.

36 McGaffey, M.E.S., Singh, A., Buote, N.J. et al. (2022). Complications and outcomes associated with laparoscopic-assisted splenectomy in dogs. *J. Am. Vet. Med. Assoc.* 260 (11): 1309–1315.

37 Maki, L.C., Males, K.N., Byrnes, M.J. et al. (2017). Incidence of gastric dilatation-volvulus following a splenectomy in 238 dogs. *Can. Vet. J.* 58 (12): 1275–1280.

38 Wendelburg, K.M., O'Toole, T.E., McCobb, E. et al. (2014). Risk factors for perioperative death in dogs undergoing splenectomy for splenic masses: 539 cases (2001-2012). *J. Am. Vet. Med. Assoc.* 245 (12): 1382–1390.

39 Wendelburg, K.M., Price, L.L., Burgess, K.E. et al. (2015). Survival time of dogs with splenic hemangiosarcoma treated by splenectomy with or without adjuvant chemotherapy: 208 cases (2001-2012). *J. Am. Vet. Med. Assoc.* 247 (4): 393–403.

40 Phipps, W.E., de Laforcade, A.M., Barton, B.A. et al. (2020). Postoperative thrombocytosis and thromboelastographic evidence of hypercoagulability in dogs undergoing splenectomy for splenic masses. *J. Am. Vet. Med. Assoc.* 256 (1): 85–92.

41 DeGroot, W., Giuffrida, M.A., Rubin, J. et al. (2016). Primary splenic torsion in dogs: 102 cases (1992-2014). *J. Am. Vet. Med. Assoc.* 248 (6): 661–668.

42 Hammer, A.S., Couto, C.G., Swardson, C. et al. (1991). Hemostatic abnormalities in dogs with hemangiosarcoma. *J. Vet. Intern. Med.* 5 (1): 11–14.

43 Panissidi, A.A. and DeSandre-Robinson, D.M. (2021). Development of perioperative premature ventricular contractions as an indicator of splenic hemangiosarcoma and median survival times. *Vet. Surg.* 50 (8): 1609–1616.

44 Lynch, A.M., O'Toole, T.E., and Hamilton, J. (2015). Transfusion practices for treatment of dogs undergoing splenectomy for splenic masses: 542 cases (2001-2012). *J. Am. Vet. Med. Assoc.* 247 (6): 636–642.

45 Goldhammer, M.A., Haining, H., Milne, E.M. et al. (2010). Assessment of the incidence of GDV following splenectomy in dogs. *J. Small Anim. Pract.* 51 (1): 23–28.

46 Grange, A.M., Clough, W., and Casale, S.A. (2012). Evaluation of splenectomy as a risk factor for gastric dilatation-volvulus. *J. Am. Vet. Med. Assoc.* 241 (4): 461–466.

47 Sartor, A.J., Bentley, A.M., and Brown, D.C. (2013). Association between previous splenectomy and gastric dilatation-volvulus in dogs: 453 cases (2004-2009). *J. Am. Vet. Med. Assoc.* 242 (10): 1381–1384.

48 Patten, S.G., Boston, S.E., and Monteith, G.J. (2016). Outcome and prognostic factors for dogs with a histological diagnosis of splenic hematoma following splenectomy: 35 cases (2001-2013). *Can. Vet. J.* 57 (8): 842–846.

49 Wirth, K.A., Kow, K., Salute, M.E. et al. (2016). In vitro effects of Yunnan Baiyao on canine hemangiosarcoma cell lines. *Vet. Comp. Oncol.* 14 (3): 281–294.

50 Lee, A., Boysen, S.R., Sanderson, J. et al. (2017). Effects of Yunnan Baiyao on blood coagulation parameters in beagles measured using kaolin activated thromboelastography and more traditional methods. *Int. J. Vet. Sci. Med.* 5 (1): 53–56.

24

Liver Biopsies

Nicole J. Buote

Department of Clinical Sciences, Cornell University, Ithaca, NY, USA

Key Points

- Hemorrhage is the most important postoperative complication of liver biopsies therefore clinicians should have access to hemostatic agents and clotting times should be evaluated before surgery if liver disease is extensive.
- Multiple biopsies should always be obtained if the abnormalities are diffuse or variable in appearance.
- Specific techniques to decrease biopsy sample artifacts should be followed to increase the diagnostic quality of samples.

Introduction

Liver biopsies can provide clinicians valuable information about a patient's underlying liver function that simply cannot be supplied by blood work or imaging alone. Biopsies of the liver can be performed by multiple methods either through an open laparotomy or laparoscopically.[1–3] Laparoscopic liver biopsies have the advantage of decreased morbidity and are recommended when only liver biopsies are required.[4] Minimally invasive liver biopsies without the use of laparoscopic equipment can also be performed. Liver biopsies taken through an open (traditional laparotomy) approach are easy to perform, and this procedure is often added to other procedures when abnormalities are seen during an abdominal explore.

Indications/Pre-operative Considerations

Liver biopsies are one of the most useful procedures a clinician can perform to determine specific prognostic information for owners regarding their pet's liver function. Understanding that agreement between ultrasound-guided fine needle aspirate and open surgical wedge biopsy is often suboptimal (30–40%), surgical biopsies are frequently considered essential. The most common reasons for liver biopsies in the author's practice are increasing liver enzymes in the face of medical treatment, persistent, or worsening changes to the architecture of the liver on ultrasound imaging, cases in which an ultrasound-guided biopsy is contraindicated, and visualization of hepatic abnormalities during abdominal exploratory (Table 24.1).

The most important preoperative consideration before proceeding with a liver biopsy is the possibility of hemorrhage. The liver is a highly vascular organ; therefore, clinicians should have access to hemostatic agents (Gelfoam®, Surgicell®, Vetigel®) to aid in hemostasis depending on the technique utilized. Patients undergoing liver biopsy for presumed liver disease may have inappropriate clotting function due to reduced synthesis of clotting factors; therefore, prothrombin time (PT) and partial thromboplastin time (PTT) should be evaluated before surgery. If coagulation function is abnormal, the procedure should be delayed while plasma is provided. A preoperative PCV/TP should always be performed to allow for a comparison postoperatively to monitor for bleeding. Depending on the illness of the patient and the number and type of biopsies, blood products should be available when performing these

Techniques in Small Animal Soft Tissue, Orthopedic, and Ophthalmic Surgery, First Edition. Edited by Kristin A. Coleman.

Companion website: www.wiley.com/go/coleman/surgeries

Table 24.1 Indications for liver biopsy.

Hepatic biochemical abnormalities
Not responding to or worsening on medical therapy
Hepatic pathology worsening on ultrasound or advanced imaging
Ultrasound-guided biopsy contraindicated
Ascites
Microhepatica
Hepatic cysts/abscesses
Vascular tumor
Cannot access specific lesions due to location
Not deemed safe to access specific lesions (too close to vessels or bile ducts)
Hepatic pathology visualized during surgery

procedures. Patients with liver disease may present with anemia (from coagulopathies, gastric ulceration), hypoglycemia (with severe hepatic insufficiency), hypoalbuminemia (which may decrease wound healing), and ascites (which may decrease tidal volume and make anesthesia more challenging). Anesthetic considerations for patients suffering from hepatic disease are discussed in detail in multiple references[1,5] and can be consulted if necessary.

Surgical Procedure

General liver biopsy tenets include the following:

1) Aiming for 1 cm × 1 cm × 1 cm tissue segment without crushing or cautery artifact to include at least six to eight portal triads.
2) For diffuse liver disease, aim for samples from at least three liver lobes but avoid the caudate lobe, because preferential perfusion to this lobe tends to make this area unrepresentative.
   a) Biopsy peripherally AND at least one central region to be sure representative samples are obtained.
3) For nodular changes or masses:
   a) If multiple nodules are all grossly identical, biopsy at least two of them.
   b) If a single mass, aim for two biopsies, avoiding very friable or necrotic areas.
   c) If multiple types of nodules, be sure to biopsy each type.
   d) If possible, target those nodules with peripheral placement, as any hemorrhage will be easier to control.
4) If quantitative copper assessment is desired, be sure to check with the particular lab for handling procedure, as they may require "fresh" tissue (biopsy placed in saline instead of formalin and refrigerated or frozen), and volume of tissue required.

Biopsy Techniques

Biopsy techniques can be separated into central or peripheral. Peripheral biopsies are performed more commonly, but in the case of specific masses/nodules, clinicians should know how to perform each type. In the case of small fibrotic livers (end-stage liver disease), caution should be taken in performing central biopsies, because the larger hepatic vessels tend to be closer to the surface due to decreased hepatic parenchyma and significant hemorrhage can occur.

Central Parenchymal Biopsy

In this technique, a 6 mm or larger skin biopsy punch (Baker's punch) is used to obtain liver tissue. The punch is gently inserted into the parenchyma and Metzenbaum scissors are used to cut the tissue at the base to remove it from the incision (Figure 24.1). Important aspects of this technique include the following:

1) Only turn the punch in one direction as see-sawing back and forth will cause artifacts to the tissue.
2) Do not grab the liver plug with forceps if possible, as this may crush the sample. Try to gently use the tips of the Metzenbaum scissors to push the sample out of the parenchyma while cutting the base.
3) Pre-cut a piece of hemostatic foam or have hemostatic gel available and apply gentle tamponade for 3 minutes after biopsy.
4) You can attempt placing a horizontal mattress suture using a 4-0 suture in the hepatic capsule if still bleeding, but the author does not find this necessary in most cases.

Peripheral Biopsy Techniques

There are multiple techniques reported for peripheral liver biopsies,[1–3] including wedge, guillotine, and laparoscopic cup forceps techniques. For open procedures, the wedge and guillotine are the most common and both provide substantial tissue for diagnosis. The guillotine method is best used when there is a tip to the liver lobe or naturally occurring fractures that allow for the suture to be well-seated (Figure 24.2a). Rounded and thickened liver lobes are not well-suited to a guillotine biopsy but cuts in the liver can be made to allow for this technique to be utilized if necessary (Figure 24.3).

Guillotine Technique

To perform the guillotine technique, pre-form a suture loop with 3-0 or 4-0 monofilament absorbable or delayed absorbable suture with a surgeon's knot and place it proximal (toward the hilus) to the liver being biopsied. It is important to tighten down the suture in one quick move, otherwise, the suture tends to "fall off" the liver lobe as it hits the capsule (Figure 24.2b,c). Complete the knot with

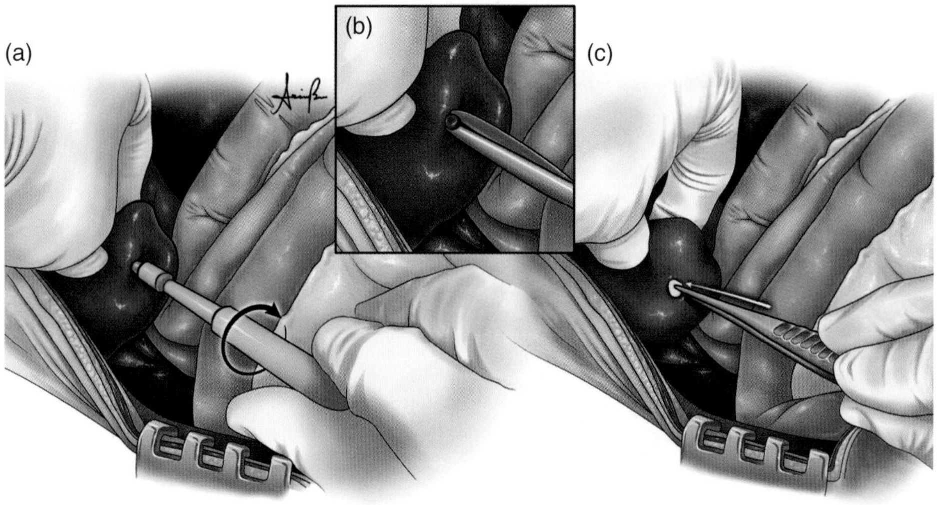

Figure 24.1 Illustration of a Baker's punch being used for a central liver biopsy. (a) The punch is inserted into the parenchyma and rotated in one direction. (b) The Metzenbaum scissors are used to cut the tissue at the base to remove it from the incision. (c) A precut plug of hemostatic foam is inserted into the biopsy site.

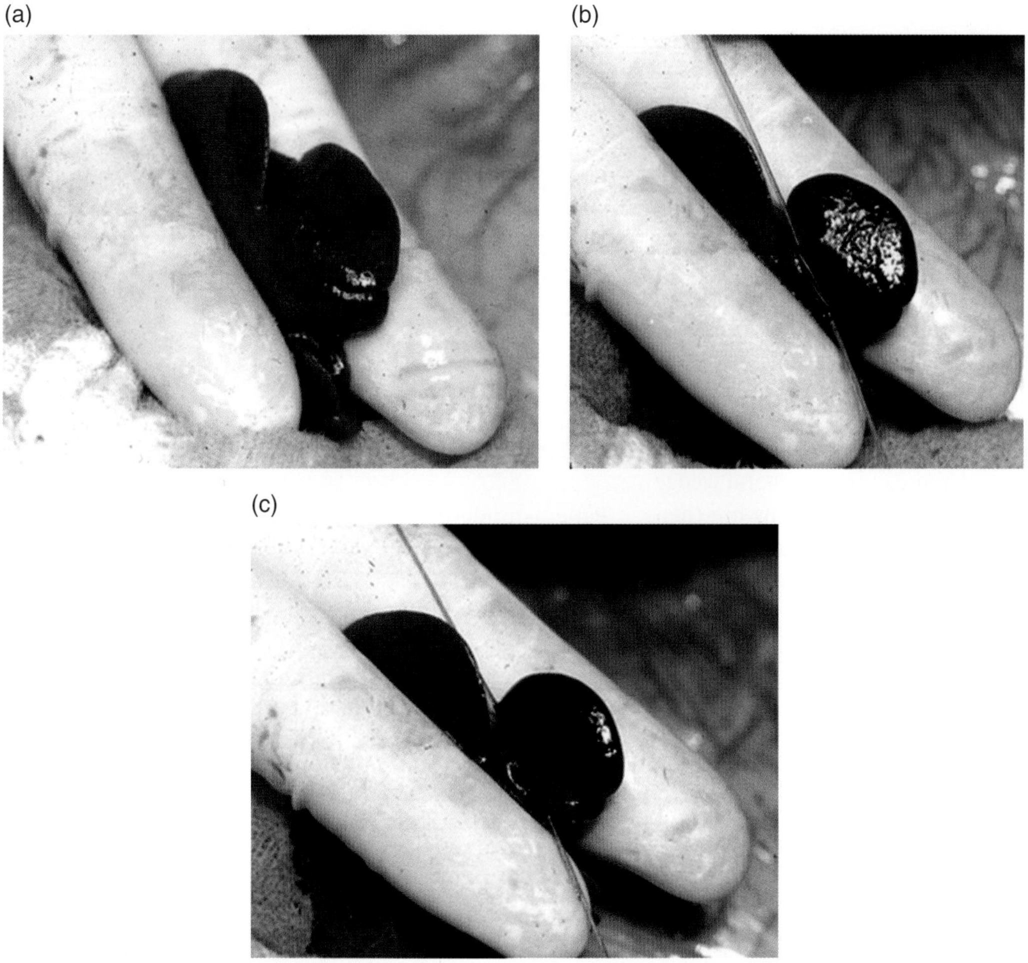

Figure 24.2 Photographs of a guillotine liver biopsy in a canine patient. (a) Liver lobe edge with naturally occurring edges that the suture will easily be seated around. (b) Pre-looped suture resting around liver edges. (c) Suture tied tightly and disappearing into liver parenchyma. *Source:* Courtesy of Dr. James Flanders.

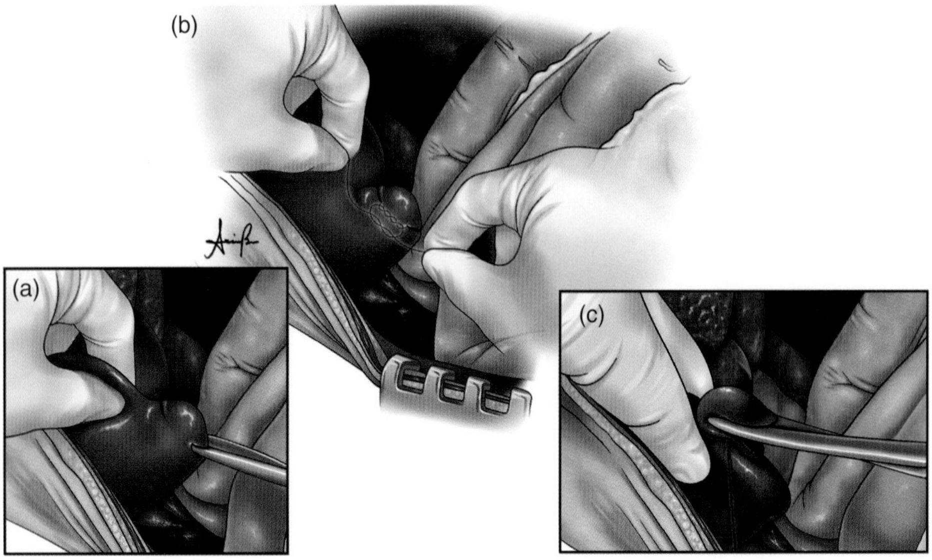

Figure 24.3 Illustration of the guillotine technique for a peripheral liver lobe biopsy. (a) Incisions being created with Metzenbaum scissors in the liver to allow the pre-formed loop of suture to be placed. (b) Pre-formed suture loop with a surgeon's knot placed within the incisions. (c) Metzenbaum scissors transecting the liver distal to the ligature after knots tied.

three additional throws, and then use Metzenbaum scissors to transect the liver distal to the ligature (Figure 24.3). Be careful not to leave too much (>2 mm) tissue distal to your ligature, as this tissue is without a blood supply and could become a nidus for inflammation or infection.

Wedge Biopsy

The wedge technique is considered by many to be the "Gold Standard." This technique results in a large sample with minimal artifact and leaves a site that can be sutured for immediate hemostasis. When performing this technique, the area of interest is transected by sharp excision with Metzenbaum scissors to remove an equilateral wedge with ~1 cm lengths. The sides of the biopsy site are then gently apposed using a horizontal mattress suture or simple interrupted sutures with 3-0 or 4-0 monofilament absorbable or delayed absorbable suture (Figure 24.4).

Potential Complications

The most common complication of liver biopsy is hemorrhage. The vast majority of times, hemorrhage is self-limiting, and if appropriate preoperative case evaluation has been performed, it is not detrimental to the patient. In cases where unexpected severe hemorrhage is encountered intraoperatively, a partial or complete liver lobectomy may need to be performed. This can be accomplished with a ligating loop (similar to the guillotine method) or stapling equipment. If concern for ongoing hemorrhage is appreciated postoperatively, the clinician can place an abdominal bandage to help with tamponade, may provide blood products, or at last resort, re-explore the patient.

Post-operative Care/Prognosis

Patients undergoing only liver biopsy could in theory be sent home the same day depending on their comfort. A postoperative PCV/TP is rechecked two hours after surgery to ensure a precipitous drop has not occurred. Do not check a PCV earlier than two hours, because fluid shifts and sequestration of red blood cells during anesthesia can produce a falsely low result. Postoperative care centers on incision care (E-collar, decreased activity) and pain medication (gabapentin 10 mg/kg PO q 8–12 hours for five days). The prognosis depends solely on the biopsy results.

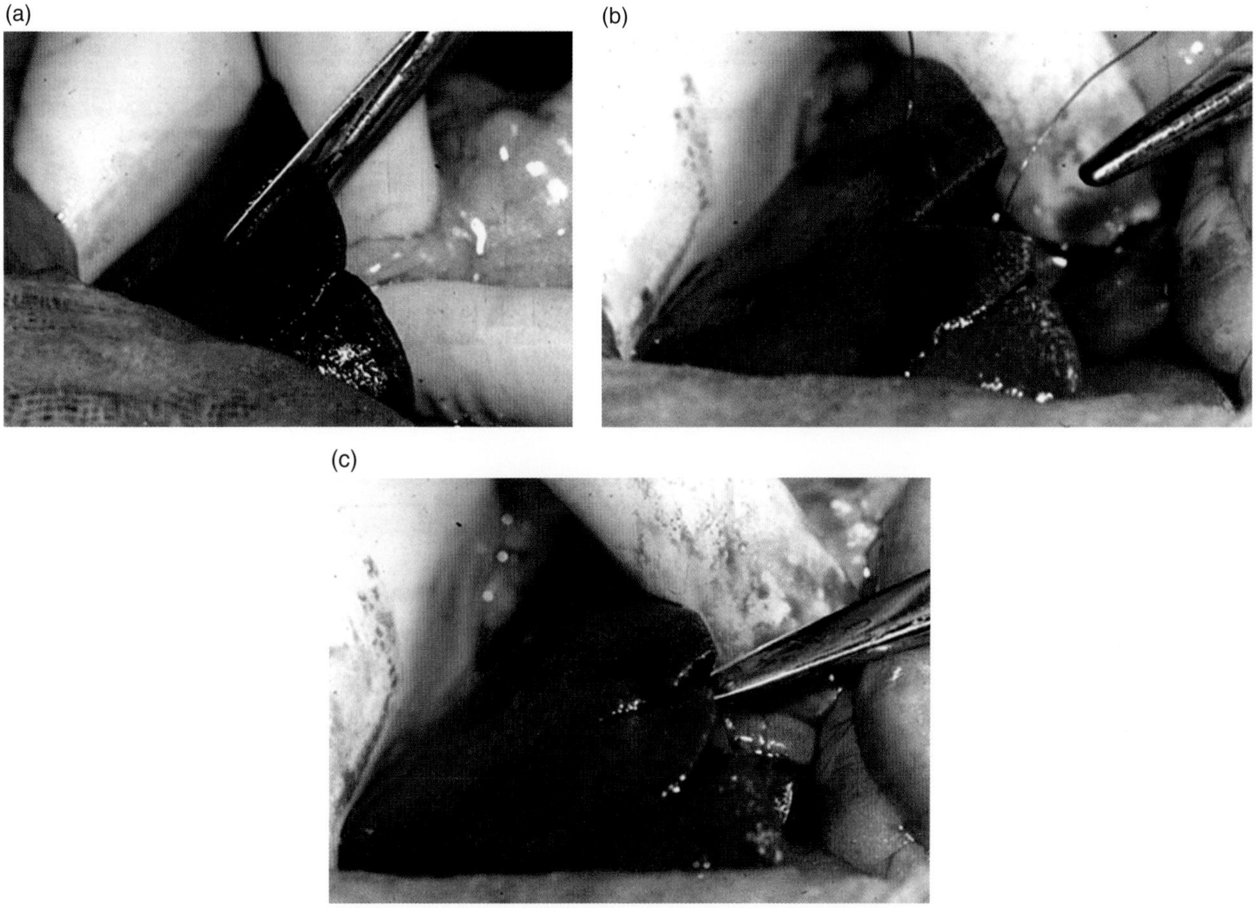

Figure 24.4 Photographs of a wedge liver biopsy in a canine patient. (a) Metzenbaum scissor being used to incise the edge of a liver lobe. (b) The first horizontal suture placed on the near side of the wedge biopsy site. (c) After the horizontal suture has been tied, an additional simple interrupted suture could be placed at the edge of this biopsy site to further impede bleeding. *Source:* Courtesy of Dr. James Flanders.

References

1 Fossum, T.W. (2018). Surgery of the liver. In: *Small Animal Surgery*, 5e (ed. T.W. Fossum), 540–570. Elsevier Health Sciences (US).

2 Case, J.B. and Alvarez, W.A. (2014). Open and laparoscopic liver biopsy. *Clinician's Brief*. https://www.cliniciansbrief.com/article/open-laparoscopic-liver-biopsy.

3 Lidbury, J.A. (2017). Getting the most out of liver biopsy. *Vet. Clin. North Am. Small Anim. Pract.* 47 (3): 569–583.

4 Buote, N.J., Loftus, J.P., and Miller, A.D. (2022). Laparoscopic twist technique has the best overall artifact profile when comparing three laparoscopic hepatic cup biopsy techniques for dogs. *Am. J. Vet. Res.* 83 (12): ajvr.22.08.0127. https://doi.org/10.2460/ajvr.22.08.0127.

5 Garcia-Pereira, F. (2015). Physiology, pathophysiology, and anesthetic management of patients with hepatic disease. In: *Veterinary Anesthesia and Analgesia, the Fifth Edition of Lumb and Jones*, 5e (ed. K.A. Grimm, L.A. Lamont, W.J. Tranquilli, et al.), 627–638. Wiley Global Research (STMS).

25

Ovariohysterectomy/Ovariectomy

Brad M. Matz

Department of Clinical Sciences, Auburn University, Auburn, AL, USA

Key Points

- Ovariohysterectomy should not be considered “routine” rather the surgeon should pay close attention to surgical principles to be sure the primary goals are achieved.
- Surgeons should consider the use of a strangle knot to ensure secure ligation of larger tissue pedicles.
- Consideration of ovariectomy is a reasonable alternative to ovariohysterectomy in the appropriate situation.

Introduction

Spaying is a very common surgical procedure in small animal veterinary practice. Ovariohysterectomy is the typical procedure taught in U.S. veterinary medical schools. This involves an abdominal approach, suspensory ligament disruption, secure ligation of both ovarian pedicles, broad ligament division, secure ligation of the uterine body and associated vasculature, and excision of the reproductive tract.

Ovariectomy, removal of both ovaries while the uterine horns and body remain, has received increased attention because the procedure can often be accomplished with a smaller incision, less tissue dissection/disruption, and no increase in long-term issues, such as pyometra and urinary incontinence.[1] However, one study did not show a difference in time to complete the surgery or pain scores between dogs undergoing ovariectomy and ovariohysterectomy.[2] Ultimately, the procedure chosen is the practitioner's decision and should be discussed with the owner. The presence of uterine pathology influences this decision; however, in young, otherwise healthy dogs, ovariectomy is a reasonable choice. It is similarly a reasonable choice in older dogs without uterine pathology.

Indications/Preoperative Considerations

The primary indication for surgery is to eliminate the potential for unwanted pregnancy and/or to eliminate reproductive behavior. Mitigation of mammary tumor development is another factor cited in favor of ovariohysterectomy. The risk of mammary tumor development has been shown to be 0.5%, 8%, and 26% when dogs were spayed before the first heat cycle, after the first heat cycle, and after the second and subsequent heat cycles, respectively.[3] Ovariohysterectomy may decrease mammary tumor recurrence under certain circumstances in dogs with mammary tumors.[4] Other indications include uterine/ovarian trauma, neoplasia, or fluid accumulation in the uterine lumen.

Preoperative considerations vary depending on patient factors and preoperative screening tests should be tailored to patient and owner factors. For example, young otherwise healthy animals may need limited blood work prior to surgery (packed cell volume, total protein, lactate, and glucose measurement) compared to an older patient with various co-morbidities. The latter might need more involved blood work (complete blood count, serum chemistry, urine analysis) and potentially imaging depending on the

Techniques in Small Animal Soft Tissue, Orthopedic, and Ophthalmic Surgery, First Edition. Edited by Kristin A. Coleman.

Companion website: www.wiley.com/go/coleman/surgeries

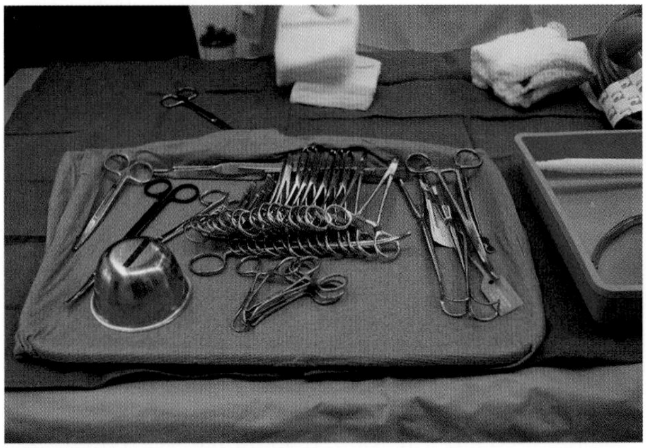

Figure 25.1 Standard instruments in a "spay pack."

reasons for ovariohysterectomy. The breed of the patient may also determine the need for additional testing prior to any surgical procedure, such as buccal mucosal bleeding time (BMBT) as a screening test for von Willebrand's disease in Doberman Pinschers.

Appropriate antiseptics, surgical consumables, such as drapes and suture material, as well as appropriate instrumentation (Figure 25.1) should be on hand. X-ray detectable sponges should be used and counted before and after surgery prior to closure.

These procedures can usually be completed by a single surgeon; however, contingencies for emergent issues (e.g., loss of pedicle control) should be in place, and it is useful to have another veterinarian or a technician practiced in aseptic technique and tissue retraction if a situation occurs. Suspensory ligament disruption is a challenging aspect of the procedure because it often takes more force than believed necessary, and the ligament is ideally disrupted deeper in the abdomen often out of the surgeon's direct sight. The ligament is broken a distance from the ovary because the physical distance from the pedicle is greater craniodorsally in the abdomen. Suspensory ligament disruption is usually needed to improve ovarian exteriorization and pedicle exposure in dogs, but not always so in cats.

Surgical Procedure

The surgical technique for ovariohysterectomy has many variations. A three-clamp technique procedure is described here with potential variations noted. Relevant differences between cats and dogs are also noted.

The clipped area should be sufficiently large enough to allow for incision extension in either the cranial or caudal direction (Figure 25.2). Clipping from immediately cranial to the xiphoid process to immediately caudal to the pubis and lateral to the nipples will result in an adequate amount of exposure.

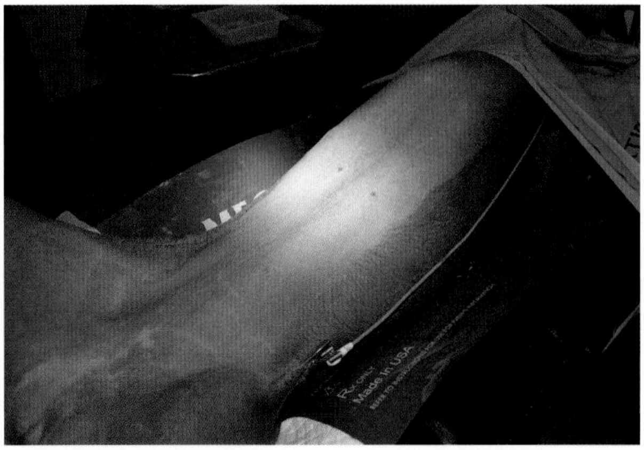

Figure 25.2 Sufficient clipping of hair should include cranial to the xiphoid process, caudal to the pubis, and lateral to the nipples.

Draping with liquid impervious quarter drapes secured with an adequate number of towel clamps to similar dimensions as the clipped area is recommended. A large over-drape is then placed and opened such that the patient is covered (Figure 25.3).

The caudal aspect of the over-drape can be attached to the instrument table or draped over it, depending on surgeon preference. This is not necessary but does create a relatively large, continuous area covered by a sterile drape. The drape is opened with scissors and a rectangle of over-drape that closely matches the quarter-draped area is removed. The over-drape can be secured to the quarter drapes with non-penetrating clamps, such as Lorna-Edna or Allis tissue forceps.

Incision length and exact location will vary depending on patient size, reproductive status, species, and exact procedure to be performed. In general, incision location and length for dogs is from immediately caudal to the umbilicus extending caudally approximately 2/3's the distance to the pubis. The incision can begin somewhat more caudally

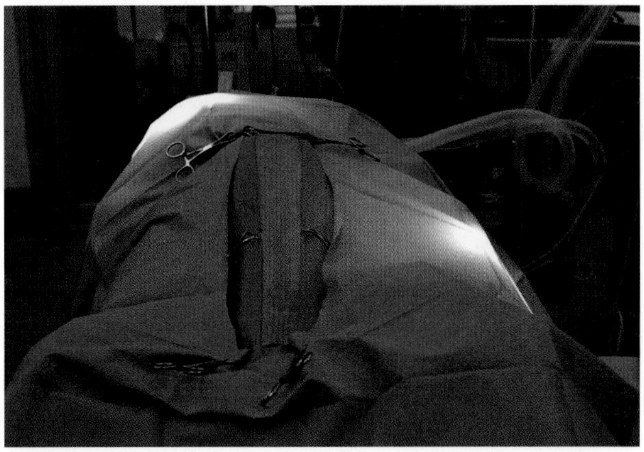

Figure 25.3 Proper draping of the ventral abdomen for open ovariectomy or ovariohysterectomy.

in cats. If an ovariectomy is to be performed, the incision can be shifted cranially and does not need to extend to the same degree caudally. If any cranial abdominal procedures will also be performed (e.g., prophylactic gastropexy), the incision will need to be sufficiently large and extend cranially to accomplish the other procedure(s). Sterile saline lavage during surgery will help limit tissue desiccation.

Ovariohysterectomy

The skin incision should be made sharply with a #10 or #15 scalpel blade with the dominant hand from cranial to caudal with the surgeon's dominant hand on the same side of the animal (right hand dominant on the animal's right side). This should be done with a smooth stroke of the blade with the thumb and first finger of the non-dominant hand tensing the skin outwardly so that the skin separates completely when incised. This will help to eliminate multiple incision attempts that result in jagged or partial incised edges. This can be continued through the subcutaneous tissues until external rectus abdominis fascia is seen. The surgeon can then use thumb forceps to grasp the subcutis, and with Metzenbaum scissors, elevate the subcutaneous tissue from the external rectus fascia as one layer of fat (Figure 25.4).

Care should be taken that this is not done laterally but in a craniocaudal or caudocranial direction to avoid excessive elevation. This can be more of an issue in cats, where the subcutaneous tissue is not as robustly attached to the external fascia as in dogs. Excision of a section of fat over the midline is not necessary and can actually be detrimental to healing in cats, where the subcutaneous tissue contains precursors necessary for woundhealing. A Brown-Adson or other thumb forceps with adequate holding ability is used to grasp the ventral midline (linea alba) and allow for controlled scalpel entry through the midline. This should not require excessive force but rather allow the sharp blade to do the work. The author recommends holding the scalpel upside down (point of a #10 blade closest to the animal) with the thumb and first finger only while allowing the "heel" of the handle to track along the abdominal wall (horizontal to the ground). This will eliminate an angled entry trajectory and hopefully limit the loss of depth control on abdominal entry. The abdominal wall incision is the same length as the skin incision, and as with any abdominal cavity entry, digital palpation of the ventral peritoneum is performed to ensure the absence of midline adhesions of viscera prior to incision. Care is then taken to stay on the ventral midline by using partially inserted thumb forceps to guide the scalpel incision. It is normal to expose rectus muscle caudally where the linea alba is narrower. A variation of this technique is preferred by some where an intentional right paramedian abdominal wall approach is made. This potentially improves exposure of the more cranially positioned right ovary; however, hemorrhage from the incised/separated rectus abdominis muscle fibers and increased post-operative discomfort may limit its utility.

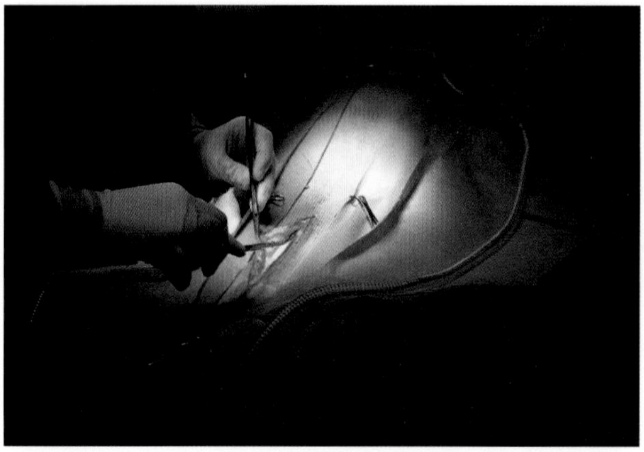

Figure 25.4 Subcutaneous tissue elevation with Metzenbaum scissors.

Uterine horn location can be done with direct visualization or with a spay hook. If a spay hook is used, it can be directed with the hook facing caudally against the interior of the abdominal wall. The instrument is then turned 90° so the hook is medially directed and gently swept medial and ventral. The surgeon should be sure to investigate what is retrieved, because misidentification and returning uterus/broad ligament to the abdomen is common. Excessive force to retrieve the hook should be avoided, since a tethered dorsally-located structure preventing easy elevation of the spay hook could be a ureter.

Once a uterine horn is located, it can be followed to an ovary. The author recommends two methods of suspensory ligament disruption. The first option is to grasp the ovarian pedicle dorsal to the ovary between the thumb and third finger of the dominant hand. This allows for the arm of the surgeon to tension the ligament caudally while the first finger is used to extend dorsally down the ligament and disrupt it while applying straight caudal pressure. The other option involves placement of hemostatic forceps on the proper ligament, caudal to the ovary, and tension the ovary ventrally and caudally while extending the first finger of the dominant hand dorsally down the ligament and disrupting as described. The surgeon should be sure their finger is directly on the ligament, and omentum or intestinal mesentery is not between the finger and the ligament. The surgeon should also be sure the ligament is tensioned while attempting disruption. If it is loose or slack, it will be more difficult to break. The surgeon should also be sure their finger stays directly on the ligament while pushing caudally. In the author's opinion, attempts at side-to-side motion or slipping off the side of the ligament with a curled finger will result in ovarian pedicle disruption (partial or complete).

This should be avoided. The suspensory ligament of the cat can be transected with scissors, taking care to avoid the vasculature, or it may be sufficiently loose to allow ovarian exposure without disruption.

A three-clamp technique can be used for ovarian pedicle ligation. A closed hemostat is directed through the broad ligament caudal to the ovarian pedicle, and the clamp is moved dorsally and ventrally to expand a "window" in the broad ligament caudal to the ovarian vasculature (Figure 25.5).

Rochester-Carmalt forceps are ideal for pedicle security because of their longitudinal serrations and should be the clamps used in the proximal and middle positions. The distal-most clamp can be a standard hemostatic forceps or a Rochester-Carmalt (Figure 25.6). The ovarian pedicle is sharply transected between the middle and distal clamps, and the ovary/uterine horn is reflected caudally (Figure 25.7).

The ovarian pedicle can be ligated with various patterns and suture types. The author typically uses monofilament, delayed absorbable suture but more rapidly absorbable suture is also acceptable. Suture size can vary significantly with patient size and the degree of fat present in the pedicle. Most mature, medium- to large-breed dogs are ligated with 2-0 to 0-sized sutures. Smaller sizes such as 2-0 to 4-0 sutures are used in small dogs and cats. Interestingly, the use of a surgeon's throw has been shown to leak at significantly lower pressures when tested on a model, and modified miller's knots have been shown to leak at physiologic blood pressure.[5] The author recommends placement of a strangle knot[5] as the first (proximal most) ligation after removing the most proximal clamp. The pedicle is then ligated with a transfixation ligation (modified Halsted or figure-of-eight), and the middle clamp is removed while holding the pedicle with thumb forceps (Figure 25.8). The site is checked for lack of bleeding while taking care to limit tension on the pedicle. Once hemostasis is assured, the pedicle is returned to the abdomen.

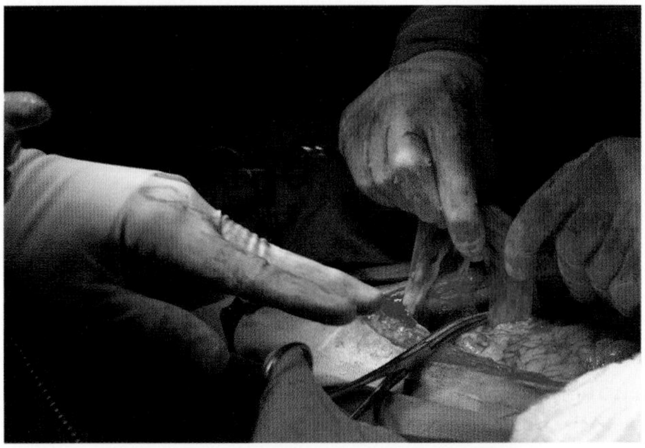

Figure 25.5 Creation of a "window" through the broad ligament.

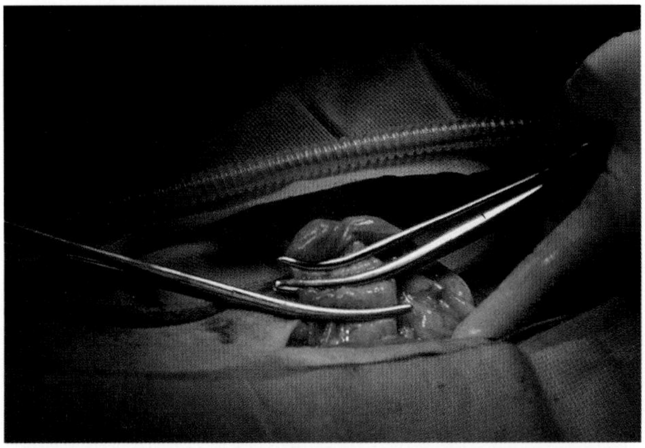

Figure 25.6 Picture demonstrating a three-clamp technique.

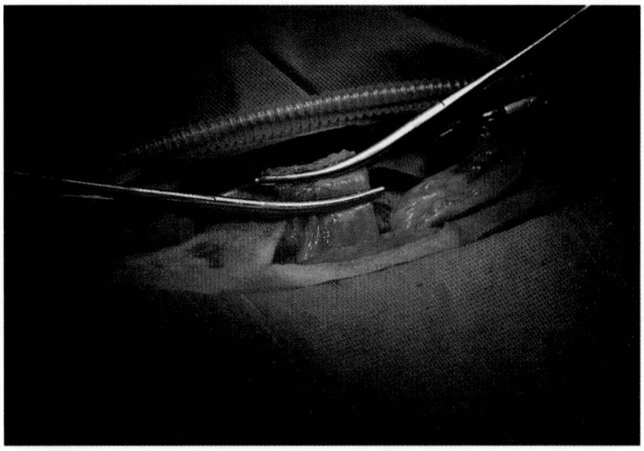

Figure 25.7 After pedicle transection, the ovary is reflected caudally.

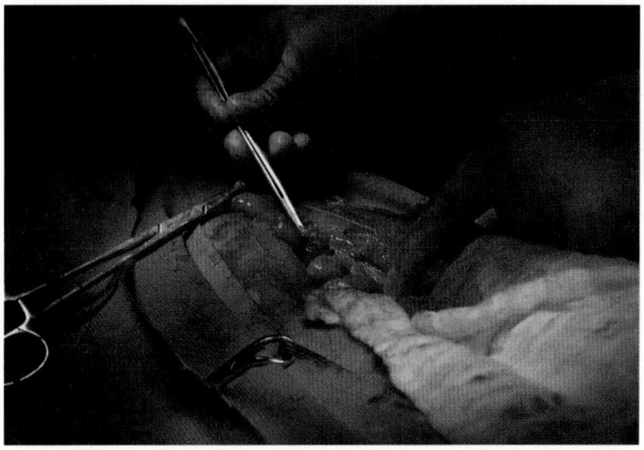

Figure 25.8 Controlled pedicle release after the final ligation.

The broad ligament is disrupted from cranial to caudal. It can be digitally torn, ligated if well-developed vasculature is present, cut sharply with scissors, or transected with electrosurgery. Alternatively, a window can be made on each side near the uterine vasculature to allow for a few fingers to be passed through. With a closed fist, bottom on the hand near the abdominal incision, the broad ligament, including the round ligament, is grasped, the wrist rotated so the closed fist is rotated to pull the round ligament through the inguinal canal and simultaneously disrupt the broad ligament. The uterine arteries/veins are ligated as described above, though the author does not typically use a three-clamp technique because it is possible to crush through the uterine tissue in both cats and dogs. Two options for uterine body ligation are commonly used. One would be to tie a transfixation ligature with the first two throws around one of the laterally-located uterine vessels at the level just cranial to the cervix, then complete the pattern by tying the remaining four throws around the caudal uterine body. This pattern is repeated on the opposite side, which essentially allows for two ligatures around the uterine body prior to transection. The other option is to separately ligate all three structures: uterine vessels and the caudal uterine body. When this method is elected, one of the three reliable friction knots (miller's knot, strangle knot, constrictor knot) according to Hazenfield et al.[5] may be used to ligate the caudal uterine body.

Each pedicle site should be evaluated for any ongoing hemorrhage and addressed if this is seen. The lateral most mesenteric structures on the right and left sides are the mesoduodenum and mesocolon, respectively. Retraction of these structures to the opposite side (to the left for the duodenum) will hold the GI tract behind the mesentery and allow for a clear line of sight to each pedicle. These maneuvers are also useful in case of loss of pedicle control during the procedure. A single hemostat can be used to gently grasp the pedicle. A single additional ligation is usually sufficient to manage any ongoing bleeding. The uterine pedicle is often located where it was replaced, but inspection dorsal to the urinary bladder is sometimes needed to locate it. Similarly, a single additional ligation is usually all that is needed to control any ongoing bleeding. If hemorrhage is encountered, visualization is often aided by extension of the incision cranially and/or caudally.

Sponge and instrument counts should be confirmed prior to closure. The abdominal wall is apposed with monofilament delayed absorbable suture, which should engage the external rectus sheath holding layer with every bite of appropriate distance from the cut edge and from the adjacent bite of suture. Simple interrupted, cruciate mattress, or simple continuous patterns are all appropriate. The subcutaneous tissue is apposed with fine, rapidly absorbable suture material in a simple continuous pattern closing dead space by occasionally taking small bites in the external fascia. The skin is apposed with skin sutures, staples, or an intradermal pattern using fine, rapidly absorbed suture material.

Ovariectomy

The initial incision is located in the same if not somewhat cranially to that described above. The caudal extent needs to be sufficient to allow adequate exposure of the uterine horns; however, it will likely not need to extend as far caudally as above since the uterine body does not require exposure. A uterine horn is located and followed to an ovary. Ovarian exposure is the same as that described above. The suspensory ligament is disrupted, the ovarian pedicle is isolated, and a three-clamp technique is used. The ovarian pedicle is ligated as described above. The uterine vasculature is ligated at the level of the proper ligament, and the ovary is excised. This is repeated for the other side. Care should be taken to ensure the entire ovary is removed, so to avoid the potential risk of ovarian remnant syndrome, it is acceptable to ligate and transect within the distal uterine horn caudal to the proper ligament.

Potential Complications

There are a number of potential complications that can be encountered during or after ovariectomy/ovariohysterectomy. One study evaluated 1880 dogs and found an overall complication rate of 7.5%.[6] Specific complications from this study included: ovarian pedicle bleeding, bleeding from the surgical site, wound-healing issues, urinary incontinence, and ovarian remnant syndrome. Anesthesia time and patient body weight were significantly associated with the development of a complication.

Hemorrhage from the ovarian or uterine pedicle sites can be due to inadequate or loose ligations. If this occurs during surgery, it can be managed by placement of additional sutures. Care should be taken during exposure of the ovaries and uterus so that excessive tension is avoided because vessel tearing can also result in hemorrhage.[7] Properly tight ligatures may be more easily attained if adequate exposure of the tissues is achieved, which means avoidance of small incisions, and if excess fat is eliminated from the perivascular area prior to suture placement.

Ovarian remnant syndrome is another important complication. Care should be taken to ensure both ovaries are removed completely. Clamping at or through ovarian tissue must be avoided. The ovarian bursa can be opened once the ovary is removed to allow for visual inspection prior to closure. Measurement of progesterone can help confirm residual ovarian tissue if suspected postoperatively.[7] Uterine remnant pyometra is only possible in a "spayed" animal when ovarian tissue remains or exogenous progesterone sources are present.

Ureteral ligation is another possible complication. Adequate incision size and confirmation of tissues removed can help minimize this issue. Care should be taken when ligating the uterine pedicle near the urinary bladder because the ureters are physically closer to the uterus in this location. One way to ensure grasping of the uterine horn and not the ureter is to follow the horn both cranially to the ovary and caudally to the uterine body, the latter of which also allows for identification of the contralateral uterine horn without the need for a spay hook.

Post-op Care/Prognosis

The prognosis following ovariectomy and ovariohysterectomy is generally excellent. The post-operative care involves activity restriction, using protective collars or shirts to deny access to the incision, and limiting self-trauma. Oral pain medications can be used for several days after surgery, and as long as aseptic technique is followed throughout the procedure, no post-operative antibiotics are necessary.

References

1. van Goethem, B., Schaefers-Okkens, A., and Kirpensteijn, J. (2006). Making a rational choice between ovariectomy and ovariohysterectomy in the dog: a discussion of the benefits of either technique. *Vet. Surg.* 35 (2): 136–143.
2. Peeters, M.E. and Kirpensteijn, J. (2011). Comparison of surgical variables and short-term postoperative complications in healthy dogs undergoing ovariohysterectomy or ovariectomy. *J. Am. Vet. Med. Assoc.* 238 (2): 189–194.
3. Schneider, R., Dorn, C.R., and Taylor, D.O. (1969). Factors influencing canine mammary cancer development and postsurgical survival. *J. Natl. Cancer Inst.* 43: 1249–1261.
4. Kristiansen, V.M., Peña, L., Díez Córdova, L. et al. (2016). Effect of ovariohysterectomy at the time of tumor removal in dogs with mammary carcinomas: a randomized controlled trial. *J. Vet. Intern. Med.* 30 (1): 230–241.
5. Hazenfield, K.M. and Smeak, D.D. (2014). In vitro holding security of six friction knots used as a first throw in the creation of a vascular ligation. *J. Am. Vet. Med. Assoc.* 245 (5): 571–577.
6. Muraro, L. and White, R.S. (2014). Complications of ovariohysterectomy procedures performed in 1880 dogs. *Tierarztl Prax Ausg K Kleintiere Heimtiere* 42 (5): 297–302.
7. Stone, E.A. (2003). Ovary and uterus. In: *Textbook of Small Animal Surgery* (ed. D. Slatter), 1487–1502. Pennsylvania: Saunders.

26

Cesarean Section

David Michael Tillson

Department of Clinical Sciences, Auburn University, Auburn, AL, USA

Key Points

- Cesarean section can be scheduled to avoid potential dystocia in at-risk breeds with good survivability in neonates.
- 60–80% of dogs and cats presenting for dystocia will require a C-section.
- Effective planning for a C-section is essential for the best outcomes.
- Anesthesia for a C-section should prioritize drugs with minimal fetal impact, reversibility, and effective analgesia for the dam.
- Ventral midline incision followed by a single hysterotomy incision on the ventral uterine body is routinely performed with fetuses advanced to the single incision.
- Hysterotomy closure can be double-layer or single-layer in a simple continuous or inverting pattern.
- Early return of the dam to the neonates is preferred, and early hospital discharge is ideal for stable patients.

Introduction

The procedure called a Cesarean section (C-section) has been around for most of human history. The term has been attributed to the legend that Julius Caesar was "cut from his mother's womb" as she died in childbirth. While a good story, its accuracy is questioned.[1] The term more likely arose from a decree from Caesar that the child of any woman dying during childbirth in Rome would be taken "by section" to maintain the population of the Empire. In veterinary medicine, a C-section is used both as an emergency procedure in patients experiencing difficulties during delivery (i.e., dystocia) and increasingly, as an intentionally planned and scheduled procedure in breeds considered to be at high risk of dystocia.

Indications

The primary indication for a C-section is anticipated or real-time difficulty in delivering fetuses at the time of birth. For this reason, a C-section can be "scheduled" or emergent. A scheduled C-section is typically used for breeds with a high risk of developing difficulties during parturition, known physical abnormalities that would negatively impact a vaginal delivery, large litter sizes, or owner preference or convenience. Neonatal survival is reportedly excellent (99%) for scheduled C-section compared to an emergency C-section (87%).[2] An emergency C-section is required when a patient is in stage 2 labor and unable to deliver a litter vaginally. This could mean a patient in active labor without producing any neonates, or it could be a partial delivery but incomplete parturition. The patient requiring an emergency C-section needs to be carefully evaluated and stabilized as effectively as possible prior to anesthesia and surgery.

Dystocia

The process of labor is divided into three stages (Table 26.1). Once the first stage of labor has begun, parturition should progress in a timely manner, and long delays without productive delivery should initiate concern.

Techniques in Small Animal Soft Tissue, Orthopedic, and Ophthalmic Surgery, First Edition. Edited by Kristin A. Coleman.

Companion website: www.wiley.com/go/coleman/surgeries

Table 26.1 Stages of labor.[3,4]

Stage 1	Silent; cervical dilation, increasing uterine contractions; typically, less than 12 h; both the bitch and queen delay the onset of labor when in unfamiliar or stressful environments; panting, restless, nesting behavior (bitch); vocalization and loud purring in the queen
Stage 2	Active contractions and process of fetal expulsion; 3–12 h in bitch; averaging a puppy/hour; queen can take longer 4–16 h but occasionally hours between kittens
Stage 3	Final stage – complete expulsion of placental membranes; often passed between fetuses

There are numerous conditions that can impair normal parturition. These conditions can be physical or physiological and are typically categorized as being of maternal or fetal origin. In dogs, roughly 3/4 of dystocias are of maternal origin, and in cats, 2/3 of dystocias are considered to be of maternal origin.[3,5] Physical issues affecting the dam or queen are related to the pelvic canal diameter, such as small pelvic size compared to fetal size, previous pelvic trauma, as well as vaginal malformation or the presence of vaginal bands that impede the passage of the fetus. More commonly occurring in the cat, uterine torsion is another potential cause of dystocia that is rare but reported. Patients with uterine torsion have been actively in stage 2 labor (contractions and straining) but without results. They can rapidly decompensate with this condition and may present to the veterinarian as depressed or moribund, tachycardiac, exhibiting poor peripheral perfusion, and have a painful abdomen on palpation. Aggressive stabilization and rapid surgical intervention are needed to salvage these patients. Other maternal factors, such as abdominal hernias or uterine prolapse, may impair the ability of the dam to generate effective abdominal pressure for labor. Similarly, the pelvic canal diameter could be compromised by soft tissue compression or non-osseous obstructions.

Physiological or medical concerns for a dystocia patient often include physical exhaustion, hypotension, hypoglycemia, and/or hypocalcemia. Primary or secondary uterine inertia may be the most common reason for dystocia.[3] Primary uterine inertia involves a failure of the uterus to begin organized, propulsive contractions. In complete primary uterine inertia, stage 2 labor is not reached, while partial primary uterine inertia results in weak, ineffective contractions only. Secondary uterine inertia can be the result of exhaustion of the uterine musculature caused by obstructions, mispositioned fetuses, or the delivery of a large litter.

Fetal causes of dystocia are typically associated with fetal positioning, fetal size, or fetal abnormalities (malformation, giantism). In some patients, problems with fetal positioning or a "stuck" fetus can be managed through sedation, lubrication, and digital manipulation; however, problems created by excessive fetal size or fetal abnormalities typically necessitate surgical intervention. Low fetal numbers or the presence of a single fetus may not stimulate progression toward stage 2 labor, resulting in extended gestation. A C-section is appropriate for gestational lengths of greater than 70 days in the dog or 71 days in the cat (day 0 being designated as the luteinizing hormone (LH) surge with ovulation happening around 48 hours after that).

Medical management can be considered when the female is in good health, there are no known physical conditions to impair fetal passage, and the cervix is adequately dilated. Imaging should be used to confirm the pregnancy and fetal positioning prior to beginning treatment.[6] Fetal heart rates should also be within normal limits, indicating no fetal stress at the time medical management is initiated. Medical management is typically supportive in nature, providing fluids, glucose, and a warm, safe, comfortable environment for parturition, as well as administration of oxytocin and calcium gluconate (Table 26.2) if the patient is hypocalcemic.

If a stuck fetus or fetal malpositioning is determined to be the cause of the dystocia, physical manipulation can be tried to see if the fetus can be removed or repositioned, allowing parturition to continue. Despite medical

Table 26.2 Drugs used in the medical management of dystocia.[3,7]

Drug	Dosage	Comment
Crystalloid fluids	2.5 mL/kg/hr (60 ml/kg/day) – standard maintenance fluid rate; additional fluid volume added to compensate for dehydration (see comments)	Bolus dose of 90 mL/kg (shock dose) can be given divided over an hour; patient should be checked every 15 min for responsiveness to resuscitation (blood pressure, heart rate, mucous membrane color, etc.) and for any signs of fluid overload.
Calcium gluconate (10%)	0.2 mL/kg IV (dog/cat) 1–5 mL per dog SQ	Intravenous administration can cause cardiac arrhythmias if given too rapidly; cardiac auscultation should be performed prior to administration and during administration. Use of calcium in queens is controversial; use with care.
Oxytocin	0.1 units/kg IM (current recommendation – dog/cat)	Other dosing includes: 0.5–2.0 U/dog or cat IM; or 5–20 U/dog IM.

intervention, it is estimated that 60–80% of dogs and cats with dystocia will still require surgical intervention.[3,5]

Fetal heart rate is important to monitor in the patient in late stage 1 or stage 2 labor. The results give the clinician vital information that will heavily influence the decision whether or not to perform an emergency C-section. The normal fetal heart rate is typically above 200 bpm (180–200 bpm).[3,7] Lower rates, between 150 and 170 bpm, are indicative of moderate to severe fetal stress, prompting the consideration of surgical intervention. Fetal heart rates of <150 bpm signal the need for immediate surgical intervention. Care should be taken when assessing fetal heart rates during labor, as uterine contractions may lower the fetal rates during an active contraction. Heart rates should be taken over 30–60 seconds and, ideally, from multiple fetuses for the best evaluation.[5]

Dogs should complete labor in 3–12 hours; averaging at least one puppy per hour. Cats can present a unique challenge since they can have extended periods of inactivity between kittens, normally completing parturition in 4–16 hours; however, it has been reported that cats can deliver a final kitten up to 42 hours after the initiation of labor.[3] Owners unfamiliar with that species-specific quirk may think their cat is experiencing a dystocia when they are, in fact, having a normal parturition. It is important that feline owners understand a queen experiencing this type of labor should not be in constant distress during this period and should not be in active labor without producing a kitten in a timely manner.

If the patient is determined to need surgical intervention, either after initial evaluation or after failed medical management, pre-anesthetic management is initiated or continued. Intravenous fluids, using a balanced crystalloid solution, are started to correct dehydration and counteract hypotension. A biochemical profile and complete blood count (CBC) should be considered. At a minimum, the patient's packed cell volume, total protein, blood urea nitrogen (BUN), lactate, glucose, and calcium should be evaluated and supplementation provided as needed. Although they are commonly encountered in dogs, neither hypoglycemia nor hypocalcemia is routinely seen in cats experiencing dystocia.[8]

When there is documented fetal death, extra care must be taken in surgery to avoid contamination of the surgical field or abdominal cavity. Patients suffering from multiple dead fetuses should be considered candidates for an "en-bloc" C-section.

Scheduled C-Section

A scheduled (i.e., "planned" or "elective") C-section is different from the dystocia-driven, emergency C-section. Scheduled C-sections are routine for breeds acknowledged to have a high risk of dystocia. These breeds include English and French Bulldogs, Boston Terriers, Pekingese, Pugs, and other brachycephalic breeds. Many other breeds have been reported to be susceptible to dystocias requiring a C-section, including Labrador and Golden Retrievers, German Shorthair Pointers, Chihuahuas, and Scottish, Yorkshire, and Dandie Dinmont Terriers, as well as giant breeds like Great Danes, Boerboels, and Mastiffs.[3,9,10–13] Cat breeds identified as being prone to dystocia include Domestic Shorthair, British Shorthair, Devon Rex, Birman, and Ragdoll cats and Oriental breeds.[7,8,11] The use of scheduled C-sections in breeds at low risk of dystocia eliminates the potential for dystocia-related complications; however, it introduces the risks associated with anesthetic, surgical, and post-operative complications.

No significant difference was found in the percentage of neonates surviving to discharge (overall 93%) between brachycephalic breeds (95%) undergoing C-sections when compared to non-brachycephalic breeds (92%).[2] The same study found that the puppies delivered by elective C-section were significantly more likely to survive discharge (99%) than puppies delivered by emergency C-section (87%).[2] A scheduled C-section can also be chosen for the convenience of the breeders and veterinarian, although the ethics of such a choice has been questioned.[13]

It is preferable to get a scheduled C-section patient as close to full-term gestation as possible to maximize neonatal survival. Gestation lengths can vary based on breed, litter size, and species. Normal gestation ranges from 57 to 72 days in the dog and 54–74 days in the cat.[4] If the decision for a C-section in a dog is to be based on breeding dates alone, it is recommended to do the C-section at full term (61–65 days) based on the last successful breeding with careful client counsel regarding breeding, ovulation, and fertilization timing (e.g., measuring LH surge). Clients should understand that in using breeding dates alone, individual variance could still potentially result in prematurity at the time of C-section.[3] Litter size can influence the duration of gestation, and larger litters tend to have a shorter gestational period. Using this criterion, puppies should be viable but there is a risk that the dam could go into labor prior to the C-section. The veterinarian should make sure the owner is aware of the clinical signs of parturition: nesting behaviors, a drop in body temperature, milk let-down, and other signs of early labor, in order for the patient to present to the veterinarian prior to the development of active labor.

The measurement of a serum progesterone level in the bitch increases the accuracy of the timing decisions associated with a scheduled C-section. Serum progesterone levels typically fall 12–24 hours prior to onset of parturition, in conjunction with the reported body temperature drop (less than 99 °F). A progesterone concentration of less than

2.0 ng/ml in a late-gestational bitch is used at the author's institution to signal the scheduled C-section should occur within the next 12–18 hours. As with all such testing, not all dogs follow the rules, and attention must also be focused on the patient for other signs of impending parturition as previously discussed.

Emergent C-Section

A dystocia-prompted C-section is considered an urgent or emergent surgical procedure. As with many surgical emergencies, the status of the patient needing the procedure can vary from anxious, yet stable, to moribund based on the duration of labor, fetal viability, and overall health status of the patient. Once it is determined that medical management is not appropriate or not working, there should be rapid progress toward surgical intervention. Considerations in when to begin anesthesia and surgery include the current health status of the dam, the stage of labor, and fetal heart rates as an indicator of intrauterine stress. Specific indications for surgical intervention in a dystocia are presented in Table 26.3.

Pre-operative management for a patient with dystocia requiring a C-section is typically aimed at making the patient a better, more stable candidate for anesthesia and surgery. Many of these measures, including fluid administration, pain management, sedation, and correcting hypocalcemia or hypoglycemia, would be undertaken during initial assessment and stabilization of the patient.

Table 26.3 Indications for surgical management of a dystocia.[6]

Maternal (majority of dystocia etiologies)	Fetal
• In stage 1 labor for more than 24 h • Have entered stage 2 labor without delivering a fetus within an acceptable period (<1 h) • Passage of green or black discharge from the vagina BEFORE delivery of the first fetus • Failure of medical management for uterine inertia • Extended period between puppies (>3 h) when additional puppies are known to remain • Visible presence of fetal membranes at the vulva without rapid passage of the fetus (10–15 min) • Significant vaginal hemorrhage • Still-born puppies • Diagnostic imaging demonstrating obstruction to fetal passage	• Fetal malpositioning • Fetal distress based on assessment of fetal heart rate • Fetal interference (two fetuses lodged at the uterine body) • Fetal abnormalities, such as malformation, giantism, or fetal monster

Table 26.4 Client communications.

Pre-operative discussions with clients are aimed at better understanding the client goals and priorities in relation to a C-section. While the goal is always to avoid operative complications, C-sections can require the veterinarian to deal with multiple issues at the same time. Adequate staffing can help temper this situation, and since many C-sections occur after-hours, staffing may be suboptimal in regards to numbers or training. As such, the veterinarian needs to have a clear insight into client priorities when dealing with unexpected complications.

Questions to clarify include:

- What are the client's priorities, mother or offspring, if an emergency should arise?
- Is the future breeding potential of the dam a priority? Is maintaining the future breeding potential of the female essential?
- Are the owners interested/willing to have the female sterilized at the time of the C-section?

Owners should not be invited into the operating room to "assist" with a C-section or with neonate resuscitation. Numerous legal actions have been pursued against veterinarians based on failing to follow this advice.

Once neonates have been delivered and stabilized, owners can be recruited to monitor the neonates – in a different room – until the procedure is completed and the mother recovered.

For all C-section patients, but especially those undergoing an emergency procedure, it is essential to have a clear understanding of the client's expectations and goals. Important questions about operative priorities must be discussed prior to the induction of anesthesia (Table 26.4). A clear understanding of the owner's expectations and priorities will assist the surgeon in making timely decisions in the event surgical findings or complications necessitate difficult intra-operative choices.

Pre-surgical Management

It is important to have a thorough patient assessment prior to C-section since the patient can be anywhere between physically normal to exhausted and agitated from prolonged labor to hypotensive, hypoglycemic, hypothermic, and borderline septic. In stable patients, minimal pre-operative management may be required, and anesthesia and surgery can proceed rapidly. In compromised patients, the goal should be to effectively resuscitate and stabilize the patient in anticipation of surgery. Rushing an unstable patient into surgery is only appropriate if aggressive stabilization efforts have failed.

Basic patient preparation includes intravenous catheterization and supportive fluid administration. Many patients in labor have had reduced fluid intake and are moderately dehydrated at presentation, making intravenous fluids appropriate. Cooperative patients can be pre-clipped along the ventral abdomen before anesthetic induction. It is also good to review instructions for puppy/kitten resuscitation to the team that will be receiving the neonates during the procedure and ensuring there is a safe, warm place for the neonates until the dam is out of surgery and recovered. This location should have supplemental oxygen and face masks available, suction bulbs, warm towels, instruments and supplies for managing the umbilical structures, and resuscitation drugs available. Radiographs may be obtained at presentation. These can be useful for evaluating puppy numbers, positioning, and documenting fetal abnormalities or death (Figure 26.1).

Anesthesia

It has been said, "There are no safe anesthetics, just safe anesthetists." This is a valid statement when considering anesthesia for a C-section. While numerous protocols exist, this section outlines several principles useful in developing

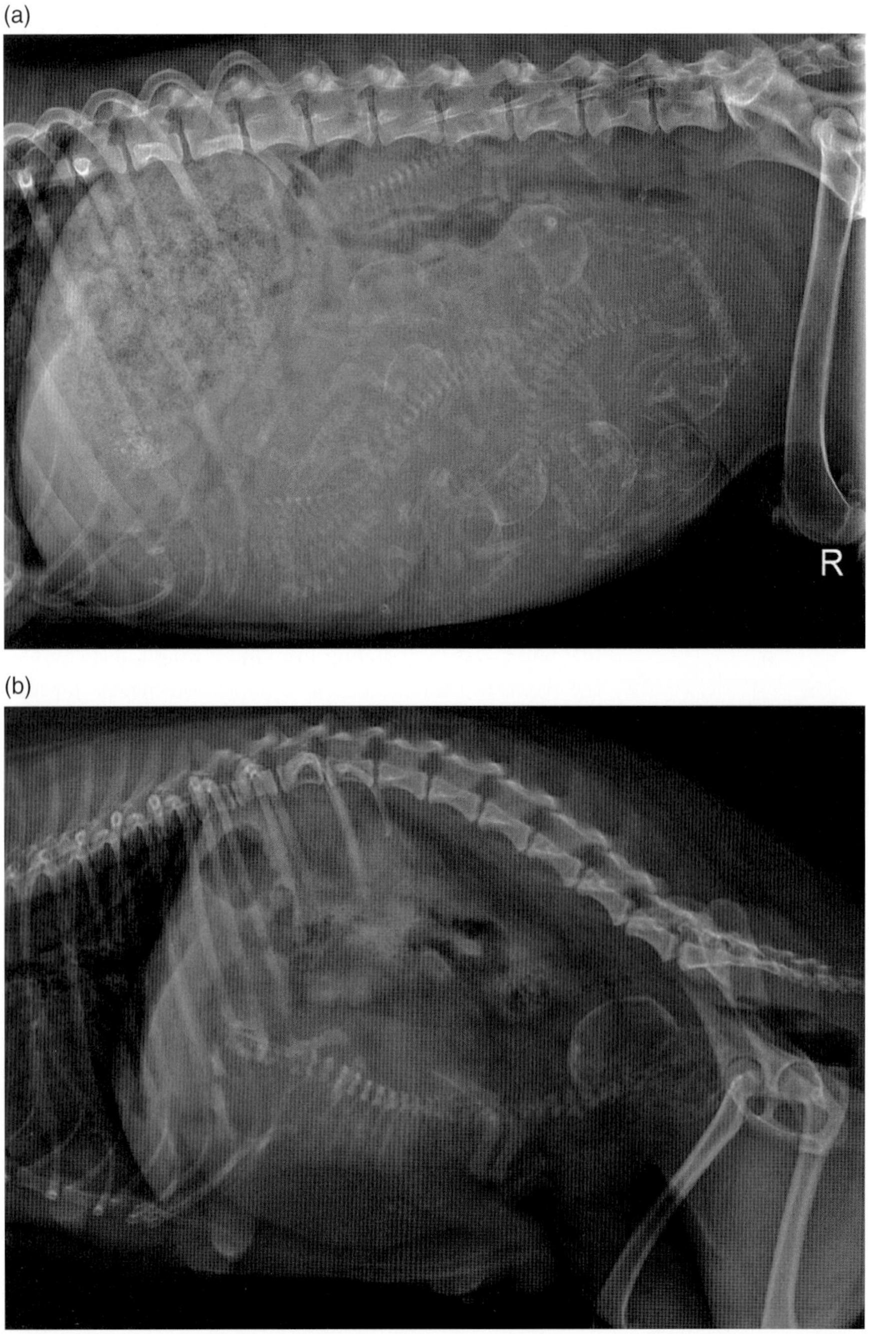

Figure 26.1 Abdominal radiographs confirm the pregnancy, permit puppy counts, and allow for the evaluation of potential dystocia concerns. (a) A lateral radiograph of a gravid female. Note: (1) the numerous puppies and (2) the full stomach. This can represent an aspiration risk if surgery is required. (b) A single puppy is seen on this lateral radiograph of a small breed dog. The large fetal size and maternal conformation make natural delivery unlikely. A C-section would be appropriate.

a protocol. It should be a goal to have all drugs, supplies, and equipment ready to move through the entire C-section procedure in a concise, timely manner. Delays in moving from one point to the next increase the risk of undesired complications and increased fetal mortality.[3,12]

Points to consider when determining the anesthetic plan include (1) minimizing negative effects of the anesthetic protocol on the neonates, (2) rapid anesthetic induction to allow immediate control of the patient's airway, thereby minimizing the potential for maternal and fetal hypoxia, (3) providing effective patient anesthesia/analgesia during the procedure, and (4) promoting a swift recovery with minimal side effects and limited residual impact on the dam. Endotracheal intubation must be included with the anesthetic protocol to maximize oxygen delivery to both the mother and the fetus and to protect the airway from aspiration events. Modification of familiar anesthetic protocols by tweaking dosages and routes or relying on reversible drugs might be safer for the practitioner than trying an entirely new protocol under difficult circumstances.

Minimal premedication drugs are used for C-sections. When the pet is compliant, intravenous catheterization, surgical site clipping, initial instrumentation, and the start of monitoring can be done without pre-meds. However, if these steps are increasing patient anxiety or the patient would benefit from sedatives or analgesics, they should be provided. Sedatives, such as acepromazine (0.02–0.05 mg/kg; SQ, IM, IV), can be used in a normotensive patient for sedation and may provide a smooth recovery. Dexmedetomidine offers good analgesia and sedation but has significant effects on cardiac output and peripheral vasoconstriction. Thus, the use of this alpha-2 agonist in C-sections is not widely embraced. A study evaluating dexmedetomidine concentrations in the amnionic fluid of puppies after IV administration showed the placental membranes to be effective barriers to the drug, even while concentrations within the placenta remained. Given this information, and with the availability of a specific reversal agent, dexmedetomidine may have a role in the anesthesia protocol for a C-section.[14,15] Premedicating with benzodiazepines can be challenging, as they can promote excitement in anxious or aggressive dogs. If they are chosen to be a part of the anesthesia protocol, give them intravenously immediately followed by anesthetic induction. Low-dose opioids can be effective for sedation and pre-operative analgesia but can cause panting, nausea, and vomiting. If analgesic needs require higher doses of opioids, they can be given IV immediately prior to or after anesthetic induction and initiation of inhalational anesthesia. Opioids are able to cross the placental barrier and can have a negative impact on neonatal respiration. When opioids are used, naloxone should be available to the neonatal team. A drop of naloxone under the tongue (transmucosal) can reverse excessive sedation and respiratory depression when resuscitating neonates. Alternatively, once all the fetuses have been delivered, additional doses of opioids or other analgesics can be given to the dam. Some anesthesiologists include pre-oxygenation in the pre-induction routine. While pre-oxygenation can be useful, the process of holding an oxygen mask over an anxious dog may create more challenges than the advantages gained. This is especially true when the anesthesia team is able to rapidly induce and intubate the patient, providing 100% O_2 via endotracheal tube, in a timely manner.

Rapid induction of unconsciousness is achieved using an intravenous induction agent, e.g., propofol (2–6 mg/kg) or alfaxalone (1–2 mg/kg), titrated to effect to allow for easy endotracheal intubation.[16] These drugs have become the preferred induction agents for C-sections and both have been shown to be safe for canine C-sections. In one study, alfaxalone was associated with better neonatal vitality for the first hour after delivery, although there was no difference beyond that point.[16] Once the patient is induced and intubated, 100% oxygen is started, and a minimal level of gas anesthetic, e.g., isoflurane or sevoflurane, is started to maintain anesthesia. The endotracheal tube is secured, and the cuff is inflated to an appropriate pressure. Typically, additional analgesics and analgesia strategies are used with a C-section to minimize the inhaled anesthetic concentrations during the neonate retrieval portion of the surgery.

A regional or local anesthesia can be administered once the patient has been intubated and stabilized under general anesthesia. An epidural of preservative-free (PF) morphine (0.1 mg/kg) and lidocaine (0.5% PF-lidocaine; 0.20–0.22 mL/kg; [max volume of 5–6 mL]) has worked well at the author's institution. This combination provides immediate anesthesia and longer analgesia for the C-section patient and allows for minimal inhalational gas concentrations during the procedure. For a routine C-section, the author's institution prefers lidocaine over bupivacaine since it is shorter-acting, typically lasting 45–90 minutes, after epidural administration. This epidural combination provides adequate time to extract puppies, after which alternative strategies can be employed, if needed, to provide surgical analgesia for the dam. In addition, an epidural with lidocaine and morphine creates comfortable post-operative patients that can be discharged from the hospital hours after the C-section. Studies have shown that the use of an epidural allowed for lower rates of opioid administration, did not exacerbate hypotension, and allowed lower concentrations of isoflurane in dogs undergoing C-section.[17,18] While initial Apgar scores were not significantly different between the dogs with or without an epidural, subsequent Apgar scores were better for neonates from the epidural group that had less exposure to isoflurane.[18] Some surgeons prefer to use line blocks with lidocaine or bupivacaine along the length of the planned incision over epidurals. The use of long-acting bupivacaine injections (Nocita®; Elanco Animal Health, Greenfield, IN) for post-operative analgesia has gained popularity to provide up to 72 hours of incisional analgesia.

Once the local or regional anesthesia has been placed, the clock is ticking. The anesthesia/surgical team should rapidly complete any additional monitoring instrumentation setup, complete the presurgical skin prep, and move to the operating room in a timely manner to take full advantage of the local anesthesia. High puppy mortality rates were reported to be associated with obstructive dystocia, i.e., a puppy lodged in the birth canal, and a longer duration of anesthesia of greater than 80 minutes.[12] Based on their results, the authors of one retrospective study suggested expediting the decision to go to surgery and an induction-to-start-surgery time of less than 30 minutes to be important for optimal puppy survival.[12]

Procedures

There are two basic techniques for performing a C-section, a hysterotomy or an "en-bloc" procedure, and each will be discussed below. For either procedure, the patient is secured in dorsal recumbency and prepared for aseptic surgery. The surgeon's goal is to minimize the time between induction of anesthesia and surgical intervention.

When positioning, the weight of the gravid uterus when the patient is placed in dorsal recumbency can compress the caudal vena cava and negatively impact venous return. This can result in decreased cardiac output and lower blood pressure; therefore, the time a C-section patient should be in dorsal recumbency should be minimized. It may also be beneficial to tilt the patient slightly to their left side in an attempt to reduce compression of the caudal vena cava. Once in position, the patient is secured, and the final skin preparation is completed. Ideally, the surgeon or an assistant is scrubbed, has set up the surgical instrument table, and is ready to begin patient draping as soon as the final prep is completed. The patient is draped broadly so the surgical incision can extend if needed to facilitate exteriorization of the uterine horns from the abdominal cavity.

Once the patient is draped, a ventral midline incision is performed. Classically, the abdominal incision extends from the umbilicus 2/3–3/4 of the distance toward the pubis. Beginning the incision cranial to the umbilicus allows for better exposure and reduces the manipulation required to exteriorize the uterine horns (Figure 26.2). The incision length can also be influenced by the puppy load; in small litters, a more modest incision may be adequate. With larger litters, it is appropriate to make the initial incision longer rather than having to extend it later. Care is taken to avoid the mammary tissue on either side of the midline incision. There are frequently substantial mammary veins coursing along the proposed incision, and some of these will anastomose across the midline. Electrocautery, if available, is useful to minimize hemorrhage and improve visualization. Otherwise, large vessels should be clamped and ligated with a small diameter, absorbable suture material (4-0 Moncryl or Vicryl; Ethicon, Somerville, NJ) for hemostasis. Minimal undermining of the subcutaneous tissue is required; however, clearing the linea will permit rapid, secure closure of the abdominal incision. The linea

(a) (b)

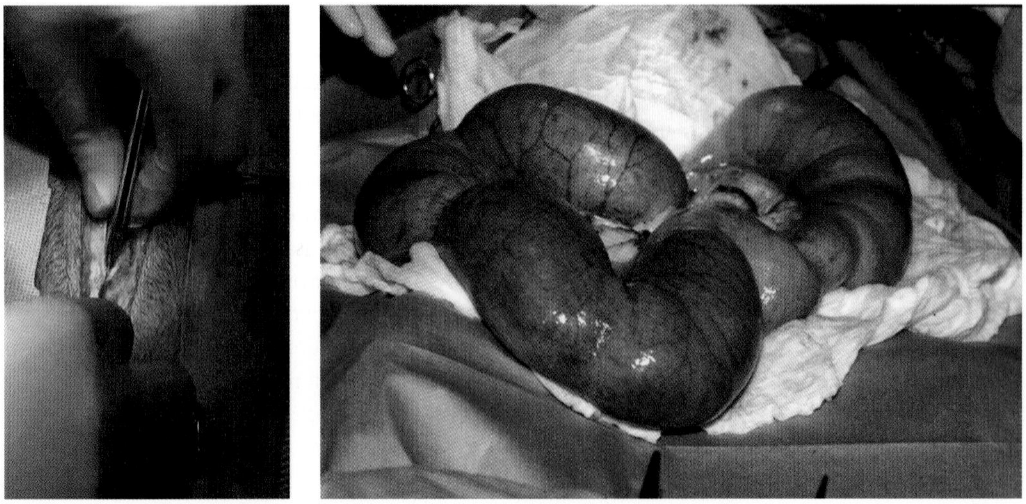

Figure 26.2 (a) The abdominal incision is made from the umbilicus to 3/4 of the distance to the pubic brim; however, the incision length is adjusted based on dam size and litter size to allow the uterus to be easily exteriorized from the incision. Cranial is at the top of the image. (b) The exteriorized uterus is lying so the dorsal side is exposed. To make a ventral incision, the uterus will need to be carefully repositioned.

is tented cranially and incised employing care to ensure there is no inadvertent surgical damage to the gravid uterus or other abdominal organs, such as the spleen or intestines, that may be displaced directly against the ventral abdominal wall. In dogs or cats with a history of previous C-section or other abdominal surgeries, the surgeon must check for ventral body wall adhesions as the initial abdominal incision is made. Once the body wall incision is completed, Balfour retractors can be placed over saline-moistened laparotomy sponges to provide adequate exposure to the abdominal cavity. The lap sponges are kept moist to prevent tissue desiccation during the procedure.

The uterus should be easily identifiable and is elevated through the abdominal incision. The surgeon must avoid grasping the uterine horns with their fingertips during exteriorization, as this can result in unintentional perforation of the distended uterus. Rather, the horns should be scooped out of the abdominal cavity using the palms of the hands. If the horns are not easily extracted, they may need to be manipulated to straighten them, as experience has shown either horn can assume unusual configuration within the abdominal cavity during gestation. Sometimes, the sterile assistant can apply gentle lateral pressure on the body wall – through the surgical drapes – to help create an upward pressure on the uterus to aid with the exteriorization of the uterine horns. Another option is a larger body wall incision, which will also facilitate easier exteriorization of the gravid uterus. Uterine tearing, rupture, and excessive hemorrhage can result from trying to pull the gravid horns through an undersized incision.

Once exteriorized, additional lap sponges or moistened surgical towels are used to isolate (pack-off) and protect the uterus. A count of all sponges and towels used is performed and recorded for later reconciliation. At this point, care should also be taken to ensure the gravid uterus does not slide off the surgical field; this is especially true with large litter sizes. Surgical assistance is beneficial for preventing this. If there is no surgical assistance available, exteriorizing one horn at a time might reduce the risk of the gravid uterus sliding off the surgical field.

Hysterotomy C-Section Procedure

The hysterotomy procedure is the classic technique for a C-section. Once the gravid uterus is exteriorized, a ventral incision is made along the uterine body moving from the bifurcation toward the cervix. Care must be taken to not injure fetuses located in the body of the uterus directly under the incision (Figure 26.3). There can be brisk hemorrhage following the uterine incision, and the use of electrosurgery, hemostats, or ligatures may be required to control the hemorrhage. Puppies (or kittens) are then individually manipulated into the incision and extracted. Rupturing

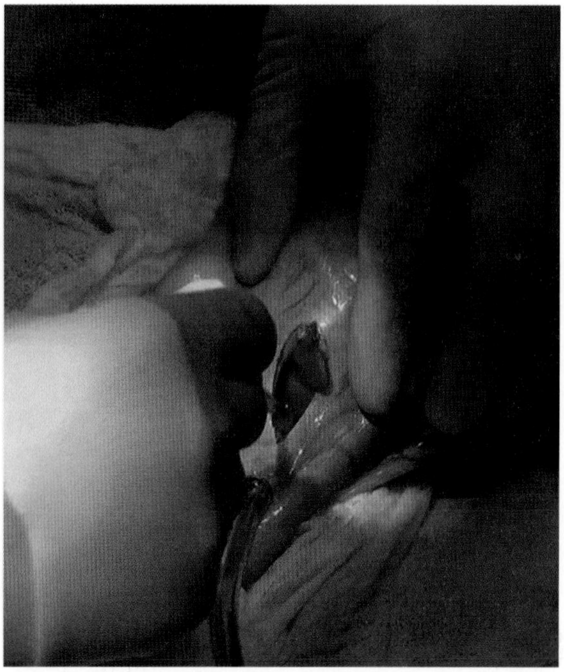

Figure 26.3 The hysterotomy incision is made on the ventral aspect of the uterine body. Care must be taken to avoid injury to any fetuses directly under the site of the incision. Notice the suction tip near the creation of the incision, which will help to limit fluid contamination into the abdominal cavity.

the outer sac (allantois) during manipulation will aid in advancing the fetus to the incision. The inner sac (amnion) is torn once the puppies have been delivered through the incision. The umbilical cord is clamped with two hemostatic forceps and then transected between them, separating the neonate from the umbilical cord. The modified technique used at the author's institution is to place a hemostat on the maternal side of the umbilical cord and place a quick ligature (2-0 silk, free-tie suture; Ethicon, Sommerville, NJ) or a vascular clip on the side of the neonate, leaving a 2–4 cm length of umbilical cord with the puppy (Figure 26.4). This will permit the umbilical vein to be catheterized if venous access is needed during resuscitation, conserves surgical instruments, and eliminates the weight of a hemostat hanging off the umbilical cord during resuscitation. The neonate is placed in a sterile surgical towel and lowered by the corners into the waiting hands of the "puppy" team. This process helps to avoid inadvertent contamination of the surgeon by the non-sterile personnel receiving the neonates. This process is continued until all of the neonates have been delivered.

After each neonate is extracted from the uterus and handed off, gentle traction is applied to the transected maternal side of the umbilical cord to separate the placenta from its zonal placentation site. This will result in mild to moderate hemorrhage from the placental site. This hemorrhage appears less and the placentas release more easily

(a) (b)

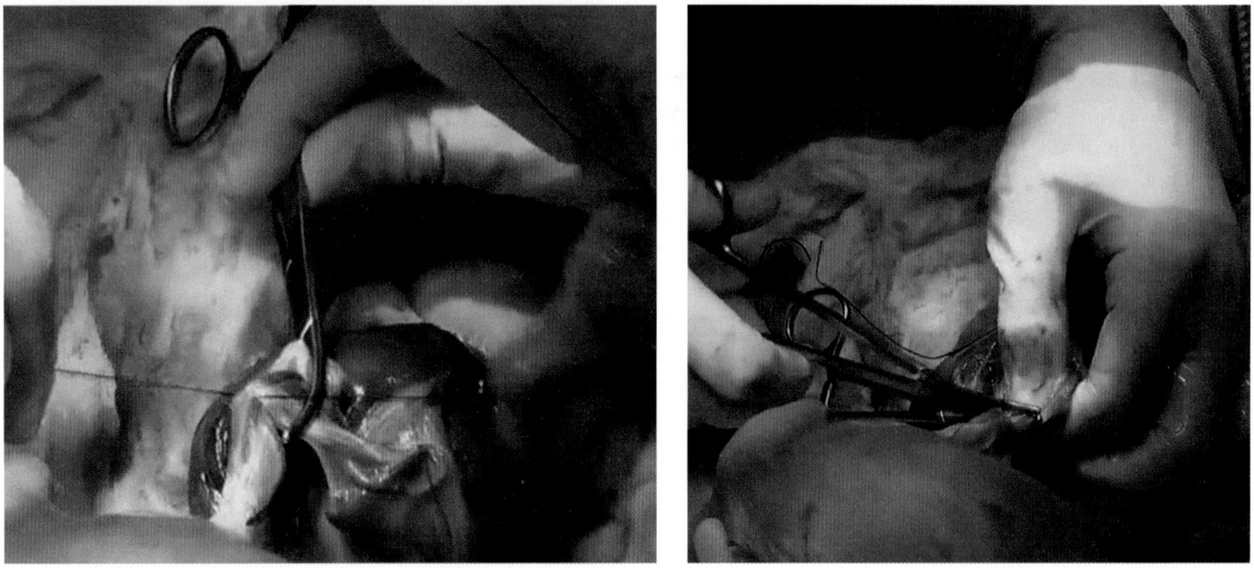

Figure 26.4 (a) A clamp is placed on the maternal side of the umbilical cord, and a silk suture is used to ligate the fetal side of the umbilical cord. (b) Scissors transect the umbilical cord, and the puppy (right) is placed in a towel and passed to a "puppy team" member.

when the dam is at full-term gestation. All placental tissue should be accounted for during surgery. Removal of the placentas also seems to ease the passage of the other feti along the uterine horn. It has been suggested that placental membranes can be left for later passage by the dam.[13] If placental membranes are left in situ, care is taken to ensure they are not trapped during hysterotomy incision closure. Close monitoring is required to ensure the fetal membranes are not retained post-operatively. Post-operative pyrexia or illness in any patient with retained fetal membranes should be investigated immediately.

Once all neonates have been delivered, the surgeon should follow each uterine horn from the cervix up to its associated ovary to ensure all neonates have indeed been extracted. At this point, an intramuscular dose of oxytocin is administered to promote uterine contraction and reduce hemorrhage from the disrupted placental sites. Prior to hysterotomy closure, any large blood clots are removed, and free blood and lavage fluid are aspirated from the uterine lumen. The hysterotomy incision is closed.

For uterine closure, a monofilament absorbable suture material (e.g., 2-0 to 4-0 Monocryl; Ethicon, Sommerville, NJ) is used. The uterus can be closed using a single-layer or a double-layer closure. For single-layer closure, a full-thickness, continuous suture pattern using either an inverting or appositional pattern is routine. Full-thickness suture placement ensures incorporation of the submucosal layer in the incision closure, providing the greatest holding strength, and a rapidly absorbable suture material should not have any long-term consequences. A simple interrupted suture pattern could be used but would require substantially more surgical time. For a double-layer closure, a continuous suture line beginning with either an inverting or appositional pattern in mucosal/submucosal layers followed by a second continuous layer in the muscularis/serosa layer can be used (Figure 26.5). Whenever a continuous pattern is used, it is ideal for the surgeon to check the suture line for excessive laxity prior to tying the final knot. After the final knot is tied, the uterus is lavaged and returned to the abdominal cavity. The positioning should be inspected to ensure there is no twisting or misplacement of the abdominal organs. Abdominal closure is outlined below.

En-bloc C-Section Procedure

An alternative to the traditional hysterotomy, the "en-bloc" C-section was widely discussed after a publication documented no significant difference between puppy survivability when the "en-bloc" procedure was compared to the more traditional procedure.[19] The "en-bloc" procedure is basically an ovariohysterectomy (OHE) of the gravid uterus with the goal of handing the uterus off to a separate group who then extract the neonates from the uterus. It gained some popularity when it was reported that puppy mortality was not significantly different from a traditional C-section and that it was a faster procedure. Advantages include the speed of the procedure, the pet is sterilized as a result of the procedure, and there is typically less blood loss compared to a routine hysterotomy with subsequent OHE. The primary disadvantage to using this procedure is all the

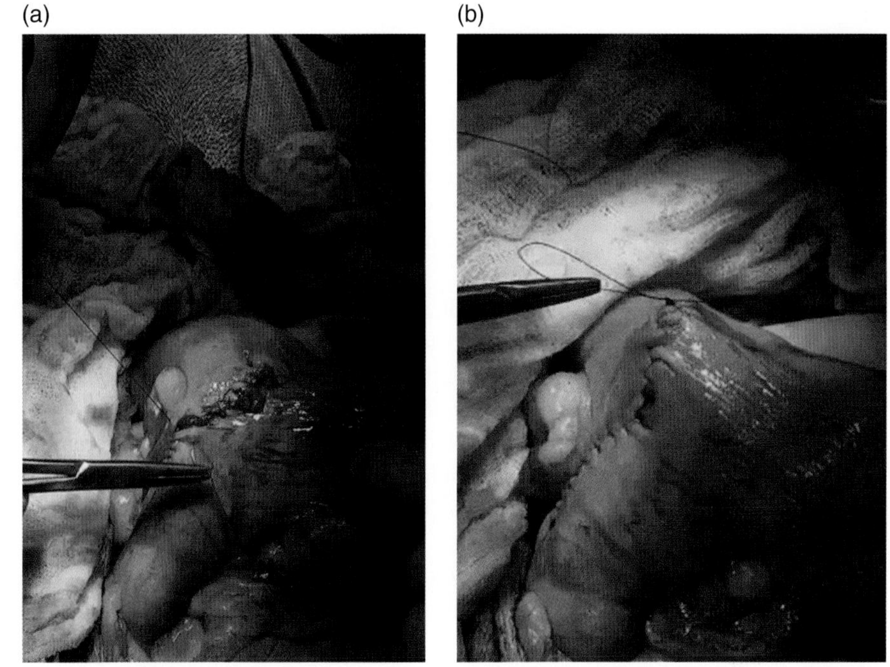

Figure 26.5 (a) The first layer of the double-layer closure has been completed, and the second layer is begun. (b) The two-layer closure is complete with a final knot. The closure was a simple continuous appositional pattern followed by an inverting (Lembert) oversew.

neonates need to be delivered at the same time. This means there must be adequate personnel available to deliver and resuscitate all the neonates once the uterus is passed from the surgical field. The theriogenology service of the author's institution prefers to have the standard delivery of puppies with a subsequent spay if that is the owner's desire.

The approach and exteriorization of the uterus is the same for the "en-bloc" procedure. Once the uterus is exteriorized, the left and right suspensory ligaments are disrupted, and the broad ligament caudal to the ovarian pedicles is fenestrated. The broad ligament is torn to the level of the uterine body, carefully avoiding or ligating any substantial vessels within the broad ligament. Any neonates that are lodged in the uterine body at the site where the clamp will be placed are gently manipulated back into a uterine horn to avoid injury. Suture material for pedicle ligations should be on the table, and there should be an adequate number of appropriately sized hemostatic clamps at the ready. A total of six to nine large hemostats (e.g., Carmalt hemostats) would be ideal for this. Finally, the surgeon should confirm that the resuscitation team is prepared to receive the uterus for puppy recovery.

With that confirmation, the first pedicle is clamped off using a two-clamp or a three-clamp technique and transected. This is immediately repeated on the opposite pedicle, relying on the clamps to occlude the pedicles. The uterine body is clamped next and then transected to free the uterus, which is handed off to a non-sterile member of the recovery team. Care should be taken during the handoff, as this step has a high risk of inadvertent contamination of the surgeon by non-sterile personnel.

Once the uterus is off the surgical field, each pedicle is securely ligated with an encircling or friction knot, employing a strangle knot or similar ligature, and appropriated sized, monofilament, absorbable suture. The author typically performs a double ligation with a proximal encircling ligature and a distal transfixation ligature on larger pedicles; however, this is truly surgeon preference if the end result is effective hemostasis. Other methods of pedicle occlusion, such as bipolar sealing devices, could be used at the preference of the surgeon. The uterine vessels are ligated next. In patients where the uterine body is enlarged or when the cervix is open with potential contamination of the uterine lumen, a single, encircling ligature is placed around the uterine body, and individual "stick-ties" are placed distally around each uterine artery and vein without encircling the uterine body again. This technique reduces the risk of entrapping a large volume of uterine tissue between the two encircling ligatures, potentially creating a complication.

At this point, each pedicle is checked for secure ligation, and the abdomen is checked for hemorrhage. Any additional vessels from the broad ligament or adjacent to the uterine body that are actively bleeding are ligated. The abdomen is lavaged, the lavage fluid aspirated, sponge counts reconciled, and abdominal wall closure is begun.

Closure

Thorough abdominal lavage is appropriate following a C-section. Uterine fluids and blood often drain into the abdominal cavity, and removal of clots and fluids is warranted. Body temperature sterile saline should be used, and all free fluid should be removed. Ideally, the lavage should be continued until the aspirated fluid runs clear. Leaving free fluid in the abdominal cavity is not appropriate and is not an appropriate method to rehydrate patients. Effective abdominal lavage may help minimize adhesion formation or severity, which is important in animals that will continue to be bred and may require future abdominal procedures.

Surgical sponges with radiopaque indicators and an accurate sponge count before the initial incision and immediately before body wall closure are essential when performing any C-section. Given the movement of personnel into and out of the operating room, the potential for substantial hemorrhage, the presence of copious uterine fluids, and the transport of neonates out of the operating room, it is very easy for sponges to get lost or left behind. If the sponge count is off, a post-operative radiograph should be obtained to confirm no sponges have been left behind during the procedure. Some clinicians also perform an instrument count as a routine part of their closing checklist when performing open procedures, such as C-sections.

Much of the body wall closure, after a C-section, is based on surgeon preference; the author's preferences are below. The ventral body wall is closed using an appropriately sized suture, typically, a long-lasting absorbable suture material (PDS; Ethicon, Sommerville, NJ) although other suture materials have and can be used. In patients with an anticipated healing concern, a non-absorbable suture material, such as polypropylene (Prolene; Ethicon, Sommerville, NJ), might be a more appropriate choice. Care is taken to include generous bites of the external sheath of the rectus abdominis muscle on each side of the incision. Body wall closure can be done with a simple continuous suture pattern, although some prefer an interrupted pattern. Each end of the incision is carefully inspected, since the gravid uterus and any extension of the midline incision can result in undercutting the linea beneath the subcutaneous tissue and skin, creating a space for potential herniation. If using a continuous pattern, the surgeon should pause and tighten the continuous suture line prior to tying the suture line. The subcutaneous tissues are apposed with a rapidly absorbing suture (3-0 or 4-0 Monocryl; Ethicon, Sommerville, NJ) using a pattern that minimizes dead space. The author completes the incisional closure using an intradermal skin closure to avoid suture tags or staples that might interfere with the nursing of the neonates (Figure 26.6).

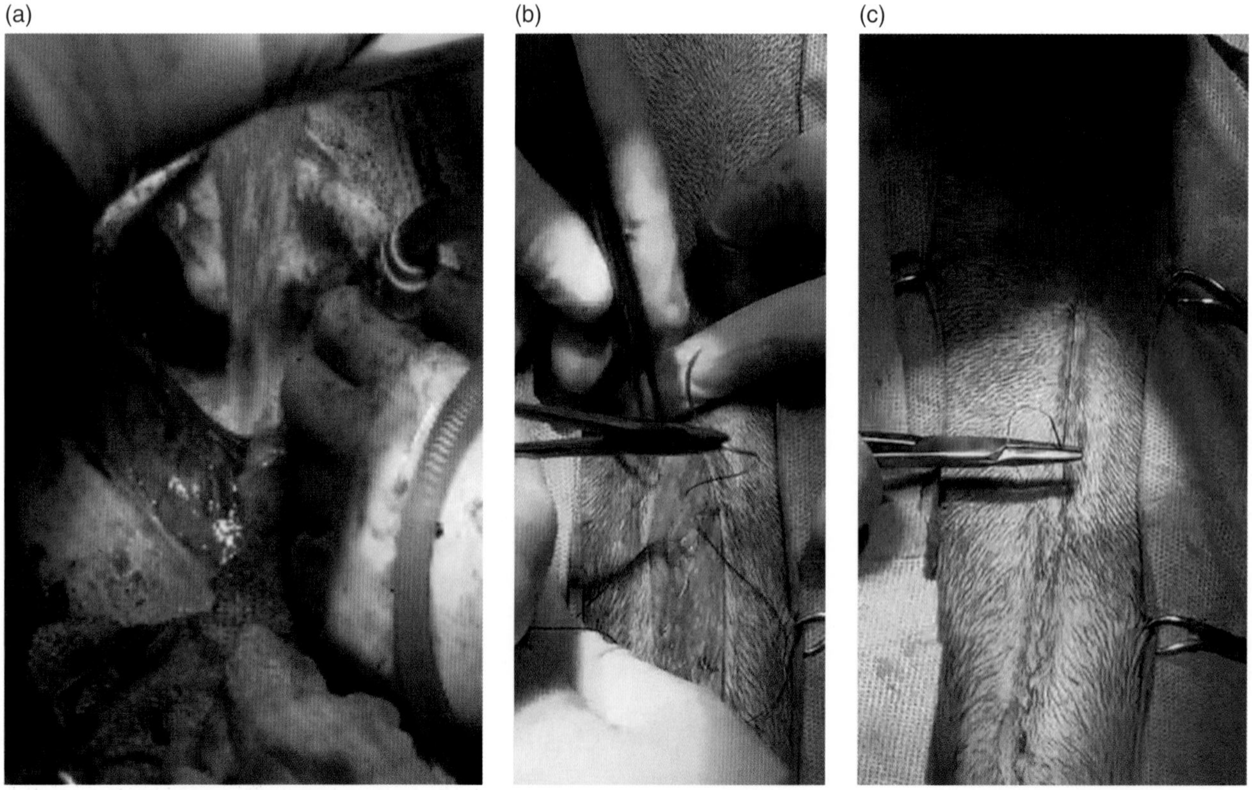

Figure 26.6 (a) After closure of the hysterotomy incision, the uterus is returned to the abdominal cavity, and a thorough lavage is performed. (b) After closure of the body wall, the subcutaneous tissues are apposed with a tacking pattern to minimize seroma formation. (c) An intradermal pattern is used to complete the procedure. In all images, cranial is at the top.

Final Thoughts

There is disagreement over the risk of a dam going through a "natural" labor if they have undergone a previous C-section, and some clinicians employ a "once a section; always a section" philosophy. Evidence for this view is not definitive; however, in one study, roughly 62% of dogs allowed to attempt normal delivery after a previous C-section required a second C-section.[13] This study included over 25 different breeds, including both brachycephalic and non-brachycephalic breeds.

The question of performing an OHE at the time of C-section is heavily discussed. Many veterinarians do not want to spay their patients during a C-section. Concerns are often focused on surgical challenges, the larger, engorged vessels, friability of the tissues, blood loss, and negative effects from the loss of ovarian and uterine hormones on the mother after the spay. The author's institution has surgeons that will perform an OHE along with a C-section if requested and others that will only perform an OHE when there is a definitive surgical indication. In an animal with a normal hematocrit, the end blood volume should not be lessened with OHE. And, as with any surgical procedure, care will need to be taken to control hemorrhage through effective ligation or vessel occlusion. In a report on mortality rates after C-section, a high mortality rate of 3.11% was reported for dogs undergoing a C-section.[20] In that report, dogs undergoing OHE at the time of C-section had an even higher mortality rate, 4.2%, compared to 2.6% for dogs with a C-section alone. The reason for the OHE in this report was equally distributed between medical necessity and owner request.[20] In a more recent review of 125 dogs undergoing C-section alone or C-section and OHE, there was no significant difference when comparing mothering abilities, operative complications, or fetal survivability for dogs.[21] While the dogs undergoing a C-section and an OHE were significantly more likely to go to surgery as an emergency were identified as more painful after surgery, were at a more advanced stage of labor at time of surgery, and had slightly longer surgical times, no maternal mortality was reported in this study.[21] This current data suggests that C-section and OHE should not have a higher risk for the bitch; however, the veterinarian must consider their comfort level and the unique surgical situation of each patient.

References

1 U.S National Library of Medicine (n.d.). Cesarean section-a brief history (Part 1). https://www.nlm.nih.gov/exhibition/cesarean/part1.html.

2 Adams, D.J., Ellerbrock, R.E., Wallace, M.L. et al. (2022). Risk factors for neonatal mortality prior to hospital discharge in brachycephalic and nonbrachycephalic dogs undergoing cesarean section. *Vet. Surg.* 51 (7): 1052–1060. https://doi.org/10.1111/vsu.13868.

3 Smith, F.O. (2012). Guide to emergency interception during parturition in the dog and cat. *Vet. Clin. North Am. Small Anim. Pract.* 42 (3): 489–499, vi. https://doi.org/10.1016/j.cvsm.2012.02.001.

4 Lamm, C.G. and Makloski, C.L. (2012). Current advances in gestation and parturition in cats and dogs. *Vet. Clin. North Am. Small Anim. Pract.* 42 (3): 445–456, v. https://doi.org/10.1016/j.cvsm.2012.01.010.

5 Traas, A.M. (2008). Surgical management of canine and feline dystocia. *Theriogenology* 70 (3): 337–342. https://doi.org/10.1016/j.theriogenology.2008.04.014.

6 Smith, F.O. (2007). Challenges in small animal parturition—timing elective and emergency cesarian sections. *Theriogenology* 68 (3): 348–353. https://doi.org/10.1016/j.theriogenology.2007.04.041.

7 Holst, B.S. (2022). Feline breeding and pregnancy management: what is normal and when to intervene. *J. Feline Med. Surg.* 24 (3): 221–231. https://doi.org/10.1177/1098612X221079708.

8 Bailin, H.G., Thomas, L., and Levy, N.A. (2022). Retrospective evaluation of feline dystocia: clinicopathologic findings and neonatal outcomes in 35 cases (2009-2020). *J. Feline Med. Surg.* 24 (4): 344–350. https://doi.org/10.1177/1098612X211024154.

9 MacPhail, C. and Fossum, T.W. (2018). Surgery of the reproductive and genital systems. In: *Small Animal Surgery*, 5e (ed. T.W. Fossum), 720–787. Mosby.

10 O'Neill, D.G., O'Sullivan, A.M., Manson, E.A. et al. (2019). Canine dystocia in 50 UK first-opinion emergency care veterinary practices: clinical management and outcomes. *Vet. Rec.* 184 (13): 409. https://doi.org/10.1136/vr.104944.

11 Fransson, B.A. Ovaries and uterus. In: *Veterinary Surgery-Small Animal*, 2e (ed. S.A. Johnson and K.S. Tobias), 2109–2130. Elsevier.

12 Schmidt, K., Feng, C., Wu, T., and Duke-Novakovski, T. (2021). Influence of maternal, anesthetic, and surgical factors on neonatal survival after emergency cesarean section in 78 dogs: a retrospective study (2002 to 2020). *Can. Vet. J.* 62 (9): 961–968.

13 De Cramer, K.G.M. and Nöthling, J.O. (2020). Towards scheduled pre-parturient caesarean sections in bitches. *Reprod. Domest. Anim.* 55 (Suppl. 2): 38–48. https://doi.org/10.1111/rda.13669.

14 Groppetti, D., Di Cesare, F., Pecile, A. et al. (2019). Maternal and neonatal wellbeing during elective C-section induced with a combination of propofol

and dexmedetomidine: how effective is the placental barrier in dogs? *Theriogenology* 129: 90–98. https://doi.org/10.1016/j.theriogenology.2019.02.019.

15 De Cramer, K.G.M., Joubert, K.E., and Nöthling, J.O. (2017). Puppy survival and vigor associated with the use of low dose medetomidine premedication, propofol induction and maintenance of anesthesia using sevoflurane gas-inhalation for cesarean section in the bitch. *Theriogenology* 96: 10–15. https://doi.org/10.1016/j.theriogenology.2017.03.021.

16 Doebeli, A., Michel, E., Bettschart, R. et al. (2013). Apgar score after induction of anesthesia for canine cesarean section with alfaxalone versus propofol. *Theriogenology* 80: 850–854.

17 Martin-Flores, M., Moy-Trigilio, K.E., Campoy, L., and Gleed, R.D. (2021). Retrospective study on the use of lumbosacral epidural analgesia during caesarean section surgery in 182 dogs: impact on blood pressure, analgesic use and delays. *Vet. Rec.* 188 (8): e134. https://doi.org/10.1002/vetr.134.

18 Antończyk, A. and Ochota, M. (2022). Is an epidural component during general anaesthesia for caesarean section beneficial for neonatal puppies' health and vitality? *Theriogenology* 187: 1–8. https://doi.org/10.1016/j.theriogenology.2022.04.015.

19 Robbins, M.A. and Mullen, H.S. (1994). En bloc ovariohysterectomy as a treatment for dystocia in dogs and cats. *Vet. Surg.* 23 (1): 48–52. https://doi.org/10.1111/j.1532-950x.1994.tb00442.x.

20 Conze, T., Jurczak, A., Fux, V. et al. (2020). Survival and fertility of bitches undergoing caesarean section. *Vet. Rec.* 186 (13): 416. https://doi.org/10.1136/vr.105123.

21 Guest, K.E., Ellerbrock, R.E., Adams, D.J. et al. (2023). Performing an ovariohysterectomy at the time of C-section does not pose an increase in risk of mortality, intra- or postoperative complications, or decreased mothering ability of the bitch. *J. Am. Vet. Med. Assoc.* 261 (6): 837–843. https://doi.org/10.2460/javma.23.01.0012.

27

Pyometra

Brad M. Matz

Department of Clinical Sciences, Auburn University, Auburn, AL, USA

Key Points

- Pyometra can be a life-threatening surgical emergency and is best addressed by prompt identification and surgical intervention.
- Surgeons should be prepared to manage the enlarged reproductive tract with care to ensure spillage of contents is avoided.
- Surgeons should avoid double ligation of the uterine pedicle to avoid retention of purulent material between the ligations.

Introduction

Pyometra is a potentially life-threatening condition seen in both dogs and cats and results in the accumulation of pus in the uterine lumen.[1] The cervix can be open or closed in this condition. If the cervix is open, purulent material can be seen coming from the vulva (Figure 27.1); however, the absence of discharge does not rule out pyometra, as the more dangerous of the two options, a closed pyometra, will not result in leaking of discharge. Treatment options include both medical and surgical management, though primary consideration is given to surgery. A range of other issues can be present and impact the systemic health of the animal secondary to the uterine infection, such as the infection systemically affecting the patient in cases of closed pyometra. This condition develops under the influence of progesterone, and *Escherichia coli* is the most common bacteria seen.[1] Lipopolysaccharides (endotoxin) associated with Gram-negative bacteria can lead to fever and systemic dysfunction.[1]

Cystic endometrial hyperplasia often precedes pyometra development. Cystic endometrial hyperplasia occurs during the diestrual phase of the heat cycle and results in cyst formation from secretory endometrial glands.[2]

Indications/Preoperative Considerations

Clinical signs at presentation vary but can include vulvar discharge, fever, polyuria/polydipsia, and vomiting.[3] Confirmation of pyometra is based on the client history and physical exam findings. Imaging with radiographs and/or abdominal ultrasound can show fluid-filled uterine horns of variable size. In open pyometra, purulent vulvar discharge is typically observed. Some animals presenting for pyometra can have serious systemic issues with signs of endotoxemia and need stabilization prior to surgical treatment. This usually involves intravenous fluid administration and antimicrobials.[4]

Surgical Procedure

Surgical treatment involves ovariohysterectomy. The incision will likely be larger than that described in the ovariohysterectomy chapter.

Laparotomy sponges are useful to help contain any spillage of uterine content (Figure 27.2). This can occur as a result of technique, tissue quality, or can come from the ovarian bursa. Access to sterile saline lavage and suction is

Techniques in Small Animal Soft Tissue, Orthopedic, and Ophthalmic Surgery, First Edition. Edited by Kristin A. Coleman.

Companion website: www.wiley.com/go/coleman/surgeries

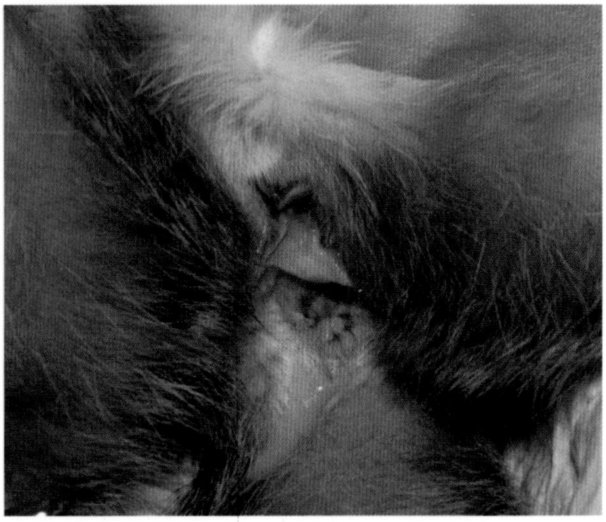

Figure 27.1 Purulent vulvar discharge from a dog with pyometra.

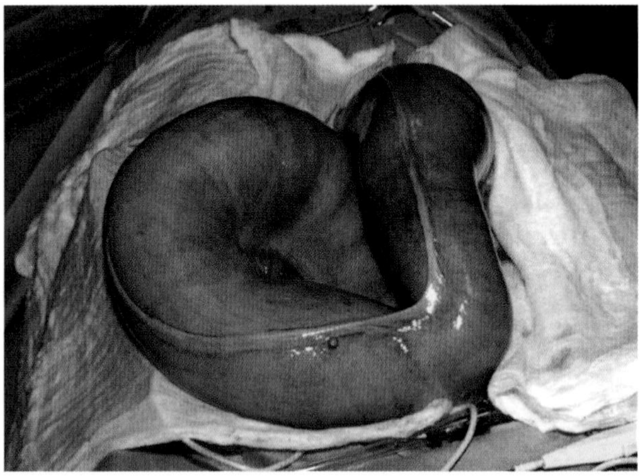

Figure 27.2 Enlarged uterine horns typical of those observed during pyometra.

recommended but not required. The author prefers to avoid a transfixation ligation in the uterus, so the pus-containing uterus is not penetrated by a needle. If the uterus/vessels are significantly enlarged, the uterine vessels can be dissected from the uterine tissue on both sides with a hemostat. This allows for the surgeon to securely ligate the uterine vasculature. This is not necessary when the uterine tissue is not excessively enlarged. The uterine tissue can be ligated with a single encircling ligation rather than being double-ligated. A strangle knot provides a very secure ligation and is one of the most reliable friction knots, and this single ligature would negate the need for additional ligation. This avoids the potential for purulent material to be trapped between two uterine ligations. Following ligation of the uterine body immediately caudal to the cervix, a large hemostat, such as a Rochester-Carmalt hemostatic forcep, is placed across the uterine body cranial to the ligature. It is recommended to place a laparotomy sponge dorsal to the uterine body at the time of transection and removal of the entire reproductive tract from the abdominal cavity, followed by local lavage and suction of the uterine pedicle.

In the editor's practice, an intra-uterine fluid sample is obtained following Ovariohysterectomy (OHE) and submitted for culture and sensitivity in most cases, especially those that are from closed pyometras or those that are systemically ill. These results are helpful in guiding antibiotic choice upon discharge from the hospital. If any masses are palpable within the uterine or ovarian tissue, the reproductive tract is submitted for histopathologic analysis.

Postoperative Care/Prognosis

Activity restriction and use of protective devices (e.g., Elizabethan collar and special protective shirts) are indicated for at least two weeks following surgery. Postoperative care and restrictions are similar to those described for other abdominal procedures.

At least two large-scale studies (>2000 dogs) reported mortality rates of approximately 3%.[5] One of these studies also showed a uterine rupture rate of 3%.[4] Prompt identification, stabilization, and surgical management will help to improve outcomes. Gentle surgical technique when handling the uterus, secure ligations, and postoperative supportive care will also help minimize periprocedural morbidity and mortality.

Injectable opioids are used for the first 12–24 hours postoperatively. The author does not routinely use postoperative antimicrobials in uncomplicated cases (non-ruptured, minimal systemic compromise), but their use is sometimes indicated and is ideally guided by culture with susceptibility testing. Postoperative pain medications are usually sent home with patients at discharge and include nonsteroidal antiinflammatory (NSAIDs) for patients (who can tolerate their use). Otherwise, oral opioids can be considered for use after discharge.

References

1 Hagman, R. (2022). Pyometra in small animals 2.0. *Vet. Clin. North Am. Small Anim. Pract.* 52 (3): 631–657.

2 Crane, B. and Kutzler, M. (2010). Diseases of the uterus. In: *Mechanisms of Disease in Small Animal Surgery*, 3e

(ed. M.J. Bojrab and E. Monnet), 454–457. Jackson, WY: Teton Newmedia.

3 Bigliardi, E., Parmigiani, E., Cavirani, S. et al. (2004). Ultrasonography and cystic hyperplasia-pyometra complex in the bitch. *Reprod. Domest. Anim.* 39 (3): 136–140.

4 Pailler, S., Slater, M.R., Lesnikowski, S.M. et al. (2022). Findings and prognostic indicators of outcomes for bitches with pyometra treated surgically in a nonspecialized setting. *J. Am. Vet. Med. Assoc.* 260 (S2): S49–S56.

5 Gibson, A., Dean, R., Yates, D. et al. (2013). A retrospective study of pyometra at five RSPCA hospitals in the UK: 1728 cases from 2006 to 2011. *Vet. Rec.* 173 (16): 396.

28

Cystotomy and Partial Cystectomy

Janet A. Grimes

Department of Small Animal Medicine and Surgery, University of Georgia, Athens, GA, USA

Key Points

- Retrograde urohydropropulsion should be performed prior to cystotomy to move urethral stones into the urinary bladder.
- Cystotomy should be performed on the ventral surface of the urinary bladder to avoid important anatomic structures located on the dorsal surface (ureters, neurovascular structures).
- Radiographic confirmation of stone removal should be performed immediately postoperatively when stones are radiopaque to ensure complete removal.
- Uroliths should be submitted for composition analysis to guide nutritional management and reduce future stone formation.

Introduction

Urinary bladder surgery is commonly performed in dogs and cats and is very feasible to be performed in general practice. In this chapter, indications and preoperative considerations for urinary bladder surgery will be discussed, including retrograde urohydropropulsion for urethral stones. Cystotomy will be covered in depth, including positioning, approach, anatomy, performing the cystotomy, removing stones, and closure of the cystotomy incision. Partial cystectomy will also be discussed. Finally, potential complications and postoperative care will be described.

Indications / Preoperative Considerations

The most common indication for cystotomy in dogs and cats is for cystolithiasis and/or urethrolithiasis. Patients with cystoliths and/or urethroliths may present with pollakiuria and hematuria and may have recurrent signs following antibiotic treatment for a presumed urinary tract infection. Urethroliths may lead to complete obstruction. Abdominal radiographs are helpful in identifying radiopaque stones, such as calcium oxalate and struvite, which are the most common stones in dogs and cats.[1,2] The other two types of stones identified with some regularity in dogs and less frequently in cats are urate and cystine stones.[2] These stones are likely to be radiolucent ("I can't CU" [cystine, urate] is a helpful mnemonic for this), although in some cases, cystine stones (less commonly urate stones) are faintly visible on abdominal radiographs.[3] Pre-operative radiographs are useful to assist in identification of the number and size of stones present and to evaluate the urethra for stones. For patients with radiolucent stones, ultrasound or double-contrast cystography may be useful for stone identification.[3] A caudal abdominal/perineal view with the pelvic limbs pulled cranially is particularly helpful for evaluation of the urethra in male dogs to avoid superimposition of the femurs with the caudal os penis, a frequent location where stones may become lodged (Figure 28.1). Other indications for cystotomy include evaluation for trauma in cases of uroabdomen or biopsy of masses.[4,5] The most common urinary bladder tumor in dogs is urothelial carcinoma (formerly known as transitional cell carcinoma), which has a very

Techniques in Small Animal Soft Tissue, Orthopedic, and Ophthalmic Surgery, First Edition. Edited by Kristin A. Coleman.

Companion website: www.wiley.com/go/coleman/surgeries

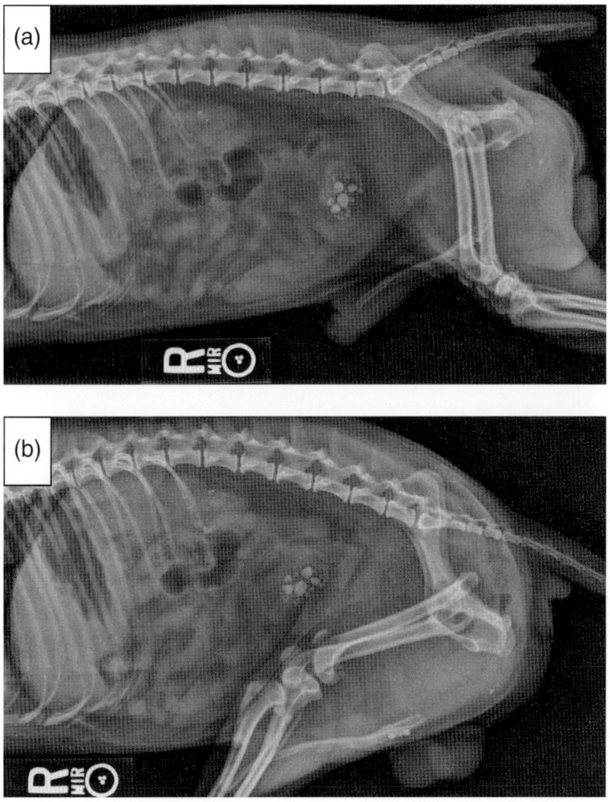

Figure 28.1 Radiographs from a male canine patient with urolithiasis and a previous right femoral head and neck ostectomy. (a) A standard right lateral abdominal radiograph is shown; (b) a caudal abdominal/perineal radiograph is shown. In (a), note how the femurs are superimposed over the caudal aspect of the os penis, making it difficult to evaluate this area for stones. In (b), note how with the pelvic limbs pulled cranially, the entire urethra can be evaluated for stones and multiple stones can be seen at the proximal aspect of the os penis. *Source:* © Janet Grimes.

high propensity for seeding and growing additional tumors on any surface the tumor cells contact; thus, biopsy of urinary bladder masses via cystotomy is rarely indicated.

Retrograde Urohydropropulsion

In patients with urethroliths, retrograde urohydropropulsion should be performed to flush the stones back into the urinary bladder to allow for cystotomy.[6] This procedure is more successful under general anesthesia due to the full relaxation of the urethral musculature that anesthesia provides compared to sedation. If the urinary bladder is distended prior to starting this procedure, it should be drained either by passing a smaller urethral catheter around the stones or by use of decompressive cystocentesis. Male dogs should be placed in lateral recumbency following induction of general anesthesia. The penis is extruded and prepped with dilute chlorhexidine or povidone–iodine solution. A sterile catheter is placed retrograde into the urethra until the obstruction is reached. This catheter should be as large as possible to assist in flushing the stones. In a sterile bowl, 1 L of saline is mixed with sterile lubricant. In large dogs, a full 5 oz tube of sterile lubricant can be used. Since this may clog a smaller diameter urethral catheter, this volume may need to be adjusted based on patient and catheter size. A 60 cc syringe (or 20–35 cc syringe in smaller patients) is filled with this saline/lubricant solution and is attached to the urethral catheter. A second assistant places a finger in the rectum and pushes down firmly onto the pubic bone to occlude the urethra. The urethral catheter is flushed with the saline/lubricant mixture (it helps to pinch the tip of the penis around the catheter with a gauze to prevent backflow of the saline/lubricant solution). The person with their finger in the rectum should feel the urethra distend caudal to their finger; when this is felt, they should release the digital pressure against the pubis to allow the fluid and stones to pass into the urinary bladder while the person injecting the saline/lubricant mixture continues to inject (Figure 28.2). The palpable distension indicates that the urethra has been dilated to allow the stone to pass back up the urethra into the urinary bladder. This process should be repeated a few times, ensuring to keep an eye on the volume of the urinary bladder and draining it as needed. If an assistant is not available to perform the rectal portion of this procedure, passing a urethral catheter until it abuts the stone and then flushing through the catheter may dislodge the stone, allowing it to flow back into the urinary bladder. If the stone does not dislodge after a few attempts, true retrograde urohydropropulsion should be performed as described above. Once the urethral catheter passes smoothly, radiographs should be taken to confirm all of the urethral stones have moved into the urinary bladder (Figure 28.3). Although this procedure is most commonly performed in male dogs, it can also be performed in female dogs and male cats. In all patients, this should be performed carefully to avoid inadvertent trauma to the urethra from the catheter.

Surgical Procedure

Patient Preparation and Positioning for Surgery

The patient should be positioned in dorsal recumbency and aseptically prepared and draped for surgery. In male dogs, the prepuce should be flushed with diluted povidone–iodine solution and the prepuce draped into the sterile field to allow for urethral catheterization. Male cats can be positioned with the pelvic limbs pulled cranially to allow for access to the penis for urethral catheterization; a towel can be placed under the caudal pelvis to increase exposure to the prepuce (Figure 28.4). In female dogs and cats,

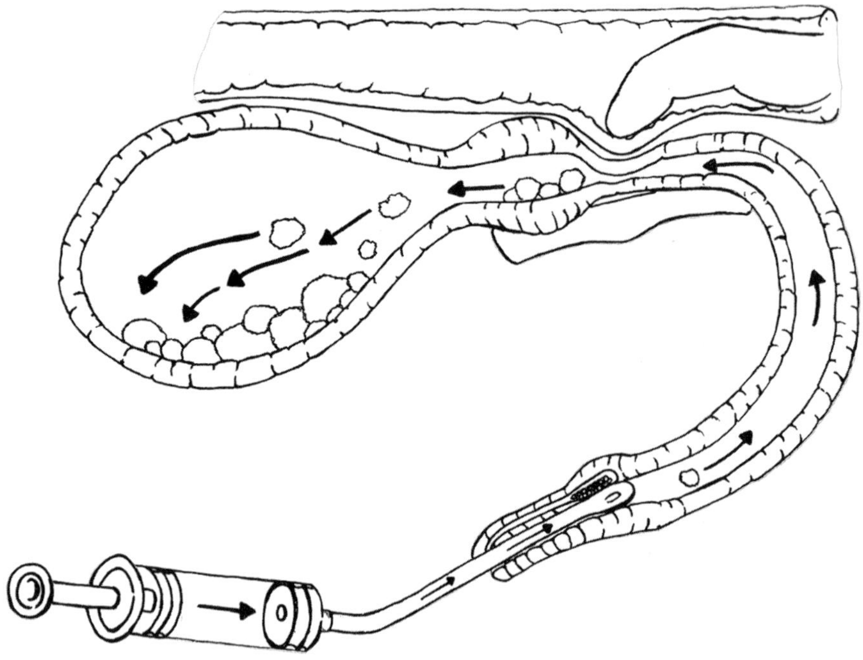

Figure 28.2 After induction of general anesthesia, the penis should be extruded and prepped with dilute chlorhexidine or povidone-iodine solution. A sterile catheter is placed retrograde into the urethra until the obstruction is reached. This catheter should be as large as possible to assist in flushing the stones. A large syringe is filled with a saline/lubricant solution and is attached to the urethral catheter. A second assistant places a finger in the rectum and pushes down firmly onto the pubic bone to occlude the urethra. The urethral catheter is flushed with the saline/lubricant mixture (it helps to pinch the tip of the penis around the catheter with a gauze to prevent backflow of the saline/lubricant solution). The person with their finger in the rectum should feel the urethra distend caudal to their finger; when this is felt, they should release the digital pressure against the pubis to allow the fluid and stones to pass into the urinary bladder while the person injecting the saline/lubricant mixture continues to inject. The palpable distension indicates that the urethra has been dilated to allow the stone to pass back up the urethra into the urinary bladder. This process should be repeated a few times, ensuring to keep an eye on the volume of the urinary bladder and draining it as needed. Once the urethral catheter passes smoothly, radiographs should be taken to confirm all of the urethral stones have moved into the urinary bladder. *Source:* Original artwork by Taylor Bergrud.

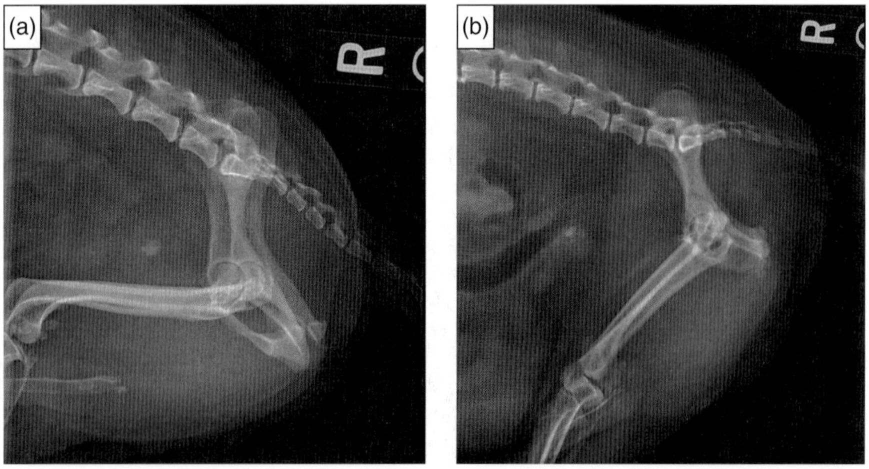

Figure 28.3 Images of a male canine patient before (a) and after (b) retrograde urohydropropulsion. Radiographs should be taken to confirm all stones have been flushed into the urinary bladder. *Source:* © Janet Grimes.

retrograde urethral catheterization is rarely necessary, but the vulva can be prepped and draped into the field, if necessary. It is recommended to drape the entire abdomen, even if the planned incision site is in the caudal abdomen over the bladder.

Surgical Approach

If the planned procedure is a cystotomy only, the abdominal incision may be just large enough to exteriorize the urinary bladder. The incision should be made directly over the palpable urinary bladder. If the urinary bladder is not palpable,

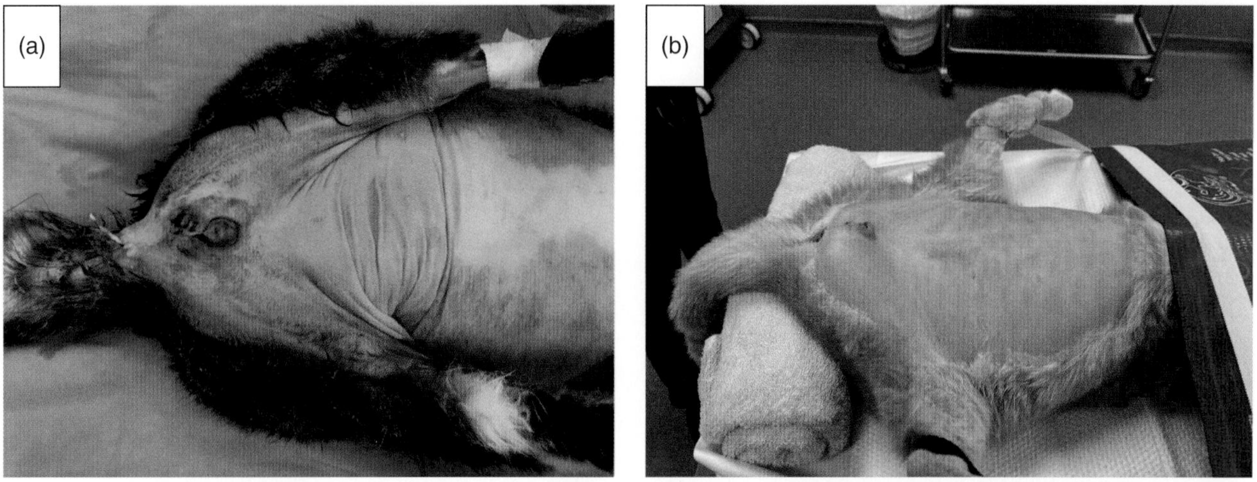

Figure 28.4 A male cat positioned for cystotomy. (a) In this image, the cat's head is to the right, and the pelvic limbs are positioned cranially to allow for access to the penis for urethral catheterization. In some cats, this positioning can make the cystotomy incision difficult due to wrinkling of the skin and subcutaneous tissues over the abdominal incision site. (b) Alternatively, towels can be placed under the pelvis to increase exposure to the prepuce if needed. (a) *Source:* © Janet Grimes. (b) *Source:* © Kristin Coleman.

the incision should be made 3–4 cm cranial to the pubis. In male dogs, the incision should be made parapreputially through the skin and subcutaneous tissues (Figure 28.5a). The prepuce and penis should then be retracted laterally and the linea alba opened on ventral midline. In female dogs and all cats, the incision should be made through the skin and subcutaneous tissues on the ventral midline, allowing for entry into the abdomen through the linea alba (Figure 28.5b). Once the abdomen is opened, the urinary bladder should be exteriorized (Video 28.1). There is often a large amount of fat in the caudal abdomen, and a distended bladder can make exteriorization difficult. If the urinary bladder is unable to be exteriorized, urine can be drained via retrograde catheterization or cystocentesis, or the abdominal incision can be extended.

Cystotomy

Once the urinary bladder has been exteriorized, it should be packed off with moistened laparotomy sponges to reduce the amount of contact with the skin (Figure 28.6, Video 28.2). The urinary bladder has three attachments to the abdominal wall (Figure 28.7). The ventral median ligament attaches the bladder ventrally to the linea alba and pelvic symphysis. In some patients, this fragile ligament may not be visible or may have been disrupted during extension of the linea incision or exteriorization of the urinary bladder. There are also paired lateral ligaments that contain fat, the distal ureters, and the umbilical arteries. A stay suture should be placed into the apex to assist with

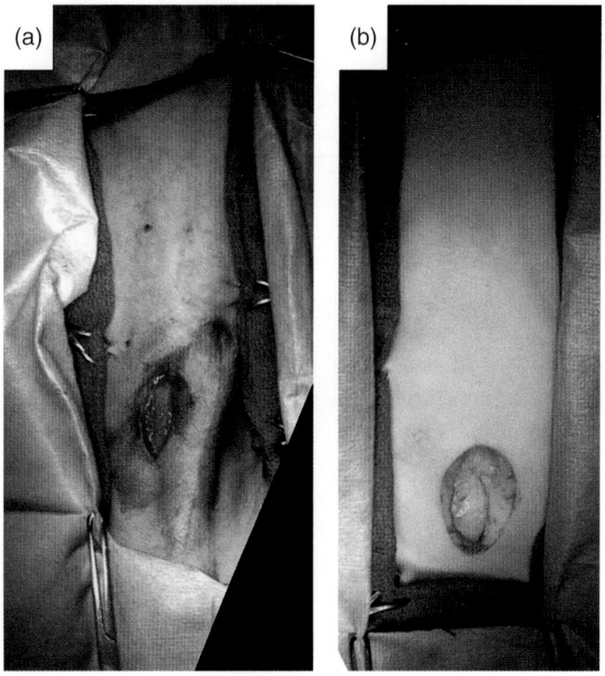

Figure 28.5 Approximate incision size and location for cystotomy in a male dog (a) or male or female cat (b). In both images, cranial is to the top of the image and caudal is to the bottom of the image. In female dogs, the incision would be made similar to as depicted for cats (b). In (a), note how the prepuce has been included in the sterile field to allow for urethral catheterization. Cats can be positioned as depicted in Figure 28.4 to allow for inclusion of the prepuce if needed. Note in both images how the entire abdomen has been aseptically prepared and draped should the incision need to be extended cranially. *Source:* © Janet Grimes.

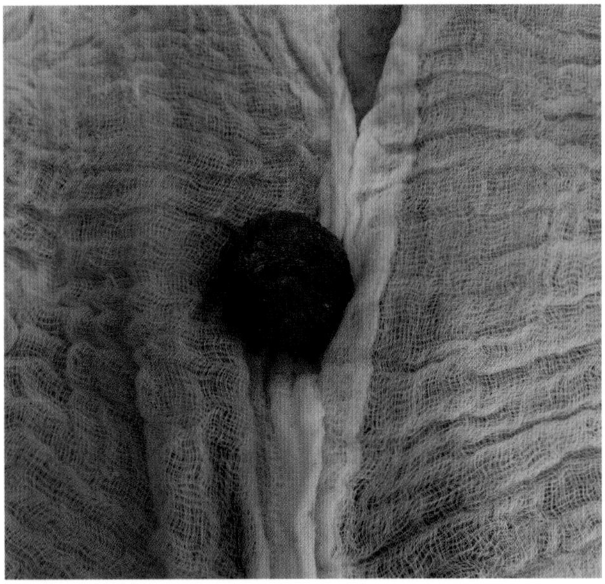

Figure 28.6 The urinary bladder has been exteriorized and packed off with laparotomy sponges. *Source:* © Janet Grimes.

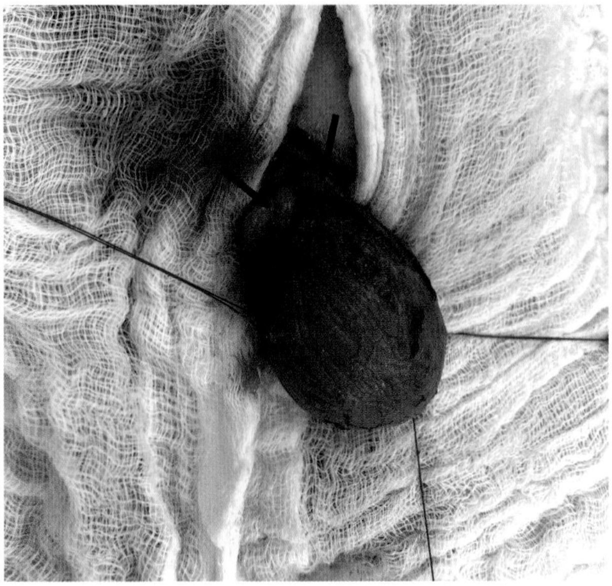

Figure 28.8 Image of the dorsal surface of the urinary bladder. The ureters enter dorsally within the paired lateral ligaments, depicted by the black arrows. Cranial is at the top in this image; the urinary bladder has been reflected caudally. *Source:* © Janet Grimes.

maintaining exteriorization of the urinary bladder. If the bladder wall is friable, a cruciate suture can be placed instead of a simple interrupted suture to provide more holding power on the stay suture.

The cystotomy incision should be performed on the ventral (uppermost) surface of the urinary bladder near the apex in an area of low vascularity. If the ventral median ligament is not already disrupted, it can be transected near the urinary bladder serosa to allow for better identification of the ventral surface of the urinary bladder. Although proposed benefits of a dorsal cystotomy are reduced risk of urine leakage due to gravity, reduced formation of adhesions to the body wall, and reduced formation of cystoliths due to gravity-dependent sedimentation separating the sediment from sutures, the need for these factors has been refuted in two studies.[7,8] Performing a cystotomy on the dorsal surface of the bladder increases the risk of damage to the ureters and neurovascular bundle (Figure 28.8). Cystotomies performed on the ventral surface are easier to perform, allow for a better view of the ureteral openings, and allow for easier access to the urethra.

Once the planned incision site is identified on the ventral surface of the urinary bladder, lateral stay sutures should be placed on either side, within 1 cm of the planned incision site (Figure 28.9, Video 28.3). Prior to incising the urinary bladder, ensure it is packed off with moistened laparotomy sponges, and have suction ready to evacuate expelled urine from the surgical site (Figure 28.10). A stab incision should be performed with a #11 or #15 blade between the stay sutures (Video 28.4). It helps to announce "you're in (urine)" at this point (personal communication, Harry Boothe). The incision should be just long enough to allow for use of the bladder spoon or for removal of the calculi, whichever is larger. In cases with numerous small stones, the incision may only be 1 cm in length

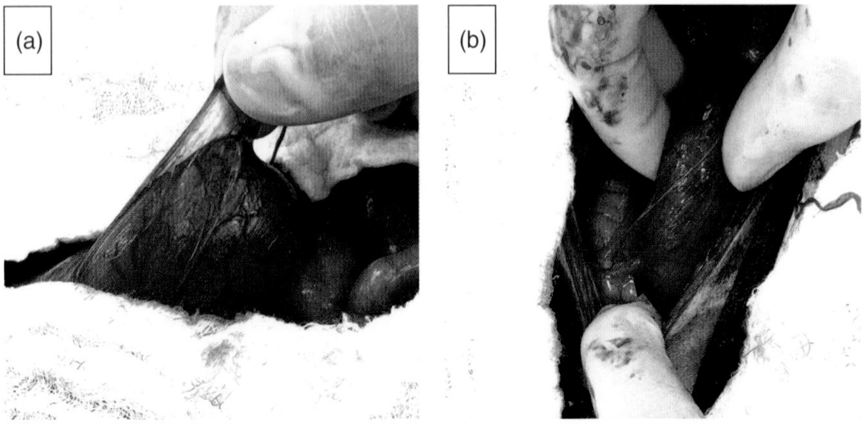

Figure 28.7 The urinary bladder has three attachments to the abdominal wall. The ventral median ligament (a) attaches the bladder ventrally to the linea alba and pelvic symphysis. This fragile ligament may not be visible or may have been disrupted during extension of the linea incision or exteriorization of the urinary bladder. There are also paired lateral ligaments (b) that contain fat, the distal ureters (arrow), and the umbilical arteries. Cranial is to the right in (a) and at the top in (b). *Source:* © Dr. Carolyn Chen.

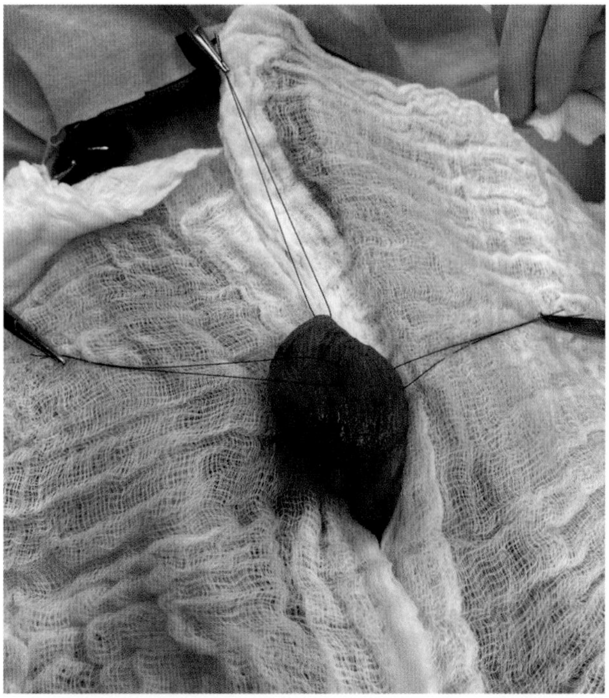

Figure 28.9 Location of stay sutures on the ventral surface of the urinary bladder prior to cystotomy. One stay suture should be placed at the apex with two additional stay sutures on either side of the planned incision site. In friable urinary bladders, a cruciate stay suture may be more resistant to pullout than a simple interrupted stay suture. *Source:* © Janet Grimes.

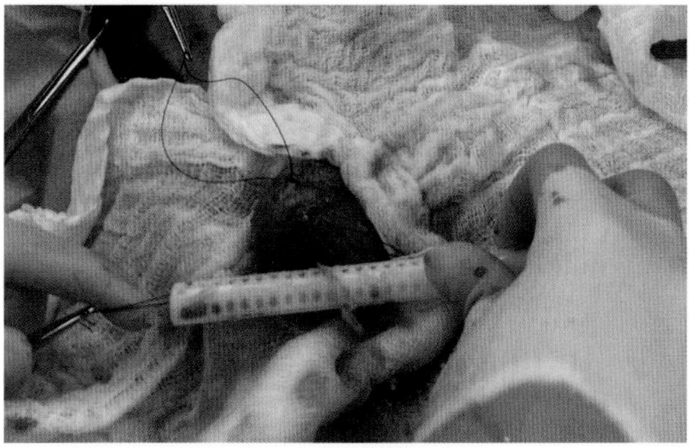

Figure 28.10 Suction should be at the ready prior to performing the cystotomy to capture any urine that is expelled during the creation of the cystotomy incision. *Source:* © Janet Grimes.

(Figure 28.11), whereas larger stones may require a larger cystotomy incision. Some surgeons prefer to make the cystotomy incision just large enough to allow for them to pass their index finger into the urinary bladder to palpate for stones. The cystotomy incision may need to be extended with the scalpel blade or Metzenbaum scissors in cases of significant urinary bladder debris (e.g., feline idiopathic cystitis), neoplasia, or a need to inspect the mucosal surface (Video 28.4). Care should be taken when nearing the

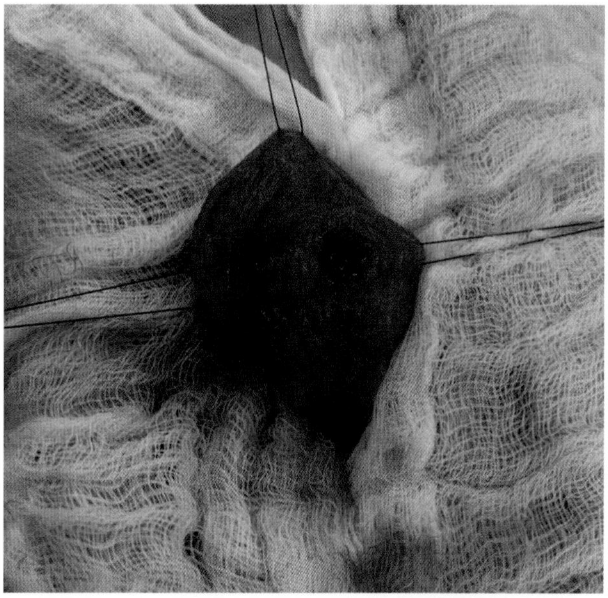

Figure 28.11 Cystotomy incision length in a patient with multiple small stones. If stones are large or inspection of the mucosal surface is required, this incision may be extended with a scalpel blade or Metzenbaum scissors. *Source:* © Janet Grimes.

trigone to ensure the ureters are identified and avoided, and this can be done by keeping the incision on ventral midline closer to the apex of the urinary bladder.

A human gallbladder spoon can be used to scoop stones out of the urinary bladder (Figure 28.12, Video 28.5). The spoon is inserted through the incision into the trigone, spun 360°, and then removed. Any retrieved stones should be collected into a sterile bowl or cup. The gallbladder spoon is used until no stones are retrieved after several attempts while attempting to insert the spoon as far as possible each time. The spoon can typically be inserted to the level of the finger grip between the two ends in most cases. If there was a countable number of stones on preoperative radiographs, removed stones are counted to determine if any stones remain, although in many cases, the stones are too numerous to count or superimposition on radiographs makes counting difficult. The urethra should be catheterized retrograde into the bladder in male dogs and also in male cats if the prepuce was draped into the surgical field (Figure 28.13). The catheter is then slowly withdrawn into the urethra, and sterile saline is flushed into the catheter to flush any stones in the urethra into the urinary bladder. The gallbladder spoon is then used to sweep the trigone area and remove any flushed stones. Some clinicians may also use digital palpation with an index finger to palpate within the lumen for any residual stones. Sweeping for stones should be repeated numerous times, until no more stones are retrieved, and retrograde passing of the catheter feels smooth. The catheter may also be passed normograde through the cystotomy incision to ensure smooth passage (Figure 28.14). The catheter should be withdrawn until it is in the proximal urethra and

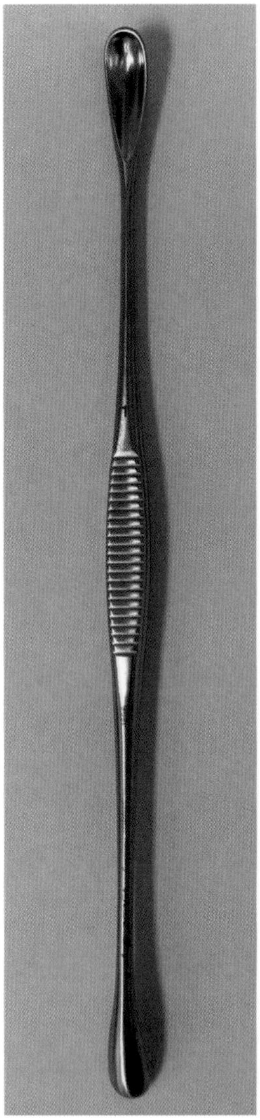

Figure 28.12 A gallbladder spoon is an ideal instrument to scoop stones out of the urinary bladder. *Source:* © Janet Grimes.

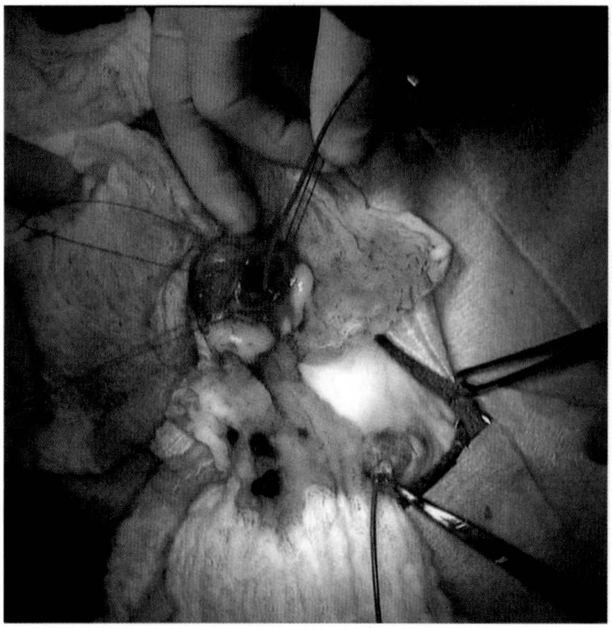

Figure 28.13 Retrograde catheterization should be performed in male dogs, which requires draping the prepuce into the surgical field. This can also be performed in cats if the prepuce is draped into the surgical field, as depicted here. Flushing should be performed as the catheter is withdrawn to flush any stones that have fallen into the urethra back into the urinary bladder for removal. Cranial is to the top left of the image. *Source:* © Janet Grimes.

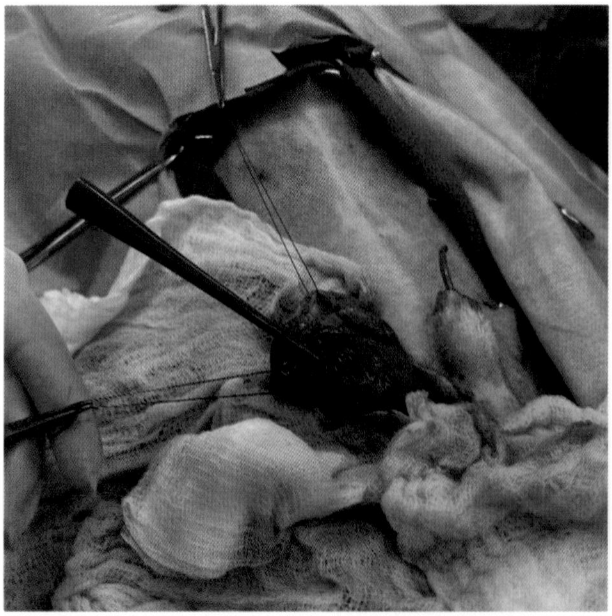

Figure 28.14 Normograde catheterization in a male dog. The catheter should pass smoothly. As the catheter is withdrawn, the catheter should be flushed to ensure an adequate urine stream is produced. Cranial is to the top left of the image. *Source:* © Janet Grimes.

then should be flushed to ensure an adequate urine stream is appreciated from the tip of the penis. In general, having three retrograde and three normograde catheterizations in which the catheter passes smoothly and no stones or mineralized debris are identified with flushing is an indication that all stones/debris have been removed and the cystotomy incision can be closed. In female dogs and cats, these steps are rarely necessary. Female cats can be retrograde catheterized relatively easy, but female dogs are difficult to retrograde catheterize. Fortunately, the female canine urethra is large enough that stones rarely lodge here, and the gallbladder spoon can often be passed fairly far down the urethra to scoop any possible stones. The bladder can also be externally digitally palpated for stones as another method to ensure complete removal, although this may be less fruitful in cases with cystitis.

Prior to closure, a small portion of urinary bladder mucosa should be excised with Metzenbaum scissors for aerobic culture and susceptibility. Submission of a stone for culture analysis can also be performed;[9] however, some clinicians feel this may not reflect an active infection as compared to urinary bladder mucosa. Use of perioperative antimicrobials does not affect culture results from samples obtained intraoperatively.[10]

Cystotomy closure is performed with monofilament absorbable suture, such as poliglecaprone 25 or polydioxanone, on a taper needle. The urinary bladder heals quickly with 100% strength in 14–21 days;[11] thus, long-lasting suture is not required. Suture size is dependent upon the patient. Recommended suture sizes are 3-0 or 4-0 suture in small dogs and cats and 3-0 suture in larger dogs. In patients with cystitis, one suture size larger than normal may be chosen. The cystotomy incision may be closed with a single-layer appositional pattern. In cases in which a short cystotomy incision was performed, a simple interrupted pattern should be used (Figure 28.15). If a longer cystotomy incision is performed, a simple continuous pattern is preferred. There is no difference in the major or minor complication rate between cystotomies closed with a single-layer appositional pattern or a double-layer inverting pattern.[12] If a double-layer closure is performed, two layers of simple continuous sutures may be preferred due to the risk of focal cystitis with an inverting pattern.[13] Suture bites should be placed evenly every 3 mm, with bites taken 3 mm back from the cut tissue edge. Sutures should be pulled snug but not strangulating or hard enough to pull through the tissues, and with a simple continuous suture pattern, tension should remain consistent along the suture line. The holding layer of the urinary bladder is the submucosa; thus, full-thickness bites through the urinary bladder wall are preferred to ensure capture of this layer. Although there is a concern for suture exposure within the lumen increasing the risk of stone formation, poliglecaprone 25 is completely absorbed in 90–120 days, and with snug apposition, little suture is exposed to the lumen.

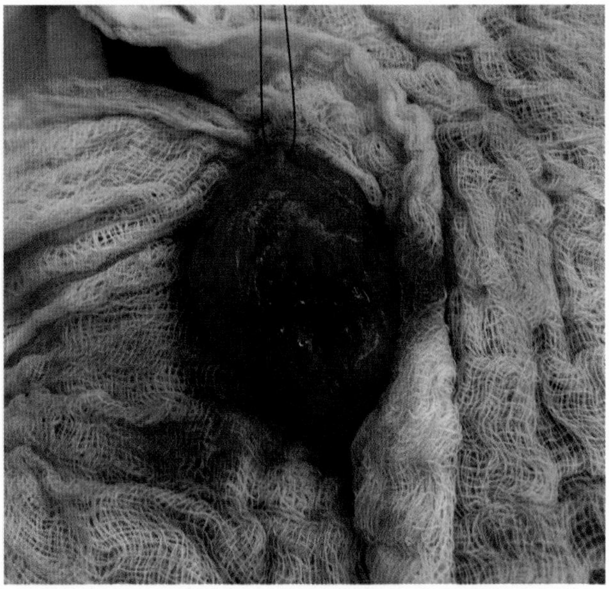

Figure 28.15 This short cystotomy incision was closed with simple interrupted sutures. A longer incision is ideally closed with a simple continuous pattern, but any appositional pattern, such as simple interrupted, is acceptable. *Source:* © Janet Grimes.

A leak test of the cystotomy closure may be performed in male patients by retrograde urethral catheterization and distension with saline (Video 28.6). A leak test is not required, but if desired, may be performed in female patients via cystocentesis and distention with saline. If leakage is noted, simple interrupted sutures should be added to reinforce a simple interrupted suture line. Simple interrupted sutures can also be added on top of a leaking simple continuous line but should not be tied tight enough to make the simple continuous line even looser around the tight simple interrupted suture. Clinicians should be aware that looseness in one region of the simple continuous line may eventually move to a different area or settle out across the entire suture line, leading to leakage. The urinary bladder should be evacuated of urine/saline prior to closure, and any urethral catheters should be removed. Local lavage should be performed (Video 28.7), and the urinary bladder should be returned to the abdomen (Video 28.8). If omentum is visible through the body wall incision, it may be placed over the cystotomy incision; if it is not visible, this is not a concern as the omentum will adhere itself even if not directly placed in the area. The abdominal wall incision is then closed in three layers (external rectus sheath, subcutaneous tissues, skin).

Immediately postoperatively, radiographs should be taken for patients with radiopaque stones to ensure complete removal. In one study, 20% (9 of 44) of dogs had incomplete urolith removal following cystotomy, emphasizing the importance of performing postoperative imaging to confirm complete removal of all stones.[14] If a residual stone(s) is/are noted, the patient should be returned to surgery and the incision reopened to complete stone removal. In patients with radiolucent stones, ultrasound may be used to determine if stone removal is complete. Excised stones should be submitted for stone analysis to assist with diet alterations or other therapies to reduce the recurrence of stone formation.

Partial Cystectomy

Partial cystectomy is performed for masses or other urinary bladder wall defects. Most urinary bladder masses are nonresectable due to their preference for the trigonal region where the ureters enter and the urethra exits. However, lesions located at the apex, ventral wall, or dorsal wall away from the ureters and urethra may be excised with partial cystectomy. Urothelial carcinoma is known to seed easily, meaning that exposure of the abdomen or abdominal incision to cells from this tumor increases the likelihood of additional tumors growing in those locations. For this reason, if a mass is known to be at the apex of the urinary bladder, excision without opening the urinary bladder may be considered.[15] In other cases, the presence of a mass or lesion that requires excision may not be known until the urinary bladder is opened. In these cases, a larger cystotomy incision may be made on the ventral surface of the bladder to allow for inspection of the mucosa. In some cases, the urinary bladder can be everted to allow for increased visibility of the dorsal mucosal surface (Figure 28.16). Once a lesion has been identified that requires excision, a stab incision should be made with a #11 or #15 scalpel blade full thickness through the urinary bladder wall. This incision may be continued with the scalpel blade or with Metzenbaum or Mayo scissors, depending on the thickness of the urinary bladder wall. For tumors, gross margins of 1 cm are excised, but the available margin may be smaller depending on the proximity of the lesion to the ureteral papillae, which should be assessed via catheterization of the ureters at the ureterovesicular junctions to identify their location. In some lesions with wall necrosis, a line of demarcation may be seen (Figure 28.16), but if not immediately visible, it is important to resect back to healthy, bleeding tissue. Once the resection has been performed, the incision is sutured as described for cystotomy above. Placing small catheters into the ureteral papillae, if not already in place, helps with identifying these structures to avoid accidentally suturing them or impinging upon them during closure.

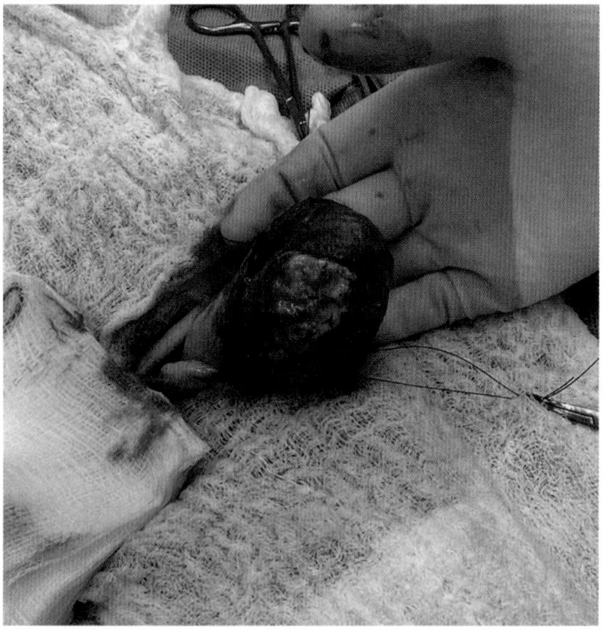

Figure 28.16 Eversion of the urinary bladder to allow for inspection of the mucosal surface. This feline patient had a large necrotic plaque present on the dorsal urinary bladder wall that was excised with partial cystectomy. Cranial is to the right in this image. *Source:* © Janet Grimes.

Potential Complications

One potential major complication following cystotomy is development of uroabdomen. Clinical signs of this are vague but include depression, vomiting, and abdominal pain. Patients may have a distended abdomen with a palpable fluid wave. Confirmation of uroabdomen is performed by several methods. An abdominal fluid creatinine greater than two times the serum creatinine concentration, abdominal fluid potassium greater than 1.4 times serum potassium, and an abdominal fluid creatinine concentration greater than four times the upper limit of the serum creatinine reference range are all consistent with a uroabdomen in dogs.[16] Other methods to diagnose uroabdomen include contrast leakage out of the urinary tract on a radiographic contrast study, such as a retrograde urethrocystogram, or surgical identification of a urinary bladder defect. Uroabdomen may be treated medically or surgically. If the leak is small, an indwelling urethral catheter can be placed for five to seven days to keep the urinary bladder decompressed and evacuate urine, allowing time for the incision to heal. Alternatively, the patient may be returned to surgery and the cystotomy incision inspected. If the tissue edges appear healthy, the incision should be resutured or patched. If the incision site appears necrotic, the edges should be debrided to healthy, bleeding tissue and sutured closed.

Other complications of cystotomy relate to the skin incision and include dehiscence, infection, and seroma formation. If postoperative radiographs are not taken to confirm stone removal, reobstruction may happen. Many patients with urolithiasis will continue to form additional stones if nutritional management is not instituted (see Postoperative Care/Prognosis section). Documentation with radiographs that all stones were removed during the cystotomy procedure is important to prove that a later diagnosis of cystoliths is not due to residual stones from the previous procedure, but rather newly formed stones.

Postoperative Care/Prognosis

Postoperatively, patients should receive appropriate analgesia such as an opioid, initially. If not contraindicated, non-steroidal anti-inflammatory drugs are helpful for analgesia from surgery and to address inflammation causing cystitis. Intravenous fluid use is patient dependent. Benefits include flushing the urinary bladder to assist in removal of any blood clots from surgery and maintaining hydration in previously obstructed patients with postobstructive diuresis. Potential negatives to intravenous fluids are that they may lead to increased distention at the cystotomy incision as the bladder fills. An indwelling urethral catheter is not necessary in these patients.

To access the videos for this chapter, please go to

www.wiley.com/go/coleman/surgeries

VIDEO 28.1 Following opening of the linea alba, the urinary bladder is exteriorized through the incision. There is often significant fat surrounding the trigonal area. In this patient, a urachal remnant was present at the apex of the urinary bladder. *Source:* © Janet Grimes.

VIDEO 28.2 Once exteriorized, the urinary bladder is packed off with moistened laparotomy sponges to prevent urine leakage into the abdomen. *Source:* © Janet Grimes.

VIDEO 28.3 Stay sutures are placed on either side of the planned cystotomy incision. In most cases, a single stay suture is also placed at the apex to assist with exteriorization of the urinary bladder. In this patient, the apex stay suture was not placed due to the urachal remnant at this location. *Source:* © Janet Grimes.

VIDEO 28.4 Following placement of stay sutures, a stab incision is made into the ventral surface of the urinary bladder with a #15 or #11 blade. Suction should be at the ready to evacuate expelled urine from the surgery site. If performing a cystotomy for stones, the incision should be just long enough to allow for use of the bladder spoon or for removal of the calculi, whichever is larger. Some surgeons prefer to make the cystotomy incision just large enough to allow for them to pass their index finger into the urinary bladder to palpate for stones. In this patient, the cystotomy incision was extended with Metzenbaum scissors to resect the urachal remnant at the apex of the urinary bladder, which was later excised entirely. *Source:* © Janet Grimes.

VIDEO 28.5 A human gallbladder spoon can be used to scoop stones out of the urinary bladder. The spoon is inserted through the incision into the trigone, spun 360°, and then removed. Any retrieved stones should be collected into a sterile bowl or cup. The gallbladder spoon is used until no stones are retrieved after several attempts, while attempting to insert the spoon as far as possible each time. The spoon can typically be inserted to the level of the finger grip between the two ends in most cases. *Source:* © Janet Grimes.

VIDEO 28.6 A leak test may be performed in male patients by retrograde urethral catheterization and distension with saline, as demonstrated in this male canine patient. Any saline used to distend the urinary bladder for a leak check should be evacuated prior to closure. *Source:* © Janet Grimes.

VIDEO 28.7 Local lavage of the urinary bladder should be performed following completion of the procedure. *Source:* © Janet Grimes.

VIDEO 28.8 The urinary bladder is returned to the abdomen and the body wall closed routinely in three layers (external rectus sheath, subcutaneous tissues, skin). *Source:* © Janet Grimes.

References

1 Bartges, J.W. and Callens, A.J. (2015). Urolithiasis. *Vet. Clin. North Am. Small Anim. Pract.* 45 (4): 747–768. https://doi.org/10.1016/j.cvsm.2015.03.001.

2 Osborne, C.A., Lulich, J.P., Kruger, J.M. et al. (2008). Analysis of 451,891 canine uroliths, feline uroliths, and feline urethral plugs from 1981 to 2007: perspectives from the Minnesota Urolith Center. *Vet. Clin. North Am. Small Anim. Pract.* 39 (1): 183–197. https://doi.org/10.1016/j.cvsm.2008.09.011.

3 Hecht, S. (2015). Diagnostic imaging of lower urinary tract disease. *Vet. Clin. North Am. Small Anim. Pract.* 45 (4): 639–663. https://doi.org/10.1016/j.cvsm.2015.02.002.

4 Grimes, J.A., Fletcher, J.M., and Schmiedt, C.W. (2018). Outcomes in dogs with uroabdomen: 43 cases (2006-2015). *J. Am. Vet. Med. Assoc.* 252 (1): 92–97. https://doi.org/10.2460/javma.252.1.92.

5 Marvel, S.J., Seguin, B., Dailey, D.D. et al. (2017). Clinical outcome of partial cystectomy for transitional cell carcinoma of the canine bladder. *Vet. Comp. Oncol.* 15 (4): 1417–1427. https://doi.org/10.1111/vco.12286.

6 Osborne, C.A., Lulich, J.P., and Polzin, D.J. (1999). Canine retrograde urohydropropulsion: lessons from 25 years of experience. *Vet. Clin. North Am. Small Anim. Pract.*

29 (1): 267–281. https://doi.org/10.1016/s0195-5616(99)50015-6.
7 Desch, J.P. and Wagner, S.D. (1986). Urinary bladder incisions in dogs comparison of ventral and dorsal. *Vet. Surg.* 15 (2): 153–155. https://doi.org/10.1111/j.1532-950X.1986.tb00195.x.
8 Crowe, D.T. (1986). Ventral versus dorsal cystotomy: an experimental investigation. *J. Am. Anim. Hosp. Assoc.* 22: 382.
9 Hamaide, A.J., Martinez, S.A., Hauptman, J. et al. (1998). Prospective comparison of four sampling methods (cystocentesis, bladder mucosal swab, bladder mucosal biopsy, and urolith culture) to identify urinary tract infections in dogs with urolithiasis. *J. Am. Anim. Hosp. Assoc.* 34: 423–430.
10 Buote, N.J., Kovak-McClaran, J.R., Loar, A.S. et al. (2012). The effect of preoperative antimicrobial administration on culture results in dogs undergoing cystotomy. *J. Am. Vet. Med. Assoc.* 241 (9): 1185–1189. https://doi.org/10.2460/javma.241.9.1185.
11 Bellah, J.R. (1989). Wound healing in the urinary tract. *Semin. Vet. Med. Surg.* 4 (4): 294–303.
12 Thieman-Mankin, K.M., Ellison, G.W., Jeyapaul, C.J. et al. (2012). Comparison of short-term complication rates between dogs and cats undergoing appositional single-layer of inverting double-layer cystotomy closure: 144 cases (1993-2010). *J. Am. Vet. Med. Assoc.* 240 (1): 65–68. https://doi.org/10.2460/javma.240.1.65.
13 Hildreth, B.E., Ellison, G.W., Roberts, J.F. et al. (2006). Biomechanical and histologic comparison of single-layer continuous Cushing and simple continuous appositional cystotomy closure by use of poliglecaprone 25 in rats with experimentally induced inflammation of the urinary bladder. *Am. J. Vet. Res.* 67 (4): 686–692. https://doi.org/10.2460/ajvr.67.4.686.
14 Grant, D.C., Harper, T.A.M., and Werre, S.R. (2010). Frequency of incomplete urolith removal, complications, and diagnostic imaging following cystotomy for removal of uroliths from the lower urinary tract in dogs: 128 cases (1994-2006). *J. Am. Vet. Med. Assoc.* 236 (7): 763–766. https://doi.org/10.2460/javma.236.7.763.
15 Milovancev, M., Scharf, V.F., Townsend, K.L. et al. (2020). Partial cystectomy with a bipolar sealing device in seven dogs with naturally occurring bladder tumors. *Vet. Surg.* 49 (4): 794–799. https://doi.org/10.1111/vsu.13395.
16 Schmiedt, C., Tobias, K.M., and Otto, C.M. (2001). Evaluation of abdominal fluid: peripheral blood creatinine and potassium ratios for diagnosis of uroperitoneum in dogs. *J. Vet. Emerg. Crit. Care* 11 (4): 275–280. https://doi.org/10.1111/j.1476-4431.2001.tb00066.x.

29

Prostatic Abscessation

Catriona M. MacPhail

Department of Clinical Sciences, Colorado State University, Fort Collins, CO, USA

Key Points

- Dogs are at risk for septic peritonitis if a prostatic abscess ruptures.
- The indication for surgery depends on the size of the prostatic abscess(-es) and the severity of clinical signs.
- The surgical treatment of choice is debridement and lavage of the prostatic abscesses followed by omentalization.

Introduction

Prostatitis refers to infection of the prostate gland, with or without abscess formation. When abscessation occurs, localized accumulations of purulent material develop within the prostatic parenchyma. Infection occurs as a result of bacteria colonizing the prostatic parenchyma. Normal host prostatic defense mechanisms may be compromised by urinary tract infection, disruption of prostatic parenchymal architecture, altered urine flow, or urine retention. Prostatic cystic hyperplasia, squamous metaplasia, prostatic cysts, and prostatic neoplasia (e.g., Sertoli cell tumor) increase the risk of infection. Abscesses may rupture, resulting in septic peritonitis.

Abscesses primarily occur in older, sexually intact males with prostatitis, squamous metaplasia, or cysts. In a cohort of dogs with prostatic disease, 7.7% had prostatic abscesses.[1] Although prostatic abscesses may occur in dogs as young as two years of age, most are older than eight years. Feline prostatic infections are rare. Dogs are usually brought in because of an acute onset of depression or lethargy, straining when urinating or defecating, hematuria, vomiting, discomfort, and polyuria/polydipsia. Other clinical signs include fever, anorexia, diarrhea, dehydration, and pelvic limb stiffness.

Physical examination may find discomfort on abdominal palpation or lumbar spine palpation. Rectal palpation is typically painful, and abscessed prostates are generally enlarged and asymmetric with fluctuant areas. Scrotal and testicular palpation may reveal masses, enlargement, or increased sensitivity. Additionally, signs of tachycardia, pale or injected mucous membranes, delayed capillary refill, and/or weak pulses may be evident if the dog is in septic shock.

Point-of-care ultrasound may reveal abdominal effusion consistent with peritonitis. Abdominal radiographic findings include prostatomegaly with indistinct borders and occasional mineralization. Ultrasonographic prostatic evaluation may reveal alterations in echogenicity and fluid-filled spaces with irregularly defined margins (Figure 29.1). Fluid within the lesion may have mixed echogenicity or a flocculent appearance. To confirm diagnosis of abscess, aspiration of fluid-filled pockets in the prostate is tempting, but the concern for rupture and resulting peritonitis is high. *Escherichia coli* has historically been the most common organism associated with prostatitis and prostatic abscessation. However, a recent study found *Staphylococcus* spp. to be the most frequently detected in prostatic aspirates.[2] This same study found that sampling the urine in dogs with prostatic disease may be consistent with bacteria isolates in the prostate. This is supported by another recent study of dogs with prostatic neoplasia;[3] however, it is unsubstantiated by a retrospective study on prostatic abscesses that found dogs with positive culture in both prostatic and urine culture agreed in only 50% of cases.[4]

Techniques in Small Animal Soft Tissue, Orthopedic, and Ophthalmic Surgery, First Edition. Edited by Kristin A. Coleman.

Companion website: www.wiley.com/go/coleman/surgeries

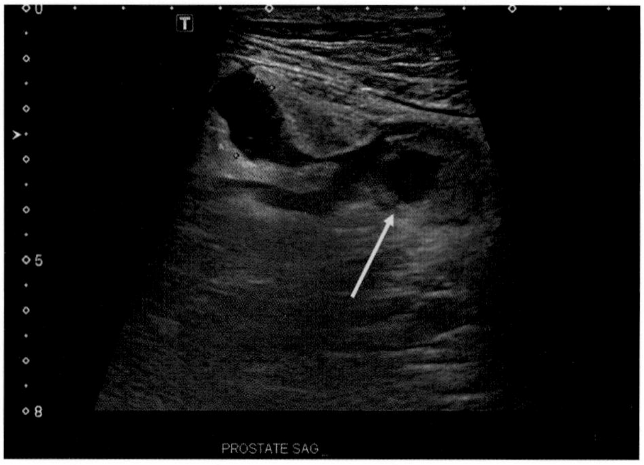

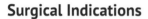

Figure 29.1 Ultrasonographic appearance of canine prostatic abscessation (arrow) with thickened urinary bladder to the left.

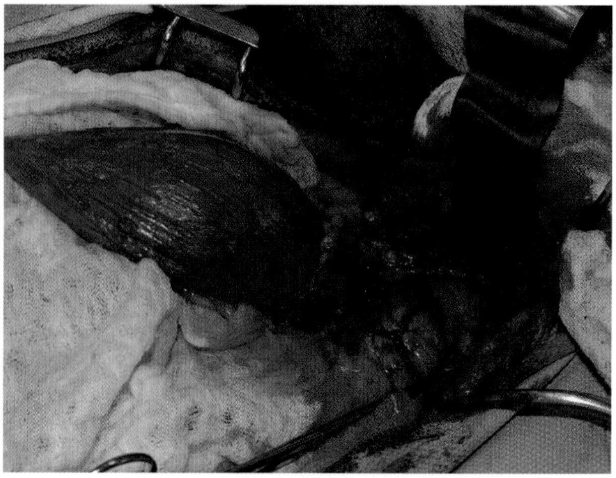

Figure 29.2 Intraoperative picture of prostatic omentalization (dog in Figure 29.1) with the urinary bladder pulled cranially using a stay suture to bring the enlarged prostate further cranially into the abdominal cavity. Cranial is to the left in this image.

Surgical Indications

Prostatitis and small prostatic abscesses (less than 1 cm) can be treated with antibiotics and fluid therapy with good success. If the animal is in a shock state, fluid replacement therapy and antimicrobials should be initiated as soon as possible. Large, untreated abscesses will eventually cause septicemia, toxemia, and death. The appropriate treatment for concurrent bacterial prostatitis and cystitis is determined by selecting an appropriate antimicrobial agent based on the results of the antimicrobial susceptibility. For empirical antimicrobial treatment, fluoroquinolones are the preferable drug category for treating prostatitis, although amoxicillin-clavulanic acid is widely used for treating bacterial prostatitis and cystitis. However, the most recent international antimicrobial use guidelines for the treatment of urinary tract disease in dogs and cats did not recommend amoxicillin-clavulanic acid for treating prostatitis.[5] For dogs with ruptured abscesses and septic peritonitis, it is appropriate to treat with both fluoroquinolones and potentiated penicillins systemically for complete antimicrobial coverage.

Drainage of prostatic abscesses is indicated when pockets are greater than 1 cm in diameter. Ultrasound-guided percutaneous prostatic drainage can be considered for pockets less than 2.5 cm in diameter.[6] Otherwise, dogs are taken to surgery for abdominal exploratory. For all cases of prostatitis, surgical castration is recommended.

Surgical Procedure

Prior to surgery, a large urinary catheter should be placed to aid identification of the urethra. The goals of surgery are to drain the abscess(-es), biopsy and culture the prostatic parenchyma, and castration. Historical options for prostatic abscess surgical intervention included placement of multiple passive drains and marsupialization. Currently, prostatic omentalization is the treatment of choice for abscess drainage. A stay suture is placed in the apex of the urinary bladder to pull the prostate cranially. Stab incisions are made in the lateral aspects of the prostate gland, and purulent material is removed by aggressive lavage and suction. The prostatic urethra is identified by palpation of the urinary catheter. Loculated abscess(es) can be digitally broken down within the parenchyma, and the stab incisions are enlarged by resecting capsular tissue (Figure 29.2). Forceps are passed through one prostatic incision and used to grasp the omentum from the opposite incision and pull it into the parenchyma. The omentum is either pulled out on the other side or wrapped around the prostatic urethra and exited through the first incision. The omentum is anchored to the prostatic capsule using absorbable, monofilament mattress sutures (Figure 29.3). A closed suction multi-fenestrated drain is placed in the caudal abdominal cavity.

Potential Complications

Potential short-term complications following surgery are hypovolemia, hypoproteinemia, hypoglycemia, anemia, sepsis, subcutaneous edema, incisional infection, and urinary incontinence. Long-term complications following omentalization include recurrent prostatitis, recurrent abscesses, urinary tract infections, and urinary incontinence. The most recent recurrence rate was reported at 12%.[4]

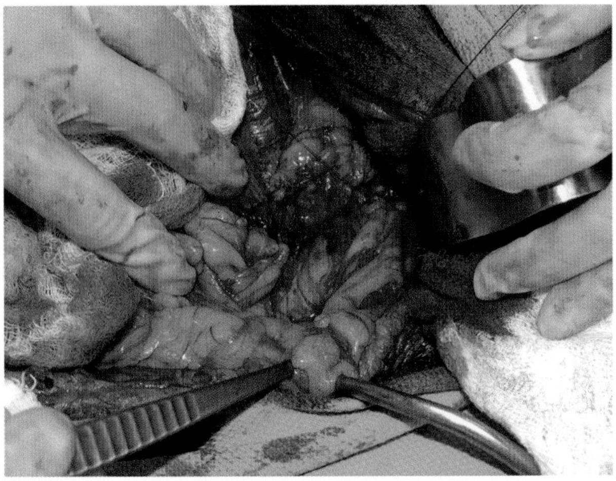

Figure 29.3 Intraoperative picture of the same dog from Figure 29.2 following omentalization of a large prostatic abscess. Cranial is to the left in this image.

Postoperative Care/Prognosis

Analgesics, antibiotics, nutritional support, and intravenous fluids are administered in the postoperative period as the dog is monitored for sepsis, shock, and anemia. Appropriate antibiotics should be given for four to six weeks postoperatively following the results of the culture. Abdominal ultrasound performed every three months is used to monitor for recurrent or persistent infection. Immediate postoperative mortality approaches 25%, but if the prostatic abscess has ruptured, mortality can approach 50%. Fair to excellent results are expected if the patient survives two weeks after surgery. In the most recent retrospective study of dogs with prostatic abscessation, the mortality rate was 11% of dogs within the first six months following diagnosis.[4]

References

1. Polisca, A., Troisi, A., Fontaine, E. et al. (2016). A retrospective study of canine prostatic diseases from 2002 to 2009 at the Alfort Veterinary College in France. *Therio* 85 (5): 835–840.
2. Phongphaew, W., Kongtia, M., Kim, K. et al. (2021). Association of bacterial isolates and antimicrobial susceptibility between prostatic fluid and urine samples in canine prostatitis with concurrent cystitis. *Therio* 173: 202–210.
3. Skorupski, K.A., Byrne, B.A., Palm, C.A. et al. (2022). Prospective comparison of prostatic aspirate culture and cystocentesis urine culture for detection of bacterial infection in dogs with prostatic neoplasia. *J. Small Anim. Pract.* 63 (12): 858–862.
4. Lea, C., Walker, D., Blazquez, C.A. et al. (2022). Prostatitis and prostatic abscessation in dogs: retrospective study of 82 cases. *Aust. Vet. J.* 100 (6): 223–229.
5. Weese, J.S., Blondeau, J., Boothe, D. et al. (2019). International Society for Companion Animal Infectious Diseases (ISCAID) guidelines for the diagnosis and management of bacterial urinary tract infections in dogs and cats. *Vet. J.* 247: 8–25.
6. Sykes, J.E. and Westropp, J.L. (2014). Chapter 89 - bacterial infections of the genitourinary tract. In: *Canine and Feline Infectious Diseases* (ed. J.E. Sykes), 871–885. W.B. Saunders.

30

Inguinal, Umbilical, and Diaphragmatic Hernias

David Michael Tillson

Department of Clinical Sciences, Auburn University, Auburn, AL, USA

Key Points

- Hernias can be static or active and can change rapidly, necessitating active surveillance until surgical repair is performed.
- Reducible hernias allow the movement of adjacent fat or organs into and out of the hernia defect; non-reducible hernias have materials that are stuck within the defect.
- Hernia repair becomes an emergency procedure if the hernia contents begin to undergo vascular compromise to the herniated tissues, leading toward tissue death.
- Umbilical hernias are typically small, congenital hernias that may or may not require any surgical management.
- Inguinal hernias are more common in small breed, female dogs, and herniation of intestinal segments or a uterine horn through the hernia will necessitate hernia repair.
- Diaphragmatic hernias are commonly associated with blunt-force abdominal trauma and require surgical repair to prevent long-term issues; however, emergency surgery is infrequently required.

Introduction

Hernias are defined as an opening in the body wall that permits the protrusion or movement of organ(s) or tissues out of the body cavity. Hernias are typically designated by anatomic location (e.g., umbilical hernia). Hernias can be congenital, traumatic, or surgical.[1] Congenital hernias are natural openings that are present at birth. Congenital hernias can have herniated tissues in the hernia when discovered or may represent a potential opening that may develop at a future date. Traumatic hernias occur when otherwise normal tissues are torn, ripped, or ruptured, creating a defect. While most traumatic hernias occur in previously normal tissues, it is possible for traumatic events to increase the size of congenital hernias, thereby, creating a traumatic hernia in a congenital location (e.g., traumatic rupture of an inguinal ring with intestinal herniation). Surgical hernias occur after technically poor incisional closure, incomplete incisional closure, or traumatic injury that reopens a perilously secured incisional closure. This chapter will focus on three commonly encountered abdominal hernias: the umbilical hernia, the inguinal hernia, and the diaphragmatic hernia.

Hernias can have three components: the hernia sac, the hernia ring, and the contents within the sac. A hernia sac is seen primarily with congenital or "true" hernias that have a peritoneal lining, such as umbilical, inguinal, and peritoneopericardial diaphragmatic hernias.[1,2] Traumatic hernias, such as pleuro-peritoneal diaphragmatic hernias or body wall ruptures, have no peritoneal lining and are called "false" hernias. As such, they have no real hernia sac, and the hernia ring tissue surrounding the protrusion is initially regular as opposed to a fibrous band in the congenital type.

Hernias are further classified as being "*reducible*" (i.e., the hernia contents can easily spontaneously return or be manipulated into the abdominal cavity) or "*non-reducible*" (i.e., the contents are not able to be replaced within the

Techniques in Small Animal Soft Tissue, Orthopedic, and Ophthalmic Surgery, First Edition. Edited by Kristin A. Coleman.

Companion website: www.wiley.com/go/coleman/surgeries

abdominal cavity). Non-reducible hernias are additionally divided into "*incarcerated*" and "*strangulated*" hernias. Incarcerated hernias have their contents trapped in the herniated location, but the contents are typically uncompromised. Strangulated hernias have the contents entrapped as well, but these hernias also have a compromised vascular supply, resulting in the questionable vitality of the herniated tissues. Incarcerated hernias can become strangulated over time due to constriction of the hernia borders around the herniated tissues, which may eventually lead to edema, vascular congestion, and/or mispositioning of the entrapped tissues within the hernia. This means incarcerated hernias must be closely monitored until definitive repair. Conversely, strangulated hernias are surgical emergencies, requiring appropriate management in an expedited manner.

It has been stated that the principles of hernia repair involve four steps.[1] First, replace the herniated contents into their original anatomic location. The next steps include securely closing the hernia ring to prevent recurrence and removing any redundant material associated with the hernia sac. Finally, the surgeon should strive to use the patient's own tissues to close the hernia whenever possible.

Umbilical Hernia

Etiology

Umbilical hernias are typically congenital and are associated with a failure of the umbilical ring to form the umbilical scar.[1–3] This can occur because the ring is too large, because there is a failure of contraction, or because the umbilicus is abnormally formed, and the result is a defect that becomes an umbilical hernia.[2] Most umbilical hernias are small and contain a small portion of falciform fat, creating a small, softly palpable mass at the site of the umbilicus.[4] Larger umbilical hernias can occur, often having intestines and abdominal fat protruding through the hernia. Omphaloceles, which are large hernias with no subcutaneous layer or skin over the herniated viscera, are rare in veterinary medicine. Until herniation, the viscera are precariously kept in the abdominal cavity by only a peritoneal sac. Most are euthanized in veterinary medicine; however, if management of an omphalocele is attempted, the peritoneal sac-enveloped viscera should be kept covered with an occlusive dressing until surgical reduction and hernia closure can be performed.

Diagnosis

The diagnosis of an umbilical hernia is made on physical examination. For neonates that are born via C-section or are presented to a veterinarian shortly after birth, the physical evaluation should include checking for large umbilical hernias. Otherwise, the initial veterinary visit for routine vaccinations may be the first time an umbilical hernia is noted.

The presence of a soft tissue mass on the ventral midline at the level of the umbilicus is diagnostic, and other diagnostic tests or imaging modalities are generally not required. It is important to document the size and the reducibility of the hernia in the medical record when first identified. The majority of umbilical hernias are small, non-painful, non-reducible masses filled with falciform or omental fat. While it is always wise to instruct owners to monitor an umbilical hernia for acute changes, these umbilical hernias are benign and are unlikely to ever be more than a minor imperfection. If desired, they are routinely addressed at the time of surgical neutering or during another abdominal procedure.

Umbilical hernias are considered heritable in several breeds, such as the Pekinese, Basenji, Poodle, Airedale terrier, and Weimaraner.[1–3] Umbilical hernias are also associated with numerous other congenital abnormalities, so the veterinarian needs to completely evaluate affected patients for other abnormalities. Large umbilical or cranial abdominal wall hernias in the Weimaraner breed should prompt thoracic films to evaluate the dog for a peritoneopericardial hernia.

Timing of Surgical Repair

Given the benign nature of most umbilical hernias, no immediate intervention is required; rather, these hernias are often repaired in conjunction with surgical neutering. If the umbilical hernia is reducible, owners should be shown how to monitor the hernia, ensuring herniated structures do not become strangulated. This should be done on a daily basis. Sudden increases in the size of the hernia, localized swelling, and/or pain on gentle palpation warrant immediate re-evaluation of the hernia. A change in a hernia from "reducible" to "non-reducible" suggests surgical correction should be forthcoming, while a strangulated hernia is an emergent situation needing immediate surgery to correct the strangulation, replace or resect damaged tissues or organs, and close the defect.

Surgical Procedure – Umbilical Herniorrhaphy

Most umbilical hernias are small and of minimal concern. They typically contain small protrusions of fat from the falciform ligament or the omentum. As such, they are at very low risk of clinically important herniations. Some umbilical hernias can be moderate to substantial in size with abdominal contents that readily herniate and then reduce spontaneously. While the smaller hernias may not necessitate repair, hernias that are easily reducible have the potential for tissues to eventually get trapped and potentially become strangulated. These hernias warrant monitoring and eventual repair. Umbilical hernias are seldom emergency procedures.

After routine patient preparation, a ventral midline incision is made. If an ovariohysterectomy or other abdominal procedure is being performed, the standard incision is extended over the umbilical hernia for an additional 2–4 cm. Care is taken to not prematurely incise into the hernia sac, which reduces the risk of damaging hernia contents during the approach. This is especially important when the hernia is large and non-reducible and is suspected to contain materials other than fat. If there is a concern, the surgeon can make their initial abdominal incision caudal to the umbilicus and use a finger to probe the hernia site to guide further incision and dissection. The hernia sac is dissected free, and the abdominal incision is continued to the level of the umbilicus. As the incision is continued cranially, the fibrous umbilical ring is removed on either side of the incision, and the incision continues as far cranially as needed. The defect created in this manner can be closed along with the rest of the ventral midline incision. Excessive skin associated with the hernia may need to be resected prior to final closure.

If the umbilical hernia is being repaired independently of other abdominal procedures, an elliptical incision is made around the base of the hernia, and the incision is deepened to the level of the external rectus fascia. The tissue surrounding the hernia is carefully undermined until the hernia sac is encountered. The overlying skin and subcutaneous tissue are removed if excessive or incised, and the hernia sac is exposed (Figure 30.1). When the hernia is reducible, the hernia contents are pressed back into the abdominal cavity, the hernia sac is opened, and excessive tissue associated with the sac is removed. This should leave the hernia ring clearly exposed. The hernia is not ready for closure.

If the hernia contents are incarcerated or strangulated, additional dissection to permit resection of the hernia contents may be required. This typically involves a larger abdominal incision extending cranially and caudally from the umbilical hernia. These adjacent incisions allow the surgeon to palpate the hernia from the visceral side and determine the extensiveness of the adhesions and the vulnerability of the hernia contents that could be damaged during surgical manipulation. While small clumps of strangulated adipose tissue offer little concern, larger volumes of compromised tissues can release vasoactive compounds if the tissues are suddenly exposed to a returning blood supply. If the tissues are compromised, an attempt should be made to isolate the damaged tissues before releasing them from their strangulated location.

Closure

Options for closure of the umbilical hernia are based on whether the hernia ring was resected and the size of the hernia defect. When the hernia ring is resected (i.e., "the

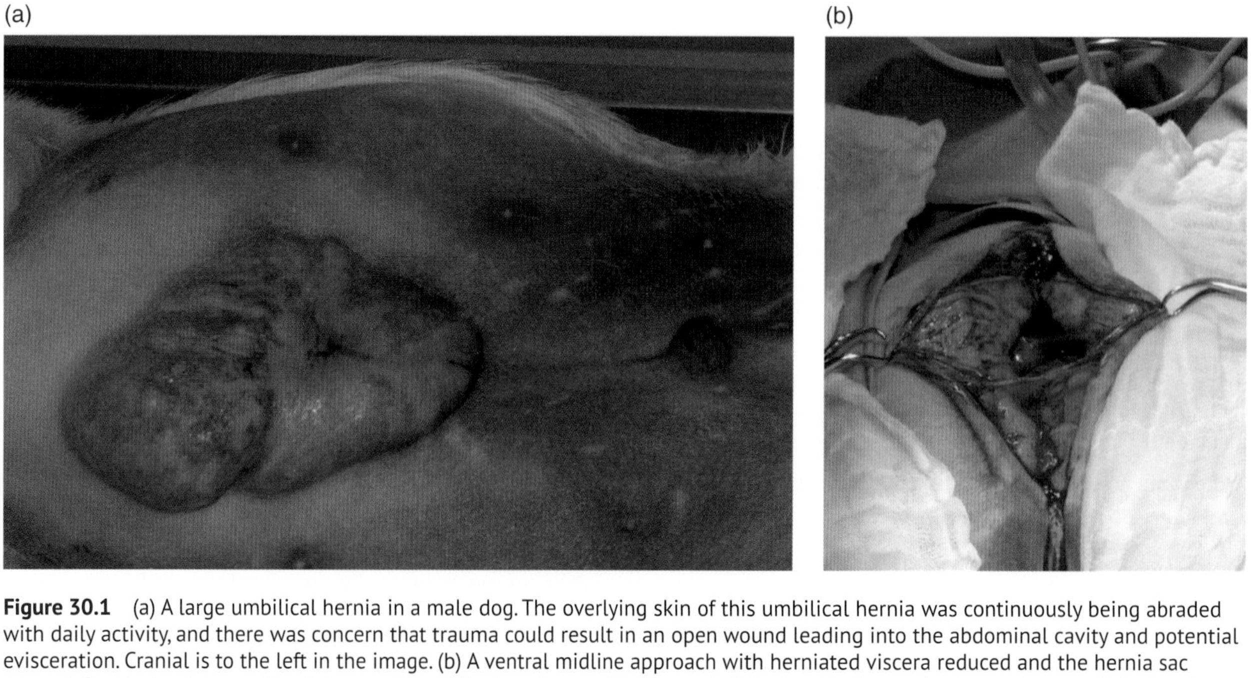

Figure 30.1 (a) A large umbilical hernia in a male dog. The overlying skin of this umbilical hernia was continuously being abraded with daily activity, and there was concern that trauma could result in an open wound leading into the abdominal cavity and potential evisceration. Cranial is to the left in the image. (b) A ventral midline approach with herniated viscera reduced and the hernia sac opened. Surgical repair would entail resection of the hernia sac, debridement of the hernia ring, and primary closure of the hernia as a part of the midline closure. Cranial is at the top of the image.

edges are freshened"), the thick fibrous ring is removed until normal tissue is exposed. This should permit primary wound healing of the body wall, including where the former umbilical hernia was located (Figure 30.2). If the hernia defect is a part of a larger incision, it is sutured as a part of the ventral midline incision closure. The author recommends closing the body wall with a simple continuous pattern. Alternatively, if the defect is small, it can be closed with the surgeon's preferred suture pattern: simple interrupted, simple continuous, cruciate mattress, or horizontal mattress sutures. A long-lasting, absorbable suture material is appropriate when the ring has been resected. If the clinician decides to not resect the hernia ring, there is a concern that the wound healing might not be sufficient to prevent reoccurrence.[5] In that situation, a non-absorbable suture material, with whichever pattern, might reduce the potential for re-herniation. The need to use a special hernia suture pattern, such as a vest-over-pants pattern, is typically not required in small animals.

In the rare situation when an umbilical defect is too large to permit primary closure, other strategies may be needed.[2] First, the surgeon can consider placing large, tension-relieving, horizontal or vertical mattress sutures to counteract the tension across the suture line, allowing tension-free, primary wound apposition. Another technique is to cover the defect with a polypropylene mesh sutured to the external sheath of the rectus abdominus muscle. Many surgeons will use omentum to cover the abdominal side of the mesh in an effort to minimize potential adhesion formation between the mesh and the

(a)

(b)

(c)

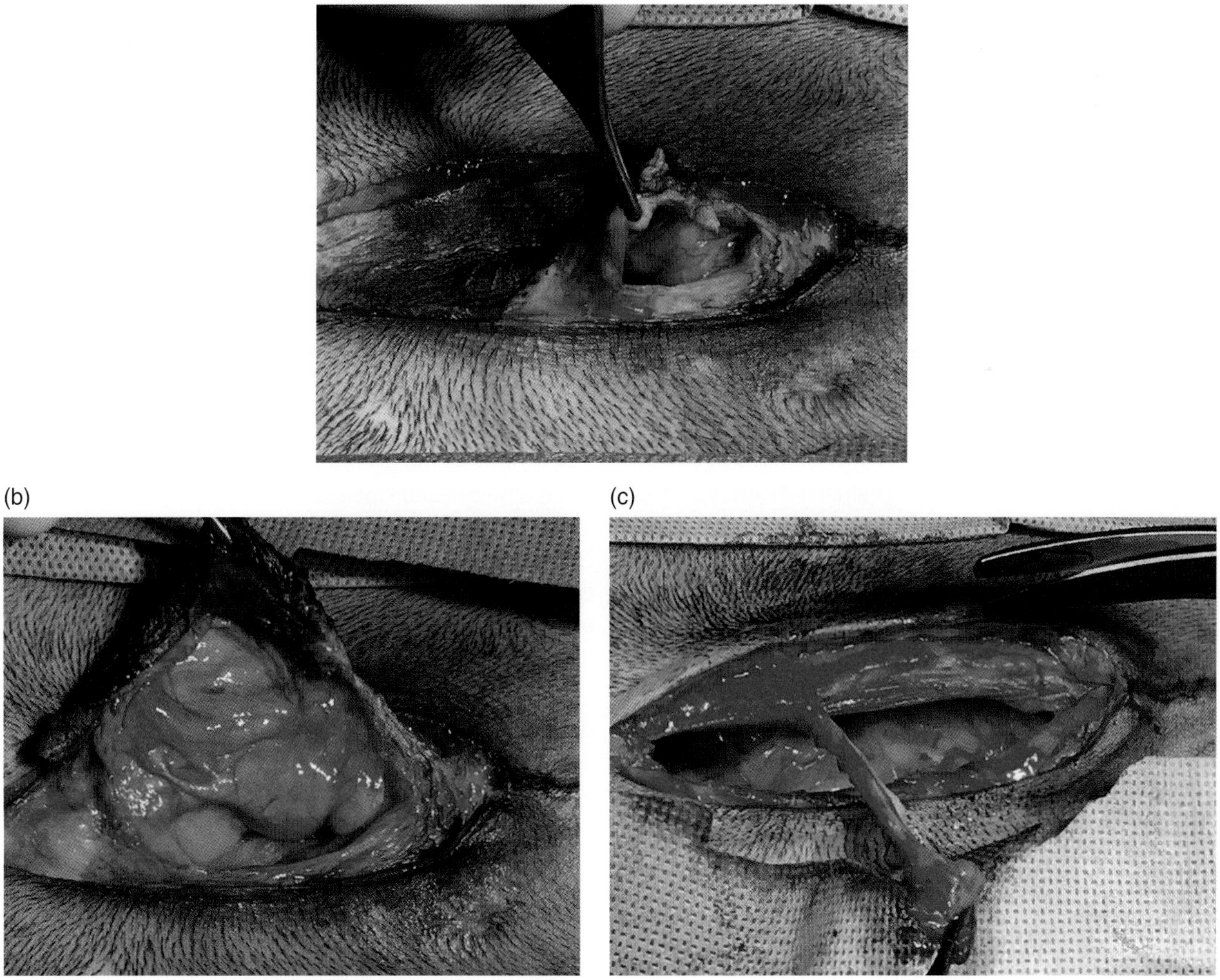

Figure 30.2 Canine patient with an umbilical hernia. Cranial is to the left in the images. (a) An elliptical incision is made around the umbilical hernia, taking care to avoid injury to any underlying or herniated tissues. (b) Dissection is continued, and the hernia sac is identified and resected. (c) After dissection and reduction of all the herniated tissues, the ring of fibrous tissue surrounding the hernia is removed to expose the external rectus fascia and rectus muscle along the hernia edge. This allows for primary closure using either a long-lasting absorbable or a non-absorbable monofilament suture material. It is important that the closure be accomplished without excessive tension along the herniorrhaphy.

abdominal viscera. A final technique for large defects is to use releasing incisions to create two bipedicle flaps from the rectus sheath, which can be advanced toward the midline for closure. Careful inspection of the flaps is needed to ensure that there is adherence of the external sheath to the underlying muscle, otherwise, this technique could create a new avenue for visceral herniation.

Once body wall closure is accomplished, the subcutaneous closure is completed, and the skin is apposed as normal.

Postoperative Management

No special postoperative care is required after umbilical hernia repair. Appropriate analgesics and a brief two-week period of exercise restriction are all that is needed. It is a good idea to encourage owners to continue to check the surgical site for recurrence, although the likelihood of such should be very small.

Inguinal Hernia

Etiology

Inguinal hernias are typically congenital; however, traumatic abdominal injuries can also cause herniation of abdominal organs through an inguinal ring. Organs that have been identified in inguinal hernia contents include the urinary bladder, intestinal segments, and the uterus.[2,3,6] Inguinal hernia is reported more frequently in female dogs compared with the males[7,8] and is very rare in cats.[6] Numerous breeds, including Basenji, Pekingese, Poodle, Basset hound, Cairn and West Highland White terriers, Cavalier King Charles spaniels, Chihuahua, Cocker spaniel, miniature Dachshund, Pomeranian, and Maltese dogs, have all been associated with inguinal hernias.[2,3,9] In addition to occurring more commonly in females and in small dogs, non-traumatic inguinal hernias seem to have a higher predilection for the left side.[9] The uterus was the most commonly herniated organ in one report, with the intestines being the second most frequently herniated organ.[9]

It can be challenging to distinguish the normal fat in the vaginal process and inguinal fat from herniated organs or abdominal fat. Occasionally, local lymphadenopathy or inguinal abscesses may mimic herniated tissue. In one case series, several cats were presented with inguinal swelling after vehicular accidents with inguinal swellings that had to be differentiated from an inguinal hernia,[10] and in another report, a dog developed an inguinal enterocutaneous fistula after intestinal adhesion at the level of the inguinal canal without apparent herniation.[11]

Traumatic episodes with subsequent increases in intra-abdominal pressure can result in inguinal hernias that may include damage to the adjacent body wall. The influence of reproductive status and the role of reproductive hormones may also be a factor in acquired inguinal hernias, since these hernias most commonly occur in intact, middle-aged female dogs during estrus or pregnancy.[1,3] Herniation of a uterine horn can occur, requiring repair prior to full gestation to prevent parturition complications. In the male dog, herniation of abdominal viscera into the vaginal process can result in a scrotal hernia. This herniation needs to the differentiated from other testicular conditions, such as testicular torsion, neoplasia, or orchitis.[8]

Surgical Anatomy

Anatomically, the inguinal canal comprises internal and external inguinal rings and the passage that connects the two. The internal and external rings are also referred to as the deep and superficial inguinal rings, respectively. The inguinal rings are typically located approximately a centimeter cranial and medial to the femoral ring. In traumatic injuries involving the inguinal canal, these two structures may merge, resulting in a larger defect for potential herniation.

The deep/internal inguinal ring is bordered medially by the rectus abdominis muscle, cranially by the internal abdominal oblique muscle, and laterally and caudally by the inguinal ligament. The superficial/external inguinal ring is a craniocaudal aperture within the aponeurosis of the external abdominal oblique muscle.[12] The inguinal canal is the passage connecting the internal and external inguinal rings.

Several structures normally run through the inguinal canal. These include the external pudendal vessels and genital nerve, which run along the caudal aspect of the inguinal canal, as well as the vaginal process, which contains fat and the round ligament in a female or the spermatic cord in the male. For this reason, a herniorrhaphy involving the inguinal canal should not close the defect entirely.

Diagnosis

Inguinal hernias are less commonly encountered compared to umbilical hernias, but they can occur together. The diagnosis of an inguinal hernia is made on physical examination. During the initial veterinary visit, there should be a careful palpation of the inguinal rings in puppies, since differentiation between inguinal fat and an inguinal hernia can be challenging.

If the inguinal mass is large or painful, additional diagnostic imaging would be appropriate to determine the contents of the hernia. Radiographs can frequently identify intestines, urinary bladder, and other viscera. Ultrasound can help determine the viability of the contents by assessing the blood flow to the various structures. Advanced imaging is seldom required, but there may be utility in some clinical situations, like a traumatic inguinal hernia with concurrent injuries.

Surgical Procedure – Inguinal Herniorrhaphy

Inguinal hernias are frequently bilateral – even if there is only active herniation on one side. The author prefers a ventral midline incision extending from the umbilicus to the pubic brim, allowing for bilateral inspection and closure of each inguinal ring. After the initial incision, the skin, subcutaneous tissues, and any mammary tissue are dissected free from the rectus fascia and retracted to expose the inguinal ring. A Gelpi or a ring retractor is useful for improved visualization when performing the procedure, especially if surgical assistance is not available. General anesthesia and the manipulations associated with surgical preparation may have reduced the herniated contents by the time the approach was made. Careful palpation will locate the inguinal hernia and determine the extent of hernia contents (Figure 30.3).

Dissection of the inguinal hernia sac can be challenging, as there are frequent adhesions between the peritoneal lining of the hernia sac and the subcutaneous fat and surrounding fascia. Delicate dissection is needed to free the sac and prevent iatrogenic injury to the herniated tissues. During dissection, the hernia sac may inadvertently be opened. This is not a major issue unless the herniated tissues within the sac are damaged.

Once the hernia sac is freed from the surrounding tissues, it is opened, and its contents are reduced back into the abdominal cavity. Since the hernia sac is frequently large, the excessive tissue is resected and ligated or sutured closed. Next, the diameter of the inguinal ring is reduced (but not completely closed) to minimize the potential for future herniation. Alternatively, when the hernia contents are easily reducible, the hernia contents can be gently pushed back into the abdominal cavity without opening the sac. The empty hernia sac is then reduced, and the herniorrhaphy is finished.

For more complex inguinal hernias, such as those with incarcerated or strangulated abdominal organs, it is preferable to extend the midline incision into the abdominal cavity as a component of the herniorrhaphy. If a non-complicated hernia is being repaired as part of an ovariohysterectomy, a celiotomy is already done but may not be a necessary part of the herniorrhaphy procedure. When performing a celiotomy, a Balfour self-retaining retractor will hold the midline incision open. The body wall can be further retracted with a towel clamp or a Green hand-held retractor to allow the

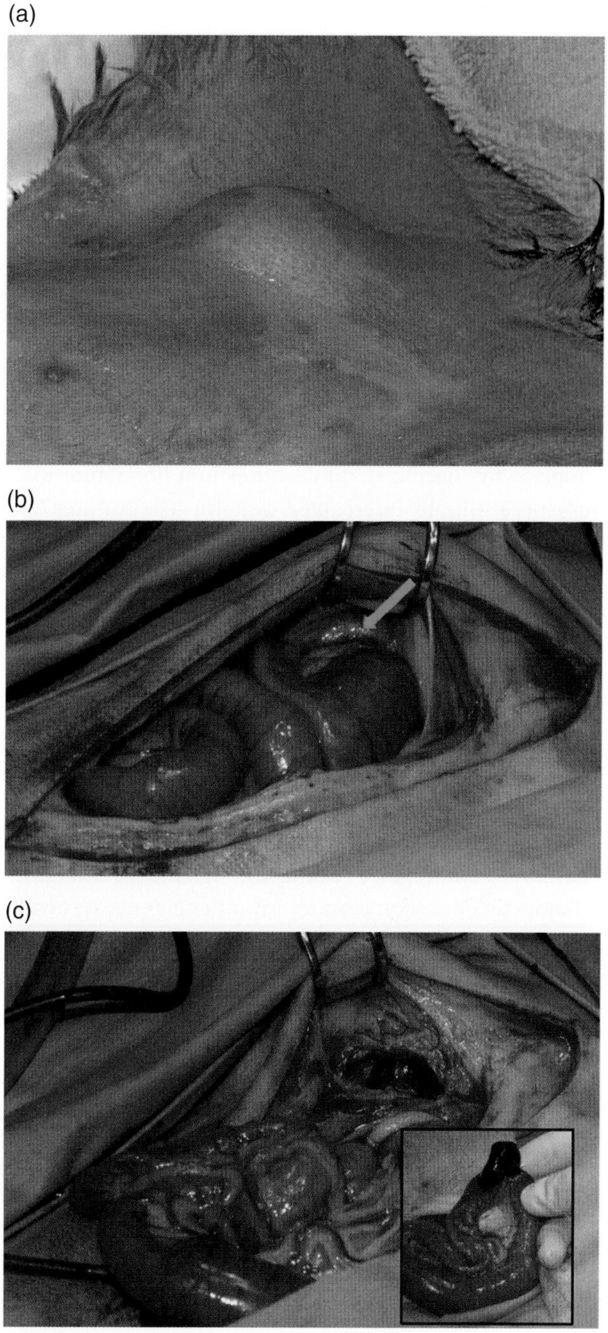

Figure 30.3 Female canine with a left inguinal hernia. Cranial is to the left in the images. (a) Left inguinal hernia that has become painful and non-reducible. (b) A midline incision was made, and obstructed intestines were identified. The intestinal obstruction could be followed to the left inguinal ring (green arrow). (c) The left inguinal hernia is exposed by dissection around the external ring. A dark tissue mass was identified. The boundaries of the inguinal ring were identified, and the abnormal tissue was dissected free. Insert: By enlarging the inguinal ring, the herniated tissue was able to be reduced into the abdominal cavity, where an intestinal resection and anastomosis were then required for the ischemic segment of the bowel.

surgeon to view the inguinal ring from the abdominal cavity. When the herniated content cannot be reduced easily, the inguinal ring should be enlarged by incising the cranial aspect of the ring until the hernia contents are reduced.

Once the contents have been reduced, hernia closure is performed. Due to the passage of the external pudendal vessels and the genital nerve through the inguinal ring, inguinal hernias are not completely closed; rather, the goal is to reduce the hernia diameter to prevent future herniation while allowing for the passage of the pudendal vessels and genital nerve.

To accomplish the closure, the inguinal borders need to be identified. If the dissection of the hernia sac was appropriate, the borders should be evident. The author prefers to pre-place the herniorrhaphy sutures in a horizontal mattress or a simple interrupted pattern. The sutures are tagged, and the effectiveness and security of the closure can be evaluated before the sutures are tied. The other advantage of pre-placing the sutures is it allows for all the sutures to be in place before the hernia ring is reduced, minimizing the blind passage of the suture needle for the final sutures. Both non-absorbable (e.g., polypropylene) and long-term absorbable (e.g., polydioxanone) sutures have been recommended, although the author prefers non-absorbable suture for this procedure.[3,8] Leaving a 5–10 mm defect at the caudal aspect is typically more than adequate for the vessels and nerves exiting through the inguinal ring.

Before final incision closure, any other planned or necessary procedures should be completed. The dissected subcutaneous tissues are sutured using a tacking pattern to reduce postoperative seroma formation, and the skin can be apposed using skin sutures or an intradermal pattern.

Postoperative Management

Postoperative management includes pain management and incision care. Limited activity is enforced for 10–14 days to allow for wound healing. It is a good idea to encourage owners to continue to check the surgical site for recurrence, although the likelihood of such should be very small.

Diaphragmatic Hernia

Types of Hernias

There are two classifications of diaphragmatic hernias (DHs): traumatic DHs and congenital DHs. In veterinary medicine, the most common congenital DH is the peritoneopericardial DH (PPDH). The traumatic DHs typically occur as the result of a rupture or tear in some portion of the muscular diaphragm secondary to blunt force trauma, and these can be referred to as pleuroperitoneal DHs. While pleuroperitoneal DH is a surgical condition, retrospective studies have reported that dogs and cats diagnosed with a non-clinical PPDH can be managed with either surgery or conservative management.[13–15] Approximately 50% of dogs and cats with PPDH are discovered as an incidental finding. In one report, a diagnosis of PPDH and the presence of clinical signs associated with displacement of the GI tract into the pericardial space, were factors that led to the recommendation of surgical correction.[15] In another report, presenting complaints were associated with respiratory or GI signs.[14] The reported mortality rate for dogs and cats undergoing PPDH repair is between 5% and 14%, and no significant difference was reported between animals treated with surgery and those managed without surgery.[13–15] The discussion in this chapter will be centered on the traumatic pleuroperitoneal DH, since many of the principles can be applied to the animal with a PPDH.

Etiology

The classic explanation for the creation of a traumatic DH comprises three actions that must occur at roughly the same moment in time. First, there needs to be an acute increase in abdominal pressure, such as the blunt force trauma of being hit by a vehicle. The second is the presence of an open glottis, which allows for air within the respiratory tract and lungs to be forced out of the thorax.[16] This results in a lack of counter-pressure to the increased abdominal pressure. The final component is the tearing of the diaphragm, which radiates parallel to the fibers of the muscular component portion or tearing and avulsing of the circumferential edge of the diaphragm away from the body wall. At this point, the hernia permits abdominal viscera to move through the hernia into the thoracic cavity, along with a reduction or equalization of the subatmospheric pressure within the thoracic cavity.

Anatomy

The diaphragm is the sheet of muscle and tendon that separates the thoracic cavity from the abdominal cavity. Contraction of the muscles of the diaphragm expands the thoracic cavity, helping to create the subatmospheric pressure that draws air into the respiratory system. Thus, respiratory function can be compromised by effectively reducing thoracic expansion, which occurs due to the loss of diaphragmatic integrity and due to the reduction in available space for pulmonary expansion with the presence of abdominal viscera in the thorax. The movement of abdominal visceral structures from the abdominal cavity into the thoracic cavity can also cause various degrees of vascular compromise to the displaced organs, resulting in organomegaly and potential ischemic tissue damage.

The three muscular portions of the diaphragm, the pars costalis, the pars sternalis, and the pars lumbalis, arise from the body wall, and the muscle fibers run centrally to attach to the central tendinous portion of the diaphragm. There are three apertures in the diaphragm with a different number of structures crossing through each, which increase in number ventral to dorsal: one through the caval foramen, two through the esophageal hiatus, and three through the aortic hiatus. The paired pars lumbalis forms the aortic hiatus, denoting the site of passage for the aorta, the azygous veins, and the cisternal portion of the thoracic duct. The esophagus hiatus is located at the ventral aspect of the pars lumbalis where the muscles attach to the central tendon, allowing the esophagus and the paired vagal nerves to pass. A slit in the central tendon, the caval foramen, allows the caudal vena cava to traverse the diaphragm and enter into the thoracic cavity.[12]

The right and left pars costalis muscles arise from the 13th rib dorsally and run cranially to the costochondral junction of the 8th or 9th ribs. The muscle fibers run inward toward the central tendon. Dorsally, the pars costalis joins the pars lumbalis. Ventrally, the pars costalis attaches to the sternum and transitions to be called the pars sternalis. Tears in the diaphragm occur at weak points, intramuscular tears, or avulsions of the pars costalis from its lateral or ventral attachments. Dorsal defects associated with the pars lumbalis are occasionally encountered.

Presentation

Animals with a traumatic diaphragmatic hernia can present anywhere along a scale from displaying no significant problems on presentation to being in severe respiratory distress.[16,17] Acutely traumatized pets may display cyanosis, tachypnea, other respiratory difficulties, concurrent bruising, and even a lack of respiratory noises on thoracic auscultation. These patients may or may not have concurrent polytrauma and orthopedic injuries, which are commonly encountered in pets with traumatic DH. Cardiac arrhythmias can also be seen in these patients.[18] Many patients will need to receive treatment for concurrent injuries, the treatment of which can be dramatically impacted if the patient also has an undiagnosed DH. This stresses the need to have DH on the differential list for any animal that has experienced trauma and obtain thoracic radiographs early in the diagnostic and treatment-planning stage. Misjudging an orthopneic patient with a DH for a painful or aggressive patient can have severe patient consequences. Heavy sedation or anesthesia can take a patient that is compensating and oxygenating normally with a traumatic DH and create a life-threatening situation of cyanosis and dyspnea, potentially leading to death. This is a major reason why when dealing with traumatized animals or those with known DH that might appear stable, the clinician needs to be prepared to rapidly intervene and gain control of the airway should a patient begin to decompensate.

Some animals with DH may appear to be "within normal limits" on their physical examination with minimal clinical signs. However, these same patients may quickly develop respiratory distress if restrained, stressed, or placed in lateral recumbency for diagnostics or treatment. Historical questioning may reveal a patient with decreased activity or reduced exercise tolerance, increased heat intolerance, or signs of positional orthopnea, and a complete history must always include questions about any previous traumatic episodes, periods outside without direct supervision, or clarification of when and how the pet came to be with the owner. It is not uncommon for a pet to have a DH of unknown duration with a history of previous trauma or being found and adopted by the new owner, frequently after seeming to have undergone some traumatic event. In these patients, the DH may be found as a part of routine diagnostics for other reasons, such as investigation of coughing, presentation for exercise intolerance, through routine thoracic imaging for older patients, or even through abdominal imaging for non-respiratory abnormalities, such as elevated liver enzymes.

Other clinical signs associated with a traumatic DH may be the result of entrapment of abdominal viscera within the thoracic cavity. The abnormal location can, through various mechanisms, result in organomegaly. This creates a "space-occupying lesion" within the thoracic cavity that can limit pulmonary expansion and, depending on the size and chronicity of the organomegaly, may cause respiratory compromise. A herniated stomach can distend with eating, resulting in mild to moderate respiratory signs, or the patient can develop gastric distention that can cause significant respiratory distress until the gastric distention is relieved. The spleen can engorge and contract within the thoracic cavity. Venous outflow compromise can result in splenomegaly, creating another type of space-occupying lesion within the thoracic cavity. Liver lobes can be compromised after being displaced through a traumatic hernia, resulting in persistently elevated liver enzymes, liver congestion, and fibrosis of the affected lobe. Rarely, a herniated liver lobe may undergo torsion. Like the spleen, liver lobes traversing a DH can develop venous congestion and start to weep a transudative fluid that can result in significant pulmonary effusion. These animals may be treated or referred for pleural effusion while the DH remains hidden, undetected due to the obscuring fluid within the pleural space. Effective removal of any pleural fluid may expose the DH, or the veterinarian may need to use other imaging modalities, such as ultrasound or computed tomography (CT) scans, to identify a DH as the underlying cause of the fluid.

Diagnosis/Diagnostics

Thoracic radiographs remain the mainstay of diagnosing a DH in dogs and cats. It is recommended for any pet that has undergone substantial trauma to have thoracic radiographs taken to assess for pulmonary lesions, pneumothorax, diaphragmatic hernia, or other abnormalities (Figure 30.4). While a DH can commonly be identified on thoracic radiographs, some cases can require additional imaging. Contrast studies, ultrasound, and CT scan may be helpful in clarifying the presence (or absence) of a DH in animals with obscuring structures or pleural effusions associated with a

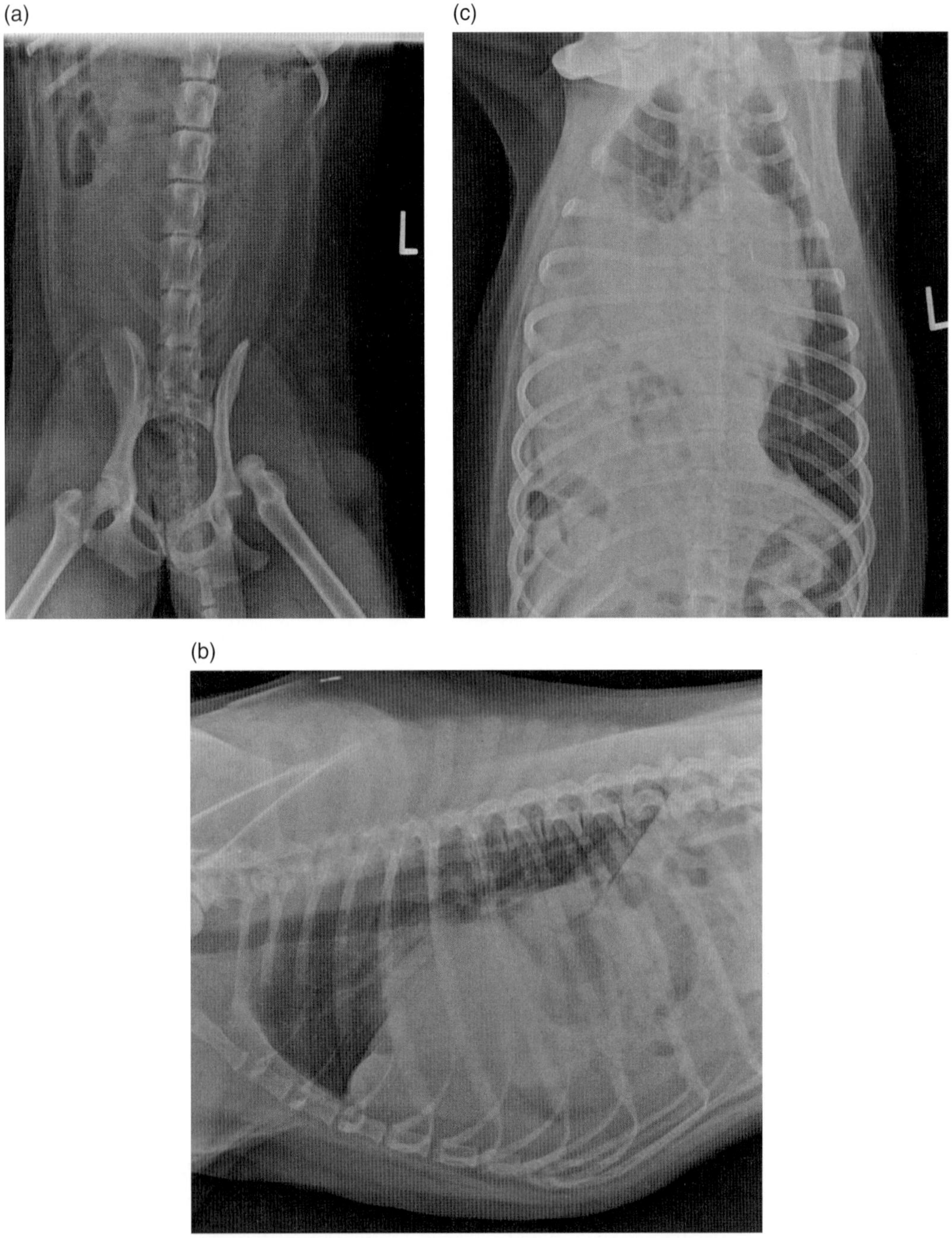

Figure 30.4 (a) A ventrodorsal pelvic radiograph of a dog with a history of being hit by a car and demonstrating a non-weight-bearing lameness of the left rear leg. Craniodorsal hip luxation is easily identifiable. It is recommended that pets with a history of traumatic injury have a thoracic radiograph to evaluate the thoracic cavity. (b,c) Lateral and ventrodorsal thoracic films were routinely obtained in this patient. Increased soft tissue opacity was noted in the caudal thorax that obscured the cardiac silhouette and the diaphragm. The presence of gas within intestinal segments confirmed the presence of GI tract segments through a diaphragmatic hernia.

DH.[19] Given that animals with DH have mild to severe respiratory impairment and can acutely decompensate, the attending clinician must be prepared to modify diagnostic procedures or intervene with respiratory support.

Surgical Procedure – Traumatic Diaphragmatic Herniorrhaphy

Anesthesia Considerations

There are a few specific challenges associated with anesthesia for the repair of a DH. Those include management of the fragile respiratory patient, pre-emptive set-up for anesthesia, and planning for ventilatory support during the procedure. Specific details and dosages for anesthesia drugs and protocols to be used in a patient with a DH are available elsewhere.[17,20]

When dealing with fragile respiratory patients, the mindset of the veterinarian and their team needs to shift to the specific needs of this type of patient. This is not a patient that can be premedicated, placed in a holding cage to "chill" while getting the rest of the anesthetic equipment together, and checking the anesthesia machine. Too often, the stable DH patient quickly destabilizes after sedation, necessitating a rapid response to ensure the patient is receiving adequate oxygen. Anticipating this possibility minimizes the impact of a patient crisis prior to induction. When planning for a DH patient's sedation or anesthetic event, all drugs and equipment needed for anesthesia induction, endotracheal intubation, and ventilation need to be in place and ready to use prior to any premedication. Ideally, the patient will already have IV access, otherwise, intravenous catheterization should be performed with as little stress as possible. The anesthesia and surgical team should have drugs drawn, endotracheal tubes, laryngoscopes, and other materials needed for intubation set out, and an anesthetic machine that is set up for manual, positive pressure ventilation. Alternatively, a mechanical ventilation unit should be immediately available. The team needs to have a trained, dedicated individual to manage ventilation if manual ventilation is needed. Once a DH patient is intubated, the anesthesia team can take control of patient ventilation and is able to manage respiratory challenges moving forward.

It is important that the primary plan (and backup plan) for ventilatory management be worked out and practiced before beginning to premedicate the DH patient. The team should be familiar with using manual ventilation, frequency of ventilations, airway pressures to be generated, and management of the pop-off valves and oxygen flush valve (don't use!). Other equipment, such as the necessary rebreathing bags and the appropriate anesthetic tubing, must be readily available. These items may not seem difficult to obtain, but the protocol for management needs to be clear; if there is an emergent situation, there should be a smooth response. The discussion of ventilatory management includes the potential for previous pulmonary trauma, which may lead to pneumothorax, the patient's potential to develop re-expansion pulmonary edema, especially with chronic hernias, and the plans for anesthesia recovery and postoperative oxygen support.

Before anesthesia, care is taken to avoid placing the patient into positions that cause additional respiratory distress or anxiety. This may include trying to preoxygenate the patient. For some patients, the face mask and associated restraint can cause them to become anxious and dyspneic. Careful patient selection is important when using this technique. Later, the anesthesia and surgical team must consider patient positioning while prepping, moving, and positioning the DH patient on the surgery table. Any position that could result in increased visceral pressure on the diaphragm or encourage additional viscera to move through the hernia into the thoracic cavity should be minimized or avoided. Once induced, the head and thorax are ideally elevated above the level of the abdomen by positioning the patient on an incline, which may be done by use of a tilt table or mat placed under the cranial aspect of the patient. Patients with gastric distention from food or water, inadvertent esophageal intubation, or aerophagia before induction will benefit from the passage of an orogastric tube to relieve gastric distention after induction and intubation. Using the tilt function on the surgery table to elevate the patient's head and thorax from induction, through clipping and prepping the abdomen and thorax, and until the procedure begins is helpful. Final positioning of the patient should only be done when the surgical team is ready to begin.

Surgical Preparation

The surgical preparation needs to be done in a timely and concise manner. It must include the potential for a more extensive procedure than planned and address any supplemental instrumentation (e.g., chest tube) that might be required. Patient clipping is started prior to anesthetic induction if the patient will tolerate it. Do not create additional patient excitement or anxiety to accomplish this goal, and avoid using excessive manual restraint. If pre-induction clipping is not tolerated by the patient, be ready to begin clipping immediately after induction. The goal is to minimize the time between induction and the start of surgery. The clipped area should begin over the sternum continuing caudally to the pubis. The more complex the DH is expected to be, the more cranial the sternum should be clipped and prepped. This allows the surgeon to extend the midline incision to include a partial or complete median sternotomy should it be required for the breakdown of adhesions or the resection of damaged tissues. If the surgeon's preference is for a postoperative chest tube, the thoracic clip is extended laterally to accommodate that preference. The surgical prep is completed in accordance with the standard preparation protocols of the practice. The patient is draped, and the procedure begins.

Abdominal Approach/Hernia Reduction

A standard ventral midline incision from the xiphoid process extending 2/3 of the distance to the pubis is begun. The linea is exposed, and the body wall incision is completed. It is important to remember that once the abdominal cavity is opened, patient ventilation using a positive pressure ventilatory technique must be initiated if not already started. The surgeon needs to communicate this with the anesthesia team. Electrocautery is used to control subcutaneous hemorrhage and to assist with the removal of the falciform ligament. The incision is covered with moistened laparotomy sponges, and a Balfour retractor is placed for visualization.

In an acute DH, the surgeon should perform a brief, complete abdominal exploratory (Figure 30.5). The timing of the exploratory is at surgeon's discretion. For some surgeons, the presence of free fluid/blood within the abdominal and thoracic cavities prompts the exploratory prior to the management of the DH. Other surgeons prefer to manage the DH first and then reassess the abdominal organs, including those removed from the thoracic cavity, immediately prior to closure. Either option is reasonable, as long as the exploratory is performed at some point.

The Balfour spoon or other hand-held retractor is useful to ventrally retract the xiphoid at the cranial aspect of the abdominal incision (Figure 30.6). This upward retraction will better expose the abdominal surface of the diaphragm, allowing for the identification of the diaphragmatic defect. Often, the diaphragmatic defect is occluded by omentum and mesentery from the herniated organs.

Reducing the herniated viscera can be challenging. Two concerns that a reduction in the original size of the diaphragmatic tear could have occurred and that the presence of adhesions to the herniated organs may be present should be foremost in the mind of the surgeon as they are thinking through the process of reducing the herniated organs. The size disparity between the existing hernia defect and the herniated organs can be challenging and intimidating. The size disparity occurs after organ herniation: a small spleen may slip through a diaphragmatic hernia, become engorged, and now, cannot be reduced back through the original defect. Similarly, the stomach and proximal small intestines could herniate into the thorax and become distended by residual gastrointestinal content, GI distention, or, in one recent patient in the author's clinic, a gastric foreign body that leads to the identification of a previously unknown DH.

In these situations, the first step to closing the diaphragmatic defect is to make it larger! This means that the

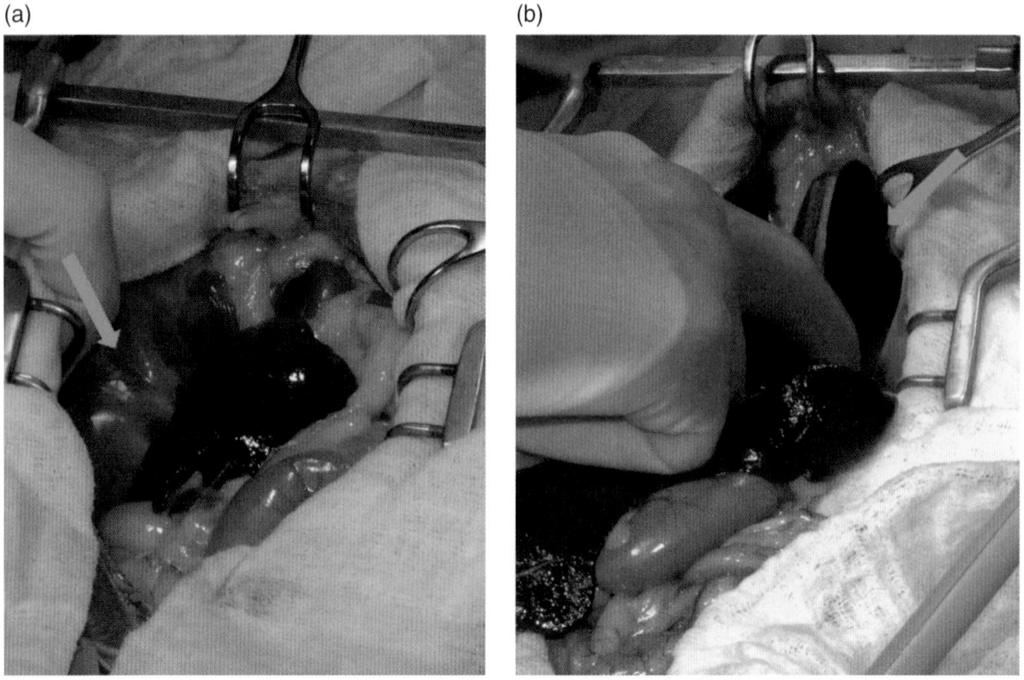

Figure 30.5 Cat with diaphragmatic hernia. Cranial is at the top in the images. (a) A feline diaphragmatic hernia upon opening the abdominal cavity. Note the bulging of the diaphragm on the right side (green arrow) from the displaced viscera. Note the abnormal position of the gall bladder and the absence of the spleen and the jejunum. (b) The abdominal viscera has been reduced, and the diaphragmatic hernia is visible (green arrow).

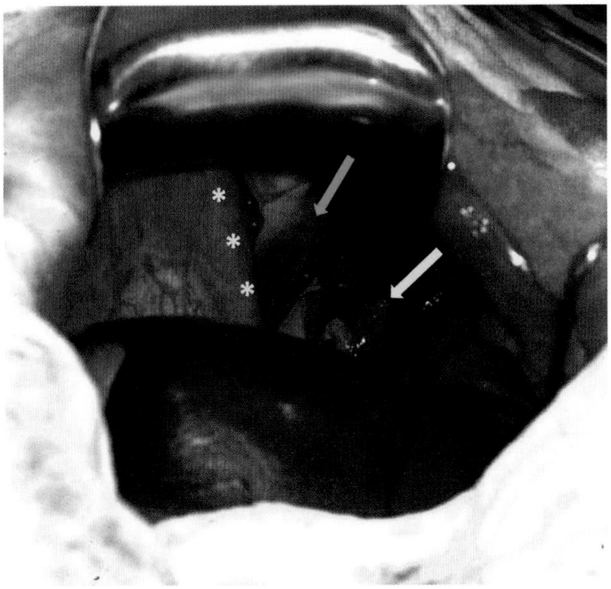

Figure 30.6 The appearance of a large combined (radial and circumferential) tear on the left side. The spoon from the Balfour abdominal retractor is being used to ventrally retract the body wall for better visualization. The central edge of the diaphragm is identifiable (yellow asterisks). Herniated viscera have been reduced back into the abdominal cavity and protected by moistened laparotomy sponges while the herniorrhaphy is performed. The heart and pericardium (green arrow) and some slowly re-inflating, atelectatic lung (yellow arrow) can be seen through the hernia.

diaphragmatic tear needs to be incised at either end to make the defect's diameter longer, allowing the surgeon to reduce the herniated organs back into the abdominal cavity. Attempting to reduce herniated, often friable, organs through a smaller defect can result in significant tissue damage and hemorrhage and prolong the surgical procedure. Enlarging the defect makes reduction much more straightforward. When enlarging the diaphragmatic tear, care must be taken to avoid inadvertent damage to major vessels or delicate tissues herniated through the defect. When possible, the extended diaphragmatic incision should parallel the muscle fibers to minimize additional tissue trauma when lengthening the defect. Some bleeding is expected, but it can be easily controlled with electrocautery. Once the incised tissue enlarges the hernia adequately, the previously herniated viscera can safely be returned to the abdominal cavity. After the viscera are returned to the abdominal cavity, they should be closely inspected for injuries that would necessitate repair or resection.

Adhesions between the herniated abdominal tissues and tissues within the thoracic cavity are another factor that can make the reduction of herniated viscera challenging. In most cases, the adhesions with traumatic DH are minimal, as dogs and cats do not form adhesions as aggressively as many other species. Thus, if the herniated tissues were not damaged at the time of herniation and have not suffered tissue trauma since herniation, there is a good chance that any adhesions encountered will be easily disrupted. However, should the herniated tissues have sustained injuries creating serosal tears or other gross tissue trauma, adhesions comprised of various degrees of severity are likely to be encountered.

Once adhesions have been identified, it must be decided if those adhesions can safely be broken down through the current diaphragmatic defect by digital, blunt, or sharp dissection or whether additional exposure, such as further expanding the diaphragmatic defect or extending the incision cranially to include a caudal sternotomy, is required to safely disrupt the adhesions. When a caudal sternotomy is performed, the insertion of Gelpi retractors will spread the sternum and provide the exposure needed to address more severe adhesions.

Diaphragmatic Herniorrhaphy

Diaphragmatic tears tend to radiate from the central tendinous portion parallel to the muscle striations (radial tear) or be around the circumference of the diaphragm adjacent to the body wall (circumferential tear). Some of the more severe tears are a combination of radial and circumferential tears. For these tears, suturing the defect is made easier by identifying the intersection between the two different tears and placing an interrupted suture between the two edges to secure this point to the ventral body wall. This action converts what seemed to be a single large tear into two smaller tears that will be simpler to suture closed. Circumferential tears can be sutured to the jagged remnant of muscle along the body wall, or the sutures can encircle the adjacent rib(s) to help secure the closure.

It is not clear as to whether or not the hernia ring needs to be debrided prior to the closure of the diaphragmatic defect. Some surgeons prefer to debride the edges of the diaphragmatic defect before they close the hernia. With an acute hernia, this is probably less important and is not required; however, in a more chronic hernia, debridement of that fibrous ring should be considered. If this decision is made to debride the hernia ring, care must be taken to avoid damaging the vena cava or other structures passing through the diaphragm adjacent to the tear. A long-lasting monofilament absorbable suture (e.g., polydioxanone or polyglyconate) is generally adequate for DH closure; however, if the hernia is chronic and there is a fibrous hernia ring around the diaphragmatic tear, it may be more prudent to suture the defect closed with a non-absorbable suture material (e.g., polypropylene). Such a choice should eliminate concerns about the hernia failing to heal and subsequently re-opening in the future.

When beginning the definitive herniorrhaphy, it is best to identify the most challenging location for defect closure and concentrate on getting this area securely closed first. Typically, this would be the most dorsal aspect of the tear near the vena cava or the central tendon. The initial suture passage is placed under the best visualization available. The suture can be placed as an interrupted pattern or as the anchor of a continuous pattern. The suture tag is left long as a stay suture to permit the deeper portions of the defect to be elevated, aiding in the accurate placement of subsequent sutures. While a wide variety of suture patterns can be used, a continuous appositional suture pattern using a size-appropriate suture is the most straightforward option to close the defect. Relying on a continuous pattern is much faster and easier than tying multiple interrupted sutures; however, mixing interrupted sutures into the suture line is appropriate when needed to improve tissue apposition, when ensuring the anchor sutures of the continuous pattern are placed in solid tissue, or when closing difficult areas where a continuous pattern might be less effective. If the surgeon is not certain the initial suture bite(s) can securely anchor a continuous line, multiple interrupted sutures are the best method for beginning the closure. Once a solid anchor point can be identified, the remaining defect can be rapidly closed using a continuous pattern. When placing the deep suture(s), care is needed to avoid placing a suture through the caudal vena cava, or other vascular, nervous, or GI structures, as they pass through the apertures of the diaphragm.

Retraction and adequate visualization are essential during all phases of the herniorrhaphy but are especially critical at the start of the closure when visualization can be difficult to achieve. The use of a self-retaining retractor, such as a Balfour abdominal retractor, Gelpi perineal retractor, or a ring retractor, or the presence of a surgical assistant who can use hand-held retractors is essential to a trouble-free procedure while repairing challenging DHs. Ribbon (malleable) retractors are very helpful for retracting liver lobes or the stomach when suturing the diaphragm. It is a good idea to cover the retracted viscera with moistened laparotomy sponges and use very limited pressure to retract parenchymal organs.

When suturing a diaphragmatic defect, it can be helpful to have long instruments, especially needle holders, thumb forceps, and scissors. These can allow for better visualization by allowing the surgeon's hands to be further away from the defect and decrease the potential obstruction. The diaphragm can easily be sutured with a taper point needle, such as a SH-type needle. A larger, taper point suture needle, such as a CT needle, may make the suturing a little easier, although, it will also make it easier to puncture the expanding lungs with each needle passage. The surgeon should coordinate the passage of the suture needle through the diaphragm with the ventilatory rate for the patient when mechanical ventilation is used. If manual ventilation is being used, the surgeon can ask the anesthetist to briefly pause ventilation during suture passage. This coordination should reduce the risk of inadvertently snagging an expanding lung and tearing a hole in the lung or incorporating lung tissue into the diaphragmatic closure.

Once the herniated organs have been reduced and the diaphragmatic defect closed, the subatmospheric pressure, or "negative pressure," within the thoracic cavity needs to be reestablished. This can be accomplished with a chest tube or by transdiaphragmatic aspiration. Placement of a chest tube is routine and has the advantage of allowing continued access after surgery. Chest tube placement is ideal when there is an expectation of continued accumulation of fluid or air into the postoperative period. It is important to realize that while an air-tight closure is ideal, it is not essential for effective diaphragmatic hernia repair since the overall goal is to prevent the herniation of abdominal organs through a defect. However, if an airtight closure can be accomplished, it will make the transdiaphragmatic aspiration of air from the thoracic cavity a viable alternative.

Transdiaphragmatic aspiration can be accomplished by placing an 18-gauge, IV catheter through the repaired diaphragm. The catheter is attached to sterile extension tubing, a three-way stopcock, and a 30 or 60 mL syringe (Figure 30.7). The syringe is used to aspirate the free air until there consistent subatmospheric pressure in the thoracic cavity. This can be confirmed by the appearance of the diaphragm; it will return to its normal concave appearance, and there should not be significant bellowing of the diaphragm during inspiration (Figure 30.8). At this point, the patient should be able to ventilate on their own, and efforts to wean the patient off the manual or mechanical ventilation can begin.

If the surgeon cannot reestablish the subatmospheric pressure within the thoracic cavity, they need to assess for any large gaps in the diaphragmatic closure or other tears that were not originally identified. These issues should be addressed prior to closure. If subatmospheric pressure is still not achievable, there could be a lung parenchymal injury. The surgeon can reopen the incision and try to find the lesion or manage the leak conservatively by placing a chest tube and attaching the patient to a continuous suction unit for the postoperative period.

When performing the transdiaphragmatic aspiration, the more air that is removed, the greater the diaphragmatic motion becomes. This can result in premature removal of the catheter from the diaphragm and be a source of frustration. To minimize this problem, the catheter should be inserted immediately adjacent to the body wall at the attachment of the diaphragm. This area has minimal movement, so dislodging of the catheter should be minimized, which should allow aspiration of the thoracic cavity to be completed more efficiently.

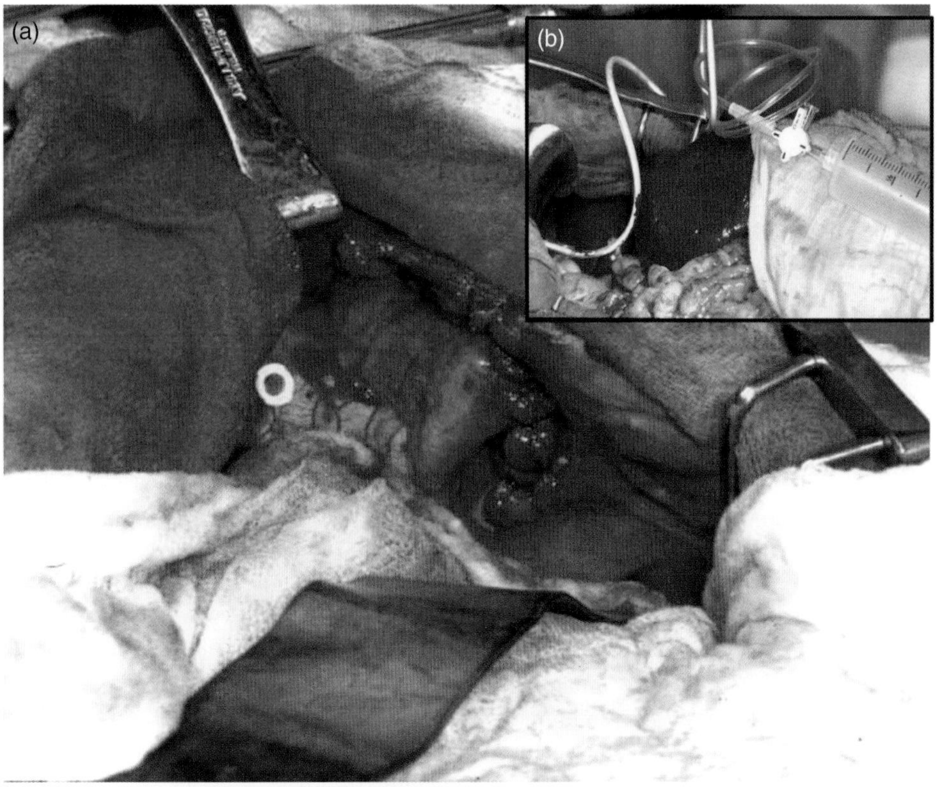

Figure 30.7 (a,b) After completing the herniorrhaphy, transdiaphragmatic thoracocentesis is performed to remove free air from within the thoracic cavity. A large bore (16- or 18-gauge) IV catheter is placed through the diaphragm, the stylet is removed, and the catheter is attached to extension tubing, a three-way stopcock, and a large syringe. Air is aspirated until the diaphragm returns to its normal conformation.

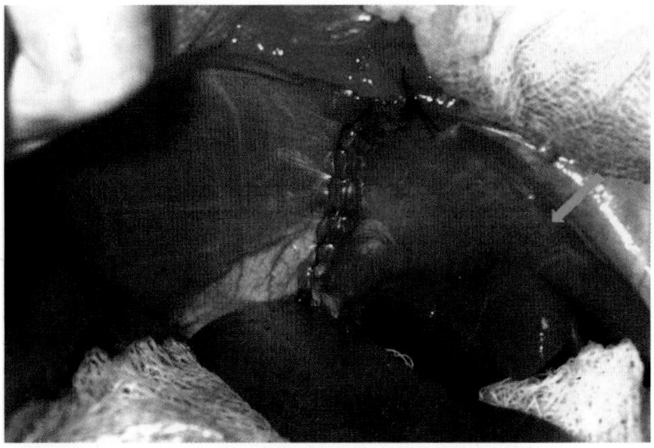

Figure 30.8 The diaphragmatic hernia has been sutured closed. A continuous, interlocking pattern with a 2-0 polydioxanone suture was used to close the radial tear that was present. The concavity of the diaphragm has been re-established, indicating that the free thoracic air has been removed (green arrow).

Another transdiaphragmatic technique is to place a fenestrated, red rubber catheter through the diaphragmatic incision immediately prior to final suture placement and closure of the defect. The catheter can then be attached to the extension set, three-way stopcock, and syringe, and air can be aspirated from the thoracic cavity as previously described. The catheter is simply pulled from the incision after the aspiration is complete, and abdominal closure is started.

Once all the residual air has been aspirated from the thoracic cavity, an abdominal exploratory is performed if not done previously, and the positioning of the reduced abdominal organs is checked to ensure no further compromise due to vascular compromise or positioning. Any concerns with the viability of the reduced organs should be addressed at this time. Once this is complete, the Balfour retractors are removed, the abdominal cavity is lavaged with warm saline to remove any blood or contamination, and the saline is aspirated. The sponge count is reconciled, and any other pre-closure activities or checklist items are completed. Routine abdominal closure in three layers follows, and the patient is taken to recovery.

When a diaphragmatic defect is too large or there has been excessive trauma to the diaphragm, the surgeon might be forced to consider alternative techniques for re-establishing the diaphragmatic separation between the abdominal and thoracic cavities. In the author's experience, this situation is extremely uncommon in dogs and cats. Despite the rarity of this need, surgeons should be aware of options in case they encounter a DH that can't be closed primarily. The most common technique mentioned for re-creating the diaphragmatic separation is the incorporation of a non-absorbable polypropylene mesh material (Prolene Mesh; Ethicon, North Brunswick, NJ) to create the separation. Perforated silicone sheets have been reported as a diaphragmatic substitute to allow drainage from the thoracic cavity into the abdominal cavity. As such, they might make a suitable diaphragmatic replacement for a hernia that cannot otherwise be closed. Omental flaps have been reported for diaphragmatic closure, but the omentum lacks any significant strength, making these flaps more appropriate as a supporting structure for other techniques. Surgeons using polypropylene mesh often choose to cover it with omentum in an effort to minimize adhesions to the mesh. Muscle flaps, created from the transversus abdominus, the rectus abdominis, and the latissimus dorsi, have been reported.[3,16]

Advancement of the diaphragmatic attachment may allow for the primary closure of a large DH. The use of autologous fascial tissues, harvested from the fascia lata and thoracolumbar fascia, has been reported to be useful for abdominal wall hernias and might be useful for diaphragmatic repair. However, the harvest of these tissues would need to occur prior to the approach for DH repair, making them less useful for spur-of-the-moment needs compared to off-the-shelf options. The author has harvested pericardial tissue to successfully close a large peritoneopericardial defect in a juvenile llama.

Postoperative Management

Supplemental oxygen may be appropriate after DH surgery. Smaller animals can be placed in an oxygen cage/tent, while larger dogs may do better with the placement of a single or double nasal cannula. The author does not use oxygen in all cases but frequently places the nasal cannulas prior to recovery, so they are in place if the patient is poorly ventilating after discontinuation of anesthesia.

Post-surgical radiographs should be obtained to document the repair prior to discharge (Figure 30.9). Some prefer to obtain films immediately after surgery. This can help document the severity of any atelectasis or residual air in the pleural space, but these factors may also reduce the diagnostic quality of the films.

Other postoperative management is routine, including incision care with daily monitoring for signs of infection or inflammation. Pain management can be achieved using a combination of short-term opioids and longer-term nonsteroidal anti-inflammatory drugs (NSAIDs). Activity is typically restricted for 10–14 days. Recheck evaluations are performed at the discretion of the clinician. As a surgeon at a referral institution, the author frequently has rechecks performed by the primary care veterinarian of the referring hospital and works with them to manage any concerns about the patient.

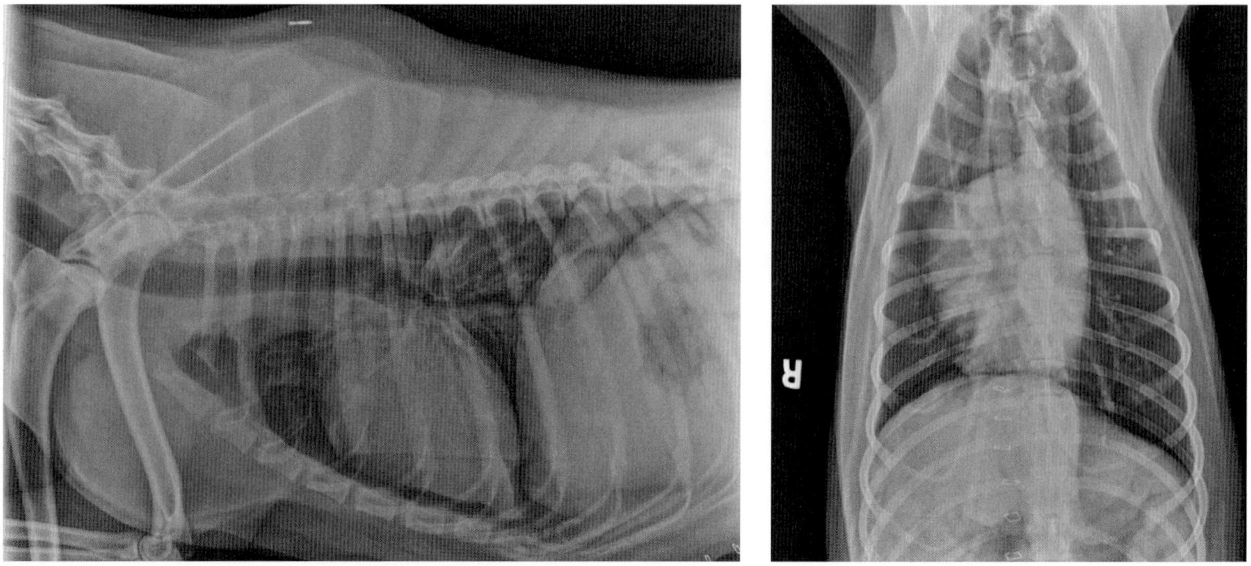

Figure 30.9 Lateral and ventrodorsal thoracic radiographs after repair of the diaphragmatic hernia. Note the small amount of air remaining within the thorax on the lateral film. Residual air, assuming there is no accumulation and there is no negative impact on respiratory efforts, can remain and be absorbed over a period of days.

References

1 Read, R.A. and Bellenger, C.R. (2003). Hernias. In: *Textbook of Small Animal Surgery*, 3e (ed. D. Slatter), 446–448. Elsevier.

2 Smeak, D.D. (2003). Abdominal wall reconstruction and hernias. In: *Veterinary Surgery-Small Animal*, 2e (ed. S.A. Johnson and K.S. Tobias), 1564–1591. Elsevier.

3 Fossum, T.W. (2018). Surgery of abdominal cavity. In: *Small Animal Surgery*, 5e (ed. T.W. Fossum), 512–539. Mosby.

4 Robinson, R. (1977). Genetic aspects of umbilical hernia incidence in cats and dogs. *Vet. Rec.* 100 (1): 9–10. https://doi.org/10.1136/vr.100.1.9.

5 Tobias, K.M. (2017). Umbilical hernia. In: *Manual of Small Animal Soft Tissue Surgery*, 2e, 93–96. Wiley.

6 de la Vega, M., Townsend, K.L., Terry, J. et al. (2018). Urinary bladder herniation through inguinal ring in a female cat. *Can. Vet. J.* 59 (10): 1085–1088.

7 Strande, A. (1989). Inguinal hernia in dogs. *J. Small Anim. Pract.* 30: 520–521. https://doi.org/10.1111/j.1748-5827.1989.tb01626.x.

8 Tobias, K.M. (2017). Inguinal hernia. In: *Manual of Small Animal Soft Tissue Surgery*, 2e, 97–102. Wiley.

9 Itoh, T., Kojimoto, A., Kojima, K. et al. (2020). Retrospective study on clinical features and treatment outcomes of nontraumatic inguinal hernias in 41 dogs. *J. Am. Anim. Hosp. Assoc.* 56 (6): 301. https://doi.org/10.5326/JAAHA-MS-7106.

10 Charlesworth, T.M. and Moores, A.L. (2012). Post-trauma inguinal seroma formation in the cat. *J. Small Anim. Pract.* 53: 301–303. https://doi.org/10.1111/j.1748-5827.2012.01188.x.

11 Kortum, A.J. and Best, E.J. (2016). Inguinal enterocutaneous fistula in a dog. *J. Small Anim. Pract.* 57: 163–166. https://doi.org/10.1111/jsap.12395.

12 Evans, H.E. (1993). *Miller's Anatomy of the Dog*, 3e, 428. Philadelphia: WB Saunders, 514, 304–307.

13 Reimer, S.B., Kyles, A.E., Filipowicz, D.E. et al. (2004). Long-term outcome of cats treated conservatively or surgically for peritoneopericardial diaphragmatic hernia: 66 cases (1987–2002). *J. Am. Vet. Med. Assoc.* 224 (5): 728–732. https://doi.org/10.2460/javma.2004.224.728.

14 Banz, A.C. and Gottfried, S.D. (2010). Peritoneopericardial diaphragmatic hernia: a retrospective study of 31 cats and eight dogs. *J. Am. Anim. Hosp. Assoc.* 46 (6): 398–404. https://doi.org/10.5326/0460398.

15 Burns, C.G., Bergh, M.S., and McLoughlin, M.A. (2013). Surgical and nonsurgical treatment of peritoneopericardial diaphragmatic hernia in dogs and cats: 58 cases (1999-2008). *J. Am. Vet. Med. Assoc.* 242 (5): 643–650. https://doi.org/10.2460/javma.242.5.643.

16 Hunt, G.B. and Johnson, K.A. (2017). Diaphragmatic hernia. In: *Veterinary Surgery: Small Animal*, 2e (ed. S.A. Johnson and K.S. Tobias), 1592–1603. Elsevier.

17 MacPhail, C. and Fossum, T.W. (2018). Surgery of lower respiratory tract: pleural cavity and diaphragm. In: *Small Animal Surgery*, 5e (ed. T.W. Fossum), 916–956. Mosby.

18 Snyder, P.S., Cooke, K.L., Murphy, S.T. et al. (2001). Electrocardiographic findings in dogs with motor vehicle-related trauma. *J. Am. Anim. Hosp. Assoc.* 37 (1): 55–63. https://doi.org/10.5326/15473317-37-1-55.

19 Sepuya, R.G., Dozeman, E.T., Prittie, J.E. et al. (2022). Comparing diagnostic findings and cost of whole body computed tomography to traditional diagnostic imaging in polytrauma patients. *J. Vet. Emerg. Crit. Care* 32 (3): 334–340. https://doi.org/10.1111/vec.13189.

20 Brainard, B. and Hofmeister, E.H. Anesthetic practices for existing conditions. In: *Veterinary Surgery-Small Animal*, 2e (ed. S.A. Johnson and K.S. Tobias), 288–308. Elsevier.

31

Canine Scrotal Ablation and Scrotal Urethrostomy

Joey A. Sapora

Department of Clinical Sciences, Colorado State University, Fort Collins, CO, USA

Key Points

- When considering a scrotal ablation and/or scrotal urethrostomy, having an understanding of the clinical indications for these procedures is required.
- Patient positioning for scrotal ablation in dorsal recumbency with the legs splayed allows for the accurate determination of skin tension.
- Preoperative owner education is important in the event a scrotal urethrostomy is required for certain challenging cases of urethrolithiasis.
- Having a grasp on the regional anatomy during surgical dissection and closure will minimize both intraoperative and postoperative hemorrhages.
- Close attention must be paid to stoma size and location in order to optimize patient outcome.
- Owner education and strict adherence to postoperative care guidelines are prerequisites for these surgical procedures to avoid major complications.

Introduction

The canine scrotum is made up of two layers, the skin and the tunica dartos, and is a potential space divided into two compartments by a median septum. The dartos forms a lining to both halves of the scrotum and also contributes to the scrotal septum.[1] The scrotum contains the testes, the epididymides, the spermatic cords, and the cremaster muscles, which are extensions of the internal abdominal oblique muscle. The external pudendal artery is the main blood vessel that supplies the scrotum, and the veins run alongside the arteries.[1]

The male canine urethra is divided into penile and pelvic components, with the pelvic component subdivided further into preprostatic and prostatic sections.[1] The penile component begins at the ischial arch, and it is surrounded by the corpus spongiosum for its entire length.[2] The urethra at the level of the scrotum is more distensible and of larger size when compared to the prescrotal urethra, its exposure is relatively straightforward, and it is surrounded by less cavernous tissue than the urethra in the perineal region.[3] There are three main reasons why the scrotal region is recommended when performing a canine urethrostomy. First, the urethra is at its largest diameter at this location, and this same diameter is continued proximally. Second, anatomically, the urethra is most superficial at this location, providing less interference from the corpus cavernosum during surgical dissection leading to less hemorrhage. Third, the urethra is widest at this location, which provides for easier urethrocutaneous apposition.

Indications for Canine Scrotal Ablation

Scrotal ablation (SA) refers to the removal of scrotal tissue. It is a procedure that can be considered at the time of neutering in older male dogs that have a large amount of scrotal tissue. This excessive tissue may pose a risk for seroma or hematoma formation postoperatively, or its removal may simply be an aesthetic request by the owner. Common

Techniques in Small Animal Soft Tissue, Orthopedic, and Ophthalmic Surgery, First Edition. Edited by Kristin A. Coleman.

Companion website: www.wiley.com/go/coleman/surgeries

medical indications for SA include the treatment of scrotal tumors and when the tissue becomes traumatized.[4] In a 2014 study that evaluated 676 canine scrotal tumors,[5] the most common scrotal neoplasms identified included round cell neoplasms (58.6%), followed by mesenchymal neoplasms (13.6%), melanocytic neoplasms (11.8%), hamartomas (7%), epithelial neoplasms (4.3%), and cysts/tumor-like lesions (4%). Mast cell tumors accounted for 54.6% (369/676) of all scrotal tumors. Utilization of the scrotum as a full-thickness skin graft has also been reported.[6]

When a patient has pathology affecting only the scrotal skin, a complete workup is indicated. Accurate owner anamnesis may increase the suspicion of scrotal trauma. Conditions that may only affect the scrotal skin include Brucellosis, Babesiosis, contact dermatitis, *Cuterebra*, *Erysipelothrix*, frostbite, hyperandrogenism, protothecosis, Rocky Mountain spotted fever, excessive UV exposure (sunburn), and neoplasia.[7] Diagnosis should be made based on a combination of cytologic evaluation (impression smears, fine needle aspirates), serologic testing, culture and susceptibility testing, as well as histopathology. The pattern of lesions may also aid in formulating differential diagnoses.[7] When neoplasia is suspected, screening for underlying tumor metastasis is recommended in the form of aspiration of superficial inguinal lymph nodes in addition to diagnostic imaging (thoracic radiographs, abdominal ultrasound, or computed tomography). Epithelial, mesenchymal, or melanocytic tumors may arise from the scrotal skin.[7] These include squamous cell carcinoma, adenocarcinoma, fibrosarcoma, myxoma, hemangioma, hemangiosarcoma, vascular hamartoma, plasmacytoma, histiocytoma, transmissible venereal tumor, malignant melanoma, and melanocytoma, with the most common tumor affecting the canine scrotum being mast cell tumor (MCTs).[5,7,8] MCTs affecting preputial, inguinal, and subungual sites have been suggested to have a more aggressive behavior,[9] however, other studies have suggested scrotal and inguinal tumors may behave similarly to MCTs in other cutaneous locations.[10–12]

Scrotal Ablation Procedure

When performing a SA, the patient is placed in dorsal recumbency, and the scrotum and surrounding fur are clipped (Figure 31.1a,b). Care should be used when clipping the scrotum to prevent iatrogenic trauma, and plucking of the fur may be less traumatic. The pelvic limbs should be allowed to abduct naturally at the level of the hip. This allows for the skin of the scrotum and inguinal region to be placed at a point of maximal tension if the patient were to sit splay-legged. When SA is combined with a routine neuter and the testes are accessible, a testicular block using 2% lidocaine with 1 mg/kg injected into each testicle is recommended for local analgesia[13,14] (Figure 31.1c). The skin and scrotum are sterilely prepped with povidone-iodine or 4% chlorhexidine and 70% isopropyl alcohol or sterile isotonic saline.[15] The patient is then draped in a routine fashion (Figure 31.2).

For an elective castration combined with SA in a healthy patient, the base of the scrotum is marked with a sterile marking pen where the thin scrotal tissue meets the thicker inguinal tissue. A routine, pre-scrotal castration is performed pushing each respective testicle up to the apex of

(a) (b) (c)

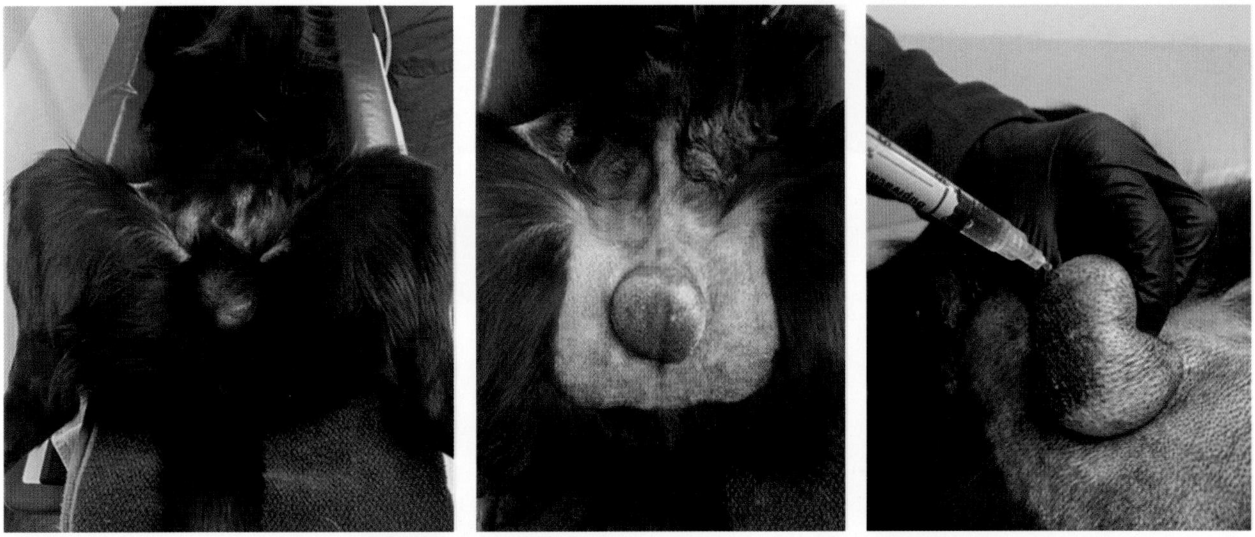

Figure 31.1 A one year old Flat-Coated Retriever presenting for elective neuter and scrotal ablation. (a) Positioning for scrotal ablation is dorsal recumbency with adequate exposure of the scrotal region; (b) amount of fur to clip for a scrotal ablation procedure; (c) testicular block with lidocaine.

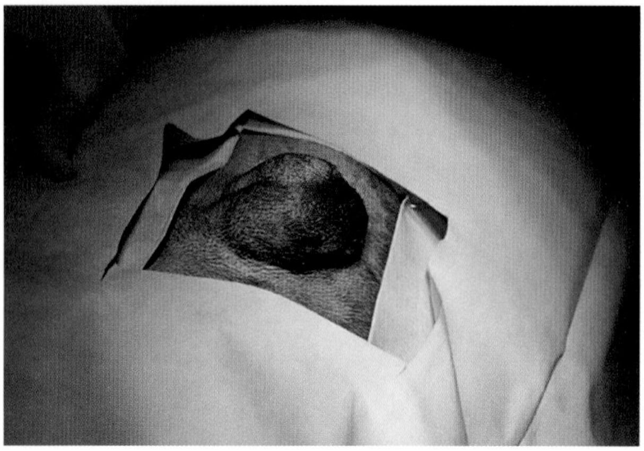

Figure 31.2 The scrotum and testes draped, and sterile field established for an elective castration and scrotal ablation procedure.

the desired SA incision. Castration prior to ablation is preferred by the author, as the vascular supply to each teste is effectively dealt with minimizing the risk of damage to the spermatic cord when later dissecting through the scrotal tissues (Figure 31.3).

Following routine castration, forceps can be placed into the right and left scrotal pouches to elevate the skin and dartos, which are to be incised along the pre-planned inked margin. This protects the underlying vascular pedicles and urethra during dissection (Figure 31.4).

Following the removal of the scrotal tissue, the underlying urethra is readily identifiable. The separate underlying fascial incisions can then be closed using an absorbable monofilament suture (Figure 31.5).

The deep subcutaneous tissue can be closed in a simple interrupted or simple continuous pattern followed by intradermal or external skin sutures (Figure 31.6a–c). The tension across the incision should be reassessed throughout the closure and at the end of the procedure with the patient undraped (Figure 31.6c). The patient is reassessed at two weeks postoperatively for appropriate tissue healing (Figure 31.7).

When severe pathology affects the scrotum in the intact patient (Figure 31.8a) or if the surgeon prefers this method for a standard SA, a more "outside-in" approach is required, as the testes are not always able to be exteriorized. The surrounding skin is inked in an elliptical shape at the point of maximal tissue resection, and the skin, subcutaneous

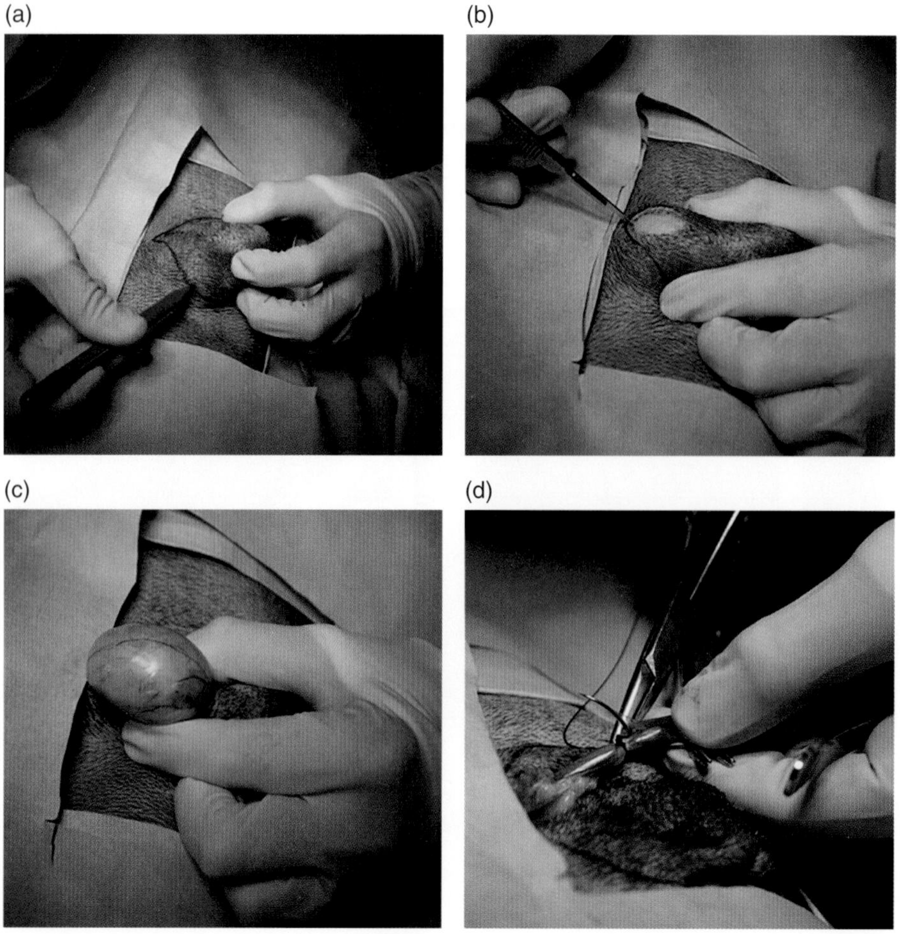

Figure 31.3 (a) Marking of the desired scrotal ablation location. (b,c) The prescrotal castration is performed by pushing the testicle to the most cranial aspect of the desired ablation incision. (d) A routine castration is performed with proximal circumferential and distal transfixation sutures on each spermatic cord.

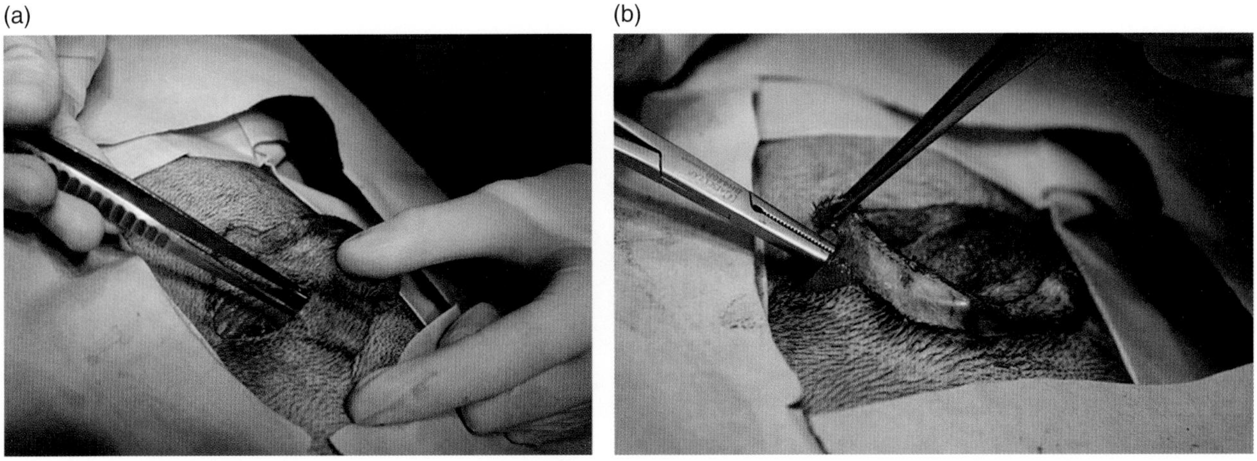

Figure 31.4 (a) Following castration, the right and left pockets of scrotal tissue are identified. (b) An instrument can be inserted into this pocket to allow for safe transection along the desired scrotal ablation incision.

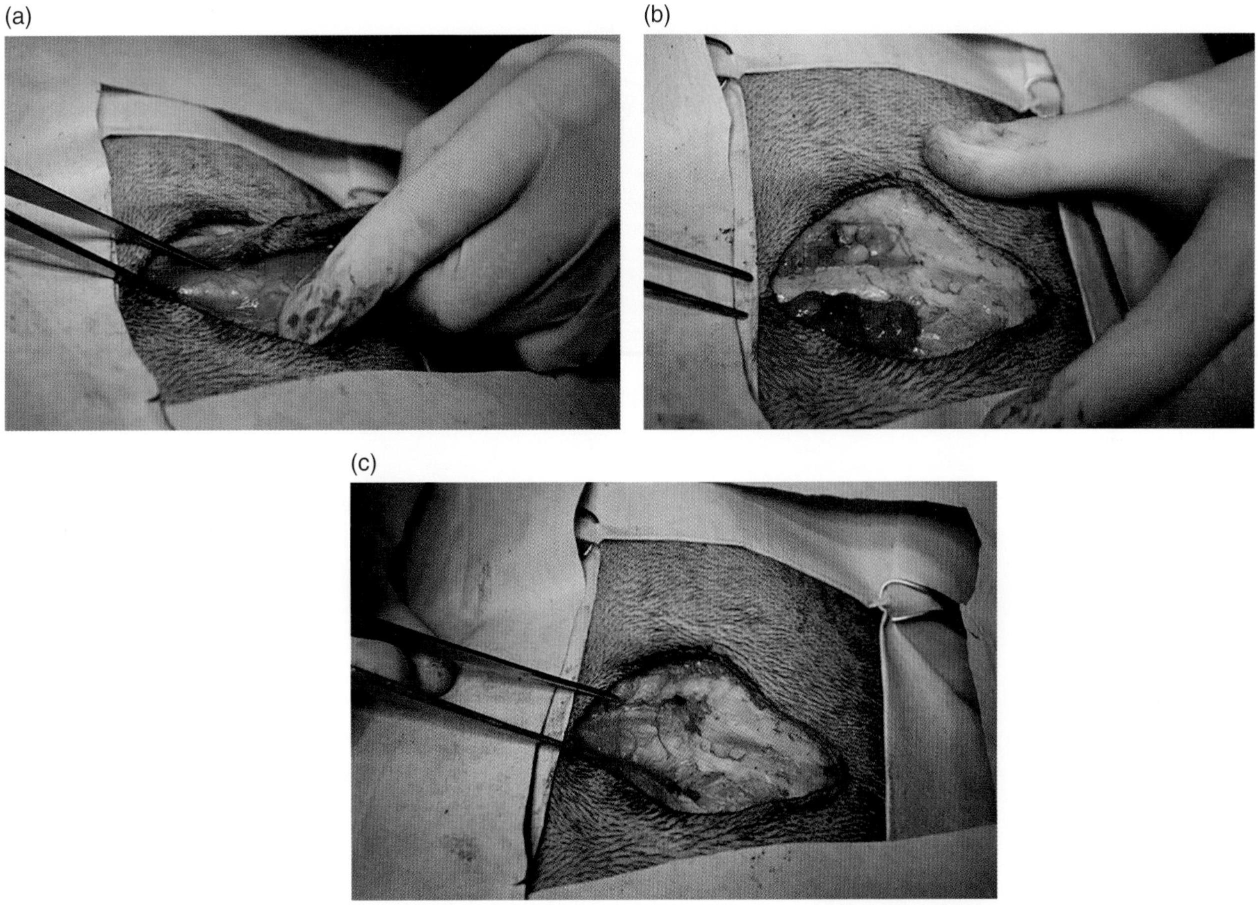

Figure 31.5 (a) Identification of the scrotal urethra. (b) The opened right and left fascial incisions. (c) Fascial incisions following closure with a simple continuous, monofilament absorbable suture.

tissues, and tunica dartos are incised (Figure 31.8b). If the patient is intact, each spermatic cord is carefully isolated, and a routine castration is performed. Identification of the spermatic cord can be challenging in the face of underlying tissue inflammation. Gentle traction on the scrotum throughout dissection and blunt dissection with right-angle forceps in parallel with the spermatic cord will aid in safe identification.

Note the degree of underlying tissue inflammation making visualization of the urethra challenging (Figure 31.8c).

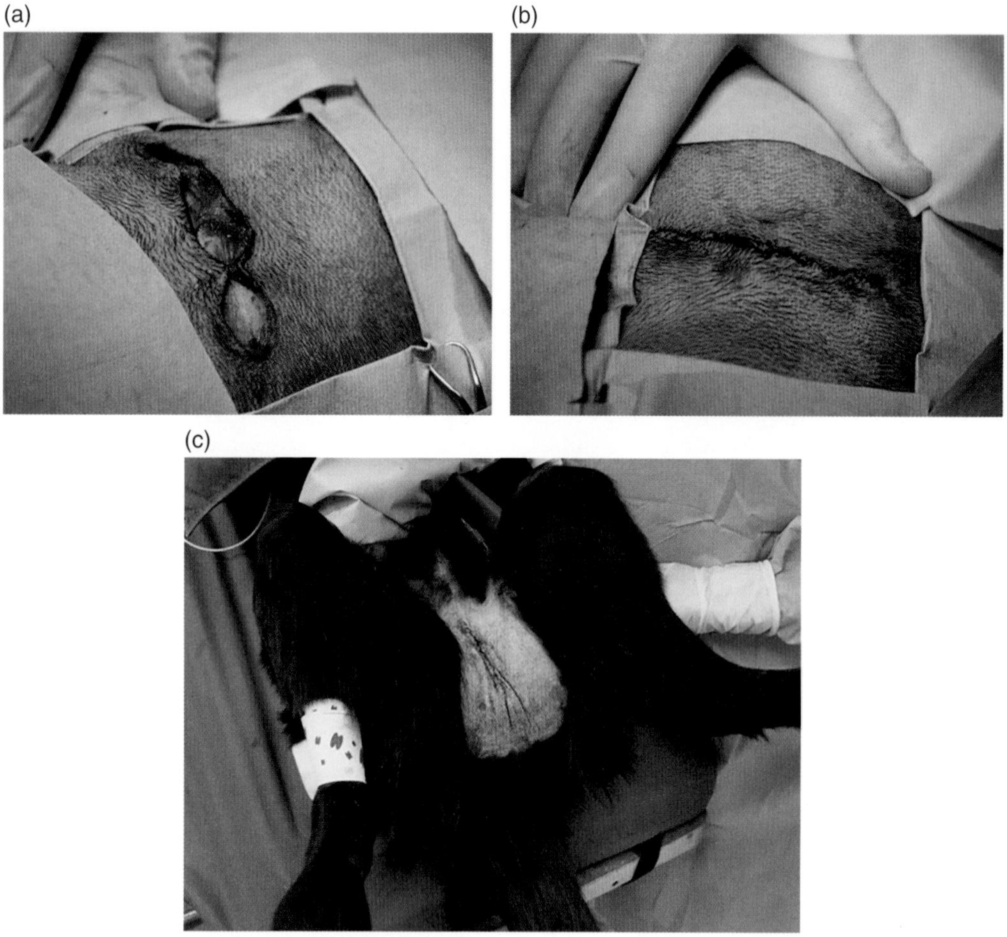

Figure 31.6 (a) Deep subcutaneous closure with buried simple interrupted, monofilament, absorbable suture. (b) Completion of an intradermal closure. (c) Assessment of incision tension following removal of surgical drapes.

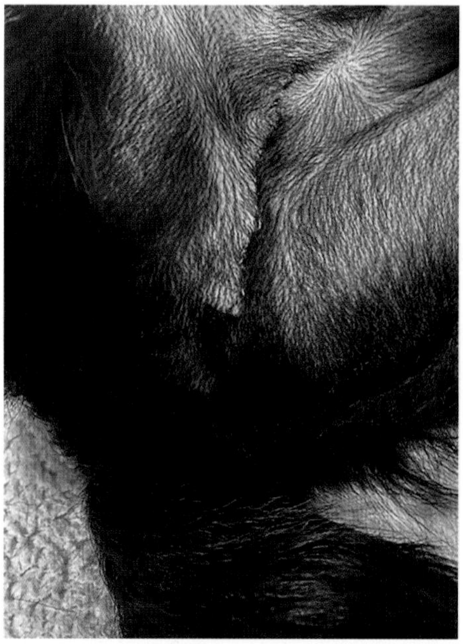

Figure 31.7 Patient two weeks postop closed castration and elective scrotal ablation.

For this reason, placement of a urinary catheter preoperatively is recommended to aid in palpation of the urethra throughout dissection. When significant subcutaneous infection is present, a closed Jackson-Pratt drain can be placed (Figures 31.8d and 31.9a).

In cases of pathology, the scrotal tissue and testicles are submitted for histopathology, and a deep tissue culture is submitted prior to closure. Similar closure is performed, taking care to not incorporate the urethra. External, tension-relieving skin sutures can be placed to reduce tension (Figure 31.9b). The patient is reassessed at two weeks postoperatively for suture removal (Figure 31.9c).

It is important to note that scrotal tumors that require wide tissue margins (i.e., MCT) of 2–3 cm and one fascial plane deep may require larger rotational skin flaps and urinary diversion to achieve complete margins. For this reason, preoperative incisional biopsies should be performed when feasible. In addition, antibiotics guided by culture and susceptibility for 7–14 days prior to the procedure may decrease inflammation and improve tissue visibility.

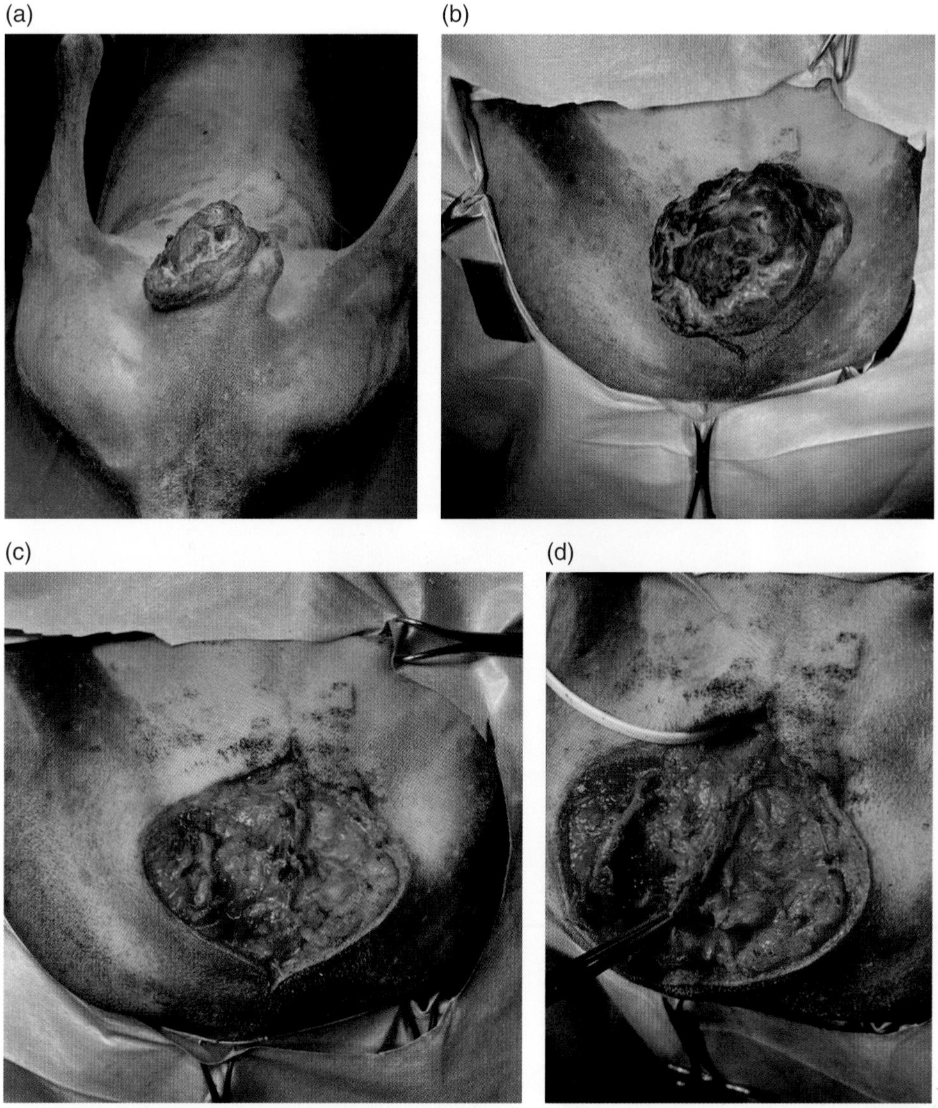

Figure 31.8 (a) Patient positioning with legs splayed. (b) Inking of the desired SA site in an elliptical shape. (c) SA site following castration. (d) The DeBakey forceps are identifying the underlying urethra, and a Jackson-Pratt drain has been placed due to deep subcutaneous abscessation with the tubing exiting to the right and craniolateral to the incision. Histopathology of the scrotal tissue revealed a narrowly excised poorly differentiated carcinoma with abscessation.

Potential Complications

Complications for SA include incisional dehiscence, superficial or deep surgical site infection, hemorrhage, urethral trauma resulting in urine extravasation or stricture, and recurrence of neoplasia.

Postoperative Care/Prognosis

Activity restriction for two to three weeks is required, in addition to an Elizabethan collar to prevent licking of the surgical site. Non-steroidal anti-inflammatories and nerve pain medication (gabapentin) for 10–14 days are recommended. Postoperative antibiotics should be reserved for patients with abscessation or infection of underlying tissues at the time of surgery, and selection should be guided by a culture and susceptibility panel. Empirical broad-spectrum antibiotics can be prescribed while awaiting culture results.

Indications for Canine Scrotal Urethrostomy

SU refers to the creation of a stoma, or permanent opening, in the urethra at the level of the scrotum to divert urine away from the pre-scrotal and penile urethra.[16]

(a) (b) (c)

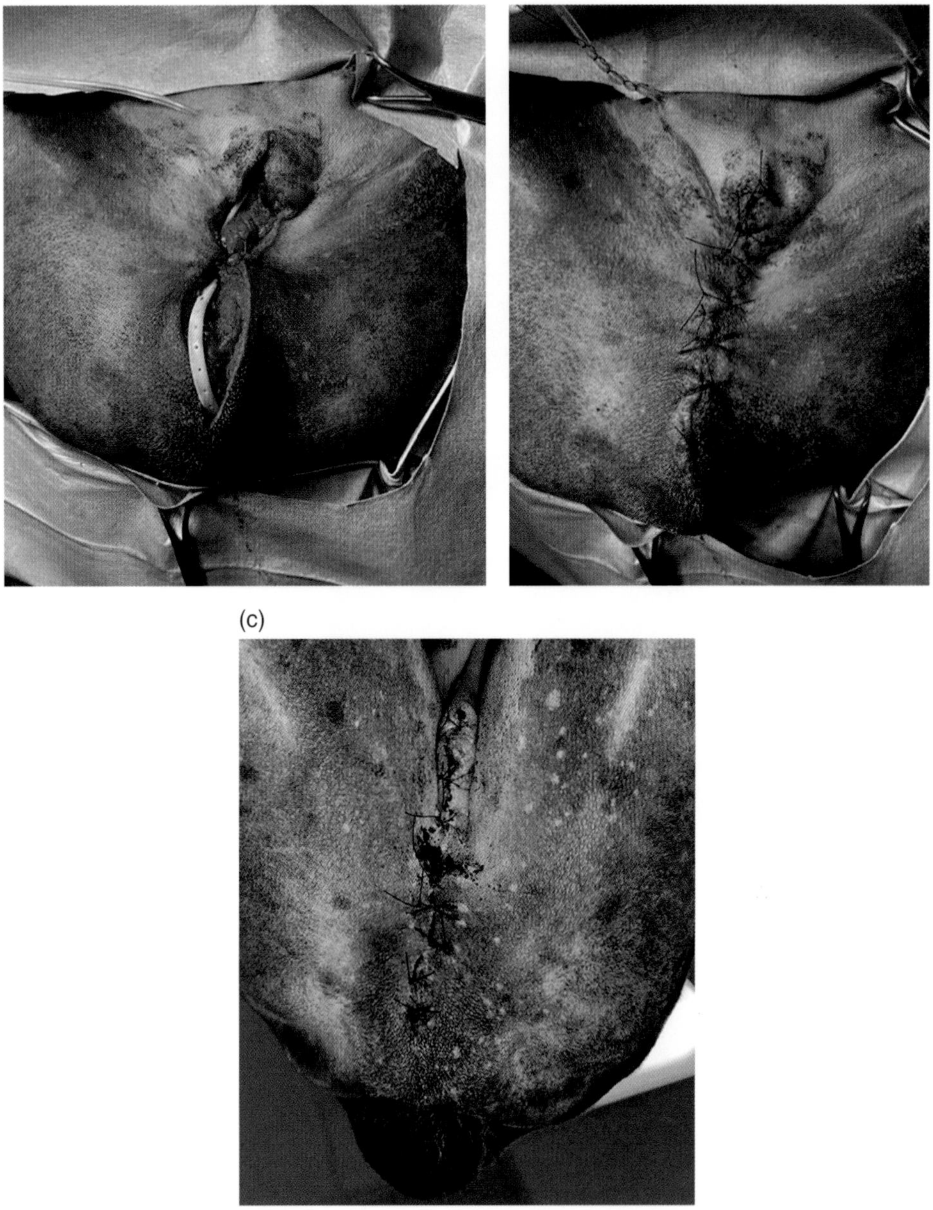

Figure 31.9 (a) Incisional closure over the Jackson-Pratt closed suction drain that was removed at three days following surgery. (b) Cruciate skin sutures placed to relieve tension across the incision site. (c) Patient at two-week postop suture removal appointment.

Indications for SU include recurrent urethral calculi unresponsive to appropriate medical therapy, obstructions in dogs that are likely to have recurrent episodes (i.e., metabolic stone-formers), severe trauma to the penile or perineal urethra, urethral strictures distal to the scrotum from trauma or previous urethral surgery, and diseases requiring amputation of the penis or prepuce including neoplasia, penile strangulation, congenital diseases such as severe hypospadias, and deficiency in penile or preputial length.[17] When related to urinary calculi, all attempts at retropulsion should be made, including *anesthetized* retrograde urohydropropulsion (Figures 31.10a, b). Prior to performing an SU, accurate localization of the urinary obstruction is required. Radiographs that should be performed include a ventrodorsal abdomen, lateral abdomen, and lateral abdomen with legs pulled cranially to better visualize the perineal and scrotal urethra (Figure 31.10c). If a stricture or radiolucent stones are suspected, a contrast cystourethrogram can be performed. The priority with preoperative imaging is to confirm that the urethral obstruction is located distal to the scrotum and that SU is appropriate.

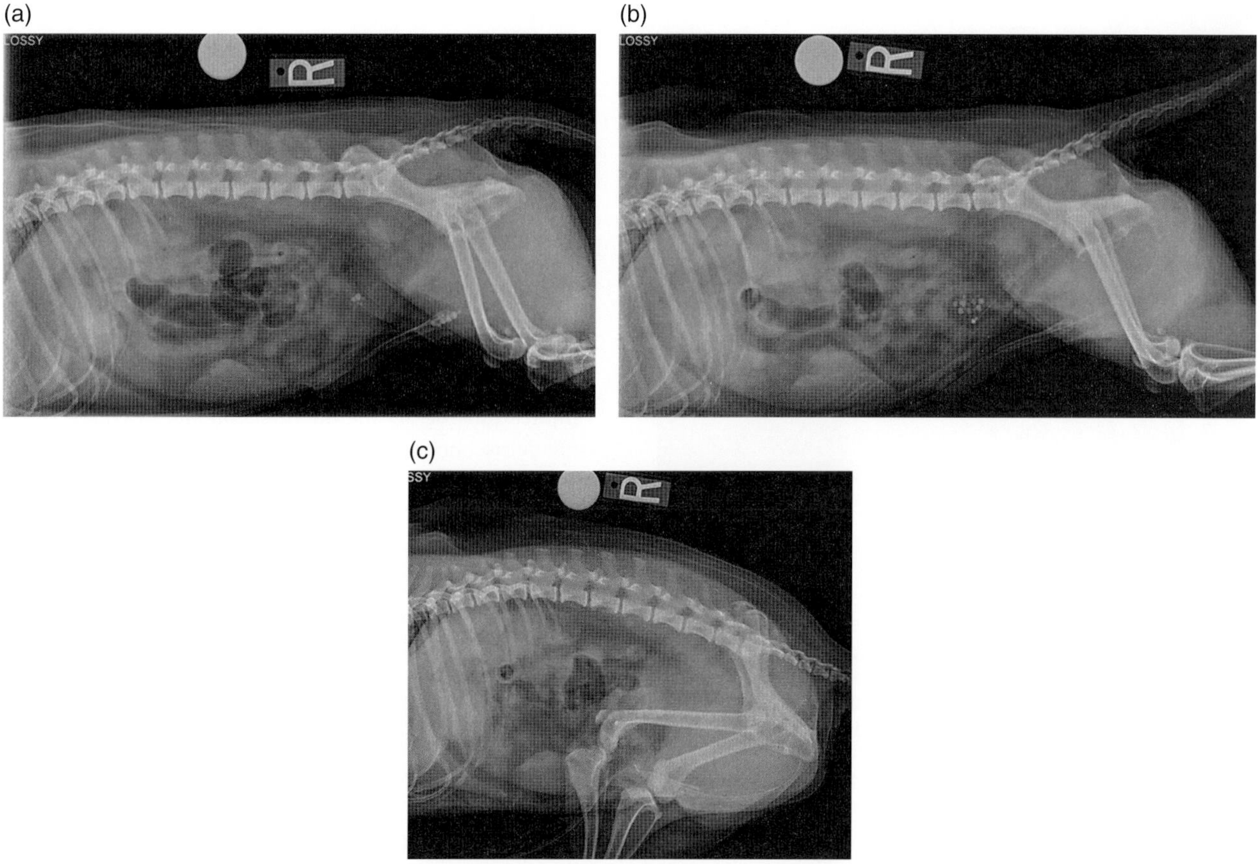

Figure 31.10 (a) Radiopaque uroliths in the urinary bladder and lodged at the base of the os penis. (b) All stones were effectively retropulsed back up into the bladder following retrograde urohydropropulsion and placement of a urinary catheter. (c) Additional radiograph with legs pulled cranially to highlight the perineal and scrotal urethra with urinary catheter in place. A cystotomy was performed for this patient following effective retropulsion.

Scrotal Urethrostomy Procedure

The patient is placed in dorsal recumbency with the legs abducted and secured to the table. A preputial flush is performed with 0.05% chlorhexidine diacetate or 1% povidone-iodine solution, and the scrotum and prepuce are draped into the surgical field. If possible, a red rubber urinary catheter is placed retrograde to aid in the identification of the urethra. An elliptical incision is then made around the base of the scrotum at the junction between the scrotal and inguinal skin, leaving enough tissue to provide a tension-free closure, and the scrotal tissue is excised. Excess tissue can be removed later in the procedure if needed. If the patient is intact, a routine castration is performed. The underlying scrotal urethra is identified (Figure 31.11), and the connective tissue along the ventral aspect of the urethra is dissected down to the paired retractor penis muscles that appear as tan bands.[17]

The retractor penis muscle is retracted laterally, and using a #15 scalpel blade, an incision is made through the ventral urethral wall over the urinary catheter. If a urinary catheter could not be placed, careful dissection is required to ensure that the dorsal urethral wall is not traumatized during the initial stab incision. The initial incision can

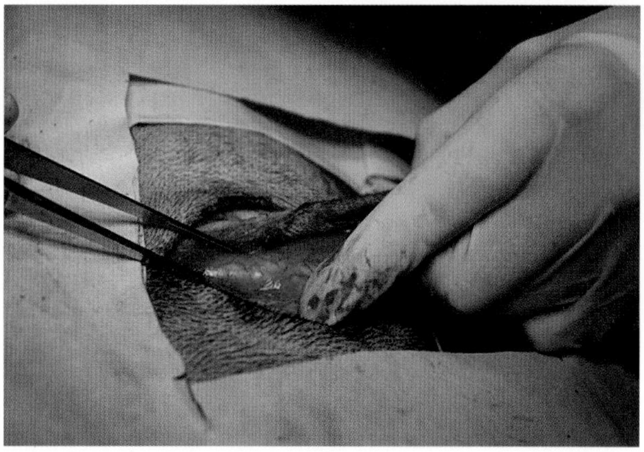

Figure 31.11 DeBakey forceps identifying the scrotal urethra while performing a scrotal ablation.

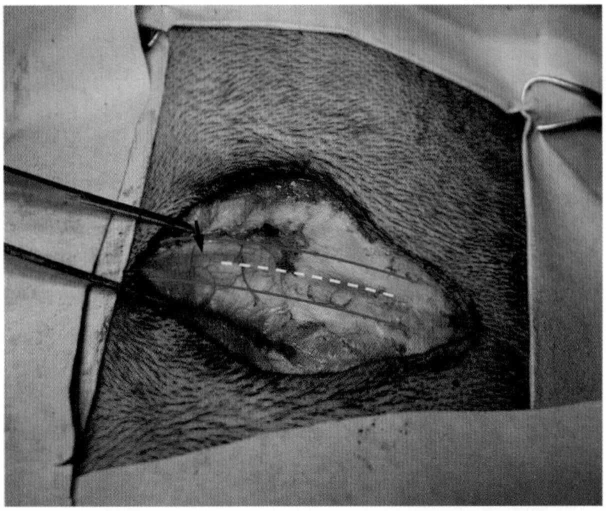

Figure 31.12 Exposure of the canine scrotal urethra with the patient in dorsal recumbency following scrotal ablation. The blue lines highlight the ventrolateral urethral margins. The yellow dotted line is the location of the desired urethrostomy incision. The black arrow is identifying the paired retractor penis muscles running along the ventral surface of the urethra. Additional dissection is required including isolation and lateralization of this retractor penis muscle prior to the urethral incision.

then be elongated with small Metzenbaum or blunted tenotomy scissors and should be 3–5 cm in length, or five to eight times the urethral diameter.[17] A large urethrostomy length is required, as the stoma will shrink by up to 50% in length as the tissues heal (Figure 31.12).

Cotton tip applicators, gauze, and digital pressure should be used to control hemorrhage. Avoid the use of an electrosurgical handpiece on the urethral tissue. The caudal extent of the incision should be extended such that urine will be directed ventrally, as the urethra begins its sweep around the ischial arch.

A 4-0 or 5-0 monofilament absorbable suture should be used on a swaged, taper-point needle. Two simple continuous suture lines have been suggested over simple interrupted bites, as they allow for the elimination of irritating knot ends and provide a better approximation of tissues.[18] It is the author's preference to place multiple simple interrupted bites to begin the urethrostomy closure for added security. Bites should be placed approximately 2 mm apart, and a three-bite closure should be implemented (Figure 31.13). The editor's preference is to start two simple continuous suture lines at the mid-point of the urethrostomy on either side. One simple continuous line is continued cranially around the drain board, while the opposite suture line is continued caudally around the stoma. They are then tied to the respective tags of the other, allowing for two knots away from the stoma. To avoid tearing the delicate urethral mucosa, re-gripping the needle with each pass and not attempting to complete all bites at once is recommended. This three-bite technique should provide gentle compression of the cavernous tissue to minimize postoperative hemorrhage.[19] The tension across the suture line should be evenly distributed and not be excessively tight. If the skin incision extends beyond that of the urethrostomy site, it is closed in a simple interrupted or intradermal fashion (Figure 31.14).

Potential Complications

Complications of SU include incision site infection, incisional dehiscence resulting in urethral stricture formation, and postoperative hemorrhage. It is important to note that if SU is indicated due to urinary calculi formation, recurrence of a calculi obstruction is possible. A urine culture in addition to urolith submission for mineral analysis is recommended for guiding appropriate medical management. If calculi become lodged proximal to the SU site, they can typically be retropulsed effectively into the bladder. If not, perineal[20] or antepubic[17] urethrostomies would need to be considered.

Postoperative Care/Prognosis

Strict use of an Elizabethan collar is required for usually three weeks postoperatively. Postoperative sedation (trazodone, acepromazine) is recommended. Petroleum gel can be placed on the skin surrounding the urethrostomy site to minimize urine-scalding immediately postoperatively. Minor hemorrhage at home can be controlled with gentle pressure and icing, however, owners should be discouraged with manipulating the SU stoma and mucosa postoperatively. Scabbing around the incision and blood clots should not be removed unless they are causing obstruction to the stoma. If they need to be removed, this should be done under sedation by the surgeon. Absorbable sutures are recommended for the procedure to avoid the need for suture removal.

Significant swelling, inflammation, and bruising of the tissues surrounding the incision in the acute recovery period may signify urine extravasation into the subcutaneous tissues. If this is noted, hospitalization and urinary diversion with an indwelling catheter for three to five days may be required to allow for second intention healing or revisional surgery for severely affected cases. The prognosis for dogs following scrotal urethrostomy is dependent upon the underlying indication for the procedure. Recurrence of obstructive calculi is possible and appropriate medical and dietary intervention is required. In a 2011 study of 18 dogs undergoing penile amputation and scrotal urethrostomy

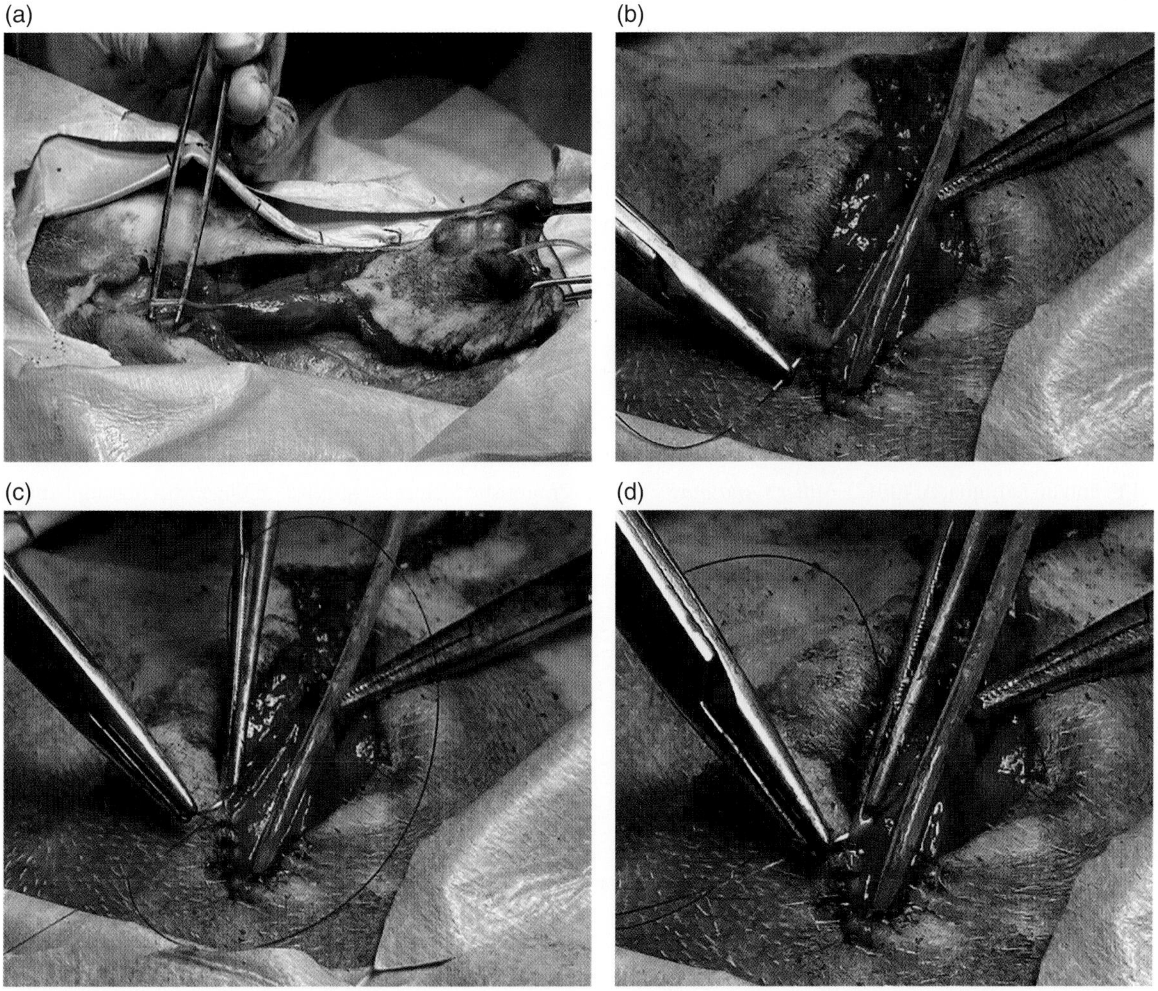

Figure 31.13 (a) Isolation of the paired retractor penis muscles in a patient undergoing a penile amputation and SU for oncologic disease of the prepuce. (b) Urinary catheter placement helps with identification of the urethral lumen throughout the procedure. Simple interrupted sutures are first placed at the apex of the urethrostomy site, with careful apposition of the urethra mucosa to the skin. The three-bite technique begins with a partial thickness bite through the skin, (c) followed by a bite through the tunica albuginea, and lastly, (d) through the urethral mucosa.

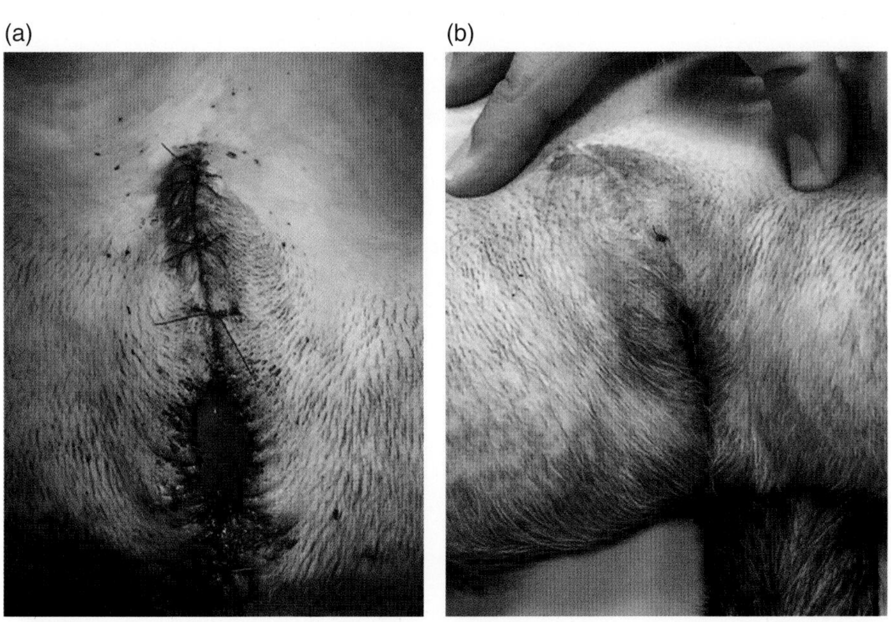

Figure 31.14 (a) Postoperative closure of a scrotal urethrostomy. Note the simple continuous closure apposing the urethral mucosa and skin in addition to the simple interrupted and cruciate sutures placed following penile amputation cranial and caudal to the urethrostomy. (b) Urethrostomy site three weeks postoperatively. Note the expected but significant contraction of the urethrostomy site. The patient was urinating well and had an uncomplicated recovery.

for various conditions, all dogs had mild postoperative hemorrhage following urination or spontaneously at home for up to 12 days after the procedure (mean 5.5 days).[10] In this same study, scrotal urethrostomy performed for non-neoplastic conditions had an excellent long-term prognosis. When performed for neoplastic conditions, local tumor recurrence and/or metastatic disease occurred within 5–12 months.

References

1. de Lahunta, A., Evans, H.E., and Miller, M.E. (2009). *Guide to the Dissection of the Dog*, 7e, 140–143, 180–183. Saunders.
2. Evans, H.E. and de Lahunta, A. (2012). *Miller's Anatomy of the Dog*, 4e, 384–385. Saunders.
3. Bojrab, J.M., Waldron, D.R., and Toombs, J.P. (2014). *Current Techniques in Small Animal Surgery*, 5e, 490–494. Teton NewMedia.
4. Harvey, C.E. (1973). Scrotal ablation and castration in the dog. *Anim. Hosp.* 9: 170–171.
5. Trappler, M.C., Popovitch, C.A., Goldschmidt, M.H. et al. (2014). Scrotal tumors in dogs: a retrospective study of 676 cases (1986–2010). *Can. Vet. J.* 55 (1): 1229–1233.
6. Wells, S. and Gottfried, S.D. (2010). Utilization of the scrotum as a full thickness skin graft in a dog. *Can. Vet. J.* 51 (11): 1269–1273.
7. Cerundolo, R. and Maiolino, P. (2002). Review cutaneous lesions of the canine scrotum. *Vet. Dermatol.* 13 (2): 63–76.
8. Bastianello, S.S. (1983). A survey on neoplasia in domestic species over a 40-year period from 1935 to 1974 in the Republic of South Africa. VI. Tumours occurring in dogs. *Onderstepoort J. Vet. Res.* 50 (3): 199–220.
9. Vail, D.M., Thamm, D.H., and Liptak, J. (ed.) (2019). *Withrow and MacEwan's Small Animal Clinical Oncology*, 6e. Saunders.
10. Burrow, R.D., Gregory, S.P., Giejda, A.A. et al. (2011). Penile amputation and scrotal urethrostomy in 18 dogs. *Vet. Rec.* 169 (25): 657. -U48.
11. Sfiligoi, G., Rassnick, K.M., Scarlett, J.M. et al. (2005). Outcome of dogs with mast cell tumors in the inguinal or perineal region versus other cutaneous locations: 124 cases (1990–2001). *J. Am. Vet. Med. Assoc.* 226 (8): 1368–1374.
12. Cahalane, A.K., Payne, S., Barber, L.G. et al. (2004). Prognostic factors for survival of dogs with inguinal and perineal mast cell tumors treated surgically with or without adjunctive treatment: 68 cases (1994–2002). *J. Am. Vet. Med. Assoc.* 225 (3): 401–408.
13. Huuskonen, V., Hughes, J.L., Bañon, E.E. et al. (2013). Intratesticular lidocaine reduces the response to surgical castration in dogs. *Vet. Anaesth. Analg.* 40 (1): 74–82.
14. McMillan, M.W., Seymour, C.J., and Brearley, J.C. (2012). Effect of intratesticular lidocaine on isoflurane requirements in dogs undergoing routine castration. *J. Small Anim. Pract.* 53 (7): 393–397.
15. Osuna, D.J., DeYoung, D.J., and Walker, R.L. (1990). Comparison of three skin preparation techniques in the dog part 1: experimental trial. *Vet. Surg.* 19 (1): 14–19.
16. Johnston, S.A. and Tobias, K.M. (2017). *Veterinary Surgery: Small Animal Expert Consult*, 2e, 2239–2240. Saunders.
17. Smeak, D.D. (2000). Urethrotomy and urethrostomy in the dog. *Clin. Tech. Small Anim. Pract.* 15 (1): 25–34.
18. Newton, J.D. and Smeak, D.D. (1996). Simple continuous closure of canine scrotal urethrostomy: results in 20 cases. *J. Am. Anim. Hosp. Assoc.* 32 (6): 531–534.
19. Waldron, D.R., Hedlund, C.S., Tangner, C. et al. (1985). The canine urethra: a comparison of first and second intention healing. *Vet. Surg.* 14 (3): 213–217.
20. Taylor, C.J. and Smeak, D.D. (2021). Perineal urethrostomy in male dogs—technique description, short-and long-term results. *Can. Vet. J.* 62 (12): 1315–1322.

32

Feline Perineal Urethrostomy

Janet A. Grimes

Department of Small Animal Medicine and Surgery, University of Georgia, Athens, GA, USA

Key Points

- Perineal urethrostomy forms an anastomosis of the urethra to the skin where the urethral diameter is wider, allowing for reduced incidence of obstructive episodes related to feline idiopathic cystitis.
- Although incidence of obstructive episodes related to feline idiopathic cystitis is reduced, continued medical management of feline idiopathic cystitis is recommended to improve patient comfort and quality of life.
- Perineal urethrostomy can be performed in dorsal or ventral recumbency and adequate dissection and meticulous mucosal/skin apposition are imperative for success of the procedure.
- The most common complications following perineal urethrostomy are stricture and recurrent urinary tract infections, although the prognosis is excellent, and owners report a very good to excellent quality of life for their cat postoperatively.

Introduction

Perineal urethrostomy is performed in male cats to alleviate urinary obstructions, most commonly associated with feline idiopathic cystitis (FIC). It is important to note that performing perineal urethrostomy reduces the risk of obstruction but does not treat the underlying disease process in cats with FIC; thus, continued medical management is strongly recommended following surgery. In this chapter, indications and preoperative considerations for perineal urethrostomy, the surgical procedure, potential complications, and outcome/prognosis will be discussed. Although perineal urethrostomy can be performed in dogs, it is not the ideal urethrostomy site (see Chapter 31 – Scrotal Urethrostomy for details) and should be avoided unless all other options have been exhausted.

Indications and Preoperative Considerations

Perineal urethrostomy is performed in male cats to create a larger urethral opening by suturing the pelvic urethra to the skin. The penile urethra in male cats is the narrowest segment of the urethra, which increases the risk of urinary obstruction in this region.[1,2] The most common indication for perineal urethrostomy in male cats is recurrent obstructive episodes related to FIC.[3,4] Other indications include inability to pass a urethral catheter in cases with obstruction, trauma, strictures, or neoplasia.[3,4] For cats with FIC, it is important for owners to understand that this procedure does not treat the underlying disease process, which requires continued medical management postoperatively. In general, perineal urethrostomy is performed after multiple obstructive episodes, but the decision as to when to

Techniques in Small Animal Soft Tissue, Orthopedic, and Ophthalmic Surgery, First Edition. Edited by Kristin A. Coleman.

Companion website: www.wiley.com/go/coleman/surgeries

perform this procedure is patient- and owner-dependent. In the vast majority of cases, perineal urethrostomy is not an emergency procedure and is performed after unblocking and stabilizing the patient; however, if a catheter cannot be passed and the patient is stable for anesthesia, perineal urethrostomy can be performed immediately. In-depth discussion of medical management of urinary obstructions will not be covered here.

Surgical Procedure

Patient Positioning

Perineal urethrostomy may be performed in sternal or dorsal recumbency. Although traditionally performed in sternal recumbency, benefits of performing perineal urethrostomy in dorsal recumbency are that no repositioning is required to perform concurrent cystotomy, improved ventilation of the patient due to reduced diaphragmatic compression by abdominal organs, reduced cranial movement of the urinary bladder to maintain adequate urethral exposure, and increased surgeon comfort.[4–7] Dorsal recumbency also provides improved exposure to the area by stretching the skin over the perineum, whereas in sternal recumbency, the prepuce and penis are sometimes more difficult to access due to the skin rolling inward if the caudal thighs cannot be externally rotated. An additional potential benefit of dorsal recumbency is that the urinary bladder may be approached for normograde urethral catheterization if retrograde urethral catheterization is not possible, although in most cases this is not necessary and the procedure can be completed without a urethral catheter. There is no difference in the length of anesthesia or surgery or the risk of short- or long-term complications between perineal urethrostomy performed in sternal compared to dorsal recumbency.[4] Cats positioned in dorsal recumbency have less vertebral canal narrowing compared to those positioned in sternal recumbency;[8] however, no differences in neurological status have been found postoperatively between cats positioned in sternal compared to dorsal recumbency.[9]

To perform perineal urethrostomy in sternal recumbency, the patient should be positioned in the perineal position with the tail taped over the back toward the head (Figure 32.1). The pelvic limbs can either hang off the table or can be frog-legged. With the limbs hanging off the table, it is important to ensure sufficient padding is present to prevent sciatic nerve deficits due to prolonged pinching of the nerve. To perform perineal urethrostomy in dorsal recumbency, the patient should be positioned with the pelvic limbs pulled upwards toward the head (Figure 32.2a,b). If exposure is inadequate, a towel may be placed under the pelvis to increase exposure to the perineal area (Figure 32.2c). The entire perineal area should be shaved, and a pursestring suture should be placed in the anus to prevent leakage due to the proximity to the surgical site (Figure 32.3).

Procedure

A sterile urethral catheter should be placed, when possible, to facilitate palpation of the urethra during the procedure, although in cases with an obstruction that cannot be relieved, a catheter is not required. An elliptical- or teardrop-shaped incision should be made encircling the scrotum and prepuce (Figure 32.4), ensuring to only incise skin at the junction of the perineal and scrotal skin. If too much skin is taken, there may be increased tension on the urethrostomy. Intact cats should be castrated routinely at this time. The subcutaneous tissues should be dissected to the level of the penis and urethra; gentle traction on the prepuce helps to facilitate this dissection (Figure 32.5,

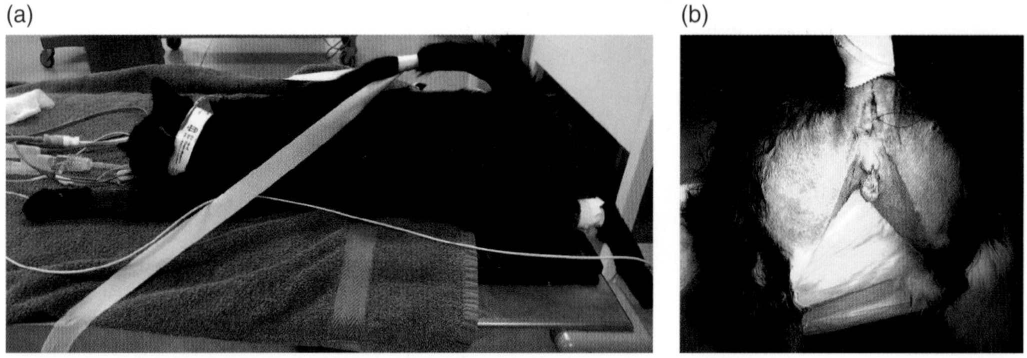

Figure 32.1 Sternal positioning for perineal urethrostomy. (a) This patient has been positioned in sternal recumbency in the perineal position. Note that the tail has been taped straight on midline over the back. In this patient, the pelvic limbs are frog-legged with the knees on the table; (b) the pelvic limbs may alternatively be allowed to hang from the table; sufficient padding should be placed under the caudal abdomen/pelvis to prevent sciatic nerve neuropraxia. *Source:* © Janet Grimes.

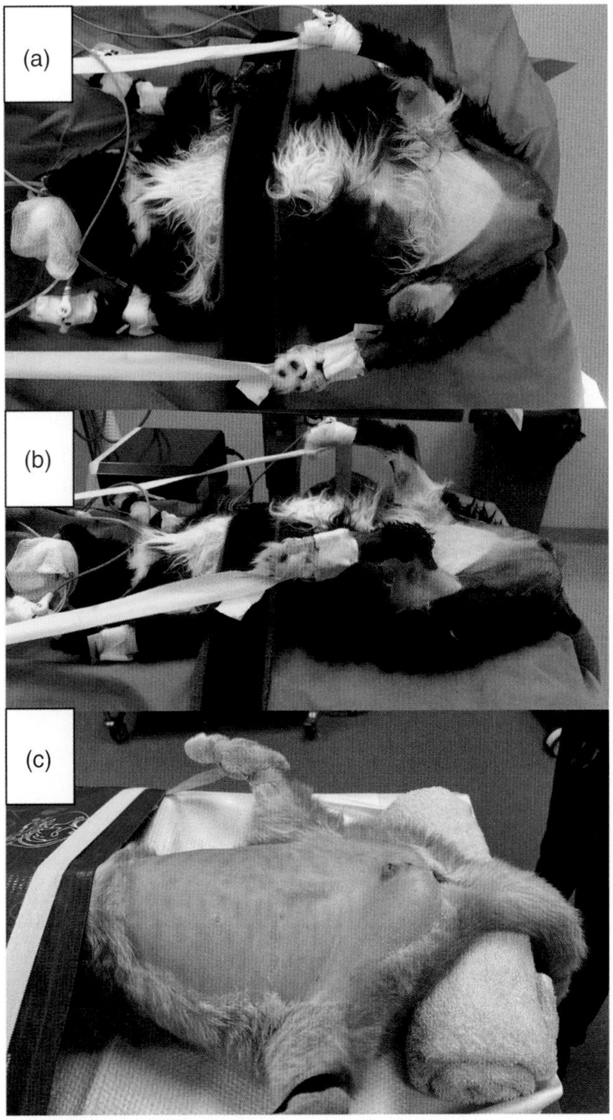

Figure 32.2 (a, b) Proper positioning of a patient in dorsal recumbency for perineal urethrostomy. The thoracic limbs may alternatively be pulled caudally, although this makes access more difficult for anesthesia. (c) If exposure is inadequate, a towel may be placed under the pelvis to increase exposure to the perineal area. (a,b) *Source:* © Janet Grimes, (c) © Kristin Coleman.

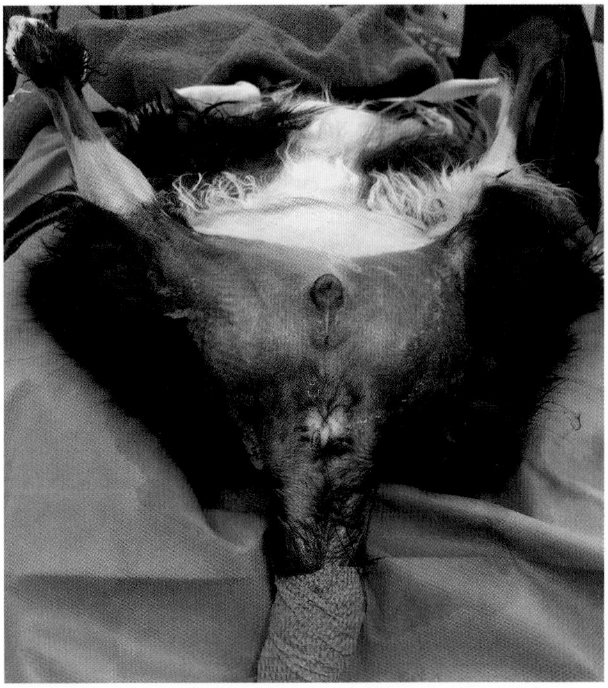

Figure 32.3 A pursestring suture has been placed in the anus to prevent leakage during this procedure. This is more essential with the patient positioned in sternal recumbency. *Source:* © Janet Grimes.

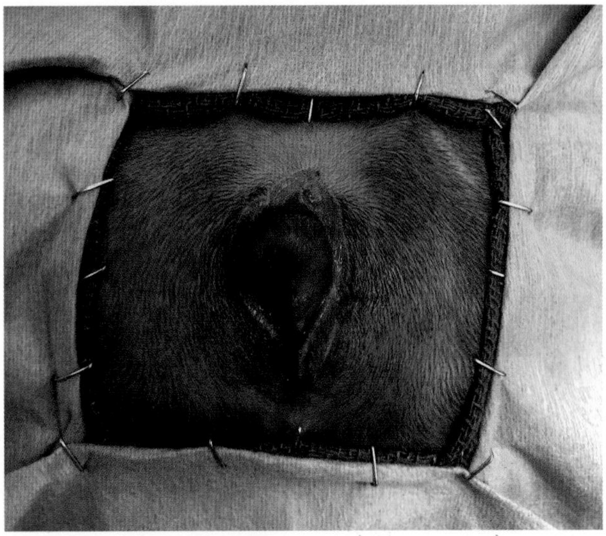

Figure 32.4 The initial skin incision should be circumferential around the prepuce and penis in an elliptical or teardrop shape. This patient is positioned in dorsal recumbency; dorsal/anus is at the bottom and ventral/abdomen is at the top of the image. *Source:* © Janet Grimes.

Video 32.1). Gelpi retractors may be placed to retract the subcutaneous tissues and assist with dissection by providing exposure and traction on the tissues. Following dissection of the caudal penis, penile attachments to the pelvis should be freed. The first attachments are the ischiocavernosus muscles, which attach the penis to the ischium (Figure 32.6a, Video 32.2). These muscles should be isolated, and an instrument should be able to be passed between the pelvis and the muscle (Figure 32.6b). Isolation can be performed with blunt dissection with curved mosquito hemostats, which are useful for isolating this muscle due to the narrow tip of the jaws. Once the muscle has been isolated, it should be transected at its attachment to the ischium (Figure 32.6c, Video 32.3). This can be performed with Mayo scissors or electrosurgery. It is important to transect this muscle at its tendinous insertion on the ischium to avoid hemorrhage. When using scissors for transection, the scissors should be laid flat against the

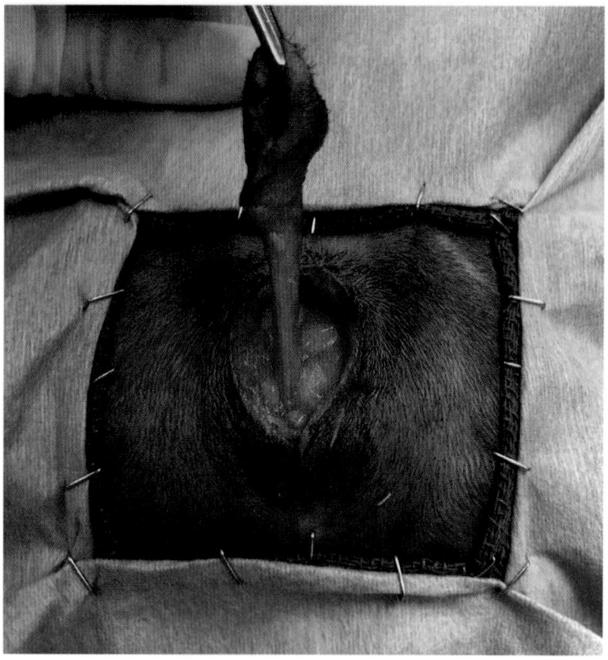

Figure 32.5 The penis is freed from the subcutaneous tissues until the only remaining attachments are those to the pelvis. This patient is positioned in dorsal recumbency; dorsal/anus is at the bottom and ventral/abdomen is at the top of the image. *Source:* © Janet Grimes.

pelvis prior to transection to ensure the tendinous insertion is transected.

Following transection of the ischiocavernosus muscles, the ventral ligament of the penis should be identified (Figure 32.7a, Video 32.4). This ligament is located on the ventral portion of the penis and attaches the penile body to the pubis. This attachment should be severed sharply at the connection with the pelvis. Once this attachment has been severed, the ventral tissues should be easily dissected with blunt finger dissection until an index finger can be passed through the pelvic canal toward the pubic brim without encountering any soft tissue attachments (Figure 32.7b, Video 32.4). Minimal dorsal and lateral dissection should be performed, as innervation to the urethra enters dorsally. Once the bulbourethral glands are identified proximal and medial to the transected ischiocavernosus muscles, dissection has proceeded to an appropriate level (Figure 32.8, Video 32.5). The bulbourethral glands are spherical glands that are more pronounced in intact males and may be a subtle rounded area in neutered males. At the level of the bulbourethral glands, the urethral diameter is adequate for perineal urethrostomy, and there will be minimal tension to suture the urethra to the skin at this level. Trying to incise the urethra more proximally will not result in a larger urethrostomy diameter; it will simply increase tension of the mucosa-skin apposition.

The retractor penis, located on the dorsal surface of the penis, should then be dissected free along the length of the penis to the bulbourethral glands with dissection using scissors or mosquito hemostats and then should be sharply transected proximal to the bulbourethral glands (Figure 32.9, Video 32.6). It is important to remove this muscle, as it overlies the urethra and will interfere with the urethrostomy apposition if not excised. Once exposure is deemed adequate, the urethra should be incised on dorsal midline. For surgeons performing this procedure in both sternal and dorsal recumbency, it is imperative to be certain which side of the urethra is dorsal prior to incising. A #11 or #15 blade should be used to initiate the incision in the mid-to-distal penis (Video 32.7). Once the catheter is identified or the urethral mucosa is identified, this incision may be continued with iris or Stevens tenotomy scissors to the level of the bulbourethral glands, at which point there will be a palpable change in the feel of cutting the urethral

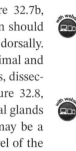

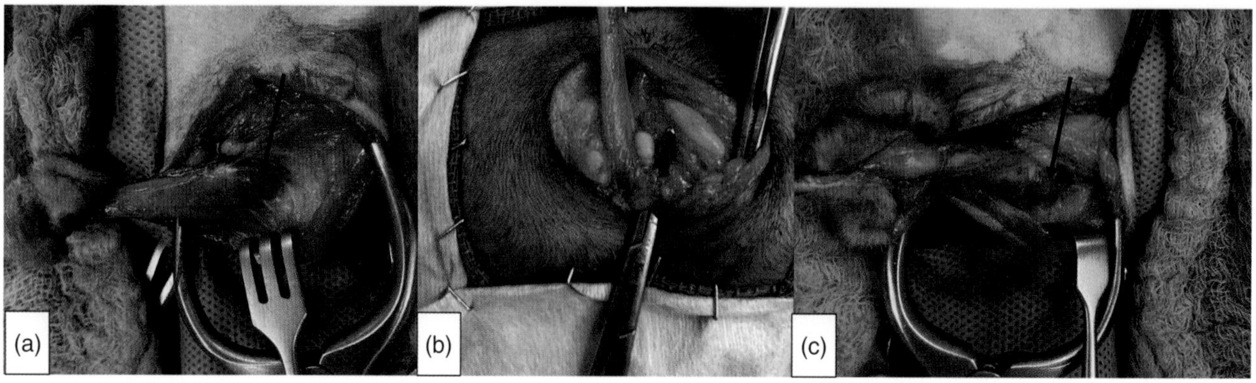

Figure 32.6 The first pelvic attachments encountered are the ischiocavernosus muscles. (a) These are paired muscles that originate on the lateral aspect of the penis and insert on the ischium. The black arrow is pointing to the left ischiocavernosus muscle; (b) the left ischiocavernosus muscle has been isolated with curved mosquito hemostats, which are under the muscle. The muscle should be transected at its pelvic attachment; (c) the left ischiocavernosus muscle has been transected with Mayo scissors at the ischial attachment. This patient is positioned in dorsal recumbency; dorsal/anus is at the bottom and ventral/abdomen is at the top of each image. *Source:* © Janet Grimes.

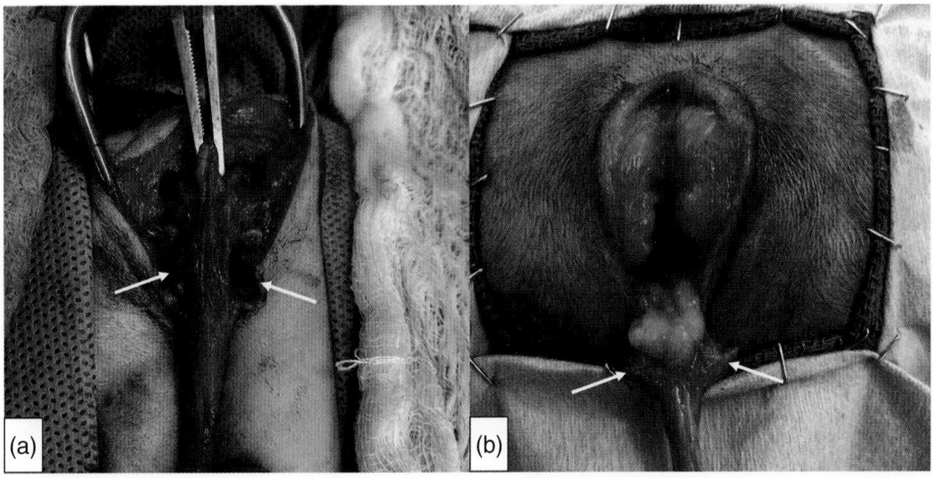

Figure 32.7 (a) The ventral ligament of the penis is within the DeBakey forceps at the top of the image. This ligament is located on the ventral aspect of the penis and attaches the penile body to the pubis; (b) this ligament has been sharply severed, and blunt finger dissection was performed to further free up the urethra within the pelvis. At this point, the surgeon should be able to pass their finger through the pelvic canal to the pubic brim without encountering soft tissue attachments from penis to pelvis on the ventral aspect. The transected ischiocavernosus muscles are denoted by the white arrows. These patients are positioned in dorsal recumbency; dorsal/anus is at the bottom and ventral/abdomen is at the top of each image. *Source:* © Janet Grimes.

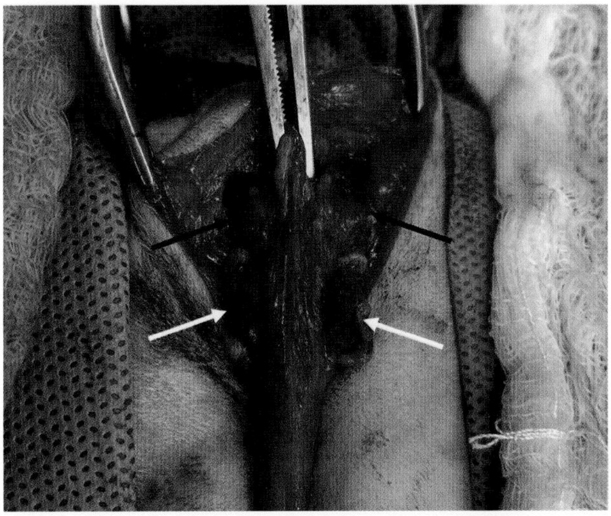

Figure 32.8 The bulbourethral glands (black arrows) are located proximally and medially to the ischiocavernosus muscles (white arrows). These glands are more pronounced in intact males and may be a subtle bulge in neutered males. This patient is positioned in dorsal recumbency; dorsal/anus is at the bottom and ventral/abdomen is at the top of the image. *Source:* © Janet Grimes.

wall with higher collagen density (Figure 32.10, Video 32.8). Hemorrhage can be quite impressive due to transection of the cavernous tissue of the penis and the extensive blood supply to the urethra. Once the incision has been made to the level of the bulbourethral glands, a mosquito hemostat should be able to be inserted easily to the level of the box lock, which indicates sufficient urethral diameter for perineal urethrostomy (Figure 32.11, Video 32.9). Alternatively, some clinicians may use an 8-Fr red rubber catheter to ensure adequate urethrostomy diameter, which can also be used to lavage the urinary bladder of any additional debris, if present, and if a cystotomy is not being performed concurrently.

Closure

Suturing the ischiocavernosus muscles to the lateral subcutaneous tissues with an interrupted cruciate or horizontal mattress suture with a monofilament absorbable suture helps to facilitate exposure of the urethra, reduce the distance from the urethra to the skin, and reduce tension on the anastomosis while suturing (Figure 32.12). The urethral mucosa should be sutured to the skin with 4-0 or 5-0 rapidly absorbed monofilament suture on a taper needle, such as poliglecaprone 25 or glycomer 631. Historically, nonabsorbable suture was used for perineal urethrostomy, but this requires suture removal two weeks postoperatively, which often requires sedation to accomplish. Use of a rapidly absorbed monofilament suture does not increase the risk of complications;[10] thus, many clinicians prefer to use absorbable suture to avoid the need for suture removal.

The dorsal-most sutures should be placed first and may be placed as stay sutures to ensure accurate apposition. These are generally placed at a 45° angle at the 10 and 2 o'clock position (with 12 o'clock being straight dorsal, Figure 32.13). It is important to ensure accurate apposition of the urethral mucosa to the skin, and the skin sutures should be aligned as an intradermal bite with the needle going through the skin and exiting in the subcuticular layer (above the subcutaneous layer). Bishop Harmon forceps are helpful for handling of the delicate tissues and surgical eye spears are an

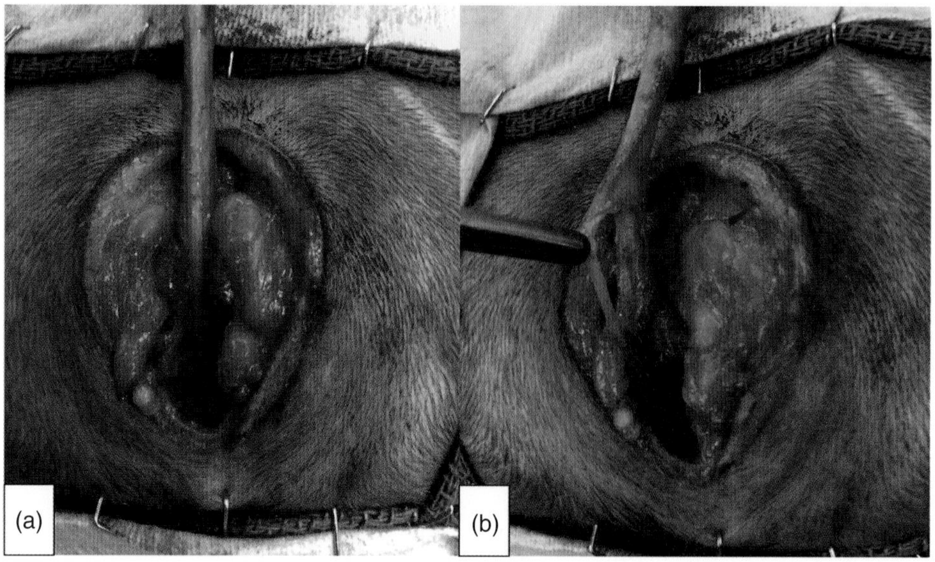

Figure 32.9 The retractor penis muscle is located on the dorsal aspect of the penis. (a) The white stripe of tissue on dorsal midline is the retractor penis muscle; (b) this muscle has been freed from the penile body. It should be dissected free up to the level of the bulbourethral glands and transected. This patient is positioned in dorsal recumbency; dorsal/anus is at the bottom and ventral/abdomen is at the top of each image. *Source:* © Janet Grimes.

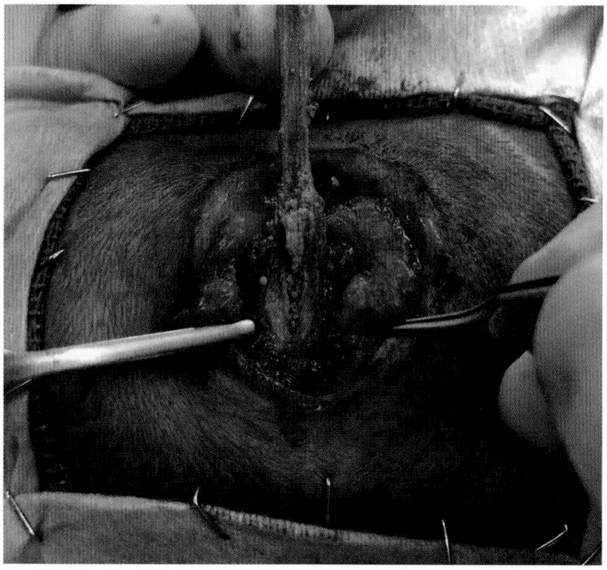

Figure 32.10 The urethral incision should be continued to the level of the bulbourethral glands. This patient underwent perineal urethrostomy due to inability to catheterize the urethra. Upon opening the urethra, a significant conglomeration of urethral calculi was noted. This patient is positioned in dorsal recumbency; dorsal/anus is at the bottom and ventral/abdomen is at the top of the image. *Source:* © Janet Grimes.

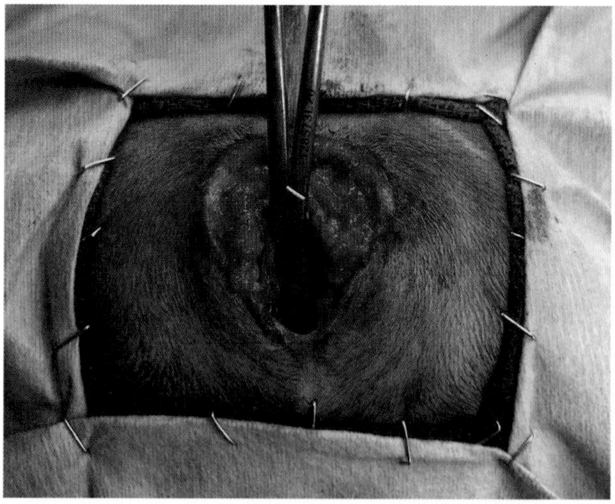

Figure 32.11 The urethral incision should be made up to the level of the bulbourethral glands. At this level, a mosquito hemostat should be able to be inserted up to the box lock, which indicates sufficient urethral diameter. Alternatively, some clinicians may use an 8-Fr red rubber catheter, which can also be used to lavage the urinary bladder of any additional debris if a cystotomy is not being performed concurrently. This patient is positioned in dorsal recumbency; dorsal/anus is at the bottom and ventral/abdomen is at the top of the image. *Source:* © Janet Grimes.

excellent tool to use for hemostasis during suturing. Once these first two sutures are tied, additional sutures can be placed on either side to form a drain board that helps to prevent urine scald and reduce the risk of stenosis. The urethra should be sutured for 1–1.5 cm in length. These sutures may be simple interrupted or simple continuous in nature; if the continuous pattern is chosen, three to four interrupted sutures are performed on each side followed by a continuous pattern for the drain board (Figure 32.14). Figure-of-eight sutures are ideal for all interrupted sutures on the anastomosis, as they keep knots away from the incision line while still

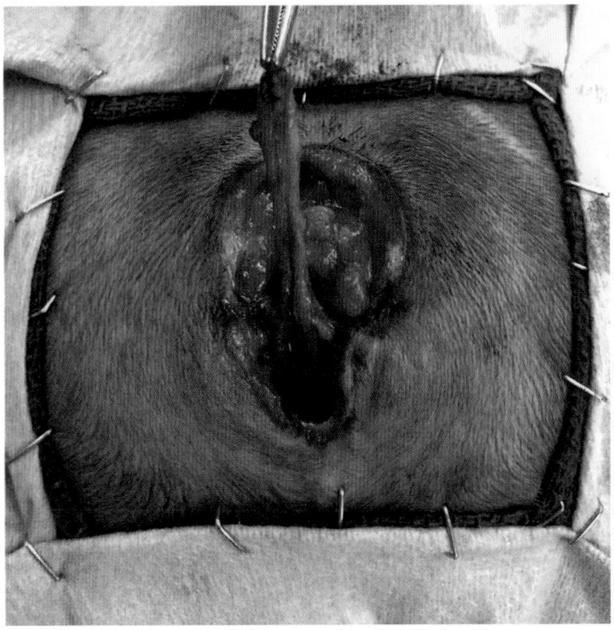

Figure 32.12 The ischiocavernosus muscles have been sutured bilaterally to the subcutaneous tissues with interrupted cruciate sutures. This helps to facilitate exposure of the urethra and brings the skin closer to the urethra to reduce tension while suturing the urethrostomy. This patient is positioned in dorsal recumbency; dorsal/anus is at the bottom and ventral/abdomen is at the top of the image. *Source:* © Janet Grimes.

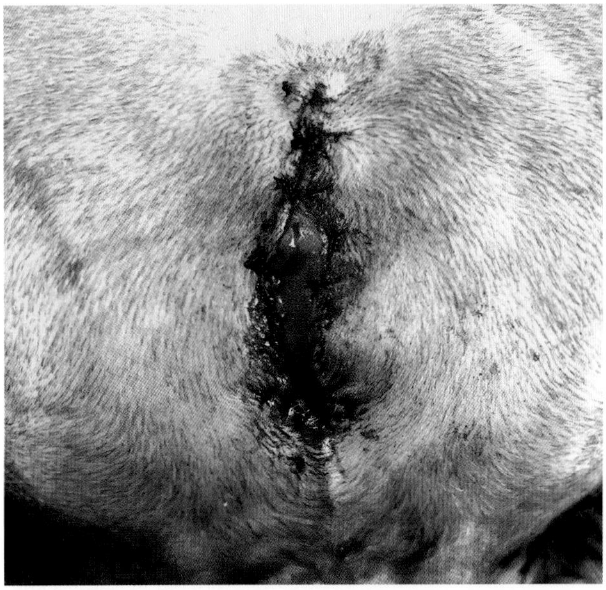

Figure 32.14 In this patient, interrupted figure-of-eight sutures were used at the dorsal aspect of the urethrostomy, followed by a simple continuous pattern down the drainboard on either side. A horizontal mattress suture was placed at the distal penis prior to amputation. The remaining ventral skin incision was closed routinely. This patient is positioned in dorsal recumbency; dorsal/anus is at the bottom and ventral/abdomen is at the top of the image. *Source:* © Janet Grimes.

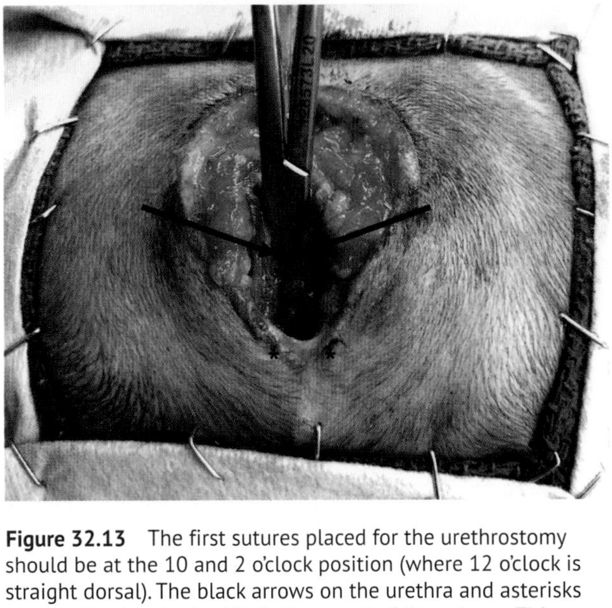

Figure 32.13 The first sutures placed for the urethrostomy should be at the 10 and 2 o'clock position (where 12 o'clock is straight dorsal). The black arrows on the urethra and asterisks on the skin denote the ideal placement of the sutures. This patient is positioned in dorsal recumbency; dorsal/anus is at the bottom and ventral/abdomen is at the top of the image. *Source:* © Janet Grimes.

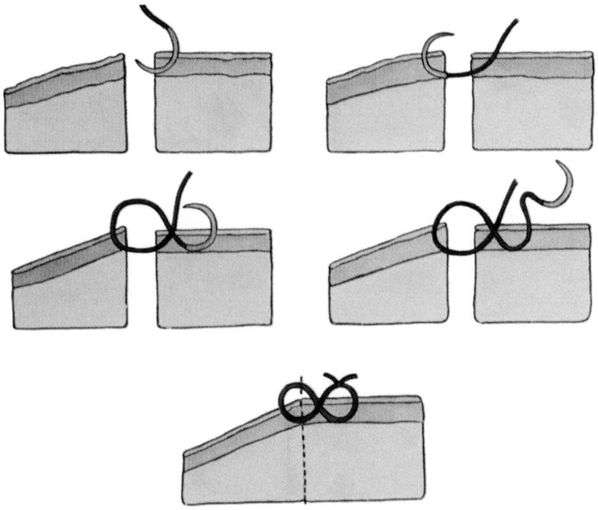

Figure 32.15 Figure-of-eight sutures are ideal as they keep knots away from the incision line while still maintaining excellent apposition. Sutures should be tied snugly to bring the urethral mucosa and skin into apposition. *Source:* Original artwork by Taylor Bergrud.

maintaining excellent apposition (Figure 32.15). Once the drain board has been established, a mattress suture is placed through the skin on one side, through the most ventral aspect of the cavernous tissues, through the skin on the opposite side, and then back through the skin on the opposite side, this time taking a bite through the dorsal-most aspect of the cavernous tissues before exiting in the skin on the side in which the suture was started (Video 32.10). The distal penis is then amputated sharply (Video 32.10).

Alternatively, a modified transfixation suture can be placed around the penile body prior to amputating the distal penis. Any skin remaining open should be closed dorsal and ventral to the urethrostomy site, as needed (Figure 32.14). In most cases, only the ventral portion of the skin incision requires separate closure.

Potential Complications

One complication following perineal urethrostomy that may require revision surgery is urethral stricture, which occurs in 3–12% of cats.[3,11] Stricture most commonly occurs in the short-term postoperative period (within four weeks) but may be a long-term complication.[3,12] The most common reason for stricture is inadequate dissection to level of the bulbourethral glands.[12] Additional reasons for stricture include poor mucosa-to-skin apposition, urine extravasation between the mucosa and skin leading to inflammation and granulation tissue formation, and trauma to the anastomosis from licking or an indwelling urethral catheter.[12,13] Another complication following perineal urethrostomy is urinary tract infection, which is most commonly a late complication.[3,13] The reason for the increased risk of urinary tract infection (UTI) following perineal urethrostomy is proposed to be the wider opening of the urethra in proximity to the anus and environment, coupled with an underlying uropathy. The recurrent UTI rate in cats undergoing perineal urethrostomy was 22% in cats with previous urethral obstruction due to FIC compared to 0% in healthy cats without FIC,[14] indicating a role of the underlying disease process in the development of UTIs. Urinary and fecal incontinence are rare following perineal urethrostomy but may occur with damage to the pudendal nerve or with aggressive dorsal dissection. Hemorrhage is an uncommon postoperative complication. Although hemorrhage during the surgical procedure can obscure the surgical field, it rarely requires treatment, as hemorrhage should abate quickly when the urethrostomy is sutured.

Postoperative Care/Prognosis

Postoperative pain is controlled initially with intravenous opioids, which can later be transitioned to oral opioids, such as buccal buprenorphine. Nonsteroidal anti-inflammatory drugs may be used in non-azotemic patients but should be used with caution in patients with recent azotemia due to potential acute kidney injury from an obstructive episode. Intravenous fluids should be continued in cats with recent obstruction and postobstructive diuresis. Postoperative antimicrobial use is not necessary in most cases as FIC is typically a sterile process. Prazosin, an $\alpha 1$-adrenergic antagonist, can be continued postoperatively to reduce urethral spasm following perineal urethrostomy for a urethral obstructive episode. There are no studies evaluating its use following perineal urethrostomy, but two randomized blinded prospective clinical studies found no difference in the rate of recurrent urethral obstruction between cats receiving prazosin or placebo for 7 or 30 days following an episode of urethral obstruction.[15,16] Although one study found that prazosin increased the rate of recurrent urethral obstruction, this was a survey-based study of veterinarians, and multivariable analysis was not performed to determine the relationship between prazosin and other variables significantly associated with recurrent obstruction (increased difficulty to unblock and a gritty feel to the urethra).[17] Because perineal urethrostomy reduces the risk of obstruction due to increased urethral diameter at the stoma, the use of prazosin may be considered. Postoperatively, all cats should be placed in a rigid Elizabethan collar for two to three weeks. Some clinicians feel the addition of a soft Elizabethan collar within the rigid collar helps to deter grooming attempts due to the noise the soft collar makes. This may be considered in cats that do not tolerate the rigid Elizabethan collar, but the soft collar should never be used alone. The sandpaper nature of their tongue causes significant trauma to the area if they are able to lick the site, increasing the risk of dehiscence and later stenosis of the site. Paper litter should also be used for two to three weeks to reduce irritation to the anastomosis site that may increase the risk of stricture. While all owners are encouraged to try the paper litter initially, a small population of cats may not readily use the paper and may instead eliminate outside of the litterbox; in these cases, the clients may resume the use of their cat's normal non-paper litter. The stoma should be left alone, as wiping off blood clots or paper litter, even if performed gently, may disturb the mucosal-skin apposition, increasing the risk of stricture. All cats undergoing perineal urethrostomy for management of obstructions due to FIC should also undergo medical management for FIC, including environmental management with increasing water intake (wet food, water fountains), urinary diets, and reduction of stress.

Outcomes for cats following perineal urethrostomy are excellent with 89–94% of owners being satisfied with the outcome of surgery.[3,11] For cats undergoing perineal urethrostomy for obstruction associated with FIC, recurrent symptoms following perineal urethrostomy occurred in only 40% of cats between 6 months and 10 years postoperatively.[11] Quality of life following perineal urethrostomy, as assessed by owner surveys, is also excellent with 89–100% of owners rating their cats as having a very good to excellent quality of life[3,11,18] and 75% of owners giving the highest possible score for quality of life postoperatively.[15] Additionally, 100% of owners felt their cat was the same (52%) or better (48%) than prior to when their cat had their urinary obstruction.[18]

To access the videos for this chapter, please go to

www.wiley.com/go/coleman/surgeries

VIDEO 32.1 The penis is freed from the subcutaneous tissues using Metzenbaum scissors until the only remaining attachments are those to the pelvis. Regular palpation of the penis is important to ensure appropriate dissection of subcutaneous tissues without disruption to the penis itself. This patient is positioned in dorsal recumbency. *Source:* © Janet Grimes.

VIDEO 32.2 Continued dissection of the subcutaneous tissues at the level of the ischium is performed to identify the ischiocavernosus muscles. These are paired muscles that originate on the lateral aspect of the penis and insert on the ischium. This patient is positioned in dorsal recumbency. *Source:* © Janet Grimes.

VIDEO 32.3 Once identified, the ischiocavernosus muscles are isolated with blunt dissection using Metzenbaum scissors or mosquito hemostats. The muscle is then transected at the ischiatic attachment using Mayo scissors. Laying the scissors flat against the ischium assists in transection of the tendinous attachment to limit hemorrhage from the muscle. In this video, this is performed on the right side of the patient and should be performed bilaterally before proceeding to the next step of the procedure. This patient is positioned in dorsal recumbency. *Source:* © Janet Grimes.

VIDEO 32.4 The ventral penile ligament is located on the ventral aspect of the penis and attaches the penile body to the pubis. Notice how digital palpation is limited by the presence of this ligament. Sharp transection of this ligament at its attachment to the pelvis allows for blunt finger dissection ventral to the penis to reduce tension on the urethrostomy site. This patient is positioned in dorsal recumbency. *Source:* © Janet Grimes.

VIDEO 32.5 The bulbourethral glands are located proximally and medially to the ischiocavernosus muscles. These glands are more pronounced in intact males and may be a subtle bulge in neutered males. This patient is positioned in dorsal recumbency. *Source:* © Janet Grimes.

VIDEO 32.6 The retractor penis muscle is located on the dorsal midline aspect of the penis. It should be dissected free up to the level of the bulbourethral glands and transected. This patient is positioned in dorsal recumbency. *Source:* © Janet Grimes.

VIDEO 32.7 The urethra is incised on dorsal midline using a #11 or #15 blade. The incision is started distally with the blade, until the urethral lumen and urethral catheter are identified. This incision can be difficult due to the hemorrhage that occurs upon incising the penis and urethra and the narrow lumen of the urethra. This patient is positioned in dorsal recumbency. *Source:* © Janet Grimes.

VIDEO 32.8 Once the urethra is identified, the urethral catheter can be removed and the urethral incision extended proximally using iris or tenotomy scissors. The incision should be extended proximally to the level of the bulbourethral glands. This patient is positioned in dorsal recumbency. *Source:* © Janet Grimes.

VIDEO 32.9 Once the urethra has been opened to the level of the bulbourethral glands, a mosquito hemostat should be able to be easily inserted to the level of the box lock. This indicates appropriate urethral diameter for the urethrostomy. Alternatively, some clinicians may use an 8-French red rubber catheter. *Source:* © Janet Grimes.

VIDEO 32.10 Following anastomosis of the urethral mucosa to the skin, a horizontal mattress suture is placed across the distal penis and then the distal penis is transected sharply. The remaining subcutaneous tissues and skin are closed routinely. *Source:* © Janet Grimes.

References

1 Cullen, W.C., Fletcher, T.F., and Bradley, W.F. (1983). Morphometry of the male feline pelvic urethra. *J. Urol.* 129 (1): 186–189. https://doi.org/10.1016/s0022-5347(17)51979-5.

2 Wang, B., Bhadra, N., and Grill, W.M. (1999). Functional anatomy of the male feline urethra: morphological and physiological correlations. *J. Urol.* 161 (2): 654–659. https://doi.org/10.1016/S0022-5347(01)61989-X.

3 Nye, A.K., Luther, J.K., Mann, F.A. et al. (2020). Retrospective multicentric study comparing durations of surgery and anesthesia and likelihoods of short- and long-term complications between cats positioned in sternal or dorsal recumbency for perineal urethrostomy. *J. Am. Vet. Med. Assoc.* 257 (2): 176–182. https://doi.org/10.2460/javma.257.2.176.

4 Bass, M., Howard, J., Gerber, B. et al. (2005). Retrospective study of indications for and outcome of perineal urethrostomy in cats. *J. Small Anim. Pract.* 46 (5): 227–231. https://doi.org/10.1111/j.1748-5827.2005.tb00314.x.

5 Goh, C.S.S. and Seim, H.B. (2014). Feline perineal urethrostomy ventral approach. *Todays Vet. Pract.* 4: 43–49.

6 Tobias, K.M. (2007). Perineal urethrostomy in the cat. *Clin. Brief.* 5: 19–22.

7 Kagan, K.G., Stewart, R.W., and Leighton, R.L. (1976). Perineal urethrostomy in male cats. *Mod. Vet. Pract.* 57 (3): 187–191.

8 Slunsky, P., Brunnberg, M., Lodersted, S. et al. (2018). Effect of intraoperative positioning on the diameter of the vertebral canal in cats during perineal urethrostomy (cadaveric study). *J. Feline Med. Surg.* 20 (1): 38–44. https://doi.org/10.1177/1098612X17709645.

9 Slunsky, P., Brunnberg, M., Lodersted, S. et al. (2019). Effect of intraoperative positioning on postoperative nueorlogical status in cats during perineal urethrostomy. *J. Feline Med. Surg.* 21 (10): 931–937. https://doi.org/10.1177/1098612X18809188.

10 Frem, D.L., Hottinger, H.A., Hunter, S.L. et al. (2017). Use of poliglecaprone 25 for perineal urethrostomy in cats: 61 cases (2007–2013). *J. Am. Vet. Med. Assoc.* 251 (8): 935–940. https://doi.org/10.2460/javma.251.8.935.

11 Ruda, L. and Heiene, R. (2012). Short- and long-term outcome after perineal urethrostomy in 86 cats with feline lower urinary tract disease. *J. Small Anim. Pract.* 53 (12): 693–698. https://doi.org/10.1111/j.1748-5827.2012.01310.x.

12 Phillips, H. and Holt, D.E. (2006). Surgical revision of the urethral stoma following perineal urethrostomy in 11 cats: (1998-2004). *J. Am. Anim. Hosp. Assoc.* 42 (3): 218–222. https://doi.org/10.5326/0420218.

13 Nye, A.K. and Luther, J.K. (2018). Feline perineal urethrostomy: a review of past and present literature. *Top. Compan. Anim. Med.* 33 (3): 77–82. https://doi.org/10.1053/j.tcam.2018.07.002.

14 Griffin, D.W. and Gregory, C.R. (1992). Prevalence of bacterial urinary tract infection after perineal urethrostomy in cats. *J. Am. Vet. Med. Assoc.* 200 (5): 681–684. https://doi.org/10.2460/javma.1992.200.05.681.

15 Reineke, E.L., Thomas, E.K., Syring, R.S. et al. (2017). The effect of prazosin on outcome in feline urethral obstruction. *J. Vet. Emerg. Crit. Care* 27 (4): 387–396. https://doi.org/10.1111/vec.12611.

16 Hanson, K.R., Rudloff, E., Yuan, L. et al. (2021). Effect of prazosin on feline recurrent urethral obstruction. *J. Feline Med. Surg.* 23 (12): 1176–1182. https://doi.org/10.1177/1098612X211001283.

17 Conway, D.S., Rozanski, E.A., and Wayne, A.S. (2022). Prazosin administration increases the rate of recurrent urethral obstruction in cats: 388 cases. *J. Am. Vet. Med. Assoc.* 260 (S2): S7–S11, 21 https://doi.org/10.2460/javma.21.10.0469.

18 Slater, M.R., Pailler, S., Gayle, J.M. et al. (2020). Welfare of cats 5–29 months after perineal urethrostomy: 74 cases (2015–2017). *J. Feline Med. Surg.* 22 (6): 582–588. https://doi.org/10.1177/1098612X19867777.

33

Rectal Prolapse

Catriona M. MacPhail

Department of Clinical Sciences, Colorado State University, Fort Collins, CO, USA

Key Points

- The main differential diagnoses for protrusion of rectal tissue from the anus are rectal prolapse and intussusception.
- Rectal prolapse is a result of significant tenesmus that is due to a variety of causes.
- The degree of surgical intervention required for rectal prolapse is dependent on the severity and duration of the condition.

Introduction

Rectal prolapse can occur in both dogs and cats. The diagnosis is straightforward due to the appearance of mucosa extending from the anus (Figure 33.1). A partial prolapse (anal prolapse) is extrusion of only mucosal tissue and is typically quite short in length, while a complete prolapse involves all layers of the rectum being exteriorized. The alternative differential is protrusion of an intussusception. These two conditions can be discerned by palpation alongside the prolapsed tissue and the anus by a blunt lubricated probe; if it passes easily, it is an intussusception, whereas a rectal prolapse will not have any space to probe in that location.

Indications/Pre-op Considerations

Prolapse of the rectum occurs to excessive straining to urinate or defecate with or without underlying anatomic defects. Causes of tenesmus include but are not limited to gastrointestinal parasitism, tumors in the lower gastrointestinal tract, perineal herniation, and inflammatory conditions of the colon, rectum, or anal sphincter. There are isolated reports of colonic duplication in both dogs and cats with rectal prolapse being a consistent clinical sign.[1–3] Diagnosing and addressing the primary problem is critical to ultimate resolution of the rectal prolapse. Intervention is required for any rectal prolapse to avoid devitalization, necrosis, or self-mutilation. The level of intervention is dependent on duration, severity, and repeated presentation.

Surgical Procedures

Animals presenting with rectal prolapse for the first time can be managed with manual reduction of the prolapse and a purse-string suture in the anus. Sedation, local analgesia (e.g., sacrococcygeal block, epidural), or general anesthesia is needed for reducing the prolapse. Reduction can be aided by using isotonic saline and lubrication. If difficulty arises, edema and swelling of the rectal mucosa can be addressed by applying any gentle osmotic agents (e.g., sugar [50% dextrose, honey]). Following reduction, a nonabsorbable monofilament suture material (e.g., 3-0 nylon) is used for a purse-string pattern in the mucocutaneous junction of the anus. The purse-string is placed loosely over a syringe, syringe case, or blood collection tube to prevent prolapse while still allowing passage of fecal material. Typically, this purse-string suture is left in place for three to five days to allow swelling to decrease and for a cause to be identified and treated.

Recurrent rectal prolapses can be addressed by colopexy or resection of the prolapsed segment, while devitalized and necrotic prolapses necessitate resection and anastomosis.

Techniques in Small Animal Soft Tissue, Orthopedic, and Ophthalmic Surgery, First Edition. Edited by Kristin A. Coleman.

Companion website: www.wiley.com/go/coleman/surgeries

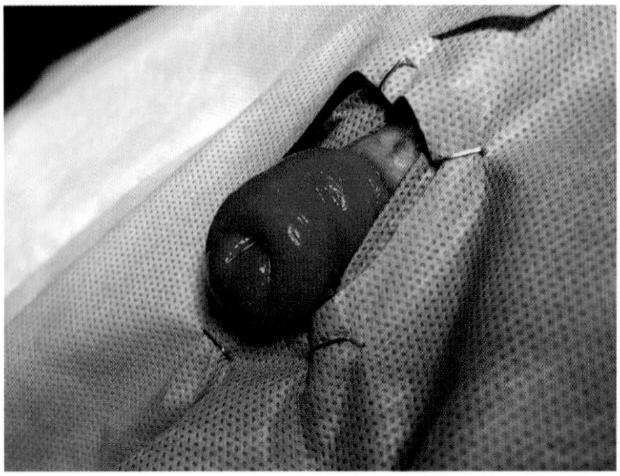

Figure 33.1 Complete rectal prolapse in an eight-week-old kitten.

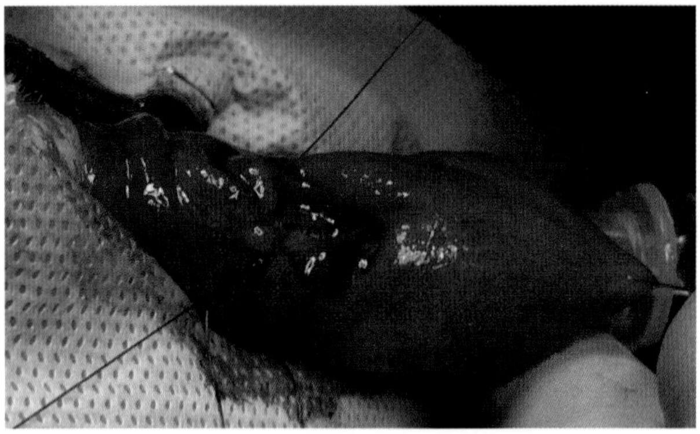

Figure 33.2 Intraoperative image of kitten in Figure 33.1 undergoing rectal resection and anastomosis. Note the syringe placed into the lumen to give the surgeon a cutting surface. Tips include placing stay sutures into the proximal tissue (closest to the patient) and only transecting one section at a time to then re-appose.

For colopexy, a caudal abdominal midline approach is performed, and the descending colon is retracted cranially to reduce the rectal prolapse. A 3–4 cm section of the descending colon is pexied to the left abdominal wall by gentle scarification of the colonic serosa and the peritoneum and transverse abdominus muscle. The colonic wall is sutured to the abdominal wall using a simple interrupted or simple continuous pattern using monofilament long-term absorbable or nonabsorbable suture. Alternatively, a partial thickness incision can be made through the seromuscular layer of the colon, although no difference in outcome has been reported.[4] Laparoscopic colopexy has also been described.[5,6]

Rectal resection and anastomosis is performed with the animal in sternal recumbency. A large syringe or blood collection tube is used to identify the lumen and provide a surface to incise against. Resection is circumferentially done in small sections approximately 1–2 cm away from the anus. Full-thickness sutures using 3-0 to 4-0 monofilament long-term absorbable suture material are placed through the remaining ends with a simple interrupted or simple continuous pattern (Figure 33.2).

Complications

The most common complication following any intervention is recurrence. Complications related to rectal resection and anastomosis are fecal incontinence, anorectal stricture, and dehiscence.

Postoperative Care/Prognosis

In the postprocedural or postsurgical period, dogs and cats should be fed a low-residue diet and treated with a laxative, such as lactulose, to achieve soft but formed stools. Rectal instillation of local analgesics (e.g., bupivacaine) prior to anesthetic recovery may provide short-term alleviation of discomfort. Systemic analgesics, such as nonsteroidal anti-inflammatory drugs, can also be administered if there are no contraindications.

If the underlying cause of a rectal prolapse is successfully addressed, resolution of the rectal prolapse is likely. However, there are no large studies reporting outcomes in dogs or cats with rectal prolapse in the veterinary literature.

References

1 Buj, E.C., Billet, J.P., Vanel, M. et al. (2020). Rectal duplication in an adult cat: a novel transanal surgical approach. *JFMS Open Rep.* 6 (1): 2055116920916956.

2 Landon, B.P., Abraham, L.A., Charles, J.A. et al. (2007). Recurrent rectal prolapse caused by colonic duplication in a dog. *Aust. Vet. J.* 85 (9): 381–385.

3 Kramer, A., Kyles, A.E., and Labelle, P. (2007). Surgical correction of colonic duplication in a cat. *J. Am. Anim. Hosp. Assoc.* 43 (2): 128–131.

4 Popovitch, C.A., Holt, D., and Bright, R. (1994). Colopexy as a treatment for rectal prolapse in dogs and cats: a retrospective study of 14 cases. *Vet. Surg.* 23 (2): 115–118.

5 Park, J., Moon, C., Kim, D.H. et al. (2022). Laparoscopic colopexy for recurrent rectal prolapse in a Maltese dog. *Can. Vet. J.* 63 (6): 593–596.

6 Zhang, S.X., Wang, H.B., Zhang, J.T. et al. (2013). Laparoscopic colopexy in dogs. *J. Vet. Med. Sci.* 75 (9): 1161–1166.

34

Perineal Hernia

Catriona M. MacPhail

Department of Clinical Sciences, Colorado State University, Fort Collins, CO, USA

Key Points

- Signalment (older intact male dogs) and clinical history (e.g., constipation, tenesmus, stranguria) should lead to a top differential of perineal herniation.
- Understanding the subtleties of canine rectal palpation is crucial to be able to confidently diagnose a perineal hernia.
- Perineal herniation can be life-threatening if urinary bladder retroflexion or small intestinal entrapment occurs.
- Multiple surgical procedures are described to address perineal herniation with an internal obturator muscle transposition flap being the most common surgery of choice for initial repair.

Introduction

Perineal herniation occurs when there is breakdown of the pelvic diaphragm and transit of intra-abdominal contents into the ischiorectal fossa of the perineum. The pelvic diaphragm consists of the levator ani muscle, coccygeus muscle, and pelvic fascia. Caudal herniation between the external anal sphincter and levator ani and coccygeus muscles is the most common of the four types. Dorsolateral herniation (between coccygeus and levator ani muscles) and lateral herniation (between coccygeus muscle and sacrotuberous ligament) can also occur. Ventral herniation with rectal sacculation occurs between the ischiocavernosus and ischiourethralis muscles and bulbocavernous muscle, and it is the most challenging type to resolve.

The most common, almost exclusive, signalment for perineal herniation is middle-aged to older, male, sexually intact canines. Inciting causes include tenesmus due to prostatic, lower urinary, or colorectal disease, hormonal alternations, and anatomic muscular weakness; however, a clear etiology often remains undetermined. A recent study found no association between perineal hernias and concurrent gastrointestinal, neurologic, or orthopedic conditions.[1] However, a separate study in adult female dogs found comorbidities to be common, including a history of trauma or chronic cough due to cardiopulmonary disease.[2] For male dogs, prostatic disease appears to be the most likely contributing factor, as a recent study investigating CT imaging of the prostate in age-matched intact males dogs with and without perineal hernias found dogs with hernias to have larger prostates, more and larger prostatic and paraprostatic cysts, and more frequent prostatic mineralization.[3] Clinical signs vary in significance and are dependent on what tissues and organs are herniated. Deviation or dilation of the rectum into the perineal region results in tenesmus and constipation. Prostatic or urinary bladder herniation results in stranguria or anuria if these organs become retroflexed and entrapped. Herniation of the small intestine is a severe but uncommon clinical scenario (Figure 34.1). Perineal hernias can be unilateral or bilateral, but with identification of an overt unilateral hernia, it is common to identify pelvic diaphragm weakness on the opposite side. One study of 31 dogs with unilateral presentation of perineal hernia found contralateral pelvic diaphragm weakness in all cases.[4]

Techniques in Small Animal Soft Tissue, Orthopedic, and Ophthalmic Surgery, First Edition. Edited by Kristin A. Coleman.

Companion website: www.wiley.com/go/coleman/surgeries

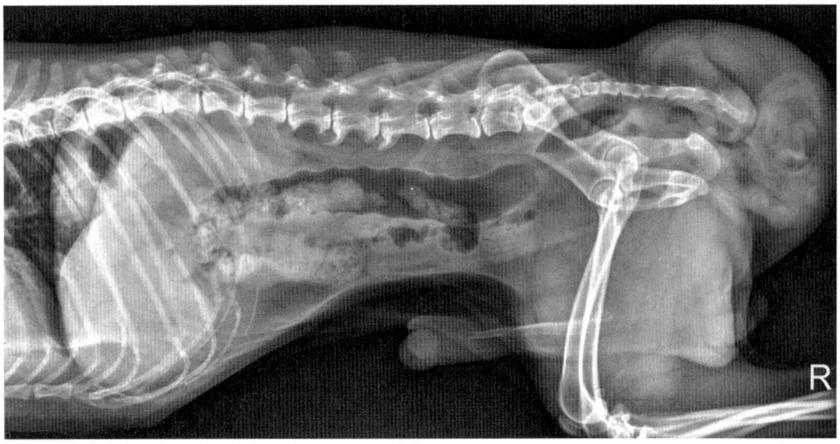

Figure 34.1 Lateral abdominal radiograph of male intact dog demonstrating severe perineal herniation of the small intestines and presumed urinary bladder due to bladder's absence in the caudal abdomen.

Indications/Pre-op Considerations

Diagnosis of a perineal hernia is confirmed by rectal palpation. Determination of the origin of hernia contents can be accomplished through abdominal radiographs and abdominal ultrasound. If there is suspicion for bladder entrapment, point-of-care ultrasound should be used immediately to determine the location of the urinary bladder. Aspiration of a fluid-filled hernia should be performed with caution; preferentially, an attempt at passage of a urethral catheter can be performed to relieve urinary obstruction.

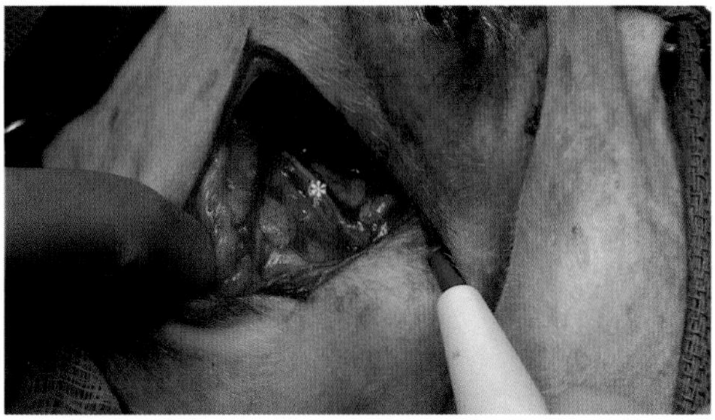

Figure 34.2 Approach to left perineal region. The left caudal rectal nerve and adjacent caudal rectal branch of the internal pudendal artery (yellow *) are avoided during the herniorrhaphy.

Surgical Procedures

Multiple surgical procedures exist to address perineal hernias. Regardless of repair technique, castration should be performed in all male intact dogs to decrease prostatic size and limit hormonal influence, in order to reduce the risk of straining and recurrence. Prior to repair, a purse-string suture is placed in the anus, and the skin and subcutaneous tissues of the perineum are carefully incised in a curvilinear dorsal to ventral direction from the base of the tail to ~1 cm ventral to the palpable ischiatic table. A tip is to stay 1–2 cm lateral to the anus in order to reduce the risk of anal sac injury. A hernia sac is commonly identified, which is a reflection of the caudal peritoneum. This tissue is breached to allow replacement of contents into the abdominal cavity. A 4×4-in. gauze square on sponge forceps can be useful to keep reduced organs in place while performing hernia repair. Important anatomical structures to avoid in this region when reducing hernia contents include the caudal rectal nerve (branch of the pudendal nerve) and caudal rectal artery (branch of the internal pudendal artery), which course together from lateral to medial near the center and dorsal aspect of the internal obturator muscle (Figure 34.2). Traditional herniorrhaphy involves the preplacement of nonabsorbable monofilament sutures (e.g., 2-0 polybutester) between the external anal sphincter and levator ani and/or coccygeus muscles. This procedure is considered outmoded due to tension across the muscular closure leading to repair failure and due to the realization that ventral support is required to minimize the chance of recurrence.

Internal Obturator Transposition

This surgical procedure is a traditional herniorrhaphy augmented with elevation and transposition of the internal obturator muscle into the repair, with or without transection of the tendon of the internal obturator muscle; currently, it is the initial surgical procedure of choice. The internal obturator muscle is elevated by first incising the caudal most attachment off the ischium through the periosteal tendinous insertion. A surgical elevator is used to lift the periosteum and muscle off the pelvis to the caudal extent of the obturator foramen, to midline of the pelvic floor, and to the lateral edge of the ischium to the point of the internal obturator muscle tendon. Care should be taken to not disrupt the sacrotuberous ligament, which inserts

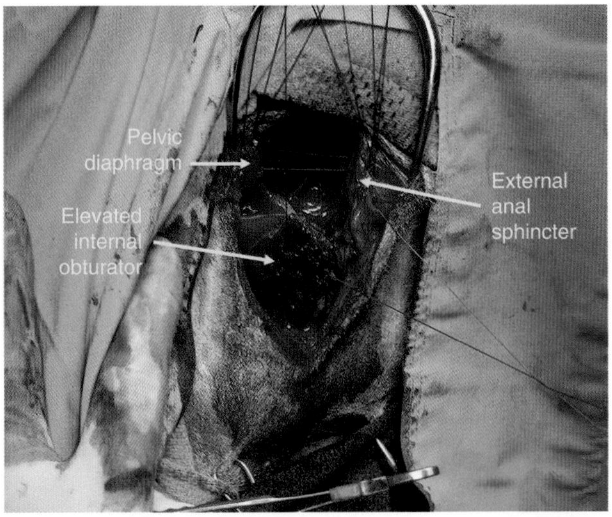

Figure 34.3 Intraoperative photograph of left-sided internal obturator transposition repair with preplaced nonabsorbable sutures placed between the internal obturator, levator ani and coccygeus, and external anal sphincter muscles.

onto the ischiatic tuberosity in dogs; this ligament is absent in cats. It is surgeon preference as to whether or not transection of the tendon of the internal obturator muscle is needed to improve mobilization of the muscle and decrease tension on the repair. The surgery proceeds as traditional herniorrhaphy but with the additional placement of sutures from the periosteal edge of the internal obturator muscle to the external anal sphincter and pelvic diaphragm musculature, creating a triangular configuration to repair the defect (Figure 34.3).

Sacrotuberous Ligament Incorporation

In dogs, if the levator ani and coccygeus muscles are too atrophied to be incorporated as a secure part of a perineal herniorrhaphy, the sacrotuberous ligament can be used instead. It is recommended to place sutures through the ligament, not around it, to avoid potential entrapment of the sciatic nerve. However, one study reports no major complications and no repair failure with sutures placed around the ligament.[5] As the sacrotuberous ligament is immobile, sutures placed from ligament to the external anal sphincter may deviate that side of the rectum cranially.

Superficial Gluteal Muscle Transposition

The superficial gluteal muscle is released from its insertion on the third trochanter, and a tip is to transect as closely as possible to the trochanter at the musculotendinous insertion to allow for eventual suturing of the tendon, which results in a more secure tissue for suturing compared to the muscle. The muscle is then rotated into the ischiorectal fossa, and the transected tendon is sutured with several preplaced encircling simple interrupted ligatures to the external anal sphincter. Alternatively, the tendon is sutured to the internal obturator muscle, and the caudal border of the muscle is sutured to the external anal sphincter. A combination of elevated internal obturator muscle and transposed superficial gluteal muscle into the perineal defect has also been reported.[6] This technique differs such that the tendon of the internal obturator muscle is transected medial to the ischiatic ridge and rotated medially to address the ventral component of the herniation. This technique may be chosen as an alternative to involvement of the sacrotuberous ligament, as there is less tension and less cranial deviation of the repair. Use of bilateral superficial gluteal muscles has been described to address ventral herniation.[7]

Semitendinosus Muscle Transposition

This aggressive technique is typically reserved for cases of recurrence and/or ventral herniation. The caudal hindlimb muscle is isolated on the contralateral side of the hernia and transected approximately midbody to allow 90–180° rotation into a ventral or lateral defect (Figure 34.4). The muscle can be sutured to any or all of the regional tissues as needed. A modification involves longitudinal splitting of the semitendinosus, leaving the lateral half of the muscle intact, providing a less redundant and more secure filling of the ventral defect.[8]

Implants

Biologic and prosthetic implants are used as a primary repair of the defect or to support other techniques. These implants include prosthetic mesh (e.g., polypropylene

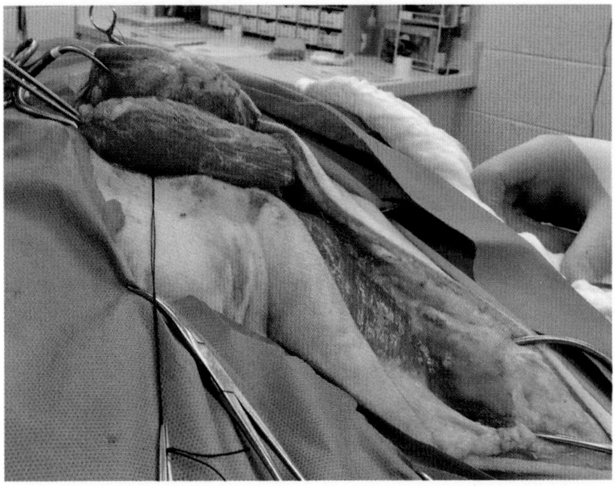

Figure 34.4 Intraoperative photograph following distal release and transposition of the right semitendinosus muscle for repair of a left-sided perineal hernia.

mesh), porcine small intestinal submucosa (porcine SIS), and autologous fascia.[9–11] Use of implants is of most use if initial muscular repair fails; however, use of the tunica vaginalis as a free autologous graft has been described with success for initial repair.[12–14]

Abdominal Organ Fixation

To address clinical signs associated with organ herniation, a caudal abdominal approach is utilized to perform colopexy, cystopexy, and/or deferentopexy. These techniques can be performed as a sole surgical procedure or in conjunction with primary repair at the level of the perineal region. An alternate technique description reports successful internal obturator transposition in conjunction with abdominal procedures with dogs in dorsal recumbency to avoid patient repositioning.[15]

For colopexy, the descending colon is retracted cranially to straighten the rectal diverticulum. A 3–4 cm section of the descending colon is sutured to the left abdominal wall by gentle scarification of the colonic serosa and the peritoneum with the underlying transversus abdominis muscle. The colonic wall is sutured to the abdominal wall using a simple interrupted or simple continuous pattern using long-term monofilament absorbable suture on a taper point needle. Alternatively, a partial thickness incision can be made through the seromuscular layer of the colon, and the apposition of the descending colon to the body wall may be created with one to two simple interrupted or simple continuous suture lines as noted above.

For cystopexy, a stay suture is placed in the apex of the bladder to facilitate manipulation and positioning of the bladder. The bladder is positioned cranially in the abdomen without excessive tension, which could potentially lead to chronic cystitis for the patient. A #15 scalpel blade is used to gently scarify the ventral bladder wall for most of the length of the body in a "hashtag" pattern. An area of similar size is created on the ventrolateral body wall just to the right or left of midline. Since this is typically performed in conjunction with a colopexy, which is performed on the left ventrolateral body wall closest to the descending colon, cystopexy is commonly performed on the right side. It is not recommended to incorporate the bladder wall in the abdominal wall closure. One or two rows of suture with a simple continuous pattern using 3-0 or 4-0 medium-term monofilament absorbable suture are placed to fix the bladder to the ventrolateral body wall (Figure 34.5). Suture should be placed partial thickness into the bladder, but absorbable suture is used in case of inadvertent luminal penetration.

For deferentopexy, each ductus deferens is located dorsal the trigone of the bladder in male dogs; this structure can be easily distinguished from the ureter, as it is freely movable and travels toward the inguinal ring instead of cranially to the renal hilus. Each ductus is transected at the level of the inguinal ring, and if castration has been performed at the same time during the surgical procedure, often the entire pedicle can be gently retracted into the abdominal cavity. Once the ductus has been isolated, it is pulled gently in a cranial direction until a small amount of tension is generated on the trigone and proximal urethra. At this level, two small transverse incisions approximately 1 cm apart are made in the transversus abdominis muscle. The ductus is fed through these incisions and then folded back on itself in a "belt-loop" type fashion. Several simple interrupted sutures of 4-0 monofilament nonabsorbable material are used to suture the end of the ductus to itself. This procedure is repeated on the other side, creating a gentle and even cranial pull of the trigone and proximal urethra.

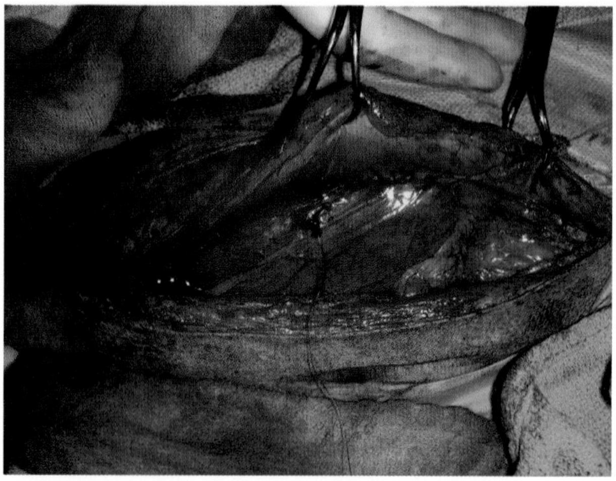

Figure 34.5 Intraoperative photograph of a cystopexy near completion. Cranial is to the right.

Postoperative Care

Immediately following surgery, a rectal examination is performed with the dog still under anesthesia to assess the repair and ensure absence of sutures within the rectum. Low-residue diets and stool softeners are recommended to decrease fecal volume and minimize straining, which could place excess tension on the surgical repair. Pain medications and optional antibiotics are sent home with the patient at the discretion of the surgeon.

Complications/Prognosis

Complications include repair failure, fecal incontinence, urinary incontinence, urinary bladder atony, tenesmus, sciatic nerve injury, rectocutaneous fistula, inadvertent prostatectomy, and incisional complications. Rates of complications, including recurrence, and thus, prognosis, are highly varied and dependent on numerous factors. Prognosis is independent of urinary bladder retroflexion.[16] When recurrence is encountered, the choice of additional procedure is dependent on the location of the hernia, the strength and viability of regional muscular anatomy, and the animal's clinical signs. It has been suggested that performing two or more procedures at the initial surgery makes recurrence uncommon.[4,6,8]

References

1 Åhlberg, T.M., Jokinen, T.S., Salonen, H.M. et al. (2022). Exploring the association between canine perineal hernia and neurological, orthopedic, and gastrointestinal diseases. *Acta Vet. Scand.* 64 (1): 39.

2 Hayashi, A.M., Rosner, S.A., de Assumpção, T.C. et al. (2016). Retrospective study (2009-2014): perineal hernias and related comorbidities in bitches. *Top. Compan. Anim. Med.* 31 (4): 130–133.

3 Åhlberg, T.M., Salonen, H.M., Laitinen-Vapaavuori, O.M. et al. (2022). CT imaging of dogs with perineal hernia reveals large prostates with morphological and spatial abnormalities. *Vet. Radiol. Ultrasound* 63 (5): 530–538.

4 Bernardé, A., Rochereau, P., Matres-Lorenzo, L. et al. (2018). Surgical findings and clinical outcome after bilateral repair of apparently unilateral perineal hernias in dogs. *J. Small Anim. Pract.* 59 (12): 734–741.

5 Cinti, F., Rossanese, M., Pisani, G. et al. (2021). A novel technique to incorporate the sacrotuberous ligament in perineal herniorrhaphy in 47 dogs. *Vet. Surg.* 50 (5): 1023–1031.

6 Carbonell Rosselló, G., Turner, A., Macias, C. et al. (2023). Combined transposition of internal obturator and superficial gluteal muscles for perineal hernia treatment in dogs: 17 cases (2017-2020). *J. Small Anim. Pract.* 64: 96–102.

7 Bitton, E., Keinan, Y., Shipov, A. et al. (2020). Use of bilateral superficial gluteal muscle flaps for the repair of ventral perineal hernia in dogs: a cadaveric study and short case series. *Vet. Surg.* 49 (8): 1536–1544.

8 Morello, E., Martano, M., Zabarino, S. et al. (2015). Modified semitendinosus muscle transposition to repair ventral perineal hernia in 14 dogs. *J. Small Anim. Pract.* 56 (6): 370–376.

9 Elkasapy, A.H., Shokry, M.M., Alakraa, A.M. et al. (2022). Prosthetic polyester-based hybrid mesh for repairing of perineal hernia in dogs. *Open Vet. J.* 12 (1): 124–128.

10 Swieton, N., Singh, A., Lopez, D. et al. (2020). Retrospective evaluation on the outcome of perineal herniorrhaphy augmented with porcine small intestinal submucosa in dogs and cats. *Can. Vet. J.* 61 (6): 629–637.

11 Bongartz, A., Carofiglio, F., Balligand, M. et al. (2005). Use of autogenous fascia lata graft for perineal herniorrhaphy in dogs. *Vet. Surg.* 34 (4): 405–413.

12 Pratummintra, K., Chuthatep, S., Banlunara, W. et al. (2013). Perineal hernia repair using an autologous tunica vaginalis communis in nine intact male dogs. *J. Vet. Med. Sci.* 75 (3): 337–341.

13 Guerios, S., Orms, K., and Serrano, M.A. (2020). Autologous tunica vaginalis graft to repair perineal hernia in shelter dogs. *Vet. Anim. Sci.* 9: 100122.

14 Heishima, T., Asano, K., Ishigaki, K. et al. (2022). Perineal herniorrhaphy with pedunculated tunica vaginalis communis in dogs: description of the technique and clinical case series. *Front. Vet. Sci.* 9: 931088.

15 Tobias, K.M. and Crombie, K. (2022). Perineal hernia repair in dorsal recumbency in 23 dogs: description of technique, complications, and outcome. *Vet. Surg.* 51 (5): 772–780.

16 Grand, J.G., Bureau, S., and Monnet, E. (2013). Effects of urinary bladder retroflexion and surgical technique on postoperative complication rates and long-term outcome in dogs with perineal hernia: 41 cases (2002-2009). *J. Am. Vet. Med. Assoc.* 243 (10): 1442–1447.

35

Anal Sacculectomy in Dogs and Cats

Arathi Vinayak

VCA West Coast Animal Emergency and Specialty Hospital, Fountain Valley, CA, USA

Key Points

- The most common non-neoplastic conditions of the anal sacs in dogs and cats include anal sacculitis, abscessation, and impaction.
- The most common neoplastic conditions of the canine anal sacs include apocrine gland anal sac adenocarcinoma, malignant melanoma, squamous cell carcinoma, perianal adenoma, perianal adenocarcinoma, lymphoma, mast cell tumor, and hemangiosarcoma.
- The most common neoplastic conditions of the feline anal sacs include apocrine gland anal sac adenocarcinoma and squamous cell carcinoma.
- If neoplasia is confirmed via cytology, staging diagnostics, including bloodwork, diagnostic imaging (i.e., thoracic radiographs, abdominal ultrasound), and/or fine needle aspiration for cytology of intraabdominal abnormalities noted on imaging, are recommended prior to surgery.
- Expression of anal sac contents and manual evacuation of the terminal rectum with either placement of an anocutaneous pursestring suture or gauze-packing are recommended pre-operatively to prevent contamination of the surgery site. Enemas are not recommended.
- Careful surgical techniques can minimize complications with low complication rates reported in dogs. While complication rates are high in cats, they tend to be self-limiting. Rectal perforation is an uncommon iatrogenic complication.
- Prognosis is good following anal sacculectomy for benign conditions. Prognosis is guarded to poor depending on the malignancy type and stage of disease.

Introduction

Anal sacs are paired sinuses consisting of a fundus and neck with a duct that opens on the anocutaneous junction at the 4 and 8 o'clock positions sandwiched between an external striated anal sphincter muscle and an inner smooth anal sphincter muscle. Non-neoplastic disease of the anal sacs occurs commonly in dogs with an incidence of 12.5–15.7% and is less common with an incidence of 0.4% in cats.[1–3] This non-neoplastic disease can be broadly divided into three categories of impaction, inflammation, and abscessation with all being on a continuum of the same disease process.[4,5] Impaction refers to a non-painful condition where the contents of the anal sac cannot be expressed. Inflammation, commonly referred to as anal sacculitis, is a swollen, painful condition that sometimes is associated with pyrexia. Abscessation refers to a painful swelling of the anal sac region associated with pyrexia and purulent and/or bloody discharge. Predisposing factors identified in a recent study included certain dermatological conditions, diarrhea, certain dog breeds (predilection in small dog breeds), male cats, and obesity in dogs.[1] Other

Techniques in Small Animal Soft Tissue, Orthopedic, and Ophthalmic Surgery, First Edition. Edited by Kristin A. Coleman.

Companion website: www.wiley.com/go/coleman/surgeries

factors identified include diet, pudendal nerve dysfunction, perianal fistulas, and inflammatory bowel disease.[6] Impaction appears to be the most common refractory problem.[1] While medical management is the mainstay for non-neoplastic conditions, anal sacculectomy is considered for refractory cases or if the client no longer wants to pursue medical management.

Surgery remains the mainstay for dogs and cats with neoplasia of the anal sacs. In dogs, apocrine gland anal sac adenocarcinoma (AGASACA) is the most common malignancy seen in this region.[7] As the name suggests, neoplastic transformation occurs in the glandular epithelial cells of the apocrine glands within the anal sacs.[8,9] While cure is seldom achieved, long-term survival can be achieved in early stages of disease and in dogs with small tumors, underscoring the importance of routine rectal examinations.

Spaniel breeds are over-represented with Cocker Spaniels having a mean relative risk estimate of 7.3.[10] Other predisposed breeds are German Shepherds, Alaskan Malamutes, Dachshunds, and Golden retrievers.[10–12] AGASACA is typically seen in middle-aged to older dogs with a median age of presentation is 9–11 years.[10–14] The more recent literature shows a relatively equal male and female prevalence.[10–14] Clinical signs associated with the tumor include perianal swelling, bloody discharge, scooting, misshapen stools, straining during defecation, and urinary incontinence.[9–16] Paraneoplastic hypercalcemia seen with this malignancy is due to production of parathyroid hormone-related protein (PTHrP) by the tumor. PTHrP functions in a manner like endogenous parathyroid hormone (PTH) by binding to receptors on renal tubular cells and osteoblasts, increasing the renal reabsorption of calcium and resorption of bone.[17] The resultant elevations in ionized and total calcium lead to inhibition of antidiuretic hormone as the mechanism behind the polyuria and polydipsia.[16] Hypercalcemia is noted in 27–53% of dogs with AGASACA.[11,12,16–19] The more recent studies in veterinary patients do not show hypercalcemia to be a negative prognostic indicator in the face of treatment.[11,20]

Other malignancies of the anal sac and perianal region include malignant melanoma, squamous cell carcinoma, perianal adenoma, perianal adenocarcinoma, lymphoma, mast cell tumor, and hemangiosarcoma.[10–14,21–26] Malignant anal sac melanoma (MASM) is an uncommon but very aggressive malignancy in dogs.[21] Bloody anal sac discharge and perianal licking are the most common presenting signs. Anal sac tumors have different prognoses depending on benign versus malignant status, tumor type, stage of disease, and treatment chosen. An in-depth discussion of the many tumor types, stages, and prognoses is not possible for the scope of this chapter, and discussion will be limited to brief discussions on prognosis after surgical excision.

Anal sac tumors in cats are uncommon and include AGASACA and squamous cell carcinoma.[27–31] Discharge and perianal ulceration were the most common clinical signs noted in cats with AGASACA and may lead to a delay in diagnosis, as the signs are similar to anal sac impaction/anal sacculitis/abscessation.[28,29] A thorough rectal examination with fine needle aspiration is warranted in cats with this presentation.[29] Paraneoplastic hypercalcemia has been reported in 1 of 5 cats in one study, and 3 of 27 cats in another study, but whether the mechanism of this hypercalcemia is due to elevated PTHrP production by the tumor is yet to be elucidated.[28,29] Squamous cell carcinoma of the anal sac in cats is a very rare disease with report of only two cats in the veterinary literature. Thus, there is little information on tumor behavior and prognosis in cats. Only one of the two cats was treated with surgery and adjuvant radiation and chemotherapy with local recurrence reported 236 days after surgery and euthanasia at 552 days post-surgery. The other cat in the report was euthanized 28 days following medical management with anti-inflammatories.[31]

Indications/Pre-op Considerations

Infections, impactions, and draining tracts need to be treated in advance of surgery to decrease the risk of complications postoperatively.[1] Untreated infection/inflammation can obscure visualization and lead to intraoperative complications, such as incomplete excision of the sac or duct, contamination of the surgical field with infection, and/or iatrogenic rectal perforation.

In cases where anal sac tumors are suspected, diagnosis is confirmed with a fine needle aspiration of the mass. If malignancy is confirmed, staging must be performed prior to proceeding with surgery. Staging diagnostics are similar for malignancies of the anal sacs in dogs and cats. Bloodwork consisting of a complete blood count, serum chemistry, urinalysis, and/or ionized calcium if total calcium is elevated is recommended. If ionized hypercalcemia is noted, PTH and PTHrP evaluation is recommended to differentiate primary hyperparathyroidism from hypercalcemia due to malignancy. Thoracic and abdominal imaging is recommended, as metastasis to the medial iliac, internal iliac (formerly known as hypogastric), and sacral lymph nodes occurs in up to 96% of affected AGASACA dogs.[11,12,20,32,33] The most recent computed tomography (CT) staging study for AGASACA revealed iliosacral lymphadenopathy in 71% and pulmonary metastasis in 11%.[34] Other less common sites of metastasis include liver, bone, and spleen.[11–13]

Markedly enlarged lymph nodes in the iliosacral or sublumbar region are more likely to be consistently detected on abdominal radiographs due to significant ventral displacement of the colon, opacity in the retroperitoneal space caudally, and lack of clear delineation of the ventral iliopsoas muscle.[35] The sensitivity and specificity of abdominal radiographs in the detection of iliosacral lymphadenopathy for general practitioners, radiology residents, and board-certified radiologists were 81/70%, 94/81%, and 75/100%, respectively.[35] Mild to moderate enlargement of the iliosacral lymph nodes may be missed on radiographs, necessitating the need for advanced imaging. Abdominal ultrasonography is routinely used for staging in veterinary medicine but has limitations, as caudally-located lymph nodes within the pelvis (such as the sacral nodes affected with anal sac malignancies) will likely be missed. When ultrasound was compared to CT for AGASACA staging, ultrasound correctly identified all affected nodes in only 30.8% of affected dogs but was able to identify at least one enlarged node in all affected dogs.[36] Another comparative study evaluating ultrasound and magnetic resonance imaging (MRI) showed that while MRI identified all abnormal lymph nodes, ultrasound only detected abnormal nodes in 33% of dogs (two of six affected dogs).[37] Thus, CT or MRI should be considered for more accurate staging for malignancies. Fine needle aspiration of any concerning findings that have the potential to represent metastasis is performed using imaging guidance for cytology. Cytology, in addition to imaging, will help identify stage, prognosis, and treatment options prior to surgery. Other tumors of the anal sacs are also staged similarly.

Open, closed, and modified closed techniques have been described.[6,38,39] The open technique is seldom used and not advocated, as this technique has a 13.67 times higher long-term complication rate when compared to a closed technique.[38] A modified closed technique pioneered by the late Dr. Phil Hobson at Texas A&M University was recently described and published.[40] The modified closed technique has an advantage over the traditional closed technique in that the entirety of the duct, including its anocutaneous opening, is excised in the case of neoplasia, thus ideally minimizing chances of tumor recurrence. Regardless of the technique chosen, care should be taken to minimize damage to the adjacent rectal wall, external anal sphincter muscle, caudal rectal nerve (branch of pudendal nerve), and caudal rectal artery (branch of internal pudendal artery).[39] If an open technique is used, care must be taken to ensure all of the sac and duct complex is excised.

The patient is placed in sternal recumbency with a towel to raise the caudal abdomen to elevate this area. The tail is gently secured cranially; over-extension of the tail is avoided to prevent nerve damage in the lumbosacral region. The anal sacs are expressed of their contents and flushed with a 22-gauge catheter, and the terminal rectum is manually evacuated of feces to prevent contamination intraoperatively. Lubricated tampon or gauze is rolled and gently inserted into the terminal rectum, and a pursestring anal suture may be placed additionally cranial to the anocutaneous anal sac duct openings. Enemas are not recommended, as liquid feces may not be contained by the gauze and pursestring suture. The pelvic limbs can be flexed at the stifles and hock such that the entire limb can be secured on the table. Alternatively, the stifle can be extended with the pelvic limbs positioned off the table, but padding between the limb and table is recommended, as there are anecdotal reports of femoral nerve damage and resultant limb paresis in the postoperative period.

Surgical Procedure

Standard Closed Technique

A mosquito hemostat or a groove director is inserted from the anal sac opening into the duct and then into the sac base. The instrument is then pushed outwards against the skin such that a curvilinear incision can be made over the sac base. This places the incision parallel to the external anal sphincter, which is then dissected from the surrounding tissues. The external anal sphincter muscle is then transected from the sac base, and care is taken to keep this dissection tight around the sac itself to prevent iatrogenic permanent damage to the muscle. Once the base is freed, the duct is traced to its opening and ligated with a small (4-0) short-term monofilament absorbable suture in a circumferential pattern near its opening. The surgical site is lavaged thoroughly. Gloves and instruments are changed. Closure is performed of the external anal sphincter, subcutaneous tissue, and the skin. Rectal sponges and pursestring suture are removed, and the rectum is palpated for any perforations not noted during dissection.

Modified Closed Technique

An incision is made over the anal sac duct and extended to the base. An instrument (hemostat or a groove director) is inserted into the duct to serve as a guide (Figure 35.1). The anal sac opening is excised in its entirety at the anocutaneous junction, and the duct is dissected from the rectal wall, including the internal sphincter muscle in cases of neoplasia. Laterally, the external anal sphincter muscle is either excised with the sac base in non-neoplastic conditions or en bloc with the anal sac tumor. Dissection is then continued ventrally and medially along the rectal wall to free up the remaining anal sac base. Instruments and gloves are changed, and the site is lavaged thoroughly. Closure is performed to appose the external anal sphincter muscle, subcutaneous tissue, and external skin. Rectal sponges and pursestring suture are removed, and the rectum is palpated for any perforations not noted during dissection.

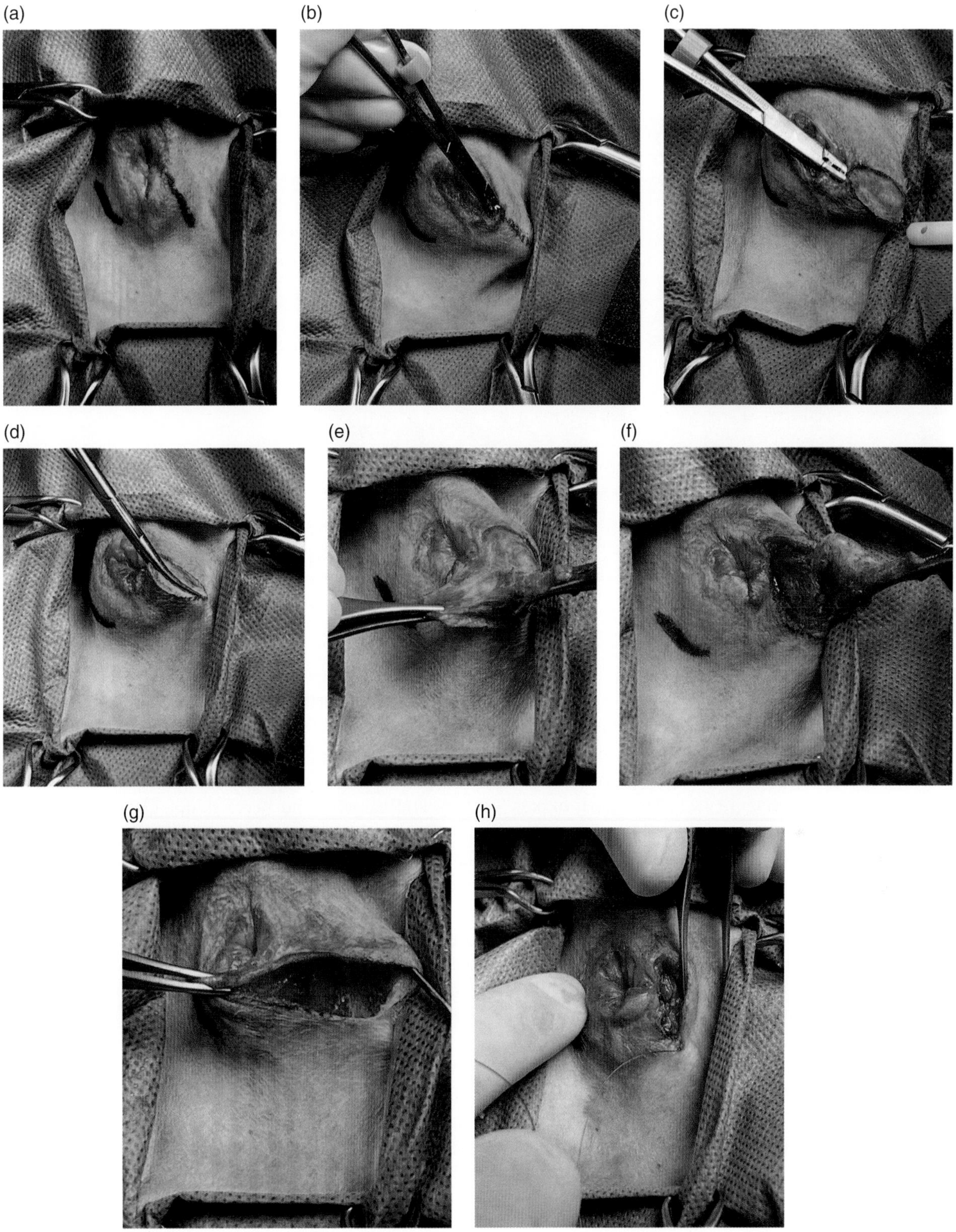

Figure 35.1 Modified closed anal sacculectomy. (a) Image shows the curvilinear incision used in the standard closed technique over the left anal sac versus the incision used in the modified closed technique parallel along the length of the duct and anal sac base. (b) A mosquito hemostat or a groove director is inserted from the anal opening into the duct and then directed into the sac base. (c) The instrument is pushed outwards against the skin, and an incision is made parallel to the instrument and perpendicular to the external anal sphincter muscle. The external anal sphincter muscle is incised on either side of the sac base. (d) A new mosquito hemostat is then inserted with one arm within the duct and one on the exterior of the duct to allow manipulation of the duct and sac. The duct opening is excised at the anocutaneous junction. (e,f) Dissection is then carried out using the hemostat to direct the sac/duct complex away from the rectal wall to allow for continued dissection ventrally and medially away from the rectal wall. Caudal traction of the sac is important to continue dissection away from the more cranially located caudal rectal nerve. (g) The surgical site is lavaged thoroughly, and gloves and instruments are changed. (h) Closure is performed of the external anal sphincter and subcutaneous tissue. (i) Skin is apposed with either non-absorbable suture that requires removal or a short-term dissolvable suture, such as poliglecaprone 25, that does not require removal (shown in the image). Rectal sponges and pursestring suture are removed, and the rectum is palpated for any perforations not noted during dissection. (j) Image of the excised anal sac and duct complex.

(i) (j)

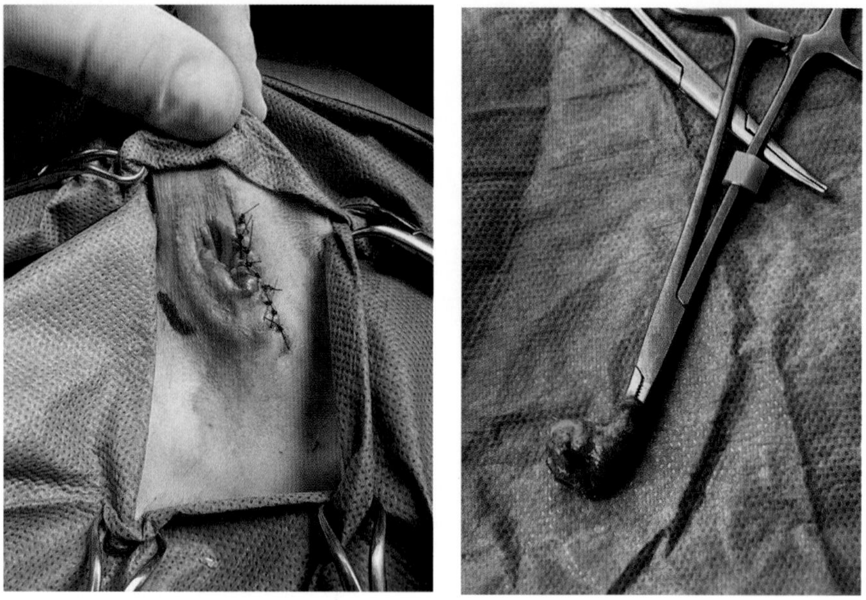

Figure 35.1 (Continued)

Anal Sac Catheter Technique

This technique for anal sacculectomy is recommended for anal sacs that may be catheterized and have a lumen, which means it is not possible with large tumors that obliterate the anal sac lumen (Figure 35.2). The idea is to pass the catheter tip balloon into the anal sac through the duct, inflate the balloon, incise the tissue around the anal sac duct (leaving a few millimeters of mucosa around the tubing), and apply traction to the catheter tubing to provide gentle traction on the anal sac as it is gradually dissected from between the internal and external anal sphincter muscles. An anal sac catheter is a Foley catheter with a short, low profile tip that continues past the balloon (compared to the longer traditional Foley catheter tips), which allows for inflation of the balloon in the anal sac. The editor prefers to use this technique with the MILA brand of anal sac catheters, which come in both 4 and 6 Fr balloons. A benefit of this technique is the en bloc excision of both anal sac and duct, as well as caudal traction during the procedure, which allows for dissection from surrounding tissues away from the neurovascular bundle in the area. If the balloon slips out during manipulation, a pursestring suture may be placed around the duct opening to secure the balloon within the lumen. Just like the other techniques, instruments and gloves are changed after removal of the excised anal sac, and the site is lavaged thoroughly. Closure is performed to appose the external anal sphincter muscle, subcutaneous tissue, and external skin. Rectal sponges and pursestring suture are removed, and the rectum is palpated for any perforations not noted during dissection.

Potential Complications

Intraoperative complications include hemorrhage, rectal wall perforation, incomplete excision of the anal sac or duct, and vascular and nerve trauma. Short-term minor complications include swelling, discharge from the incision line, seroma, infection, scooting, tenesmus, and dyschezia.[39] Long-term complications are seldom reported in dogs with fecal incontinence, fistulae, strictures, and continued licking reported in 1.1–14.7% of dogs.[39,41] If the caudal rectal nerve is severed during surgical dissection, innervation from the contralateral side occurs within a few weeks after unilateral surgery, contributing to the low rate of permanent incontinence.[6,38] If fecal incontinence is noted greater than three to four months postoperatively, this is often a permanent sequela and likely due to bilateral single-stage surgery and/or excessive trauma to the external anal sphincter or the caudal rectal nerve.[38,42]

In a study of cats with non-neoplastic anal sac conditions, the rate of short-term postop complications was high in 50% of cats; however, all resolved without further intervention and were, thus, considered minor. Fecal incontinence was not reported as a permanent sequela.[43]

Infection can occur due to contamination during surgery as well as fecal contamination of the incision site in the postop period. Wound care with lavage, surgical debridement, antibiotic therapy, and open wound management generally allows for successful resolution of a surgical site infection. Draining tracts in and around the surgery site should raise the concern for gland/ductular remnants and

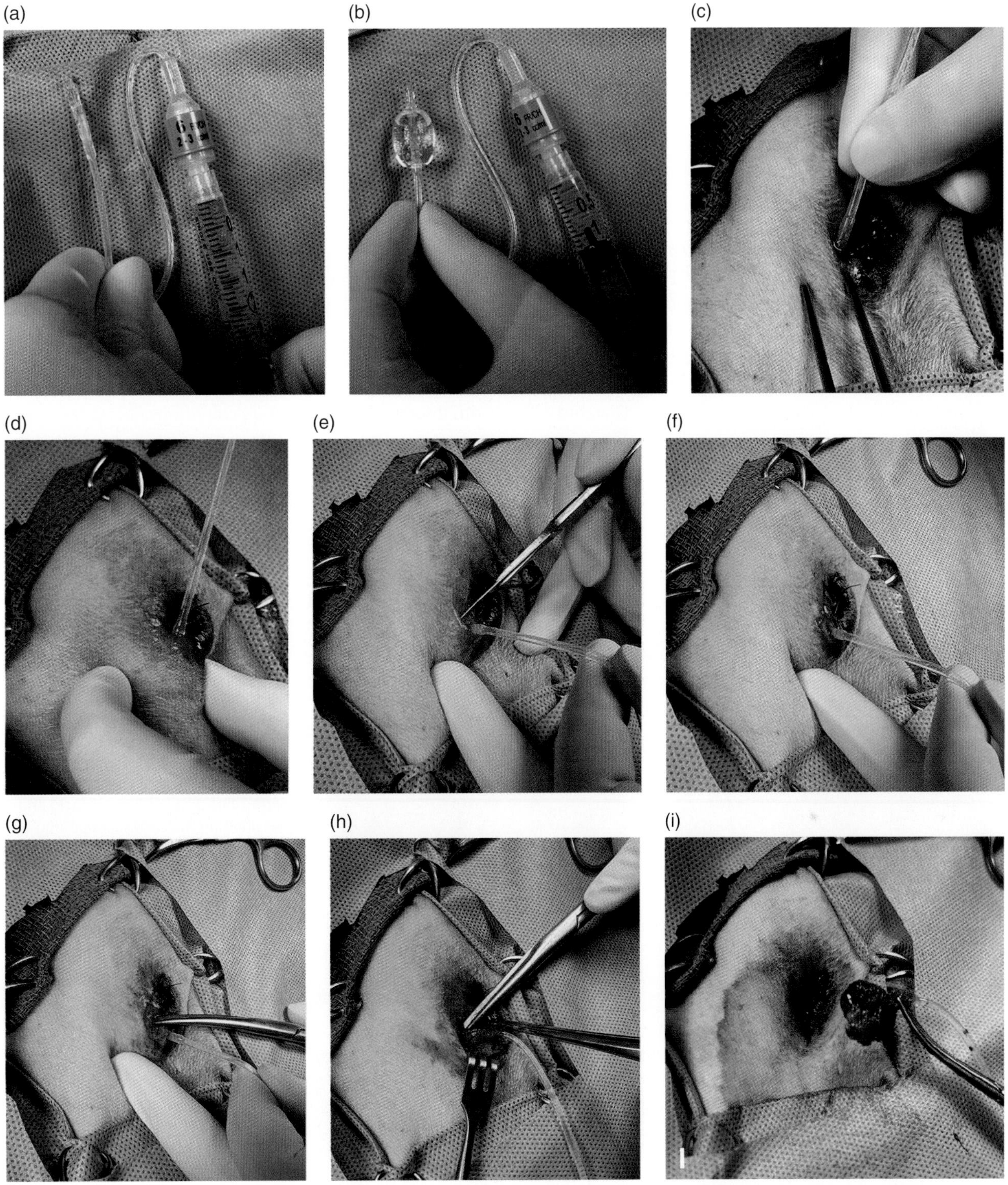

Figure 35.2 Anal sac catheter anal sacculectomy technique. (a) Following placement of the pursestring suture and sterile draping of the area, the anal sac catheter should be chosen based on size of the patient and the anticipated anal sac lumen: 4 Fr (up to 1 mL saline to be instilled into balloon) or 6 Fr (up to 3 mL saline to be instilled into balloon). (b) A syringe of saline should be attached and used to inflate the catheter balloon to assess for leakage prior to placement into the patient. (c) The lubricated tip of the catheter is passed into the anal sac duct. (d) Saline is infused into the catheter balloon until the point of allowing tension on the catheter tubing without the balloon being pulled out of the anal sac lumen. While this particular catheter balloon had a maximum capacity fill of 3 mL, only 2 mL was needed for infusion. Filling to the maximum capacity could result in rupture of the balloon or the anal sac wall. (e,f) A scalpel blade (#11 or #15) is used to make a circumferential incision around the anal sac duct opening, leaving a few millimeters of tissue for manipulation of the catheter. If too little tissue is left around catheter, the anal sac duct may be widened to the point of the balloon slipping out during application of tension. (g) Curved Metzenbaum scissors are used for small careful bites to dissect the anal sphincter muscles from the anal sac. (h) Dissection is continued circumferentially with the dominant hand while traction is being applied to the tubing with the non-dominant hand. (i) After the anal sac is removed, hemostasis is confirmed, the region is lavaged, gloves and instruments are changed, and routine closure is performed. *Source:* © Kristin Coleman.

require a revision surgery if remnants are suspected. Iatrogenic rectal perforation if noted intraop is addressed and can also present similar to a surgery site infection; however, discharge with fecal elements is an indication for a thorough gentle exploration of the adjacent rectal wall to ensure this is addressed.

Rectal perforations addressed in surgery or after surgery with primary repair of the rectal wall tend to recur, as the rectal wall seldom retains the sutures (Figure 35.3). This complication can be managed by surgically opening the entire dehiscence tract to the rectal perforation, and the site is then managed by hydrotherapy several times a day to keep the area as clean as possible from fecal contamination that will inevitably occur after defecation. Diarrhea, if present concurrently, will need to be managed to prevent constant contamination of the site. Second-intention healing will occur with appropriate care, and the site generally heals within two to three weeks postoperatively.

Post-op Care

Infiltration of the tissues at the time of closure with liposome-encapsulated bupivacaine is helpful for pain management. Postoperative narcotics and anti-inflammatory medications are used as part of multimodal pain management. Antibiotics are considered in patients with infectious/inflammatory conditions necessitating the

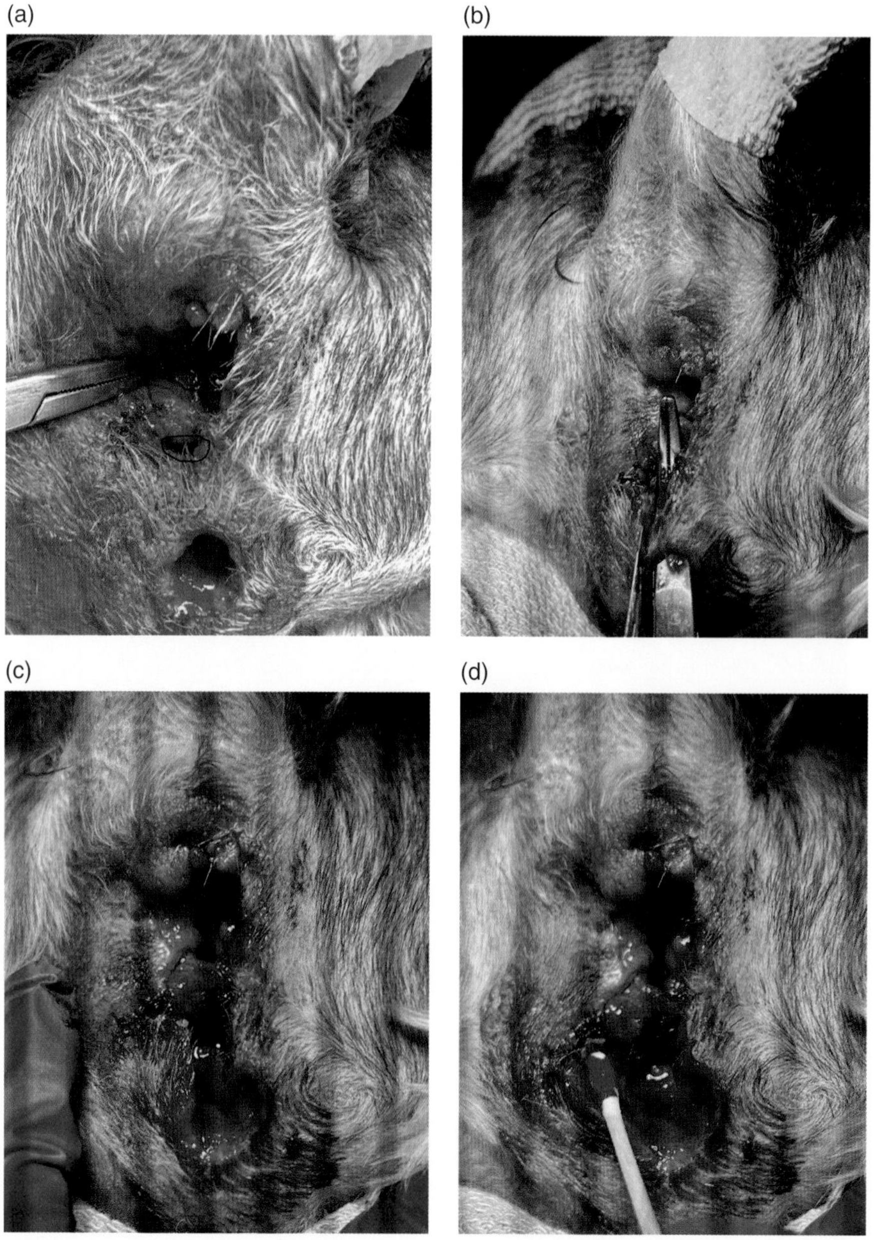

Figure 35.3 Rectal perforation following anal sacculectomy in a 10-year-old spayed female dog for chronic anal sac abscessation. The rectal wall site had been repaired primarily four days postop when fecal material was noted oozing from the incision site after defecation. A Penrose drain had been placed at the same time as primary rectal wall repair. Three days following the repair, fecal material was noted to be exiting the Penrose drain site. (a) Image shows dehiscence of the rectal perforation site (circled in black) and the draining tract with an opening at the Penrose drain site ventral to the perforation. A hemostat indicates the anal opening and terminal rectum. (b) A new mosquito hemostat is inserted into the tract to exit at the level of the rectal perforation, and a #15 blade is then used to incise overlying skin and expose the draining tract. (c) The tract is now contiguous with the rectal perforation without closed areas for fecal accumulation. (d) The surgery site is then managed with hydrotherapy to heal by second intention.

anal sacculectomy, or if contamination of the surgery field occurs intraoperatively. Modification to the diet to include fiber to make the stools bulky allows for a more complete emptying of the rectum and may prevent fecal contamination of the incision site from loose stools. Stress colitis must be managed immediately. Elizabethan collars are a must for all dogs and cats to prevent self-mutilation of the surgery site with subsequent dehiscence and infection. Scooting must be prevented to avoid injury to the site. This can be managed with sedation, confinement in a crate or run to limit access to rough surfaces, and an abdominal sling to lift up during walks if scooting were to occur.

Prognosis

Prognosis after anal sacculectomy for benign disease is excellent.

Prognosis for early-stage, non-metastatic AGASACA in dogs with a primary tumor size of <3.2 cm with surgery only is favorable with a median survival time of 1237 days reported.[9] Local recurrence rates are low and generally between 12% and 22%.[9,32,44] Wide-margin excisions are not feasible in this region due to the tumors wedged against the rectal wall and infiltrating the external and internal anal sphincter muscles. In dogs with metastatic lymph nodes, surgical excision of the primary anal sac tumor in addition to the metastatic nodes can lead to prolonged survival times ranging between 713 and 1035 days.[41,44]

In dogs with squamous cell carcinoma of the anal sacs, local progression appears to be the leading cause of death in dogs.[22] In dogs with MASM, regardless of treatment, prognosis was guarded to poor with a mean overall survival time of 107 days, and most dogs are euthanized due to locoregional or distant disease progression.[21] Earlier diagnosis of MASM may improve survival times, as the one dog in the report with a small tumor and complete excision survived more than a year after surgery.[21]

In cats undergoing anal sacculectomy for apocrine gland anal sac adenocarcinoma, local recurrence appears to be the life-limiting factor (11 of 30 cats) with local recurrence more frequently noted with an incomplete excision and high nuclear pleomorphic scores.[29] This highlights the need for early detection and wide margins obtained in surgery. The overall median disease-free interval and survival time were 234 and 260 days.[29] The poor prognosis is likely due to a more advanced stage of local disease from a lack of routine rectal examinations in cats, complicated by the rare occurrence of both benign and malignant diseases in feline anal sacs with similar clinical signs. Adjuvant radiation and chemotherapy for this disease needs further evaluation. In the report of two cats with squamous cell carcinoma of the anal sacs, one of the two cats was treated with surgery and adjuvant radiation and chemotherapy with local recurrence noted at 236 days after surgery, and euthanasia due to disease progression at 552 days post-surgery.[31] The other cat in the report was medically palliated with anti-inflammatory therapy and euthanized 28 days after diagnosis.[31]

References

1 Corbee, R.J., Woldring, H.H., van den Eijnde, L.M. et al. (2021). A cross-sectional study on canine and feline anal sac disease. *Animals* 12 (1): 95. https://pubmed.ncbi.nlm.nih.gov/35011201.

2 Halnan, C.R.E. (1976). The frequency of occurrence of anal sacculitis in the dog. *J. Small Anim. Pract.* 17 (8): 537–541.

3 Halnan, C.R.E. (1976). Therapy of anal sacculitis in the dog. *J. Small Anim. Pract.* 17 (10): 685–691.

4 Frankel, J.L., Scott, D.W., and Erb, H.N. (2008). Gross and cytological characteristics of normal feline anal-sac secretions. *J. Feline Med. Surg.* 10 (4): 319–323.

5 Duijkeren, E. (1995). Disease conditions of canine anal sacs. *J. Small Anim. Pract.* 36 (1): 12–16.

6 Matthiesen, D.T. and Marretta, S.M. (1993). Diseases of the anus and rectum. In: *Small Animal Surgery*, 2e (ed. D. Slatter), 627–645. Philadephia: Saunders.

7 Berrocal, A., Vos, J.H., van den Ingh, T.S.G.A.M. et al. (1989). Canine perineal tumours. *J. Vet. Med. Ser. A* 36 (1–10): 739–749.

8 Pradel, J., Berlato, D., Dobromylskyj, M. et al. (2018). Prognostic significance of histopathology in canine anal sac gland adenocarcinomas: preliminary results in a retrospective study of 39 cases. *Vet. Comp. Oncol.* 16 (4): 518–528.

9 Skorupski, K.A., Alarcón, C.N., de Lorimier, L.P. et al. (2018). Outcome and clinical, pathological, and immunohistochemical factors associated with prognosis for dogs with early-stage anal sac adenocarcinoma treated with surgery alone: 34 cases (2002–2013). *J. Am. Vet. Med. Assoc.* 253 (1): 84–91. https://pubmed.ncbi.nlm.nih.gov/29911942.

10 Polton, G.A., Mowat, V., Lee, H.C. et al. (2006). Breed, gender and neutering status of British dogs with anal sac gland carcinoma. *Vet. Comp. Oncol.* 4 (3): 125–131. https://pubmed.ncbi.nlm.nih.gov/19754809.

11 Bennett, P.F., DeNicola, D.B., Bonney, P. et al. (2002). Canine anal sac adenocarcinomas: clinical presentation and response to therapy. *J. Vet. Intern. Med.* 16 (1): 100–104.

12 Williams, L.E., Gliatto, J.M., Dodge, R.K. et al. (2003). Carcinoma of the apocrine glands of the anal sac in dogs: 113 cases (1985-1995). *J. Am. Vet. Med. Assoc.* 223 (6): 825–831.

13 Polton, G.A. and Brearley, M.L. (2007). Clinical stage, therapy, and prognosis in canine anal sac gland carcinoma. *J. Vet. Int. Med.* 21 (2): 274–280.

14 Goldschmidt, M.H. and Zoltowski, C. (1981). Anal sac gland adenocarcinoma in the dog: 14 cases. *J. Small Anim. Pract.* 22 (3): 119–128. https://pubmed.ncbi.nlm.nih.gov/7230749.

15 Ross, J.T., Scavelli, T., and Matthiesen, D. (1991). Adenocarcinoma of the apocrine glands of the anal sac in dogs: a review of 32 cases. *J. Am. Anim. Hosp. Assoc.* 27: 349–355.

16 Repasy, A.B., Selmic, L.E., and Kisseberth, W.C. (2022). Canine apocrine gland anal sac adenocarcinoma: a review. *Top. Compan. Anim. Med.* 50: 1–10. https://pubmed.ncbi.nlm.nih.gov/35792243.

17 Bergman, P.J. (2012). Paraneoplastic hypercalcemia. *Top. Compan. Anim. Med.* 27 (4): 156–158. https://pubmed.ncbi.nlm.nih.gov/23415382.

18 Gröne, A., Weckmann, M.T., Blomme, E.A.G. et al. (1998). Dependence of humoral hypercalcemia of malignancy on parathyroid hormone-related protein expression in the canine anal sac apocrine gland adenocarcinoma (CAC-8) nude mouse model. *Vet. Pathol.* 35 (5): 344–351.

19 Rosol, T.J., Nagode, L.A., Couto, C.G. et al. (1992). Parathyroid hormone (PTH)-related protein, PTH, and 1,25-dihydroxy vitamin D in dogs with cancer-associated hypercalcemia. *Endocrinology* 131 (3): 1157–1164.

20 Hoelzler, M.G., Bellah, J.R., and Donofro, M.C. (2001). Omentalization of cystic sublumbar lymph node metastases for long-term palliation of tenesmus and dysuria in a dog with anal sac adenocarcinoma. *J. Am. Vet. Med. Assoc.* 219 (12): 1729–1731. https://pubmed.ncbi.nlm.nih.gov/11767923.

21 Vinayak, A., Frank, C.B., Gardiner, D.W. et al. (2017). Malignant anal sac melanoma in dogs: eleven cases (2000 to 2015). *J. Small Anim. Pract.* 58 (4): 231–237.

22 Esplin, D.G., Wilson, S.R., and Hullinger, G.A. (2003). Squamous cell carcinoma of the anal sac in five dogs. *Vet. Pathol.* 40 (3): 332–334.

23 Mellett, S., Verganti, S., Murphy, S., and Bowlt, K. (2015). Squamous cell carcinoma of the anal sacs in three dogs. *J. Small Anim. Pract.* 56 (3): 223–225. https://pubmed.ncbi.nlm.nih.gov/25208811.

24 Sfiligoi, G., Rassnick, K.M., Scarlett, J.M. et al. (2005). Outcome of dogs with mast cell tumors in the inguinal or perineal region versus other cutaneous locations: 124 cases (1990–2001). *J. Am. Vet. Med. Assoc.* 226 (8): 1368–1374.

25 Choi, E.W. (2019). Deep dermal and subcutaneous canine hemangiosarcoma in the perianal area: diagnosis of perianal mass in a dog. *BMC Vet. Res.* 15 (1): 1–5.

26 Kosanovich Cahalane, A., Payne, S., Barber, L.G. et al. (2004). Prognostic factors for survival of dogs with inguinal and perineal mast cell tumors treated surgically with or without adjunctive treatment: 68 cases (1994-2002). *J. Am. Vet. Med. Assoc.* 225 (3): 401–408. https://pubmed.ncbi.nlm.nih.gov/15328716.

27 Parry, N.M.A. (2006). Anal sac gland carcinoma in a cat. *Vet. Pathol.* 43 (6): 1008–1009.

28 Shoieb, A.M. and Hanshaw, D.M. (2009). Anal sac gland carcinoma in 64 cats in the United Kingdom (1995-2007). *Vet. Pathol.* 46 (4): 677–683.

29 Amsellem, P.M., Cavanaugh, R.P., Chou, P.Y. et al. (2019). Apocrine gland anal sac adenocarcinoma in cats: 30 cases (1994–2015). *J. Am. Vet. Med. Assoc.* 254 (6): 716–722.

30 Elliott, J.W. and Blackwood, L. (2011). Treatment and outcome of four cats with apocrine gland carcinoma of the anal sac and review of the literature. *J. Feline Med. Surg.* 13 (10): 712–717.

31 Kopke, M.A., Gal, A., Piripi, S.A., and Poirier, V.J. (2021). Squamous cell carcinoma of the anal sac in two cats. *J. Small Anim. Pract.* 62 (8): 704–708.

32 Emms, S.G. (2005). Anal sac tumours of the dog and their response to cytoreductive surgery and chemotherapy. *Aust. Vet. J.* 83 (6): 340–343. https://pubmed.ncbi.nlm.nih.gov/15986909.

33 Turek, M.M., Forrest, L.J., Adams, W.M. et al. (2003). Postoperative radiotherapy and mitoxantrone for anal sac adenocarcinoma in the dog: 15 cases (1991-2001). *Vet. Comp. Oncol.* 1 (2): 94–104. http://www.ncbi.nlm.nih.gov/pubmed/19379321.

34 Sutton, D.R., Hernon, T., Hezzell, M.J. et al. (2022). Computed tomographic staging of dogs with anal sac adenocarcinoma. *J. Small Anim. Pract.* 63 (1): 27–33.

35 Murphy, M.C., Sullivan, M., Gomes, B.J. et al. (2020). Evaluation of radiographs for the detection of sublumbar lymphadenopathy in dogs. *Can. Vet. J.* 61 (7): 749–756.

36 Palladino, S., Keyerleber, M.A., King, R.G., and Burgess, K.E. (2016). Utility of computed tomography versus abdominal ultrasound examination to identify iliosacral lymphadenomegaly in dogs with apocrine gland adenocarcinoma of the anal sac. *J. Vet. Intern. Med.* 30 (6): 1858–1863.

37 Anderson, C.L., Mackay, C.S., Roberts, G.D., and Fidel, J. (2015). Comparison of abdominal ultrasound and magnetic resonance imaging for detection of abdominal lymphadenopathy in dogs with metastatic apocrine gland adenocarcinoma of the anal sac. *Vet. Comp. Oncol.* 13 (2): 98–105. https://pubmed.ncbi.nlm.nih.gov/23432735.

38 Hill, L.N. and Smeak, D.D. (2002). Open versus closed bilateral anal sacculectomy for treatment of non-neoplastic anal sac disease in dogs: 95 cases (1969–1994). *J. Am. Vet. Med. Assoc.* 221 (5): 662–665. https://avmajournals.avma.org/view/journals/javma/221/5/javma.2002.221.662.xml.

39 Baines, S.J. and Aronson, L.R. (2018). Rectum, anus, and perineum. In: *Veterinary Surgery Small Animal*, 2e, vol. 2 (ed. S.A. Johnston and K.M. Tobias), 1783–1827. St. Louis, MO: Elsevier.

40 Chen, C.L., Lapsley, J.M., and Selmic, L.E. (2022). Minimal complications observed with a modified surgical approach for treatment of canine anal sac neoplasia. *J. Am. Vet. Med. Assoc.* 260 (S1): S59–S64.

41 Hobson, H.P., Brown, M.R., and Rogers, K.S. (2006). Surgery of metastatic anal sac adenocarcinoma in five dogs. *Vet. Surg.* 35 (3): 267–270. https://pubmed.ncbi.nlm.nih.gov/16635006.

42 Marretta, S.M. and Matthiesen, D.T. (1989). Problems associated with the surgical treatment of diseases involving the perineal region. *Probl. Vet. Med.* 1 (2): 215–242.

43 Jimeno Sandoval, J.C., Charlesworth, T., and Anderson, D. (2022). Outcomes and complications of anal sacculectomy for non-neoplastic anal sac disease in cats: 8 cases (2006–2019). *J. Small Anim. Pract.* 63 (1): 56–61.

44 Barnes, D.C. and Demetriou, J.L. (2017). Surgical management of primary, metastatic and recurrent anal sac adenocarcinoma in the dog: 52 cases. *J. Small Anim. Pract.* 58 (5): 263–268.

36

Caudectomy

Kristin A. Coleman[1] *and Trent T. Gall*[2]

[1] *Gulf Coast Veterinary Specialists, Houston, TX, USA*
[2] *Gall Mobile Veterinary Surgery, Longmont, CO, USA*

Key Points

- The goal of a caudectomy (i.e., tail amputation) is to treat a traumatic injury or to remove a diseased (non-traumatic) portion of the tail.
- A partial caudectomy is any amputation of the tail distal to the third coccygeal vertebra or distal to the perineum.
- Brachycephalic breeds of dogs, particularly English Bulldogs, may have an anatomic deformity of their tail, known as "screwtail," "ingrown tail," "twisted tail," or "corkscrew tail," that can lead to a painful condition called intertriginous dermatitis, which may be surgically addressed via caudectomy.

Introduction

A caudectomy (partial or full) is a procedure that has many different variations and is performed for several reasons, most of which are in an effort to increase the comfort of the patient. A caudectomy, also known as "high tail amputation" or "complete tail amputation," is removal of the tail at the sacrococcygeus junction, at a level even with or proximal to the perineum, or at a level with or proximal to the second to third coccygeus intervertebral disc space. Any tail amputation caudal to these parameters is deemed a partial caudectomy.

Anatomy

The tail is a continuation of the vertebral column that contains coccygeal or caudal vertebrae of differing numbers depending on the species, breed, and individual with a normal range of 6–23 vertebrae.[1] These vertebral bodies are separated by intervertebral discs, are surrounded by several muscles, and are supplied by five different arteries. For the length of the tail, there are two main dorsal (sacrocaudalis dorsalis lateralis and medialis), two main ventral (sacrocaudalis ventralis lateralis and medialis), and two main lateral (intertransversarius dorsalis caudalis and ventralis caudalis) muscles, and the muscles of the pelvic diaphragm attach to the first few coccygeal vertebrae. These muscles, the levator ani and coccygeus, as well as the rectococcygeus muscle, only insert onto the proximal aspect of the tail and should rarely, if ever, be encountered during a caudectomy. The blood supply courses along the lateral aspects (lateral caudal artery), dorsal aspect (small dorsolateral caudal artery), and ventral aspect (median caudal and ventrolateral caudal arteries). The lateral caudal arteries are branches of the caudal gluteal artery, which is a branch of the medial sacral artery. The tail's venous supply feeds into the caudal vein, which goes into the right internal iliac vein, which then merges with the right external iliac vein to start the caudal vena cava.[1,2]

As with many anatomic variations among dog breeds, brachycephalic breeds can have an abnormal configuration of their tail as it deviates inward on itself, known by many names but most commonly as an "ingrown tail," "screwtail," "twisted tail," or "corkscrew tail," that may appear similar to the shape of a cinnamon bun in the dorsal plane. This abnormal tail conformation causes issues due to the deep skin folds created by the characteristic twisting of the tail, which can lead to skin fold dermatitis, pyoderma, and intertrigo caused by the decreased ventilation within the tail fold pocket and proliferation of surface bacteria.[3]

Techniques in Small Animal Soft Tissue, Orthopedic, and Ophthalmic Surgery, First Edition. Edited by Kristin A. Coleman.

Companion website: www.wiley.com/go/coleman/surgeries

This condition can lead to a vicious cycle of treating with systemic antibiotics and surface cleansing wipes, infections within the tail pocket penetrating the deeper layers of tissue, and discomfort to the patient, all of which result in continued inflammation and resistant infections. The treatment for this end-stage condition is often tail amputation to remove the screwtail.

Indications/Pre-operative Considerations

Caudectomy, both complete and partial, has many clinical indications and can be grouped in multiple ways: traumatic versus non-traumatic or therapeutic versus non-therapeutic. In dogs and cats, the most common indication for partial caudectomy is a wound sustained to the mid-distal tail,[4,5] and in 80% of the cat tail wounds in one study, these were degloving injuries caused by the appendage being stuck in a door.[4]

If using the therapeutic versus non-therapeutic classification, the latter basically entails just cosmetic docking. All other reasons for caudectomy would be grouped as "therapeutic" and would include amputating for trauma, "happy tail," chronic non-union fractures, infection (bone or soft tissue), severe dermatitis/painful tail skin fold pyoderma that is refractory to medical management (e.g., screwtail), paralysis (e.g., "tail pull" injury) or neuropathy,[6] severe tail deformities that result in pain, and neoplasia.[4,7–9] Some small masses may be marginally excised from a tail, but if too much tissue is removed circumferentially, there is a risk of excessive tension leading to a tourniquet effect of the tail. Therefore, if wide margins for particular neoplasms are desired (e.g., 2 cm lateral margins and a fascial plane deep for a mast cell tumor excision, 3 cm lateral margins and two fascial planes deep for a sarcoma excision), a tail amputation is often the recommended procedure to achieve adequate margins and a tension-free closure.

The level at which the surgeon decides to amputate depends on the reason for amputation. A "caudectomy" is also known as a "total" or "high tail amputation," and this generally means amputation at or anywhere proximal to the third coccygeal vertebra (or simply, cranial to the perineum). A "partial caudectomy" is an amputation anywhere more distal to this point. While this chapter is going to focus on dogs and cats, complete or partial caudectomies may be performed in a variety of animals, including ferrets (Figure 36.1).

Instruments needed for a tail amputation include an IV stand to hang the tail for sterile preparation in the operating room, sterile self-adhesive bandaging (e.g., VetWrap), a standard "soft tissue surgery pack," a sterile marker, gauze (radiopaque or non-radiopaque), and bone-cutting forceps (e.g., Liston). Optional tools include monopolar electrosurgery and equipment for a tourniquet depending on both availability and surgeon preference.

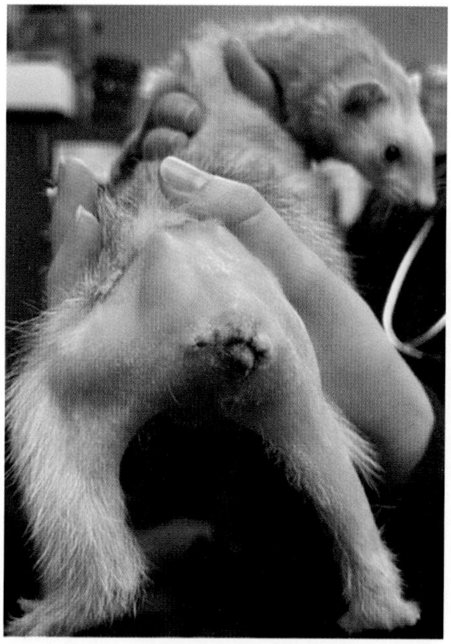

Figure 36.1 Ferret that presented two weeks postoperatively following a high tail amputation for completely excised sarcoma. *Source:* © Kristin Coleman.

Surgical Procedure

Partial Caudectomy

Positioning

After general anesthesia is induced, the tail, perineum, and dorsal pelvic area are clipped. The most distal portion of the tail may be covered with an exam glove and then covered proximally with self-adhering bandaging to secure it to the tail, since the portion to be amputated does not need to be fully clipped but should be covered in surgery. It is then important to place a purse-string suture around the anal orifice to reduce the risk of fecal contamination during the procedure. For partial caudectomies close to the distal portion of the tail, purse-string sutures in the anus are not necessary.

Patients are frequently positioned in sternal recumbency and at the edge of the table with the pelvic limbs hanging freely over the edge (Figure 36.2). It is essential to provide plenty of padding over the edge of the table intraoperatively for the patient's comfort during postoperative recovery, especially since the edge of the table can cause trauma to the hindlimb vasculature, sciatic nerve, or femoral nerve if not properly padded. For the padding, there are several options: multiple beach towels, a pool noodle over the sharp edge, or several blue pads to name a few. An alternative position would be to pull the patient forward with the pelvic limbs abducted and supported by the table.

The tail is suspended with tape or a towel clamp to an IV stand or pole (or similar object) to allow a hanging-type preparation and draping technique a few centimeters

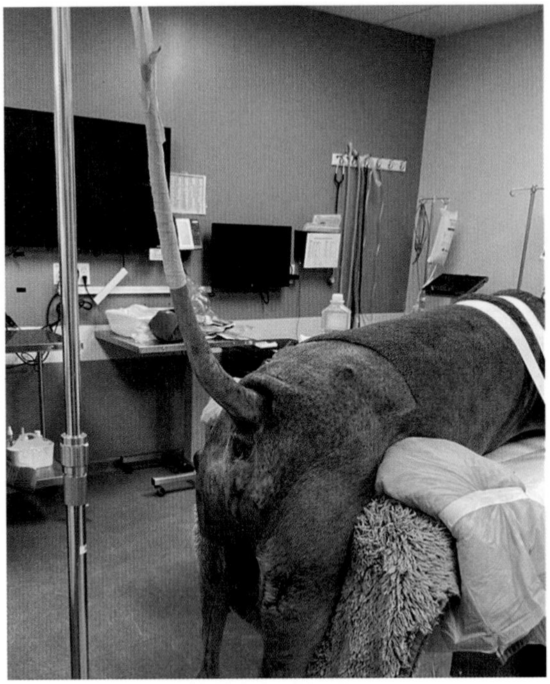

Figure 36.2 Proper patient positioning for partial caudectomy for neoplasia in a Mastiff. The patient is in sternal recumbency with padding in his caudal abdominal region and cushioning the edge of the table, and his tail is suspended with the use of an IV pole. *Source:* © Kristin Coleman.

proximal to the proposed incision. Quarter-draping is either performed on the proximal aspect of the tail or around the dorsal pelvic and perineal region. An impermeable drape or sterilized aluminum foil should be used to grab the distal aspect of the tail (the portion that has not been aseptically prepared), followed by application of a sterile self-adhering bandage (e.g., VetWrap) to cover the distal portion of the tail. The surgeon should be careful to not contaminate themselves during this portion of draping (Video 36.1).

A tourniquet may or may not be placed around the proximal aspect of the tail to decrease bleeding during the procedure. The duration of tourniquet application depends on its tightness. Loosening and replacing the tourniquet every 20–30 minutes may be necessary to avoid soft tissue and vascular injury.[9] The authors do not use tourniquets for tail amputations and prefer to ligate or cauterize blood vessels as they are encountered at the time of dissection.

Incision

After draping is completed and prior to making an incision, the sterile marker should be used to draw on the patient's tail at the level of the intended amputation. This is important for surgical planning to avoid tension of the final closure, maintain symmetry, and create a cosmetic incision with the dorsal aspect being slightly longer than the ventral aspect. The first step is to choose the area of amputation and mark the corresponding joint space. If desired, a hypodermic needle may be used as an alternative to identify the location of the intervertebral space.[9] The next step is to make an incision in the shape of a "fishmouth with an overbite," and it consists of two arches drawn on the dorsal and ventral aspects of the tail. The "corners of the fishmouth" are on the lateral aspects, and the proposed incision should be at least one coccygeal vertebra distal to the desired intervertebral amputation site to allow for a tension-free closure (Figure 36.3).

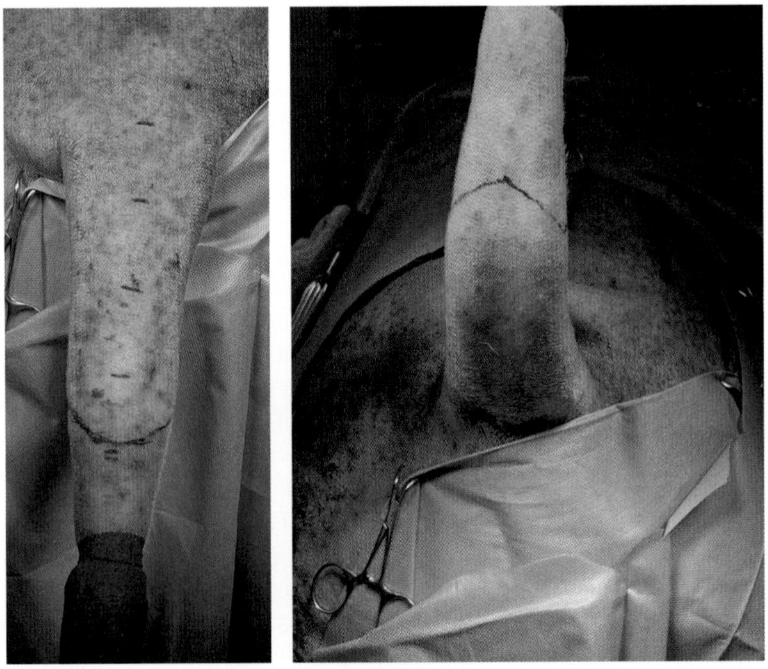

Figure 36.3 Dorsal aspect of tail with lines denoting the palpable dorsal spinous processes of the coccygeal vertebrae to allow for identification of the intervertebral amputation site. The distal transverse line is the arch of the "fishmouth" drawn approximately one vertebral body length distally from the desired amputation site and is where the skin incision will be made (left image). Ventral aspect of tail is marked with the arch of the "fishmouth" (right image). *Source:* © Kristin Coleman.

Dissection

After making an incision through the skin and subcutaneous layers (Figure 36.4), the tissues are dissected to the level of the desired intervertebral space for disarticulation. While the muscles may be sharply transected, there are several vessels that require ligation, especially in large patients. The lateral caudal arteries are located dorsal to the coccygeal transverse processes in the proximal aspect of the tail and are located ventral to the processes in the distal aspect of the tail, and depending on patient size, they may either be ligated with suture (short-acting monofilament absorbable), hemoclip, or monopolar electrosurgery (if the vessel is <2–3 mm in diameter). If a nerve block was not performed pre-operatively, nerves may be locally blocked with a local anesthetic as they are encountered and sharply transected (Figure 36.5).

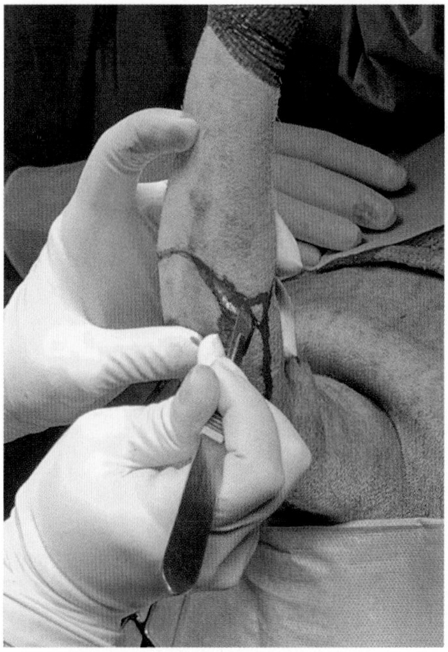

Figure 36.4 A #10 blade is used to make the incision through the skin and subcutaneous layers. After completing this step, the skin is retracted proximally to begin dissection through the musculature at the point of desired amputation. *Source:* © Kristin Coleman.

Ligation/Transection

The intervertebral disc space to be transected is confirmed, and the joint space is disarticulated with a #10 blade, Mayo scissors, or bone-cutting forceps (Figure 36.6). After the tail is removed, the remaining cartilage from the caudal aspect of the proximal vertebral end-plate is removed with rongeurs. If a tourniquet was used, it should be released prior to closure to assess for hemostasis.

Closure

Following lavage, closure should start with a buried simple interrupted suture using a short-acting monofilament absorbable synthetic suture on midline to bring the dorsal and ventral aspects of the subcutaneous tissue over the exposed coccygeal vertebra. This may continue a few more times to symmetrically bisect the deep subcutaneous tissues before routine closure of subcutaneous tissue and skin (Figure 36.7). If any of the edges have appreciable tension, an additional coccygeal vertebra should be removed. While a non-absorbable suture in a cruciate mattress pattern is ideal for skin closure, an intradermal pattern is chosen in aggressive patients (Figures 36.8 and 36.9).

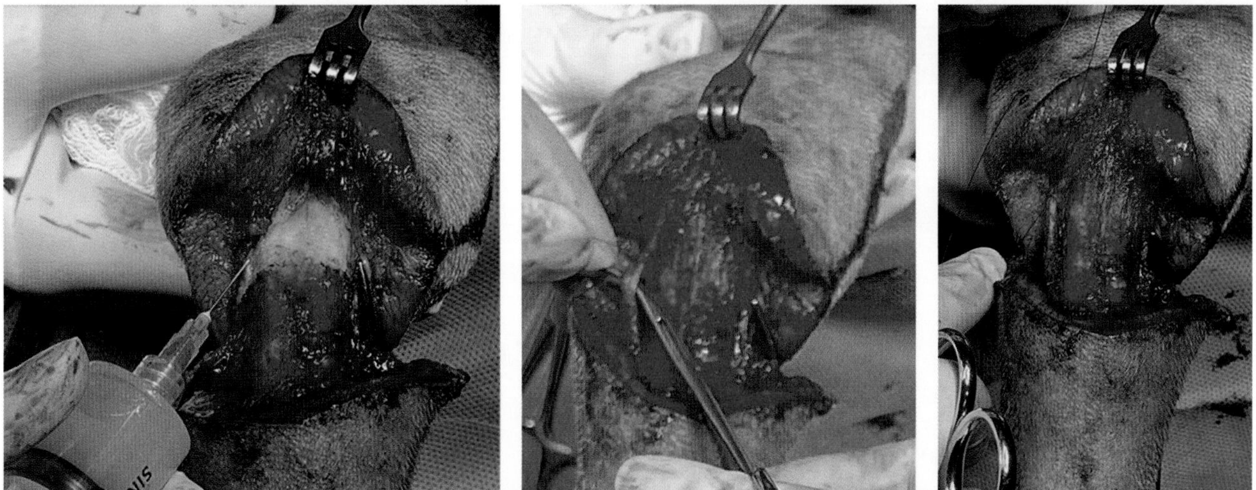

Figure 36.5 As nerves are encountered, they should be injected with a local anesthetic using a 25-gauge needle (bevel up) (left image). Whichever ligation strategy is chosen, the lateral caudal arteries should be isolated (center image), ligated (right image), and then transected. *Source:* © Kristin Coleman.

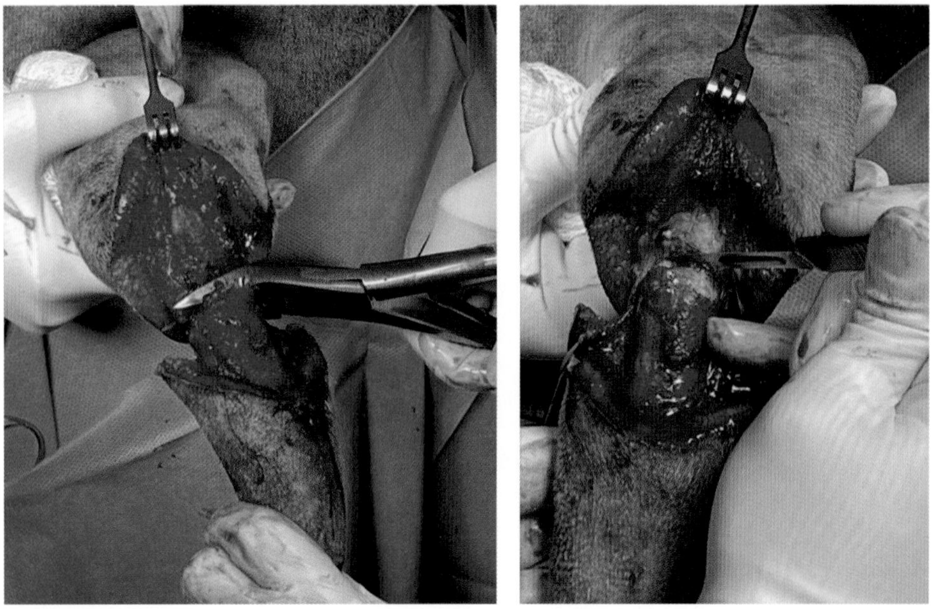

Figure 36.6 Once all soft tissues have been dissected from the intervertebral disc space or vertebral body to be transected, Liston bone-cutting forceps, Mayo scissors, or a #10 or #11 blade may be used to complete the amputation by disarticulation. If the skin is appreciated as having too much tension after removal of the tail, an additional vertebral body should be amputated. *Source:* © Kristin Coleman.

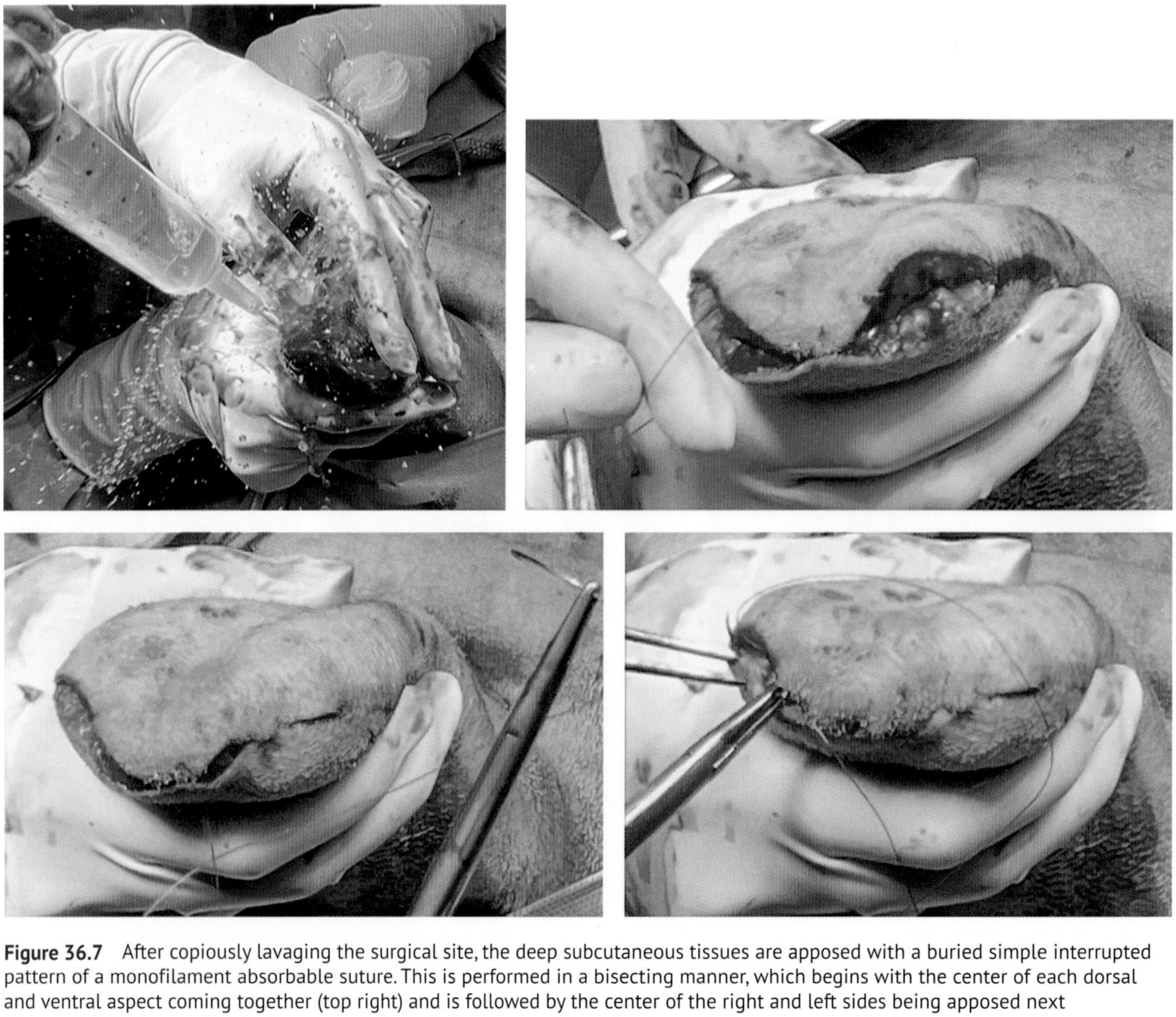

Figure 36.7 After copiously lavaging the surgical site, the deep subcutaneous tissues are apposed with a buried simple interrupted pattern of a monofilament absorbable suture. This is performed in a bisecting manner, which begins with the center of each dorsal and ventral aspect coming together (top right) and is followed by the center of the right and left sides being apposed next (bottom left). The superficial subcutaneous layer is then apposed in a simple continuous pattern with short-term monofilament absorbable suture. *Source:* © Kristin Coleman.

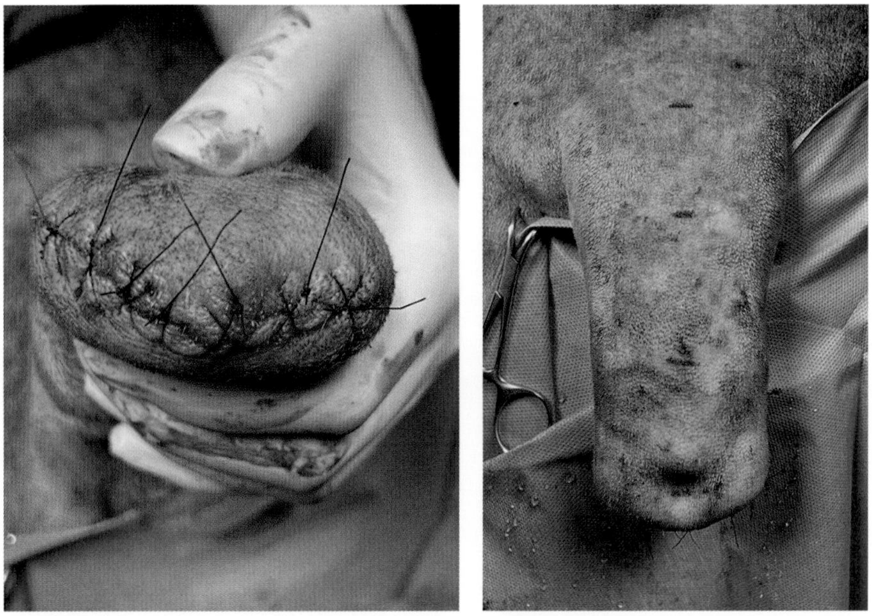

Figure 36.8 Closure of skin with non-absorbable monofilament suture (3-0 nylon) in a cruciate mattress pattern (left image). Note the tension-free closure with soft tissue apposed approximately 1/2 vertebral body length from the visible end of the bone (right image). *Source:* © Kristin Coleman.

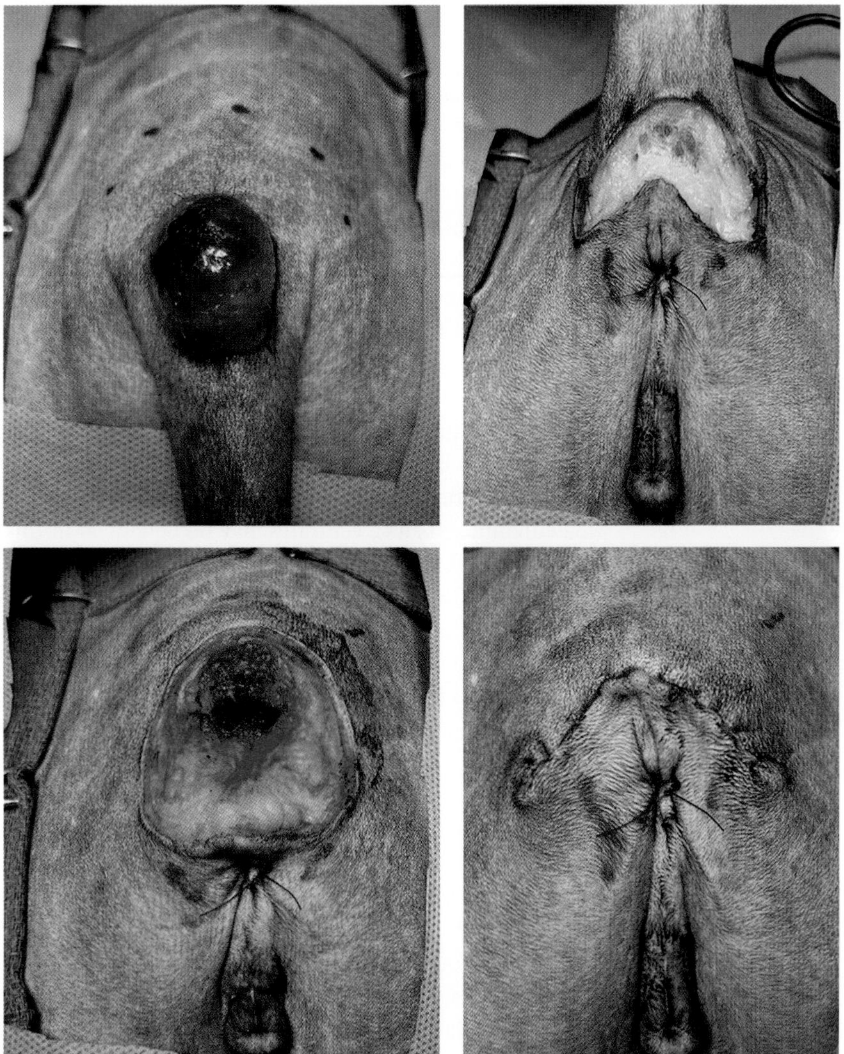

Figure 36.9 Feline patient with a peripheral nerve sheath tumor of the dorsal proximal tail. A high tail amputation (i.e., complete caudectomy) was performed to attain the recommended 3 cm lateral margins and two deep fascial planes. The patient was healed in two weeks and had no intra- or postoperative complications. *Source:* © Kristin Coleman.

Caudectomy for Screwtail

Positioning

The patient is placed in sternal recumbency with the hind limbs hanging off the end of the table. Care must be taken to place substantial padding under the patient's caudal abdomen/inguinal region and over the edge of the table, since the edge of the table can cause trauma to the hind limb vasculature, sciatic nerve, or femoral nerve if not properly padded. For padding, a rolled towel or even pool noodle works well. A purse-string suture is placed around the anus with either gauze or tampon in the caudal rectum to prevent fecal contamination during the procedure, and some kind of marker should be placed on the patient, on the anesthetist's clipboard, on the O.R. checklist, etc. to remind everyone that this purse-string is present and requires removal postoperatively. A caudal or sacrococcygeal epidural can be performed to help with pain during and after the procedure, though not absolutely required.

For this procedure, it is advisable to use monopolar electrocautery due to the vascular nature of the tissues surrounding the tail skin folds. These tend to be quite vascular due to chronic inflammation of the skin. It is possible to perform this procedure without the use of electrocautery, but there will be blood contamination in the surgical field with the need to ligate bleeding vessels. Once the patient is in position and the purse-string suture is placed, a surgical scrub is performed (at least three times), trying to clean the deep skin folds of the tail pocket as best as possible. However, the surgical technique described below will hopefully avoid any contact of the surgeon or incision with the deep portions of the chronically infected skin fold.

Incision

An elliptical incision is performed around the tail base and around the tail skin fold (caudal aspect of the sacrum) with the points of the ellipse on the lateral aspects. For added precision to attain a symmetrical incision, a sterile marker may be used to plan the incision and draw on the skin prior to cutting (Figure 36.10). The incision is made between the anus and the ventral skin fold, being sure to leave as much skin possible dorsal to the anus, staying out of the skin fold, and incorporating all of the skin folds into the elliptical incision. The goal is to remove the coccygeal vertebrae and skin folds all en bloc.

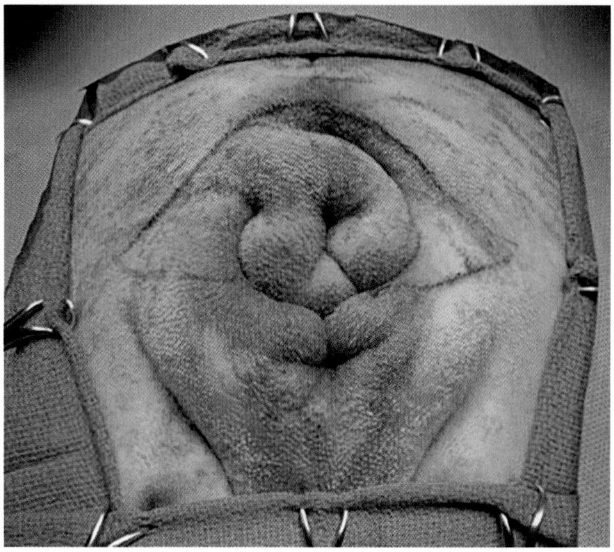

Figure 36.10 The patient is positioned with hindlimbs hanging over the end of the surgical table. Dorsal is at the top of the image, and ventral is at the bottom of the picture. A sterile surgical marker was used to make the outline of the elliptical incision. Dorsal margin is the caudal aspect of the sacrum, and the ventral margin is proximal to the anus. *Source:* © Kristin Coleman.

Dissection/Ligation/Transection

The subcutaneous tissue is then dissected down to the level of the palpable coccygeal vertebrae dorsally, ventrally, and on both lateral aspects to the area of the "twist" in the vertebrae (Figure 36.11). This can be challenging because the surgeon should ideally stay just outside of the subcutis of the offending tail folds/tail pocket without entering the infected area. If the pocket or folds cannot be appreciated during dissection, an instrument, such as a Kelly hemostat, should be placed into the pocket area as a landmark. Remember that whatever instrument is passed into the tail fold depth is considered contaminated and should not be handled by the surgeon on the portion contacting the skin.

When dissecting ventrally to the vertebrae, be very careful not to stray away from the vertebrae, since the rectum is directly below the dissection area. Blunt dissection (i.e., with a finger), opposed to sharp dissection (i.e., Metzenbaum scissors), ventrally may be beneficial in this region to avoid inadvertent penetration into the rectum. Once the "twist" in the vertebrae has been reached, the coccygeal and levator ani muscles are severed at their tendinous insertion onto the vertebrae, and any bleeding vessels are cauterized or ligated. After the bone of the coccygeal vertebrae is exposed, a bone-cutting forcep or Gigli wire is used to transect the bone at the level of the vertebral body or cut in the intervertebral disc space at the level of the "twist." Any soft tissue connections that are remaining can be dissected away (Figure 36.12).

Closure

The twisted coccygeal vertebrae and skin fold are then removed en bloc. It is possible to remove the entire piece in one conglomeration without touching or going into the soft tissue envelope of the skin fold, which helps decrease the risk of contamination. The surgical field is lavaged with

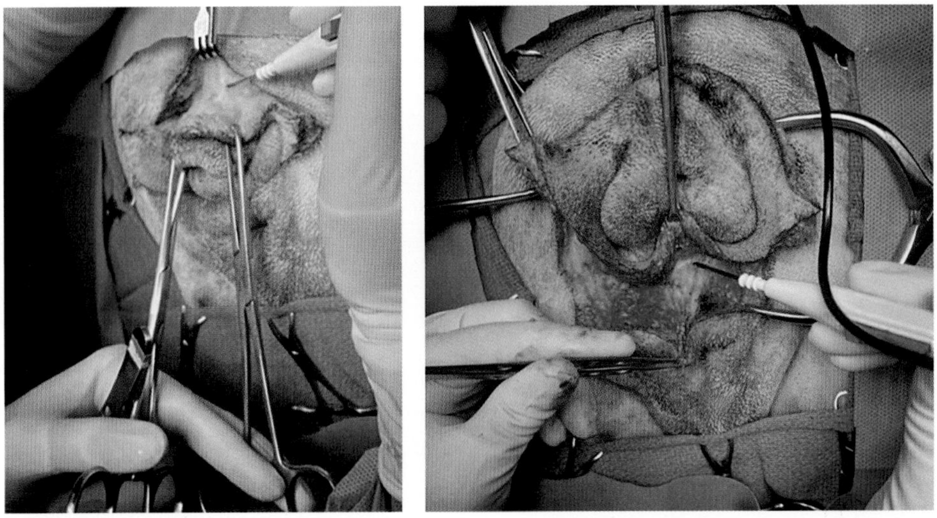

Figure 36.11 Dorsal dissection is performed in the left image. The use of retractors (Senn and Gelpi) is very helpful to visualize the chosen plane of dissection. Allis tissue forceps are also essential for handling of the infected tail fold tissue to retract and manipulate the tail segment. In the right image, ventral dissection is performed to stay close to the ventral aspect, and care must be taken NOT to breach the rectum. Dissection is continued completely around the skin fold and coccygeal vertebrae. *Source:* © Kristin Coleman.

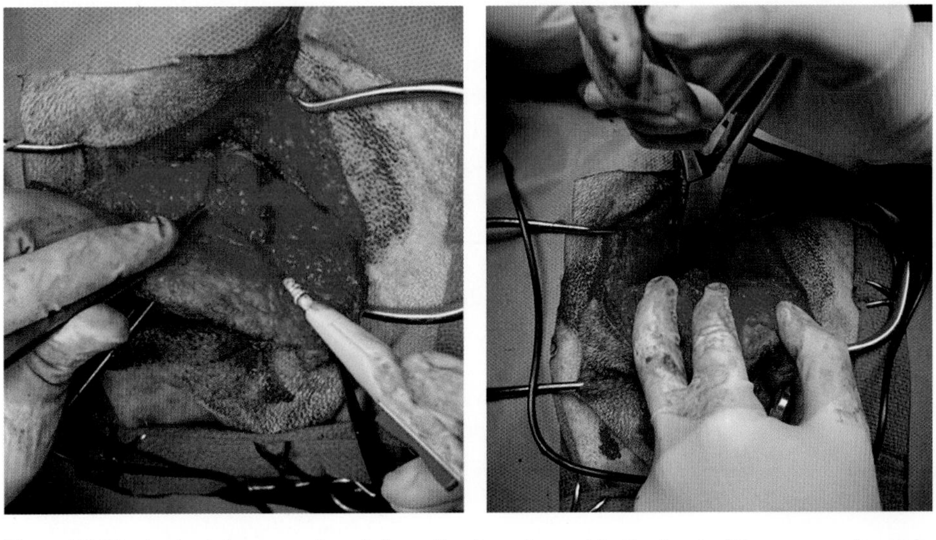

Figure 36.12 In the left image, dorsal dissection is performed to the level of the coccygeal vertebrae at the level of the "twist" or just dorsal to the "twist" in the vertebrae. In the right image, Liston bone-cutting forceps are used to transect the intervertebral disc space just cranial to the abnormality and palpable cranial end to the tail pocket once all soft tissues have been dissected from the area. Note the two Gelpi perineal retractors and assistant retracting the dorsal tissues with a Senn retractor for aiding in visualization. *Source:* © Kristin Coleman.

copious amounts of sterile saline, and a culture is obtained by either a swab or a small piece of tissue to assess for deep-seated infection within the surgical site from the chronically infected tail pocket. If the muscles surrounding the vertebrae are robust enough, these get apposed with a fascial closure over the cut end of the vertebrae. In the authors' experiences, these muscles are often too small for a fascial closure over the vertebral end. If there is redundant skin, it can be excised at this time. The deep subcutaneous tissue is closed with a long-term absorbable monofilament suture in a bisecting fashion to close the ellipse in a buried simple interrupted pattern, which allows the closure to remain symmetrical. The author likes to start in the center of the incision with a deep subcutaneous ligature and then place a ligature in the center of each of the sides (Figure 36.13). The superficial subcutaneous tissue is closed with a short-term absorbable monofilament suture in a simple continuous pattern. The skin is closed routinely. At this time, REMOVE THE PURSE-STRING SUTURE AND GAUZE-PACKING/TAMPON! Digitally palpate the rectum to make sure it has not been breached during the procedure (Figure 36.14).

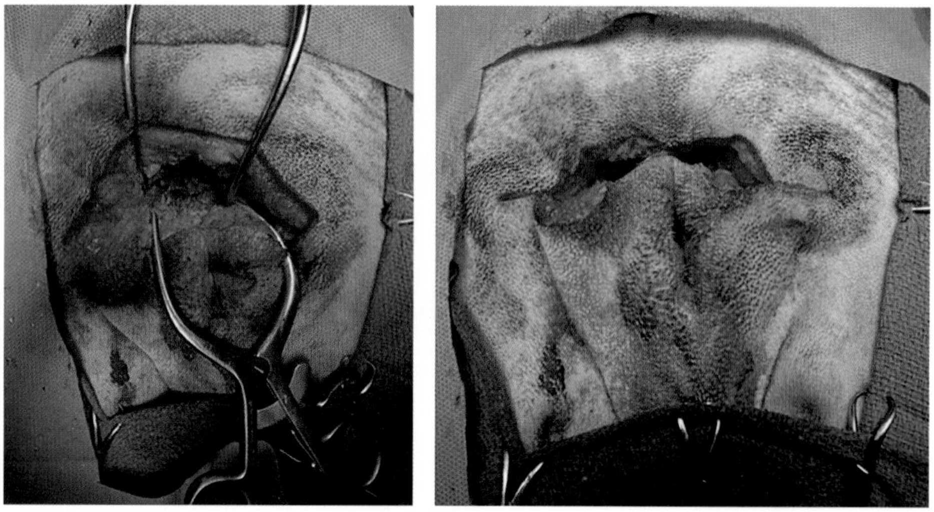

Figure 36.13 In the left image, the caudectomy has been performed, and the site is now inspected for signs of rectal perforation, remaining hair or skin, and success of hemostasis. The muscles often cannot be closed over the cut end of the vertebra in this area. If this is the situation, close deep subcutaneous tissues as in the right image. *Source:* © Kristin Coleman.

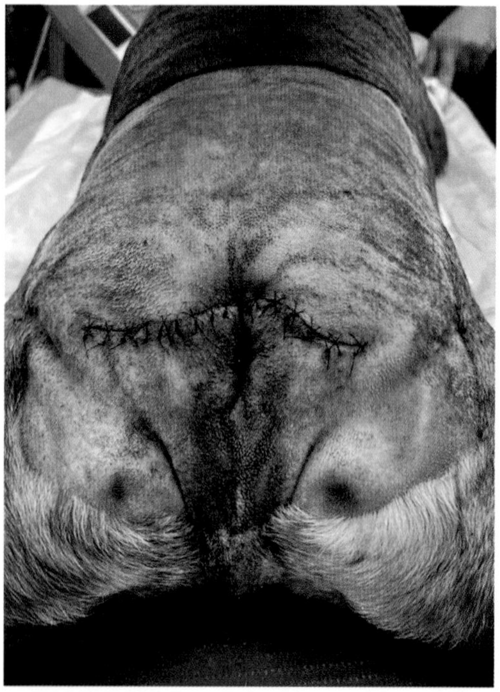

Figure 36.14 Immediate postoperative picture of skin closure with cruciate mattress sutures of 3-0 nylon. Be sure to REMOVE THE PURSE-STRING SUTURE AND ANY PACKED GAUZE FROM THE RECTUM!!! *Source:* © Kristin Coleman.

Potential Complications

In cases of both complete and partial caudectomy, the same potential complications exist intra- and postoperatively as with any surgery with an incision, including but not limited to death under anesthesia, bleeding, nerve damage, infection, dehiscence, or seroma formation. In addition, complications associated with caudectomy also include fecal incontinence, self-trauma, tension leading to dehiscence or incisional irritation, and neuroma formation, particularly those secondary to tail-pull injuries or high tail amputations.[3,9] With higher tail amputations comes an increased number of potential complications, which may include decreased rectal sensation with adequate anal tone, failure to posture to defecate, and post-op draining tracts immediately after surgery (12% in one study) and delayed wound healing, persistent tail chasing behavior, and temporary changes in defecation habits at the time of suture removal (13% in one study).[3]

There are several tips for reducing the risks of complications. Peri-operative antibiotics are recommended with a 22 mg/kg IV dose of cefazolin being given 30–60 minutes prior to skin incision and repeated every 90 minutes throughout the procedure. In cases of screwtail caudectomy or in cases of infection or trauma as the reason for caudectomy, antibiotics are continued postoperatively. In cases where the infected or traumatized tissue has been removed with caudectomy with no culture obtained, empirical antibiotics are continued for approximately seven days. In cases of screwtail where the risk of deep-seated infection exists and a culture was obtained, broad-spectrum antibiotics should be dispensed until the culture and sensitivity results are finalized, at which point the authors dispense appropriate antibiotics for an additional one to two weeks.[3] Neuroma formation may have decreased risk if individual nerves encountered during surgery are sharply transected with scissors or a blade (NOT with electrosurgery) and if local anesthetics are used to infuse the area around the nerves.

Postoperative Care/Prognosis

In cases of partial caudectomy, the patient often remains hospitalized only until recovered from anesthesia and then may be discharged from the hospital, which is often the same day as surgery. Due to the more invasive nature of a screwtail caudectomy in a brachycephalic breed of dog, these patients are kept overnight for monitoring of both surgical site comfort and respiratory watch. Once these patients are discharged, they are advised to wear a hard cone collar for two weeks until their recheck appointment with suture removal/incision check. With partial caudectomies, a longer than normal cone collar may need to be sent home to reduce ability for self-mutilation of the site. Pain medications dispensed typically include gabapentin and, if not contraindicated, a non-steroidal anti-inflammatory drug (NSAID). Some surgeons recommend that the client applies triple antibiotic ointment or a petroleum-based product (e.g., Vaseline) to the incision two to three times daily for the first two weeks postoperatively. The purpose is to prevent contaminants, particularly fecal material, from directly contacting the incision as it is healing, and if the owner notices contaminants stuck to the ointment, they may simply wipe it away. The patients should be kept in a small room without carpet (to reduce the risk of scooting behavior) with no running, jumping, or playing and should only be taken out on a leash for short walks. After two weeks, the incision should be healed, and the patient may resume normal activity (Figure 36.15).

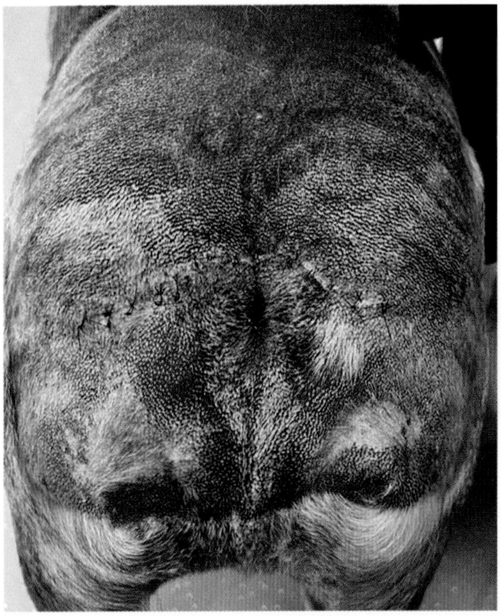

Figure 36.15 Two-week postoperative status prior to suture removal. *Source:* © Kristin Coleman.

Due to the surgical site's proximity to the anal orifice and possible reason for performing surgery being infection in cases of screwtail caudectomy, antibiotics are often initiated or simply continued from their preoperative course in the authors' cases. One study had 76% of their postoperative screwtail amputation patients continue antibiotic therapy after surgery for an average of 13.5 days.[3] In this study of caudectomy in brachycephalic dogs with screwtails, surgery resolved clinical signs with no long-term complications.

To access the videos for this chapter, please go to

with website **www.wiley.com/go/coleman/surgeries**

VIDEO 36.1 Appropriate sterile-draping of a hanging tail prior to partial caudectomy in a dog. *Source:* © Kristin Coleman.

References

1. Evans, H.E. (1993). *Miller's Anatomy of the Dog*, 3e. Philadelphia, PA: Elsevier.
2. Dyce, K.M., Sack, W.O., and Wensing, C.J.G. (2002). *Textbook of Veterinary Anatomy*, vol. 3. Philadelphia, PA: Elsevier.
3. Knight, S.M., Radlinsky, M.G., Cornell, K.K. et al. (2013). Postoperative complications associated with caudectomy in brachycephalic dogs with ingrown tails. *J. Am. Anim. Hosp. Assoc.* 49 (4): 237–242.
4. Simons, M.C., Ben-Amotz, R., and Popovitch, C. (2014). Post-operative complications and owner satisfaction following partial caudectomies: 22 cases (2008 to 2013). *J. Small Anim. Pract.* 55 (10): 509–514.
5. Diesel, G., Pfeiffer, D., Crispin, S. et al. (2010). Risk factors for tail injuries in dogs in Great Britain. *Vet. Rec.* 26: 812–817.
6. Grubb, T. (2010). Chronic neuropathic pain in veterinary patients. *Top. Compan. Anim. Med.* 25: 45–52.
7. Bellah, J.R. (2006). Tail and perineal wounds. *Vet. Clin. North Am. Small Anim. Pract.* 36: 913–929.
8. Schoen, K. and Sweet, D.C. (2009). Canine and feline tail amputation. *Lab. Anim.* 38: 232–233.
9. Risselada, M. (2022). Therapeutic tail amputation. *Clinician's Brief* (issued January 2022).

37

Preparing for Orthopedic Procedures

Ivette Juarez, Christine A. Valdez, and Marbella Lopez

Department of Small Animal Surgery, Gulf Coast Veterinary Specialists, Houston, TX, USA

Key Points

- Learn thorough preparation of an operating room for a standard orthopedic procedure.
- Learn appropriate preparation of the patient, including surgical clip, scrubbing, positioning, and draping.
- Learn about setting up instrumentation for a standard orthopedic procedure.
- Review postoperative orthopedic care.

Introduction

This chapter focuses on the detailed preparation of the patient, operating room setup, instrumentation setup, and intraoperative and postoperative considerations when managing basic orthopedic procedures.

The setup for all advanced orthopedic procedures is beyond the scope of this chapter.

Preoperative Steps

Equipment Preparation

Immediately prior to an orthopedic surgery, the operating room is established with the appropriate equipment and instrumentation depending on the type of orthopedic procedure (Box 37.1, Figure 37.1). Creating a list of commonly used instruments and each surgeon's preferences for a variety of procedures may help with efficiency when setting up an operating room (Figure 37.2). Heating systems are turned on. Intravenous fluids are spiked and primed. Anesthetic machines are checked for leaks (Figure 37.3), and an induction area is prepared with the necessary materials.

At this point, the appropriate diagnostic tests, including blood work, have been performed on the patient, and an intravenous catheter has been placed. When placing an intravenous catheter, consideration of the affected limb undergoing surgical intervention should be taken. For example, if performing surgery on the right radius/ulna, the IV catheter should be placed on the opposite forelimb or hindlimb. Depending on the patient's signalment and history, a preoperative ECG should be performed to assess for an arrhythmia.

After the patient has been placed under general anesthesia, they can generally be positioned in lateral recumbency for preparation of the skin (side will depend on the laterality of the affected limb). Monitoring equipment can then be attached, including but not limited to electrocardiogram, pulse oximetry, non-invasive blood pressure, and a capnometer. If a patient's position needs to be adjusted at any point, it is ideal to disconnect the breathing circuit from the patient's endotracheal tube to prevent extubation or tracheal damage.

Skin Preparation

If performing an elective surgery (e.g., medial patella luxation repair), it is advised to check the skin over the proposed surgical area, preferably before the patient is under general anesthesia. This can help determine if surgery needs to be delayed until the possible infection is cleared to minimize the risk of post-surgical site infection.

Techniques in Small Animal Soft Tissue, Orthopedic, and Ophthalmic Surgery, First Edition. Edited by Kristin A. Coleman.

Companion website: www.wiley.com/go/coleman/surgeries

Box 37.1 Examples of Equipment and Instrumentation Needed for an Orthopedic Surgical Procedure

- Suction unit, hose, and canister
- Electrosurgical unit with equipment (e.g., monopolar cautery pen, bipolar cautery pen, foot switch, ground plate, cautery tip cleaner)
- Orthopedic surgery pack (image within this box) (e.g., surgical gowns, large patient drape, adhesive surgical drapes, adhesive transparent drape, cohesive bandage wrap, bulb syringe, needle counter box, radiopaque gauze)

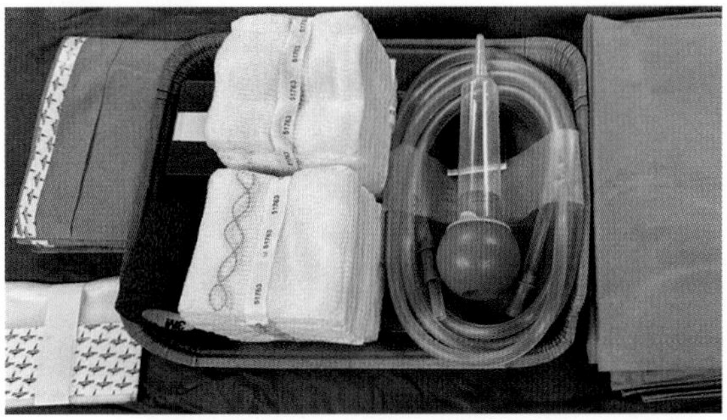

- Orthopedic instrument tray (e.g., towel clamps, scalpel handles, needle holders, thumb forceps, periosteal elevators, bone holding forceps, dissecting scissors, suture cutting scissors, tissue forceps, hemostatic forceps, bowl)
- Orthopedic implants and power equipment (e.g., bone plates and screws, pins, wire, interlocking nail, external fixators)
- Suction tip (e.g., Frazier, Yankauer)
- Retractors (e.g., Senn, Army-Navy, Hohmann, Gelpi)
- Stapling equipment (e.g., skin staples)
- Light handles
- Sterile gloves (e.g., orthopedic gloves)
- Suture
- Blades (#10, #11, #15)
- Other instruments (e.g., antimicrobial incise drape, curettes, rongeurs, osteotomes with mallet, Jacob's hand chuck, pin cutters, wire twisters, Bovie holster)
- C-arm fluoroscopy and table

Since the duration of anesthesia correlates with infection rates, preoperative preparation should be thorough but efficient. Clipping should be performed outside of the operating room to minimize contamination. The technician should wear exam gloves while clipping. With a #40 clipper blade, shave the entire circumference of the affected limb in the region that includes the proximal and distal bone or joint relative to the affected bone or joint (Table 37.1). In some cases, the distal portion of the limb may remain unclipped (Figure 37.4). If a wound is present around the surgical area, sterile lube can be applied to the wound prior to clipping to prevent hair from entering the wound site. If a bone autograft is needed, confirm with the surgeon which additional sites need to be clipped. Be sure to watch the temperature of the clipper blade. If the blade becomes palpably hot, either replace the blade or spray with a cooling lubricant. In areas with friable, thin skin, it is advised to have steady movements to reduce the risk of unwanted abrasions. After clipping is completed, a vacuum can be used to pick up loose hair.

If there is an unclipped portion of the limb remaining, it can now be covered. Wrap the limb using an exam glove, covering all hair. Next, cover and secure the glove with tape until the glove is no longer visible. Be careful not to overstress the tape, cutting off blood circulation. Covering the foot this way will later allow the surgical limb to be scrubbed and included into the sterile field (Figure 37.5).

The technician should replace their exam gloves for the "dirty" scrub. Have two stacks of non-woven gauze set aside. Keep one stack dry and the other one mildly dampened with water (Figure 37.4). Lightly pour chlorhexidine scrub onto the dampened gauze. Begin scrubbing from the center of the expected incision site and continue moving outward in a spiral course until the shaved region has been covered. Avoid an aggressive scrubbing motion to reduce the risk of skin irritation and inflammation. Follow it with the dry gauze to clear excess lather. This combination is repeated a minimum of three times or until the gauze no longer contains visible debris. If the foot was clipped, debris can be better removed by soaking it in a diluted chlorhexidine solution. For long-haired patients, water or ultrasonic gel can be used to push the hair down to keep it away from the surgical field.

Preoperative Considerations

Local incisional anesthesia, an epidural, and a regional nerve block are all acceptable pain management strategies (Figure 37.6). If the doctor or technician plans on administering the epidural or nerve block, it can be done after the "dirty" scrub. Adding an intravenous constant rate infusion of an analgesic is another good strategy that can be applied if none of the above-mentioned is possible.

If the anus is in close proximity to the proposed surgical area, a purse-string suture technique can be applied to protect the surgical site from potential fecal contamination. Manual deobstipation and expression of the anal glands should be done prior to the purse string placement.

(a)

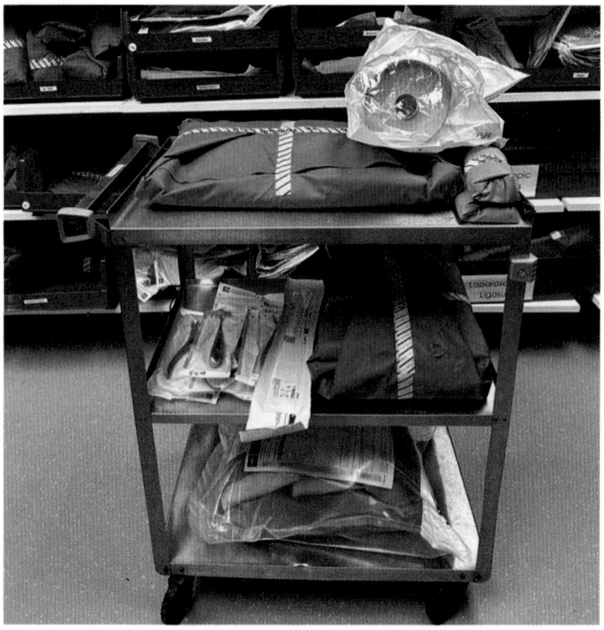

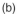

(b)

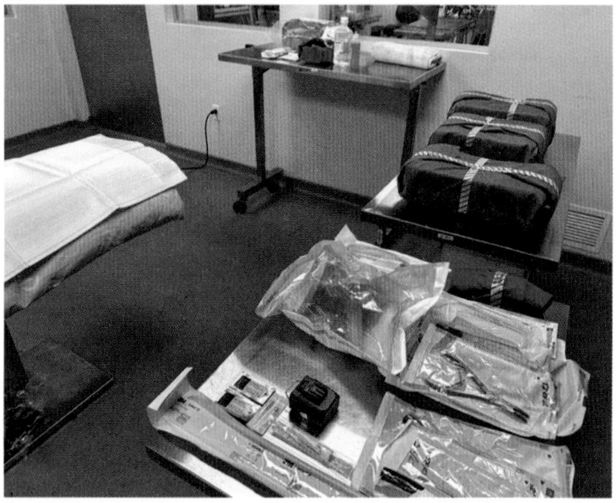

Figure 37.1 (a) Instrumentation for an orthopedic surgery is pulled from sterile supply and placed onto a cart. (b) Equipment and instrumentation in the operating room.

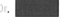

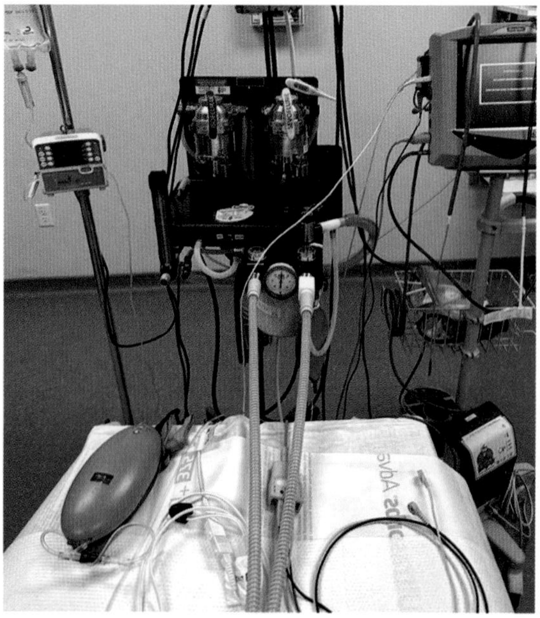

Figure 37.3 Anesthetic machine, intravenous fluids, monitoring equipment, and heating systems ready to be used.

Table 37.1 General shave margins for various orthopedic procedures.

Bone or joint	Shaving margins (approximate depending on the procedure)
Metacarpus/phalanges	Proximal radius/ulna to entire distal foot
Radius/ulna	Proximal humerus to metacarpal region
Humerus	Proximal scapula to distal antebrachium
Pelvis	Lumbar region to perianal region, dorsal midline to distal femur
Femur	Lumbar region to ischiatic tuberosity, dorsal midline to tarsus
Stifle	Proximal femur to distal tarsus or metatarsal region
Tibia/fibula	Proximal femur to metatarsal region
Metatarsus/phalanges	Proximal tibia/fibula to entire distal foot

Medial Patella Luxation Repair (MPL)

- Knee pack/cautery/light handles/hoister
- Gelpis
- Point-to-point reduction forceps
- Small osteotomes
- Single-action rongeur
- Single bone rasp
- Pin cutters
- Spools of wire/wire twisters
- Power and battery
- Sagittal saw

+/– Hobby saw
+/– Countersink
+/– Beaver blade 6400 and handle

Dr. [redacted]

- Reciprocating saw
- 4 pack of towels if unilateral

Dr. [redacted]

- Spiral bone rasp
- Flat hobby saw (no handle)
- (2) Sm gelpi and (1) med gelpi

Position: Like a TPLO. Lateral Recumbency for WW when unilateral
Reminder: Additional AP Femur radiograph if getting a TPLO/ Have "Stryker box" in O.R

Figure 37.2 Example of a procedure instrument list.

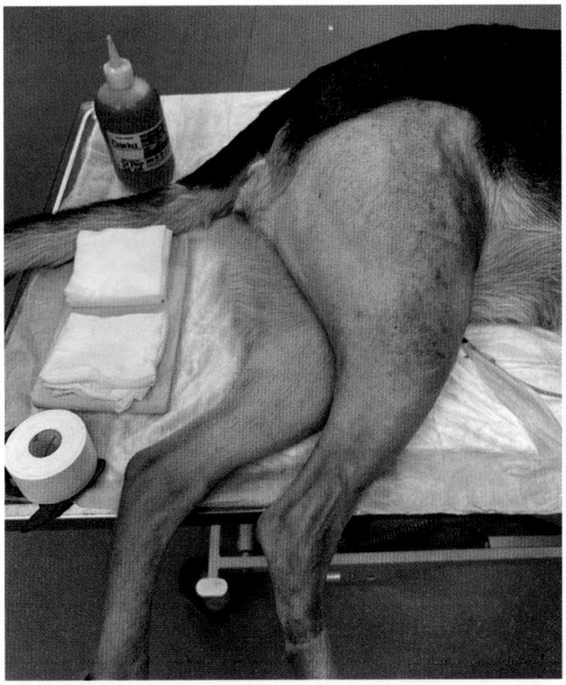

Figure 37.4 Shaving margins for a stifle. Distal foot has been left unclipped, so it is wrapped with an exam glove and adhered to the skin with either white tape or self-adherent bandaging.

Radiographs

Radiographs are an integral part of orthopedic surgery. Radiographs should be obtained before moving into the operating room if they have not been obtained prior to the day of surgery. The bone proximal and distal to the surgical bone should be included in the radiographic view. A radiographic reference ball should be included in all views near and at the same level as the bone or joint of interest in order for the surgeon to template for implants (Figure 37.7). Confirm with the surgeon if contralateral radiographs are needed.

Transportation into the Operating Room

Using a gurney is recommended as the safest method of patient transportation. The patient is moved to the operating table and is placed in lateral, sternal, or dorsal recumbency depending on the surgery. The breathing circuit is once again connected to the patient, with oxygen and anesthetic gas turned back on. If the anesthesia machine has both sevoflurane and isoflurane capabilities, be sure the correct gas is selected. Monitoring equipment, intravenous fluids, and heat support can be applied to the patient (Figure 37.8). The anesthetist can administer the prophylactic antibiotic injection around this step or 30–60 minutes before the incision is made.

Positioning

Depending on how the surgeon plans to approach the incision, positioning of each patient can vary. For the majority of orthopedic surgeries, the affected limb will need to be suspended in order to achieve a proper sterile scrub. In some cases, a surgical bean bag can be used as an alternative to hanging the limb (Figure 37.9). An intravenous stand pole can be used by adding strips of tape to the wrapped foot and extending the limb by looping the tape over the pole (Figure 37.10). If the foot and digits need to be clipped, prepped, and part of the surgical field, a towel clamp may be used to grasp the nail or interdigital webbing in order to suspend the foot. The other limbs can be secured to the table with tape, rope, or leashes. Distal limb perfusion is improved by spreading the forces applied circumferentially to the extremities. Caution should be exercised to prevent over-tightening of the limb.

Positioning of the instrument table is something that also needs to be considered. If the affected limb is positioned toward the end of the operating table, the instrument table

(a) (b) (c)

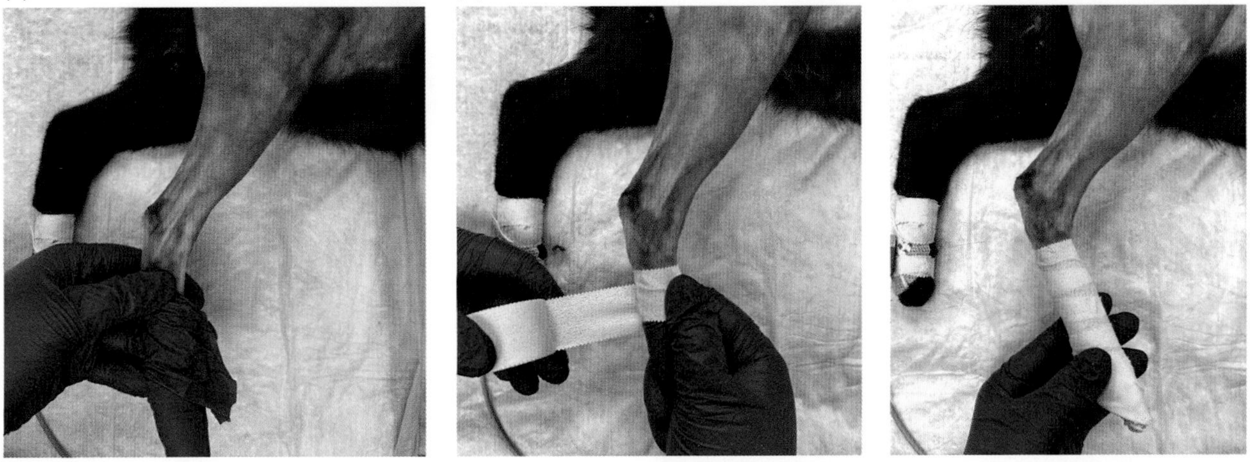

Figure 37.5 (a) A glove is placed on the unclipped foot. (b) The glove is being secured with tape. (c) The glove is completely covered.

(a) (b)

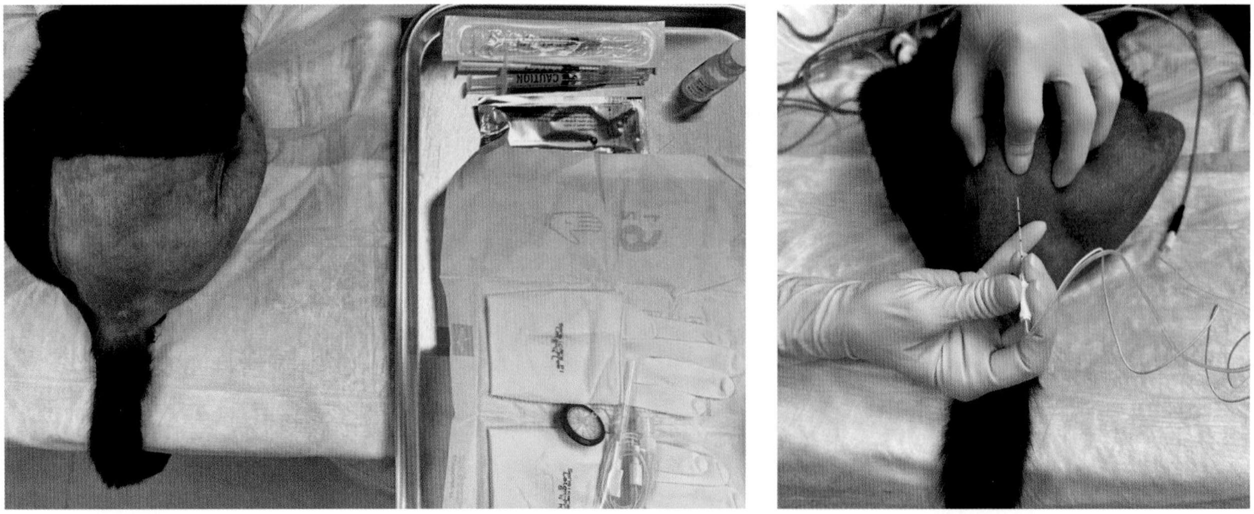

Figure 37.6 (a) The patient is positioned for an epidural. (b) Administration of the epidural.

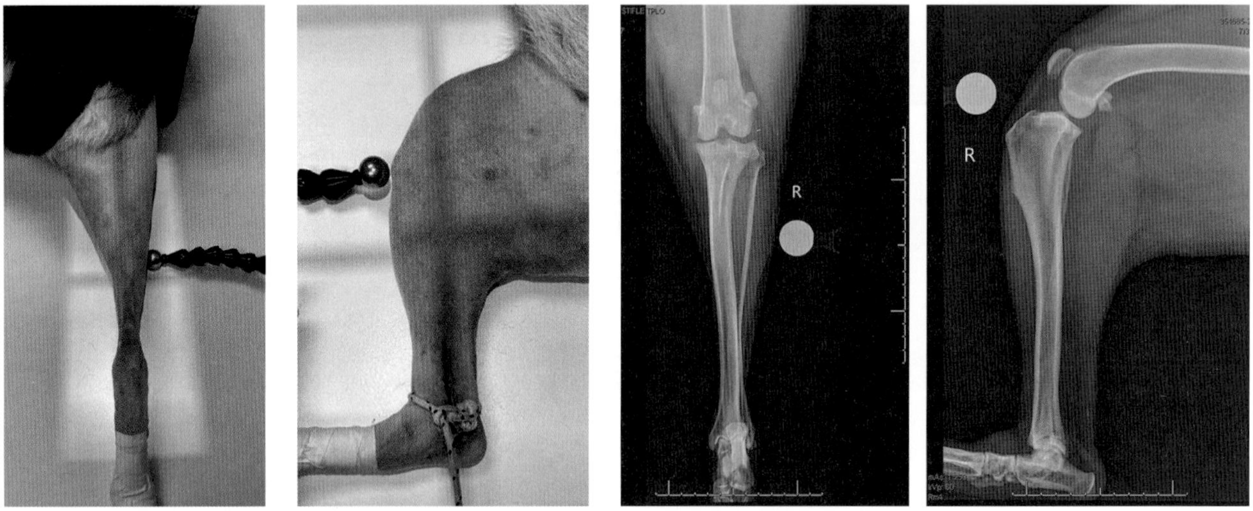

Figure 37.7 Example of right stifles two-view radiographs that include a reference ball.

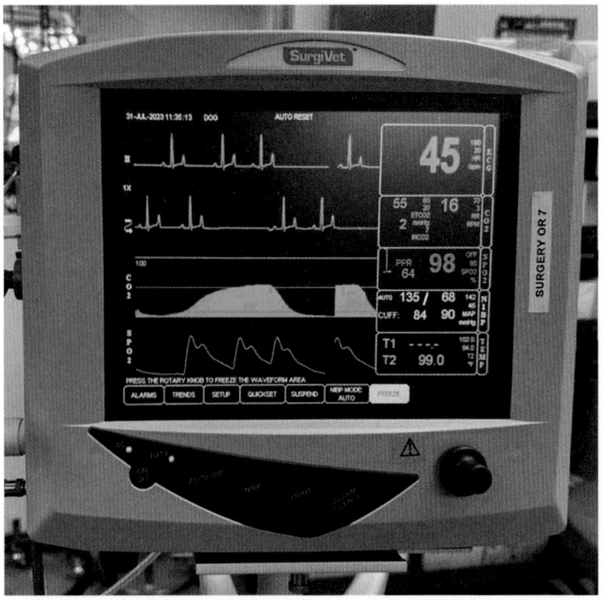

Figure 37.8 The patient's vital signs are seen on the monitoring screen.

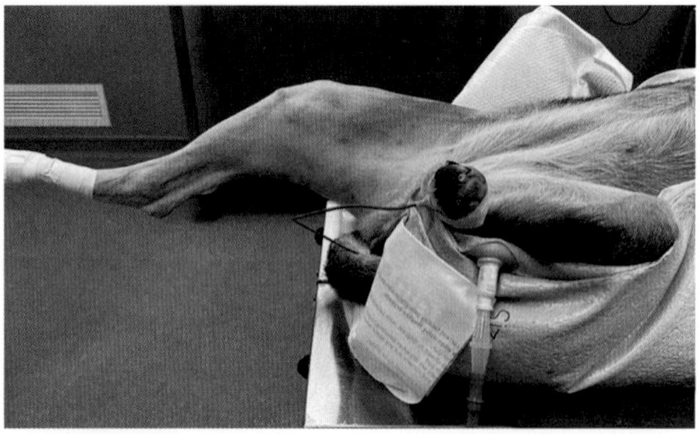

Figure 37.9 A surgical bean bag is holding a surgical limb in place. Therefore, hanging assistance is not needed.

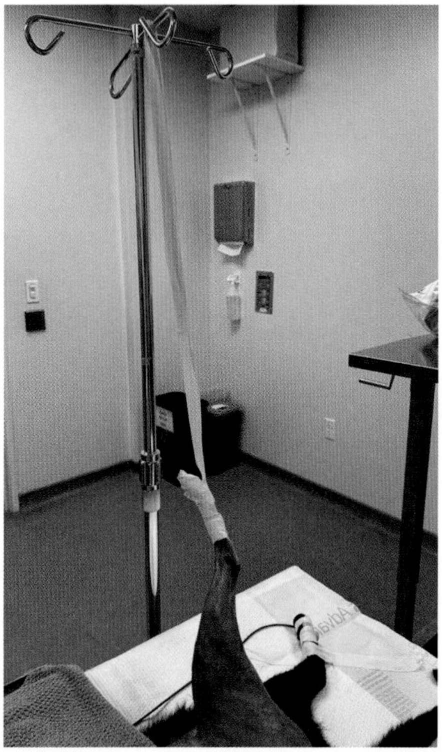

Figure 37.10 The surgical limb is hanging from an intravenous pole by the use of tape.

can either be moved cranially over the patient (Figure 37.11), remain caudal to the patient and draped with the patient, or caudal to the patient but not connected to the patient and draped separately.

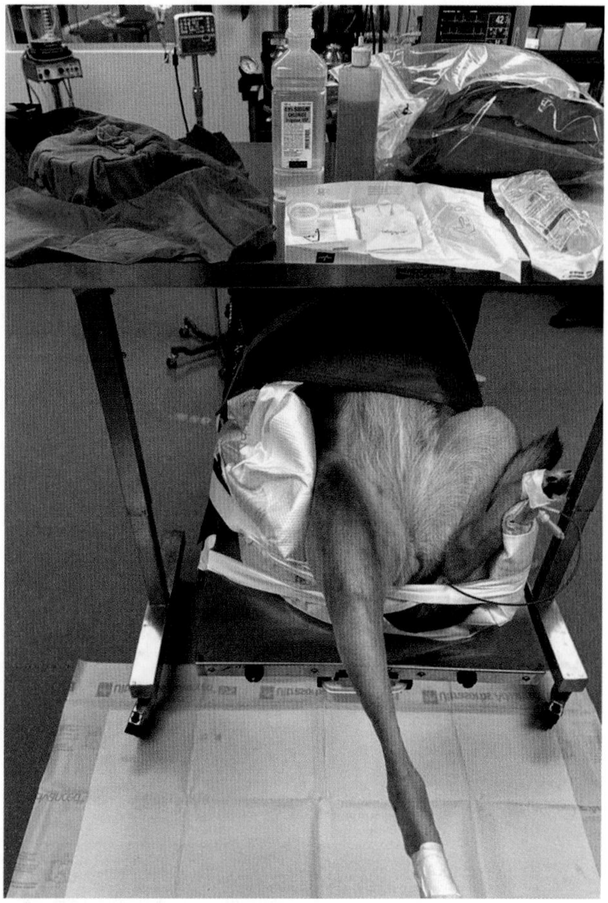

Figure 37.11 The instrument table is positioned cranially over the patient. Supplies for a sterile scrub are laid out.

Sterile Scrub

Patient is now ready for sterile preparation. Remove the cap from the sterile saline bottle and have chlorhexidine scrub to the side. Open a sterile bowl containing a stack of sterile non-woven gauze. Apply a sterile glove to the dominant hand only. Split the sterile gauze into two stacks with the dominant hand, leaving one stack inside the bowl and keeping the other stack dry outside of the bowl. With the non-sterile hand, pour sterile saline into the bowl until the gauze is well dampened. Lightly pour chlorhexidine scrub onto the dampened gauze. With the dominant hand, begin scrubbing at the center of the expected incision site and continue moving outward in a spiral course until the shaved region has been covered (Figure 37.12). Each chlorhexidine swipe should last approximately 60 seconds to allow adequate contact time before wiping off with the sterile dry gauze. This combination is repeated a minimum of three times. If hair is touched, restart the count.

Allow chlorhexidine scrub to fully dry if planning on using 3M™ DuraPrep™ solution, which is an antimicrobial surgical prepping solution that also enhances drape adhesion. DuraPrep™ should not be used on open wounds (Figure 37.13).

Draping

Open the orthopedic surgery pack (seen in Box 37.1) and orthopedic instrument tray. Lay out a sterile gown and gloves for the person scrubbing in. From this point, each of the following tasks should be performed with the intent of avoiding contamination. Using sterile surgical towels or sterile adhesive drapes, a "four-quarter-drape" technique will be used on the affected limb. Stepping away from the sterile field, open and hold the adhesive drape up with both hands, folding the top of the longest side, away from the sterile assistant. Peel off the adhesive protector and position each hand on the corners and wrap the adhesive drape around them, creating a cuff (Figure 37.14). This will protect the sterile glove from contacting the patient while draping.

While making sure the surgical gown does not touch the unsterile part of the table, place an adhesive drape cranially, caudally, and then laterally on both sides. Placement of the adhesive drapes should be approximately 1-inch

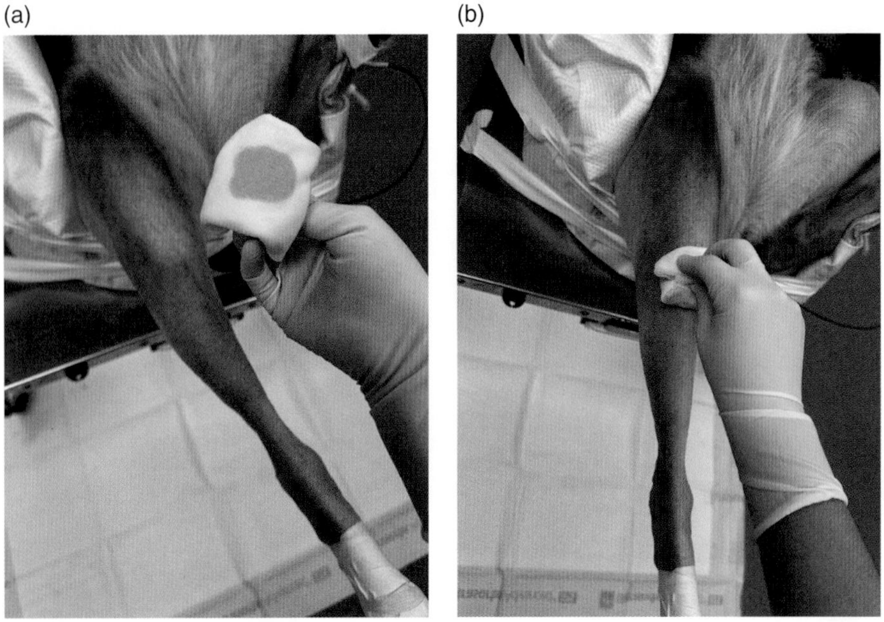

Figure 37.12 (a) Chlorhexidine scrub is applied to the sterile gauze. (b) Sterile scrub is started from the center of the proposed incision site.

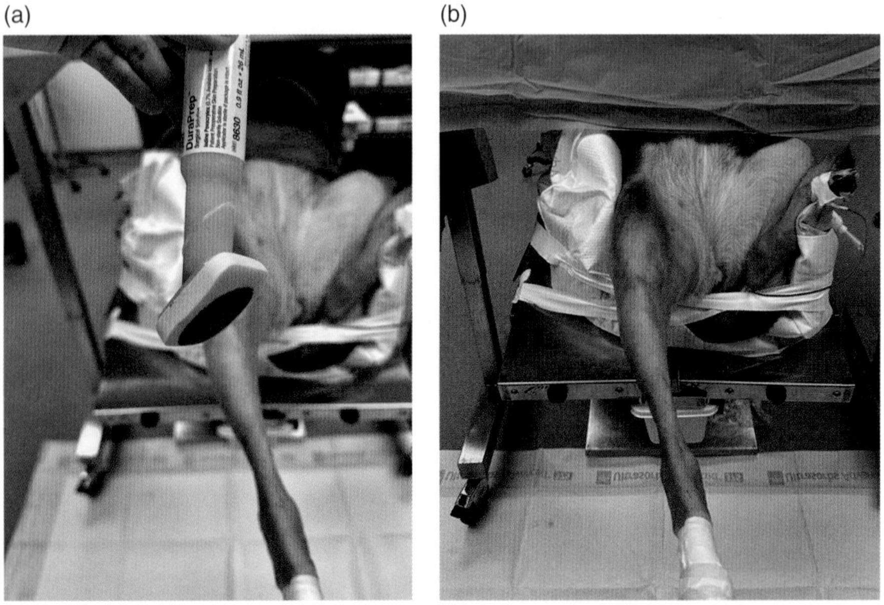

Figure 37.13 (a) 3M™ DuraPrep™ solution (iodine and isopropyl alcohol as antiseptic agents) has been snapped to allow fluid to flow into the sponge. (b) Surgical limb has been "painted" with DuraPrep™.

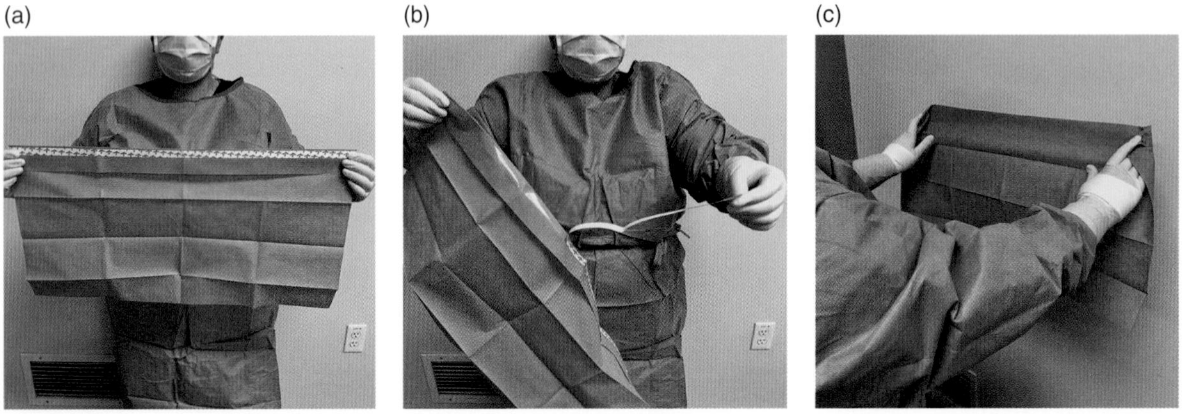

Figure 37.14 (a) Adhesive drape is opened and folded. (b) The adhesive protector is peeled off. (c) Each hand is wrapped around the drape.

from the clipped hair. The corners where the adhesive drapes meet should overlap each other. When using sterile adhesive drapes, the choice of using towel clamps is optional. Next, if using towel clamps, place them on the corners or about 5 mm from the lateral aspects of the drape where needed, penetrating both towel and epidermis. Each towel clamp should only be tightened to the first ridge. Drapes should be even and taut to prevent hair from entering the sterile field. If the surgical limb is suspended from a pole, use a sterile clear adhesive drape and/or sterile cohesive bandage wrap (e.g., Vetrap™) to cover the foot. This creates a sterile barrier, allowing the entire limb to be manipulated in the sterile field. Once the foot is halfway draped, the circulating technician will release the tape to allow the sterile assistant to complete coverage of the foot (Figure 37.15).

A large patient drape sheet is then placed on top of the patient. Keeping one hand on the patient drape, start unfolding cranially and caudally, including the sterile instrument table to create one big sterile field. Open the drape toward the person setting up. Next, use both hands to spread open the rest of the drape. If the instrument table is not connected to the patient, a separate drape sheet can be used to cover each table. Refrain from cutting a hole in the patient drape until instrumentation has been set up to reduce skin exposure.

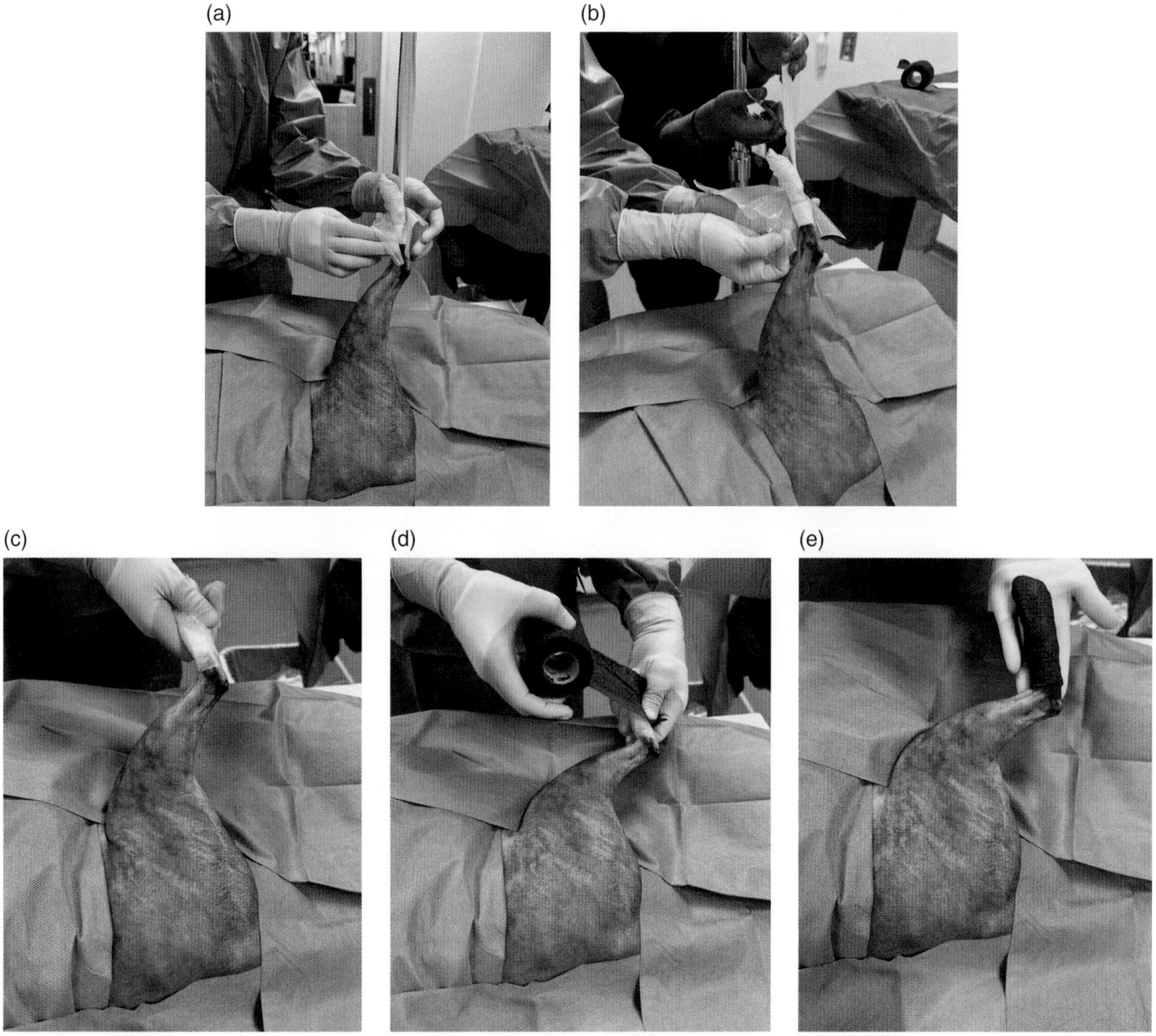

Figure 37.15 Using a sterile technique to include the limb into the surgical field. (a) A sterile clear adhesive drape is wrapped around the foot. (b) The circulating technician uses bandage scissors to release the tape attached to the foot. (c) The foot is completely covered with the sterile clear adhesive drape. (d) The sterile assistant starts to cover the foot with a sterile cohesive bandage wrap. (e) The foot is now completely covered with sterile cohesive bandage wrap.

Instructions on how to properly drape the patient are presented in Chapter 1, Figure 1.14.

Surgical Instrument Table

The patient and surgical instrument table should now be draped. Before an extra protective layer is added on top of the instrument table with a huck towel, any cables (e.g., monopolar cautery and power cords; Figure 37.16) can be laid out and passed off to the circulating technician toward the back of the table to be plugged into their respective power sources. The towel drape will help the cords stay hidden and prevent them from getting in the way intraoperatively (Figure 37.17). If suction or any other connections are at the front end of the patient table, secure them with a spare traumatic forcep, like an Allis tissue forcep.

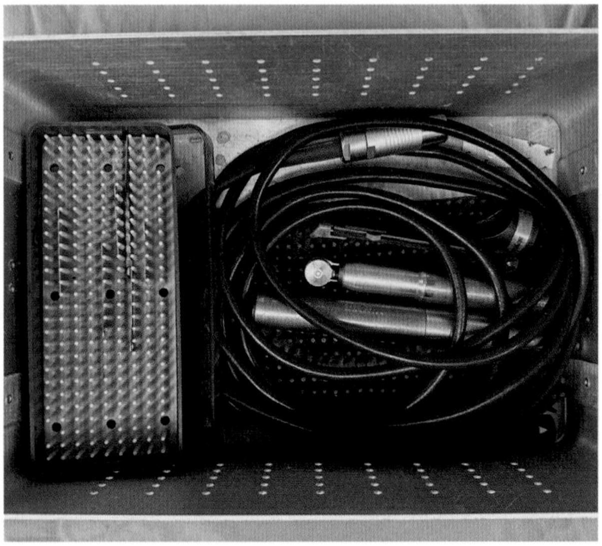

Figure 37.16 Sterile sagittal power and cord.

Avoid using an atraumatic forcep, like a mosquito hemostatic forcep, to prevent the more delicate instruments from being damaged.

The orthopedic instrument tray (Figure 37.18) can now be placed on the instrument table with the rings of the instruments facing the surgeon. Instrumentation should be set out in the order that it will be utilized (Figure 37.19), and dexterity of the surgeon should be considered (i.e., left- versus right-handed).

The circulating technician may then begin opening more instruments (i.e., implants, power equipment, antimicrobial incise drape, and light handles) that are specific to the procedure being performed. Scalpel blades should be dropped last. Create a hole in the patient drape to expose the center of the four-quarter drape. Carefully reach into the cut-out hole, grab the sterile foot, and pull the limb into the surgical field. A sterile antimicrobial incise drape (e.g., 3M™ Ioban™) can be placed. Ioban is designed to help reduce the risk of surgical site infection by delivering broad-spectrum antimicrobial activity throughout the surgical procedure. The incise drape should be smooth over the proposed incision site (Figure 37.20). This completes the instrument table and patient setup (Figure 37.21).

If the C-arm fluoroscopy was requested, it can now be draped with a plastic sterile cover. The sterile assistant and a circulating technician must assist each other in draping the C-arm. The sterile assistant will open up the C-arm drape while the circulating technician helps grab the inner, unsterile, portion of the drape and pull down until the C-arm is completely covered (Figure 37.22). The sterile assistant may now move and position the fluoroscopy where it is needed. If the procedure requires the fluoroscopy table, the table will also require draping. The table must be completely covered on all sides to allow the C-arm to be positioned between the patient and the table.

(a)

(b)

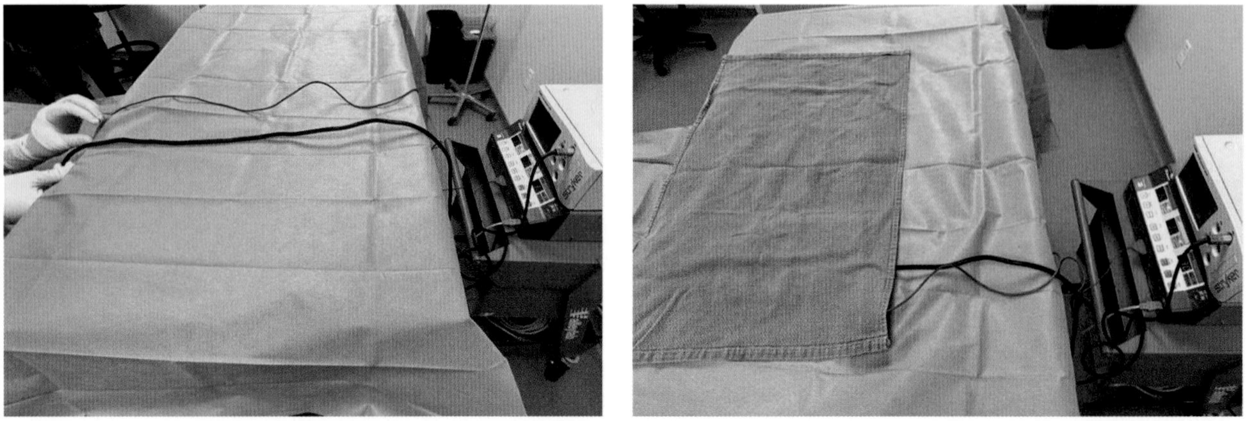

Figure 37.17 (a) Monopolar cautery and power cords are passed off. (b) A towel drape is laid on top of the cords.

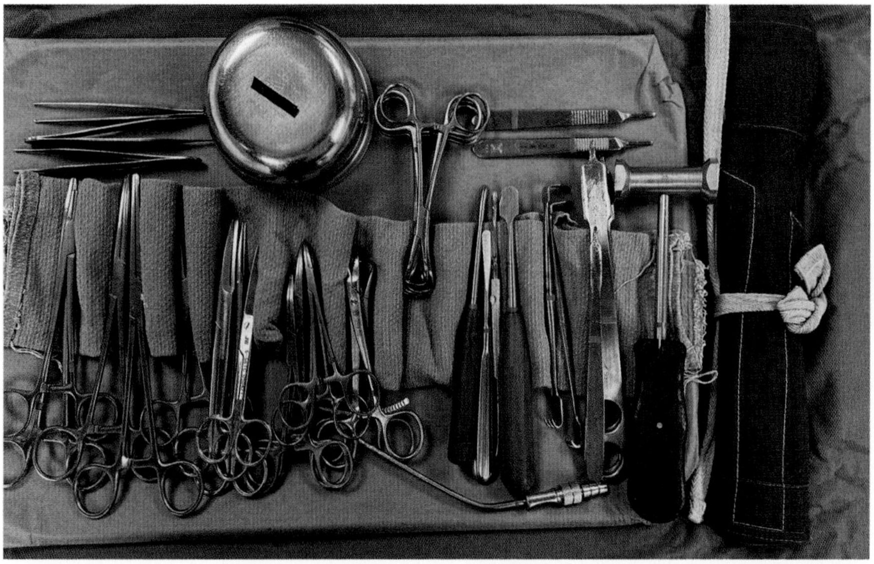

Figure 37.18 An orthopedic tray.

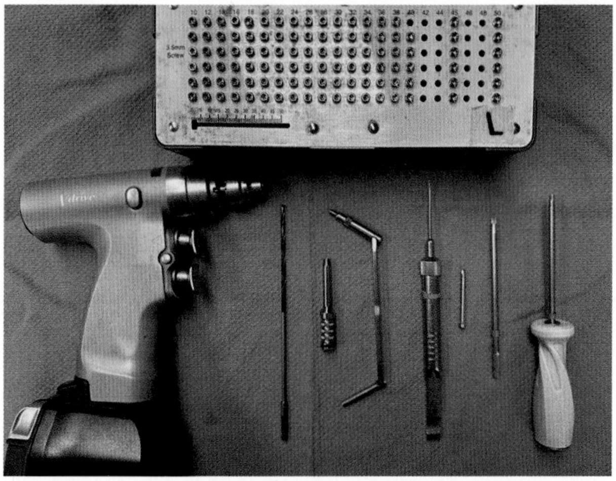

Figure 37.19 (Top) Sterile bone screw rack. (Bottom) Power tool, drill bit, locking drill guide, double drill guide, depth gauge, bone screw, power screw driver quick-release attachment, and handheld screw driver.

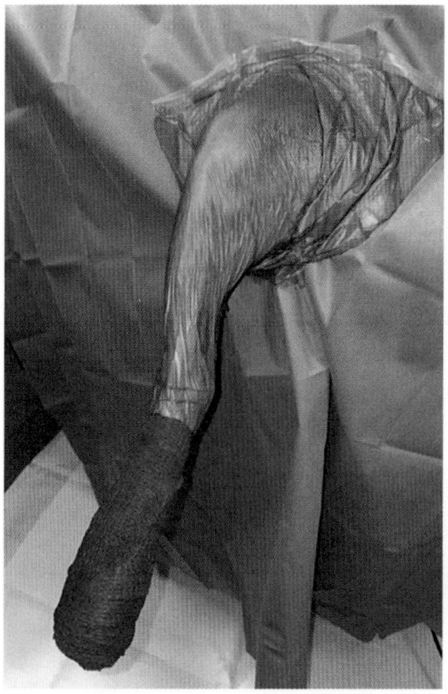

Figure 37.20 The limb is included in the surgical field and an antimicrobial incise drape is placed.

Intraoperative Considerations

Checklist

Before the surgeon starts the incision, people in the operating room should introduce themselves and a technician will recite a safety checklist. A checklist helps ensure important information has been gathered and reduces the potential for medical errors, thus improving patient care (Figure 37.23). It is important for orthopedic procedures to have preoperative radiographs ready and displayed for the surgeon (Figure 37.24).

The operating table should be adjusted to the surgeon's height to ensure good posture. The technician circulating should pay attention to the procedure and proactively anticipate the surgeon's needs throughout the entire surgery. Gauze and saline may be to be refilled and additional instrumentation may be needed. The circulating technician should be prepared to refill and retrieve these items. All personnel should be cognizant of the operating room and respect the sterile field. The room should be kept clean and organized. The scrub assistant should ensure tidiness of the instrument table. All orthopedic implants used should be taken into account for documentation purposes.

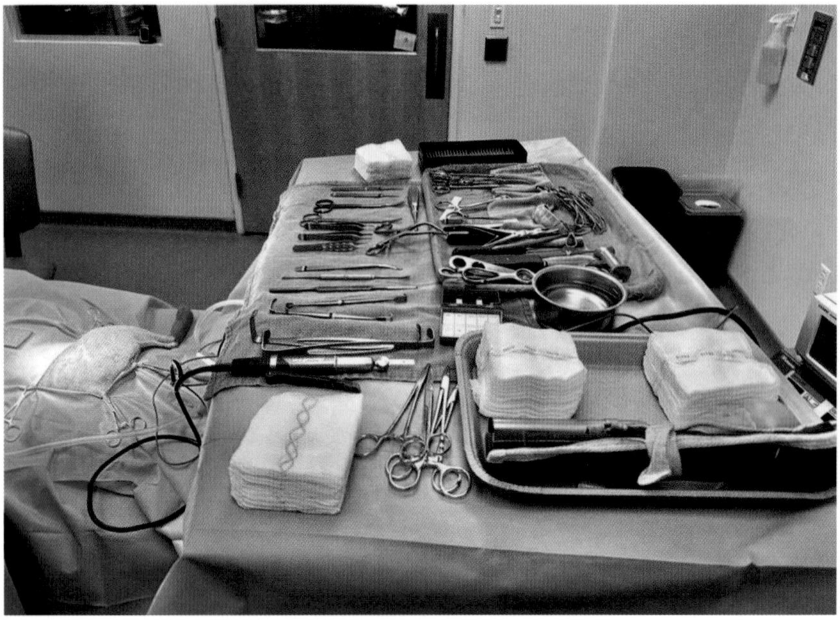

Figure 37.21 Complete instrument setup.

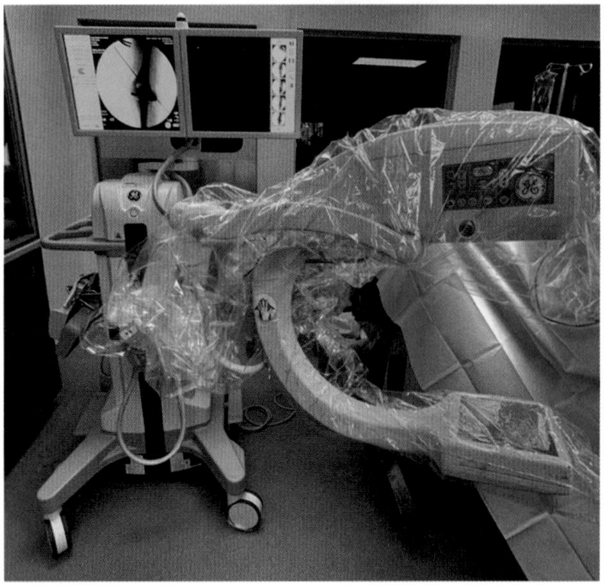

Figure 37.22 C-arm fluoroscopy is completely covered with a sterile C-arm drape.

The anesthetist should monitor and record vital signs on a medical record every five minutes (Figure 37.25). It is important to communicate with the surgeon if a patient's vital signs are abnormal or if the patient's plane of anesthesia changes and intervention is needed. An emergency drug sheet tailored to the patient's weight should be readily available in the case of an emergency. The anesthetist may repeat administration of antibiotic injection if needed. The patient's eyes should be lubed every 30 minutes to reduce the risk of corneal ulceration.

Postoperative Considerations

After surgery is finished, sharp objects should be removed from the surgical field and all dirty instruments put away for cleaning. Gently remove the large patient drape and huck towels or adhesive drapes, being mindful of towel clamps.

If the foot was covered, ensure wrap is removed safely with proper bandage scissors. Clean around the incision site with saline. Once dry, apply an adhesive wound dressing (e.g., Primapore) to protect the incision for the first 24 hours after surgery. If a purse string suture was placed on the anus, it can be removed. All patients who had orthopedic implants inserted (and some other patients per surgeon discretion) should have postoperative radiographs to ensure proper placement was achieved. Before the patient is transported out of the operating room, ensure there is a radiology room and recovery area ready (Figure 37.26). Once radiographs are obtained and have been approved by the surgeon, the patient may now be moved to a recovery area. Before the anesthetic gas is completely turned off, confirm with the doctor if they prefer the patient to stay unconscious for treatment (i.e., bandage application and urinary catheter placement). Bandage material should be readily available if needed postoperatively (Figure 37.27).

In cases where a patient received an epidural, the patient's bladder should be expressed manually or with the use of a red rubber catheter. Surgeons may consider keeping a urinary catheter postoperatively for bandage protection, for an aggressive patient who requires limited contact, or if strict cage rest without walks is deemed necessary.

Recovery period can vary per patient, and it should never be rushed. Keep the patient warm, moisten the tongue, and

SURGERY SAFETY CHECKLIST

PRE-OP (Before Surgeon arrives)

- ☐ CPR ___ DNR _____
- ☐ CPR sheet
- ☐ Confirm patient / Procedure / Positioning
- ☐ Print signed est. _____ $? _____
- ☐ Allergies? _____ Owner food?_____
- ☐ Owner Meds?________________
- ☐ Radiograph request submitted: Pre-op_____ Post-op _____
- ☐ BW Requested ___ Submitted ___
- ☐ Reviewed By: ___________
- ☐ Anesthetic protocol complete?
- ☐ Confirm surgical site: __________
- ☐ Check skin or N/A

  Anesthesia machine check
- ☐ Prep _______ OR _______
- ☐ Antibiotic given or HOLD
- ☐ Pre-op Text sent
- ☐ RTC Time ____________
- ☐ Open Dr. WW Operating Report

INTRA-OP (To be read to surgeon)

Date:
Procedure: ____________________
Surgeon: ____________________
Anesthetist: ____________________

- ☐ Anesthetic monitoring devices
- ☐ Specific equipment available
- ☐ Essential imaging displayed
- ☐ Gauze: #_____ Soft: #_____ or N/A
  Sponge: # _____
  Hemoclips: #___________
- ☐ Patient name/ Procedure/ Site/State
- ☐ Inform surgeon of CPR status
- ☐ Blades dropped

Patient Label

POST-OP

- ☐ Sponge count complete or N/A
  Hemoclips used: #____________
- ☐ Marked stapling equipment
- ☐ Scope/C-arm images iPad ___ Server ___
- ☐ Scope Tower: Buttercup / Blossom / Bubbles
- ☐ Confirm charges / Implants
- ☐ Sharps safely removed
- ☐ Equipment problems recorded
- ☐ Remove surgical footwrap or N/A
- ☐ Purse string/ Tampon removed or N/A
- ☐ Recovery concerns: ________ or none
  IMC vs ICU
- ☐ Express bladder or N/A (i.e. Epidural)
- ☐ Nail trim
- ☐ 1st IVC Plan: IVF ___ CRI ___ Flush ___
  2nd Flush ___ Pull____
- ☐ Specimens submitted to: ______________
  by:_________ EVP-Ezyvet charge_______
- ☐ Remove ART line / Pressure wrap
- ☐ Cage card/Smartflow reflects patient's CPR status

Figure 37.23 An example of a surgery safety checklist.

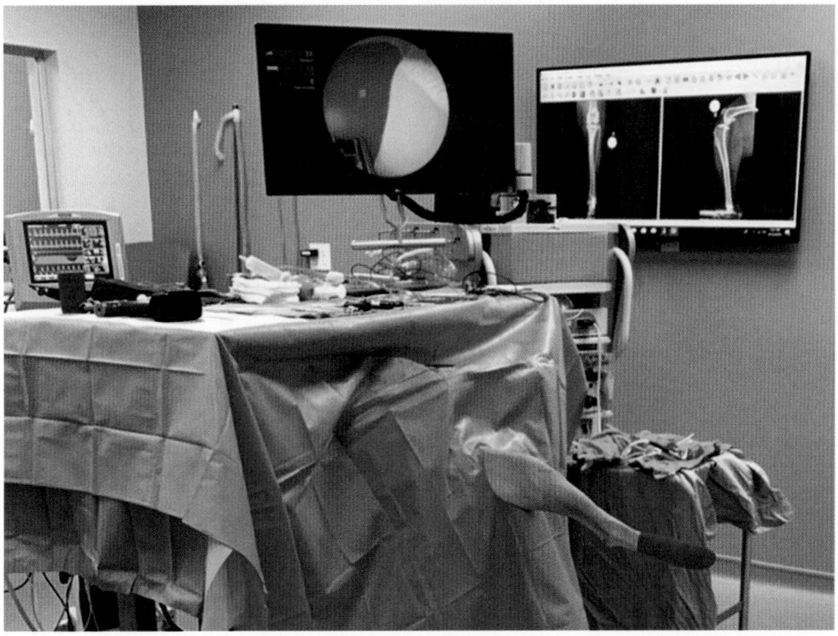

Figure 37.24 Preoperative radiographs displayed for the surgeon.

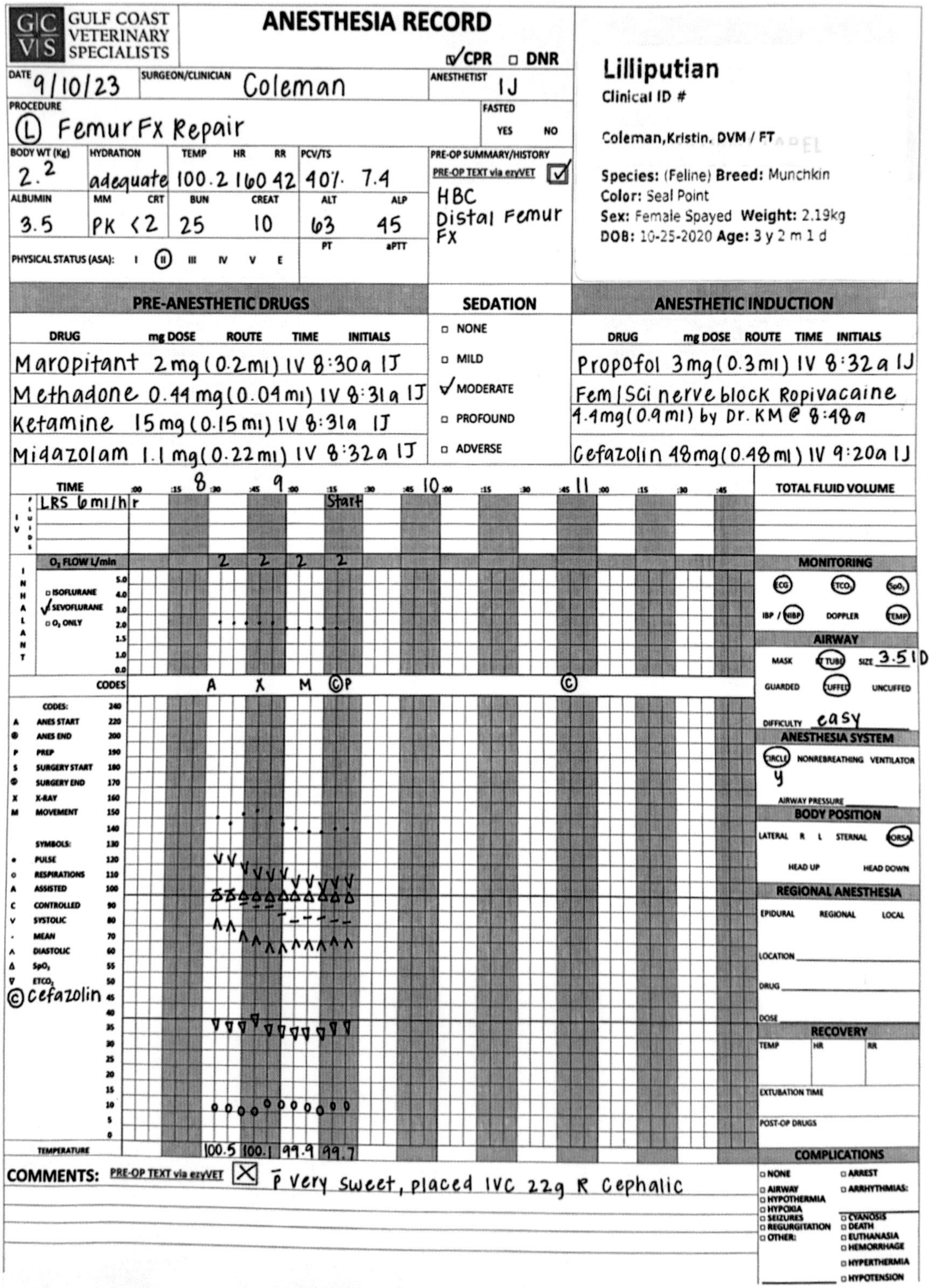

GULF COAST VETERINARY SPECIALISTS

ANESTHESIA RECORD

☑ CPR ☐ DNR

DATE 9/10/23 | SURGEON/CLINICIAN Coleman | ANESTHETIST IJ

PROCEDURE Ⓛ Femur Fx Repair | FASTED YES NO

Lilliputian
Clinical ID #
Coleman, Kristin, DVM / FT
Species: (Feline) Breed: Munchkin
Color: Seal Point
Sex: Female Spayed Weight: 2.19kg
DOB: 10-25-2020 Age: 3 y 2 m 1 d

BODY WT (Kg)	HYDRATION	TEMP	HR	RR	PCV/TS	
2.2	adequate	100.2	160	42	40%	7.4

ALBUMIN	MM	CRT	BUN	CREAT	ALT	ALP
3.5	PK	<2	25	10	63	45

PT aPTT

PHYSICAL STATUS (ASA): I Ⓘ III IV V E

PRE-OP SUMMARY/HISTORY
PRE-OP TEXT via ezyVET ☑
HBC
Distal Femur Fx

PRE-ANESTHETIC DRUGS

DRUG	mg DOSE	ROUTE	TIME	INITIALS
Maropitant	2mg (0.2ml)	IV	8:30a	IJ
Methadone	0.44 mg (0.04ml)	IV	8:31a	IJ
Ketamine	15mg (0.15ml)	IV	8:31a	IJ
Midazolam	1.1 mg (0.22ml)	IV	8:32a	IJ

SEDATION
☐ NONE
☐ MILD
✓ MODERATE
☐ PROFOUND
☐ ADVERSE

ANESTHETIC INDUCTION

DRUG	mg DOSE	ROUTE	TIME	INITIALS
Propofol	3mg (0.3ml)	IV	8:32a	IJ
Fem/Sci nerve block Ropivacaine 4.4mg (0.9ml) by Dr. KM @ 8:48a				
Cefazolin	48mg (0.48ml)	IV	9:20a	IJ

TIME :00 :15 8 :30 :45 9 :00 :15 :30 :45 10 :00 :15 :30 :45 11 :00 :15 :30 :45 | TOTAL FLUID VOLUME

FLUIDS: LRS 6ml/hr — Start

O₂ FLOW L/min: 2 2 2 2

INHALANT: ☐ ISOFLURANE ✓ SEVOFLURANE ☐ O₂ ONLY (5.0, 4.0, 3.0, 2.0, 1.5, 1.0, 0.0)

CODES: A X M ©P ©

CODES: A ANES START; ● ANES END; P PREP; S SURGERY START; ● SURGERY END; X X-RAY; M MOVEMENT

SYMBOLS: • PULSE; o RESPIRATIONS; A ASSISTED; C CONTROLLED; V SYSTOLIC; · MEAN; ^ DIASTOLIC; Δ SpO₂; ▽ ETCO₂

© cefazolin

TEMPERATURE: 100.5 100.1 99.9 99.7

MONITORING: ECG, ETCO₂, SpO₂, IBP / NIBP, DOPPLER, TEMP

AIRWAY: MASK, ET TUBE, SIZE 3.5 ID; GUARDED, CUFFED, UNCUFFED; DIFFICULTY easy

ANESTHESIA SYSTEM: CIRCLE, NONREBREATHING, VENTILATOR; y; AIRWAY PRESSURE

BODY POSITION: LATERAL R L, STERNAL, DORSAL; HEAD UP, HEAD DOWN

REGIONAL ANESTHESIA: EPIDURAL, REGIONAL, LOCAL; LOCATION; DRUG; DOSE

RECOVERY: TEMP, HR, RR; EXTUBATION TIME; POST-OP DRUGS

COMPLICATIONS: ☐ NONE ☐ ARREST ☐ AIRWAY ☐ ARRHYTHMIAS: ☐ HYPOTHERMIA ☐ HYPOXIA ☐ SEIZURES ☐ CYANOSIS ☐ REGURGITATION ☐ DEATH ☐ OTHER: ☐ EUTHANASIA ☐ HEMORRHAGE ☐ HYPERTHERMIA ☐ HYPOTENSION

COMMENTS: PRE-OP TEXT via ezyVET ☒ p̄ very sweet, placed IVC 22g R Cephalic

Figure 37.25 An intra-operative anesthesia medical record. See Chapter 1 (Figure 1.23) for an example of a blank anesthesia record.

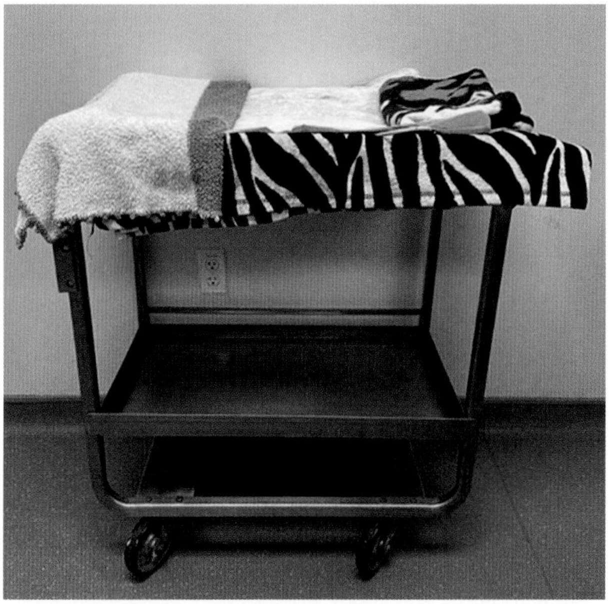

Figure 37.26 Example of a postoperative gurney for patient transportation.

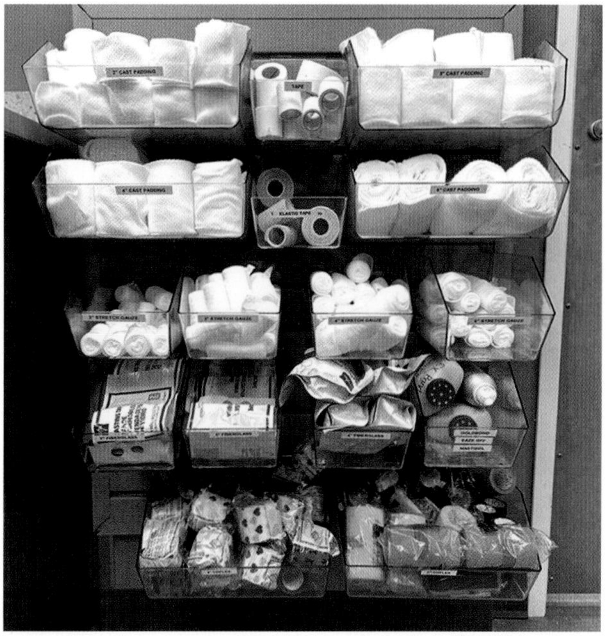

Figure 37.27 Various bandage materials.

apply lube to the eyes one more time. Before the anesthetic gas is completely off, ensure the patient has not regurgitated and needs attention. At this point, the patient's nails can be trimmed, anal sacs expressed, and ears cleaned if the patient is not in a critical state. Oxygenate the patient for five minutes after inhalant gas has been turned off. To prepare for extubation, the endotracheal tube's cuff should be completely deflated and untied. The technician should be prompt to react if the patient wakes up in a dysphoric state and needs protection from hurting themselves. The patient should be kept in the recovery area until the doctor is comfortable with the postoperative vital signs.

Before the patient is moved to its recovery kennel, ensure the kennel is prepared. Examples of a well-prepared kennel include having clean and comfortable bedding, non-slip mats, heat support, infusion pumps, and an Elizabethan collar. Icing the incision is a good postoperative practice and should be done for 5–10 minutes every 6 hours to reduce postoperative swelling. A support sling should be used to assist the patient when walking. Ideally, two technicians should assist with sling walking for better support and control on larger patients. The patient should be kept safe, comfortable, and relaxed; have oral sedation orders ready (i.e., trazodone). The doctor's postoperative treatment plan should be followed and monitoring continued until the patient is discharged into their owner's care.

38

Principles of Fracture Repair

Seth Bleakley

CARE Surgery Center, Phoenix, AZ, USA

Key Points

- Surgical fixation often better restores anatomy than conservative management.
- Surgical fixation allows a more rapid return to function often without the need for external coaptation and associated morbidity.
- Biological osteosynthesis refers to minimizing the impact of fracture treatment on the healing potential of the fracture zone.
- A trend toward biological osteosynthesis has led to less invasive approaches to fracture repair.
- Minimally invasive osteosynthesis (MIO) refers to approaching a fracture with the goal of preserving healing potential and includes minimally invasive plate osteosynthesis (MIPO), minimally invasive nail osteosynthesis (MINO), external skeletal fixation (ESF), and percutaneous pin/screw fixation.

Introduction to Fractures

A bone fracture can be defined as a partial or complete break in a bone. Fractures can occur in long or flat bones. Most fractures in healthy bones are due to trauma, where a force is communicated either extrinsically or intrinsically, excessive to the bone's ability to resist deformation. The type of fracture is dependent on patient age, injury location, and type of inciting force.

Patient age affects the composition and mechanical properties of bone. Bone is comprised of collagen rich connective tissue and a mineralized matrix supporting a diverse regenerative cellular population that includes osteoblasts, osteocytes, osteoclasts, and white and red blood cells. Young patients have a higher ratio of collagen rich connective tissue to mineralized matrix, as well as a collagen-dense periosteum. As such, there may be greater plastic deformation before yield in juvenile fractures; or, in layman's terms, more bending of bone before it breaks. This has led to the coining of the phrase "greenstick" fracture, where in a juvenile long bone there may be bending or incomplete cortical disruption, or a lack of overlap of fracture ends due to an intact thick periosteum. Mature bone has a high proportion of mineralized cortical bone and, as a result, is more brittle and prone to complete cortical disruption.

Another consideration in juvenile fractures is physeal involvement. The physis is defined as a hyaline cartilage plate in the metaphysis of each end of a long bone and is responsible for growth, hence the synonymous term, growth plate. Hyaline cartilage is not mineralized but converted to bone through the process of endochondral ossification. This junction between soft cartilage and hard bone creates mechanical weakness, predisposing the physis to fracture.

* Please see Chapter 39 for more details about "Orthopedic Implants," which complements this chapter well for an in-depth understanding of orthopedic implants and their ideal applications.

Techniques in Small Animal Soft Tissue, Orthopedic, and Ophthalmic Surgery, First Edition. Edited by Kristin A. Coleman.

Companion website: www.wiley.com/go/coleman/surgeries

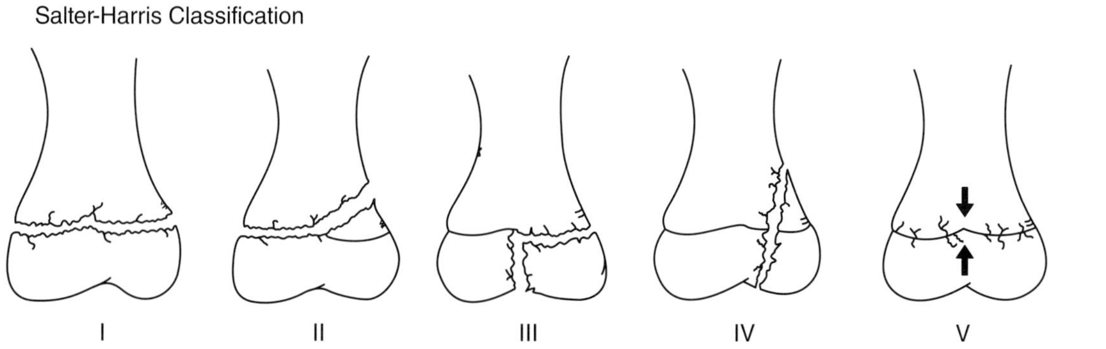

Figure 38.1 The five basic fracture types of the Salter-Harris classification are shown. A S-H type I fracture is a separation through the physis. A S-H type II fracture enters the plane of the physis and exits through the metaphysis. A S-H type III fracture enters the plane of the physis and exits through the epiphysis. A S-H type IV fracture crosses the physis, extending from the metaphysis to the epiphysis. A S-H type V fracture is a crushing injury to the entire physis, resulting in the destruction of further growth.[1] A S-H type VI fracture (not shown in this diagram) involves partial crushing of the physis.

The incidence of physeal involvement in juvenile fractures is attested by the existence of the classification scheme described by Robert Salter and William Harris in 1963 leading to physeal fractures being known as "Salter-Harris" fractures[1] (see Figure 38.1).

Injury location and type of inciting force also affect the resultant type of fracture. The diaphysis of mature long bone has a higher proportion of mineralized cortical bone to collagen so is more prone to comminuted fractures than the epiphysis/metaphysis or flat bones. Higher energy extrinsic trauma, such as from vehicular or ballistic impact, results in a higher incidence of bony comminution (e.g., Figure 38.19) than low energy or intrinsic trauma, such as from a fall (e.g., Figures 38.9 and 38.10).

Fractures may be described using the following terms:

- **Complete**: fracture with complete loss of cortical integrity
- **Incomplete**: fracture with incomplete loss of cortical integrity (e.g., "greenstick" fracture)
- **Transverse**: fracture line largely perpendicular to the long axis of the bone
- **Short oblique**: fracture line at a slight angle to the long axis of the bone
- **Long oblique**: fracture line at a very acute angle to the long axis of the bone, resulting in a relatively long fracture line
- **Spiral**: fracture where at least one part of the bone has been twisted
- **Segmental**: fracture involving three sequential pieces
- **Comminuted**: fracture involving more than three pieces
- **Open**: fracture with a wound communicating through the skin
- **Traumatic**: fracture secondary to extrinsic or intrinsic force
- **Pathologic**: fracture in a bone made weak by intrinsic disease, such as a lytic bone tumor or osteomyelitis
- **Displaced**: fracture ends deviate from anatomical alignment
- **Articular**: fracture with disruption of the hyaline cartilage articular surface of a joint

General Principles and Physiology of Fractures

Fracture management has made rapid advances in recent decades largely thanks to a greater understanding of physiology and technological advances in instrumentation. A key contributor has been the AO Foundation (*Arbeitsgemeinschaft für Osteosynthesefragen*, German for "working group for bone fusion issues"). Founded as a group in Switzerland in 1958 dedicated to improving fracture management, they described what have become known as the *AO* Principles,[2] which have become tenets of clinical decision-making ever since. The *AO principles* can be summarized as follows:

- Restoration of anatomy
- Establishment of stability
- Preservation of blood supply
- Early mobilization[2]

Restoration of Anatomy

Anatomical reduction of a fracture will restore bone length and alignment in all three planes. Planes used to describe long bones include the frontal, sagittal, and transverse. Lateral deviation in the frontal plane is known as valgus (Figure 38.2a), while medial deviation is known as varus (Figure 38.2b). Cranial deviation in the sagittal plane is known as recurvatum, while caudal deviation is known as procurvatum (Figure 38.2a). Deviation in the transverse plane is known as torsion and may be internal or external. Bone-healing with deviation from anatomical origin is known as malunion and can have variable consequences depending on the bone in question. Generally speaking, varus, valgus, and torsional deformities of long bones can have the most significant clinical consequences due to asymmetrical joint-loading, increased load on ligaments, and gait abnormalities. Therefore, in many cases, diligently restoring skeletal anatomy may offer the best chance of return to normal function.

Another major factor in considering anatomical restoration is articular involvement. Fractures involving articular surfaces carry the risk of degenerative joint disease if reduction is not anatomical. A gap in the articular surface will lead to fibrocartilaginous remodeling. A step or irregularity will lead to abnormal joint mechanics, which can wear hyaline cartilage and accelerate osteoarthritis. Consequently, anatomical reduction and rigid fixation is often paramount for favorable long-term prognosis in fractures involving articular surfaces.

Establishment of Stability

An explanation of the need for fracture stability requires a description of strain.

Strain has been defined as change in length relative to initial length:

$$Strain = \frac{Change\ in\ length}{Original\ length}$$

Softer tissues tolerate more strain than bone. Soft callus will tolerate 100% strain and still be able to form/heal (e.g., during the first few weeks of fracture healing, this initial soft callus will form despite movement in the fracture zone). Fibrocartilage will tolerate 10–30% strain (e.g., as the soft callus becomes denser, less movement is tolerated). Bone will only form in low strain environments of $<2\%$ (e.g., bone will not form until motion is almost eliminated).

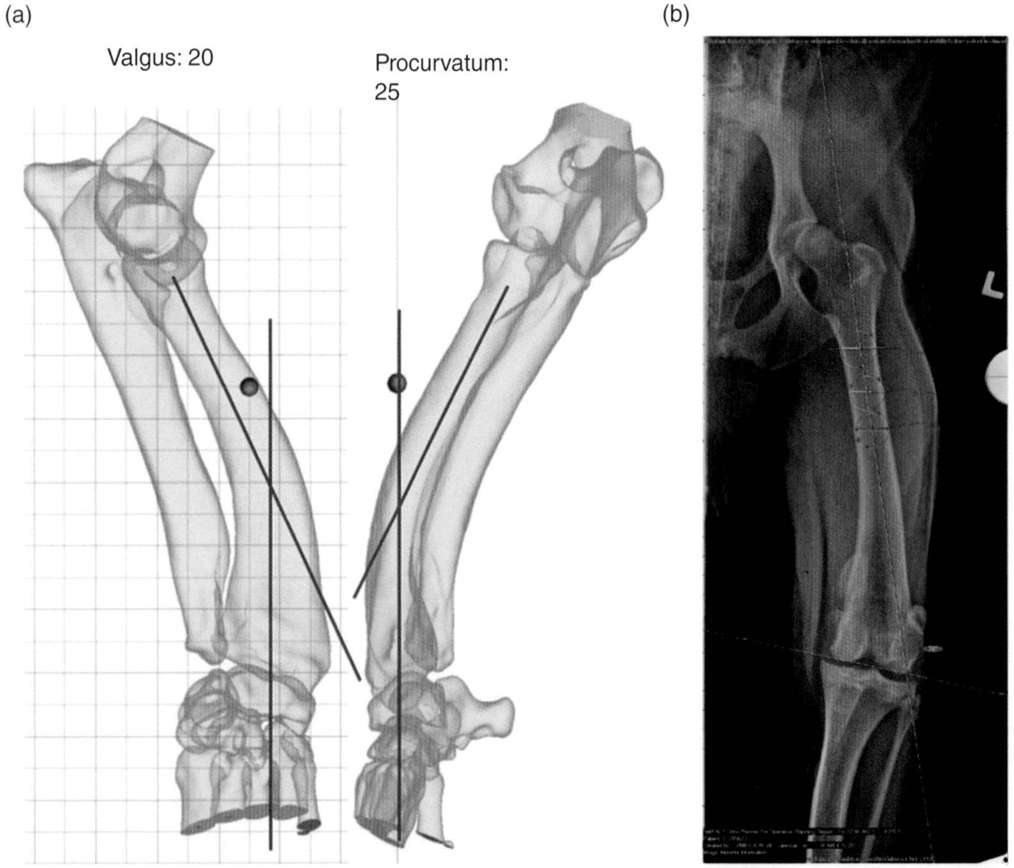

Figure 38.2 Demonstrations of angular limb deformities. (a) CT reconstruction of a canine antebrachium demonstrating lateral deviation in the frontal plane (=valgus) and caudal deviation in the sagittal plane (=procurvatum). (b) Cranio-caudal radiograph of a canine femur demonstrating medial deviation in the frontal plane (=varus). *Source:* © Seth Bleakley.

Strain is concentrated in small fracture gaps. Biologically speaking, unstable fractures heal by producing strain-tolerant tissues, such as soft callus that eventually mineralizes (becoming visible on radiographs), until enough stability is present to produce strain-intolerant bone. A fracture gap fills with a hematoma followed by fibrous connective tissue laying down cartilage and osteoid, also known as callus. This connective tissue forms rapidly, and proliferation exceeds the radius of the bone beyond anatomical origins. As the area moment of inertia of a cylinder is directly proportional to the radius to the power of 4 $\left(I = \frac{\pi(ro4 - ri4)}{4}\right)$ where I is area moment of inertia, ro is the outer diameter, and ri is the inner diameter), a small increase in radius creates a large increase in resistance to bending, and, therefore, rapid increase in stability. This lowers the strain, allowing formation of osteoid and bony remodeling until normal cortical bone can be formed, a process known as Haversian remodeling.[3] This entire process is known as secondary bone-healing and is the mechanism by which unstable fractures heal. However, if fracture instability is such that strain remains excessive for callus formation and biological stabilization to ever materialize, a nonunion will occur.

If fracture stability can be surgically achieved with a low strain environment <2%, primary bone-healing can occur without intermediate bone callus.[3] This requires very rigid fixation, often coupled with anatomical reduction. Interfragmentary compression is also often required to reduce strain sufficiently for primary bone-healing. The goal of achieving primary bone-healing has led to advances in internal fixation instrumentation and techniques.

Preservation of Blood Supply

Blood supply is critical to the healing of any tissue including bone.[4] Healthy bone requires a substantial blood flow to supply the requisite oxygen and nutrients and to eliminate carbon dioxide, acid, and other metabolic waste products.[4] Oxygen plays a critical role in the formation of collagen, the growth of new capillaries, and the control of infection. Sources from which fractures recruit their blood supply include endosteal vessels, periosteal vessels, muscles and surrounding soft tissues. Disruption of these sources can lead to delayed union or nonunion of bone. Successful fracture management must include a careful balance between anatomical reduction, rigid fixation, and preservation of blood supply. There is often a trade-off among the three. Zealous efforts to achieve anatomical reduction can disrupt the fracture hematoma, strip soft tissues, and reduce vital blood supply. While adding implants may improve fracture stability, each comes at the cost of blocking blood supply, especially where periosteal compression is involved. On the other hand, withholding implants to preserve blood supply can have negative consequences if the construct is not strong enough and subsequently fails. Achieving this balance requires appropriate decision-making, knowledge of the local anatomy of the soft tissue structures surrounding the fractured bone, and surgical skill for success in treating fractures.

Early Mobilization

That the AO Group started in Davos, Switzerland could be attributed to proximity to Alpine skiing-related injuries and long bone fractures. Historically, such injuries were managed conservatively with traction and immobilization with casting or limb-hanging. Disadvantages of such an approach included muscle atrophy, joint stiffness, decreased bone density, and a prolonged rehabilitation period before full function could be (if ever) established. Bone responds to immobilization according to Wolff's law, which states that it will adapt to the load under which it is placed, or conversely, will become less dense and weaker under decreased load.[5] Joint immobilization has been reported to lead to stiffness, replacement of hyaline cartilage with bone, and decreased ligament and tendon strength.[6,7]

On 17 September 1908, Orville Wright crashed the infamous *Wright Flyer* and suffered severe injuries that included femoral, pelvic, and rib fractures. His injuries were cared for in the conservative manner of the day at Fort Myer Army Hospital in Arlington, Virginia. He wasn't discharged until 1 November 1908, almost three months later. His injuries reportedly never fully healed, he suffered pain in his pelvis and ribs for the rest of his life, and his time as a pilot was subsequently greatly reduced.[8] Some of the most obvious benefits of modern fracture management include short hospitalization time, early mobilization, and early return to function. Early mobilization is both prerequisite to, and a benefit of, successful fracture management.

Minimally Invasive Osteosynthesis and the *Carpenter* Versus *Gardener* Paradigm

Successful fracture management must include a careful balance between anatomical reduction, rigid fixation, and preservation of blood supply. A bias in this balance has been described paradigmatically as the "*Carpenter*" versus the "*Gardener*" approach.

Simplistically, the "*Carpenter*" will be more concerned with anatomical reduction and the appearance of the repair visually and radiographically. This will be reflected in the invasiveness of the approach and the number of implants necessary to achieve such, often with bone plates, lag screws, and cerclage wires applied with the goal of interfragmentary compression. This can offer many of the aforementioned benefits, including restoration of anatomy/alignment, rigid fixation, early return to function, and the potential for primary bone-healing.

However, there is often a biological cost. Draining the fracture hematoma through open reduction and internal fixation has been shown to delay healing.[9] In experimentally-induced femoral fractures in rats, drainage of the fracture hematoma led to approximately 50% bending rigidity of the fracture callus at four-weeks post-fracture compared to the intact hematoma controls.[9] The effect was even more detrimental when drainage of the hematoma was delayed by two or four days, with intact hematoma fractures being 5–10 times stronger at four weeks.[9] The intact hematoma has been shown to provide growth factors and mesenchymal cells vital to rapid angiogenesis and fibrocartilaginous callus.

Application of implants directly to bone involves both stripping surrounding soft tissues, such as muscle, and compressing periosteal vasculature. The result is reduced blood supply to the bone for maintenance and healing. Cortical bone beneath compressed implants becomes devitalized,[10] and bone-healing may be delayed or impaired. Delayed bone-healing will increase the amount of time and subsequent cyclic-loading forces on the construct and implants. This can increase the incidence of screw loosening, material fatigue, and implant failure. Ironically, a stronger, more rigid construct can have a higher incidence of failure if there is a threshold detriment to the biological component of fracture healing. If the application of implants robs the fracture zone of its ability to heal quickly, the construct will have to resist fracture forces longer and may fail.

Simplistically, the "*Gardener*" will be more concerned with the preservation of soft tissues and blood supply than anatomical reduction and rigid fixation. Surgical approaches will be less invasive than those of the "*carpenter*," and, therefore, less disruptive to soft tissues and periosteum. Implants will be more minimalistic and more focused on spanning the fracture zone rather than reconstructing it. Fragments and interfragmentary compression will often be ignored, with the assumption that the body will integrate and remodel fragments through biological processes. Biological osteosynthesis will occur more rapidly due to the preservation of fracture hematoma and soft tissues providing blood supply.

There are both mechanical and biomechanical costs to bias toward the "*Gardener*" approach. Implants distant to the axis of the bone will reduce the stiffness of the construct. A minimalistic blood supply-friendly construct may have reduced load-sharing with bone, be less mechanically adequate, and may create a risk of early failure. Since primary bone-healing requires a low-strain environment, a repair without rigid fixation and interfragmentary compression can only result in secondary bone-healing with intermediate callus. Excessive micromotion may even lead to delayed or nonunion. Lack of attention to anatomical reduction can lead to malunion and angular deformities with subsequent clinical consequences.

Table 38.1 Summary of clinical data related to the treatment of human femoral fractures over three decades.

Variable	**Group 1 (1970s)**	**Group 2 (1980s)**	**Group 3 (1990s)**
Number of plate holes	12	14	15
Plate length (cm)	22	26	28
Number of plate screws	11	11	7
Plate screw density	95%	84%	45%
Primary bone graft	16%	30%	4%
Implant failures	*19%*	*10%*	*4%*
Delayed unions	*14%*	*7%*	*0*
Nonunions	*10%*	*3%*	*4%*
Malunions	*10%*	*7%*	*0*
Re-operations	*43%*	*31%*	*13%*
Clinical union (months)	5	5	3
Success rate	**62%**	**83%**	**87%**

As surgical techniques evolved toward biological osteosynthesis, complication, and revision rates significantly decreased, while bone-healing time and success rates significantly improved.
Source: Adapted from Rozbruch et al. [11]

As one would expect, neither paradigm is superior, and successful fracture management necessitates a careful balance between the "*Carpenter*" and "*Gardener*" approaches. Every fracture must be critically evaluated, taking mechanical, biological, and patient and client factors into account before making a treatment decision. Nevertheless, there has been a historical trending toward more minimally invasive fracture repair to promote biological osteosynthesis with data showing an improved clinical union success rate.[11]

As demonstrated in Table 38.1, over a period of ~30 years, a trend toward reducing plate holes, increasing plate length, and decreasing screw number and density, there has been a decrease in implant failures, delayed unions, malunions, and surgical revisions. While there may be a list of variables affecting these outcomes, repairs that better preserve biological osteosynthesis have an improved prognosis.

Fracture Forces

Discussing fracture repair options first necessitates an understanding of fracture forces. Repair choice will affect which forces are resisted and is a factor of both fracture configuration and the mechanical competencies of each

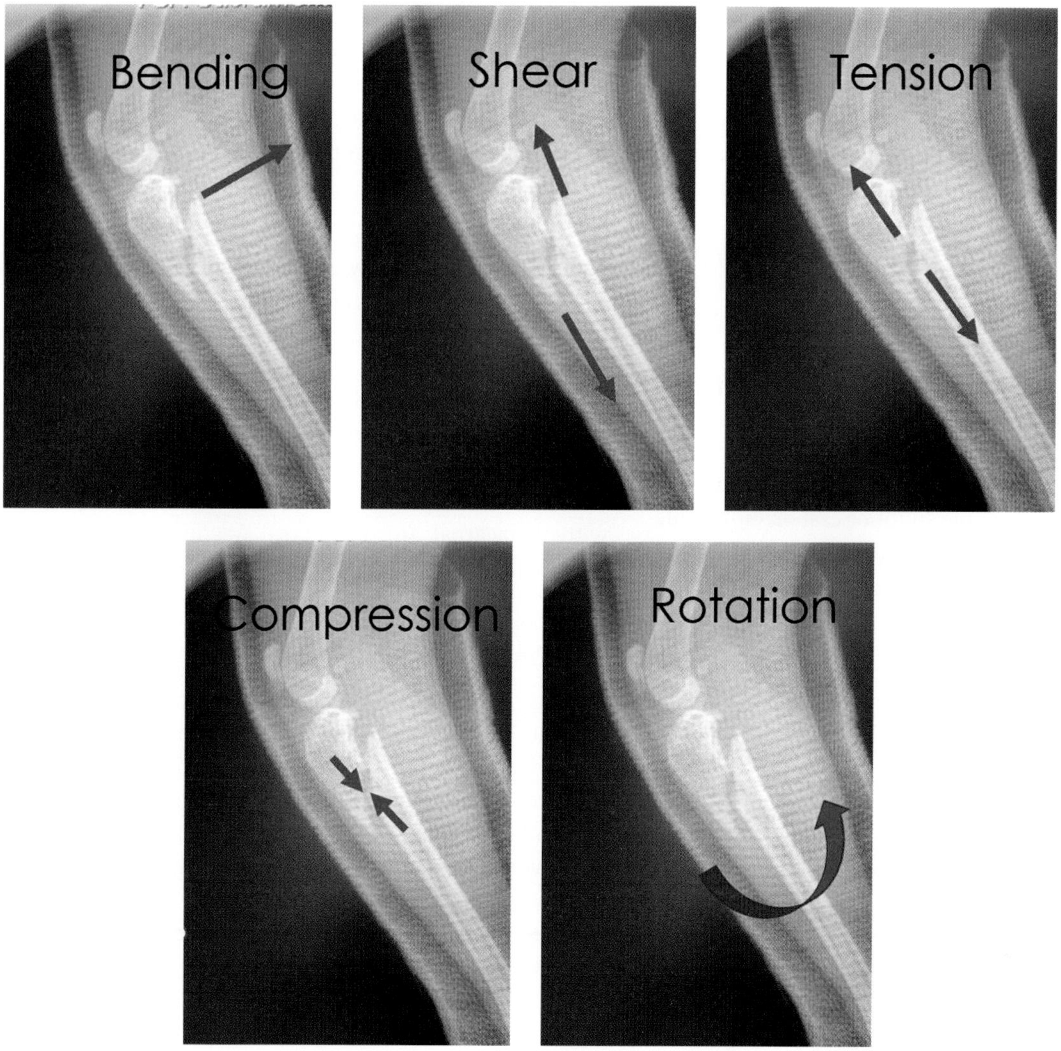

Figure 38.3 Fracture forces demonstrated by an oblique proximal tibial fracture in a feline. *Source:* © Seth Bleakley.

device or treatment option. Forces relevant to fractures include bending, shear, tension, compression, and rotation (Figure 38.3).

The rigid fixation will resist all fracture forces, resulting in the biggest reduction in strain and the best chance of primary bone-healing. A fracture with motion in any plane can only heal with secondary bone-healing with intermediate callus formation. Understanding fracture forces will aid clinical decision-making.

Fracture Treatment Options

The following fracture treatment options have been listed in ascending order of invasiveness (or impact on the biology of the fracture zone). This order is simplistic and does not reflect superiority but rather serves as a guide for decision-making with biological osteosynthesis in mind.

- External coaptation
- External skeletal fixation
- Minimally invasive osteosynthesis (MIO)
  - Percutaneous pin/screw fixation
  - Minimally invasive nail osteosynthesis (MINO)
  - Minimally invasive plate osteosynthesis (MIPO)
- Open reduction and internal fixation
  - Open but do not touch approach
  - Interlocking nail
  - Bone plate and screws
  - Pin and cerclage wire
  - Plate-rod, screw, cerclage combinations

External Coaptation

In the context of fractures, external coaptation involves attempted closed reduction (where indicated) and circumferential application of soft and rigid materials to a limb with the goal of providing support and preventing further displacement. External coaptation can also help reduce swelling and reduce discomfort associated with fractures in the acute and sub-acute periods. External coaptation has the advantages of avoiding surgery and any detriment to the biology of the fracture zone. The fracture hematoma is preserved, as are all soft tissues surrounding the fracture zone. However, while ligamentotaxis permits some control of fracture position, the closed reduction does not permit anatomical reduction and only allows for limited control of alignment. From a mechanical standpoint, external coaptation provides minimal resistance to fracture forces. External coaptation can provide resistance to bending forces but only in mid-diaphyseal fractures in appendicular long bones. As resistance to bending is a function of force and distance, the length of the splint or cast on either side of the fracture will determine efficacy. As such, external coaptation is less effective in femoral and humeral fractures, juxta-articular fractures, and in small chondrodystrophic breeds with short limbs.

External coaptation can provide limited resistance to rotational forces if a joint, such as the tarsus, is included in the splint or cast, but care must be taken to avoid sores on such bony prominences. There is a trade-off between adding additional cast padding to prevent sores and mechanical stability, as thick padding will result in increased motion within the cast (Figure 38.4). Depending on fracture configuration, external coaptation will only poorly resist shear, tension, and compression forces. Fractures most amenable to external coaptation include:

- Transverse mid-diaphyseal long bone fractures that permit load-sharing.
- Minimally displaced fractures that require minimal reduction.
- Fractures of distally located appendicular long bones, such as the tibia, radius, and ulna.
- Fractures in young animals with an intact periosteum that will heal rapidly.
- Fractures in compliant patients with compliant owners.

External coaptation may also be useful for fracture management post-operatively. A soft-padded bandage in the immediate postoperative period (one to two weeks) can be used to help manage peri-operative swelling and improve patient incisional compliance (e.g., to help prevent licking). A splint or a cast may also be used to protect a tenuous surgical repair such as when implants are deliberately undersized or anatomical limitations preclude rigid fixation, such as with metacarpal and metatarsal fractures (Figure 38.5). See Chapter 40 for external coaptation details.

External Skeletal Fixation (ESF)

External skeletal fixation involves the application of pins to bone adjacent to a fracture zone and connecting said pins with bars and/or rings to build a frame that spans a fracture, external to soft tissues. External skeletal fixation can be built to resist all fracture forces and is one of the most versatile methods of fracture fixation because of the ease of modification at any stage of the repair or healing process. The frame may be modified to increase or decrease rigidity or even lengthen the bone, such as in distraction osteogenesis. External skeletal fixation involves closed reduction without disrupting the biology of the fracture zone but permits more accurate alignment and

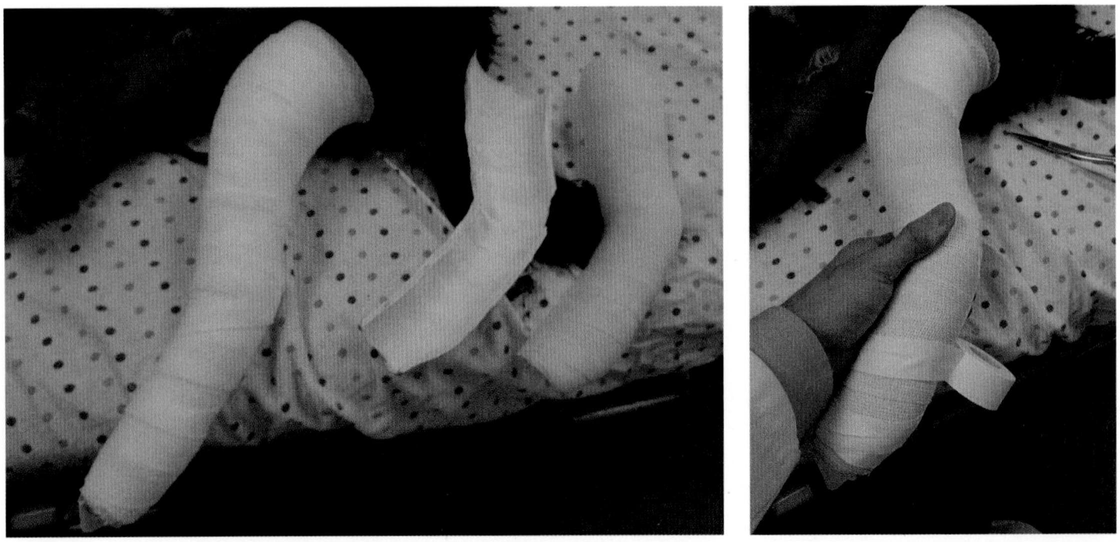

Figure 38.4 Example of external coaptation with a bivalved cast for a canine tibial fracture. Adequate cast padding is applied to minimize the risk of sores while still minimizing micromotion. The cast has been molded close to a standing angle and is secured with cotton tape. *Source:* © Seth Bleakley.

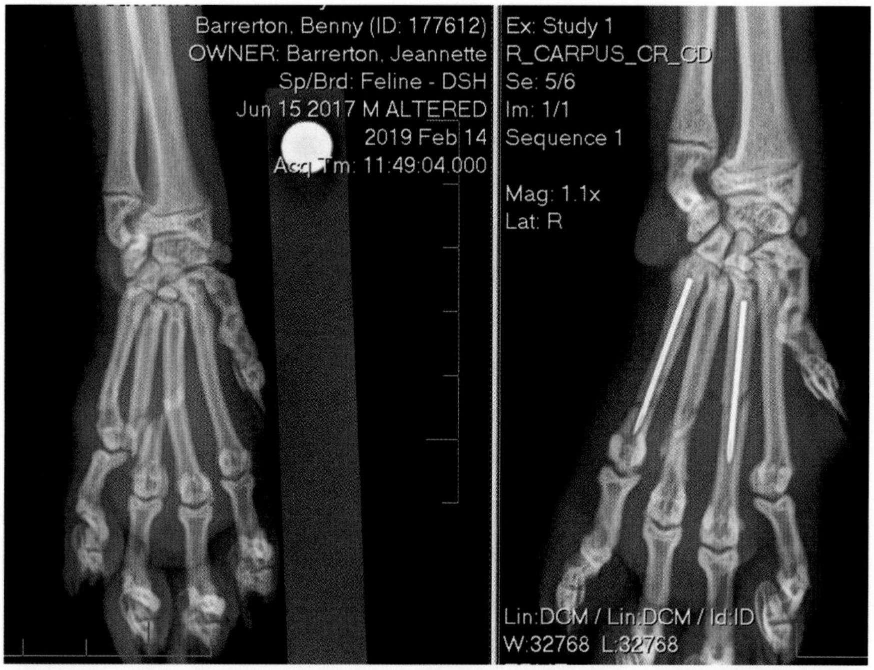

Figure 38.5 Open reduction and internal alignment of feline metacarpal fractures with intramedullary Kirschner wires. These bones were considered too small for more rigid fixation techniques, and therefore, external coaptation is required in the postoperative period until the clinical union is achieved. *Source:* © Seth Bleakley.

appositional correction through manipulation of the pin and connecting bar position.

External skeletal fixation can be classified as **linear**, **ring**, or combination, known as **hybrid**. Connecting bars can be made of steel, titanium, polymers, carbon, or custom-molded acrylic. Linear fixators can be applied to any bone that accepts pins, while ring-shaped fixators can be applied to distal long bones only. U-shaped fixators increase versatility around joints and even spinal fractures. Linear external skeletal fixation is classified as follows:

- Type 1a = unilateral, uniplanar
- Type 1b = unilateral, biplanar
- Type 2 = bilateral, uniplanar (Figure 38.6)
- Type 3 = bilateral, biplanar

Ring fixators have the advantage of requiring minimal bone purchase using tensioned Kirschner wires so are particularly useful for juxta-articular fractures where there is limited room for multiple pins or screws (Figure 38.6).

Another advantage of external skeletal fixation is all implants are temporary. All pins will be removed and can be removed in stages to allow the dynamization of the fracture, which can stimulate bone-healing. The main disadvantage of external skeletal fixation is increased aftercare compared to internal fixation methods. The frame and pin tracts through soft tissues need to be carefully monitored and cleaned to avoid infection. Pins and the frame are bandaged to avoid trauma to the patient and furniture. Owner preference for internal implants may be a factor in the decision to pursue external fixation. That the fixator will have to be removed in subsequent procedures in every case is a disadvantage for some and needs to be discussed with the client prior to application.

Minimally Invasive Osteosynthesis (MIO)

MIO involves the application of implants for fracture stabilization without making an extensive surgical approach to expose the fracture site. The bone segments are reduced using indirect reduction techniques without direct manipulation of the bone at the fracture site. As stated previously, advantages include more rapid biological osteosynthesis through preservation of the fracture hematoma and blood supply. Disadvantages include less control of anatomical reduction, lack of interfragmentary compression, and, therefore, promotion of secondary (not primary) bone-healing.

Intraoperative imaging is essential to guide fracture reduction and implant introduction. Fluoroscopic guidance is the gold standard with a variety of commercially available devices designed for intraoperative use in various shapes and sizes, many with C-arm designs that permit draping and facilitate aseptic repositioning (Figure 38.7). Intraoperative fluoroscopy has major advantages including real-time visualization of fracture reduction and implant placement without extensive surgical approaches. The main disadvantage is operator exposure to radiation, which must be mitigated with personal protective equipment, dosimeter monitoring, and observation of radiation safety protocols.

The simplest form of fixation in the category of minimally invasive osteosynthesis is **percutaneous pin or screw fixation.**[12] The fracture zone is not approached surgically

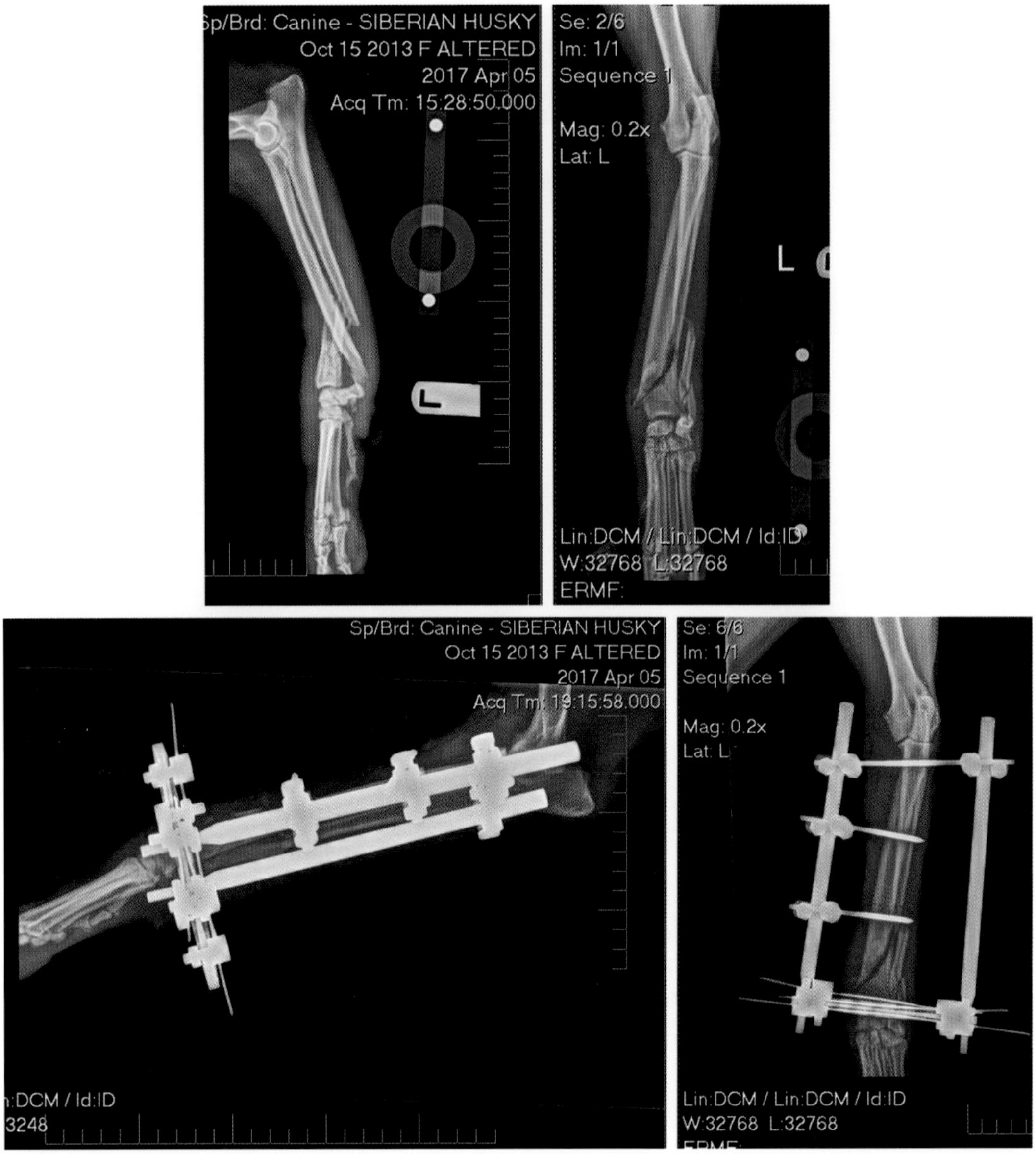

Figure 38.6 Juxta-articular radial/ulnar fracture in a large breed canine repaired via external skeletal fixation with a type II hybrid fixator (bilateral, uniplanar, combining linear, and ring components). The tensioned Kirschner wires in the distal ring permit stable purchase in the small distal bone fragment where space for screw fixation with a plate or interlocking nail would be limited. *Source:* © Seth Bleakley.

beyond small skin incisions to permit the introduction of implants. Sometimes, the incision is limited to that made by a large bore needle, which can serve as a drill guide for Kirschner wires. Incisions can be extended as needed to facilitate reduction and implant placement, but generally, the fracture zone is not approached.

Examples of fractures amenable to percutaneous pin or screw fixation include:

- Salter-Harris fractures of the distal radius with cross pins.
- Humeral condylar fractures with a lag screw and anti-rotational pin combinations (Figures 38.9 and 38.10).[13,14]
- Salter-Harris fractures of the proximal humerus with pins or screws.
- Supraglenoid tubercle fractures of the scapula with pins +/− tension band.[15]
- Salter-Harris fractures of the distal femur with cross pins (Figure 38.8).
- Salter-Harris fractures of the tibia with cross pins (Figure 38.11).[16,17]
- Capital physeal fractures of the femur with pins (Figure 38.12).[18]
- Sacroiliac luxation reduction and stabilization with lag or headless compression screw +/− pin combination.

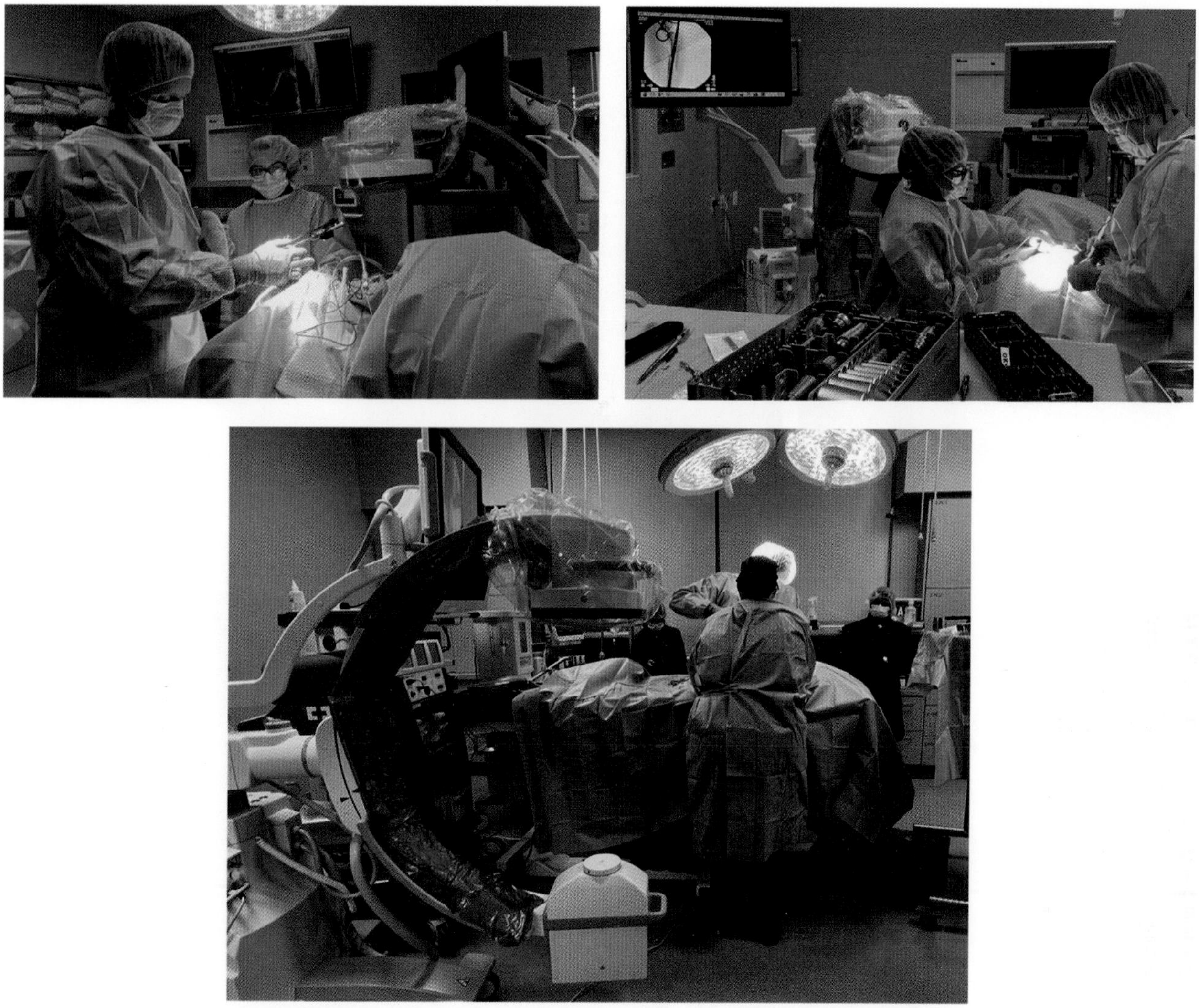

Figure 38.7 Intraoperative use of fluoroscopy to guide reduction and fixation during minimally invasive nail osteosynthesis. Intraoperative imaging permits a less invasive approach but necessitates personal protective equipment for all personnel present in accordance with local radiation safety guidelines. *Source:* © Seth Bleakley.

Only acute fractures evaluated within the first 48 hours after trauma are selected for percutaneous pinning. Reduction is performed with careful manipulation of the fracture to minimize the trauma to the growth plate. Depending on the anatomic location, the pins are cut flush with the bone or bent. The main advantages of this technique are minimal surgical trauma and lower perioperative morbidity.[12,19]

Minimally Invasive Nail Osteosynthesis (MINO)

Minimally invasive nail osteosynthesis (MINO) involves closed reduction and fixation of a fracture through the introduction of an interlocking nail implant.[20–25] Amenable long bones include the humerus, tibia, and femur. In certain cases, an interlocking nail may be introduced into the ulna. The procurvatum and articular anatomy of the radius generally preclude interlocking nail fixation. If applied correctly, an interlocking nail will resist all fracture forces. The axially located implant has excellent resistance to bending in all planes, and bolts locking into the nail stabilize against shear, tension, compression, and rotation. Newer implants with threaded bolts, known as angle-stable interlocking nails, have further enhanced construct stability for better resisting all fracture forces.[26–29] As no implants are fixed to the periosteum, periosteal blood supply is preserved, which is particularly important in some species, such as varanids, who rely on their periosteal blood supply for fracture healing.

Incisions necessary for the introduction of interlocking nails are often limited to access incisions associated with nail and bolt introduction. Approaching the fracture zone is often not necessary, therefore, the fracture hematoma,

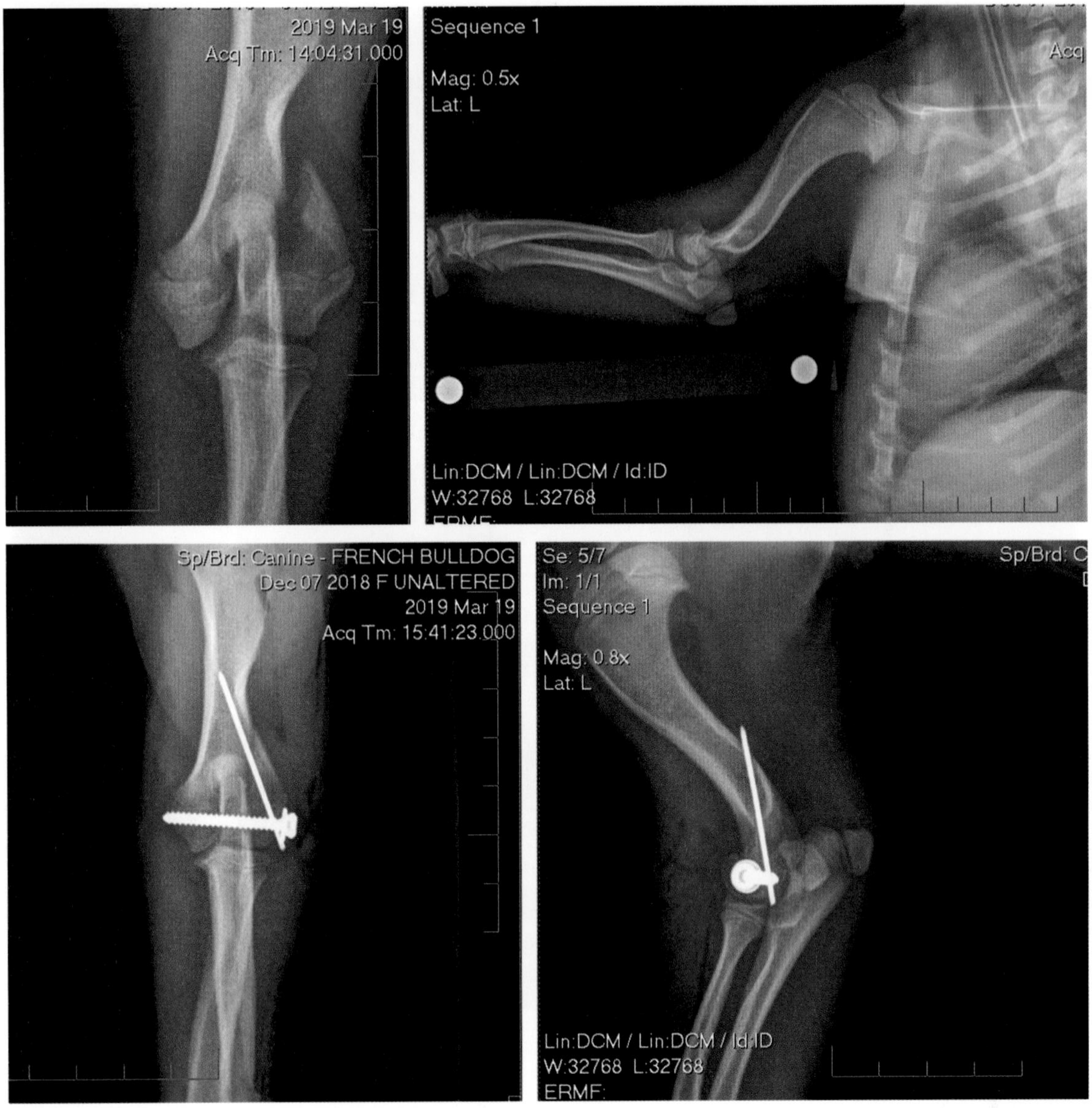

Figure 38.8 Cross-pin fixation of a Salter-Harris I fracture of a feline distal femur. *Source:* © Seth Bleakley.

soft tissues, and overall healing potential can be better preserved. Intraoperative imaging with fluoroscopy may or may not be necessary, although it is recommended to aid fracture reduction, and implant placement, and help avoid technical challenges with bolt engagement. While the introduction of the nail will straighten long bones in the frontal and sagittal planes, care must still be taken to avoid malalignment. Torsion must be carefully judged to ensure the paw is not internally or externally rotated following nail introduction. Additionally, making a long bone as straight as a nail is not always desirable in bones such as the tibia and femur that have a natural procurvatum. Straightening the natural distal recurvatum of the tibia can increase the tibial plateau angle, which can have clinical consequences such as increased incidence of cranial cruciate ligament disease. In such cases, anatomical alignment is still feasible by carefully bending the interlocking nail at the center of rotation of angulation (CORA) to match the anatomy of the bone prior to introduction.

The many advantages of minimally invasive nail osteosynthesis have made this approach the gold standard for most long-bone fracture repair in people and is becoming more standard of care in dogs and cats. The stable, strong construct introduced through a minimally invasive approach permits reduced pain and swelling, early return to function, rapid healing, and good clinical outcomes compared to open approaches (Figures 38.13, 38.14, 38.15, 38.16, and 38.17).[29,30]

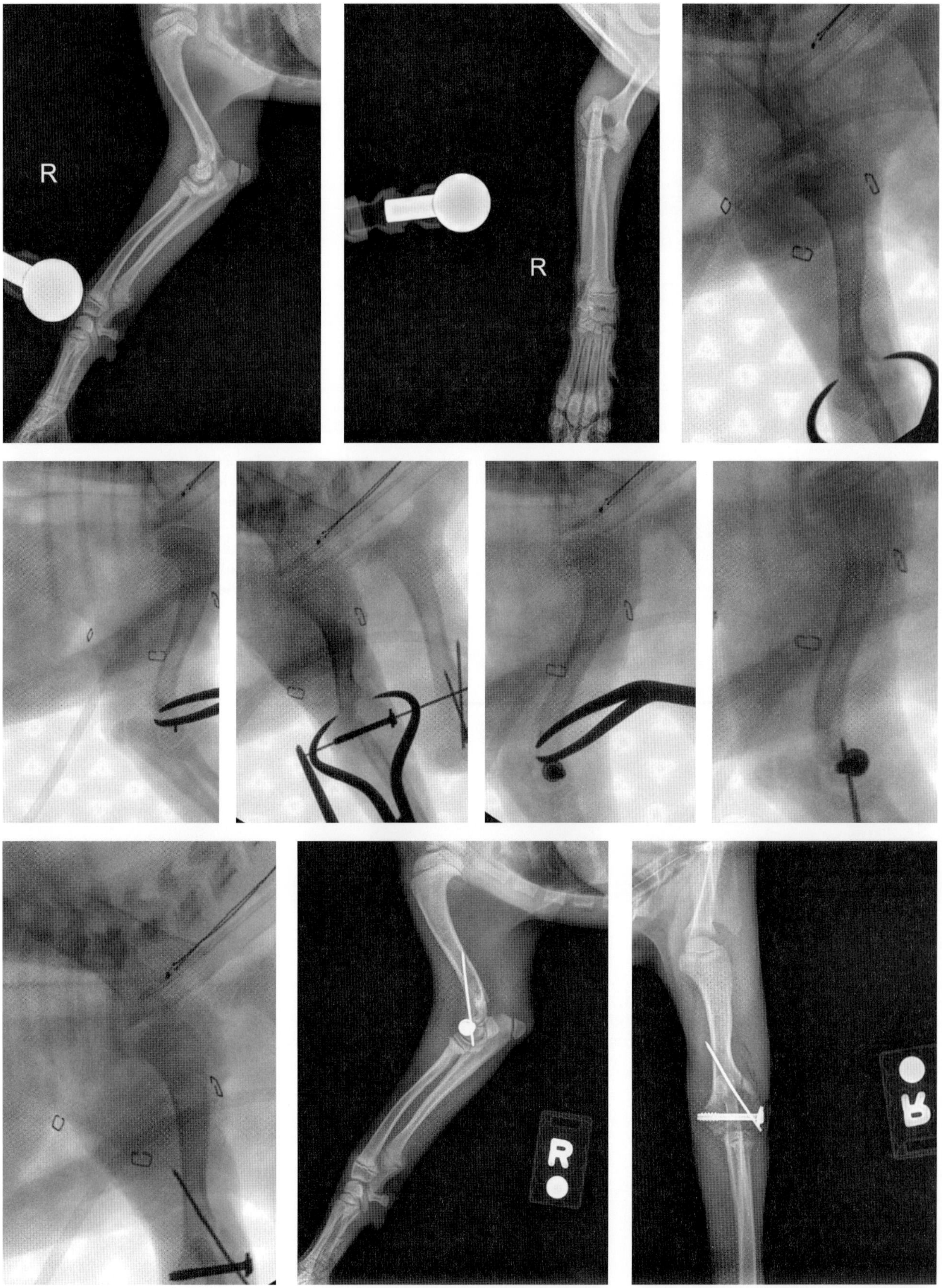

Figure 38.9 Percutaneous/minimally invasive repair of a lateral humeral condylar fracture in a French Bulldog with a lag screw and washer and anti-rotational pin applied with fluoroscopic guidance. *Source:* © Seth Bleakley.

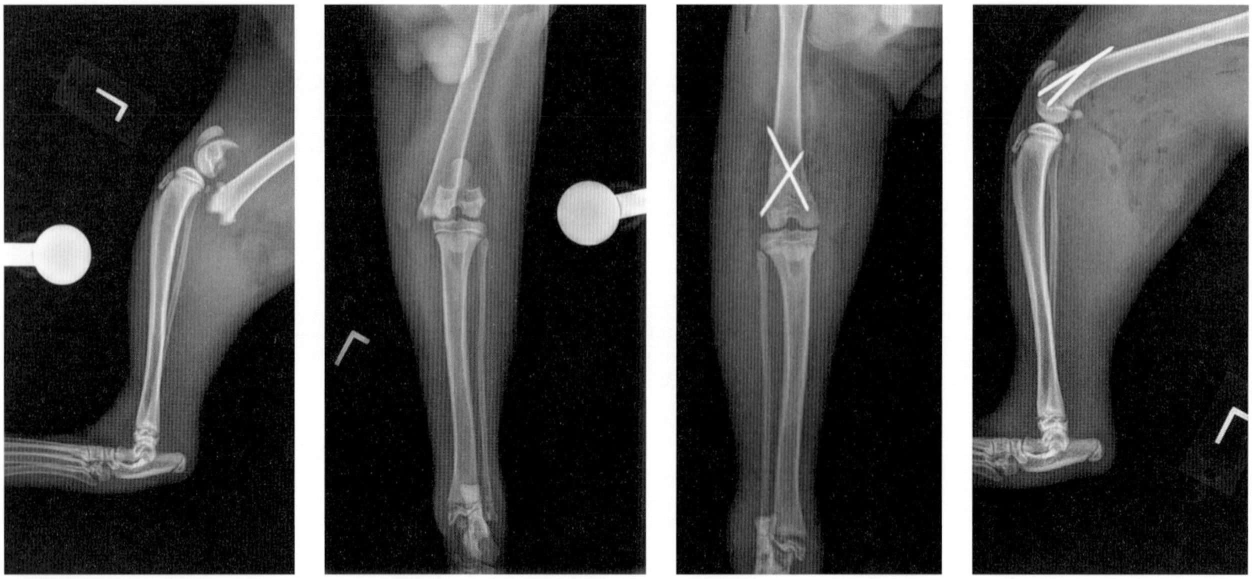

Figure 38.10 Percutaneous/minimally invasive repair of a lateral humeral condylar fracture in a French Bulldog with a cannulated lag screw and washer and anti-rotational pin applied with fluoroscopic guidance. *Source:* © Seth Bleakley.

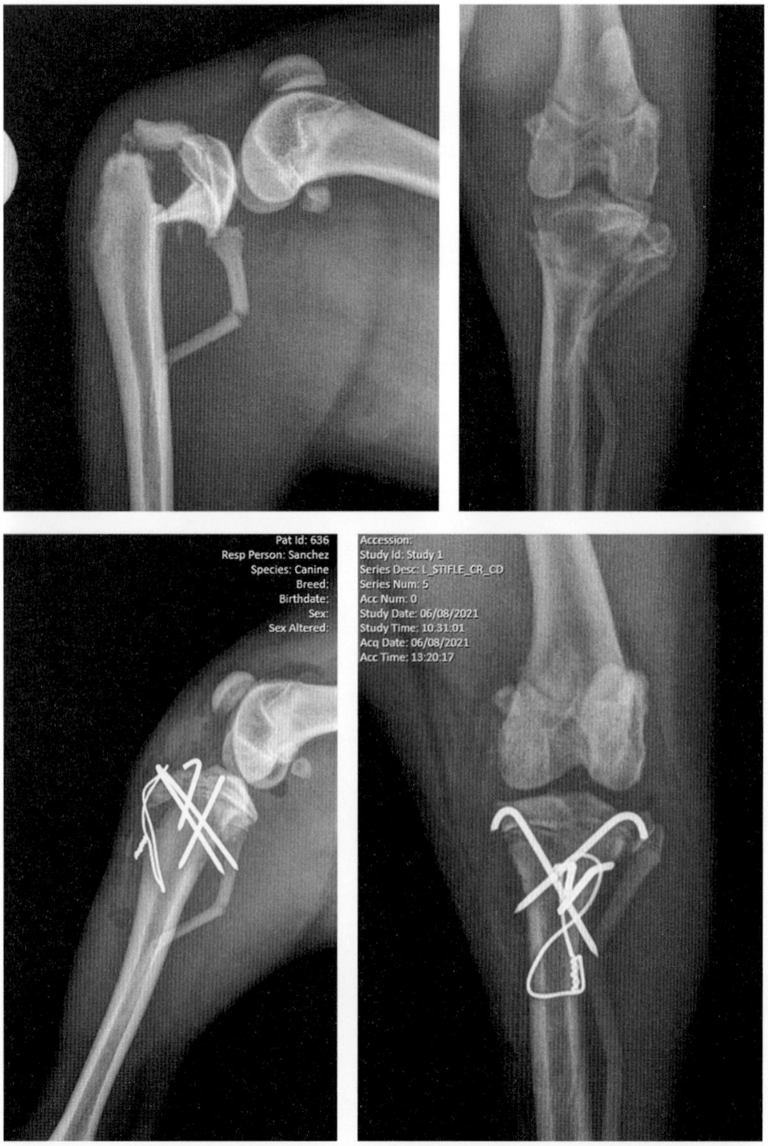

Figure 38.11 Open reduction and internal fixation of a tibial plateau fracture in a juvenile canine with a tension band and cross pins. *Source:* © Seth Bleakley.

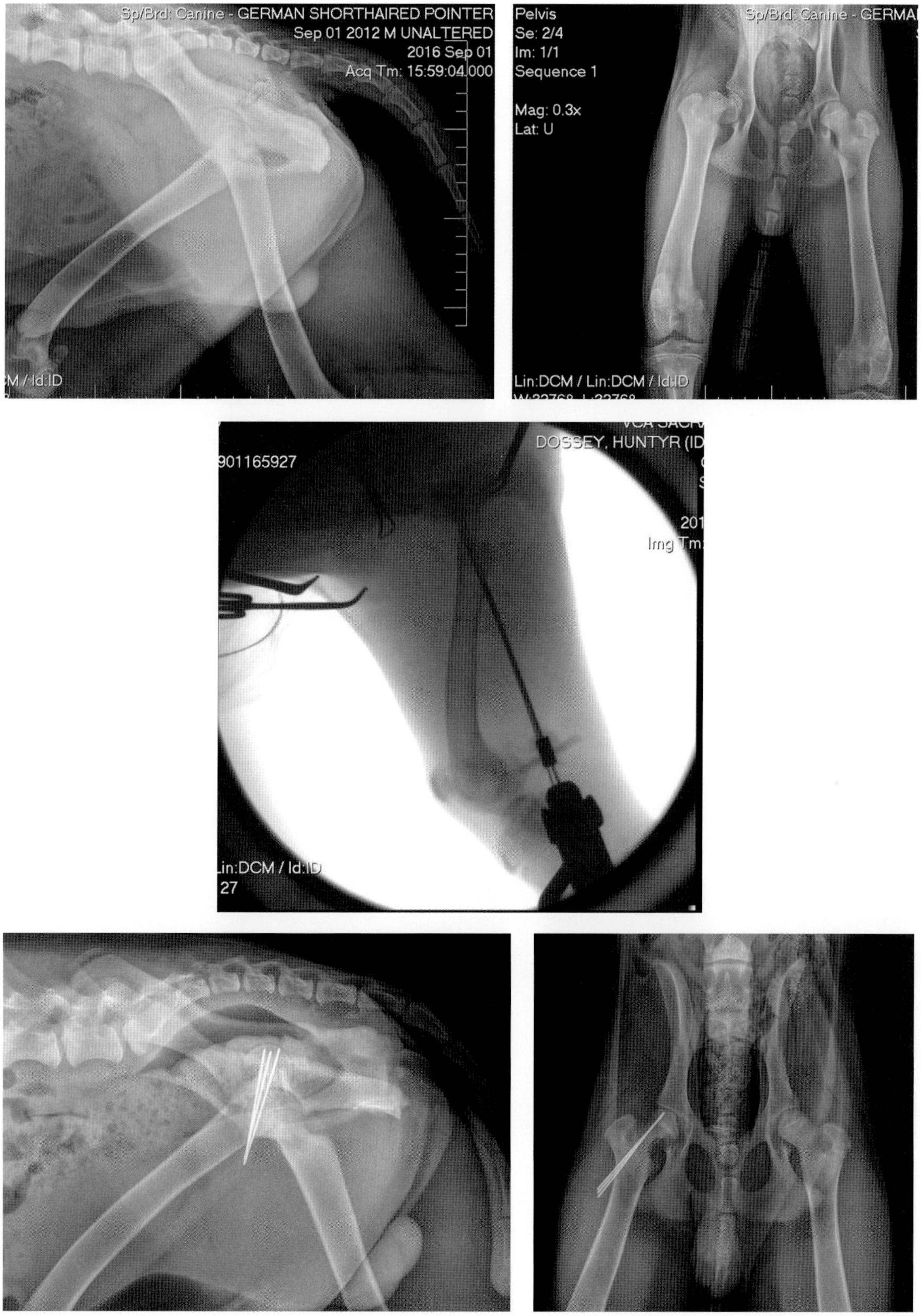

Figure 38.12 Minimally invasive/percutaneous repair of a canine capital physeal fracture with temporary Kirschner wire fixation applied with fluoroscopic guidance. *Source:* © Seth Bleakley.

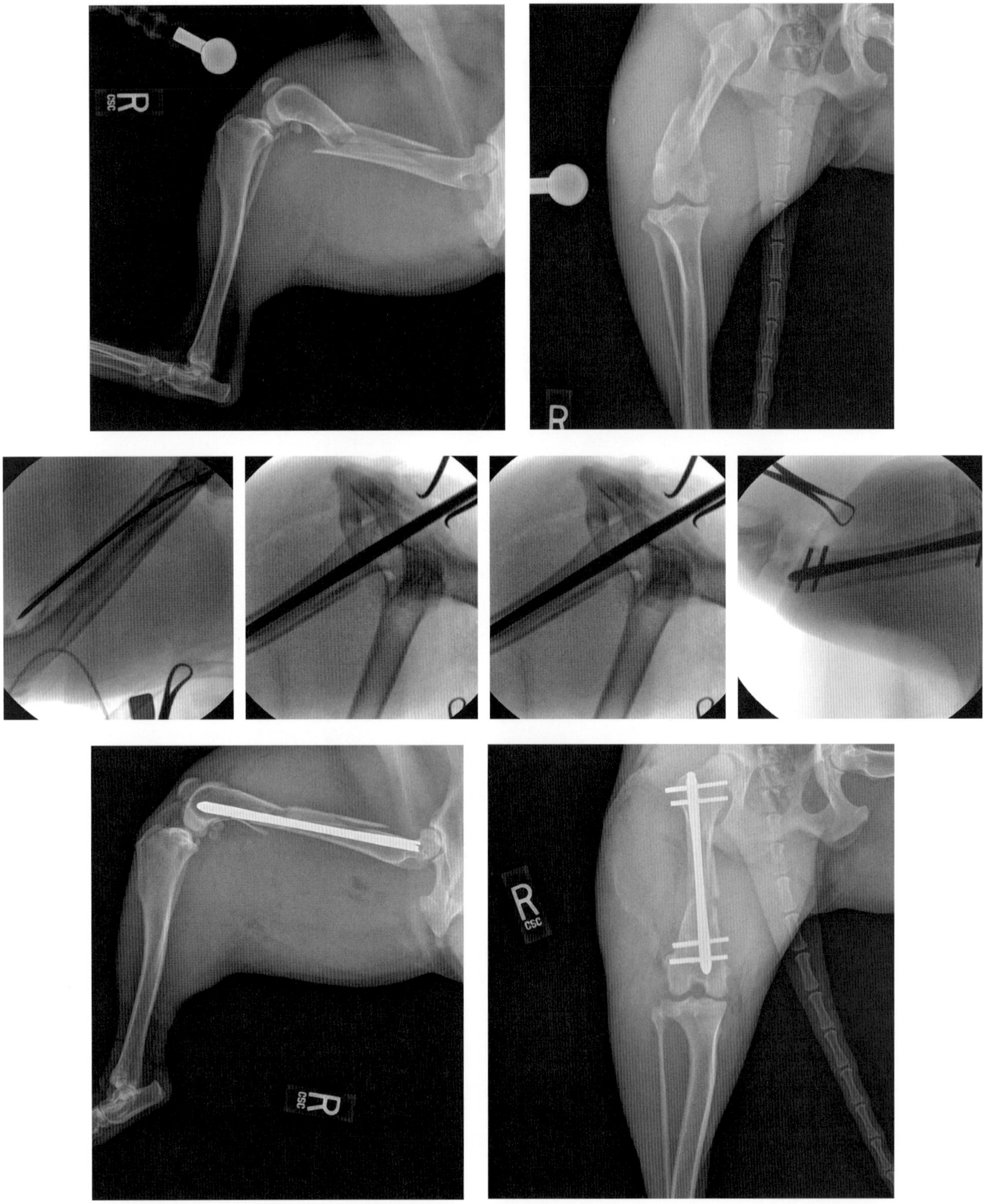

Figure 38.13 Minimally invasive nail osteosynthesis of a closed comminuted mid-diaphyseal right femoral fracture in a canine with fluoroscopic guidance. *Source:* © Seth Bleakley.

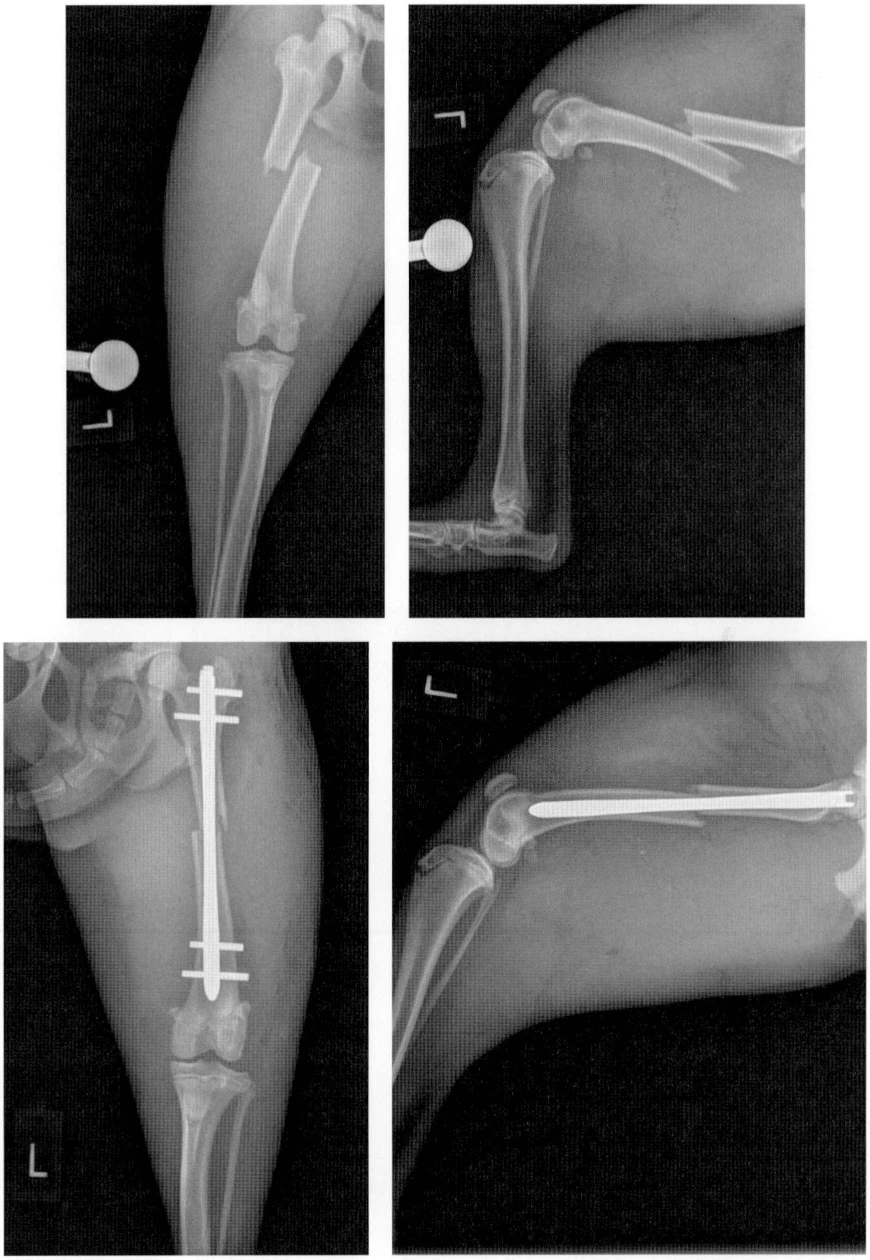

Figure 38.14 Minimally invasive nail osteosynthesis of a closed transverse caudomedially displaced mid-diaphyseal left femoral fracture in a canine with fluoroscopic guidance. *Source:* © Seth Bleakley.

Plate Fixation and Minimally Invasive Plate Osteosynthesis (MIPO)

Plate fixation is a very versatile method of fracture repair and can provide excellent resistance to all fracture forces. Plate fixation permits accurate fracture reduction, early return to function, rapid healing, and usually excellent clinical outcomes. Morbidity associated with external coaptation can be avoided, as fractures repaired via plate fixation are often stable enough for weight-bearing without a cast or splint.

An in-depth description of open reduction and internal fixation techniques is beyond the scope of this chapter and is well described in AO manuals of fracture management.[2]

A bone plate and screws are typically applied across a fracture zone and combined with other implants as judged necessary to stabilize the fracture depending on reconstructability. A "reconstructable" fracture is defined by the possibility of reconstructing load-sharing across the fracture zone. For example, a transverse, spiral, or short oblique fracture without comminution can be reconstructed with plate fixation alone to permit load transmission through the bone that will decrease the strain on implants (Figure 38.18). Long oblique, segmental, or fractures with large butterfly fragments may be considered reconstructable with additional implants that provide interfragmentary compression, such as lag screws and cerclage wire.

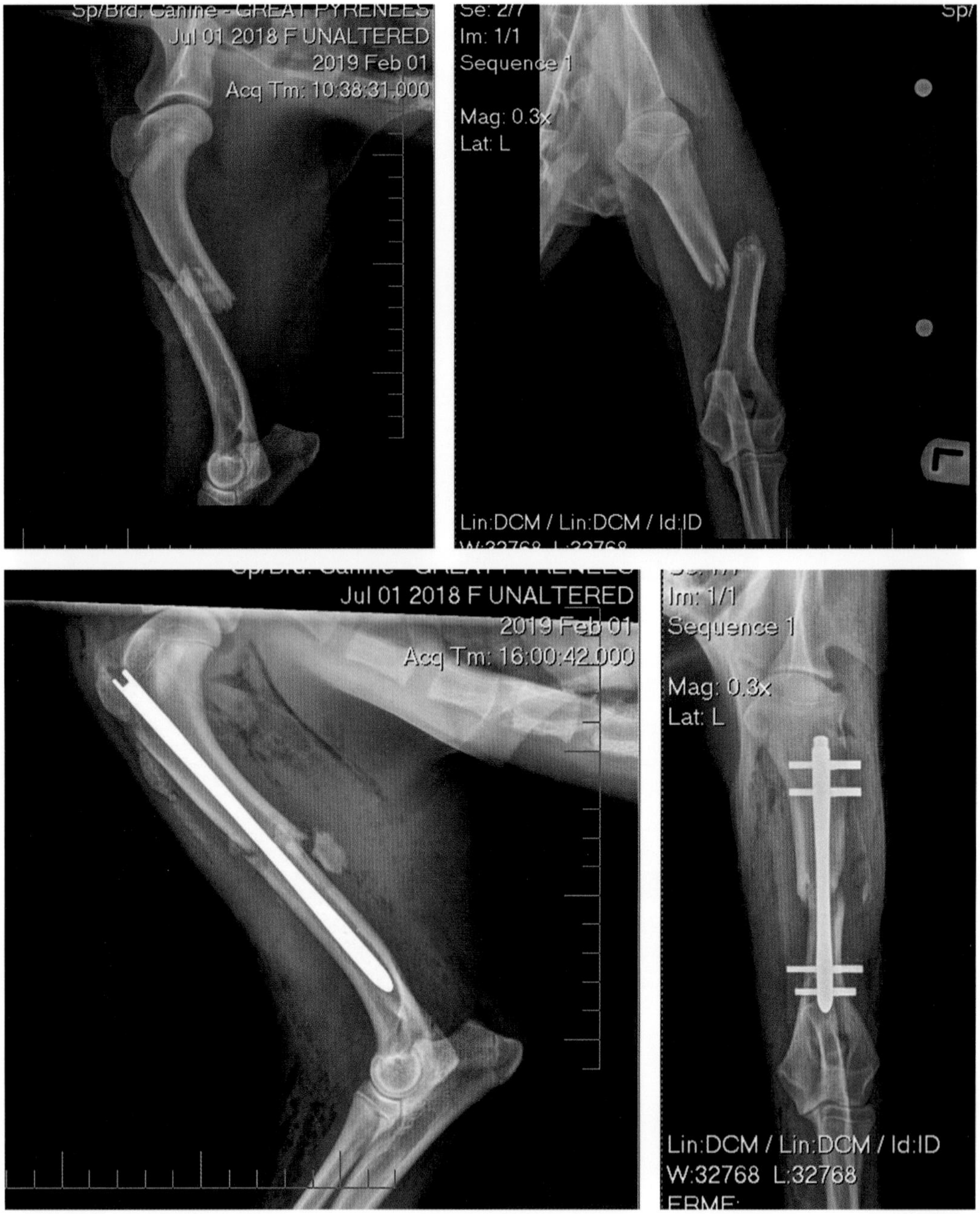

Figure 38.15 Minimally invasive nail osteosynthesis of a closed transverse craniolaterally displaced mid-diaphyseal canine left humeral fracture. Interlocking nail fixation is particularly helpful with humeral fractures where neurovascular structures surrounding this long bone can present a challenge to a safe surgical approach. *Source:* © Seth Bleakley.

A "nonreconstructable" fracture is typically too comminuted to permit load-sharing, so fixation requires a "bridging" construct or a "buttress" construct if near the joint (Figure 38.19). Implant size and strength must be selected accordingly, ensuring adequate strength and stability to support the entire load. Larger plates or multiple plates (e.g., stacked or orthogonal) may be used. The inclusion of an intramedullary pin is common in both reconstructable and nonreconstructable fracture repairs but is especially advantageous in bridging or buttress constructs. In a fracture gap model, the inclusion of an intramedullary pin in a plate-rod construct has been shown to reduce stress on a plate twofold while increasing the fatigue life 10-fold.[31]

A better understanding of the biological cost of plate fixation has led to the evolution of plate design, application technique, and minimally invasive techniques. Biomechanical studies of plate fixation in sheep have demonstrated the impact of the bone plate interface on cortical bone, with

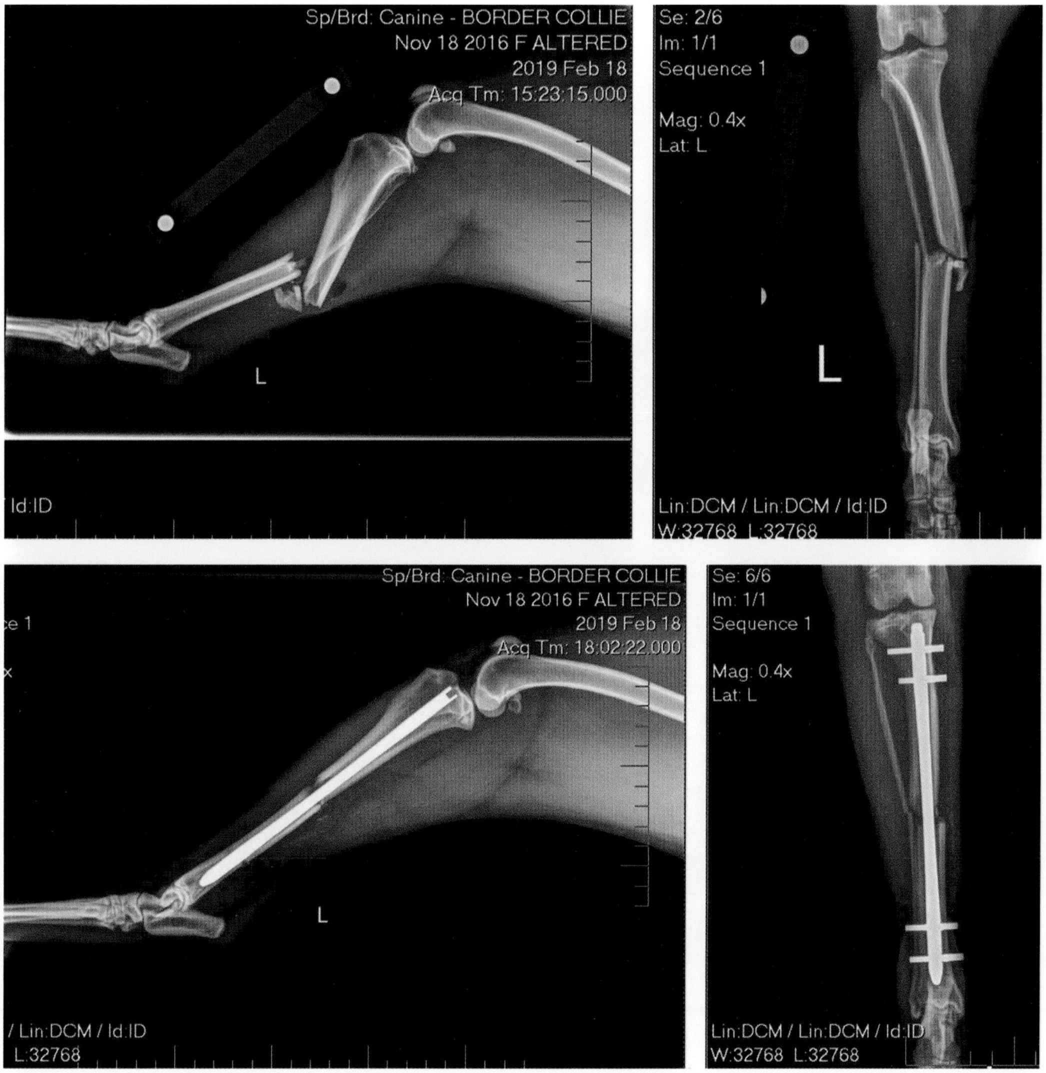

Figure 38.16 Minimally invasive nail osteosynthesis in an open canine transverse craniolaterally displaced mid-diaphyseal left tibial fracture. *Source:* © Seth Bleakley.

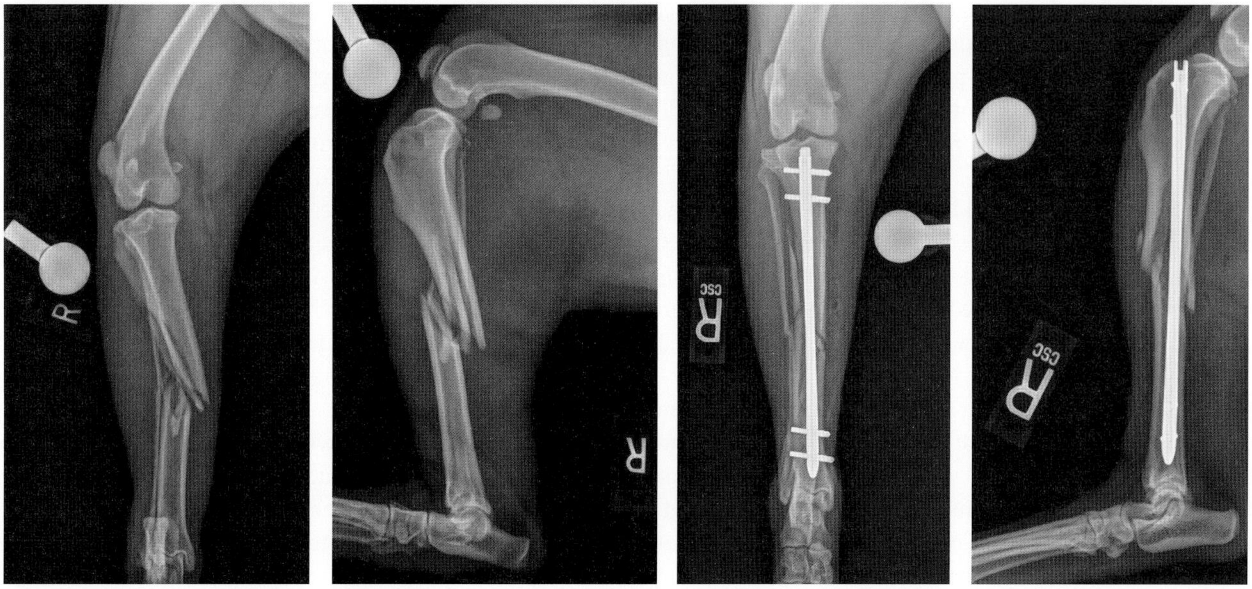

Figure 38.17 Minimally invasive nail osteosynthesis in a closed canine comminuted craniolaterally displaced mid-diaphyseal right tibial fracture. *Source:* © Seth Bleakley.

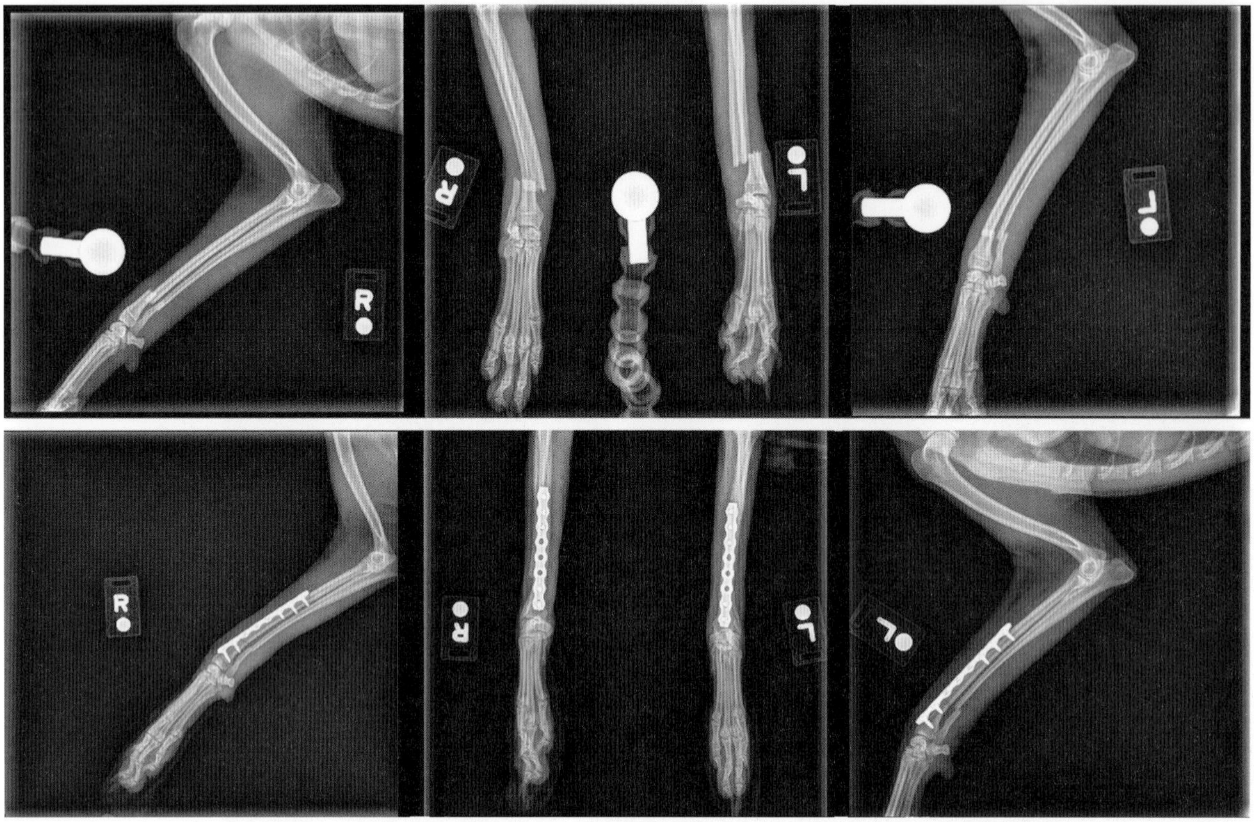

Figure 38.18 Bilateral distal radial/ulnar fractures in a small breed canine openly reduced and internally fixated with titanium advanced locking plates. These are examples of "reconstructable" fractures where the load is shared between bone and implants. *Source:* © Seth Bleakley.

reduced blood supply leading to bony resorption and necrosis-induced remodeling.[10] This has led to re-engineering of plate design to reduce plate contact and periosteal compression. Examples include the point contact fixator (PC-fix), limited contact dynamic compression plate (LC-DCP), string-of-pearls plate (SOP), locking compression plates (LCP), and the advanced locking plate system to name a few (Figures 38.19, 38.20, 38.21, 38.22, 38.23, and 38.24).

These plates are designed to provide space beneath the bone plate to preserve periosteal blood supply and reduce compression on bone, which would cause cortical necrosis with a standard plate applied with cortical screws. When coupled with locking screws, they can be considered "internal fixators," where a locking screw plate interface permits application without compression on periosteum and cortical bone. The result has been faster healing and lower infection rates.[10,32–34] Additionally, the concept of the internal fixator has facilitated plate placement through less invasive means. With locking screws, plates do not need to be anatomically contoured to ensure screw head compression or rely on friction at the plate-bone interface for stability. Smaller surgical approaches become feasible. Fewer bicortical screws are necessary. In general, the purchase of greater than five cortices or at least three bicortical screws proximal and distal to a fracture zone is typically recommended for a conventional nonlocking plate. Bicortical screws provide the compression necessary to maintain friction between the plate and bone to avoid screw loosening. As a locking construct does not require this compression and failure by screw-loosening is unlikely, monocortical screw fixation may be considered adequate with locking plates, and typically, only a minimum purchase of three cortices is required for stable fixation in cortical bone.[35,36] This reduced screw density better preserves blood supply and may be a factor in improved healing potential in fractures repaired with locking plate constructs.[11]

It should be noted that while implant failure by screw-loosening in locking constructs is rare, a locked screw-plate interface does increase shear stress and risk of screw fracture. Most manufacturers recognize this and have compensated by increasing the core diameter and, therefore, the area moment of inertia of locking screws to reduce

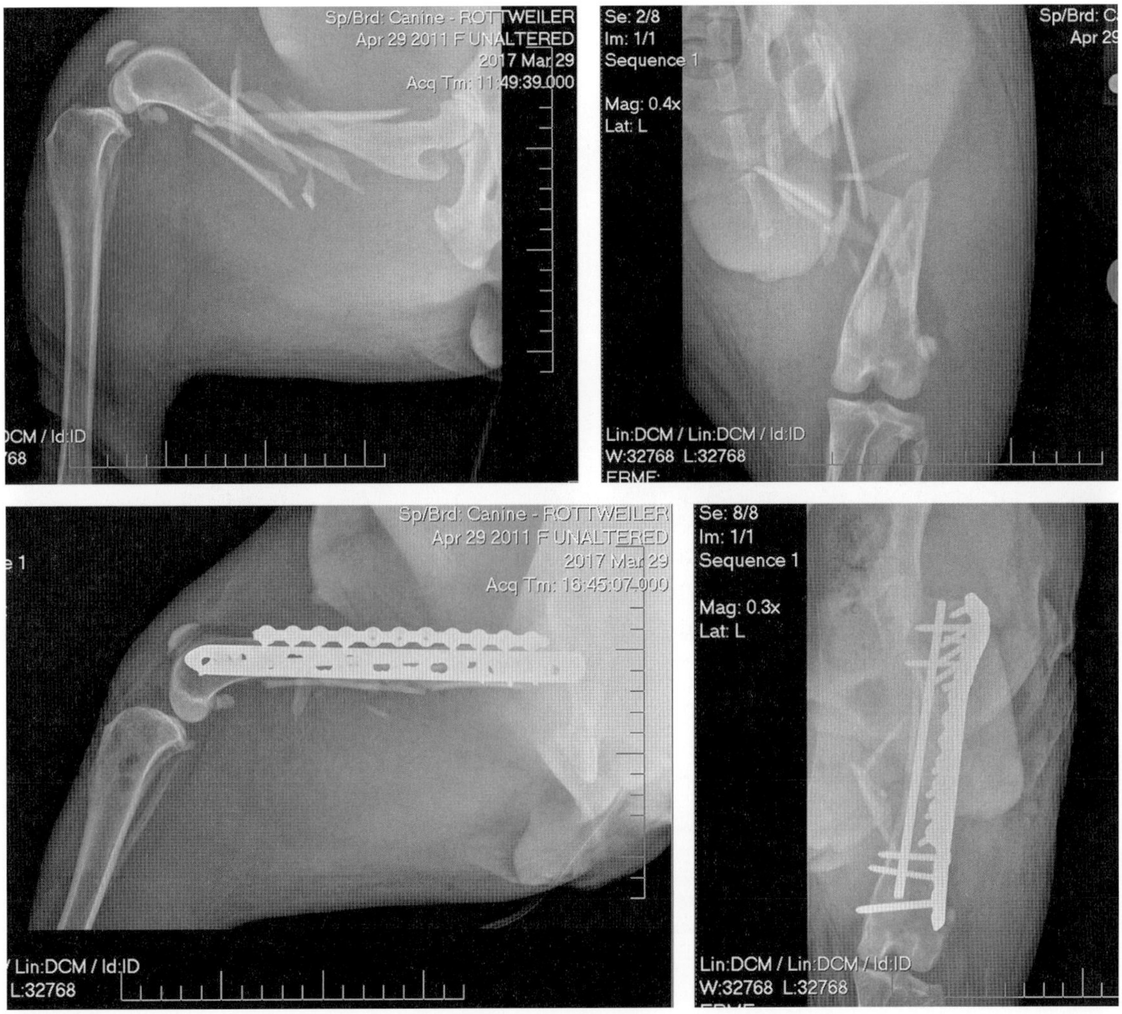

Figure 38.19 Example of a nonreconstructable closed canine comminuted femoral fracture repaired via open reduction and internal fixation with a bridging construct with a double plate-rod combination with a locking compression plate and a string-of-pearls plate. Note the bone-grafting tunnels in the proximal tibia where autologous cancellous bone graft was harvested to improve healing potential in the fracture zone. *Source:* © Seth Bleakley.

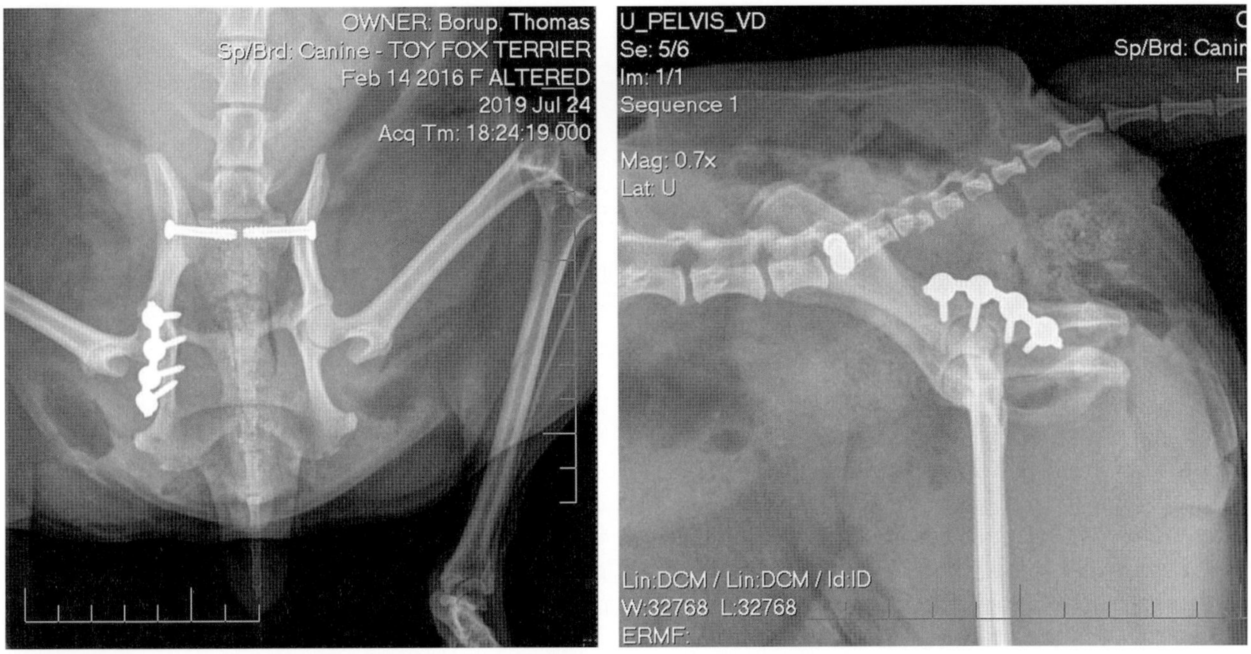

Figure 38.20 Use of a String-of-Pearls (SOP) plate applied as an internal fixator across an acetabular fracture in a dog. String-of-Pearls plates permit locking constructs with conventional screws. In this patient, a bilateral sacroiliac luxation has also been stabilized with bilateral cortical screws placed in a lag fashion. *Source:* © Seth Bleakley.

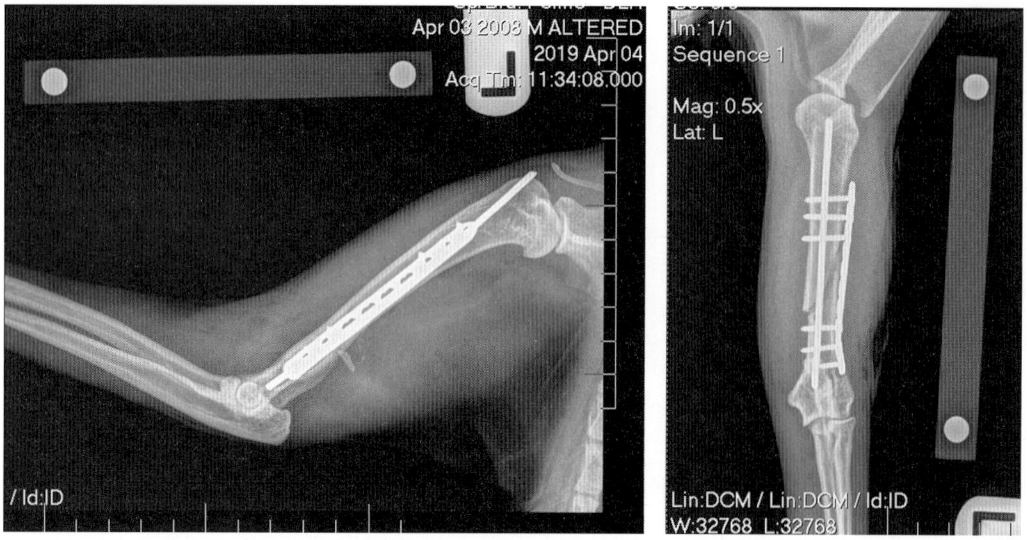

Figure 38.21 Open reduction and internal fixation of an oblique mid-diaphyseal left humeral fracture in a dog with an intramedullary pin and a locking compression plate. *Source:* © Seth Bleakley.

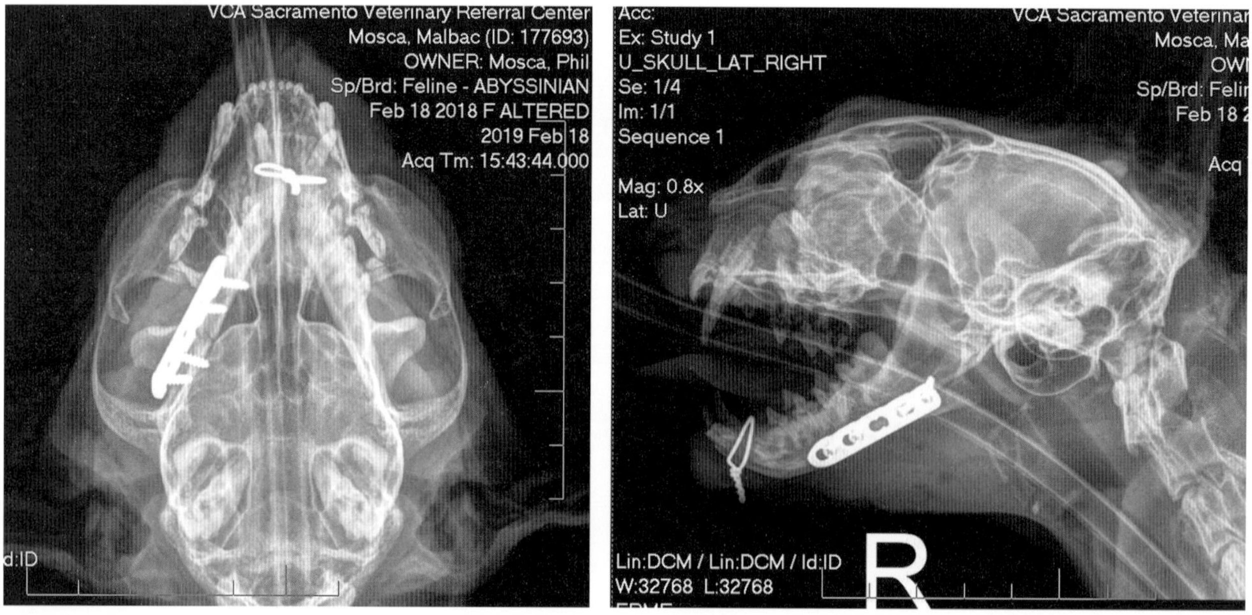

Figure 38.22 Right mandibular fracture repair in a cat with a locking compression plate and a cerclage wire applied to the rostral mandible for symphyseal stabilization. *Source:* © Seth Bleakley.

the risk of screw fracture. However, an understanding of the different biomechanical properties of locking and nonlocking implants is important for success with plate fixation.

The simplest change from open reduction and internal fixation with a bone plate to a less invasive approach is known as an **open but do not touch approach**. An open incision to the bone receiving the plate is performed but manipulation of the fracture zone is kept to a minimum to avoid disturbance to the blood supply and healing potential of the fracture zone.[19] Preserving the fracture hematoma is often not possible, but the reduced impact on the periosteum and regional musculature favors early fracture healing.[19]

The trend toward a less traumatic method of bone-plating is referred to as **minimally invasive plate osteosynthesis** (MIPO), or percutaneous plating.[37] During MIPO fracture stabilization, plates are inserted through

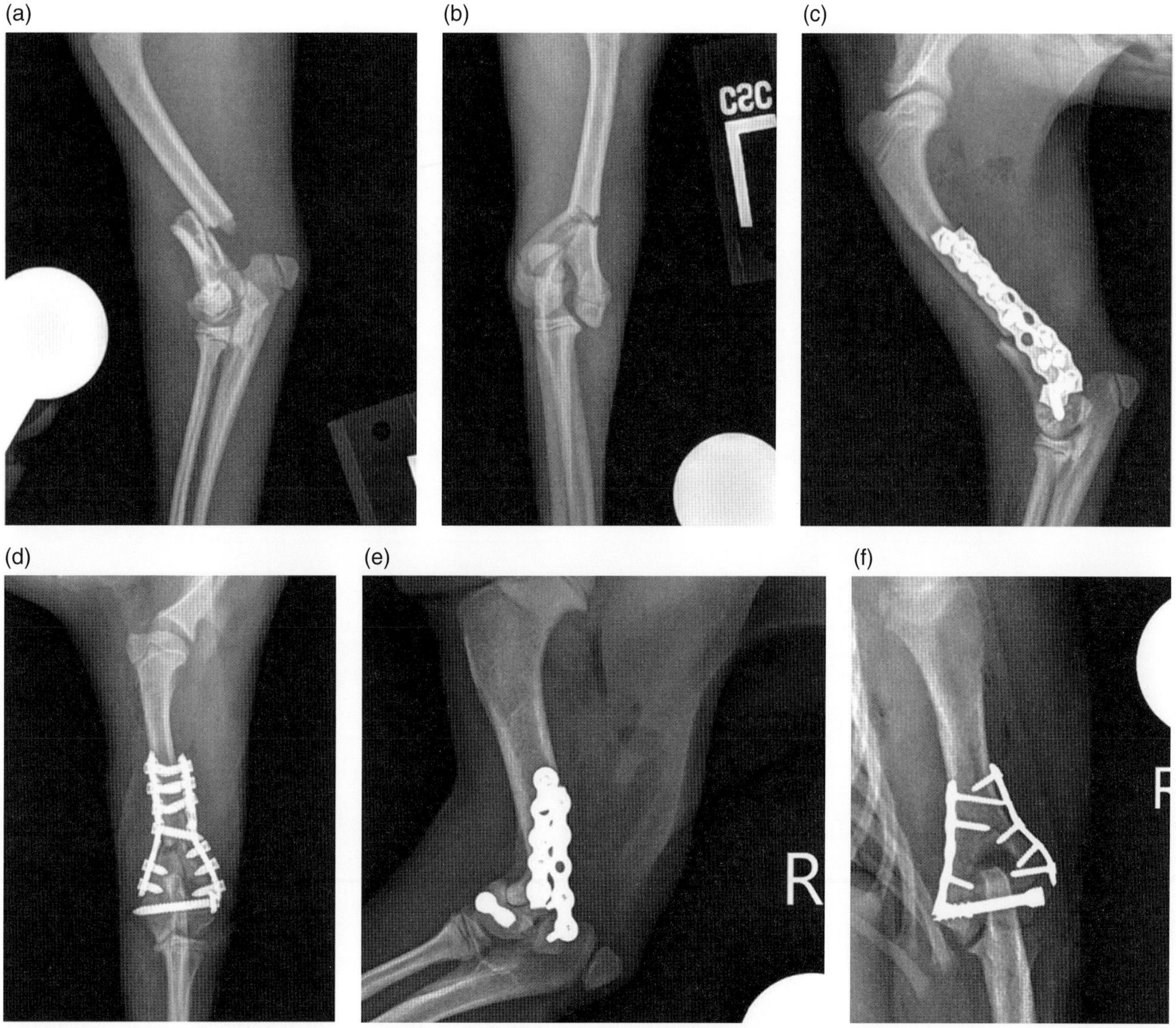

Figure 38.23 Images (a–d) are the pre-operative and immediate post-operative radiographs of open reduction and internal fixation of a left dicondylar (Y) humeral fracture in a small breed canine with a lag screw and two titanium advanced locking plates. Images (e,f) show the same type of fracture with a slightly different stabilization utilizing a 2.4 mm headless compression screw and two titanium 1.7 mm Fixin locking plates in a 4-month-old spayed female French Bulldog. In certain fractures, an invasive approach may be necessary to adequately reduce and stabilize a challenging articular fracture. (a–d) *Source:* © Seth Bleakley. (e,f) *Source:* © Kristin Coleman.

short incisions and a communicating epiperiosteal tunnel. Typically, bone plates applied to long bones in this fashion have a bridging function and may be combined with an intramedullary pin. The IM pin serves as a reduction aid and decreases strain on the plate while increasing the fatigue life of the construct.[31]

As stated previously, the advent of locking screws has facilitated MIPO, as anatomically contouring the plate is not necessary with an internal fixator. Reduction and implant placement are often facilitated by intraoperative imaging, such as fluoroscopy, to help reduce the need for surgical exposure. Plates are often placed with a long "working length," defined as the distance between the proximal and distal screw in closest proximity to the fracture. This increases the elasticity of the construct and subsequent strain at the level of the fracture zone, promoting secondary bone-healing. Combined with better preservation of blood supply, the result is a more rapid clinical union and lower complication rate in appropriately selected cases.[19,37] Less pain and faster return to function are also expected when compared to an open approach (Figures 38.25, 38.26, and 38.27).

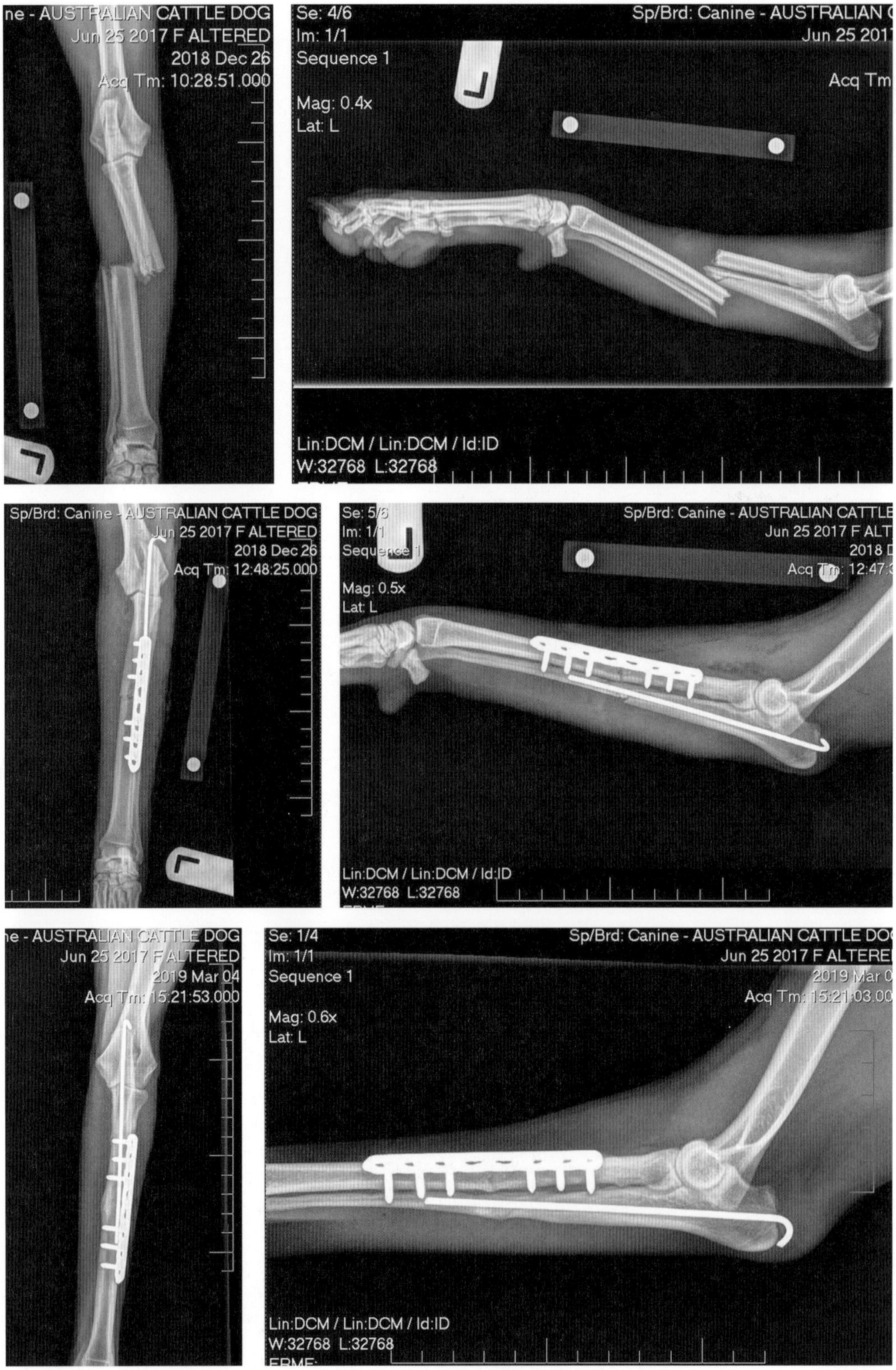

Figure 38.24 Open reduction and internal fixation of a closed canine transverse caudolaterally displaced mid-diaphyseal left radial/ulnar fracture with an ulnar intramedullary pin and a radial locking compression plate. Clinical union demonstrated at three months post-operatively. *Source:* © Seth Bleakley.

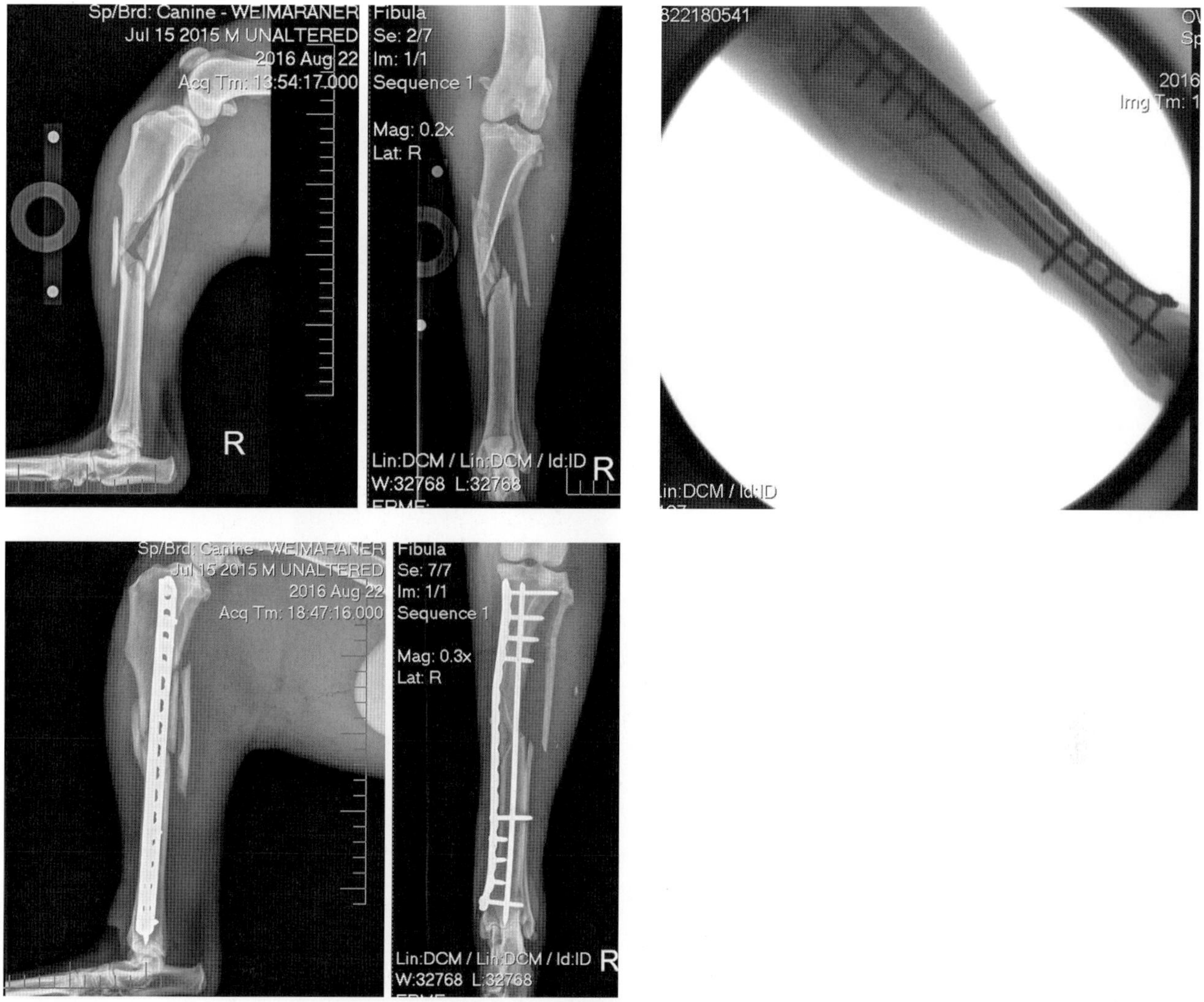

Figure 38.25 Minimally invasive plate osteosynthesis in a canine nonreconstructable comminuted mid-diaphyseal right tibial fracture with an intramedullary pin and locking compression plate applied with fluoroscopic guidance. Note the monocortical locking screws are distally applied due to interference with the IM pin but compensated for with additional screws. *Source:* © Seth Bleakley.

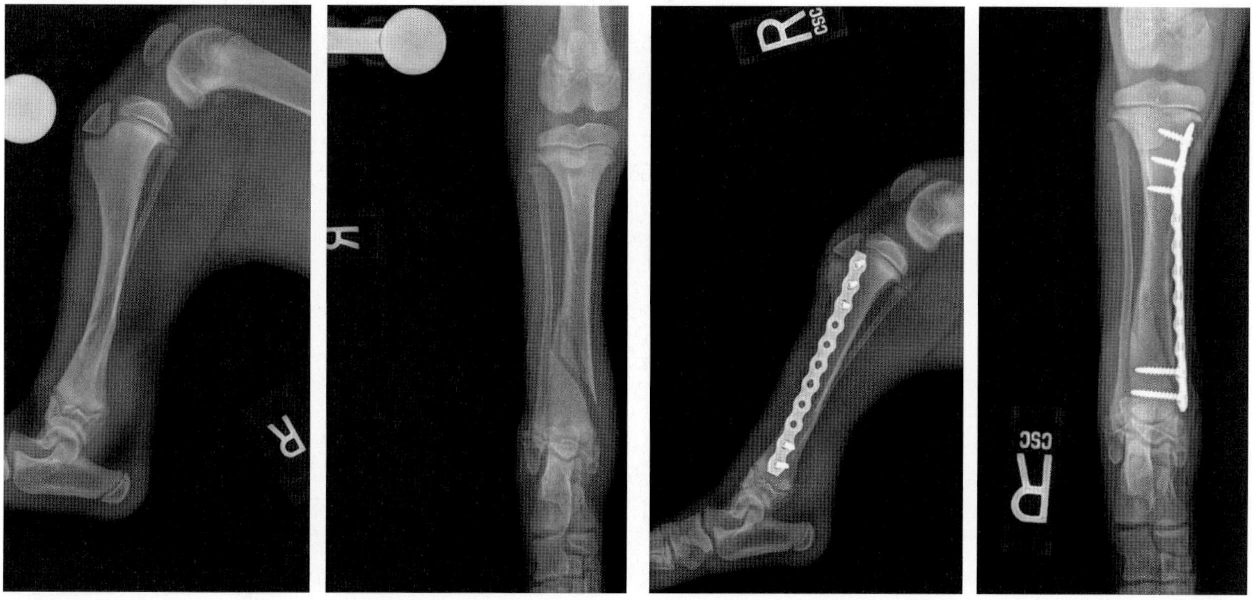

Figure 38.26 Minimally invasive plate osteosynthesis of a juvenile comminuted minimally laterally displaced right distal diaphyseal tibial fracture with a titanium advanced locking plate. Note the lack of an intramedullary pin (deemed unnecessary with an intact fibula) to avoid trauma to the physes. Likewise, screw fixation has been applied proximal and distal to the physes to avoid morbidity that could affect growth. *Source:* © Seth Bleakley.

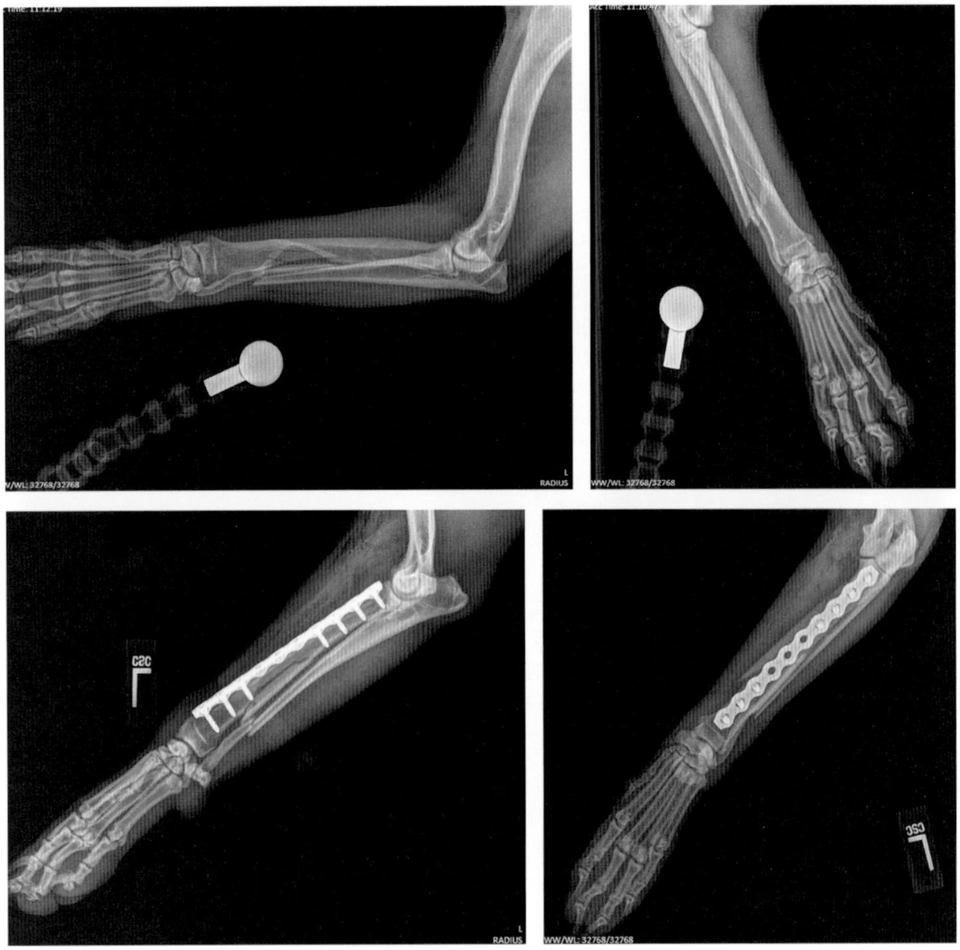

Figure 38.27 Minimally invasive plate osteosynthesis of left radial (comminuted mid-diaphyseal) and ulnar (short oblique distal diaphyseal) fractures in a large breed canine with a titanium advanced locking plate spanning the dorsal radius. *Source:* © Seth Bleakley.

Conclusion

It has been said that success in surgery is 20% skill and 80% decision-making, and such an adage is certainly relevant to fracture repair. Principles are stated here with the goal of aiding clinical decision-making to improve chances of success. They are not exhaustive, neither are all fracture repair options listed. A trend toward less invasive approaches favoring biological osteosynthesis has been shown to offer advantages but may not be the correct approach for every fracture. Careful consideration of the nature of the fracture, available implant options, the patient, and the client are essential in clinical decision-making and successful fracture management.

References

1 Cepela, D.J., Tartaglione, J.P., Dooley, T.P. et al. (2016). Classifications in brief: Salter-Harris classification of pediatric physeal fractures. *Clin. Orthop. Relat. Res.* 474 (11): 2531–2537.

2 Johnson, A.L., Houlton, J.E.F., and Vannini, R. (2005). *AO Principles of Fracture Management in the Dog and Cat.* Davos Platz: Thieme.

3 Marsell, R. and Einhorn, T.A. (2011). The biology of fracture healing. *Injury* 42 (6): 551–555.

4 Marenzana, M. and Arnett, T. (2013). The key role of the blood supply to bone. *Bone Res.* 1: 203–215.

5 Wolff, J. (1986). *The Law of Bone Remodeling.* Berlin Heidelberg, New York: Springer.

6 Hettrich, C.M., Gasinu, S., Beamer, B.S. et al. (2013). The effect of immobilization on the native and repaired tendon-to-bone interface. *J. Bone Joint Surg. Am.* 95 (10): 925–930.

7 Campbell, T.M., Reilly, K., Laneuville, O. et al. (2018). Bone replaces articular cartilage in the rat knee joint after prolonged immobilization. *Bone* 106: 42–51.

8 McCullough, D. (2016). *The Wright Brothers.* New York, NY: Simon & Schuster.

9 Grundnes, O. and Reikeras, O. (1993). The importance of the hematoma for fracture healing in rats. *Acta Orthop. Scand.* 64: 340–342.

10 Perren, S.M. (2002). Evolution of the internal fixation of long bone fractures. *J. Bone Joint Surg.* 84 (8): 1098–1109.

11 Rozbruch, S.R., Müller, U., Gautier, E. et al. (1998). The evolution of femoral shaft plating technique. *Clin. Orthop. Relat. Res.* 354: 195–208.

12 Kim, S.E., Hudson, C.C., and Pozzi, A. (2012). Percutaneous pinning for fracture repair in dogs and cats. *Vet. Clin. North Am. Small Anim. Pract.* 42 (5): 963–974.

13 Cook, J.L., Tomlinson, J.L., and Reed, A.L. (1999). Fluoroscopically-guided closed reduction and internal fixation of fractures of the lateral portion of the humeral condyle: prospective clinical study of the technique and results in ten dogs. *Vet. Surg.* 28 (05): 315–321.

14 Maritato, K.C. and Rovesti, G.L. (2020). Minimally invasive osteosynthesis techniques for humerus fractures. *Vet. Clin. North Am. Small Anim. Pract.* 50 (01): 123–134.

15 Kulendra, E.R., Beer, A.J.C., Hockley, G.C.A. et al. (2019). Outcome of Supraglenoid tubercle fractures in 12 dogs. *Vet. Comp. Orthop. Traumatol.* 32 (4): 341–350.

16 von Pfeil, D.J.F., Megliolia, S., Malek, S. et al. (2021). Tibial apophyseal percutaneous pinning in skeletally immature dogs: 25 cases (2016-2019). *Vet. Comp. Orthop. Traumatol.* 34 (2): 144–152.

17 von Pfeil, D.J.F., Glassman, M., and Ropski, M. (2017). Percutaneous tibial physeal fracture repair in small animals: technique and 17 cases. *Vet. Comp. Orthop. Traumatol.* 30 (4): 279–287.

18 de Moya, K.A., Kim, S.E., and Guiot, L.P. (2022). Closed reduction and fluoroscopic-guided percutaneous pinning of femoral capital physeal or neck fractures: thirteen fractures in 11 dogs. *Vet. Surg.* https://doi.org/10.1111/vsu.13867.

19 Pozzi, A., Lewis, D.D., Scheuermann, L.M. et al. (2021). A review of minimally invasive fracture stabilization in dogs and cats. *Vet. Surg.* 50: O5–O16.

20 Browner, B.D. (1996). *The Science and Practice of Intramedullary Nailing*, 2e. Baltimore: Williams and Wilkins.

21 Dueland, R.T., Johnson, K.A., Roe, S.C. et al. (1999). Interlocking nail treatment of diaphyseal long-bone fractures in dogs. *J. Am. Vet. Med. Assoc.* 214: 59–66.

22 Duhautois, B. (1995). L'enclouage verrouille veterinaire: etude clinique retrospective sur 45 cas. *Prat. Med. Chir. Amin. Comp.* 30: 613–630.

23 Durall, I., Diaz, M.C., and Morales, I. (1993). An experimental study of compression of femoral fractures of an interlocking intramedullary pin. *Vet. Comp. Orthop. Trauma* 6: 93–99.

24 Durall, I., Diaz, M.C., and Morales, I. (1994). Interlocking nail stabilization of humeral fractures. Initial experience in seven clinical cases. *Vet. Comp. Orthop. Traumatol.* 7 (1): 3–8.

25 Muir, P., Parker, R.B., Goldsmid, S.E. et al. (1993). Interlocking intramedullary nail stabilization of a diaphyseal tibial fracture. *J. Small Anim. Pract.* 25: 397–406.

26 Déjardin, L.M., Cabassu, J.B., Guillou, R.P. et al. (2014). In vivo biomechanical evaluation of a novel angle-stable interlocking nail design in a canine tibial fracture model. *Vet. Surg.* 43 (3): 271–281.

27 von Pfeil, D.J.F., Déjardin, L.M., DeCamp, C.E. et al. (2005). In vitro biomechanical comparison of a plate-rod combination–construct and an interlocking nail–construct for experimentally induced gap fractures in canine tibiae. *Am. J. Vet. Res.* 66 (9): 1536–1543.

28 Déjardin, L.M., Lansdowne, J.L., Sinnott, M.T. et al. (2006). In vitro mechanical evaluation of torsional loading in simulated canine tibiae for a novel hourglass-shaped inter-locking nail with a self-tapping tapered locking design. *Am. J. Vet. Res.* 67 (4): 678–685.

29 Dejardin, L.M., Guiot, L.P., and von Pfeil, D.J.F. (2012). Interlocking nails and minimally invasive osteosynthesis. *Vet. Clin. North Am. Small Anim. Pract.* 42: 935–962. https://doi.org/10.1016/j.cvsm.2012.07.004.

30 Marturello, D.M., Perry, K.L., and Déjardin, L.M. (2021). Clinical application of the small I-Loc interlocking nail in 30 feline fractures: a prospective study. *Vet. Surg.* 50 (3): 588–599. https://doi.org/10.1111/vsu.13594.

31 Hulse, D., Hyman, W., Nori, M. et al. (1997). Reduction in plate strain by addition of an intramedullary pin. *Vet. Surg.* 26 (6): 451–459.

32 Tepic, S., Remiger, A.R., Morikawa, K. et al. (1997). Strength recovery in fractured sheep tibia treated with a plate or an internal fixator: an experimental study with a two-year follow-up. *J. Orthop. Trauma* 11 (1): 14–23.

33 Stephan, A., Eijer, H., Schlegel, U. et al. (1999). Influence of the design for fixation implants on local infection: experimental study of dynamic compression plates versus point contact fixators in rabbits. *J. Orthop. Trauma* 13 (7): 470–476.

34 Eijer, H., Hauke, C., and Arens, S. (2001). PC-fix and local infection resistance–influence of implant design on postoperative infection development, clinical and experimental results. *Injury* 32 (2): 38–43.

35 Field, E.J., Parsons, K., Etches, J.A. et al. (2016). Effect of monocortical and bicortical screw numbers on the properties of a locking plate-intramedullary rod configuration. An in vitro study on a canine femoral fracture gap model. *Vet. Comp. Orthop. Traumatol.* 29 (6): 459–465.

36 Bleakley, S., Palmer, R., Miller, N. et al. (2021). Biomechanical comparison of tibial plateau leveling osteotomy performed with a novel titanium alloy locking plate construct vs. an established stainless-steel locking plate construct. *Front. Vet. Sci.* 8: 698159.

37 Hudson, C.C., Pozzi, A., and Lewis, D.D. (2009). Minimally invasive plate osteosynthesis: applications and techniques in dogs and cats. *Vet. Comp. Orthop. Traumatol.* 22 (3): 175–182.

39

Orthopedic Implants

Rebecca J. Webb

VetSurg, Ventura, CA, USA

Key Points

- A range of orthopedic implants are available for the surgical fixation of fractures that can be largely grouped into internal implants, such as Steinmann pins, Kirschner-wires (K-wires), orthopedic wire, bone plates, and interlocking nail (ILN), and external implants, such as external skeletal fixator (ESF).
- Each implant has distinct advantages and disadvantages and has appropriate clinical situations for its use.
- Familiarization with the implants available and their appropriate uses is important for any clinician who is surgically repairing fractures.
- Continuing education courses for many implant systems occur frequently, and clinicians should consider pursuing these educational opportunities to develop comfort with a new system and achieve positive clinical outcomes.

Introduction

Fractures are common in veterinary medicine and often require surgical fixation for the return of limb function. The fixation of fractures requires implants, which can either be internal (Steinmann pins and Kirschner wires [K-wire], bone plates, and interlocking nails [ILNs]) or external (external skeletal fixators [ESFs]). Internal fixation has the benefit of providing stable fixation to the fracture due to the proximity of the implants to the bone. Depending on the construct, either primary or secondary bone healing will occur. Internal fixation, however, requires a surgical approach to place, which can damage the surrounding tissues and lead to delays in healing. In comparison, ESFs have the advantage of being able to be placed without a surgical approach to the fracture, which has a distinct advantage for preserving the soft tissues and vasculature of the fracture site. They can be modified easily postsurgery and are relatively simple to remove when they are no longer needed. Due to their external nature, they are not as stiff and strong as other internal fixation options, such as plates, and complications, such as pin loosening, can occur over time. External fixators require more intensive postsurgical care in the form of bandaging, which may not be tolerated by some patients and clients.

In this chapter, we will discuss the appropriate use and application of each type of implant along with tips and tricks for the smooth application of each.

Steinmann Pins/Kirschner Wires

Steinmann pins and Kirschner wires (K-wires) are long pins made of 316L stainless steel. These pins and wires come in a variety of sizes, and, typically, Steinmann pins refer to pins larger than 0.062 in. and K-wires refer to pins 0.062 in. and smaller (Figure 39.1). These implants are very

* Please see Chapter 38 for more details about the "Principles of Fracture Repair," which complements this chapter well for an in-depth understanding of orthopedic implants and their ideal applications.

Techniques in Small Animal Soft Tissue, Orthopedic, and Ophthalmic Surgery, First Edition. Edited by Kristin A. Coleman.

Companion website: www.wiley.com/go/coleman/surgeries

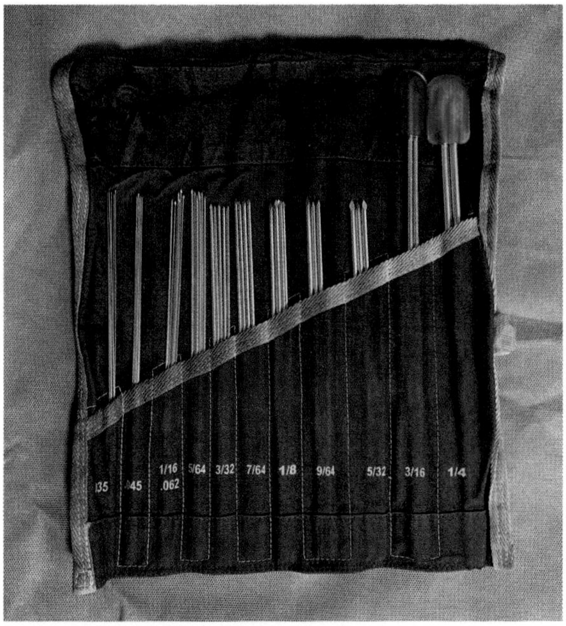

Figure 39.1 Kirschner wires and Steinmann pins of various sizes within an autoclavable cloth bag. *Source:* © Rebecca Webb.

versatile and have a wide range of uses for orthopedic fixation. These pins can be used as intramedullary implants to resist bending at the fracture site, to secure small fragments by skewering them, in a cross-pin fashion, to maintain temporary reduction of the fracture while a stronger primary fixation is applied, or as components of an external skeletal fixation. Pins are mostly used to resist bending forces, and the strength of a pin is calculated by the radius of the pin to the fourth power. Due to this, small increases in the size of a pin will have a significant increase in the strength of the pin when resisting bending.

Intramedullary Pin (IM Pin)

Pins can be placed within the intramedullary canal to provide resistance to bending forces. Placement of these pins can either be performed in a retrograde (advancing the pin from within the fracture site to the outside of the bone, then redirecting across the fracture site) or a normograde (advancing the pin into the intramedullary canal from the proximal aspect of the bone and across the fracture site) manner. The bones that are amenable to intramedullary pinning include the humerus, femur, tibia, ulna, and metacarpal and metatarsal bones. Intramedullary pinning of the radius is contraindicated due to the risk of carpal joint injury.

The size of the pin used will be determined by the medullary canal size of the patient's bone. Clinicians should aim for at least 70% fill of the medullary canal when the IM pin is the only device within the intramedullary canal. Pins can also be used in conjunction with a plate to increase the overall strength of the construct (see "Plates - Bridging Plates"). In these instances, the size of the pin needs to be reduced to allow bi-cortical screw purchase, so clinicians should aim to fill 35–40% of the medullary canal in these cases (Figure 39.2).[1] The size of the medullary canal can

(a) (b)

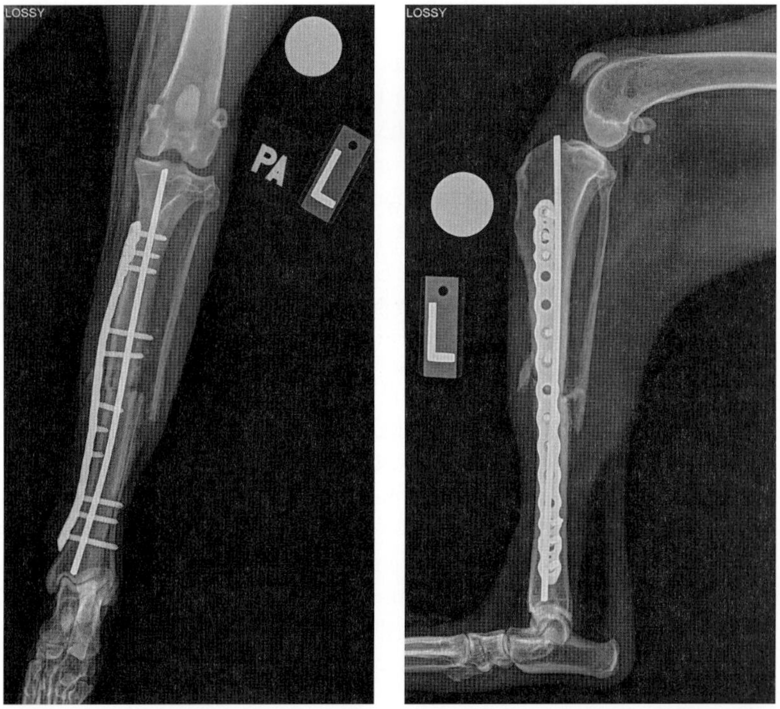

Figure 39.2 Postoperative craniocaudal (a) and lateral (b) radiographs of internal fixation of a left chronic comminuted tibia fracture with a 2.8 mm IM Steinmann pin and a 3.0 mm Arthrex® OrthoLine™ plate. *Source:* © Rebecca Webb.

either be judged at the time of surgery or using calibrated radiographs to make measurements of the canal for pre-surgery fixation planning.

IM pins will resist bending forces but have limited strength against rotational or compressive forces. For this reason, IM pins are rarely used alone as a fixation, and they are commonly combined with additional implants, such as cerclage wire, plates, or as part of an external fixator, to counteract these other fracture forces. The use of multiple IM pins, referred to as "stacked pinning," was historically used to improve the resistance to rotational forces; however, it was found that multiple IM pins provided no improvement in resistance when compared with a single pin, so the application of stacked pinning is no longer recommended. [2] Prior to the wide availability of plating systems, intramedullary pinning, in addition to placement of cerclage wire, was historically used frequently for fracture repair. While this can be an efficacious treatment option, careful case selection is imperative to its success. This type of fracture fixation is suitable only for reconstructable long oblique or spiral fractures. In these fracture types, there must be complete reconstruction of the bony column; this provides load-sharing between the IM pin and cerclage and the bone and gives stability to the overall construct.

The placement of an intramedullary pin can be in either a normograde or retrograde manner. Pins placed within the tibia are typically normograde to avoid accidental injury to the stifle joint surface. Placement within the other bones mentioned above can be performed in either a normograde or retrograde fashion. Normograde is typically preferred when possible, as there is less disruption of the fracture callus for insertion of the pin. However, normograde insertion can be challenging to accurately perform if visualization of the entry point cannot be visualized, such as in the femur. It is important prior to placement of the pin that the surgeon has two pins of the same length so that one of the pins can be used as a comparison measuring pin to monitor how deep the pin in the bone is being inserted. The pin can be advanced into the fracture fragments with either a hand-driven Jacobs chuck or with power equipment. Using a hand chuck typically will give the surgeon a better feel for the insertion of the pin and help the surgeon judge if they are still within the medullary canal by the ease with which the pin is advanced. Power equipment can also be used, but surgeons are more likely to over-advance the pin or penetrate through the cortex when it is used, as there is little feedback through the power equipment for the surgeon.

Once the pin is visualized at the fracture site, the pointed tip of the pin can be cut off to help prevent accidental penetration through the cortex into the distal joint. The surgeon should be aware that if the tip is removed from the IM pin being placed, the reduction in length is taken into consideration when using the comparison measuring pin (or the measuring pin reduced by a similar amount in length to make them the same again) to judge penetration into the distal fragment. The fracture is then reduced, and the pin advanced into the distal fragment. Once the pin starts to engage within the distal metaphyseal bone, the pin will become subtly more difficult to advance again. This is a good indicator to the clinician that the pin length is sufficient. Pin length should be checked against the measuring pin one more time, and the distal joint should be put through a range of motion to feel for crepitus. The presence of crepitus or restricted range of motion of the joint indicates joint penetration and should be rectified prior to leaving the OR. If this is noted, the pin should be withdrawn from the distal fragment and advanced again in a new position within the intramedullary canal. Simply pulling the pin back and away from the joint without redirecting it is not advised, since with micromotion at the fracture site, the pin will likely just advance back through the hole and into the joint again postsurgery.

Once the additional fixation (plate, external fixator, or cerclage) has been applied to stabilize the construct, the tip of the pin should be cut as short as possible. This is most easily performed by dissecting away some of the soft tissue from the exposed pin length to advance the pin cutters to cut the pin as close to the bone as possible. If it is not possible to apply the pin cutters close to the bone, the surgeon can withdraw the pin 1–2 cm from its insertion within the bone. To be accurate during the withdrawal, it is recommended to score the pin with pin cutters so the clinician can tell how much of the pin has been withdrawn from the bone. Once the pin is slightly withdrawn, the surgeon can cut the pin shorter than before. The pin should be cut as close as possible to the insertion, then the pin is advanced back into its original location within the distal metaphysis with a pin punch (Figure 39.3). This method allows for a shorter length of pin exposed, which is important, as leaving the end of the pin too long will lead to complications, such as seroma, muscular trauma, pin loosening/migration, poor use of the limb, and nerve damage (e.g., in femoral fractures with sciatic nerve impingement).

Small Fragment Fixation

Small K-wires are used for the fixation of small bony fragments. This is commonly performed when repairing avulsion fractures, such as tibial tuberosity avulsions or olecranon fractures (Figure 39.4). When placing these pins, the pins should be placed with a bridge of bone separating them, and when used alone as the fixation, the pins should be slightly angled away from each other to improve fixation strength. More than one pin, typically two, should be placed, or the small fragment will just rotate on the

(a) (b) (c)

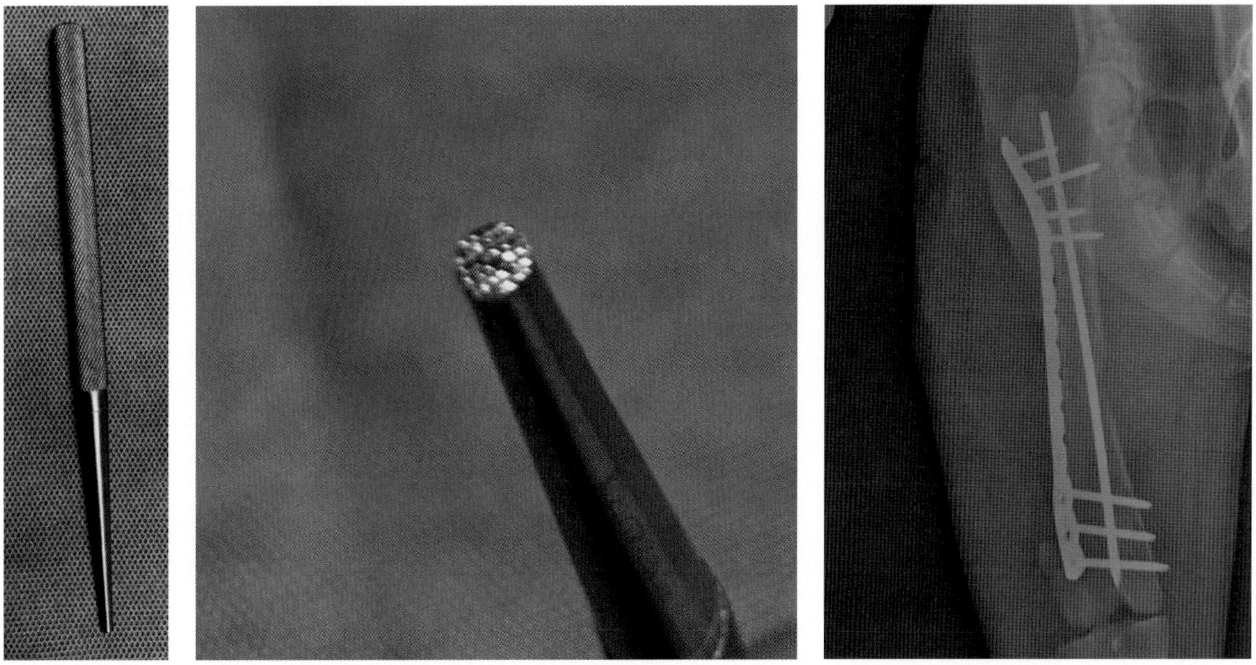

Figure 39.3 (a,b) Pin punch. The tip of the punch is roughened to allow it to capture the head of the pin. A mallet is used on the other end to advance the pin within the bone. (c) Craniocaudal radiograph of a postoperative femur fracture repair with an IM pin and lateral 3.5 mm Synthes LCP® plate. Note the IM pin is well-seated within the femur with no pin protruding past the greater trochanter. *Source:* © Rebecca Webb.

(a) (b)

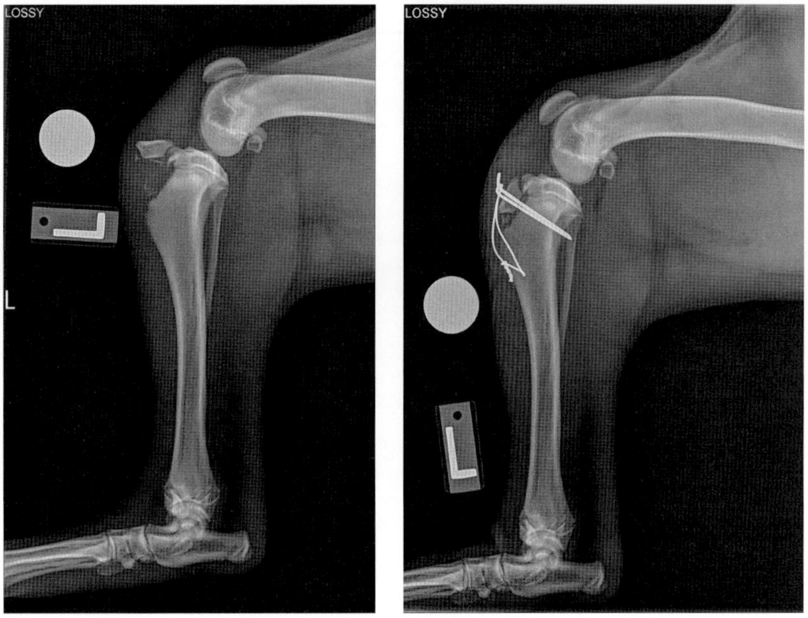

Figure 39.4 (a) Pre- and (b) postoperative radiographs of an immature dog with a left tibial tuberosity avulsion fracture. Small 0.045″ K-wires have been placed with a 20-gauge figure-8 tension band to secure the tuberosity bone fragment. *Source:* © Rebecca Webb.

singular pin. When placing pins to repair growth plate fractures, the ideal angle is typically perpendicular to the growth plate, so that any further remaining growth from the growth plate can occur (Figure 39.5).

The ends of the pins should be bent to prevent migration and cut short. There are multiple ways to achieve a bend in a K-wire, including commercially available pin benders, a metal Frazier suction tip, Jacobs chuck, or needle drivers (Figure 39.6). Most commonly, a "Z-bend" technique is utilized, which uses two bends to achieve an acute angle. To perform the bend, the bending instrument is applied over the K-wire as close as possible to its insertion on the bone,

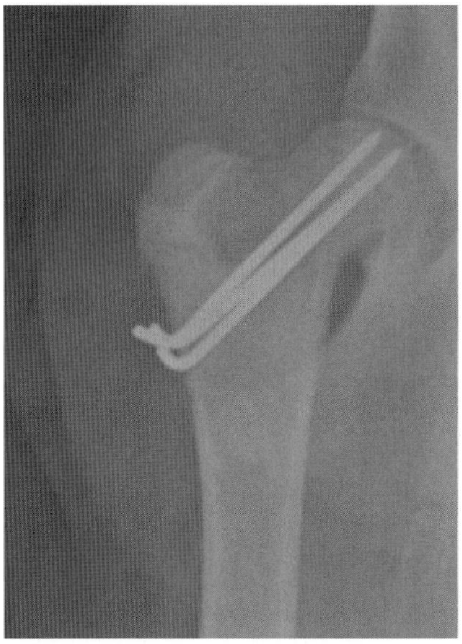

Figure 39.5 Postoperative craniocaudal radiograph of surgical repair of a capital physeal fracture in a medium-sized dog. Note the pins are placed perpendicular to the physis to help limit any impact on further physeal growth. *Source:* Courtesy of Dr. Desmond Tan.

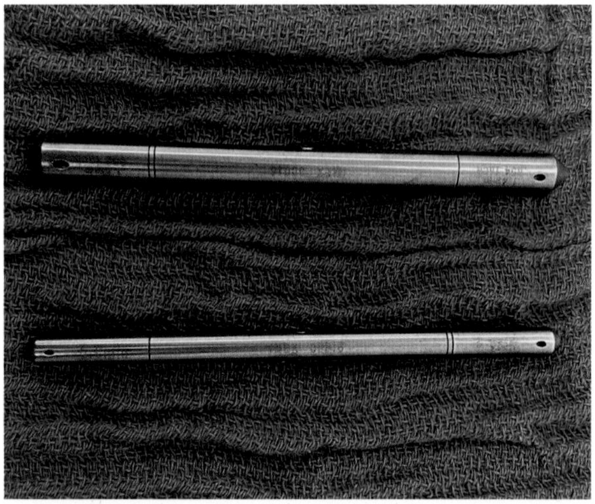

Figure 39.6 IMEX® Veterinary K-wire benders. These can be useful for bending small K-wires at acute angles. If these are not available, the surgeon can use a metal Frazier tip suction piece, Jacob's chuck, or needle drivers. *Source:* © Rebecca Webb.

and the K-wire is bent as acutely as the instrument will allow. The bending instrument is then withdrawn slightly further up the K-wire, and a second bend is performed in the opposite direction (to form the "Z"). Most commonly, this second bend is created by the surgeon pushing the instrument toward the floor and medially or laterally away from the bone (Video 39.1; Figure 39.7).

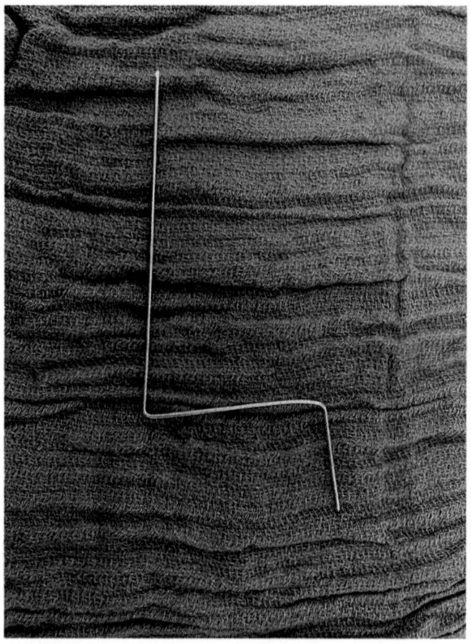

Figure 39.7 The K-wire placed in Video 39.1 was subsequently removed from the bone to demonstrate the "Z-bend" within the wire. The wire at the bottom of the image was placed within the bone, the two bends performed to create an acute bend on the K-wire are shown in the remaining pin. *Source:* © Rebecca Webb.

Cross-Pinning

For fractures in the distal metaphysis with only a small amount of bone stock for implant purchase, cross-pinning is an appropriate technique. Depending on the size of the patient (and, therefore, the size of the bone), either K-wires or Steinmann pins can be used. The overall strength of this fixation is low, and due to that, this technique is best suited to patients who are expected to have rapid healing (young, otherwise healthy patients). To place these pins, the fracture is reduced, and a pin is placed from the distal segment in a lateral-to-medial direction and a second pin in a medial-to-lateral direction. It is important for both pins to penetrate the far cortex to give stability to the construct. The pins should cross within the metaphyseal segment and not within the fracture (Figure 39.8). Occasionally, during the placement of cross pins, the pin will fail to penetrate the far cortex and, instead, start to travel up the shaft of the bone. This has been termed a "Rush-pin" technique and has been found to have less stability than traditional cross-pinning.[3] This typically occurs when the angle of placement is acute and a small pin is used, allowing it to bend instead of penetrating the far cortex. This fixation is commonly used to repair physeal fractures. Given that the pins are not placed perpendicular to the growth plate, there is some concern that they will impede further growth from the physis. However, it is important to note that the physis has already been significantly damaged during the incident causing the fracture, so it is challenging to determine if the physeal disturbance is secondary to the trauma or the

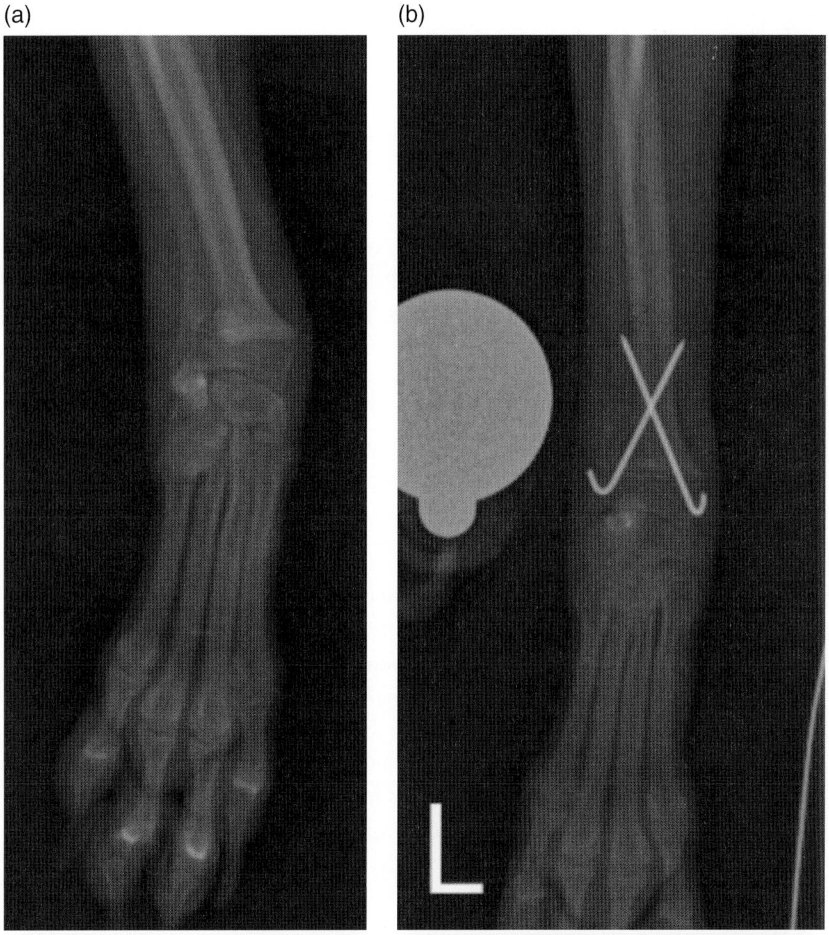

Figure 39.8 (a) Pre- and (b) postoperative radiographs of a left distal radial Salter-Harris type II fracture and distal ulna greenstick fracture in a Yorkshire terrier. The postoperative image shows two 0.035″ K-wires placed in cross-pin fashion. Note that the pins cross within the metaphyseal bone and not within the fracture site. *Source:* © Rebecca Webb.

repair. When these fractures occur in superficial locations, pin removal once the fracture is healed can be considered if there is evidence of physeal dysfunction.

Orthopedic Wire

Orthopedic wire is often used in conjunction with pins or a plate in reconstructable fractures. It is made from 316L stainless steel, which has been fashioned into a malleable wire that comes in a range of sizes from 16- to 24-gauge (Figure 39.9). The wire comes in two different forms, either gauge wire, which is straight wire that comes on a spool, or loop wire, which has an eye created in one end. Orthopedic wire can be used in a variety of techniques, including cerclage, tension band, hemicerclage, and interfragmentary. As cerclage and tension bands are the most common uses, we will focus on their application in this chapter. Orthopedic wire resists loads aligned with the wire well but has very little bending strength; due to this, it needs to be applied correctly for the construct to gain strength from the wire. As with IM pins, the strength of orthopedic wire is calculated by its radius to the fourth power, which leads to a dramatic increase in the strength of the wire for a small increase in wire size. It is recommended to use the largest size that appears appropriate for the size of the bone of the patient. In the author's practice, a general guideline for size selection is 16-gauge wire for patients over 40 kg, 18-gauge

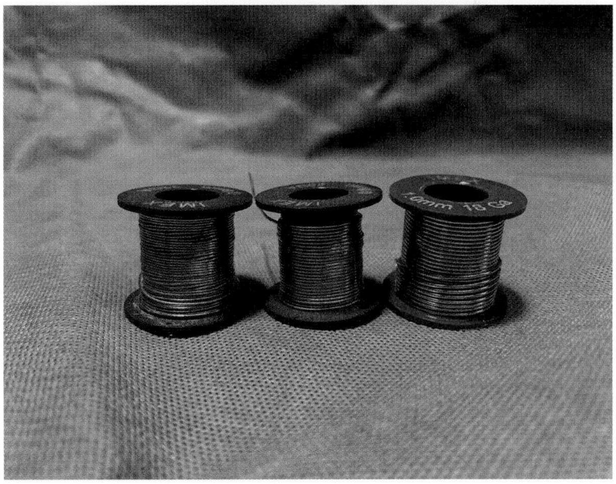

Figure 39.9 Orthopedic wire of different sizes on spools: 18G, 20G, and 22G. *Source:* © Rebecca Webb.

wire for patients over 20 kg, 20-gauge wire for patients weighing 10–20 kg, and 22- and 24-gauge for small dogs and cats. However, ultimately, the size chosen will depend on the bone size and the forces applied to it.

Methods of Securing Orthopedic Wire

Orthopedic wire can be secured in a variety of ways, and in veterinary patients, twist knot, single-loop knot, and double-loop knot are most commonly used. The twist knot is the most common, since the two types of loop knots require a tensioner for placement. When the three-knot types were compared biomechanically, the double loop cerclage had a higher tension capacity than twist and single loop knots and was able to resist a greater load.[4] Clinically, any of these knots can be used with success so long as the principles of placement are adhered to.

- **Twist knot** – The twist knot can be created with wire twisters or an old pair of needle drivers. It is most important when performing this knot that the ends of the wire both wrap around each other rather than one wire wrapping around another (Figure 39.10). To start the twist, the two ends of the wire should be twisted around each other by hand for two to three twists, this helps to ensure that the wire ends both continue to wrap around each other. The jaws of the wire twister are then centered in the middle of the twist and the clinician continues to twist the wire while pulling firmly away from the bone (Figure 39.11). The twist is then cut, leaving three twists remaining. It is important to note that any manipulation of the twist following placement will reduce the tension that the wire will maintain,[4] which includes cutting and bending of the twist.[5] This is most important to consider when the wire is being used as a cerclage, since tension within the wire imparts its function. This is less important when the wire is being used as a tension band, since the tension within the wire is less crucial for its function. Typically, when a twist knot is used to secure cerclage, it is cut short and not bent over to maintain its tension, whereas when it is used for a tension band, it can be laid flat during the last twist of the wire to help minimize the loss of wire tension during bending.
- **Single loop fixation** – Single loop fixation uses orthopedic wire with a prebuilt eye in one end. The wire is passed around the bone, the loose end of the wire is threaded through the eye, then it is tightened with a single-loop wire tightener. Within the wire tightener, the wire is threaded around a crank and rotated to tighten the wire. Once adequate tension is achieved, the free end of the wire is bent over the eye to secure the loop. To fully secure it with an acute bend in the loop, the tightener is loosened from the wire, slid up the wire approximately an inch, retightened to the wire, and the wire is pushed against the bone to fully secure the loop. The wire tightener is then removed, and the wire cut.
- **Double loop fixation** – For double loop fixation, a single piece of straight wire is folded in half to create a loop,

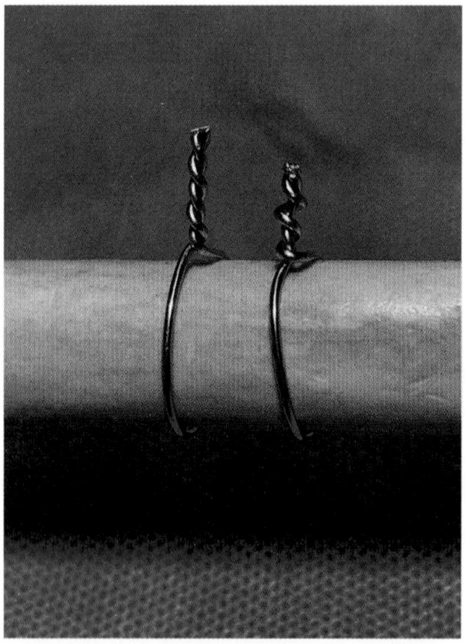

Figure 39.10 Twist knot using 18-gauge orthopedic wire. The twist knot on the left exhibits the correct application of a twist knot: note how the two strands are both twisted around each other. The twist knot on the right shows the incorrect application of a twist knot with one strand wrapped around the other. This gives the appearance of a "snake on a pole" and is not an appropriate twist. If this occurs, the knot should be restarted with a new piece of wire, and the surgeon should focus on applying traction to the wire as the wire is twisted. *Source:* © Rebecca Webb.

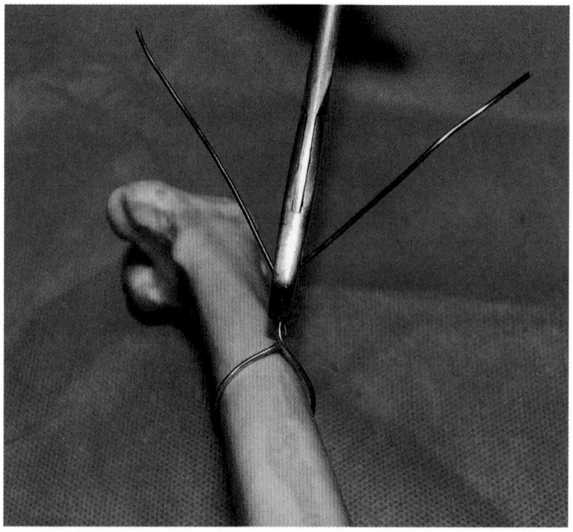

Figure 39.11 Jaws of the wire twister centered in the middle of the twist. To complete the twist, the surgeon pulls firmly away from the bone while continuing to twist the wire ends. *Source:* © Rebecca Webb.

the two free ends are passed around the bone and both free ends are inserted into a double loop wire tightener device. The wires are both tensioned at the same time by turning the cranks of the tightener device and secured by folding over the wire as for the single loop.

Cerclage

Cerclage is a technique that involves wrapping orthopedic wire around the bone tightly to apply compression to the fragments and give stability (Figure 39.12). This technique is only useful when the fracture is reconstructable and should only be used in long oblique or spiral fractures or to protect a fissure from propagating. Cerclage is only functional when the fracture fragments contact each other, and the bone column is reconstructed. If the fragments are poorly reduced or the fragments shift at all following placement, the wire will become loose and fail to function. When well-placed, cerclage should not impair fracture healing.[6] However, when cerclage is placed poorly or the fragments shift following placement, it becomes loose. It is thought that the loose wire impedes the formation of blood supply to the fracture and subsequently impairs healing.

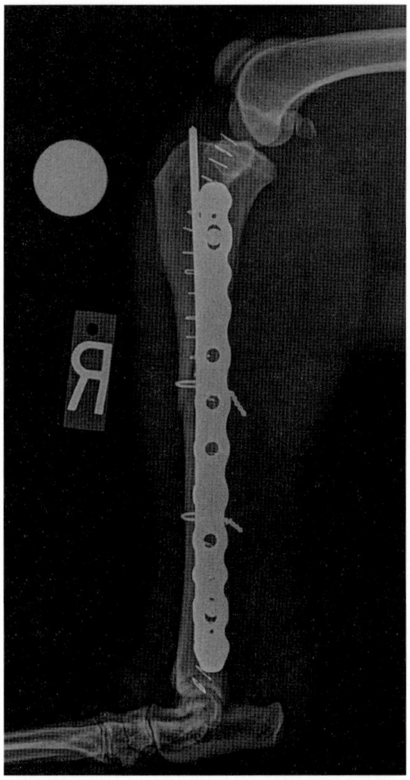

Figure 39.12 Postoperative lateral radiograph of a right long oblique tibial fracture that has been stabilized with an IM pin and a 3.5 mm Arthrex® OrthoLine™ locking plate. 18-gauge cerclage wire was used to prevent the propagation of fissures noted pre-operatively proximally and distally. *Source:* © Rebecca Webb.

Guidelines for appropriate cerclage wire placement are as follows:

1) Cerclage wires may be applied to long oblique or spiral fractures if the length of the fracture is 2–3x the medullary canal width.
2) The fracture must be anatomically reduced.
3) At least two wires must be used, preferentially three.
4) Wires should be spaced approximately half a bone diameter apart from each other at a minimum.
5) All wires should lie directly on the bone without any interposing soft tissue.
6) Cerclage wire should not be used as the only form of fracture fixation. Placement of a secondary implant to stabilize the fracture (e.g., IM pin, bone plate, ILN, or external fixator) is required for final fixation.
7) Cerclage wire can be placed temporarily to help reduce fractures while a secondary implant, such as a plate, is placed. Once the secondary implant is placed, the cerclage is typically removed so that the plate can sit closer to the bone.
8) In patients with fissures present, cerclage wire may be placed to help stabilize these fissures and prevent propagation during the placement of additional implants.

During the placement of cerclage wire around the bone, it is important that there is no interposing soft tissue. If there is soft tissue underneath the wire, the pressure of the wire after tensioning will cause necrosis of the underlying soft tissue, leading to loosening of the wire. To avoid this, a cerclage wire passer can be used to create a circumferential tunnel around the bone while excluding the surrounding soft tissue. Through the wire passer, the wire is then placed, enabling placement without entrapping soft tissue. In the absence of this instrument, a curved hemostat can be used in a similar manner.

Tension Band

Avulsion fractures occur in regions where muscles originate or insert onto bone. The avulsed bone fragment is typically reduced with two or more K-wires. The pull of the muscle that attaches to the bone fragments creates tension on the repair, which must be counteracted. In these cases, a tension band wire is placed to counteract the tension force and convert it into a compressive force across the fracture line. To place a tension band, the fragment is reduced with two or more K-wires. These K-wires should be placed perpendicular to the fracture line to be more effective and should be placed parallel to each other. A hole is drilled transversely across the main bone fragment to create a bone tunnel to pass the orthopedic wire. The placement of this tunnel is approximately equidistant below the fracture line, as the pins are above the fracture line.

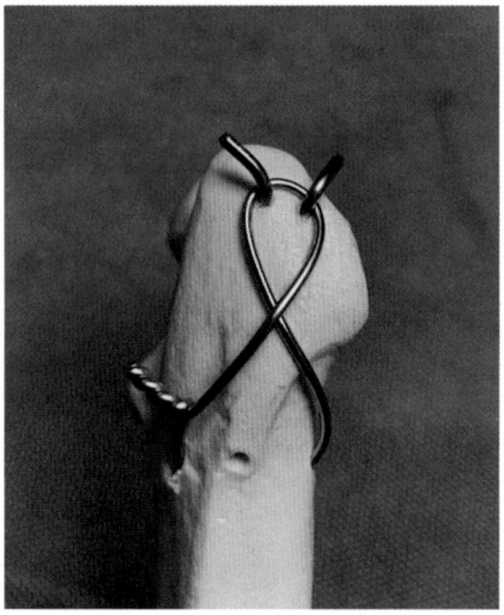

Figure 39.13 16-gauge orthopedic wire used for figure-of-8 tension band placement on a greater trochanter model with one twist knot. Two smooth 0.062″ K-wires are placed to secure the fragment followed by the tension band. *Source:* © Rebecca Webb.

The orthopedic wire is threaded through this tunnel, and the ends cross over each other. One end is then looped around the pins to create a figure-of-8 pattern. The two ends are then tightened, typically with a twist knot, and the pins are bent and cut short as previously described (Figures 39.4 and 39.13). As the orthopedic wire makes a few sharp turns, it is important for the clinician to eliminate the slack as the wire is passed through each turn. This helps to ensure that the wire is tight on the bone and will be effective in its function. In larger gauge wire, this becomes more challenging to do. In these cases, the use of two twist knots, one on either side, can be helpful to eliminate the slack (Figure 39.14).

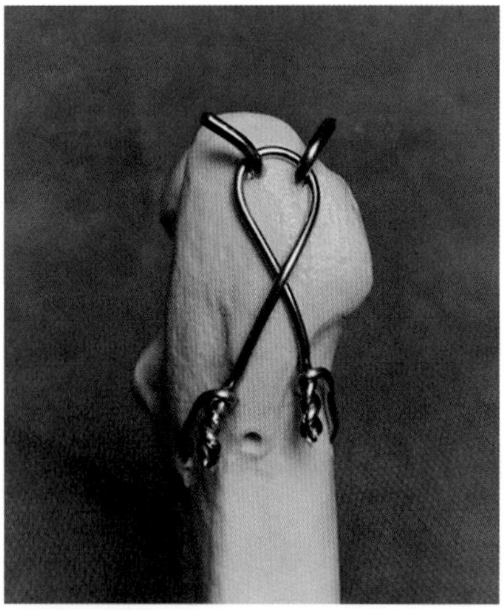

Figure 39.14 16-gauge orthopedic wire used for figure-of-8 tension band placement on a greater trochanter model with two twist knots. Two smooth 0.062″ K-wires are placed to secure the fragment followed by the tension band. To create the second twist knot, a loop is made in the wire between the pins in the first section of the figure-of-8 pattern. The ends of the wire are twisted as normal to create two twist knots. *Source:* © Rebecca Webb.

Bone Plates and Screws

Plates and screws are commonly used in orthopedic surgery to provide stability to fractures. Locking and nonlocking implants are available with locking plates being preferred by many surgeons, particularly in comminuted fractures due to increased stability with their use. Recent advances in plate design include scalloping of the underside of the plate to decrease cortical bone contact and preserve periosteal blood flow, development of compression holes, combination locking and compression holes, variable angle locking screws, and the use of new materials, such as titanium alloys.

Plates and screws can be used alone or in combination with other implants to stabilize complex fractures. The appropriate application of these implants depends on the fracture configuration and the method in which the plate is being used. In this chapter, we will discuss the basics of these implants and their uses, however, it is important to note that there are subtle nuances to each system and their application. Clinicians should be aware that there are many continuing education courses on these implants and their appropriate application, which can be of great benefit when starting to use a system that is unfamiliar to the clinician.

Screws

Screws are versatile implants and can be used in multiple ways. Screws can be categorized in one of two ways. First, they are characterized by the type of screw (e.g., cortical, cancellous, locking, cannulated, and self-tapping). Second, screws can be categorized as to how the clinician uses them in the patient (e.g., plate screw, positional screw, and lag screw). Screws are commonly made from 316L stainless steel. Titanium alloy screws are now available, but they should be reserved for use with titanium plates.

Cortical Screws

Cortical screws are threaded along their length and are designed for implantation into dense cortical bone. The pitch of a screw describes the distance between the threads and is a common descriptor for the different types of screws. The pitch of a cortical screw is typically shorter than that of a cancellous screw but longer than that of a locking screw, and the depth of the threads is typically shallower than that of a cancellous screw but deeper than

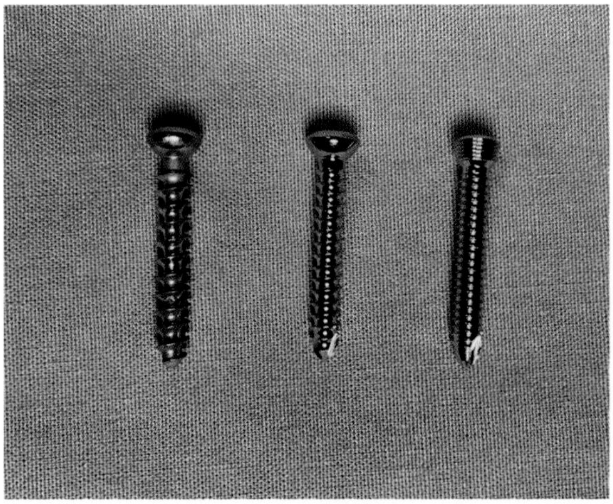

Figure 39.15 From left to right: 4.0 mm cancellous screw, 3.5 mm cortical screw, and 3.5 mm locking screw. Note that the pitch of the threads is the smallest for the locking screw, followed by the cortical, then the cancellous screw. The depth of the threads of the cancellous screw is deepest, followed by the cortical, then the locking screw. *Source:* Courtesy of Christine A. Valdez.

that of a locking screw (Figure 39.15). When cortical screws are implanted within a plate, they function by compressing the plate to the bone, and this creates friction between the bone and the plate to give stability to the construct. Due to this, it is important that when these screws are placed within a plate, they are tightened appropriately, or their function will be impaired. When using cortical screws, the clinician should be cautious that the plate is sitting flush against the bone prior to placement of the screw, as a large gap between the plate and bone will result in the screw pulling the bone toward the plate, disrupting the prior reduction of the fragments.

Cancellous Screws

In comparison to cortical screws, cancellous screws have a thinner core diameter (compared with cortical screws of the same size) but wider and deeper threads (Figure 39.15). This increases the holding power of these screws within the trabecular bone of the metaphysis. These screws come in either completely threaded or partially threaded variations. The fully threaded variant functions like a cortical screw when placed in a plate. The partially threaded version can have a "lag effect" when placed in the traditional manner (see "Screw uses: Lag screw"), so long as the threads only engage the far fragment.

Locking Screws

Locking screws are screws that physically engage or "lock" into a plate. The locking mechanism to achieve this varies for different plating systems. Commonly, the screw head is threaded, and these threads engage into either matching threads within the plate (Locking compression plate [LCP®] by Synthes, OrthoLine™ by Arthrex®) (Figure 39.15) or to cut their own threads into the plate (PAX® Polyaxial locking system by Securos Surgical®). Additional locking systems include the FIXIN® (Intrauma®) and String of Pearls (SOP™) (Orthomed) systems. The FIXIN® system uses a threaded bushing within the screw hole and a conical taper to the screw head to lock the screw into the plate. The String of Pearls system uses cortical screws to lock into the plate hole or "pearl" using a thread at the base of the screw hole as well as a contact ridge within the screw hole.

Locking screws give strength to a plate construct in a different manner than cortical screws. As the head of the screw is "locked" into the plate, they form a fixed angle construct, meaning that their position in relation to the plate and bone is fixed. These constructs do not rely on close contact between the bone and plate to create friction and give strength as cortical screws do. Instead, the forces created during the loading of the bone in locking constructs are converted into compressive forces at the screw-bone interface to give strength (see "Locking plate systems").[7]

Cannulated Screws

Cannulated screws are screws with a central hole within the screw (Figure 39.16). Through this hole, a K-wire can be threaded through. These screws are placed by first passing a K-wire into the proposed location for the screw. This K-wire acts as a guide for the final placement of the screw. Over this K-wire, a cannulated drill bit is used to drill into the bone for the screw hole. The cannulated screw can then be placed over the K-wire and into position. These screws are most helpful for reconstruction of metaphyseal or epiphyseal fractures. Achieving the appropriate angulation of screws for fixation of these fractures can be challenging. Cannulated screw systems give the clinician the ability to have multiple attempts to achieve the correct screw placement with the K-wire prior to drilling the screw hole, which makes these screw systems invaluable for the repair of fractures where there is limited bone stock for implantation (Figure 39.17).

Headless Compression Screws

Compression screws are placed across a fracture line and function to compress the near and far cortices together. They typically achieve compression across the fracture line due to a change in the pitch diameter of the threads of the screw with a wider pitch in the leading threads of the screw and a narrower pitch near the head of the screw. This means that when the screw is placed, it travels more quickly through the bone with the leading threads of the

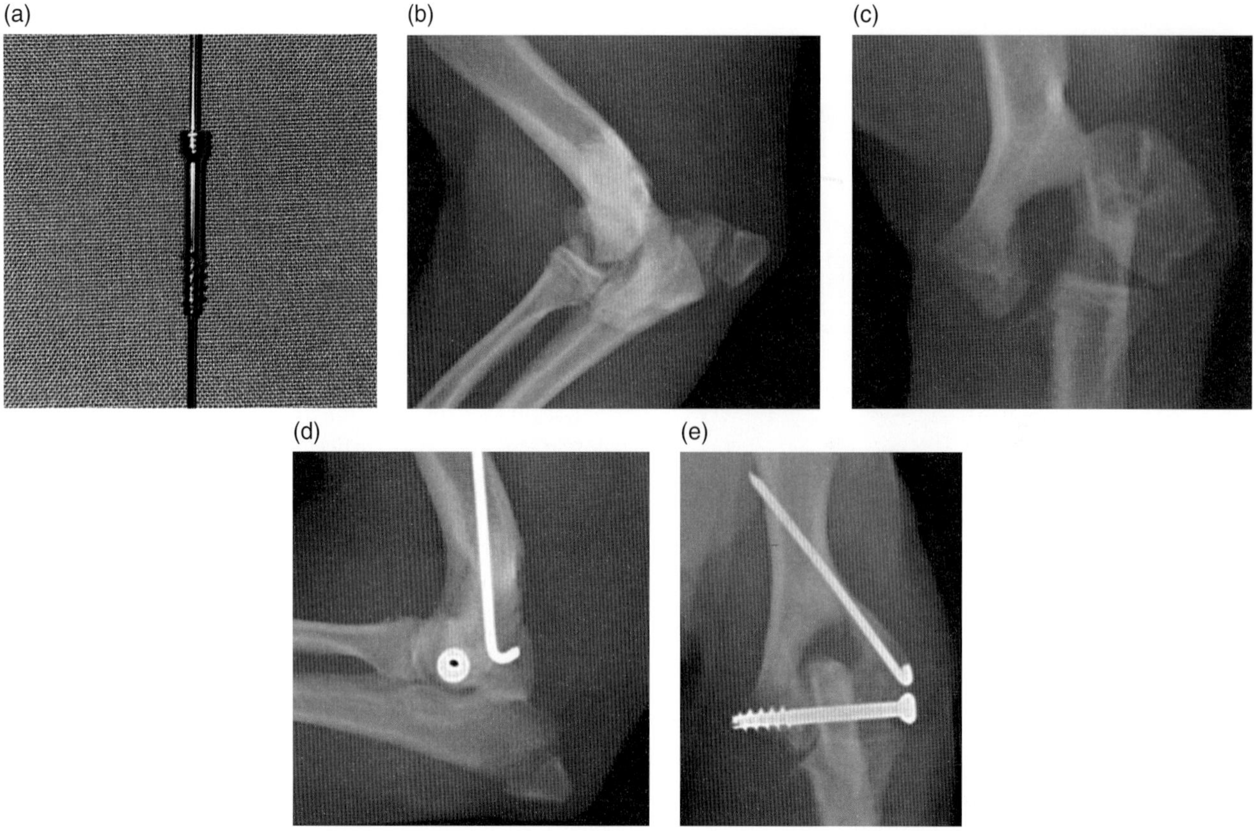

Figure 39.16 (a) A cannulated 3.0 mm headless compression screw with a K-wire going through the center of the screw. Typically, the K-wire is placed first, a cannulated drill bit is threaded over the K-wire to drill the hole, and the screw is then placed over the K-wire. (b,c) Pre-operative (b) lateral and (c) craniocaudal radiographs of a juvenile canine patient with a lateral humeral condylar fracture. (d,e) Postoperative (d) lateral and (e) craniocaudal radiographs of the same patient postfixation with a 4.0 mm cannulated, partially threaded screw (Synthes) and an epicondylar 0.062″ K-wire. (a) *Source:* Courtesy of Christine A. Valdez; (b–e) *Source:* Courtesy of Dr. Desmond Tan.

screw and then more slowly with the threads near the head. The change in the thread pitch results in compression between the two cortices during placement, similar to a screw placed in "lag fashion" (see "Screw uses: Lag screw") (Figure 39.18).

Screw Placement

The general steps for screw placement are as follows:

1) An appropriately sized drill brit for the screw being placed is loaded in a drill. A drill guide, which is appropriate for the size of the screw, is selected to achieve appropriate angulation during placement and protect the soft tissues from damage secondary to the drill bit. The bone is drilled with the drill bit through the drill guide under lavage.
2) A depth gauge is used to measure the depth of the bone in this location, and an appropriately long screw is selected for placement. If the exact length of the screw measured is not available for implantation, the surgeon should select the next longer screw.
3) For non-self-tapping screws, an appropriately sized tap is used to cut the threads within the hole to fit the screw being placed. Self-tapping screws have a cutting flute at the end of them, which acts to cut the threads as the screw is placed. This mostly eliminates the need for a tap in small animal patients, unless the screw is being implanted into particularly hard or brittle bone. Clinicians should be aware that the presence of the cutting flute at the end of the screw reduces the screw-bone interface in this region. Due to this, the cutting flutes should extend 2 mm beyond the far cortex of the bone to achieve similar stability to a non-self-tapping screw.[7] Typically, this corresponds to a 2 mm increase in screw length chosen for these screws.
4) A screwdriver with a tip that is of the appropriate type for the screw is used to implant the screw. The type of screwdriver is dependent on the screw being placed and is typically different for different implant systems. Power equipment can be used during this process with the addition of a torque-limiting device specific to the size of the screw being used. Manual tightening of the screws is suggested following this to ensure the screws

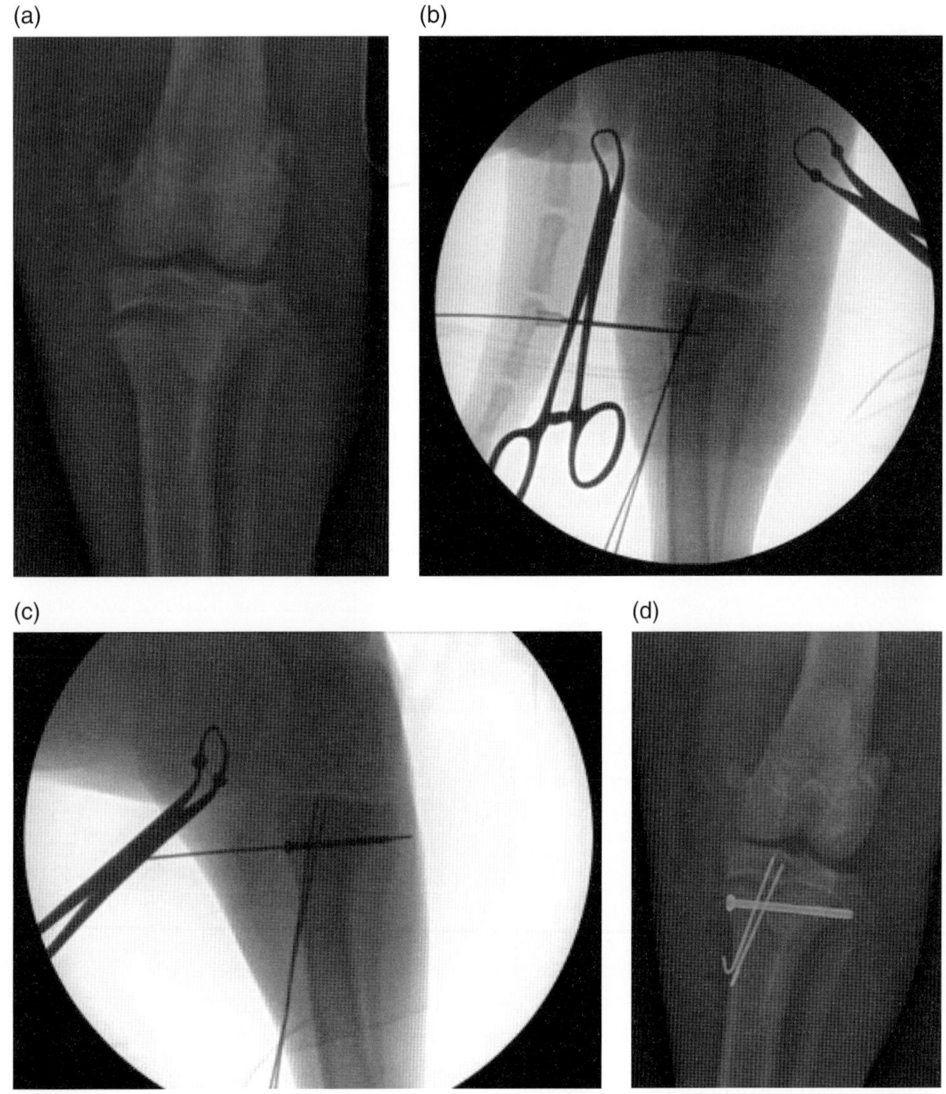

Figure 39.17 Fixation of a Salter-Harris type II fracture of the proximal tibia using a cannulated screw and K-wires. (a) Pre-operative craniocaudal radiograph of a young canine with a Salter-Harris II fracture. (b) Intraoperative fluoroscopy was utilized in this case to perform the repair in a minimally invasive manner. In this image, a K-wire is being placed from medial to lateral. Two additional small (0.045″) K-wires have been placed in this case from distal to proximal to give additional fixation and secure the segment while the medial-lateral screw is placed. (c) Once the surgeon was satisfied with the trajectory of the medial-lateral K-wire, the K-wire was over-drilled with a cannulated drill bit, and a 3.5 mm cannulated screw was placed. (d) Postoperative craniocaudal radiograph showing the final fixation with the medial-lateral cannulated screw and the two distal-proximal K-wires. *Source:* © Rebecca Webb.

are adequately tight within the construct. Tightness recommendations have been suggested for a few screw sizes as follows; two fingers for a 2.0 mm screw, three fingers for a 2.7 mm screw, and the whole hand for a 3.5 mm screw.[8]

Screw Uses

Lag Screw

The term "lag screw" relates to a method of screw placement and not a particular type of screw. In fact, any screw can function as a lag screw, as long as its threads only engage the far cortex. Since the threads of the screw only engage the far cortex, when the head of the screw contacts the near cortex and is then tightened, this creates compression across the two fragments in this region. This effect can be achieved using screws that are partially threaded or placing a fully threaded screw in a screw hole where the near cortex has been over-drilled so that the threads do not engage the bone. This is called a "glide hole". These screws need to be placed at a right angle to the fracture line to create compression across the fracture. This limits their effective use to fractures where the length of the fracture is greater than 1.5x the diameter of the bone. The following

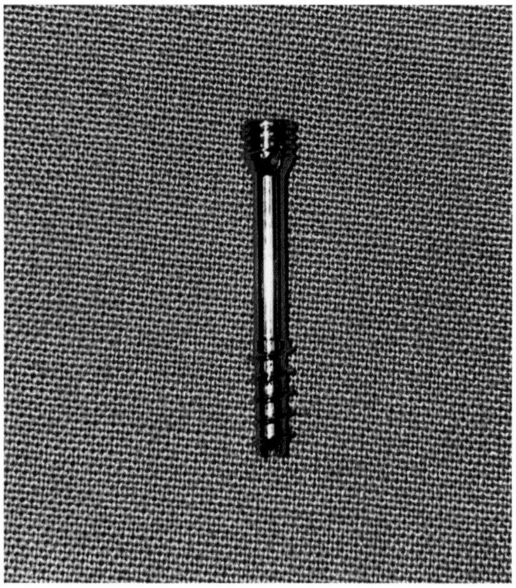

Figure 39.18 A 3.0 mm headless compression screw. Note the wider pitch in the leading threads of the screw and a narrower pitch near the head of the screw, which function to apply compression across a fracture line or osteotomy. *Source:* Courtesy of Christine A. Valdez.

steps outline the placement of a fully threaded screw as a lag screw.

1) Once the fragments are apposed, a drill bit of the same width (or slightly larger) as the screw threads are used to drill the near cortex. The size of this drill hole will be the same size as the screw threads, preventing them from engaging the bone in this region. This creates the "glide hole."
2) A drill guide with an outer diameter the size of the glide hole and an inner diameter the size of the core diameter of the screw is placed within the glide hole. A drill bit the size of the core diameter of the screw is used to drill the far cortex.
3) The screw hole is measured, and the appropriate length screw is selected. The far cortex is tapped with the appropriate size tap (if a self-tapping screw is not used).
4) The lag screw is placed. The screw threads engage the far cortex, and the head engages the near cortex. Further tightening creates compression across the fragments.

Positional Screw

A positional screw is used to secure a fragment back into position for reconstruction of a fracture. Positional screws are typically used when the placement of a lag screw would lead to the fragment collapsing into the medullary canal. To place these screws, the bone fragment is held in apposition with bone reduction forceps, and the screw hole is drilled in a traditional manner. Once the screw is placed, apposition of the fragments should be maintained. Unlike a lag screw, the threads of these screws engage both the near and far fragments. However, this is overall a less stable construct than a lag screw. These screws are typically used to reconstruct complex articular fractures.

Plate Screw

A plate screw is a screw placed to secure a plate to the bone. The size of the screw used to affix the plate will depend on the size of the plate (see "Plates").

Plates

Bone plates are most commonly made from 316L stainless steel, with some newer plates now made with titanium alloys. Bone plates are available in many different styles, each with their advantages and disadvantages. One of the biggest divisions in plating systems is between the nonlocking plates and the locking plates. Nonlocking plates, when placed, bring the plate in close contact with the bone. The contact between the bone and plate creates friction, and this friction creates stability to allow healing. Due to this, it is important that the plate is well-contoured to the bone surface and that there is no soft tissue between the plate and bone.

Locking plates function differently than nonlocking plates, and they instead create a fixed angle construct, which functions like an external fixator placed close to the bone. These plates do not rely on direct contact between the plate and the bone to create stability for healing. Locking plates are thought to create a stronger and stiffer construct compared with traditional plates.[9] This may reduce the number of cortices needed for a stable construct. The angle-stable nature of the screws also allows any monocortical screws placed to provide more benefit to the stability of the construct than nonlocking monocortical screws.[9] Although locking plates are less reliant on accurate contouring for strength when compared to nonlocking plates, excessive gaps between a locking plate and the underlying bone will weaken the construct and are to be avoided. Bone plates are typically labeled by the size screw that the holes accept. The most common sizes include 1.5, 2.0, 2.4, 2.7, 3.5, and 4.5 mm, although other sizes are available in different plating systems. The most common shape for a bone plate is the straight plate. The manufacturers typically produce a range of different length plates in each size to minimize the need to cut the plates intraoperatively. Aside from the straight plates, a range of other shaped plates are produced, including the T-plate, curved plates (for acetabular repair), and procedure-specific plates, such as the pancarpal or pantarsal arthrodesis plates, distal femoral osteotomy plates, anatomic-specific plates, such as the humeral condylar plate, tibial osteotomy plates, and pelvic osteotomy plates, among others.

Functions

Depending on the fracture configuration and how a plate is applied to the bone, plates can function in several fashions.

Neutralization Plate

In long oblique, reconstructable fractures, a lag screw may be used to provide interfragmentary compression. However, this lag screw is not strong enough on its own to withstand all the forces applied to the fracture site. Neutralization plating is where a bone plate is applied in addition to a lag screw(s) to protect the lag screw(s) from failure, and it remains "neutral" by not applying compression to the fracture site. The neutralization plate protects the screw(s) from all rotational, bending, and shear forces.

Bridging Plate

In nonreconstructable fractures, the plate is applied as a bridging plate. As the fracture has not been reconstructed, there is no load-sharing between the plate and the bone, which means that the forces that enter the distal segment of the bone are transmitted from those distal screws and through the locking plate to the screws within the proximal segment of bone. The forces basically bypass the fracture zone, and the plate alone carries the full force in this location. Due to this non-load-sharing construct, the plate must withstand all forces until a mature callus forms. The plate-rod combination can be particularly effective for these fractures, as the intramedullary pin is effective in protecting against bending forces and the plate is effective in protecting against axial compression and rotation. Typically, when an IM pin is used in combination with a plate, it is recommended that it fills 35–40% of the medullary canal.[1] This size reduces strain on the plate and increases its fatigue life while still allowing microstrain within the fracture, which is beneficial for callus formation.[1] In addition, the IM pin can also be helpful for the clinician to both re-establish spatial alignment of the limb in comminuted fractures, as well as maintain reduction while the bone plate is placed. In these cases, the IM pin is placed first, followed by the plate. As the IM pin is occupying a portion of the medullary canal, some screws may need to be monocortical (only engaging one cortex). Due to this, the plate-rod technique lends itself more to locking plates than nonlocking plate constructs. Additional methods for increasing the plate strength when used in a bridging fashion include selecting a larger plate, shortening the working length of the plate (by placing screws closer to the fracture site) or by adding an additional implant (such as an IM pin as previously discussed or a second plate).[10]

Buttress Plate

During weight-bearing in metaphyseal shear fractures, there are compressive forces which occur. These can lead to a collapse of the articular surface. Buttress plates are placed to prevent this collapse. This method of plate use is uncommon in veterinary patients, as these fractures tend to be infrequent in our patients.

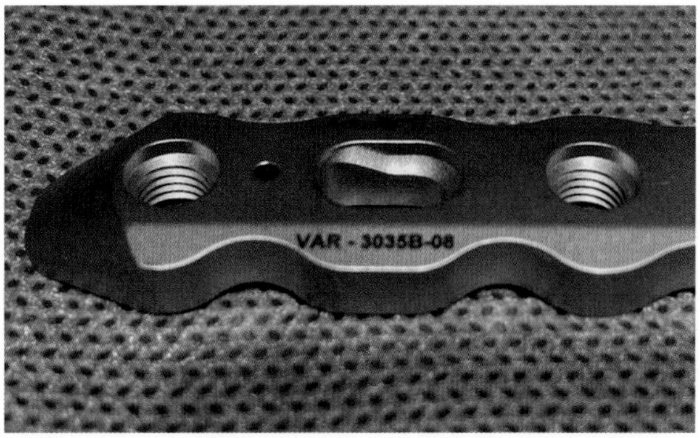

Figure 39.19 An Arthrex® OrthoLine™ 3.5 mm broad plate. The second hole from the left is a compression hole. Note the sloped nature of the hole. When the clinician wishes to apply compression to the fracture site, the hole for the screw is drilled at the higher end of the hole (to the left of the image). Then, as the screw is tightened, the bone underlying the plate slides along the plate to apply compression. *Source:* © Rebecca Webb.

Compression Plate

Specific compression plates can be used to apply a compressive force across a fracture gap. This function should only be applied to transverse fractures; application of a compressive force across an oblique fracture will lead to a shear force across the fracture fragments, and this could lead to fragment displacement and loss of reduction. Compression plates have specifically designed holes that are oval rather than the traditional round holes. In addition, the hole is sloped, the slope is higher away from the fracture site and lower toward the fracture (Figure 39.19). The clinician drills an eccentrically placed hole (away from the fracture, at the high side of the sloped hole), and as the screw is tightened, the head slides down the slope to the lower end of the hole. During this, the bone fragment the screw is engaging also moves with it, thus creating compression at the fracture site. Compression can be applied from both sides of the fracture. The amount of compression applied is plate system and plate size specific. For example, in the Synthes dynamic compression plate (DCP) system, 1.0 mm of compression is applied for each compression hole in the 3.5 and 4.5 mm systems and 0.8 mm in the 2.7 mm plate system. After the insertion of one compression screw, additional compression can be applied by applying a second compression screw. This is performed by applying the second compression screw before the first is fully tightened. Compression is mostly used when reconstructing transverse fractures and during plating osteotomy procedures.

Nonlocking Plates

As previously discussed (see "Cortical screws"), nonlocking plates are affixed to the bone with cortical screws. These screws compress the plate down to the bone. The friction created by the contact between the plate and the bone provides stability to the healing fracture. Nonlocking plates were some of the first bone plates produced, and they are typically less stiff and strong than their locking counterparts.[9] Due to this, anatomic reconstruction of the fracture is usually recommended when using them, so that load-sharing can occur between the bone and the plate construct, giving more stability to the fracture site and decreasing the risk of early implant failure. As these plates rely on bone-to-plate contact for stability, they need to be accurately contoured to the bone surface, so that when the cortical screws are applied and tightened, the bone fragments do not shift out of reduction. Nonlocking plates can have additional functions, such as compression holes, which are used to apply compression to the fracture or osteotomy site.

Dynamic Compression Plate (DCP)

The DCP is a nonlocking plate with the ability to apply compression to the fracture site. The plate was first introduced in 1969.[11] The oval shape of the holes allows 25° of angulation of the screw in the longitudinal plane and 7° in the transverse plane. This plating system comes with three different drill guides. The green (neutral) drill guide will apply the drill hole centrally within the screw hole and produce a neutral screw (without angulation or compression). The gold (compression) drill guide will produce a drill hole that is offset from the center of the plate hole. When the screw is applied, this will apply compression to the fracture site. The gold (compression) drill guide has a small arrow on its surface, and this arrow should be pointing in the direction that compression is to be applied. The universal drill guide will allow the clinician to angle the screw within the screw hole. Further advances in plating technology have led to these plates being largely replaced by the limited contact dynamic compression plates (LC-DCPs) (see below). Typical sizes available include 1.5, 2.0, 2.4, 2.7, 3.5, and 4.5 mm. Each size comes in a range of different lengths.

Limited Contact Dynamic Compression Plate (LC-DCP)

The previously described DCP was further refined into the LC-DCP (Figure 39.20). The underside of the LC-DCP is scalloped rather than solid (as for the DCP). This modification addresses two primary issues with the DCP plating system. First, the scalloping of the undersurface of the plate reduces the area of the plate in direct contact with the bone, and this is thought to improve the vascularity of the area compared with the DCP system.[12] In addition, the scalloping of the plate reduces the stiffness of the solid section of the plate, making it more closely match the stiffness of the section with holes. Since the stiffness is more closely matched, stress is not concentrated at the screw

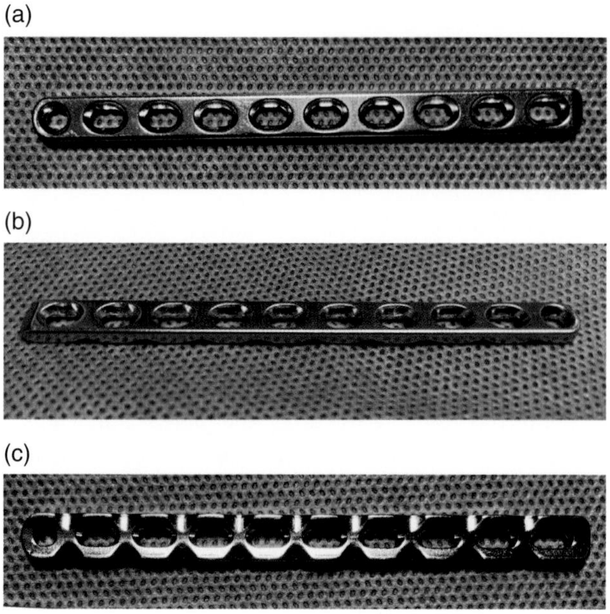

Figure 39.20 Synthes 2.4 mm limited contact dynamic compression plate. (a) The superficial surface with oval compression holes. (b) A side view with the sloped compression holes. (c) The deep surface, which is in contact with the bone. The scalloped edges of this surface decrease the area in contact with the bone and have multiple benefits as described in the text. *Source:* © Rebecca Webb.

holes, as it is for the DCP system. The scalloping also has the added benefit of allowing any contour introduced to the plate with bending to be more evenly distributed along the plate, rather than concentrated at the screw holes as it is for the DCP system.

As discussed, the scalloping of the undersurface of the plate has many benefits; however, it is important to note that the reduction in stiffness by scalloping reduces the strength of the plate when compared with the size equivalent DCP.[13] Since the optimal strength and stiffness of a plate are currently unknown, it is unclear if this decrease in strength is of any clinical significance. In addition to the scalloping, the underside of the plate hole of the LC-DCP plate system has been enlarged compared with the size equivalent DCP, and this allows the screw to be angled to a greater degree in the longitudinal plane (up to 40° for the LC-DCP) than the DCP system (25° of longitudinal angulation). As for the DCP system, the LC-DCP system allows screws to be inserted in neutral, in compression, and in an angled fashion, and it has similar drill guides. The LC-DCP plating systems come in a range of sizes including 1.5/2.0, 2.0/2.4, 2.7, 3.5, and 4.5 mm. They are available in a range of lengths and available in titanium and stainless steel.

Veterinary Cuttable Plate (VCP)

The veterinary cuttable plate comes in two sizes: 1.5 mm (which can accept 1.5 and 2.0 mm screws) and 2.0 mm

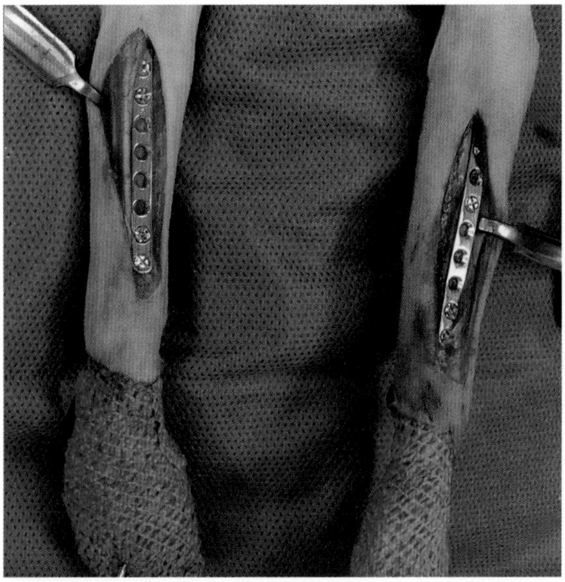

Figure 39.21 A juvenile toy breed canine patient with bilateral radius and ulna fractures. A craniomedial approach has been performed to expose both fracture sites, and the radial fractures have been plated with 2.0 mm veterinary cuttable plates with two 2.0 mm cortical screws proximally and distally on either side. *Source:* © Rebecca Webb.

(which can accept 2.0, 2.4, and 2.7 mm screws) (Figure 39.21). Each plate is 50 holes in length and can be cut to size depending on the length that is required. These plates have round holes, which do not allow for compression at the fracture site as discussed above. The number of holes per unit length of the plate is significantly higher than that of the LC-DCP and DCP plates. Given that it is a cuttable plate, the stiffness and strength of the plate are quite low. This can be increased by stacking a second plate on top of the first.[14,15] Given the low strength of this plate, it is best suited to reconstructed fractures where there is load-sharing between the bone and plate or in immature patients where rapid healing is expected.

Locking Plates

As discussed previously (see "Locking screws"), locking plates provide an "angle-stable" construct between the screw, plate, and bone. As the screw is locked into the plate at a specified angle, these plates function more closely to external fixators than nonlocking plates. Due to this, they have also been named "internal fixators." When compared with external fixators, these plates are much closer to the bone, increasing their mechanical strength. There are both fixed angle constructs, where the screw is locked into the plate at an angle specified by the manufacturer, as well as variable angle constructs, which allow a small amount of variation in the angle of the screw to the plate. Stability in both constructs is provided by the locking mechanism between the screw and the plate, which can be different for different systems. Due to the locking nature, the plate does not rely on direct bone contact for strength as the nonlocking plates do. This means that accurate plate contouring is less crucial for these systems. The reduction in contact between the bone and the plate may also improve the underlying blood supply and reduce bone resorption under the plate.[16] In addition, the locking nature of the screws prevents bone fragment displacement during placement. Overall, locking plates give greater stability than standard, nonlocking plates.[9,17] Due to the above improvements on the nonlocking plates, locking plates are more suited for bridging (see previously) and biological osteosynthesis where there is limited load-sharing between the bone and plate. In contrast to more traditional plating techniques, which typically prioritize reconstruction of the fracture site for load-sharing, biological osteosynthesis seeks to enhance healing by maintaining the biologic properties of the fracture. The biological properties are maintained by minimizing surgical intervention at the fracture site and not attempting anatomical reconstruction of the fracture. The goal of biological osteosynthesis is to achieve relative stability of the fracture site and secondary bone healing. This method of osteosynthesis has advanced over time and now includes the minimally invasive application of locking plates to adhere to the principles of biological osteosynthesis more closely.[18] The angle-stable nature of the implants increases the strength of any monocortical implants when compared with nonlocking systems. This makes them helpful for the reconstruction of articular fractures, such as the acetabulum, carpus, and tarsus if a screw is inadvertently aimed at the joint surface. They are also beneficial when performing "double-plating" (i.e., orthogonal plating) and when using a plate as part of a plate-rod construct, as some screws may need to be monocortical to avoid interference with the additional implants. To decrease the plate strain and likelihood of plate failure, recommendations have been suggested for the use of locking plates in human medicine. These include spanning a long section of bone (greater than three times the length of the fractured segment), limiting the screw-to-hole ratio to less than 0.5 and limiting the distance between the plate and bone to less than or equal to 2 mm.[19,20] Locking plate constructs can be made stiffer by selecting a larger sized plate, adding additional implants (an IM pin or second plate), or by shortening the "working length" of the plate (i.e., by placing screws closer to the fracture site).[10,21] Two screws per fracture segment are the minimum required when using locking systems. There is a minimal advantage to placing more than three screws per segment and placing the third screw toward the fracture site increases stiffness.[22]

Fixed Angle Locking Plates

Locking Compression Plate (LCP; Synthes)

The locking compression plate (LCP; Synthes) is a locking plate made from 316L stainless steel (Figure 39.22a), and it comes in a range of sizes, including 1.5, 2.0, 2.4, 2.7, 3.5, 4.5, and 5.5 mm, each with a range of lengths and shapes. The LCP plate has a combination hole or "combi hole" (Figure 39.22b), which can accommodate either a conventional nonlocking screw or a locking head screw. The end that accepts a nonlocking screw is a compression hole, which allows the clinician to apply compression to the fracture site. The locking end of the hole is threaded. The threads on this hole accept the threads of the locking head screw to create a locking mechanism. Given the combi hole allows both compression and locking to be applied to the fracture, the LCP plate can be used as a compression plate, as a locking plate, or using components of both features. The LCP plate also has a scalloped underside, like the LC-DCP plate, with the same advantages as such. There are two drill guides for each size. For the locking screws, a locking drill guide is used. This guide is threaded and screwed into the threads of the plate at a fixed angle. In this way, the screw hole is drilled so that the angle is appropriate to allow the threads of the screw and plate to match and lock together. The other guide is a universal guide that can be used to apply a nonlocking screw in either compression or neutral modes.

(a)

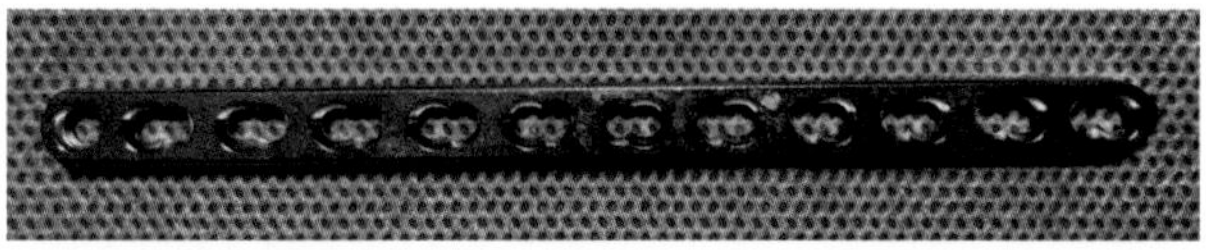

(b)

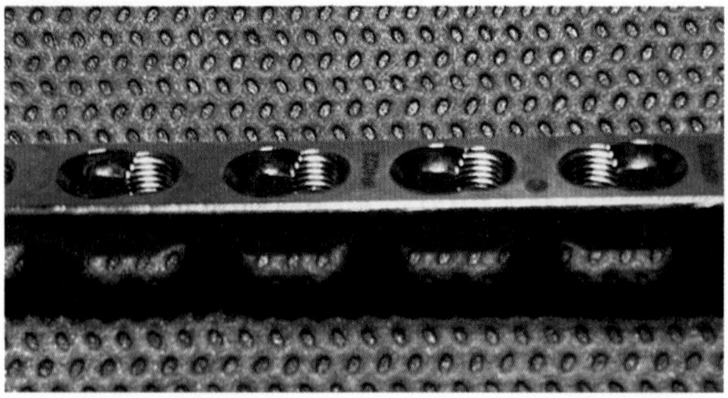

Figure 39.22 (a) A 2.4 mm locking compression plate (LCP®; Synthes). (b) A close-up image of the holes of the plate in image (a), showing the combination plate hole, or "combi" hole. The hole has a compression end (to the left side of the plate hole) and a locking end (to the right side of the plate hole). *Source:* © Rebecca Webb.

String of Pearls (SOP™; Orthomed)

The String of Pearls plate or SOP™ plate is unusual in comparison to the other locking systems discussed here, as it uses standard cortical nonlocking screws. They are available in 2.0, 2.7, and 3.5 mm sizes in 316L stainless steel and titanium and can be cut to length (Figure 39.23). The plate consists of spherical "pearls," which accept cortical nonlocking screws. The pearls are connected to each other with cylindrical sections or "internodes." The screw head press fits within the "pearl" using a thread at the base of the screw hole as well as a contact ridge within the screw hole. The plate can be contoured in multiple planes, including medial to lateral bending, cranial to caudal bending, and torsion at the internode. To prevent the pearls from becoming deformed during the bending and twisting, bending tees are placed within the holes of the 2.7 and 3.5 mm plates (Figure 39.24). These plates can withstand a

(a)

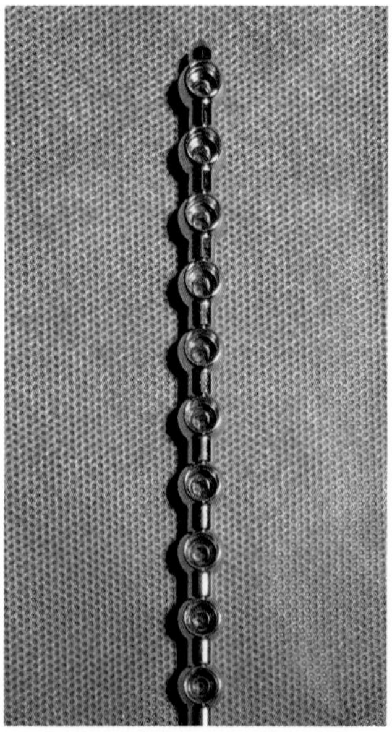

(b)

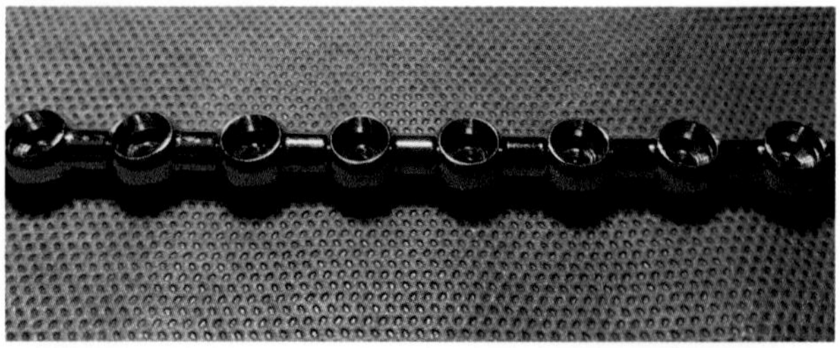

Figure 39.23 A 3.5 mm String of Pearls (SOP™; Orthomed) plate in 316L stainless steel. Images show the top (a) and side views (b) of the plate without screws. The spherical "pearls" accept cortical nonlocking screws. The cylindrical "internodes" connect between the pearls and can be contoured in six degrees of freedom. *Source:* © Rebecca Webb.

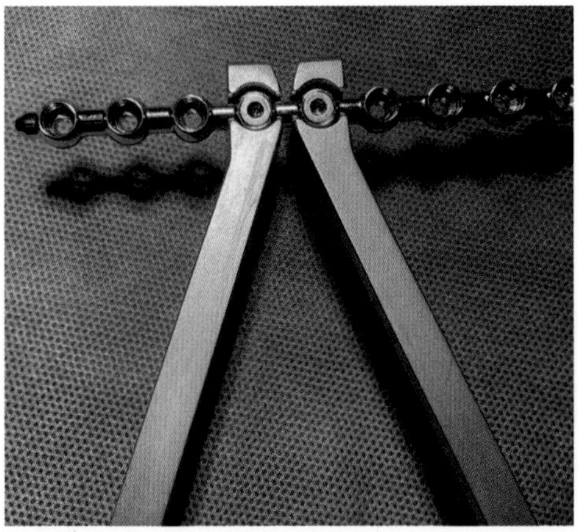

Figure 39.24 A 3.5 mm String of Pearls (SOP™; Orthomed) plate in 316L stainless steel. The bending irons have been applied across two pearls of the plate. The two pearls of the plate which are going to be bent have been filled with bending tees to prevent deformation of the plate holes during bending. *Source:* © Rebecca Webb.

high degree of contouring, giving them an advantage over other plating systems (Figure 39.25). However, these plates can be bulky in comparison to a similarly sized LCP plate, so their use is limited in regions with minimal soft tissue coverage.

FIXIN® (Intrauma)

The FIXIN® system is a locking system that comes in three size ranges. The Micro Series (1.3–1.7 mm, developed for toy breed dogs and cats weighing 3–4 kg), the Mini Series (1.9–2.5 mm, developed for small dogs and cats weighing up to 10 kg), and the Large Series (3.0–3.5–4.0 mm, developed for large dogs weighing 15–70 kg). The plates are constructed from 316L stainless steel, and the screws are a titanium alloy and come in a range of straight plates and contoured plates. While historically there has been concern for galvanic corrosion when mixing two different types of materials for implants, this is suspected to not be a clinical problem when mixing titanium and stainless steel.[23] The FIXIN system uses a threaded bushing within the screw hole and a conical taper to the screw head to lock the screw into the plate (Figure 39.26). In this system, the bushing screws into the plate and acts as an intermediary between the screw and the plate. Locking is achieved between the screw head and the bushing. The advantage of this system is the ease of removal if required. In other locking mechanisms, if the screw has been cold welded to the plate or if the screw head is unable to engage with the screwdriver, removal can be challenging. In comparison, the FIXIN® can be removed more easily, as the bushing is able to be easily removed. The addition of the bushing also increases the screw's resistance to shear forces and allows for a thinner plate design. This allows more elasticity, promotes early callus formation, and can be easily used in regions with limited soft tissue coverage. The plates also come with K-wire holes, which can be helpful for temporary fixation of the plate while screws are drilled.

Variable Angle Locking Plates

There are currently two locking plate systems which feature variable angle locking screws. In both systems, the locking mechanism can be maintained with a slight angulation to the screws. The ability to angle these screws is beneficial for complex fractures where screws need to be angled away from joint surfaces, other implants, or fracture lines. In traditional locking plate systems, the angulation of placement would necessitate the use of a

Figure 39.25 (a) Pre-operative lateral radiograph of a long oblique distal femoral fracture in a canine patient. (b) Postoperative lateral radiograph of a long oblique femoral fracture postfixation with a 9/64″ IM pin and a lateral 3.5 mm SOP™ plate (Orthomed) with six screws placed distally and five proximally. *Source:* Courtesy of Dr. Desmond Tan.

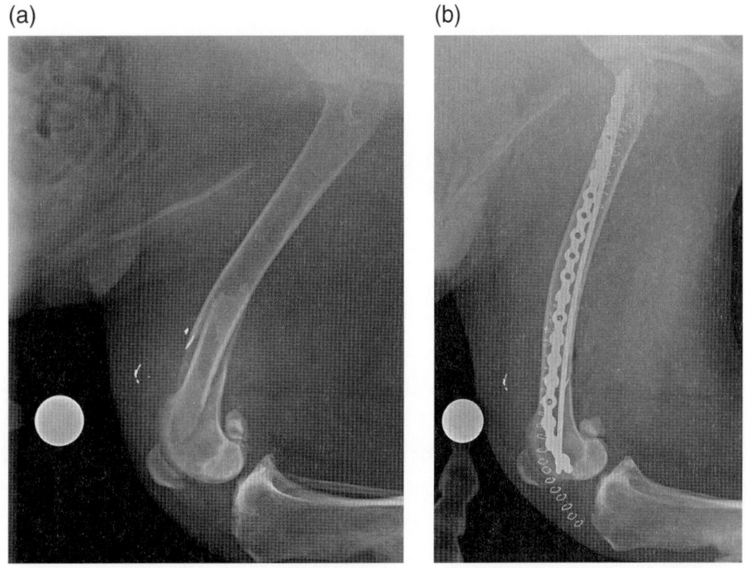

(a) (b)

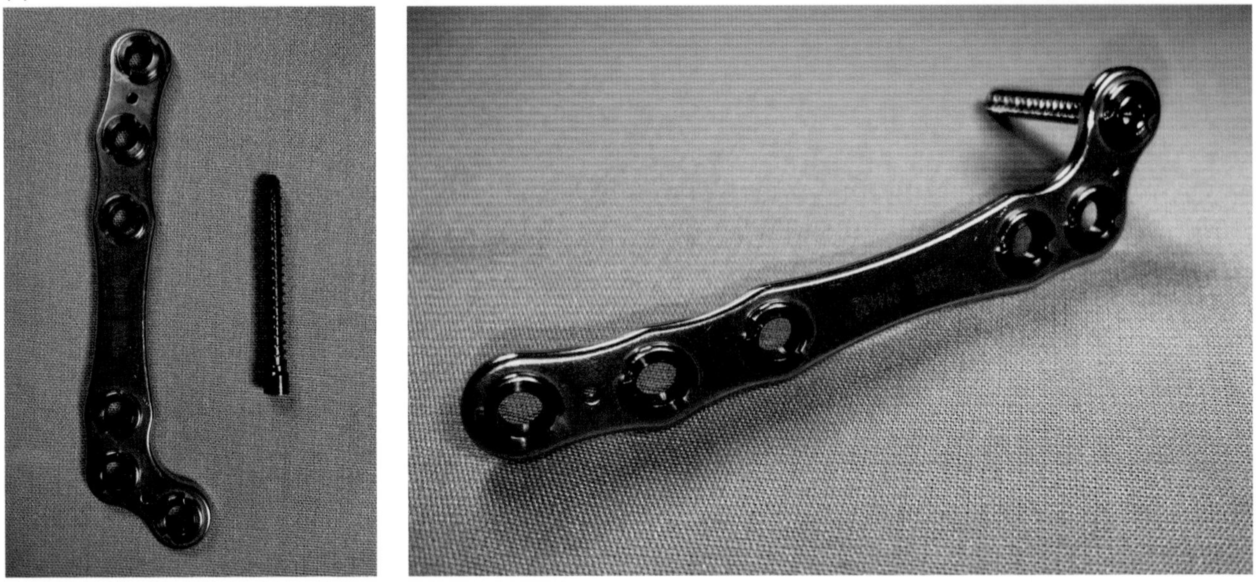

Figure 39.26 (a) FIXIN® 3.0–3.5–4.0 mm series L support long plate with a 3.5 mm autolocking screw, note the blue-colored bushings in the plate holes. (b) The FIXIN® plate from image (a) with the autolocking screw inserted into the distal most screw hole. *Source:* Courtesy of Christine A. Valdez.

cortical screw, which isn't as strong. It is less ideal to use a cortical screw in these situations if there isn't appropriate contact between the plate and the bone at the required screw hole location. The ability to angle a locking screw slightly while still maintaining the locking mechanism with the below systems can be very useful, particularly in these scenarios.

OrthoLine™ System (Arthrex® Vet Systems)

The Arthrex® OrthoLine™ system comes in a range of sizes, including 1.6, 1.6 broad, 2.0, 2.4, 3.0, 3.5, and 3.5 broad/4.0 mm. The plates in the 1.6–3.0 mm range are made of titanium, and the larger plates are made of 316L stainless steel. The plates come in a range of straight plates (Figures 39.19 and 39.27), T-plates, and TPLO plates, as well as distal humeral condyle plates (Figure 39.28). The straight plates are designed to have a higher screw density toward the ends of the plate and have a central bridge within the middle of the plate with fewer holes to help span transverse and short oblique fractures; this means that a screw hole is less likely to be left open over the fracture line. The plates feature compression, slide, and locking holes.

The plates were designed to allow multiple methods of temporary K-wire fixation to the bone. As discussed for the FIXIN® system, it can be very helpful to temporarily stabilize the plate to the bone with K-wires while the screw holes are drilled. In the OrthoLine™ system, the K-wires can be placed within the K-wire holes of the plate, through a

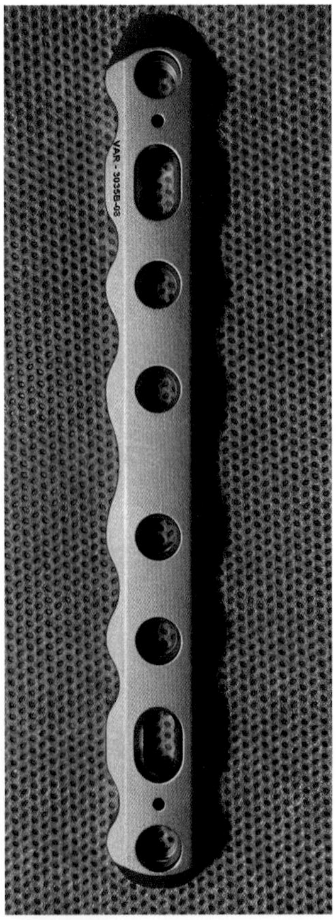

Figure 39.27 A 3.5 mm stainless steel broad 8-hole Arthrex® OrthoLine™ plate. Note the small K-wire holes for temporary fixation. *Source:* © Rebecca Webb.

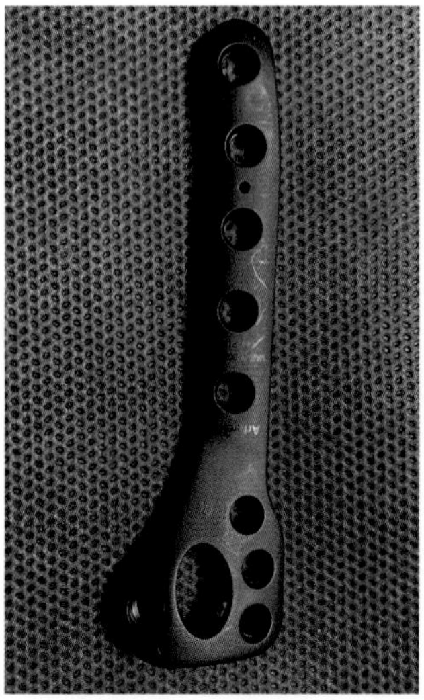

Figure 39.28 A 3.0 mm titanium right-sided distal humeral condylar plate. The plate is pre-contoured so that it fits the distal humeral condyle. The screw holes of this plate accept conventional locking, variable locking, and cortical screws. Note the small K-wire holes for temporary fixation. *Source:* © Rebecca Webb.

bending plug, which fits within one of the locking screw holes, or using a Bb-Tak (Arthrex®), which is a specific K-wire with a small cylinder attached that can be drilled into the screw holes. Like the LCP and LC-DCP™ plates, the underside of the OrthoLine™ plates is scalloped on the underside to limit contact with the bone surface, which is thought to improve periosteal blood supply. The plates can accept cortical, standard locking, and variable locking (titanium sizes only) screws. The standard locking screw is applied using a standard locking guide that screws into the threads of the locking screw hole, similar to the LCP (Synthes) system. The standard locking screws are angled at a fixed angle from the plate. The variable angle locking screws are available for the titanium plates only and allow the clinician to place them with up to 12° of angulation in any direction. To place the variable angle screw, a conical drill guide is used, which allows the clinician to angle the drill bit within a fixed 12° range. The system also comes with a 4.0 mm locking screw, which can be used in the 3.5-mm and 3.5-broad plates. Due to the larger core diameter of the 4.0 mm screw, this size further increases the strength of the construct for large and giant dog breeds. The T-plates within this system have been designed with the locking screws angled away from the joint surface by 7.5° to enable safer placement close to joint lines.

PAX® System (Securos Surgical®)

The polyaxial locking plate system (PAX®) is a titanium plating system that comes in sizes 2.0, 2.4, 2.7, and 3.5 mm. The plates come in reconstruction plates, lengthening plates (with a central region without screw holes), T- and L-plates. The screws can be angled up to 10° from vertical. The PAX® system functions by using different titanium alloys for the screw and the plate. The alloy used for the screw head is approximately twice as strong as that of the plate. This allows the screw to cut its own threads into the plate as it is inserted, at angles of up to 10° from vertical. Generating adequate torque when inserting these screws is important to ensure that the variable locking mechanism functions appropriately.

Interlocking Nail (ILN)

ILNs are used primarily in long bone fractures of the humerus, femur, and tibia, and occasionally, in the ulna of very large dogs. As with IM pins, their use is contraindicated in the radius. They consist of an intramedullary nail, which comes in a range of sizes (3, 4, 5, 6, 7, 8, and 10 mm in diameter), each with a range of lengths (Figure 39.29). These nails typically have two holes on either end, which accept either screws or bolts. These screws or bolts affix the intramedullary nail to the cortical bone of the proximal

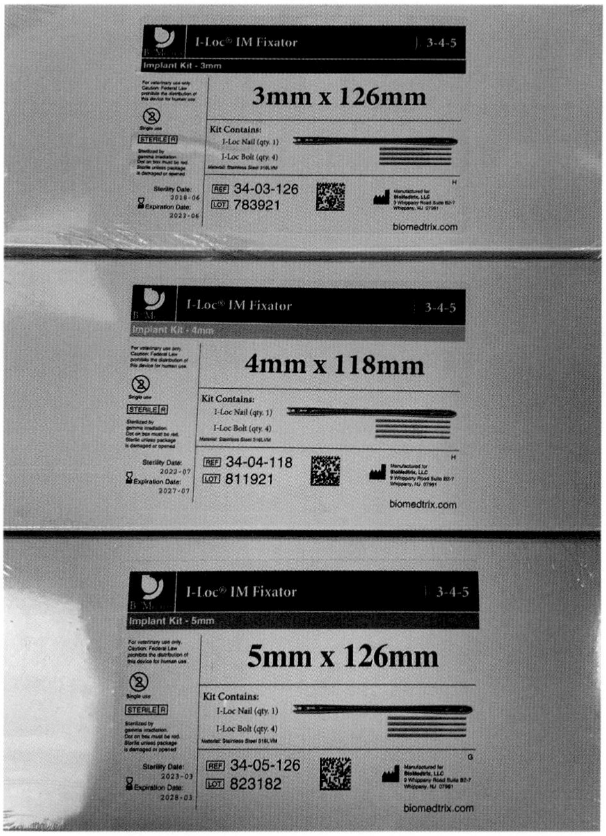

Figure 39.29 BioMedtrix® I-Loc® interlocking nails in 3, 4, and 5 mm widths of various lengths. *Source:* Courtesy of Christine A. Valdez.

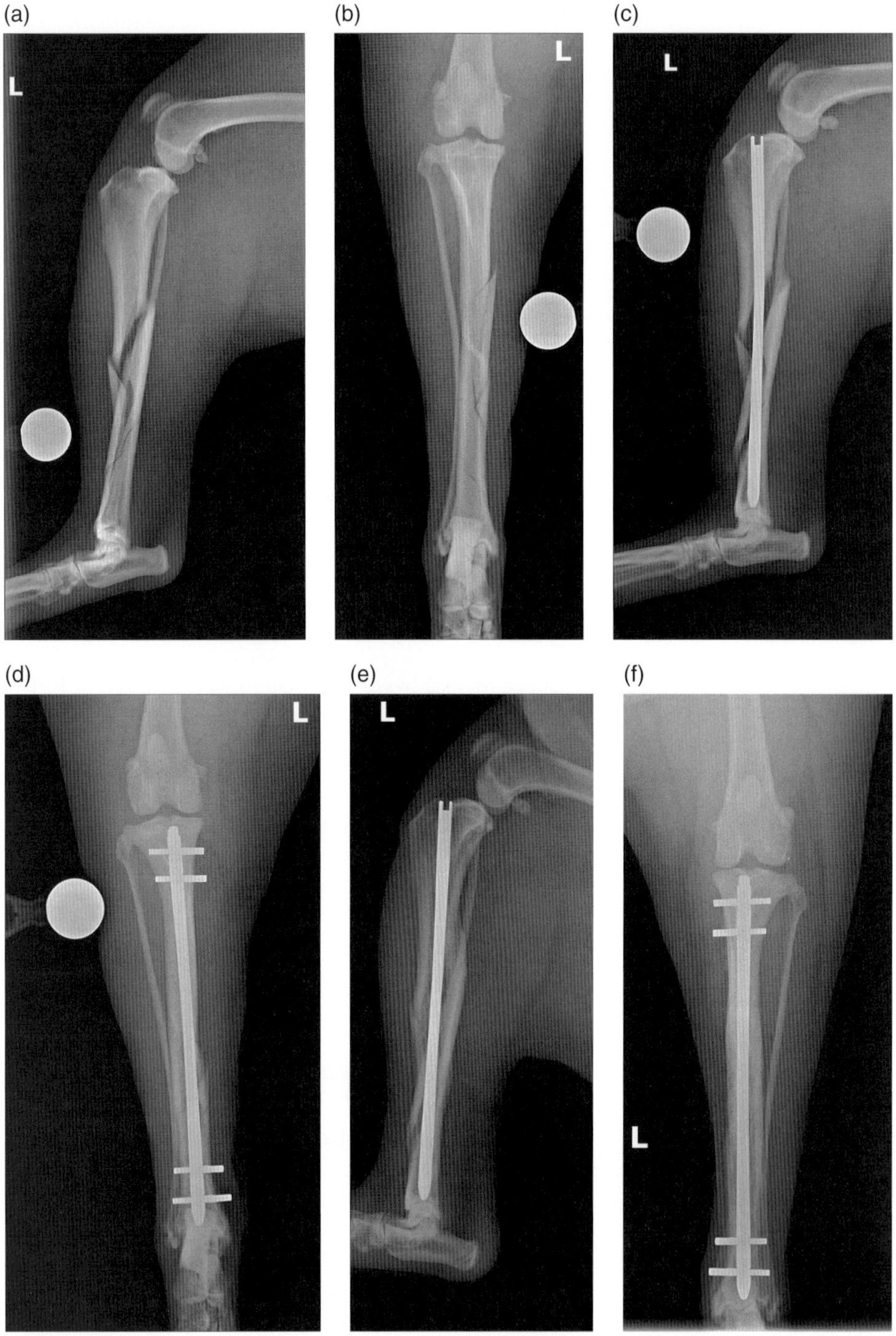

Figure 39.30 (a,b) Pre-operative lateral and craniocaudal radiographs of a canine patient with a left comminuted tibial diaphyseal fracture. (c,d) Immediate postoperative lateral and craniocaudal radiographs of the same patient postplacement of a 172 mm long, 6 mm I-Loc® interlocking nail (Biomedtrix®) with two bolts proximally and distally. (e,f) Six-week postoperative lateral and craniocaudal radiographs of the same patient showing a marked progression in healing callus. *Source:* Courtesy of Dr. Desmond Tan.

and distal fragments and give stability to the construct (Figure 39.30).

ILNs resist all forces placed upon a fracture. The intramedullary nail resists bending and compression, and the fixation bolts provide axial and rotational support. ILNs have some biomechanical advantages over conventional bone plates. As they are placed near the neutral axis of the bone, they tend to be subjected to more compressive forces during ambulation.[24–27] In comparison, bone plates are placed eccentrically from this axis and are subjected to more bending forces.[28,29] The bending forces that plates experience can predispose them to fatigue failure at lower

(a) (b)

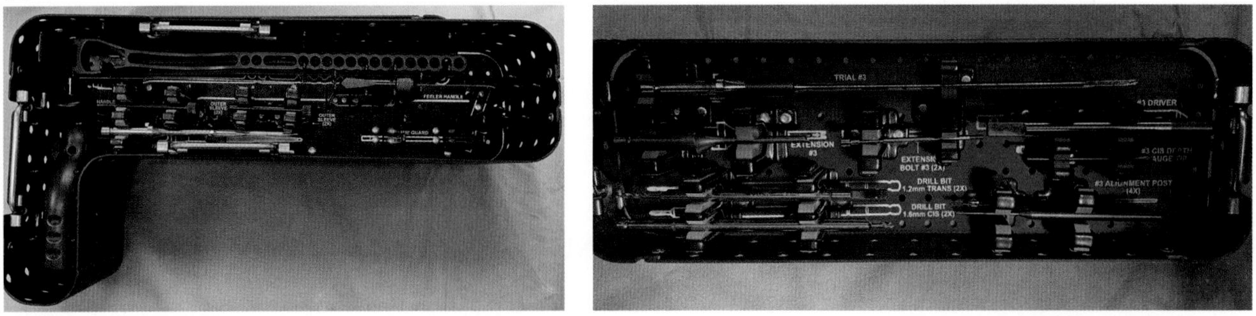

Figure 39.31 Instrument set for a 3 mm I-Loc® system. (a) General I-Loc® instruments. (b) Instruments specific to the 3 mm size I-Loc® system. *Source:* Courtesy of Christine A. Valdez.

loads compared with ILN, especially in fractures with large, comminuted segments.[30,31] In addition, the intramedullary placement of the ILN prevents it from being subjected to screw pull-out, which can be seen in plates, particularly when placed in weak bone. There are multiple ILN systems, which use either screws or bolts to stabilize the fragments. While these implants primarily provide axial and rotational support to the fragment, earlier implant systems using screws would fail secondary to the bending of the screw. Due to their larger core diameter, bolts are more resistant to bending forces compared with screws, and their use is preferred to reduce the risk of implant failure. This chapter will focus primarily on the I-Loc® IM Fixator system (BioMedtrix®) (Figure 39.31). This system uses threaded tapered bolts that screw into threaded cannulations in the nail. As discussed previously with the other implant systems, there are regular continuing education courses that clinicians can pursue for more in-depth knowledge of and training for the system they will be using. These courses are essential for achieving successful clinical results with the ILN.

The ILN is typically used in diaphyseal fractures of the bones listed previously, provided there is enough cortical bone in the proximal and distal fragments to accept two fixation screws or bolts. The screws or bolts should be placed a length of at least 1–2x the bone diameter away from the fracture site to prevent the development of fissures.[32,33] The clinician should pay particular attention to the presence of any fissures on the pre-operative radiographs, which may preclude ILN placement. The proper use and application of ILN involves selecting a nail of appropriate size and length, drilling a hole in the bone to allow the nail to be passed into the medullary canal, and locking the nail in place with screws or locking bolts. The ILN can be placed either in an open approach or in a minimally invasive manner with the use of fluoroscopy. The use of fluoroscopy and minimally invasive placement of the ILN does not disturb the fracture site and leads to improved fracture site biology, promoting early healing for these patients.

Implant Selection

Based on calibrated pre-operative radiographs, the width of the medullary canal at its narrowest point (i.e., the isthmus) is measured. This is easiest to perform on the contralateral (noninjured) limb. The width of the nail chosen should be the largest nail without exceeding 70–90% of the isthmus, which reduces the risk of iatrogenic fracture during insertion.[24,25] To limit stress-shielding with the I-Loc (BioMedtrix), a limit of 75% of the isthmus is suggested.[34] Typically, nails 3–4 mm in diameter are appropriate for use in cats and small dogs (5–15 kg), the 6 mm nail is appropriate for mid-sized dogs (15–30 kg), the 7 mm nail is usually appropriate for large dogs (up to 40 kg), and 8–10 mm nails are usually used for giant breed dogs (>40 kg).[9] The length of the nail should span most of the length of the bone. Similar to the selection of the width of the nail, this is most easily measured from radiographs of the nonfractured contralateral limb.

Application

The ILN is applied in a normograde manner to allow the use of an aiming guide for placement. The first step in application is gaining entry to the medullary canal of the fractured bone. This is typically performed using a Steinman pin. Following this, the medullary cavity is prepared to allow the ILN to pass within it. The cavity must be prepared to the appropriate width and length for the selected nail, and this is typically performed with a series of dedicated awls.

The ILN to be inserted is attached to an extension piece, which is then attached to a handle. The handle is used to insert the ILN. Once the ILN is inserted, an aiming jig is attached to the handle to align the drilling of the locking bolts with the holes of the ILN (Figure 39.32). It is of great importance at this point in the fixation to accurately assess the alignment of the joints proximal and distal to the fracture fragment. While anatomic reconstruction of the

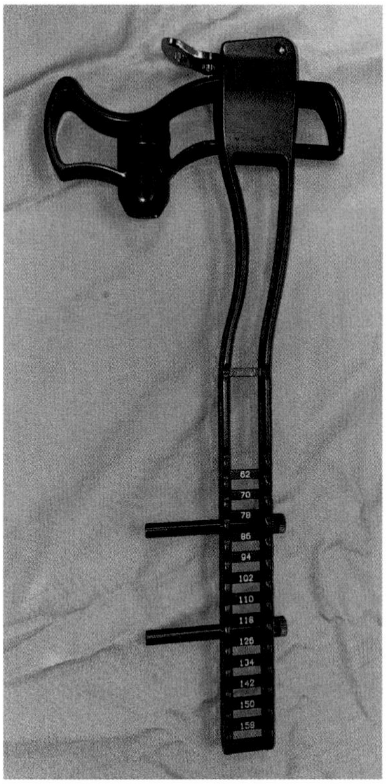

Figure 39.32 The handle (horizontal piece) is connected to an aiming jig (vertical piece). The aiming jig has measurements on it, which correspond to the locations of the ILN holes for different ILN lengths. In the clinical case, the interlocking nail would be attached to the handle on the left-hand side of the image via an extension piece. *Source:* Courtesy of Christine A. Valdez.

fracture fragments is not necessary for this technique to be successful, it is of vital importance that the joints are accurately aligned, or an angular limb deformity will result. For each locking bolt, there will be two drill bits to be used to place it. There will be a drill bit for the cis-cortex (i.e., near) and a separate drill bit for the trans-cortex (i.e., far). Once the cis-cortex has been drilled, a feeler handle is used to palpate within the medullary canal for the threads of the ILN within. This helps the clinician to confirm that the drilling has accurately targeted the hole of the ILN within. Careful drilling and assessment of these holes are very important to ensure that the bolt is passing through the ILN hole.

Prior to drilling, it is important to tighten the connections between the aiming jig and the nail to ensure they are not loose, as this can potentially lead to missing the ILN hole during drilling. Using a sharp drill bit can also be helpful to maintain the trajectory of the aiming jig. Following this, the trans-cortex is drilled, and the hole is filled with an alignment post. The remainder of the holes are drilled in the same manner. Once the holes have been drilled, one alignment post is removed at a time, and a specialized depth gauge is used, which gives a reading for both the cis- and trans-cortical lengths for the bolt. A bolt is then cut to length on both the cis- and trans-ends and applied to the ILN. The remainder of the bolts are placed sequentially, usually proximally to distally. Finally, the handle and extension piece are removed from the ILN.

External Skeletal Fixation (ESF)

ESFs are external devices that are attached to the bone through percutaneously placed implants to stabilize fractures, to temporarily immobilize a joint, or to correct bone deformities. ESF consists of fixation pins or wires (Figure 39.33), connecting clamps (Figure 39.34), and connecting bars (Figure 39.35). ESFs are commonly used in open fractures, fractures with soft tissue damage, or in comminuted fractures. ESF has some unique advantages compared with conventional plating. They can be applied in a closed, or open but do not touch manner, making them helpful for biological osteosynthesis.[35–37] By avoiding an approach to the fracture site or performing minimal disruptions of the fracture site at the time of surgery, the local soft tissues and vasculature can be preserved. In addition, the implants make minimal contact with the periosteum, further limiting damage to the vascular supply of the fracture. The implants aim to align the joint surfaces and adequately stabilize the fracture fragments to enable secondary bone healing to occur. This may speed up overall

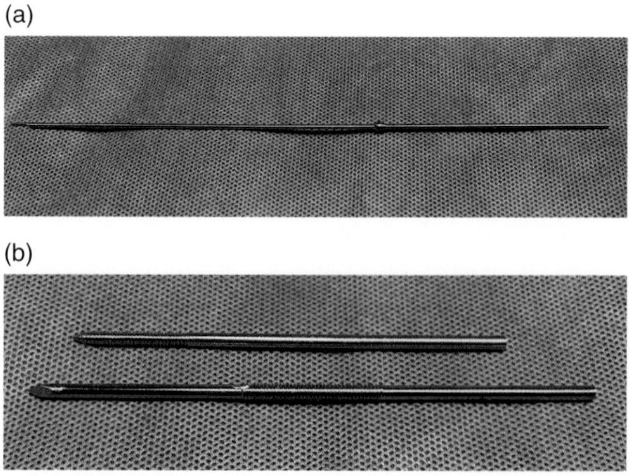

Figure 39.33 Fixation pins and wire. (a) 1.6 mm Stopper Fixation Wire (IMEX®). This wire features a special cutting point that increases accuracy in placement. The bead on the wire contacts the bone surface when placed to prevent migration of the bone along a smooth wire. (b) Top: 2.5 mm Duraface Fixation Half-Pin, NP (No-point) (IMEX®); bottom: 2.5 mm Centerface Fixation Full-Pin (IMEX®). Both implants are fixation pins. The threaded sections are placed within the bone, then the smooth sections are secured with a connecting clamp. *Source:* © Rebecca Webb.

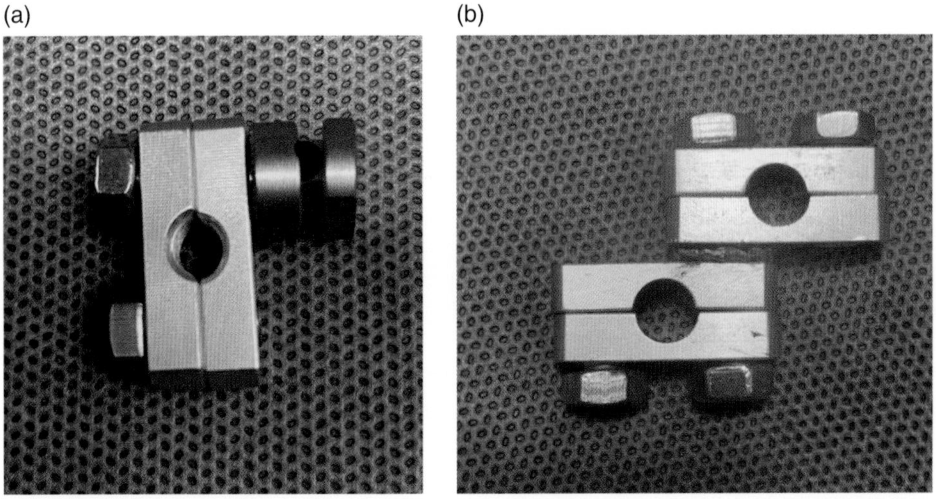

Figure 39.34 (a) Small SK® ESF Clamp, Single (IMEX®). The pin-gripping bolt is visualized on the right. Through this, the fixation pin is secured. Centrally, the open hole is designed to fit the connecting bar. The bolts on the left side of the image are used to secure and tighten the gripping bolt (top) and the connecting bar (bottom). (b) Small SK® ESF Double Clamp (IMEX®), the double clamp is required for attaching two connecting bars to each other (one through each of the central holes). *Source:* © Rebecca Webb.

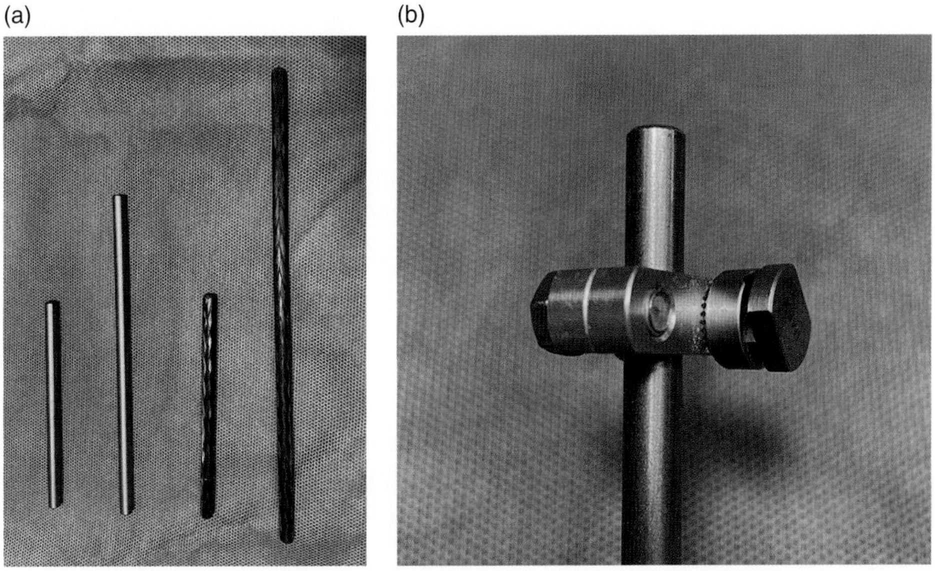

Figure 39.35 (a) Connecting bars come in a range of different lengths and are made in different materials. All connecting bars in the image are 6.3 mm in diameter and are designed for the Small SK® ESF system (IMEX®). The two connecting bars on the left are made of titanium and the two on the right are carbon fiber rods. Each are shown in 100 and 150 mm lengths. (b) A 6.3 mm diameter titanium connecting bar with a Small SK® ESF Single Clamp attached (IMEX®). The gripping bolt, which holds the fixation pin, is visualized on the right of the image. *Source:* © Rebecca Webb.

healing compared with more invasive internal fixation methods.[35,37,38]

The external position of the implants makes them very useful for stabilizing open fractures associated with large wounds or contamination of the fracture site. In these cases, access to the wounds and contaminated regions is maintained, so the wounds can be adequately treated while the fracture heals. In addition, for cases with heavy contamination, the use of an external frame, which is eventually removed, is helpful when compared with internal implants. With internal implants, there is a potential for biofilm formation in infected regions, often necessitating future surgical implant removal. However, with the ESF, implants are typically removed easily under sedation when healing is appropriate. Another advantage of ESF is that the rigidity of the ESF system can also be altered (typically decreased throughout the healing process). As a fracture callus forms and starts providing some stability to the fracture site, the initial level of rigidity is no longer necessary. Individual components can then be gradually removed, in a process called dynamization, to approximate the physiologic needs of the fracture site more closely.[39–41]

There are several disadvantages to the ESF systems that should also be noted. First, closed application, although it is beneficial to preserve the biological environment of the fracture, is best performed with intra-operative imaging, which is not always widely available. Alternatively, the clinician can use pre-operative calibrated radiographs to measure and help approximate implant placement locations, use a limited open approach, or can use a sterile hypodermic needle to help delineate the bone edges in each region. Second, given that the fixation pins and wire are placed percutaneously, they can act as a tract for ascending bacterial contamination. Pin tract infections occur with some frequency and can lead to early pin loosening. Appropriate postoperative pin tract care is important to minimize this complication. They are also not ideal for every bone, such as the femur, which would involve pins traversing a large mass of muscle to reach the affected bone.

When compared with conventional plates, the connecting bars of an ESF are eccentric to the central axis of the bone. This places them at a mechanical disadvantage when compared with bone plates, which can lead to pin loosening over time. If this pin loosening occurs before the fracture is healed, the construct will become weaker and may not be able to adequately stabilize the fracture for healing. Due to this, ESF systems are not designed for long-term use or for use when delayed healing is anticipated. Lastly, the postoperative care is more intensive on the owner, patient, and veterinary staff for ESF. Regular bandage changes are required in the postoperative period to prevent pin tract infections, which may not be tolerated by some patients or clients. There is also a risk of the external frame injuring the patient or client at home.

It is important to recognize the advantages and disadvantages of ESF when choosing a surgical stabilization method. There are several types of fixators available, including linear, circular, hybrid, and acrylic systems. For each of the systems, there are a range of brands. The proper use and application of ESF involve selecting pins or wires of appropriate size and strength for the patient, drilling holes in the bone to allow the pins or wires to pass through, and securing the pins or wires to the frame or external bar with proper tension. ESF can be used alone or in combination with other implants (such as intramedullary pins).

Linear External Skeletal Fixation

Components

- **Pins** – Pins used in combination with an external fixator are referred to as fixation pins. Smooth pins were used in early ESF but had a high rate of pin loosening compared with threaded pins, so their use is uncommon now. The threaded pins are classified into positive profile and negative profile pins. Positive profile pins have a solid shaft throughout the pin and threads are rolled onto the pin, leading to a larger diameter in the threaded portion. Negative profile pins have threads cut into the solid shaft to create the threaded portion, so they have a smaller core diameter in the threaded location. The transition zone in the negative profile pins is important to its overall strength. In the early models, the transition zone from threaded to nonthreaded portions of the pin was abrupt, which was found to make this region prone to failure.[42] Due to this, a tapered transition between the threaded and nonthreaded portions was developed (Duraface pins by IMEX®) (Figure 39.33b). The tapered transition avoided the stress-riser effect of the previous abrupt transition and overall enlarged the core diameter of the pin, increasing its strength. The use of these pins in particularly complex fractures, in fractures with short segments, and in ESF with long working lengths (e.g., femur fractures) may be helpful, as they have been shown to be stiffer and stronger than the corresponding sized positive profile pin.[43]
  Pins can be classified as either half- or full-pins. Half-pins penetrate the soft tissues on only one side, leaving one end exposed for incorporation into the ESF frame. In comparison, full-pins penetrate the soft tissue on both sides of the limb and have pin ends exposed on both sides, which can be incorporated into the ESF frame. Anatomically safe corridors for pin placement have been described and should be referenced when placing fixation pins.[44,45] Pins should be placed as centrally within the bone as possible to maximize stability and pull-out resistance. The half-pins should be placed so that the threads engage both cortices and the tip of the pin is protruding slightly into the soft tissue. If the pin is placed too far into the soft tissue, then the clinician should note that retracting the pin will degrade the quality of the engagement of the pin with the bone. Therefore, clinicians should pay close attention to appropriate initial placement.
- **Clamps** – ESF clamps are used to attach the fixation pins to the connecting bar. The clamps come in different sizes and are specific to the connecting bar width to be used with them. Depending on the size of the clamp, it will accept a particular size range of fixation pins. Clamps are available as single clamps, which attach a fixation pin to a connecting bar, and double clamps, which can attach one connecting bar to a second connecting bar (Figure 39.34). Other linkage devices are available, such as bolts or acrylic, and the reader is directed to other texts for information about these supplies.

- **Connecting bars** – Connecting bars come in a range of sizes and materials, such as titanium, stainless steel, carbon fiber, aluminum, and acrylic. The sizes of the connecting bars vary for different-sized clamps, so the size of the connecting bar chosen will dictate the clamp size to be used. Connecting bars come in a range of lengths so that an appropriate length can be chosen for the patient. The thicker the connecting bar, the stiffer the frame will be. However, the weight of the connecting bar can then become a limiting factor for small patients. Due to this, titanium, carbon fiber, aluminum, and acrylic bars were developed to be of a lighter weight than the original stainless steel connecting bars.

Classification

Classification of ESF frames can be helpful to document the surgical procedure performed, as well as to help predict the mechanical performance of the frame. The classification scheme initially classifies based on whether a construct is unilateral (has a connecting bar on one side only) or bilateral (connecting bars on both sides) (Figure 39.36). It then considers whether the frame is uniplanar (pins placed in a single plane) (Figure 39.37) or biplanar (pins placed in more than one distinctly different plane). This results in four different classification types, which are ranked in order of weakest to strongest (Figure 39.38). As the complexity of the frame increases, so does the stiffness and strength of the construct.[46,47] However, the added strength should be balanced with the increase in biological compromise by the added pins. The anatomical safe corridors that were mentioned previously are very important when planning a construct. It is also important to note that there are very few locations where there are safe corridors on both sides of the limb, therefore, any full-pin will invade into at least one unsafe corridor. For this reason, traditional type II frames (which use only full pins) are rarely used. Over time, ESF systems have been refined and the pins, clamps, and connecting bars improved, so that type Ia or type Ib frames now provide sufficient stability for bone healing. Due to this, the need for full pins and more complex frames is reduced.[48]

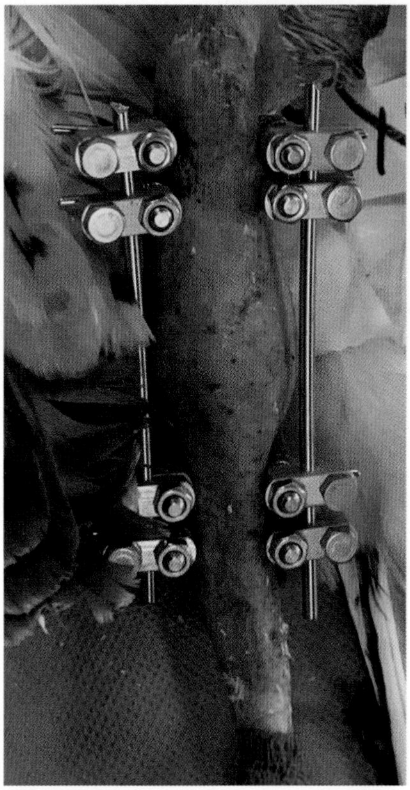

Figure 39.36 An avian patient postoperative for a short oblique tibiotarsus fracture. The fracture has been stabilized with a type II ESF. Proximal is to the top of the image, distal is to the bottom of the image. *Source:* © Rebecca Webb.

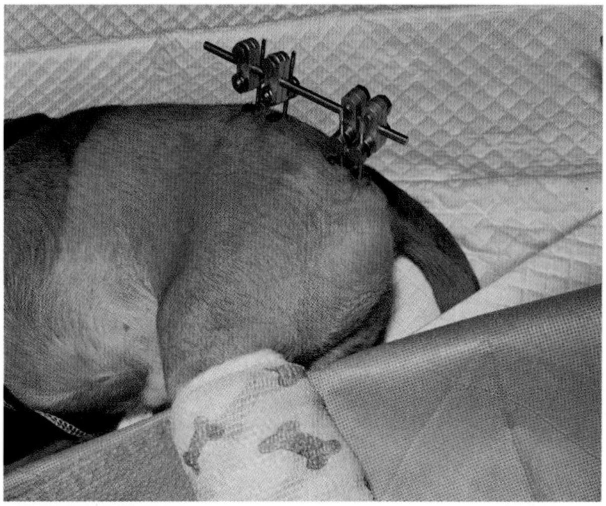

Figure 39.37 A juvenile canine patient with a type I ESF placed on the lateral aspect of the left ilium for a caudal ilial fracture. This is an uncommon use for the ESF system, which was chosen in this patient due to the young age of the patient and chronicity of the fracture. The head is to the left of the image. *Source:* © Rebecca Webb.

Pin-Bone Interface

The pin-bone interface is the most common location of failure of an ESF. Failure at this location leads to pin loosening, which may prevent healing or may require removal of the frame prior to bone healing. This could result in additional surgery to stabilize the limb. Due to this, several techniques have been devised to help maintain this interface, and therefore, extend the longevity of the ESF frame.

Type	Pins (Full versus half)	Connecting bar number	Pin geometry
I-A	Half	1	Unilateral, uniplanar
I-B	Half	2	Unilateral, biplanar
II, Modified	Half with 2 full	2	Bilateral, uniplanar
II	Full	2	Bilateral, uniplanar
III	Half and full	3	Bilateral, biplanar

Figure 39.38 Four different classification types listed in order of weakest to strongest.

Tips and techniques used to preserve the pin-bone interface include:

- Use appropriately sized pins: the threaded portion of the pin should be approximately 20–30% of the bone diameter.
- Adhere to appropriate pin placement: central placement of the pin within the bone.
- Predrilling: predrilling with a drill bit 0.1 mm smaller than the pin shaft prior to pin placement is recommended to decrease thermal necrosis.
- Slow insertion speed: use <300 rpm when inserting the ESF pins.
- Threaded pins should be used over smooth pins.[49,50]

ESF Placement

Generally, three to four pins are placed per bone segment on either side of the fracture. The stiffness of the fixation can be increased by increasing the number of pins placed; however, the additional stiffness achieved in placing more than four pins per fragment does not offset the increase in morbidity of placing more pins. The first pins placed are the two that are farthest from the fracture site. Once these are placed, a connecting bar is added, and the alignment and reduction are altered as needed. Once the alignment and reduction are adequate, the pins closest to the fracture site are placed to maintain the alignment. Following this, additional pins are placed between the two pins on either side of the fracture to increase the stiffness of the construct. Generally, pins are placed half a bone diameter from the fracture site and ¾ of a bone diameter from the adjacent joints to obtain maximal bone purchase and avoid joint penetration.

Acrylic External Skeletal Fixation

Acrylic ESF is ESF where the clamps and connecting bars have been replaced by an acrylic (typically methyl methacrylate or epoxy resin) column (Figure 39.39). These are also called free-form skeletal fixators, as the construct is custom-molded for the patient. Different-sized pins can be

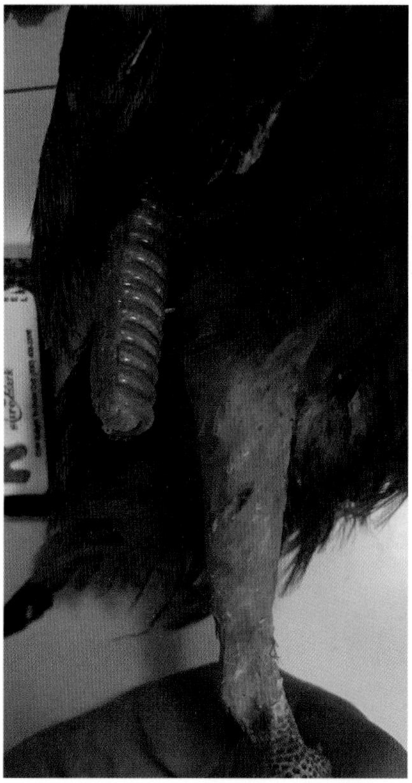

Figure 39.39 A type I acrylic frame on an avian femoral fracture. Not visualized is an intramedullary pin, which has been incorporated into the acrylic frame to increase construct strength for this patient. Proximal is to the top of the image, distal is to the bottom of the image. *Source:* © Rebecca Webb.

used in the fixator, and the shape of the connecting bar does not have to be linear. The acrylic columns have the benefits of being strong, lightweight, and economical. Due to their lightweight nature, their use is common in small breeds and exotics. The significant drawback of the acrylic fixator is the inability to alter the fixation postcuring of the acrylic. This also limits the staged disassembly of the construct as previously described. In acrylic fixators, disassembly can be achieved by cutting a pin or cutting the connecting bar between pins of a fracture segment to decrease stability.[51] The strength of the acrylic construct can be increased by increasing the size of the acrylic column.[52] The effect that bending the fixation pins and incorporating them within the acrylic (like rebar) has on the strength of the construct has not been studied; however, it is thought to help increase pin purchase within the acrylic and may help to prevent pin pull-out.

Circular External Skeletal Fixation

A circular external skeletal fixation (CESF) frame uses rings and tensioned wires instead of larger bone pins to secure the bone fragments. The wires pass through the bone and then are secured to a ring on either side with bolts instead of clamps (Figure 39.40). Rings are placed around the proximal and distal fragments and are then connected with connecting rods to create the final construct. Circular components are particularly useful with small juxta-articular fragments due to their ability to use wires instead of pins for fixation. Wires allow axial micromotion to occur during the loading of a fracture. This micromotion is limited and has been shown to stimulate osteoblasts and bone healing.[53] The appropriate amount of wire tension is crucial for this effect to occur, and a tensioning device is recommended to achieve it.

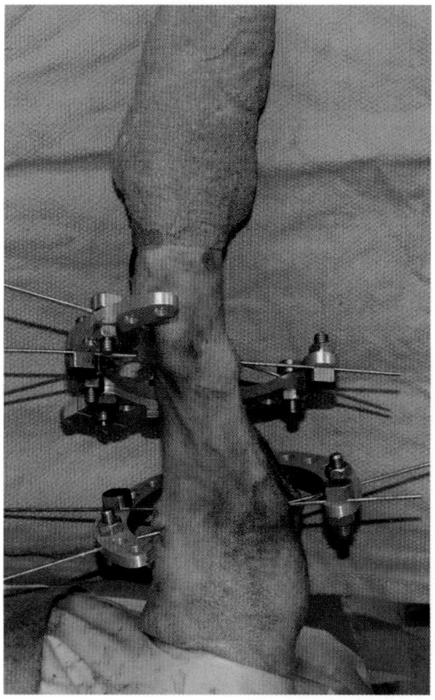

Figure 39.40 Intra-operative photograph of a patient with an antebrachial angular limb deformity. A Stretch Ring has been placed in line with the joints proximally and distally and secured with two Stopper fixation wires (IMEX®) in each section. Once a closing wedge resection is performed to correct the deformity of the radius, connecting bars will be attached to the rings, the limb straightened, and the circular ESF will be used as a form of temporary stabilization prior to plate placement. Distal is to the top of the image, proximal is to the bottom of the image. *Source:* © Rebecca Webb.

Components

- **Rings** – Rings are made of aluminum, stainless steel, or carbon fiber and have multiple holes around the circumference for placement of additional components. They are named for their internal diameter and come in a range of sizes. There are several types, including full rings, arches, and stretch rings (Figure 39.41). Stretch rings look like a horseshoe and are partial rings with straight segments on either side. These rings accommodate challenging locations, such as near joints. In frames that are stabilized only with fixation wires, the ring size is the primary determinant of stiffness.[54,55]
- **Fixation elements** – Most commonly, wires are used to affix the bone to the rings. The fixation wires come in both a smooth wire and a stopper wire (Figure 39.33a). The wires have a cutting point on their tip to help with accurate placement. Typically, two wires can be attached to a ring, one above the ring and one below. If the wires are placed at a 90° angle from each other, both wires will resist translation of the bone fragment along the other wire. Realistically, placing wires at 90° angles from each other is rarely possible, but the clinician should aim for as close to this as possible. The stopper wires have a small bead of metal, which also resists the translation of the bone fragment. These wires are driven so that the stopper is pressed against the cortex. The use of two stopper wires, with a stopper on either opposing cortex, will resist translation further. Wires

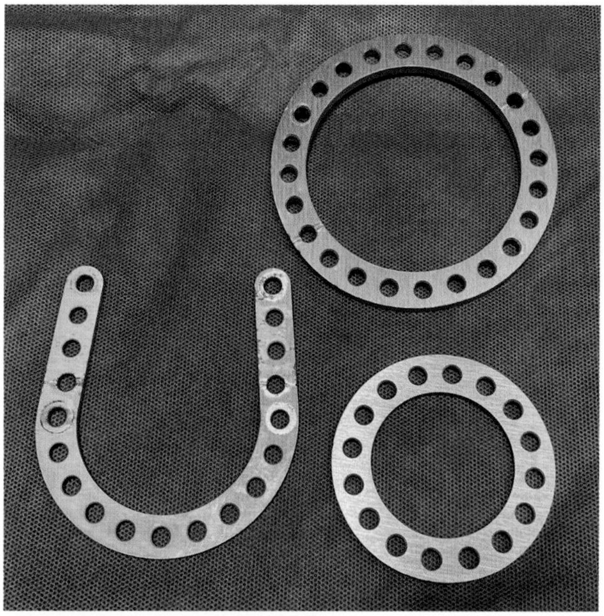

Figure 39.41 A range of circular ESF components. The ring on the left is a Stretch Ring. The two rings on the right are two different sizes of Full Rings (50 and 84 mm) (IMEX®). *Source:* © Rebecca Webb.

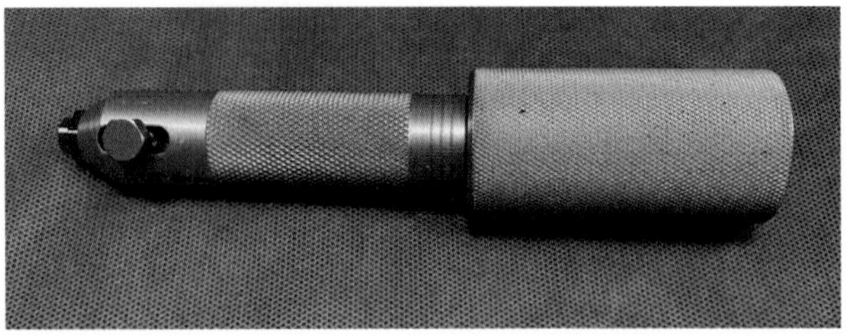

Figure 39.42 A wire tensioner is used to appropriately tension wires in the circular section of the ESF (IMEX®). *Source:* © Rebecca Webb.

are tensioned against the ring to increase their strength with a wire tensioner (Figure 39.42). The amount of tension applied to the wire is a function of the size of the ring it is being tensioned against, so it is important to use a wire tensioner to achieve the appropriate tension level. By tensioning a 1.6 mm wire using the tensioning device, it becomes as strong as a 4 mm pin.[53,56,57] Additional wires can be added to the ring called "drop wires" by using a post to raise or lower the attachment point of the fixation wire. Fixation pins can also be used and attached to the ring; however, mixing fixation wires and pins is controversial. Wire fixation creates an environment of axial micromotion, which can be helpful for callus formation. However, stability is required to maintain the pin-bone interface of the fixation pin, and pins will loosen prematurely if used in addition to wires on the same bone fragment.[58]

- **Clamps** – A range of clamps are used to attach the fixation elements to the ring. A wire fixation bolt (Figure 39.43) can be used to fix wires either above or below the ring. The wires can either be passed through the central cannula of the bolt or can be attached using the slot on one side of the fixation bolt. Half-pin fixation bolts (Figure 39.44) can be used if fixation pins are being used instead of wires for the fixation element. The pin is passed through the central cannula in the bolt, and the bolt is affixed to the ring with a hex nut.
- **Connecting bars** – Rings are typically fixed to each other using connecting bars. The connecting bars can be fixed at a 90° angle from the rings or can be angled either by using spherical nuts and washers (to allow up to 7.5° of angulation), the IMEX® Universal SK® Hybrid adaptor (up to 30° of angulation), or the IMEX® VariBall locking hybrid rod (up to 100° of angulation) (Figure 39.45).

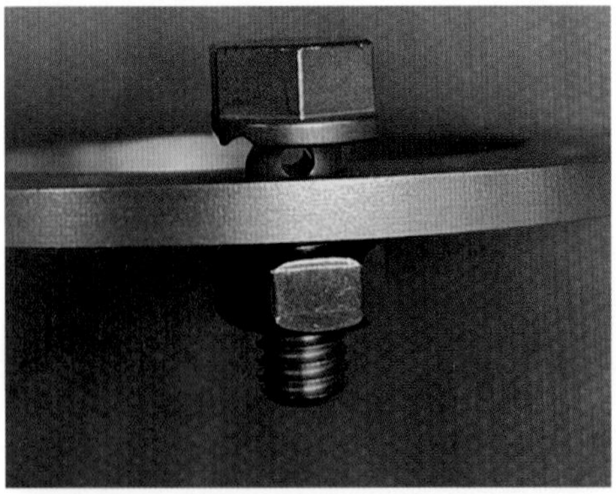

Figure 39.43 A slotted wire fixation bolt (IMEX®) attached to a circular ring. Wires can be passed through the bolt in two locations, through the central cannula of the bolt or through the slot on the underside of the head of the bolt (visualized on the left side of the bolt in the image). *Source:* © Rebecca Webb.

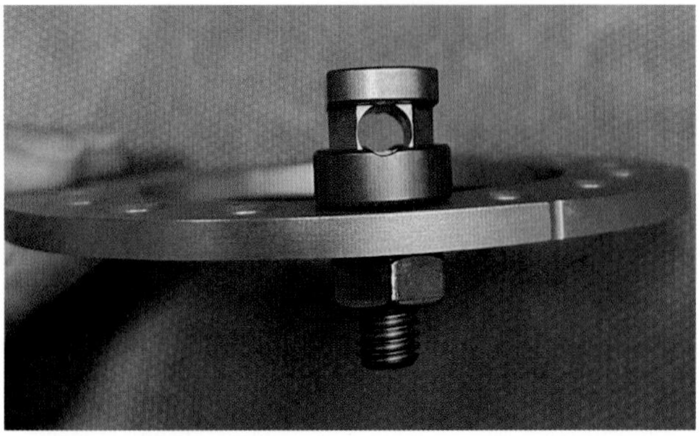

Figure 39.44 A half-pin fixation bolt can also be applied to the ring to allow fixation pins to be secured to the ring instead of a wire. The fixation pin is passed through the central cannula of the bolt (IMEX®). *Source:* © Rebecca Webb.

Hybrid External Skeletal Fixation

Hybrid external fixators are fixators with a circular component on one end of the fracture and a linear component on the other end of the fracture (Figure 39.46). These fixators

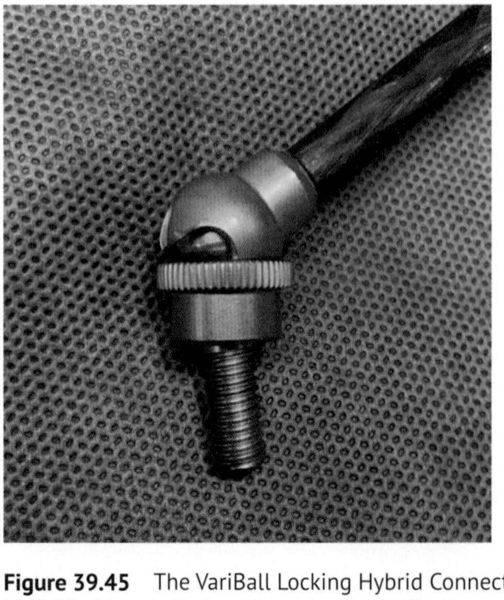

Figure 39.45 The VariBall Locking Hybrid Connecting Rod (IMEX®). The multi-directional locking ball is integrated with a 6.3 mm carbon fiber rod. *Source:* © Rebecca Webb.

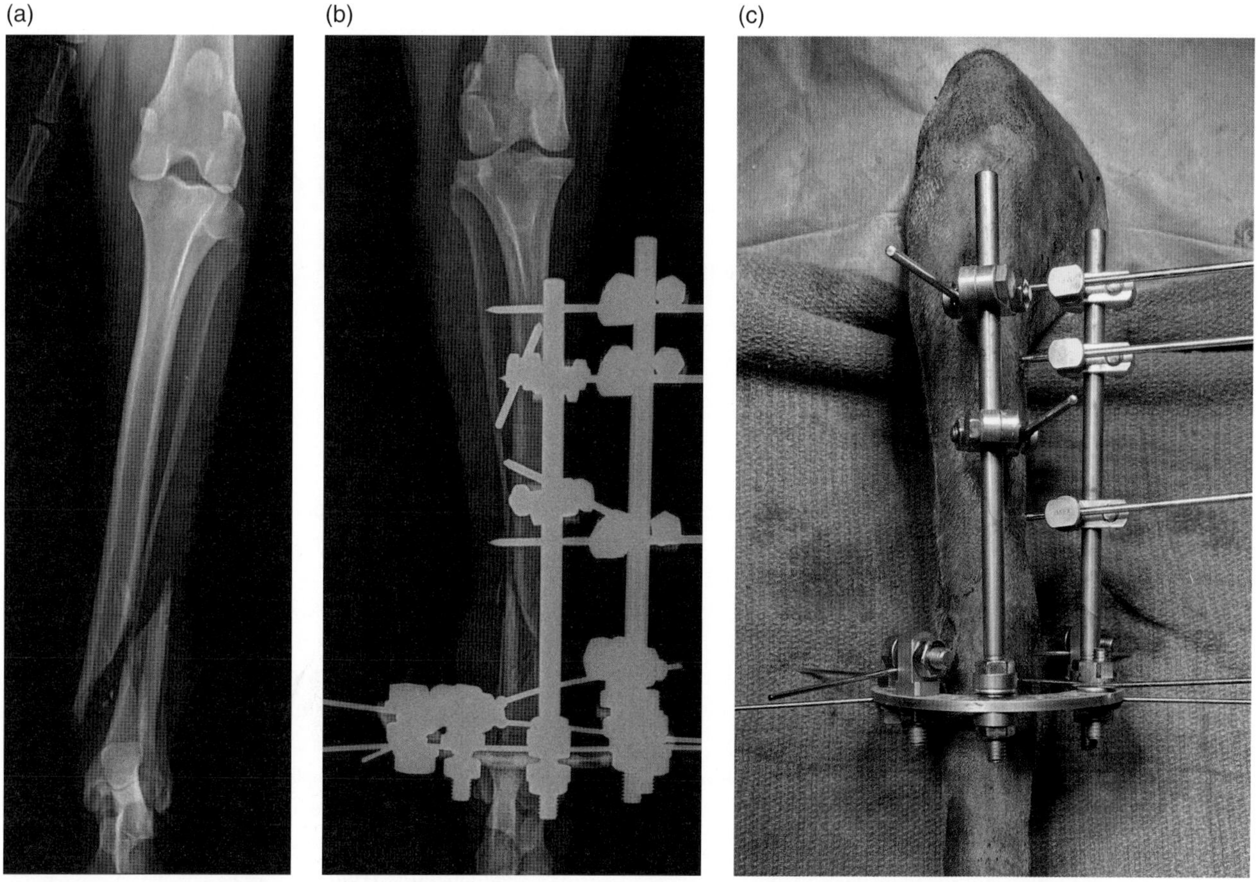

Figure 39.46 (a) Pre-operative craniocaudal radiograph of a canine patient with a distal tibial comminuted open fracture. (b) Postoperative craniocaudal radiograph of the same patient postsurgical repair with a hybrid I-B small SK ESF frame (IMEX®). (c) Postsurgical repair of the right tibial fracture with a hybrid I-B small SK ESF frame (IMEX®) showing the components. Following confirmation of appropriate fixation on postoperative radiographs, the pins were then cut to the level of the clamp, and the wires were bent to prevent injury and cut to the level of the ring. *Source:* © Rebecca Webb.

are most commonly used when there is a small juxta-articular fragment, and the circular component is used to gain adequate fixation of the small fragment. The hybrid ESF then takes advantage of the ease of application and preservation of safe corridors of the linear system for the other, larger bone fragment. Biomechanically, they exhibit characteristics of both the static axial stiffness of the linear ESF and the dynamic micromotion of the circular system.[59] Using a similar classification system as for the linear ESF, the connecting bars can be placed in a type IA (unilateral, uniplanar), a type IB (unilateral, biplanar), or a type II (bilateral, uniplanar) configuration.

Frame Destabilization and Removal

Stabilization of fractures with highly stiff constructs can lead to a delay in bone healing. In some cases, such as very comminuted fractures with minimal load-sharing, a very stiff construct is required in the early stages of fracture healing. However, as a fracture callus forms, the level of stability that the fracture requires is decreased, and continued stabilization with a stiff frame at this point can actually slow bone healing. In these cases, staged, partial disassembly can be performed to destabilize the construct and help improve bone healing. During the healing process, regular radiographs should be taken, which will help guide when destabilization is appropriate. This should be coupled with palpation of the fracture site for stability with the frame slightly loosened. There must be sufficient stability present at the fracture site to tolerate the destabilization, or destabilization could lead to delayed union or implant failure. Generally, the timing for destabilization is 4–6 weeks following placement for young dogs, 6 weeks following placement for adult dogs, and 8–10 weeks following original ESF placement for older dogs and cats.[40] There are multiple options for destabilization, including pin removal (pins that are causing patient morbidity [discharge, infection, or loosening] should be prioritized for this), removal of the "near" pins (those closest to the fracture site), removal of one connecting bar and associated pins (in a type Ib and higher construct), downsizing the clamps, removing augmentations (tie-in IM pins or diagonal connecting bars) and connecting bars, or replacing aluminum or titanium connecting bars with carbon fiber.

To access the videos for this chapter, please go to

www.wiley.com/go/coleman/surgeries

VIDEO 39.1 Video demonstrating the "Z-bend" technique of bending K-wires.

References

1. Hulse, D., Ferry, K., Fawcett, A. et al. (2000). Effect of intramedullary pin size on reducing bone plate strain. *Vet. Comp. Orthop. Traumatol.* 13 (4): 185–190.
2. Vasseur, P.B., Paul, H.A., Crumley, L. et al. (1984). Evaluation of fixation devices for prevention of rotation in transverse fractures of the canine femoral shaft: an in vitro study. *Am. J. Vet. Res.* 45 (8): 1504–1507.
3. Sukhiani, H.R. and Holmberg, D.R. (1997). Ex vivo biomechanical comparison of pin fixation techniques for canine distal femoral physeal fractures. *Vet. Surg.* 26: 398–407.
4. Roe, S.C. (1997). Mechanical characteristics and comparisons of cerclage wires: introduction of the double-wrap and loop/twist tying methods. *Vet. Surg.* 26: 310–316.
5. Wahnert, D., Lenz, M., Schlegel, U. et al. (2011). Cerclage handling for improved fracture treatment. A biomechanical study of the twisting procedure. *Acta Chir. Orthop. Traumatol. Cech.* 78 (3): 208–214.
6. Wilson, J.W. (1991). Vascular supply to normal bone and healing fractures. *Semin. Vet. Med. Surg. Small Anim.* 6 (1): 26–38.
7. Murphy, T.P., Hill, C.M., Kapatkin, A.S. et al. (2001). Pullout properties of 3.5-mm AO/ASIF self-tapping and cortex screws in a uniform synthetic material and in canine bone. *Vet. Surg.* 30 (3): 253–260.
8. Johnson, A.L., Houlton, J.E.F., and Vannini, R. (2005). *AO Principles of Fracture Management in the Dog and Cat.* AO Publishing.
9. Johnston, S.A., von Pfeil, D.J.F., Dejardin, L.M. et al. (2018). Internal fracture fixation. In: *Veterinary Surgery Small Animal*, 2e (ed. S.A. Johnston and K.M. Tobias), 654–690. Missouri, USA: Elsevier.
10. Pearson, T., Glyde, M.R., Day, R.E. et al. (2016). The effect of intramedullary pin size and plate working length on plate strain in locking compression plate-rod constructs under axial load. *Vet. Comp. Orthop. Traumatol.* 29 (6): 451–458.
11. Perren, S.M., Russenberger, M., Steinemann, S. et al. (1969). A dynamic compression plate. *Acta Orthop. Scand. Suppl.* 125: 31–41.
12. Field, J.R., Hearn, T.C., and Caldwell, C.B. (1997). Bone plate fixation: an evaluation of interface contact area and force of the dynamic compression plate (DCP) and the limited contact-dynamic compression plate (LC-DCP) applied to cadaveric bone. *J. Orthop. Trauma* 11 (5): 368–373.
13. Little, F.M., Hill, C.M., Kageyama, T. et al. (2001). Bending properties of stainless-steel dynamic compression plates and limited contact dynamic compression plates. *Vet. Comp. Orthop. Traumatol.* 14 (2): 64–68.
14. Rose, B.W., Pluhar, G.E., Novo, R.E. et al. (2009). Biomechanical analysis of stacked plating techniques to stabilize distal radial fractures in small dogs. *Vet. Surg.* 38 (8): 954–960.
15. Bichot, S., Gibson, T.W.G., Moens, N.M.M. et al. (2011). Effect of the length of the superficial plate on bending stiffness, bending strength and strain distribution in stacked 2.0-2.7 veterinary cuttable plate constructs: an in vitro study. *Vet. Comp. Orthop. Traumatol.* 24 (6): 426–434.
16. Borrelli, J., Prickett, W., Song, E. et al. (2002). Extraosseous blood supply of the tibia and the effects of different plating techniques: a human cadaveric study. *J. Orthop. Trauma* 16 (10): 691–695.
17. Gardner, M.J., Brophy, R.H., Campbell, D. et al. (2005). The mechanical behavior of locking compression plates compared with dynamic compression plates in a cadaver radius model. *J. Orthop. Trauma* 19 (9): 597–603.
18. Strauss, E.J., Schwarzkopf, R., Kummer, F. et al. (2008). The current status of locked plating: the good, the bad, and the ugly. *J. Orthop. Trauma* 22 (7): 479–486.
19. Ahmad, M., Nanda, R., Bajwa, A.S. et al. (2007). Biomechanical testing of the locking compression plate: when does the distance between bone and implant significantly reduce construct stability? *Injury* 38 (3): 358–364.

20 Vaughn, D.P., Syrcle, J.A., Ball, J.E. et al. (2016). Pullout strength of monocortical and bicortical screws in metaphyseal and diaphyseal regions of the canine humerus. *Vet. Comp. Orthop. Traumatol.* 29 (6): 466–474.

21 Delisser, P.J., McCombe, G.P., Trask, R.S. et al. (2013). Ex vivo evaluation of the biomechanical effect of varying monocortical screw numbers on a plate-rod canine femoral gap model. *Vet. Comp. Orthop. Traumatol.* 26 (3): 177–185.

22 Stoffel, K., Dieter, U., Stachowiak, G. et al. (2003). Biomechanical testing of the LCP: how can stability in locked internal fixators be controlled? *Injury* 34: B11–B19.

23 Hol, P.J., Molster, A., and Gjerdet, N.R. (2007). Should the galvanic combination of titanium and stainless steel surgical implants be avoided? *Injury* 39 (2): 161–169.

24 Roush, J.K. and McLaughlin, R.M. (1999). Using interlocking nail fixation to repair fractures in small animals. *Vet. Med.* 94: 46.

25 Dueland, R.T., Berglund, L., Vanderby, R. Jr. et al. (1996). Structural properties of interlocking nails, canine femora, and femur-interlocking nail constructs. *Vet. Surg.* 25 (5): 386–396.

26 Kyle, R.F. (1985). Biomechanics of intramedullary fracture fixation. *Orthopedics* 8 (11): 1356–1359.

27 Wheeler, J.L., Stubbs, W.P., Lewis, D.D. et al. (2004). Intramedullary interlocking nail fixation in dogs and cats: biomechanics and instrumentation. *Compend. Contin. Educ. Pract. Vet.* 26 (7): 519–529.

28 Hulse, D., Ferry, K., Fawcett, A. et al. (2000). Effect of intramedullary pin size on reducing bone plate strain. *Vet. Comp. Orthop. Traumatol.* 13 (4): 185–190.

29 Hulse, D., Hyman, W., Nori, M. et al. (1997). Reduction in plate strain by addition of an intramedullary pin. *Vet. Surg.* 26 (6): 451–459.

30 Bernardé, A., Diop, A., Maurel, N. et al. (2002). An in vitro biomechanical comparison between bone plate and interlocking nail. *Vet. Comp. Orthop. Traumatol.* 15 (2): 57–66.

31 Bernardé, A., Diop, A., Maurel, N. et al. (2001). An in vitro biomechanical study of bone plate and interlocking nail in a canine diaphyseal femoral fracture model. *Vet. Surg.* 30 (5): 397–408.

32 Bucholz, R.W., Ross, S.E., and Lawrence, K.L. (1987). Fatigue fracture of the interlocking nail in the treatment of fractures of the distal part of the femoral shaft. *J. Bone Joint Surg. Am.* 69 (9): 1391–1399.

33 Dueland, R.T., Johnson, K.A., Roe, S.C. et al. (1999). Interlocking nail treatment of diaphyseal long-bone fractures in dogs. *J. Am. Vet. Med. Assoc.* 214 (1): 59–66.

34 Déjardin, L.M. (2015). I-Loc IM fixator. BioMedtrix Workshop. The Ohio State University, Columbus, OH.

35 Palmer, R.H. (2012). External fixators and minimally invasive osteosynthesis in small animal veterinary medicine. *Vet. Clin. North Am. Small Anim. Pract.* 42 (5): 913–934.

36 Palmer, R.H. (1999). Biological osteosynthesis. *Vet. Clin. North Am. Small Anim. Pract.* 29 (5): 1171–1185.

37 Palmer, R.H., Hulse, D.A., Hyman, W.A. et al. (1992). Principles of bone healing and biomechanics of external skeletal fixation. *Vet. Clin. North Am. Small Anim. Pract.* 22 (1): 45–68.

38 Johnson, A.L., Egger, E.L., Eurell, J.A.C. et al. (1998). Biomechanics and biology of fracture healing with external skeletal fixation. *Compend. Contin. Educ. Pract. Vet.* 20 (4): 487–500.

39 Auger, J., Dupuis, J., Boudreault, F. et al. (2002). Comparison of multistage versus one-stage destabilization of type II external fixator used to stabilize an oblique tibial osteotomy in dogs. *Vet. Surg.* 31 (1): 10–22.

40 Egger, E.L., Histand, M.B., Norrdin, R.W. et al. (1993). Canine osteotomy healing when stabilized with decreasingly rigid fixation compared to constantly rigid fixation. *Vet. Comp. Orthop. Traumatol.* 6 (4): 182–187.

41 Larsson, S., Kim, W., Caja, V.L. et al. (2001). Effect of early axial dynamization of tibial bone healing: a study in dogs. *Clin. Orthop. Relat. Res.* 388: 240–251.

42 Palmer, R.H. and Aron, D.N. (1990). Ellis pin complications in seven dogs. *Vet. Surg.* 19 (6): 440–445.

43 Griffin, H., Toombs, J.P., Bronson, D.G. et al. (2011). Mechanical evaluation of a tapered thread-run-out half-pin designed for external skeletal fixation in small animals. *Vet. Comp. Orthop. Traumatol.* 24 (4): 257–261.

44 Marti, J.M. and Miller, A. (1994). Delimitation of safe corridors for the insertion of external fixator pins in the dog 1: hindlimb. *J. Small Anim. Pract.* 35 (2): 16–23.

45 Marti, J.M. and Miller, A. (1994). Delimitation of safe corridors for the insertion of external fixator pins in the dog 2: forelimb. *J. Small Anim. Pract.* 35 (2): 78–85.

46 Brinker, W.O., Verstraete, M.C., and Soutas-Little, R.W. (1985). Stiffness studies on various configurations and types of external fixators. *J. Am. Anim. Hosp. Assoc.* 21: 801–808.

47 Egger, E.L. (1983). Static strength evaluation of six external skeletal fixation configurations. *Vet. Surg.* 12: 130.

48 White, D.T., Bronson, D.G., and Welch, R.D. (2003). A mechanical comparison of veterinary linear external fixation systems. *Vet. Surg.* 32: 507–514.

49 Egger, E.L., Histand, M.B., Blass, C.E. et al. (1986). Effect of fixation pin insertion on the bone-pin interface. *Vet. Surg.* 15 (3): 246–252.

50 Anderson, M.A., Mann, F.A., Kinden, D.A. et al. (1996). Evaluation of cortical bone damage and axial holding power of non-threaded and enhanced threaded pin placed with and without drilling a pilot hole in femurs from canine cadavers. *J. Am. Vet. Med. Assoc.* 208 (6): 883–887.

51 Störk, C.K., Canivet, P., Baikad, A. et al. (2003). Evaluation of nontoxic rigid polymer as a connecting bar in external skeletal fixators. *Vet. Surg.* 32: 262–268.

52 Shahar, R. (2000). Relative stiffness and stress of type I and type II external fixators: acrylic versus stainless-steel connecting bars a theoretical approach. *Vet. Surg.* 29: 59–69.

53 Lewis, D.D., Lanz, O.I., and Welch, R.D. (1998). Biomechanics of circular external skeletal fixation. *Vet. Surg.* 27 (5): 454–464.

54 Bronson, D.G., Samchukov, M.L., Birch, J.G. et al. (1998). Stability of circular external fixation: a multivariable biomechanical analysis. *Clin. Biomech.* 13 (6): 441–448.

55 Lewis, D.D., Bronson, D.G., Cross, A.R. et al. (2001). Axial characteristics of circular external skeletal single ring constructs. *Vet. Surg.* 30 (4): 386–394.

56 Cross, A.R., Lewis, D.D., Murphy, S.T. et al. (2001). Effects of ring diameter and wire tension on the axial biomechanics of four-ring circular external fixator constructs. *Am. J. Vet. Res.* 62 (7): 1025–1030.

57 Lewis, D.D., Radasch, R.M., and Beale, B.S. (1999). Initial clinical experience with the IMEX(TM) circular external skeletal fixation system. Part I. Use in fractures and arthrodeses. *Vet. Comp. Orthop. Traumatol.* 12 (3): 13–22.

58 Lewis, R.A., Lewis, D.D., Anderson, C.L. et al. (2016). Mechanics of supplemental drop wire and half-pin fixation elements in single ring circular external fixation constructs. *Vet. Surg.* 45 (4): 471–479.

59 Hudson, C.C., Lewis, D.D., Cross, A.R. et al. (2012). A biomechanical comparison of three hybrid linear-circular external fixator constructs. *Vet. Surg.* 41 (8): 954–965.

40

Principles of External Coaptation

Seth Bleakley

CARE Surgery Center, Phoenix, AZ, USA

Key Points

- Bandages, splints, casts, and other supportive devices can be used to support fractures, joint injuries, and other musculoskeletal disorders in small animal practice.
- External coaptation can be used in place of surgery or ancillary to surgical treatment.
- An understanding of mechanical principles will not only improve efficacy but will help prevent abrasions, sores, and other morbidity associated with external coaptation.
- Longer casts and splints are mechanically superior, decrease pressure, and lower incidence of bandage sores when compared to short casts and splints.
- Elastic bandage materials create high tension and risk of ischemic injury and should never be used as a contact layer or applied before padding.
- Lateral and medial splint placement allows for a more rigid construct than cranial and caudal splint placement.
- Constructs can be custom-made using commercially available materials or purchased pre-fabricated with a variety of adaptive devices now available.

Introduction

External coaptation is defined as the use of bandages, splints, casts, or other materials to provide support, compression, and sometimes analgesia. Indications for use include fractures and wounds. In fractures, the goal of external coaptation may be

1) Primary fixation
2) Ancillary support of a surgical repair
3) Temporary support pending definitive treatment

In cases of primary fixation, the goal of external coaptation is to prevent displacement of fractured bone so as to increase chances of secondary bone healing with close to anatomical alignment as well as to reduce discomfort from swelling and moving fracture fragments. In cases of ancillary support of a surgical repair, the goal of external coaptation is to reduce forces on the repair that could be detrimental to construct stability and implant integrity, as well as manage swelling and pain. In cases of temporary fixation, the goal is to improve alignment and reduce pain from moving fracture fragments and swelling until definitive treatment can be pursued. With regard to wound management, external coaptation is used to prevent contamination, aid hemostasis, reduce desiccation of tissues, absorb exudate, reduce swelling, aid thermoregulation, maintain wound contact layers, and promote moist wound healing. Wound management is discussed briefly in Chapter 18 and is described in detail in separate texts, the most recent one being: *Textbook of Wound Management* (edited by Dr. Nicole Buote). The purpose of this chapter is to describe mechanical principles of external coaptation for orthopedic indications.

The Hippocratic phrase “first, do no harm” applies to decision-making with external coaptation. One of the

Techniques in Small Animal Soft Tissue, Orthopedic, and Ophthalmic Surgery, First Edition. Edited by Kristin A. Coleman.

Companion website: www.wiley.com/go/coleman/surgeries

major disadvantages of external coaptation in small animal practice is morbidity, which can take the form of sores, ischemic injury,[1] muscle atrophy, flexor tendon laxity/weakness,[2] joint stiffness, decreased ligament strength,[2] cartilage loss,[3] and gait miseducation. Figure 40.1 shows examples of abrasions and ischemic injuries associated with external coaptation in dogs. In a study of nine dogs and two cats that suffered from ischemic injury secondary to bandaging, five animals required skin grafts, three required digit amputations, and two required limb amputations.[1] Avoiding such morbidity with external coaptation requires appropriate case selection, padding, tension, protection from the elements, and patient and owner compliance. A secondary goal of this chapter is to help the veterinary practitioner avoid bandage morbidity through an understanding of the mechanical principles of external coaptation.

Mechanical Principles

Three-Point Corrective System

When a transverse force is applied to a fixed longitudinal structure, the resultant reaction is known as bending moment and is directly proportional to the product of the force and the distance from the pivot. An unconstrained longitudinal structure, such as a limb, will require application of at least three forces, one opposing the other two, to create bending moment. A simplistic example of this is bending or breaking a pencil (Figure 40.2). Three forces are required, two in opposition to a central force. Less force is required if the distance between them is increased. It is challenging to bend and break a pencil if it is held with fingers close together, or in other words, more force is required as distance decreases.

In the context of external coaptation, forces are applied by the immobilized limb against the soft or rigid materials applied to constrain the joint from flexion. Forces involved are a factor of the patient's weight, the ground reactive force, and the position of the applied materials. Figure 40.3 demonstrates this in the canine hindlimb. Without muscle resistance, weight bearing will lead to extension of the paw, flexion of the tarsus, flexion of the stifle, and flexion of the hip (Figure 40.3a). Subsequently, the paw will displace cranially, the tarsus caudally, the stifle cranially, and the hip caudally. In the context of external coaptation, immobilization of a limb will involve application of corrective forces (CFs) in three locations. In the hindlimb, this would involve caudal forces on the paw and the tibia, and a cranial force on the tarsus (Figure 40.3b). Clinical relevance of this principle is clear when examining bandage sores (Figure 40.1), which, in the hindlimb, are typically associated with the digits, the caudal tarsus, and the cranial tibia. Careful padding of these locations is essential to prevent morbidity, but the length of the construct also becomes relevant due to the aforementioned formula for bending moment. A shorter bandage will decrease the distance between the CFs, and as ground reaction force is constant, the force to resist bending moment will be subsequently greater (Figure 40.3c). This, coupled with decreased surface area (which is inversely proportional to pressure), will lead to a higher incidence of sores and ischemic injury. This has been demonstrated experimentally. In a prospective study of 13 dogs, Iodence et al. demonstrated through pressure mapping with sensors underneath casts applied to the pelvic limbs that a short cast significantly increased pressure on the calcaneus and proximal tibia (Figures 40.4, 40.5, 40.6, 40.7, and 40.8).

The principle of the three-point corrective system will guide clinical application of external coaptation by creating awareness of the effect of construct length and location. Generally speaking, the longer the bandage, splint, or cast, the more effectively it will resist limb movement and lower the chance of bandage sores and ischemic injury. In practicality, external coaptation should **include the paw** and extend **as proximally as possible** – to the level of the stifle in the hindlimb and to the level of the elbow or above in the forelimb. Attention should be paid to the location of subsequent CFs. For example, padding should be adequate around the paw, caudal calcaneus, and proximal tibia in the hindlimb and around the paw, carpus, and proximal antebrachium/elbow in the forelimb, to correspond with CFs as demonstrated in Figures 40.3, 40.4, 40.5, 40.6, 40.7, and 40.8. Rigid materials should be trimmed or adapted in these locations to mitigate pressure and abrasions, especially over bony prominences. Thoughtful application will help ensure morbidity of external coaptation does not become a bigger problem than the presenting complaint.

Area Moment of Inertia and Rigid Materials

Area moment of inertia is a cross-sectional property used to predict the resistance of an object to bending and deflection. A basic understanding of area moment of inertia aids clinical decision-making with external coaptation by helping ensure adequate strength and rigidity while balancing padding and weight (Figure 40.9).

This formula becomes relevant in the context of ensuring mechanical adequacy of a cast. A small increase in cast thickness through application of additional material will lead to a large increase in resistance to bending (specifically, the increase in cast thickness to the power of 4). There is also relevance in application of cast padding. Adequate cast padding is desired to prevent sores, but excessive padding can increase motion within the cast

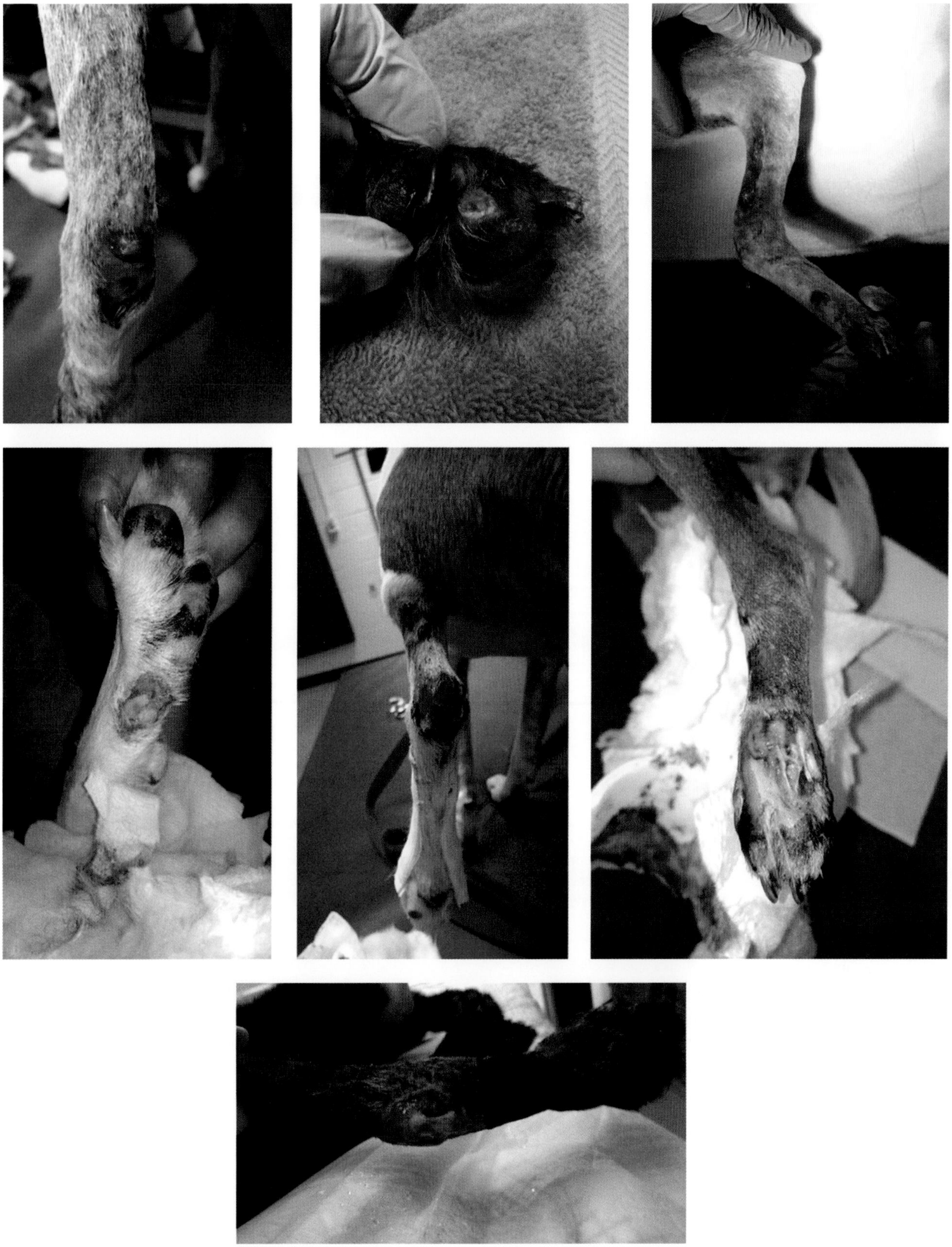

Figure 40.1 Examples of abrasions and ischemic injuries associated with and secondary to external coaptation in dogs. *Source:* © Seth Bleakley.

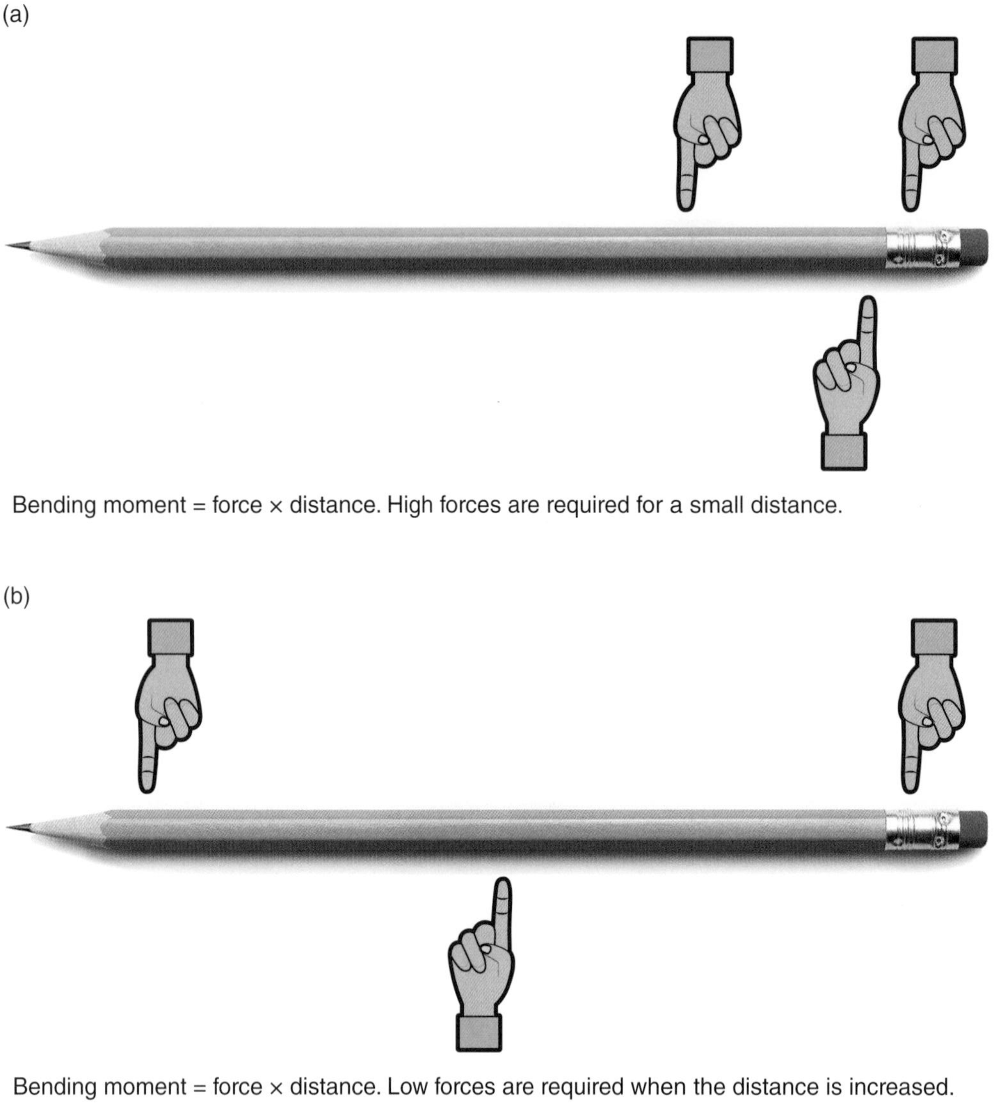

(a)
Bending moment = force × distance. High forces are required for a small distance.
(b)
Bending moment = force × distance. Low forces are required when the distance is increased.

Figure 40.2 The principle of bending moment can be demonstrated simplistically by bending/breaking a pencil. Three forces are required and are represented by the finger icons. Increasing the distance between the forces as in part (b) makes it easier to bend/break the pencil when compared to the more narrowly distributed forces demonstrated in part (a).

(reducing immobilizing function), as well as affect the rigidity of the cast. With a fixed volume of cast material, a wider cast diameter will decrease the thickness and, therefore, resistance to bending of the cast. Thus, additional rolls of cast material may be needed in casts with wider diameters to ensure mechanical adequacy.

This formula (AMI of a cuboid) has relevance to splinting. If a splint is applied caudally or cranially, resistance to bending will be proportional to the thinnest section of the splint to the power of 3. This would be akin to bending a ruler (Figure 40.10) when it is flat; intuitively not very rigid, as h becomes the thickness of the ruler while b remains the length. If a splint is applied laterally or medially, h becomes the width of the splint, and area moment of inertia is increased to width of the splint to the power of 3. Similarly, bending a ruler turned on its side is intuitively challenging; explained by the width of the ruler becoming h in the formula while b remains the length. Therefore, splints will be much stronger and more resistant to bending when applied laterally or medially.

Pressure

In the context of external coaptation, pressure is directly proportional to bandage tension and inversely proportional to the radius of the limb and the bandage width.[1]

$$P = \frac{T}{RW}$$

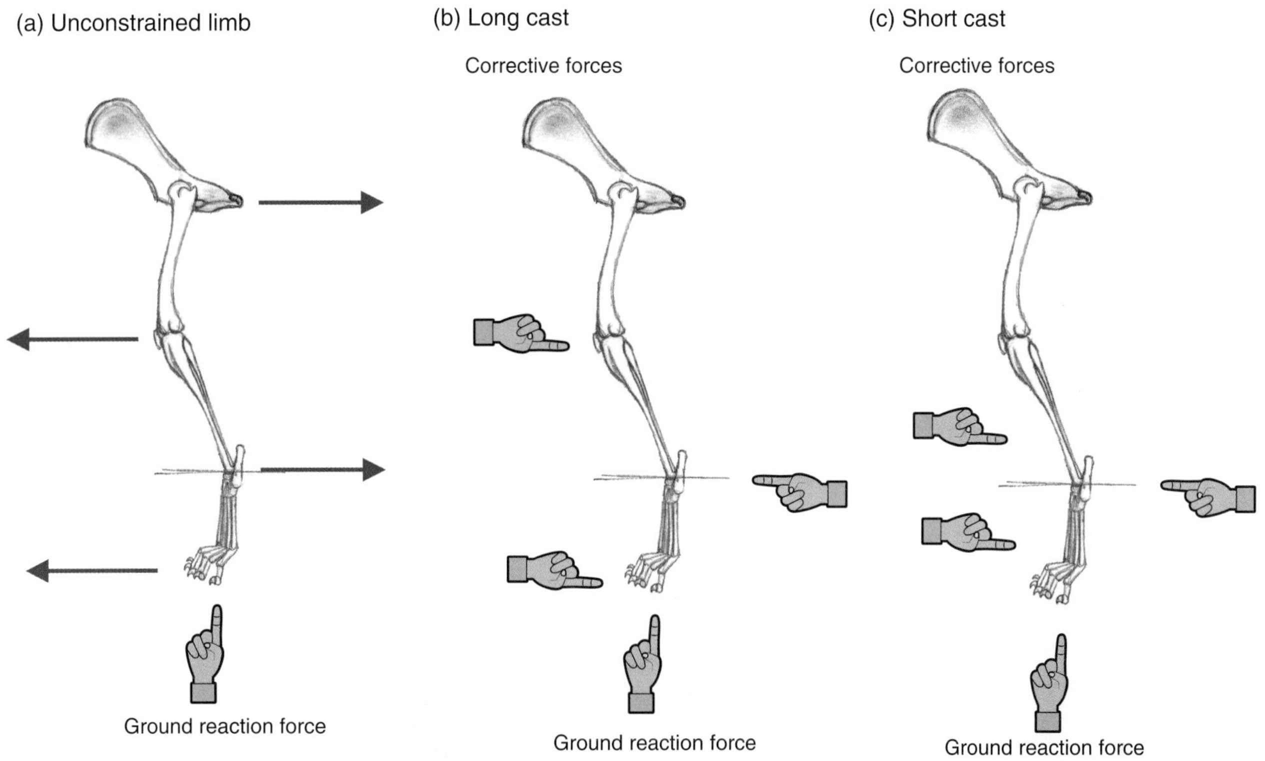

Figure 40.3 Schematic of the canine hindlimb demonstrating the principle of the three-point corrective system. (a) demonstrates the direction of joint movement during flexion of the unconstrained limb in response to ground reaction force; (b) demonstrates application of three corrective forces (CFs) to resist flexion, such as in a long cast; (c) demonstrates how a short cast would alter the proximal CF, decreasing the distance. As ground reaction force is constant, the force to resist bending moment will be subsequently greater. This, coupled with decreased surface area (which is inversely proportional to pressure), will lead to a higher incidence of sores and ischemic injury.

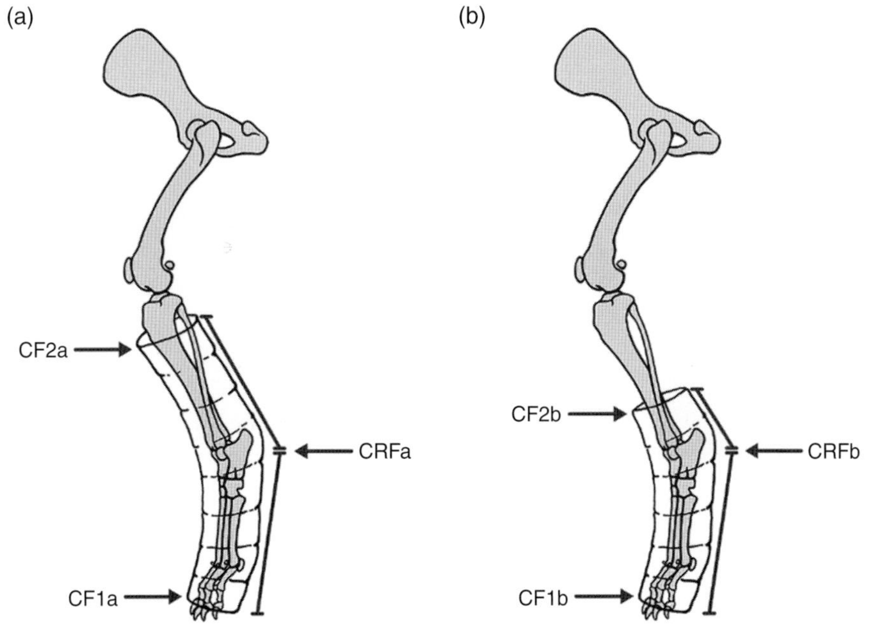

Figure 40.4 Schematic diagram that depicts the concept of the three-point corrective system for a tall cast (a) and short cast (b) applied to a pelvic limb of a dog. The force acting at the calcaneus is the corrective reaction force (CRF) for the tall (CRFa) and short (CRFb) casts. For the tall cast, the two opposing CFs are acting at the points where the cast terminates on the cranial surface of the proximal portion of the tibia (CF2a) and digits (CF1a). For the short cast, the two opposing CFs are acting at the points where the cast terminates on the cranial surface of the distal portion of the tibia (CF2b) and digits (CF1b). For both cast configurations, the forces of both CFs are expected to equal the force applied at the CRF location. The extended lever arm associated with the tall cast configuration results in lower pressures at CF2a and CRFa, compared with the pressures at the corresponding locations (CF2b and CRFb) with the short cast configuration. *Source:* Iodence et al.[4] published with permission from Dr. Felix Duerr.

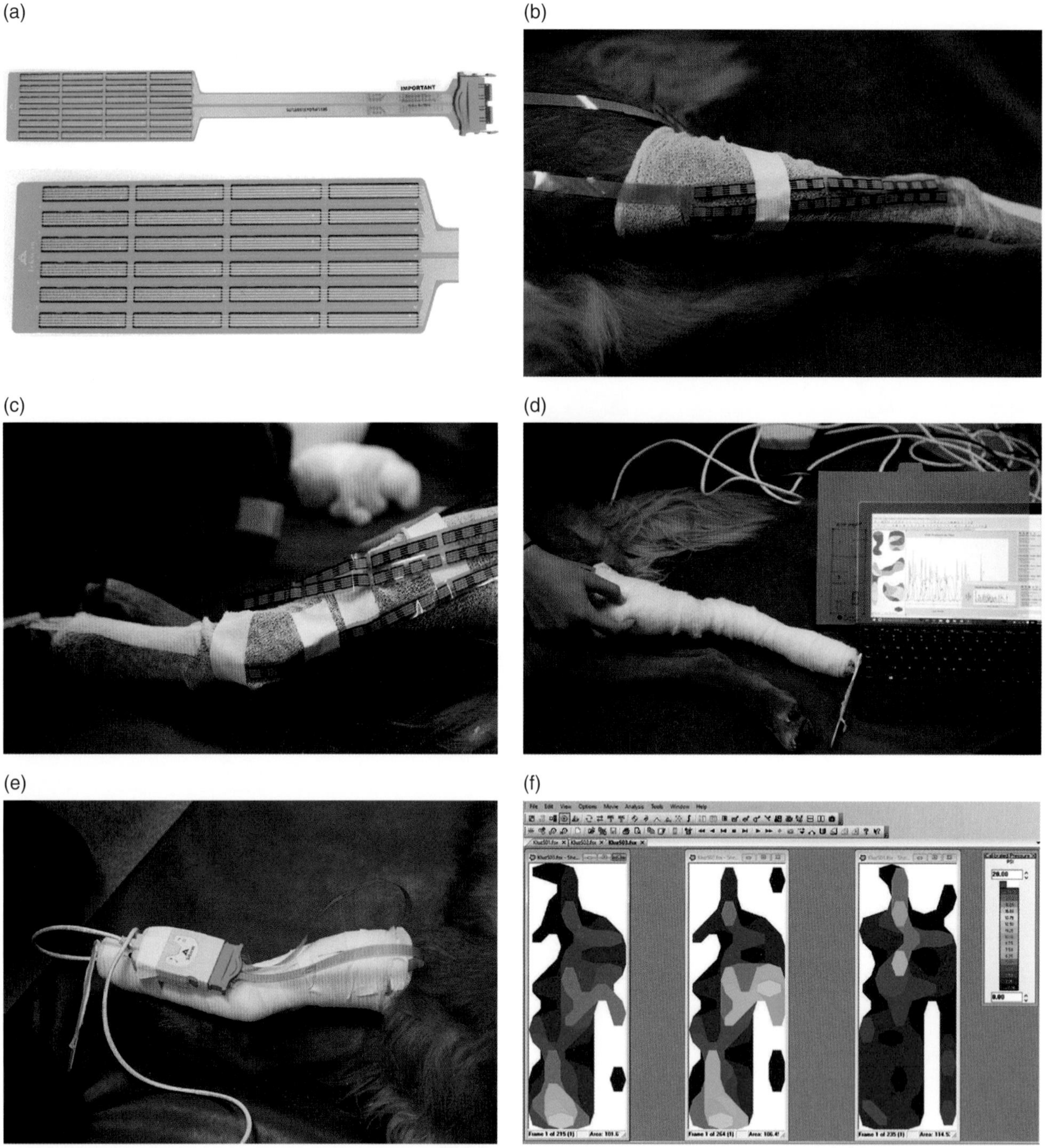

Figure 40.5 Photographs of a pressure sensor, application of the pressure sensors to a pelvic limb of a dog, and outputs from the sensor. (a) Photographs of the pressure sensor (top) and a magnified view of the six sensor columns (bottom). (b) Photograph of three sensor columns positioned (starting proximally at the tibial tuberosity) over the cranial aspect of the pelvic limb of a dog. (c) Photograph of one sensor column positioned over the calcaneus. Notice that the two other sensor columns in the photograph are positioned outside the area to be evaluated (i.e., outside the calcaneus). (d) Photograph of the screen overlay for the pressure-mapping software. Notice that the investigator is applying direct pressure to the area to be evaluated to record its location on the screen overlay for subsequent use in data analysis. (e) Photograph of the final positioning of the sensors, cast padding, and fiberglass cast on a pelvic limb. The sensor cuff is affixed to the exterior of the cast over the tarsus. The sensor wires attach directly to the pressure-mapping system. (f) Photographs of the screen overlays of three recorded pressure measurements. Notice that areas of lower pressure appear dark blue, whereas areas of higher pressure appear yellow or green. *Source:* Iodence et al.[4] with permission from American Veterinary Medical Association.

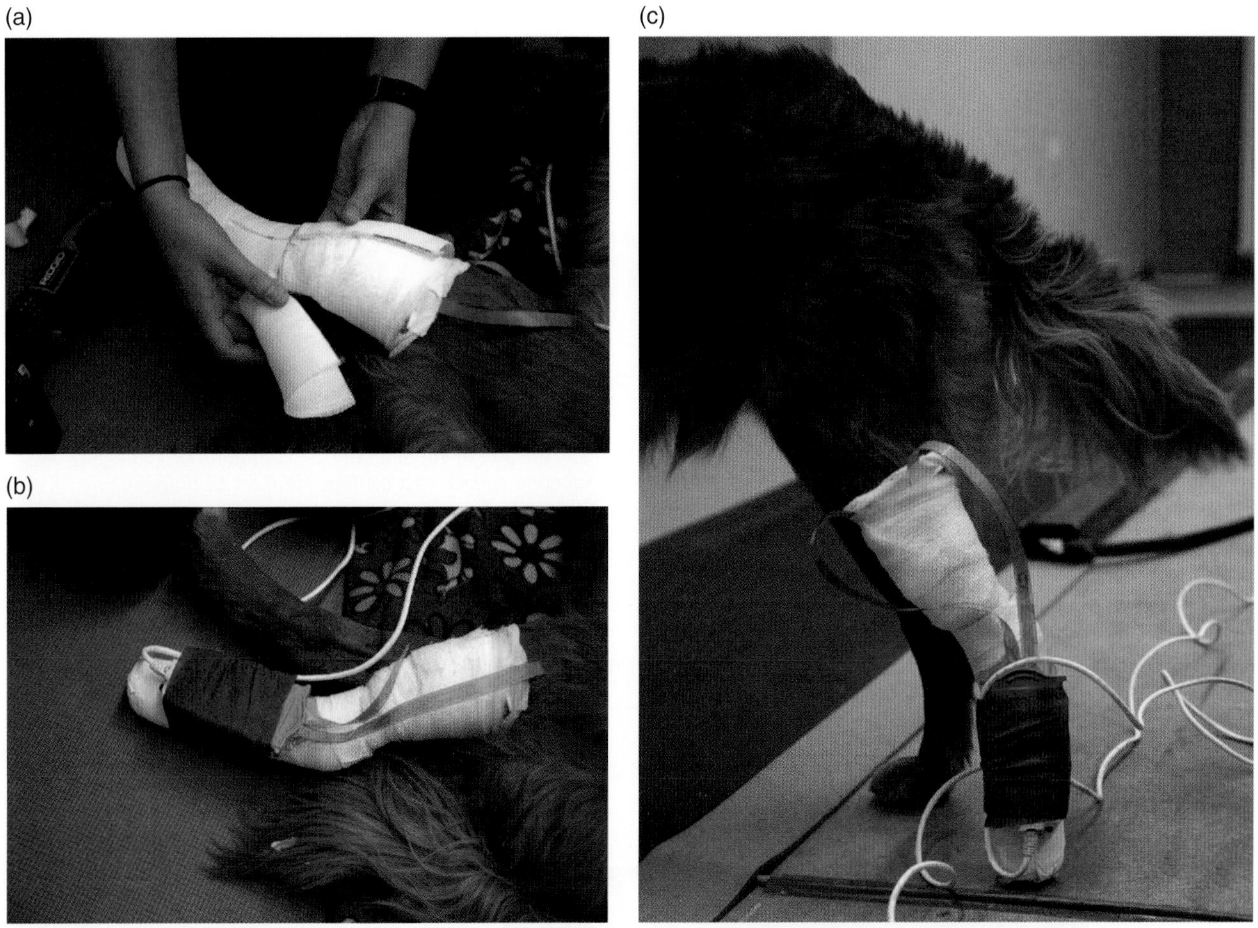

Figure 40.6 Photographs of procedures for the application of a short cast configuration. (a) Photograph of the longitudinal transection of a short cast on the lateral and medial aspects of the limb by use of a battery-operated oscillating saw. (b) Photograph of a short cast on the pelvic limb. Notice that the two halves of the cast have been aligned, fully compressed, and taped together circumferentially. (c) Photograph of the final positioning of a short cast with the sensors, cast padding, and short cast in place. The sensors and padding were not removed to ensure there was no change in sensor placement. The sensor cuff is affixed to the exterior of the cast over the tarsus. The sensor wires attach directly to the pressure-mapping system. *Source:* Iodence et al.[4] with permission from American Veterinary Medical Association.

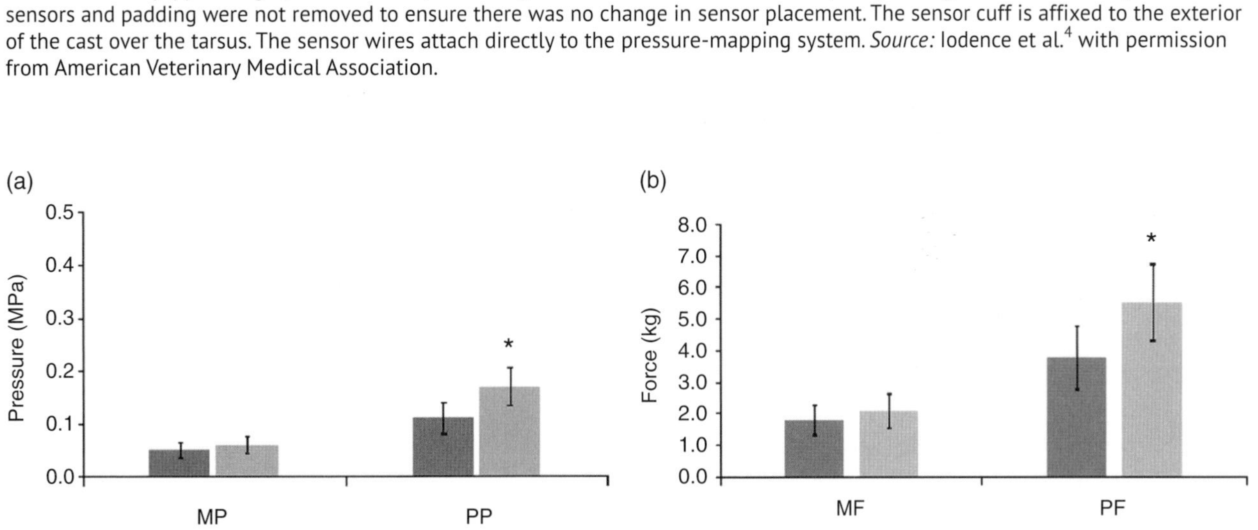

Figure 40.7 Mean and 95% confidence intervals for the mean pressure (MP) and peak pressure (PP) (a) and mean force (MF) and peak force (PF) (b) of a tall cast configuration (dark gray bars) and a short cast configuration (light gray bars) at the level of the calcaneus for 13 dogs. *Within a variable, the value for the short cast configuration differs significantly ($P \leq 0.05$) from the value for the tall cast configuration. *Source:* Iodence et al.[4] published with permission from Dr. Felix Duerr.

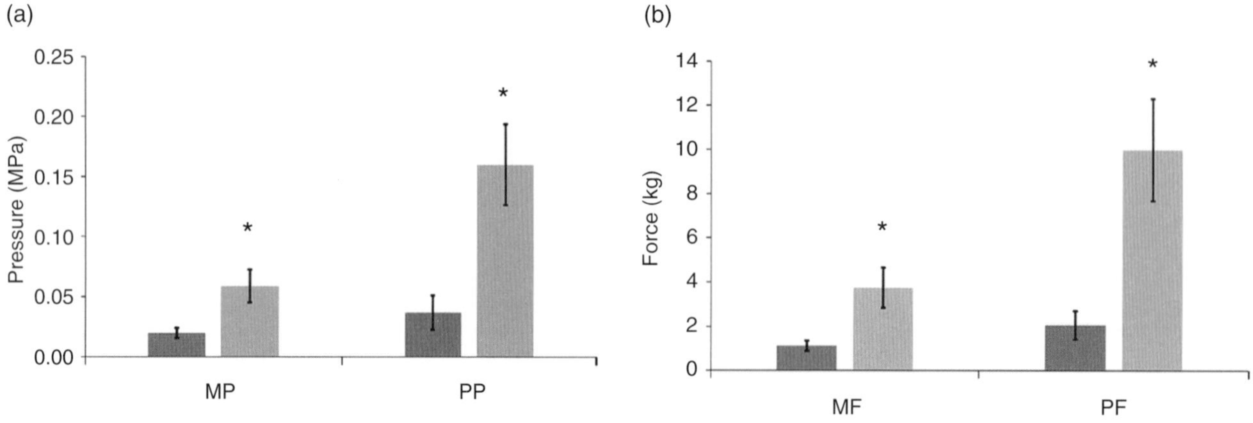

Figure 40.8 Mean and 95% confidence intervals for the MP and PP (a) and MF and PF (b) of a tall cast configuration (dark gray bars) and a short cast configuration (light gray bars) at the level of the proximal edge of each cast configuration for 13 dogs. See Figure 40.7 for remainder of key. *Source:* Iodence et al.[4] published with permission from Dr. Felix Duerr.

(a)

$$I = \frac{\pi(ro4 - ri4)}{4}$$

Where *I* represents area moment of inertia, *ro* represents the outer radius of the cylinder, and *ri* represents the inner radius of a cylinder.

(b)

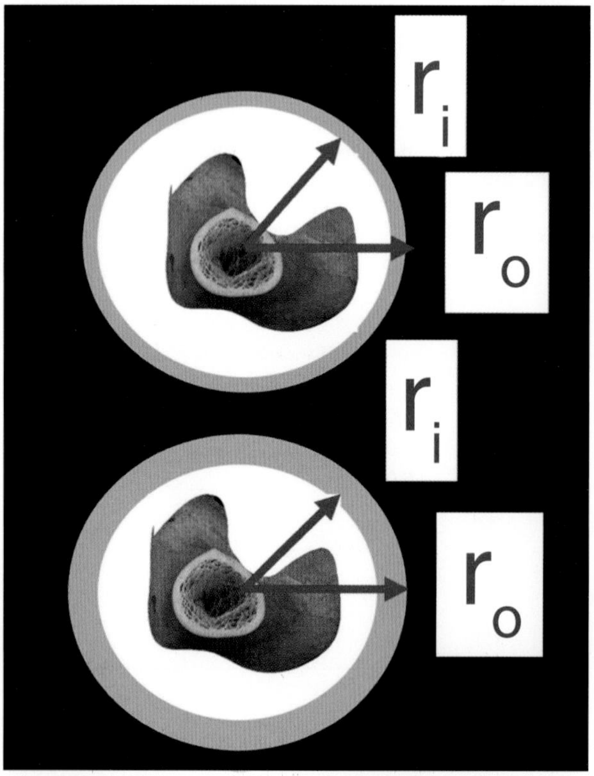

Figure 40.9 (a) The formula for area moment of inertia of a cylinder. (b) Schematic demonstrating application of the formula to cast thickness.

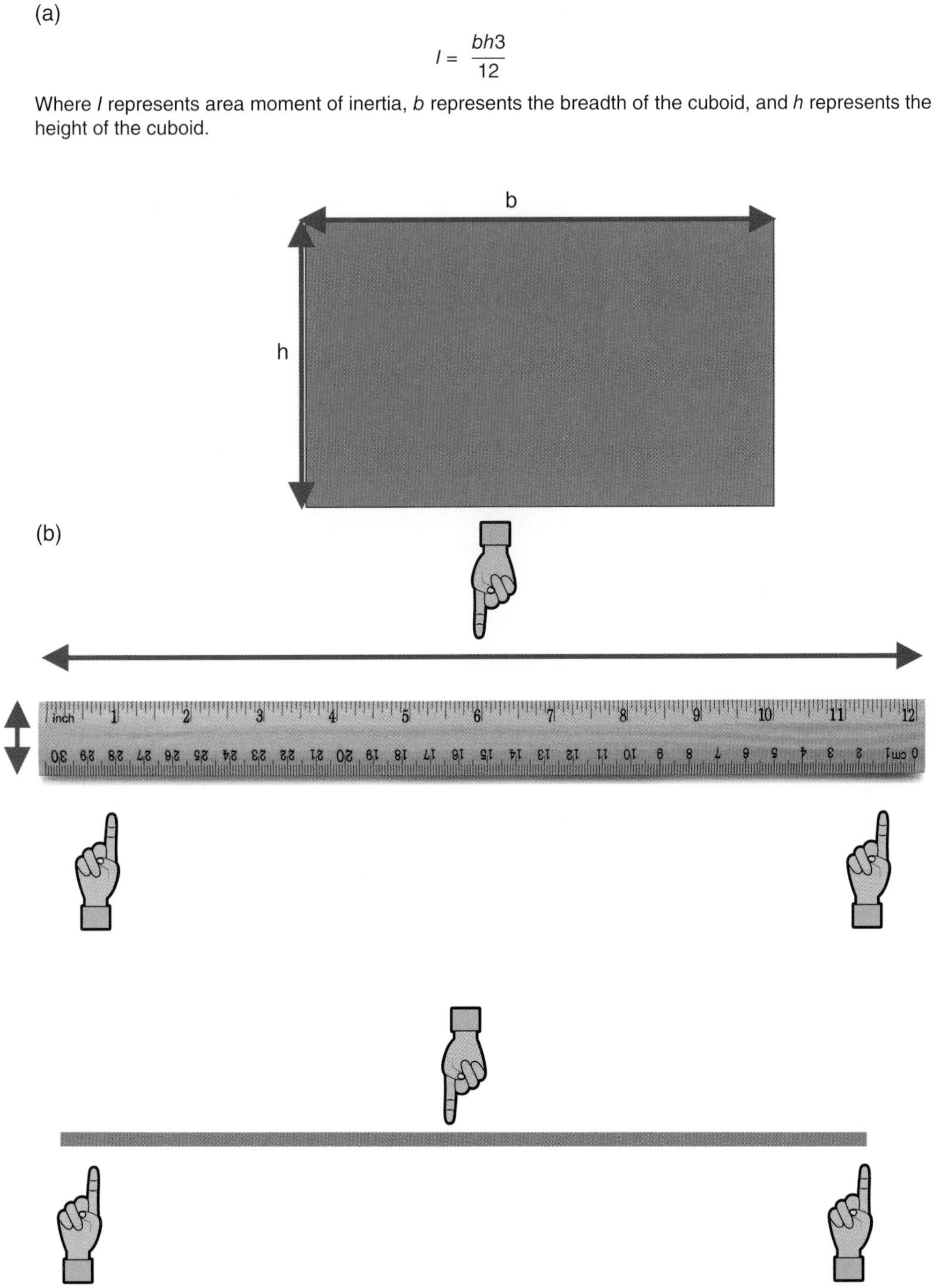

(a)
I = bh3/12
Where I represents area moment of inertia, b represents the breadth of the cuboid, and h represents the height of the cuboid.
b
h
(b)
inch

Figure 40.10 (a) The formula for area moment of inertia of a cuboid. (b) Schematic representing relevance with regard to splint placement using a ruler as an example. *Source:* Kenishirotie/Adobe Stock.

Where P = pressure, T = bandage tension, R = radius of limb, and W = bandage width.

Pressure is dependent on the material used. Cotton has very low tension even at 100% extension; therefore, it is extremely unlikely to cause excessive pressure with cast padding. Elastic material has high tension even at 40–50% extension so **should not be used as a primary layer in external coaptation**. Pressure is also exacerbated by limb flexion, which should be taken into account, especially when applying elastic material around joints.

As pressure is inversely proportional to the radius of the limb, care must be taken in **small dogs that may be more susceptible to ischemic injury** (Figure 40.1), both because of increased pressure and because of decreased bandage length and, therefore, proportional CF.

As pressure is inversely proportional to bandage width, increasing padding is one of the surest ways to decrease pressure and avoid morbidity.

External Coaptation Technique

The above principles are applied and coupled with standard bandaging techniques to ensure success with external coaptation while avoiding morbidity. External coaptation typically involves the following steps:

Tape stirrups (Figures 40.11 and 40.22). Cotton or equivalent tape stirrups serve to help prevent the bandage/cast/splint from falling off while walking, as well as reducing sliding motion that could contribute to abrasions. The conical shape of the limb of a dog or cat coupled with motion from limb flexion and extension will frequently result in slipping and loss of material over time, especially in the absence of tape stirrups. Tape stirrups should be applied to either side of the limb where possible (i.e., when bilateral placement is not inhibited by an incision or wound). Temporary fixation of free tape to a tongue depressor distal to the paw can be helpful in controlling the tape during application of bandage materials. Another tip is to leave the tape in place where it is attached to the limb and trim it distally in subsequent changes, and simply reapply new stirrups over the original portion on the limb. This will avoid an uncomfortable waxing-like event for the patient when removing the tape during each bandage change.

Contact layer where necessary. If there is a closed incision or wound present, a sterile non-adherent semi-occlusive contact layer is desired to help prevent infection and adherence of soft bandage materials. Contact layers associated with open wounds are discussed briefly in Chapter 18 and in more detail in other texts.

Cast padding (Figures 40.12 and 40.22). Regardless of the construct, padding is essential and should be the primary layer other than a wound contact layer. Cotton or equivalent synthetic cast padding material has a very low tension even at 100% extension so is extremely unlikely to cause excessive pressure even when unrolled while stretched. Elastic material has high tension even at 40–50% extension so should not be used as a primary layer in external coaptation. The amount of cast padding applied is a case-dependent matter of clinical judgment. Generally speaking, enough padding should be applied that application of conforming gauze leads to compression and shaping of said padding, as well as a certain amount of restriction/support. Multiple rolls are usually required depending on patient size and roll diameter. Cast padding is typically applied starting at the toes and unrolling proximally with greater than 50% overlap with each pass around the circumference of the limb. An even layer is desirable, but padding can be increased around the paw, joints, bony prominences, and proximal aspect of the construct (see Principle of Three-Point Corrective System). Cast padding should be applied as proximally as limb anatomy permits, with at least a joint above the region to be supported. Cast padding should extend beyond the level of the planned cast or splint.

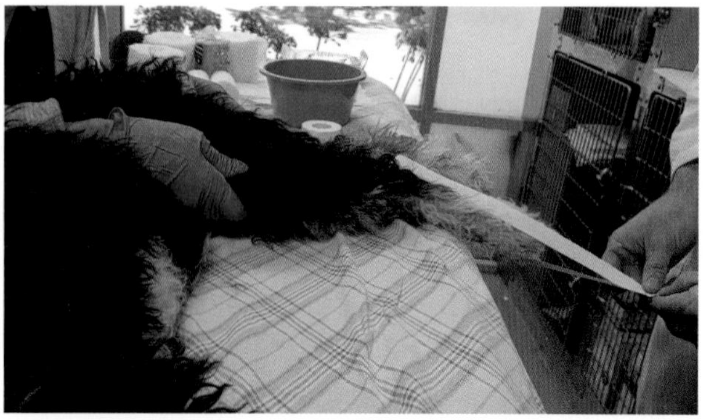

Figure 40.11 Application of cotton tape stirrups in a canine hindlimb. *Source:* © Seth Bleakley.

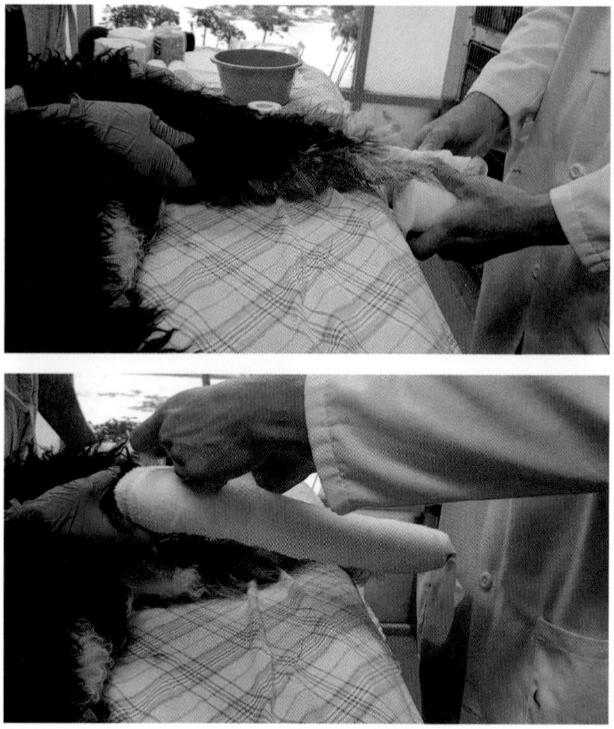

Figure 40.12 Application of cotton cast padding in a canine hindlimb. It is helpful to place the cast padding tightly and starting at the distal aspect with two to three passes circumferentially in the same spot, after which each subsequent circumferential pass should proceed proximally with ~50% overlap per pass. *Source:* © Seth Bleakley.

Conforming stretch gauze (Figures 40.13 and 40.22). This will compress the cast padding layer to both add shape and some support. Appropriate tension is a matter of

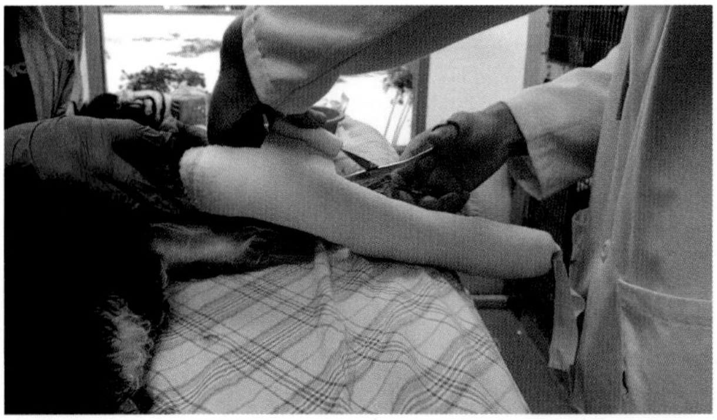

Figure 40.13 Application of conforming stretch gauze in a canine hindlimb. Notice how only one layer of the conforming gauze is applied, and after reaching the proximal aspect of the bandage, it is cut and tucked into itself or taped in place. *Source:* © Seth Bleakley.

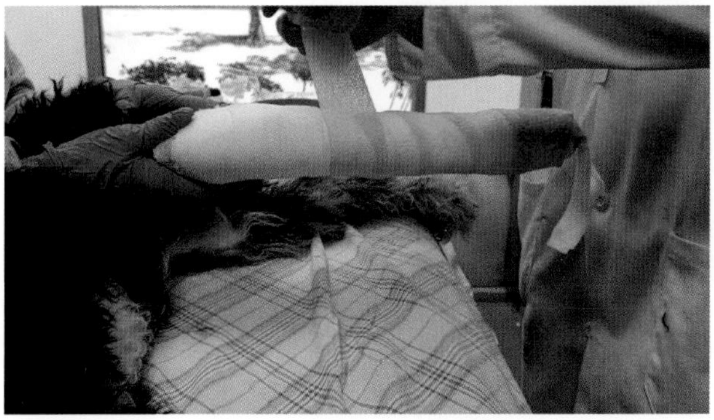

Figure 40.14 Application of Coban (3M) to serve as a non-stick layer prior to cast application. *Source:* © Seth Bleakley.

clinical judgment and depends on the thickness of cast padding, the size of the limb (larger limbs will tolerate more tension without ischemic injury than small ones), and the configuration and purpose of the bandage. Conforming stretch gauze should be applied from distal to proximal, starting at the toes and unrolling with greater than 50% overlap with each pass around the circumference of the limb. Conforming stretch gauze can be used to compress the limb and help move swelling proximally, but care must be taken to not overtighten and cause ischemic injury, especially around joints and vulnerable structures.

Optional non-stick layer (Figures 40.14 and 40.22). Where cast or splint material is to be applied, a non-stick layer here can facilitate the first bandage changes rather than allowing stretch gauze and cast material to adhere to the setting cast or splint. Options include elastic cohesive bandage (VetWrap/Coban 3M) or even tissue paper. Since this layer is only a covering to prevent adherence, the principle of greater than 50% overlap does not apply here.

Rigid cast or splint materials (Figures 40.15 and 40.22). With advances in material science, casts are now generally molded by unrolling fiberglass casting tape rather than plaster-based products. Most commercially available

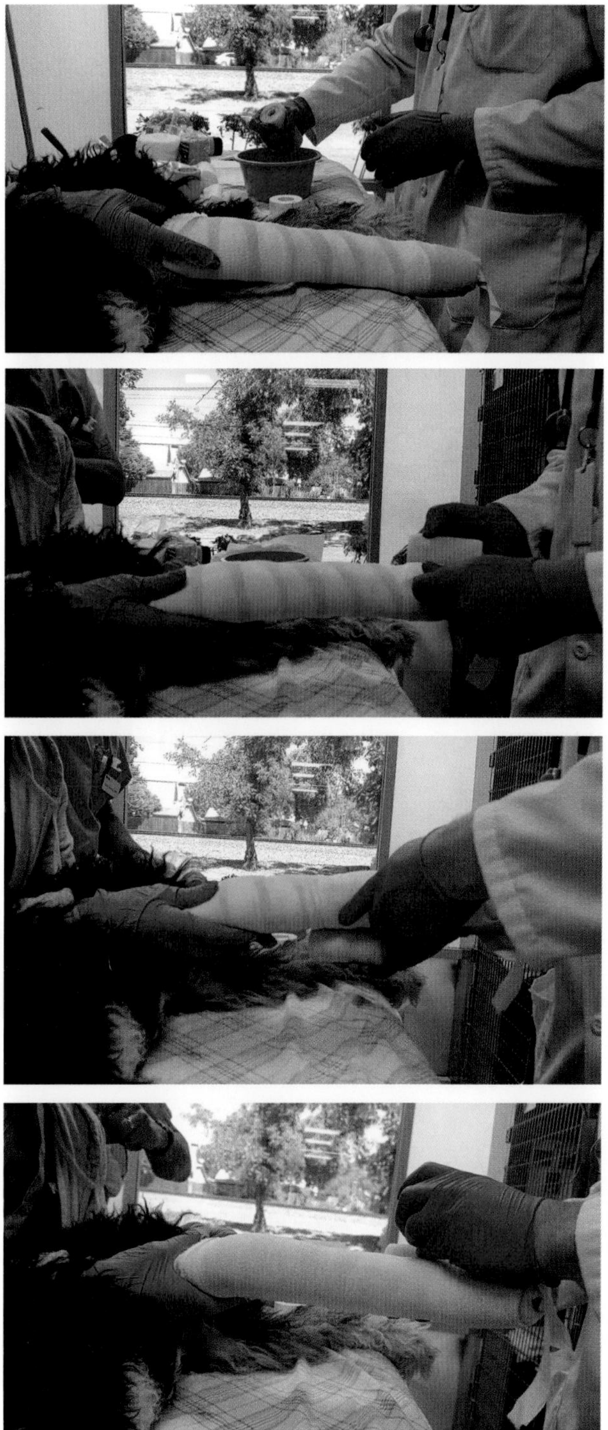

Figure 40.15 Application of fiberglass casting tape (ScotchCast, 3M). *Source:* © Seth Bleakley.

fiberglass casting tape (e.g., ScotchCast, 3M, or equivalent) has a self-adhesive activated by water. It is lighter and cleaner to work with than previous plaster-based materials, as well as faster setting and easier to cut. The roll should be thoroughly submerged and squeezed in water to ensure all adhesive is activated. Increasing the temperature of the

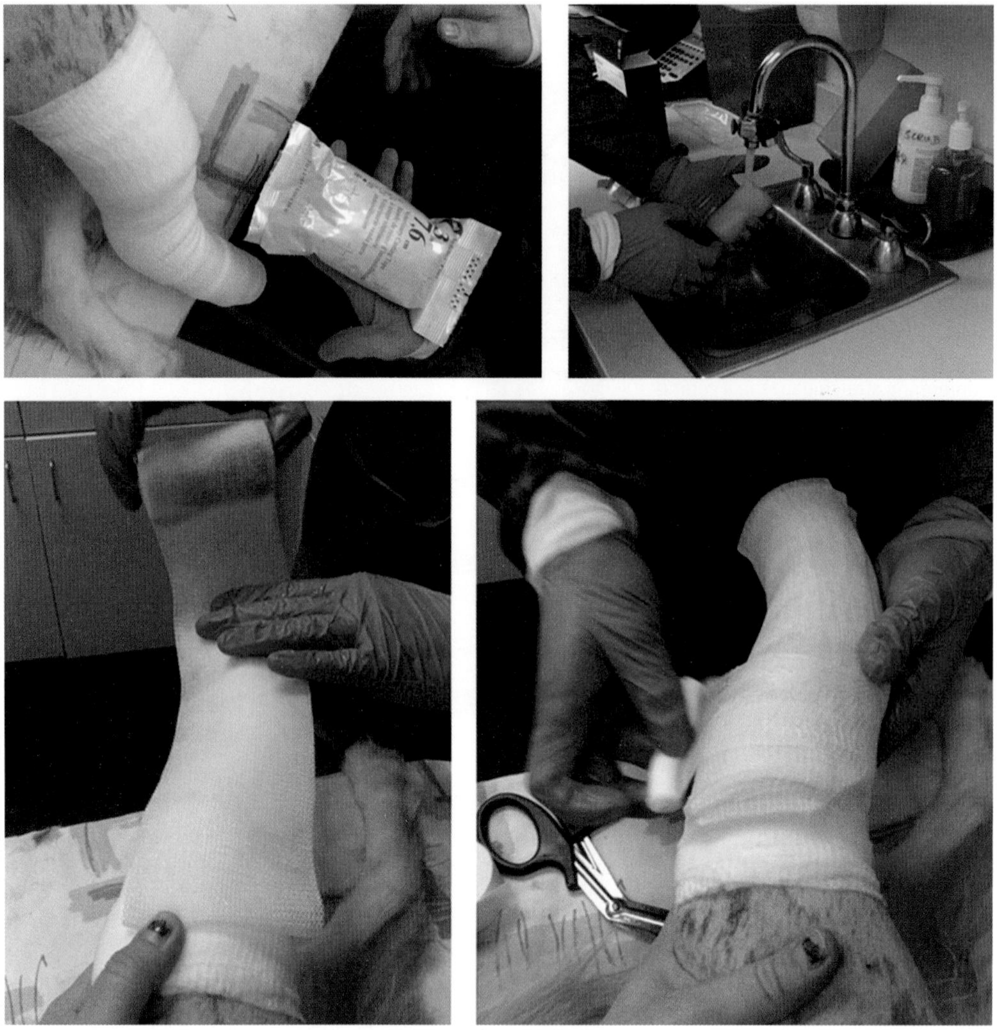

Figure 40.16 Custom lateral splinting in a canine hindlimb using 3″ fiberglass tape (ScotchCast, 3M). *Source:* © Seth Bleakley.

water will speed up activation time, resulting in less time for the cast or splint to harden, although care should be taken that the roll does not harden too quickly or before unrolling and shaping. Fiberglass casting tape is unrolled from distal to proximal with greater than 50% overlap with each pass around the circumference of the limb, starting at the toes and ending just distal to the end of the cast padding proximally. Fiberglass casting tape should not be applied in unpadded regions where a hard, sharp edge could cause abrasion to unprotected skin. Fiberglass casting tape should conform tightly to underlying layers but not increase tension, especially around the toes and joints where a tight cast could cause discomfort or sores. Attention should be paid to the joint angles. A standing angle or slight limb extension is desired to permit standing/walking in a cast. Care should also be taken to avoid folding the cast in an effort to achieve more flexion after unrolling, as such could create pressure around the joint. Fiberglass casting tape will dry and harden rapidly depending on temperature. Depending on the material used, the curing process is exothermic, so feeling heat from a curing cast is normal.

A custom splint can be molded from layered fiberglass casting tape, thermomoldable plastics, or other commercially available materials. Material is most commonly applied laterally or caudally, depending on the limb. There are mechanical advantages to lateral application (see area moment of inertia of a cuboid, Figure 40.10). As opposed to circumferential casting, where unrolled or thermomoldable material is allowed to set, custom splints are typically immediately molded while still pliable via application of conforming stretch gauze (Figures 40.16 and 40.17). Again, ensuring a standing angle or only mild extension is desirable from a limb function standpoint. Adequate conforming stretch gauze is important to ensure the hard material will not loosen, move, and cause sores.

There are commercially available spoon and lateral splints (Figure 40.18), which can be selected and trimmed according to size and applied instead of a custom molded splint.

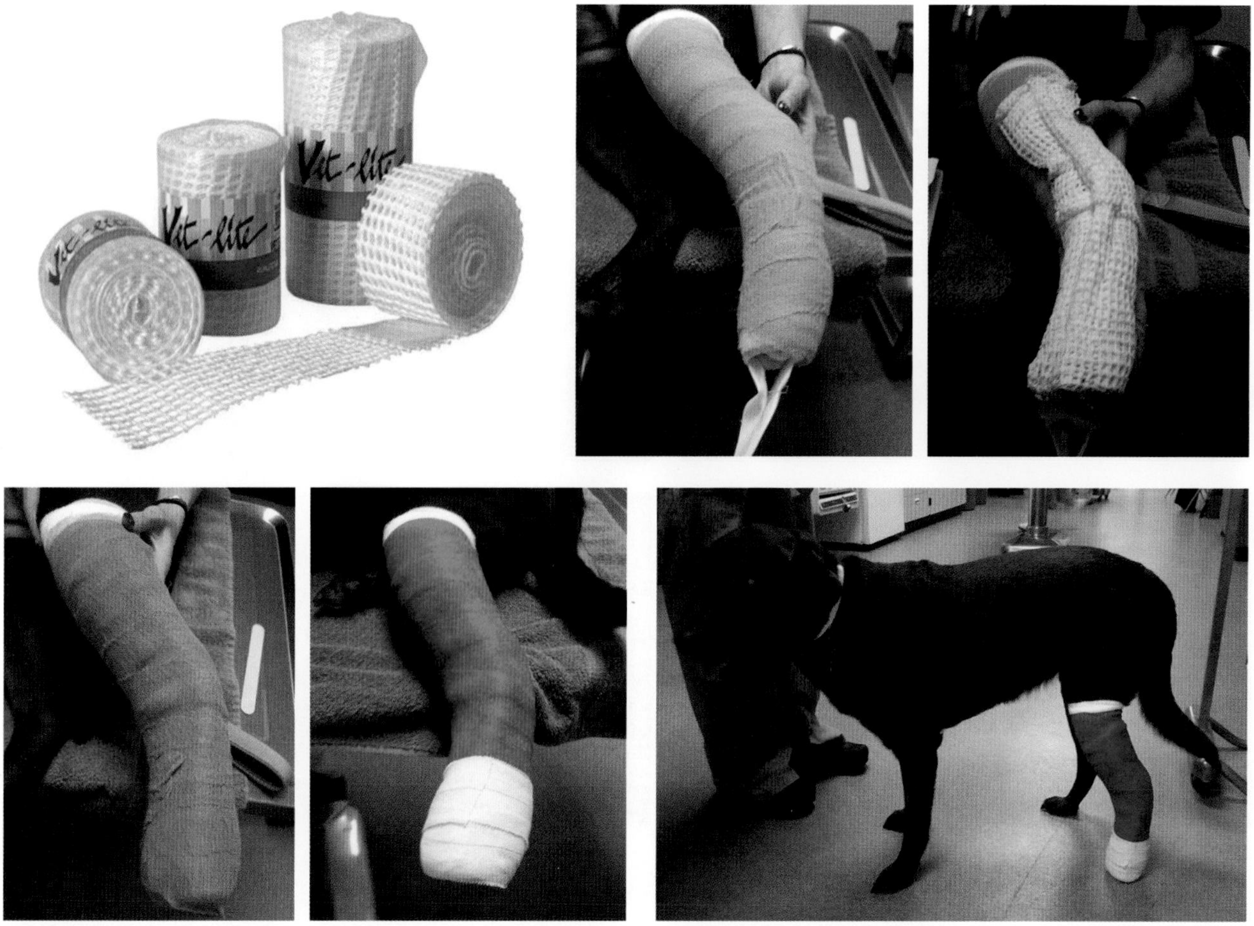

Figure 40.17 Use of a thermomoldable plastic (Vet-Lite) in lateral splinting of a canine hindlimb. A benefit of this material is that it can be re-molded if necessary using a hairdryer or bowl of hot water to soften the material. *Source:* © Seth Bleakley.

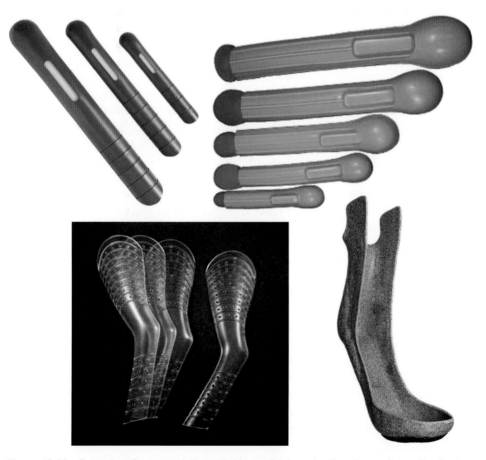

Figure 40.18 Examples of commercially available pre-fabricated splints for use in small animal external coaptation.

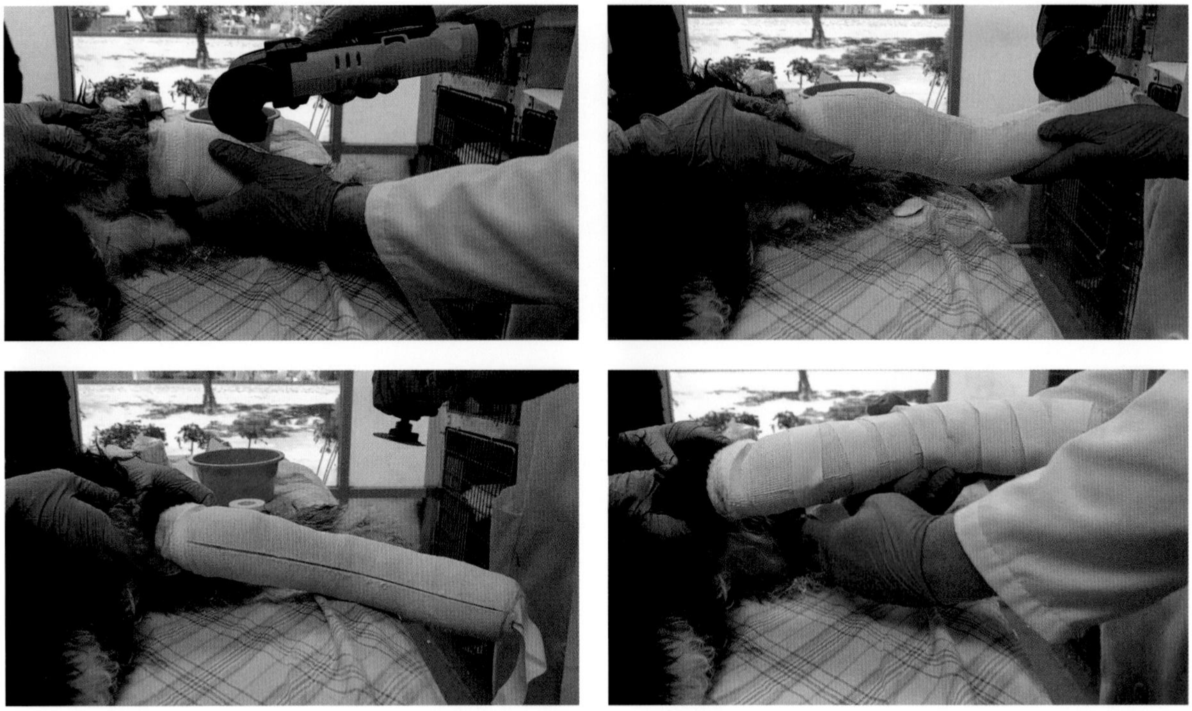

Figure 40.19 Trimming and bivalving a fiberglass cast using an oscillating saw. The cast is then re-secured using cotton tape, and stirrups are secured to help prevent slipping. *Source:* © Seth Bleakley.

Adequate padding is still important, and adequate conforming stretch gauze is important to secure these splints so that the hard material will not loosen, move, and cause sores.

Bivalving and trimming (Figures 40.19, 40.20, and 40.22). Most indications for external coaptation will involve a number of weeks of maintenance to permit healing. As cast padding will wear (especially if soiled or moistened), it must be changed frequently to prevent sores; usually weekly depending on the case. Bivalving involves cutting a cast in half and facilitates replacement. An oscillating saw is typically used, as its mechanism is largely atraumatic to underlying soft materials, as well as the patient's soft tissues. However, an oscillating saw can be loud, and the vibrations stressful to an unsedated patient. Therefore, bivalving a cast at the time of application is desirable if the patient is sedated or under anesthesia, which is common in cases requiring closed fracture reduction or simply for improved patient compliance in cast fabrication.

In addition to bivalving the cast, it can be trimmed and modified with the saw to reduce chances of abrasion and pressure sores (Figure 40.20). For example, it can be trimmed/shortened caudally in the hindlimb or cranially in the forelimb to reduce the chance of it rubbing on the caudal thigh or cranial humerus with stifle or elbow flexion, respectively. Windows can be created in the cast material over bony prominences, such as the olecranon or calcaneus. Trimming of sharp edges and modification of the cast or splint can be made at the time of application or at any future bandage change as needed to prevent and manage sores.

After bivalving a cast, it will need to be re-secured. Cotton tape or equivalent is typically used, applied either in a spiral fashion across the length of the cast or in a multifocal cerclage fashion. The tape stirrups should be reflected and secured at this point.

Final protective layers (Figures 40.21 and 40.22). Elastic cohesive bandage (VetWrap/Coban 3M, or equivalent) is typically applied as one of the final layers. As stated previously, it should never be applied as an early contact layer due to high tension leading to a risk of pressure-induced ischemia, even at minimal extension. The purpose of an elastic cohesive bandage is to provide one more layer of protection to the bandage, not to shape it or provide any support. Use for support has a high risk of creating a tourniquet effect in small animals, especially during joint flexion. Elastic cohesive bandage may be somewhat water-repellent, but it is not waterproof. A secondary benefit of elastic cohesive bandage is esthetics, as it covers casts and splints and is available in a very wide range of colors and designs.

Elastic tape (Elastikon, Johnson and Johnson, or equivalent) is another protective layer useful in late stages of bandaging. Elastic tape is thick, robust, and has a strong adhesive. It can be used to reinforce vulnerable sections of a bandage. It is particularly useful distally around the paw and bottom of a cast, as it can protect a cast or splint from wear on hard ground, as well as provide some traction to

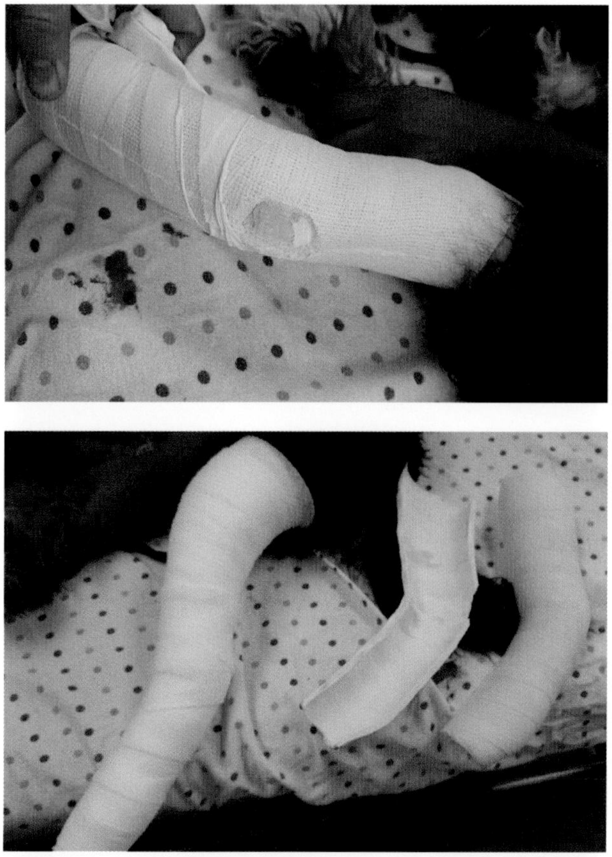

Figure 40.20 Examples of bandage changes of a bivalved cast in a canine hindlimb. Note the window in the cast material made caudal to the calcaneus to reduce pressure and risk of sores. A tip is to label the two sides of a bivalved cast with regard to laterality and/or side of the limb, as this can sometimes become confusing on certain bones. *Source:* © Seth Bleakley.

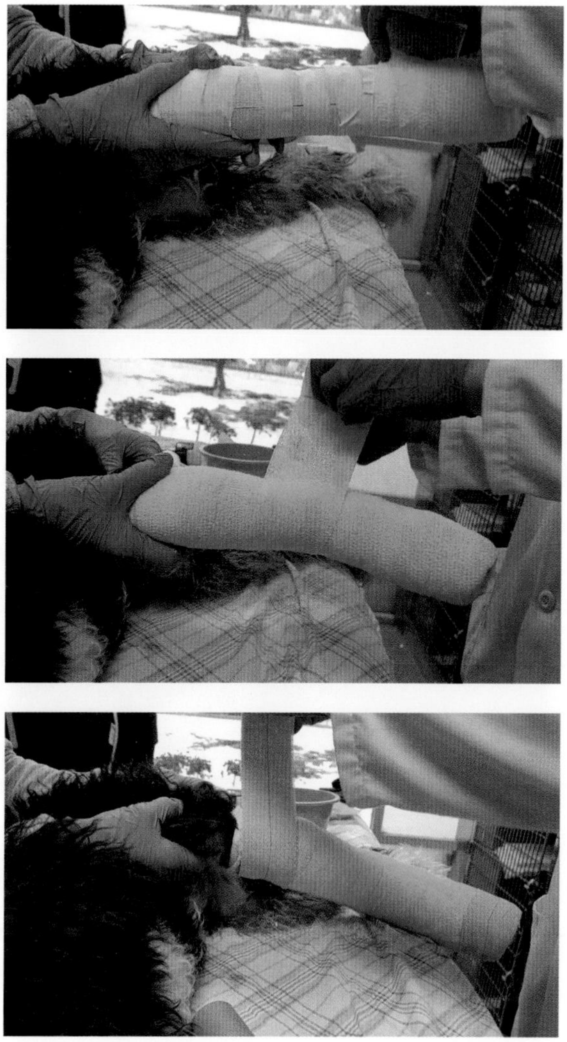

Figure 40.21 Application of Coban (3M) and Elastikon (Johnson & Johnson) as final protective layers. *Source:* © Seth Bleakley.

the patient during ambulation. Elastic tape can be used to secure a bandage directly to a patient, notably the proximal aspect if slipping is a concern; however, care should be taken to avoid use of elastic tape on sensitive skin, and repeatedly reapplying elastic tape to skin with bandage changes can lead to irritation.

Specific Types of Bandages

Robert Jones

Robert Jones was a Welsh orthopedic surgeon who practiced in the 1870s and 1880s, and he has been called the "Father of modern orthopedics."[5] His name is well known for a specific type of soft bandage used for temporary stabilization following an orthopedic injury, such as a fracture. A true Robert Jones bandage is primarily made of cotton and is extremely bulky (Figure 40.23). It is only used for temporary stabilization to provide compression, to provide analgesia (from reduced fracture fragment movement), and to control effusion and bleeding. A Robert Jones bandage should not be used as a definitive treatment for fractures and should be replaced with surgical repair or rigid coaptation within 24–48 hours after placement.

A Robert Jones bandage begins similarly to the previously described external coaptation technique. Tape stirrups are recommended to help secure the bandage. As a Robert Jones bandage has to be bulky enough to provide significant compression and immobilization, a thick cotton wool roll is typically used. Previous principles of bandage length apply, and the bandage should extend from the toes to at least the joint proximal to the injury. After applying a very thick (usually one to two times the limb diameter) even layer of cotton circumferentially, compression is provided with conforming stretch gauze. Conforming stretch gauze is unrolled and wrapped tightly, starting at the toes and unrolling proximally with >50% overlap per circumferential pass. As many rolls of conforming stretch gauze

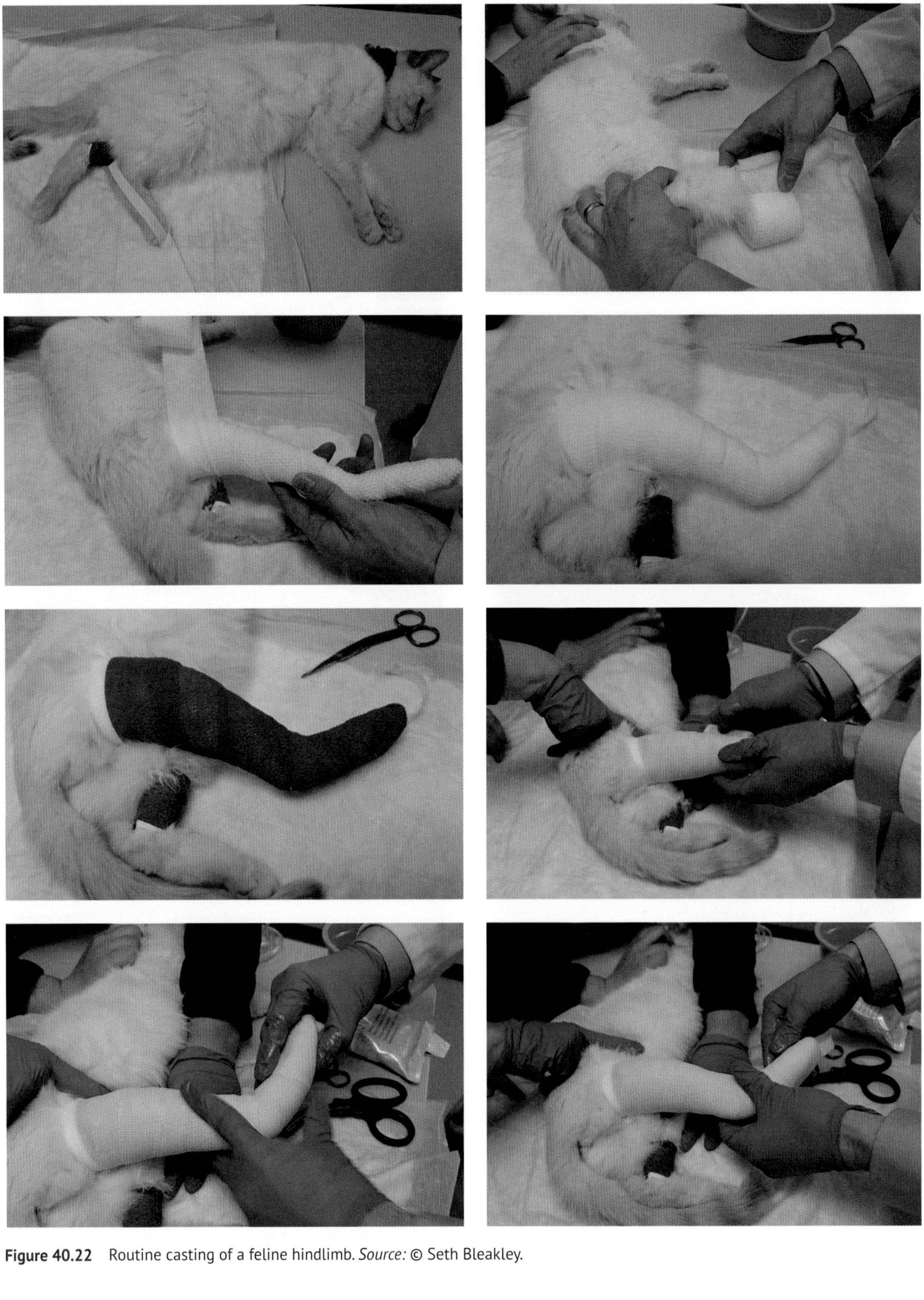

Figure 40.22 Routine casting of a feline hindlimb. *Source:* © Seth Bleakley.

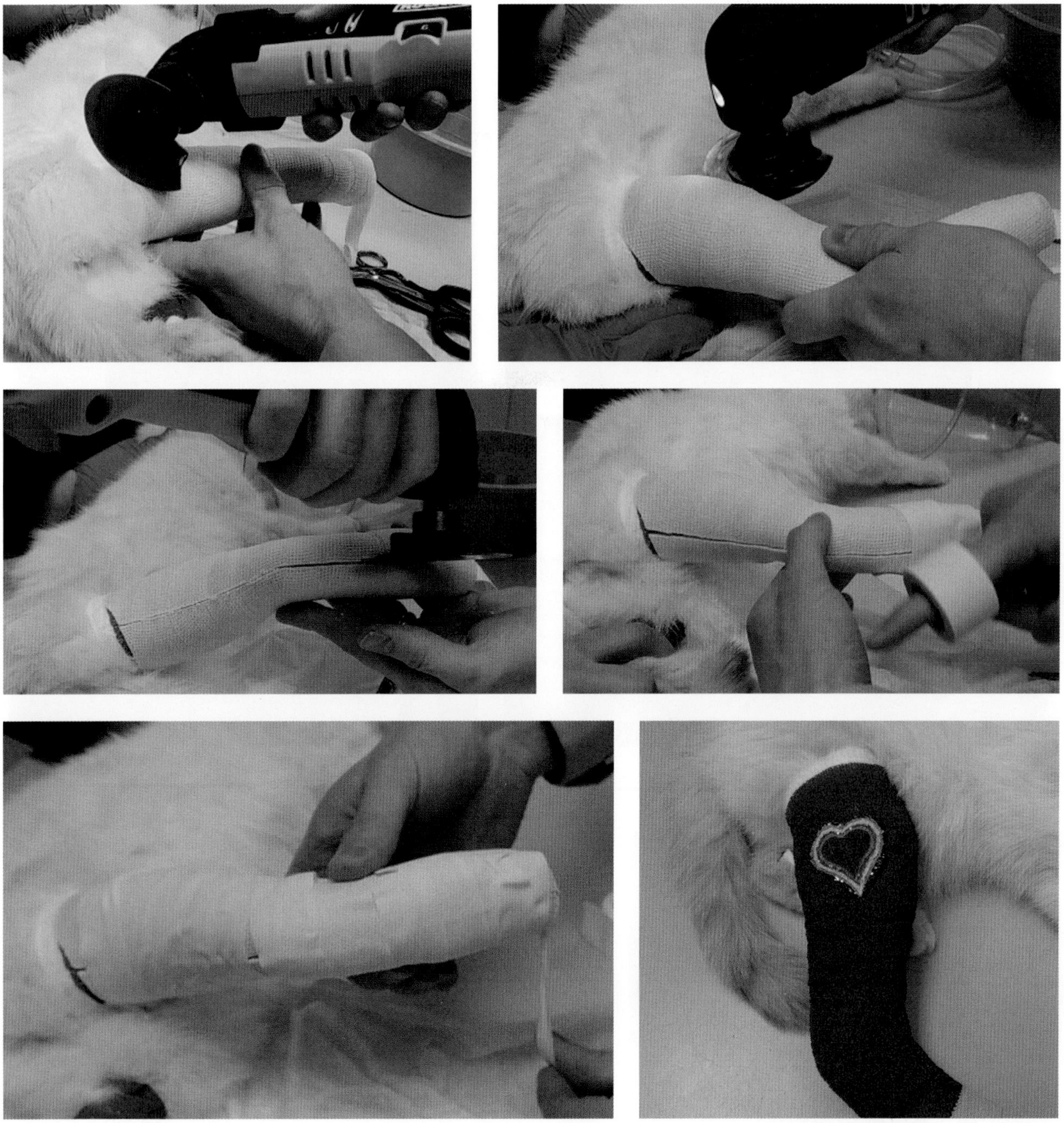

Figure 40.22 (Continued)

are applied as is necessary to create a firm construct. It has been said when a Robert Jones bandage is appropriately compressed, it should make a dull sound when flicked with a finger, like the "sound of a ripe watermelon." After conforming stretch gauze has been applied, the stirrups are reversed and secured. The bandage is protected routinely with elastic cohesive bandage (VetWrap/Coban 3M, or equivalent) and elastic tape (Elastikon, Johnson and Johnson, or equivalent).

Modified Robert Jones

A variation of the Robert Jones bandage using cotton or synthetic cast padding rather than cotton wool roll has come to be known as a "modified" Robert Jones bandage (Figure 40.24). It is less bulky and provides less compression. It is not appropriate for fracture stabilization but rather is used to address post-operative swelling or cover wounds.

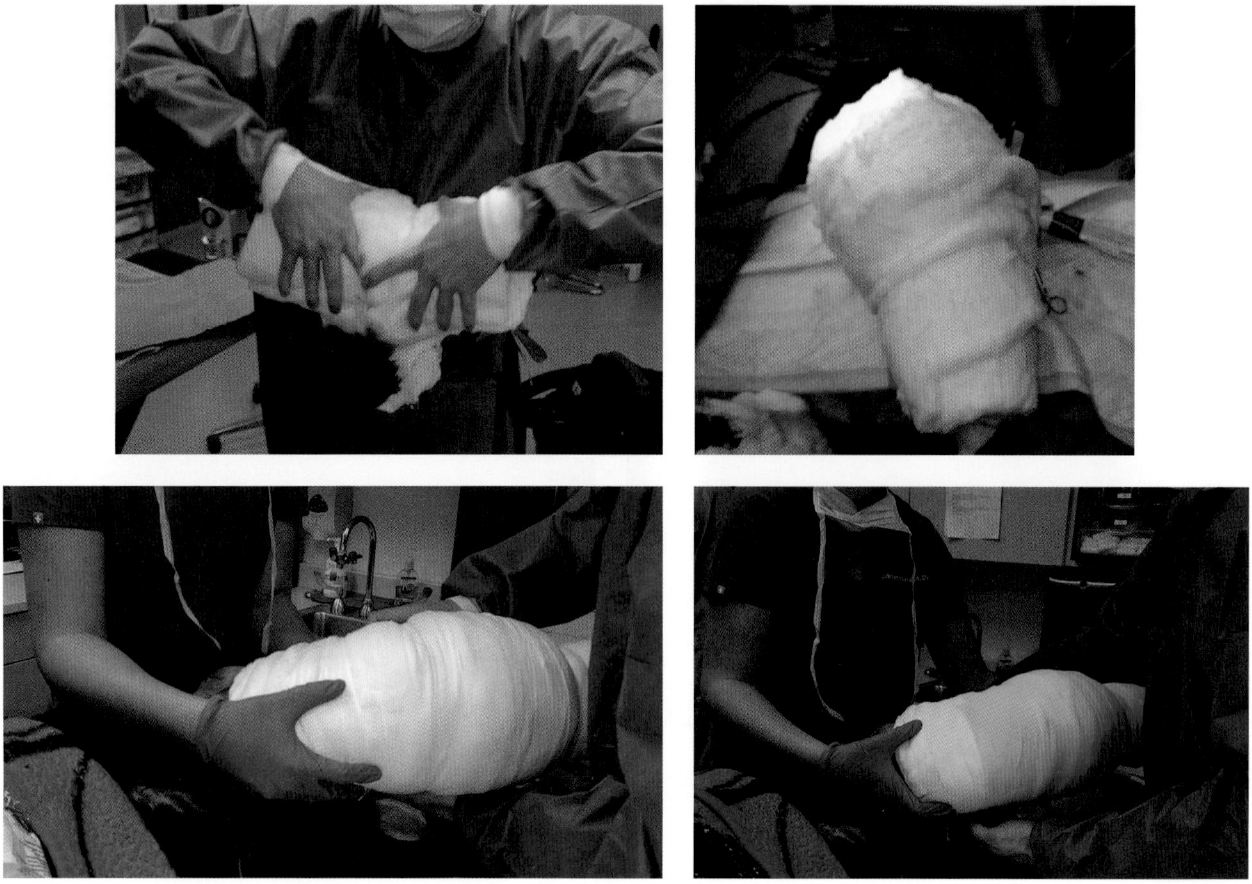

Figure 40.23 Application of a Robert Jones bandage. *Source:* © Seth Bleakley.

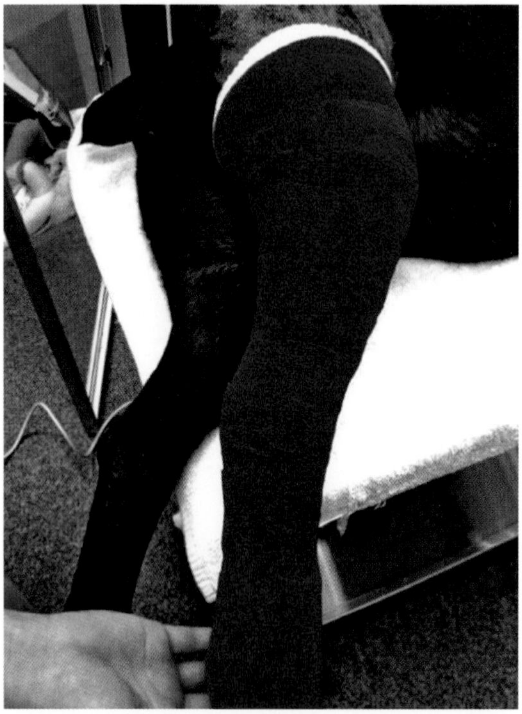

Figure 40.24 A modified Robert Jones bandage or soft-padded bandage. *Source:* © Seth Bleakley.

Reinforced Robert Jones Bandage

A reinforced Robert Jones bandage involves incorporating the use of rigid cast material, splints, aluminum, or thermomoldable plastics into a modified Robert Jones bandage (Figures 40.16, 40.17, 40.18, and 40.25). This expands the utilization of application of the construct, which can now be rigid enough for either temporary stabilization or long-term stabilization, including definitive treatment of orthopedic injuries. The rigid material is incorporated into a bandage as described in the external coaptation technique. As stated previously, the bandage should be changed at least weekly to prevent sores.

Spica Splint

While anatomical limitations in small animals result in most bandages and splints only extending to the stifle or elbow, a Spica splint (Figure 40.26) allows immobilization to extend proximally to the shoulder or hip. The bandage and rigid material are applied from the toes to the torso on either the forelimb or hindlimb. Cast padding and conforming gauze are applied circumferentially around the limb and trunk. The rigid splint material

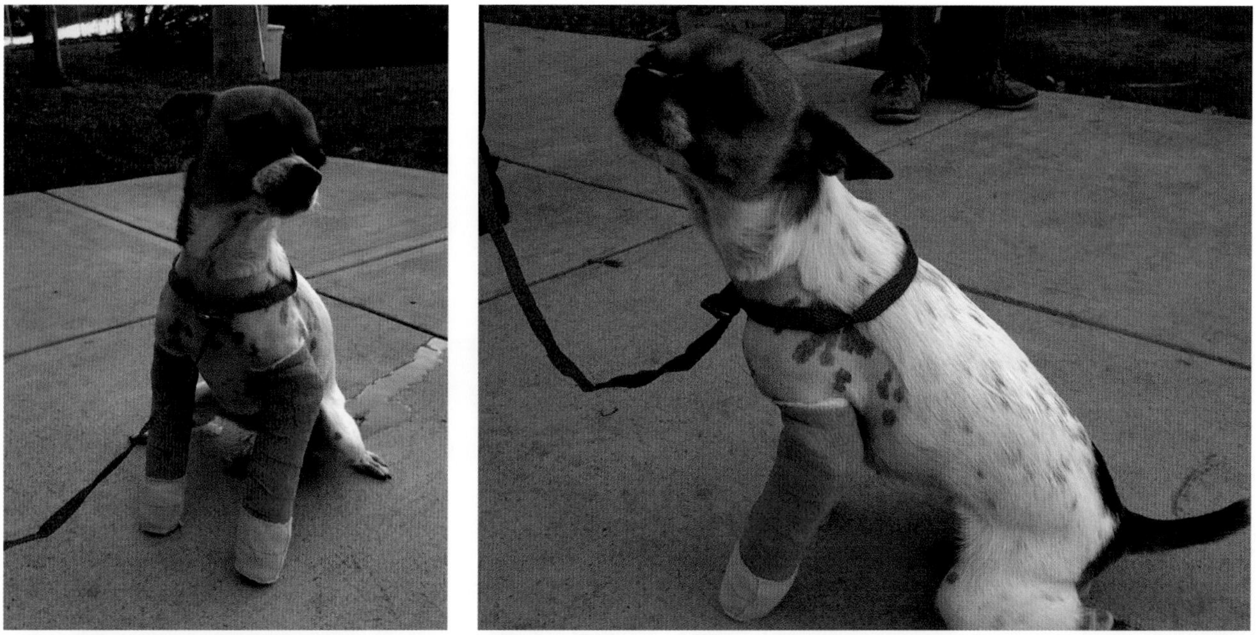

Figure 40.25 Example of reinforced Robert Jones bandages applied to a canine with bilateral antebrachial fractures. *Source:* © Seth Bleakley.

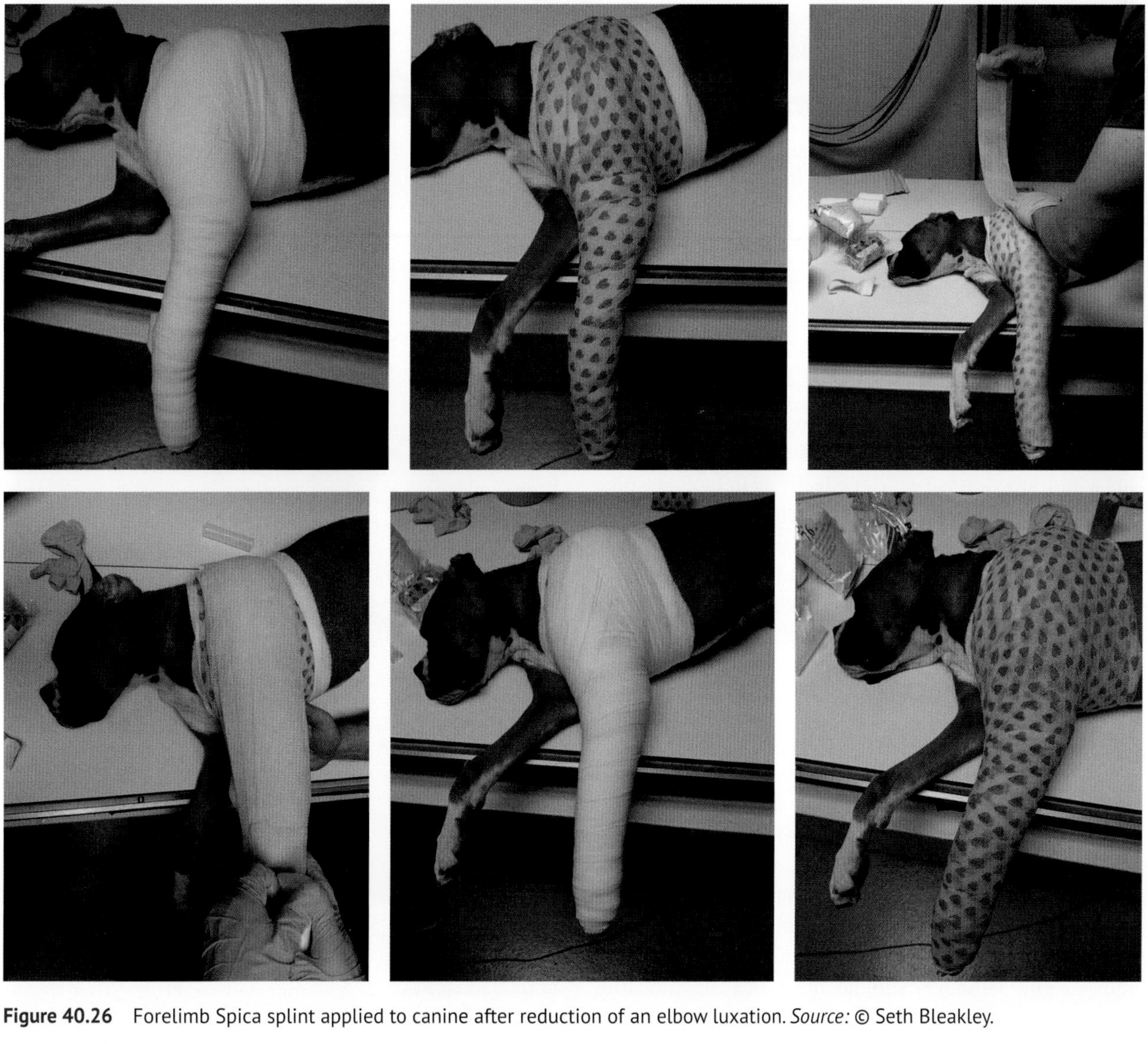

Figure 40.26 Forelimb Spica splint applied to canine after reduction of an elbow luxation. *Source:* © Seth Bleakley.

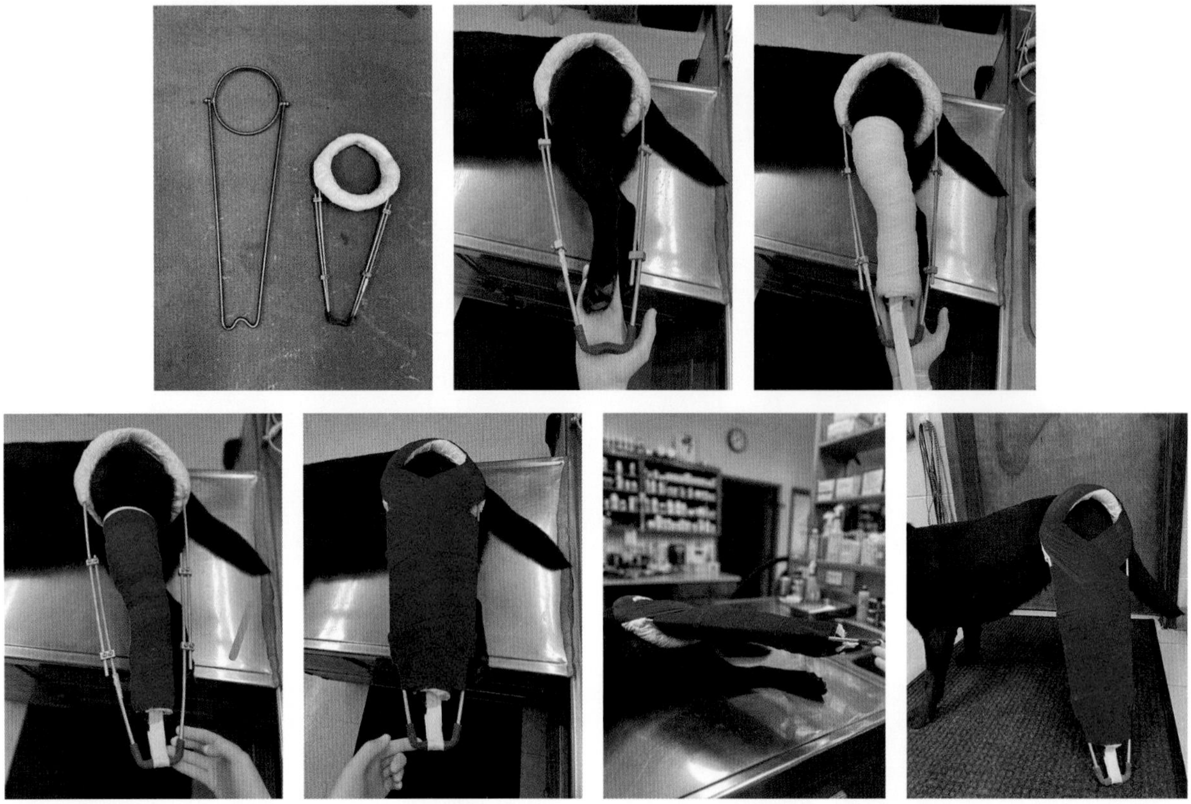

Figure 40.27 Example of Schroeder-Thomas splint application to a canine pelvic limb. The frame is constructed from aluminum rods and a ring, surrounded by rubber distally for grip, and padded proximally to avoid sores. The frame is secured to the limb with cotton tape stirrups, cast padding, conforming gauze, and elastic cohesive bandage. This splint design completely unloads weight bearing from the digits and pes. *Source:* © Dr. Jess Work.

extends from the toes to past the dorsal midline. As stated previously, the bandage should be changed at least weekly to prevent sores.

Schroeder-Thomas Splint

This wire-framed construct can effectively immobilize distal long bones, especially when weight bearing through the distal limb is unwanted for part of the healing process (Figure 40.27), but this technique has largely been superseded by splints and casts in the small animal world of orthopedics.

Non-weight-bearing Bandages

Described bandages/slings that prevent weight bearing altogether include a carpal flexion bandage, a Velpeau sling, a Robinson sling, and an Ehmer sling.

A carpal flexion bandage involves applying cast padding from the toes to the antebrachium and then wrapping with conforming gauze with the carpus in flexion (Figure 40.28). The flexion angle should be adapted for patient comfort (i.e., if a carpal range of motion is reduced, the bandage should not force it into full

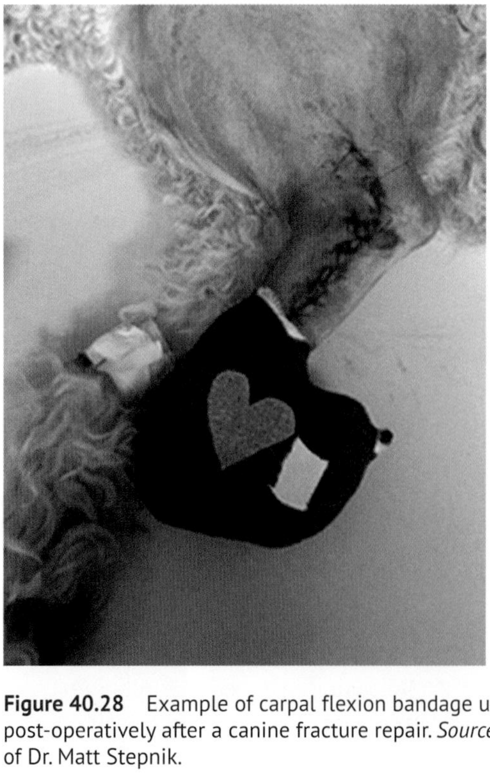

Figure 40.28 Example of carpal flexion bandage used post-operatively after a canine fracture repair. *Source:* Courtesy of Dr. Matt Stepnik.

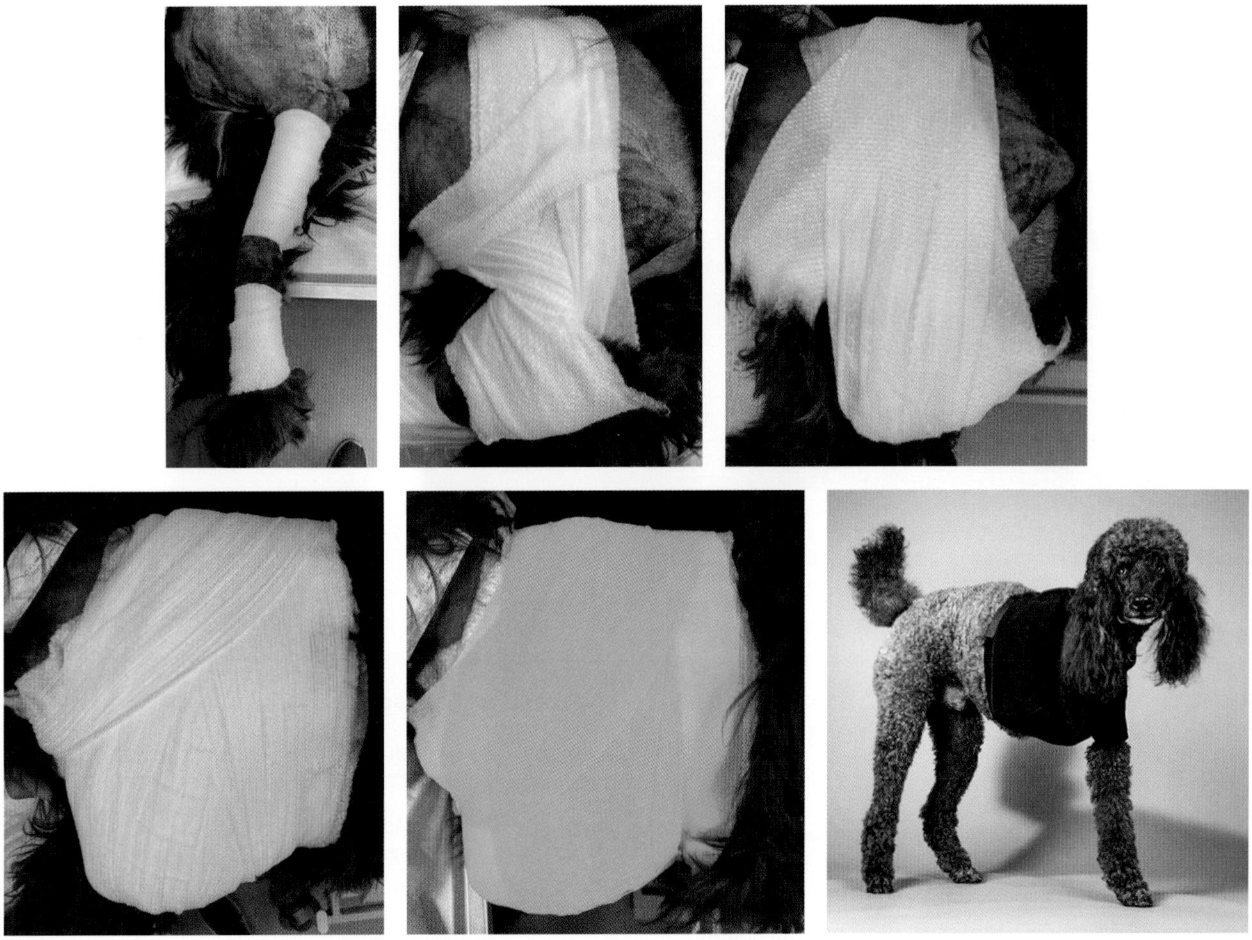

Figure 40.29 (a) Example of Velpeau sling bandage being applied for conservative management of a left supraglenoid tubercle fracture in a one-year-old castrated male Poodle mix. *Source:* Courtesy of Dr. Meghan Lancaster. (b) Example of a commercially available Velpeau Sling (DogLeggs). *Source:* dogleggs.com.

flexion). The minimum of 90° of flexion is acceptable, the principle being to discourage weight bearing only. Adequate padding should also be ensured to prevent discomfort or ischemic injury. Additionally, the patient should be carefully monitored, as many animals may attempt weight bearing on the dorsal aspect of the immobilized carpus in time. Indications for this bandage include injuries of the mid- to proximal forelimb for which any weight bearing would be detrimental.

A Velpeau sling prevents weight bearing in the forelimb but is primarily used for shoulder immobilization. Indications for applying this bandage include select cases of medial shoulder instability (either for conservative management or as an adjunctive treatment following surgery), stabilization following reduction of a shoulder luxation, and conservative management of some scapular fractures. A Velpeau sling can be made out of traditional bandage materials with cast padding, conforming stretch gauze, elastic cohesive bandage (VetWrap/Coban 3M), and elastic tape (Elastikon, 3M) or commercially-available neoprene and Velcro material (DogLeggs) (Figure 40.29).

The forelimb is wrapped in cast padding and conforming stretch gauze, then the forelimb and cranial thorax are wrapped with the carpus, elbow, and shoulder in gentle flexion. As dogs are known to free themselves from the sling by pulling the forelimb out cranially, the author has found reverse tape stirrups useful, starting at the manus, extending along the metacarpus, and reversed at the level of the carpus to be secured along the metacarpus. The limb and thorax are wrapped with conforming stretch gauze as needed until secure, after which elastic cohesive bandage is applied. Security is increased by the addition of elastic tape, while being mindful to not excessively compress the thoracic cavity during bandaging.

An Ehmer sling is a non-weight-bearing sling designed to maintain coxofemoral hip reduction following craniodorsal luxation and closed reduction and to assist in

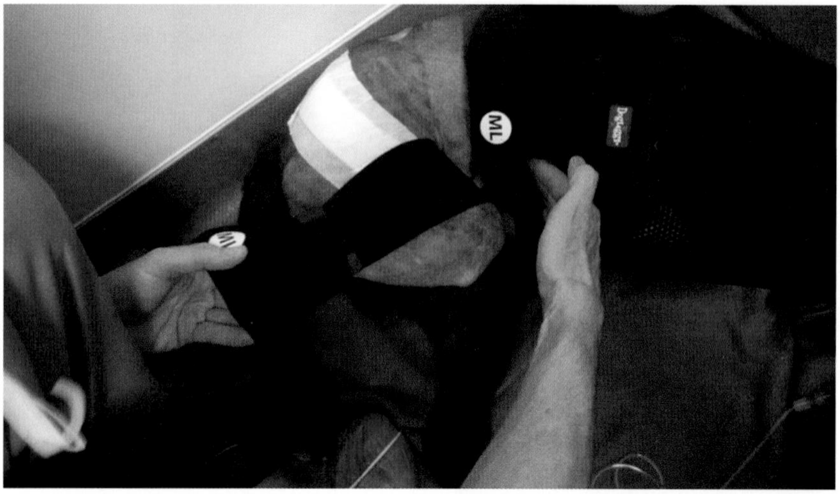

Figure 40.30 Use of a commercially available Ehmer Sling (DogLeggs) post-operatively in a canine with craniodorsal hip luxation and subsequent reduction. *Source:* © Seth Bleakley.

post-operative management of some types of femoral fractures (e.g., femoral neck) or acetabular fractures for which weight bearing is not ideal for the first few weeks after surgical repair (Figure 40.30).

After reduction, the metatarsus is padded, and the tarsus, stifle, and hip are flexed with slight abduction and internal rotation of the hip, which allows for healing of the presumably injured joint capsule. The metatarsus is secured to the thigh with circumferential application of cotton then non-elastic tape. This band is then secured to the abdomen to maintain hip flexion, with circumabdominal application of cotton then non-elastic tape.

Commercially available neoprene and Velcro Ehmer slings are available (DogLeggs).

Orthotic Devices

Veterinary orthotic and other adaptive devices have become more and more available in a wider range of constructs (Figure 40.31). Custom devices generally have a higher efficacy and a lower incidence of morbidity, although fabrication may be more costly. Similar to routine external coaptation, orthotic devices can be prescribed as a primary mode of stabilization or as ancillary support of a surgical repair. They are particularly useful in ligamentous and tendinous injuries. Unlike casts and splints, orthotic devices can be modified and adjusted to increase the range of motion as clinically dictated over time. They also do not require frequent bandage changes with replacement of cast padding, and they can be donned and doffed by the owner on a prescribed schedule. The same principles of the three-point corrective system apply, and care must be taken to avoid associated sores.

Frequency of Bandage Changes

The timing of changing any of these bandages is often dependent upon the reason for which the bandage is being applied. In the case of wound management, some types of primary contact layers require changing of the bandage more than once per day, whereas those applied for orthopedic stability, particularly while awaiting definitive surgery or treating a fracture conservatively to allow healing, may only require once weekly bandage changes. A good rule of thumb is to keep a list of patients who have bandages applied, since clients may not understand the dire circumstances that may result from neglecting the recommended bandage changes (Figure 40.32). If a list is kept, clients who have skipped a bandage change appointment may be contacted. Another tip is to have a standard "Bandage Care" document that is sent home with clients whose pet has a bandage applied, which will allow them to understand monitoring of their pet's bandage (e.g., to have it changed when wet, to never replace the bandage on their own, to watch for toes spreading).

A Note on Post-operative Use of External Coaptation

Factors affecting the decision to apply external coaptation following fracture repair include the nature of the fracture, the stability of the repair, the presence of wounds, the patient temperament, and ultimately, clinician preference. However, whether or not bandaging benefits post-operative swelling more than other rehabilitation therapy modalities has been investigated. In a prospective study of dogs undergoing tibial plateau leveling osteotomy, Unis et al. demonstrated no significant difference in swelling between the

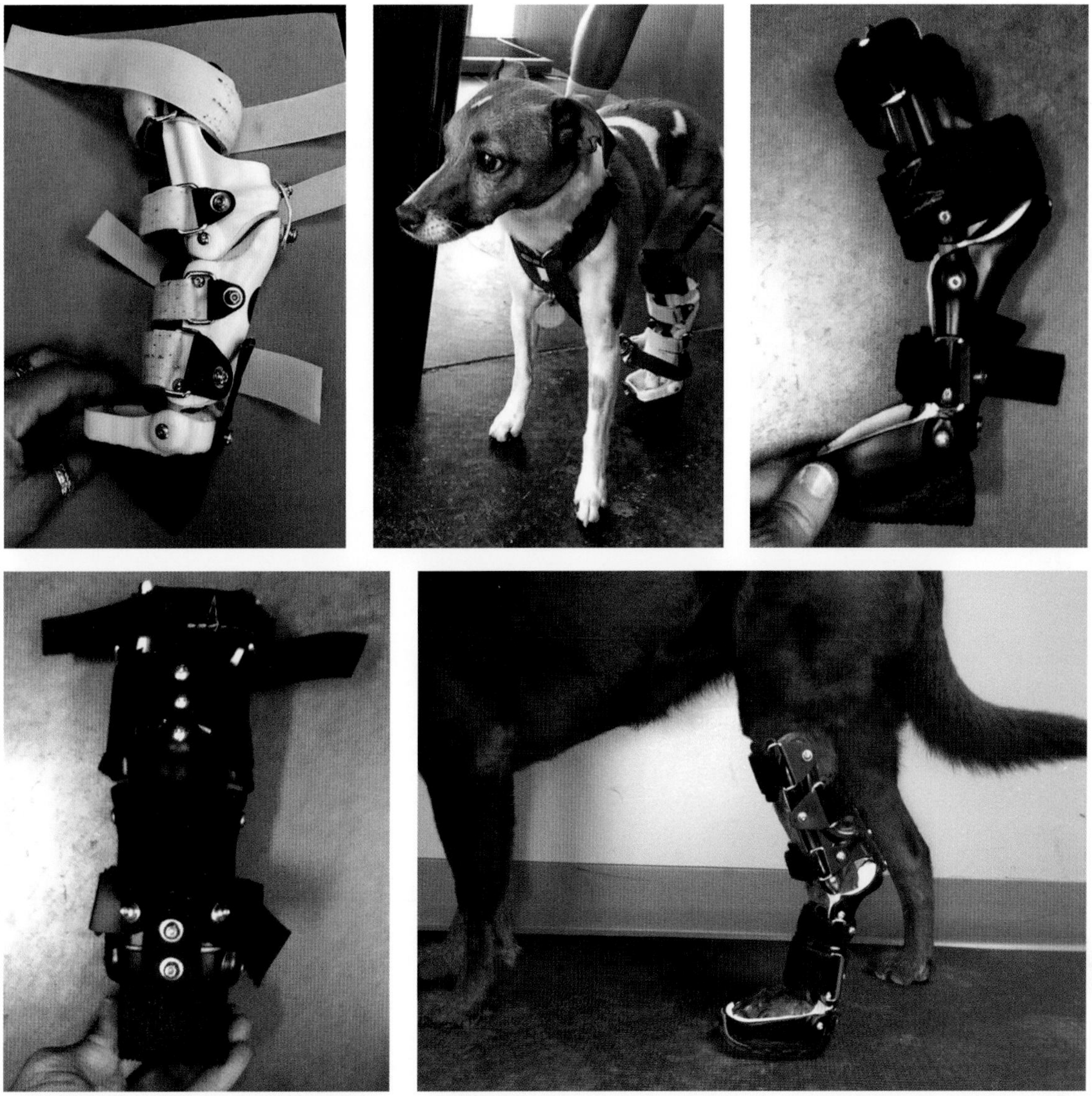

Figure 40.31 Examples of canine hindlimb custom orthotic devices (OrthoPets), which provide support while permitting control of joint motion through adjustable articulation. *Source:* © Seth Bleakley.

bandaged and unbandaged groups.[6] In a study of 24 dogs undergoing surgery for cranial cruciate ligament rupture, Rexing et al. assessed limb girth with cold compression, versus a modified Robert Jones bandage, versus cold compression with a bandage, versus microcurrent electrical therapy. Limb girth was assessed around the femur, stifle, and tarsus. Of the four groups, the modified Robert Jones bandage had the least effect with swelling at the level of the femur being significantly greater compared to the other groups. There was also greater swelling at the level of the stifle and tarsus, although measurements here were not statistically significant.[7] In a study of 21 dogs undergoing tibial plateau leveling osteotomy, Kieves et al. assessed weight bearing, stifle range of motion, and post-operative swelling at 12, 24, and 36 hours after cold compression, placement of a modified Robert Jones bandage, or a combination. There was no significant difference in weight bearing, range of motion, or limb swelling among the three groups. Although not statistically significant, the cold compression group, with or without a bandage, seemed to bear more weight.[8]

While stifle surgery may not reflect the variety of fracture repairs for which post-operative external coaptation may be pursued, a lack of benefit to post-operative swelling demonstrated in these studies may translate and aid decision-making following other surgeries. It would appear where there is stable fixation and a closed wound, forgoing external coaptation may be beneficial inasmuch as such permits access to the limb for cold compressive therapy. Other benefits of limb access include the opportunity for a

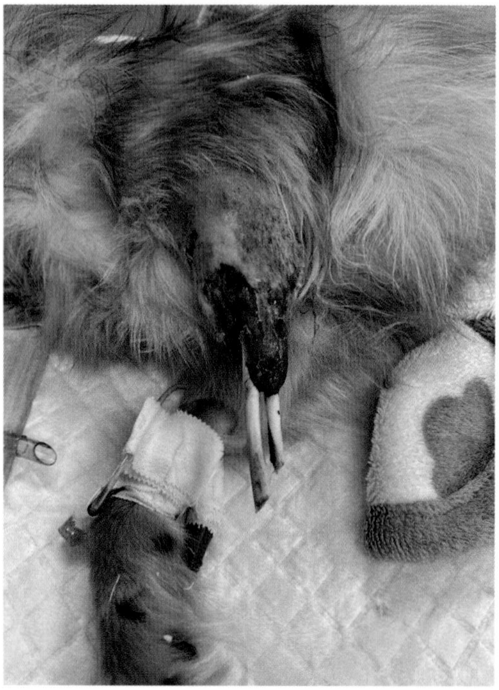

Figure 40.32 A two-year-old castrated male Chihuahua mix was presented to his primary care veterinarian for a closed left short oblique distal diaphyseal radius/ulna fracture, at which point a splint bandage was applied. No bandage changes were performed for two months. After eight weeks, the patient was presented to a specialty center for evaluation of fracture healing and bandage removal, and the distal aspect of the limb came off with the bandage. Bottomline: emphasize weekly bandage changes for soft tissue assessment, even if attempting to heal a fracture with external coaptation. *Source:* © Dr. Stephen C. Jones.

range of motion exercises, massage, therapeutic exercise, cold laser therapy, microcurrent electrical therapy, and other emerging rehabilitation modalities. Other benefits of avoiding post-operative external coaptation where possible include reduced muscle atrophy, reduced joint stiffness, and improved joint homeostasis. Ultimately, such benefits must be weighed against factors, such as fracture repair stability, patient compliance (sometimes a bandage is easier to maintain than an Elizabethan collar for incision protection), owner compliance, and clinical preference.

References

1 Anderson, D.M. and White, R.A. (2000). Ischemic bandage injuries: a case series and review of the literature. *Vet. Surg.* 29 (6): 488–498.

2 Hettrich, C.M., Gasinu, S., Beamer, B.S. et al. (2013). The effect of immobilization on the native and repaired tendon-to-bone interface. *J. Bone Joint Surg. Am.* 95 (10): 925–930.

3 Campbell, T.M., Reilly, K., Laneuville, O. et al. (2018). Bone replaces articular cartilage in the rat knee joint after prolonged immobilization. *Bone* 106: 42–51.

4 Iodence, A.E., Olsen, A.M., McGilvray, K.C. et al. (2018). Use of pressure mapping for quantitative analysis of pressure points induced by external coaptation of the distal portion of the pelvic limb of dogs. *Am. J. Vet. Res.* 79 (3): 317–323.

5 Tham, W., Sng, S., Lum, Y.M. et al. (2014). A look back in time: Sir Robert Jones, 'Father of Modern Orthopaedics'. *Malays. Orthop. J.* 8 (3): 37–41.

6 Unis, M.D., Roush, J.K., Bilicki, K.L. et al. (2010). Effect of bandaging on post-operative swelling after tibial plateau levelling osteotomy. *Vet. Comp. Orthop. Traumatol.* 23 (4): 240–244.

7 Rexing, J., Dunning, D., Siegel, A.M. et al. (2010). Effects of cold compression, bandaging, and microcurrent electrical therapy after cranial cruciate ligament repair in dogs. *Vet. Surg.* 39 (1): 54–58.

8 Kieves, N.R., Bergh, M.S., Zellner, E. et al. (2016). Pilot study measuring the effects of bandaging and cold compression therapy following tibial plateau levelling osteotomy. *J. Small Anim. Pract.* 57 (10): 543–547.

41

3D-Printing in Orthopedics

Paul Schwarzmann

Tierklinik Schwarzmann, Rankweil, Austria

Key Points

- 3D-printed patient specific guides (3DP-PSG) allow for an accurate execution of a surgical plan.
- The production of a 3DP-PSG consists of four steps: diagnostic imaging, 3D-data acquisition, guide design, and 3D-printing.
- The guide should be planned in a position where the interference to the soft tissue is minimal.
- In surgery, a correct "press-fit" of the guide on the bone is essential to achieve accuracy.
- Good knowledge of the performed surgery is needed to recognize a defective guide and continue the surgery conventionally.

Introduction

The use of three-dimensional (3D) printing, also referred to as "rapid prototyping" or "additive manufacturing," in a medical setting began in the 1980s in human medicine.[1] To the author's best knowledge, the use of 3D-printing in veterinary medicine was first described in 2003 for the assessment and preoperative planning for the treatment of bilateral pelvic limb deformities in a German Shepherd dog.[2] Nowadays, 3D-printing in veterinary surgery is used for several applications; while patient-specific saw guides are mainly used for deformity correction of long bones,[3–8] 3D-printed drill guides have various applications, such as the treatment of vertebral instability,[9–18] humeral intracondylar fissure,[19] ununited anconeal process (UAP),[20] and other procedures.

The basic concept of a 3D-printed, patient-specific surgical guide (3DP-PSG) is mostly the same: a negative imprint of the bone surface is created, which sits "press-fit" on the bone like a key in a keyhole. For instance, drill guides or saw guides direct either a drill or a saw in the preoperatively planned direction and thereby allow accurate execution of a surgical plan. In general, the production of a 3DP-PSG consists of four steps: obtaining imaging data of the patient through computed tomography (CT) or magnetic resonance imaging (MRI),[21] 3D-data acquisition from the obtained diagnostic imaging, guide design, and 3D-printing. Since 3D-printers are more affordable by now, a newer application of 3D-printing in veterinary medicine is surgical education and training.

The following chapter describes the development and process of a patient-specific, 3D-printed drill and saw guide, its use during surgery, the advantages and disadvantages of 3DP-PSGs, and the use of 3D-printing in surgical education and training.

Techniques in Small Animal Soft Tissue, Orthopedic, and Ophthalmic Surgery, First Edition. Edited by Kristin A. Coleman.

Companion website: www.wiley.com/go/coleman/surgeries

Production of a 3D-Printed Guide

Imaging and 3D-Data Acquisition

For the 3D-planning of a specific procedure and the design of a 3DP-PSG, it is necessary to obtain an accurate 3D model of the desired bone. It is possible to gain 3D-data from CT or MRI although CT has a higher accuracy for bone models and is, therefore, recommended.[22] For the CT scan, the desired bone should be positioned perpendicular to the CT gantry to avoid artifacts in the resulting 3D model. The slice thickness should be as thin as possible to get the highest resolution. Higher radiation settings in CT result in a higher accuracy of the resulting bone model.[23] The imaging data is exported as Digital Imaging and Communications in Medicine (DICOM) file format.[21]

The process of obtaining a 3D bone model from DICOM images is called segmentation. Several commercial and free open-source software programs are available to perform this task. Commonly used commercial software programs for segmentation of CT data are Mimics (Materialise, Leuven, Belgium),[5,7,24,25] and OsiriX (Pixmeo, Bernex, Switzerland).[6,8,14,15,19,26] A free, open-source software commonly used for segmentation is 3D slicer (https://www.slicer.org).[27,28] Other free, open-source software used by the author is the software Horos (https://horosproject.org) and ITK-SNAP (http://www.itksnap.org).[20,29] The main differences between the mentioned software programs are the user friendliness, the tools available for segmentation, and the operating system it runs on. The decision of which software to use should be based on the needs, experience and personal preference of the user, the computing power and the operating system of the personal computer (PC), and the costs of the software.

With most of these software programs, bones can be either automatically or manually segmented. For automatic segmentation, a region of interest (ROI) needs to be selected and certain structures can be isolated based on their gray value (threshold).[30] The higher the threshold is set, the brighter the gray value of the pixels that are selected. Some software offers threshold presets for bone in CT scans, which may be sufficient in most cases but can possibly lead to insufficient accuracy of the resulting bone model since the gray value of bone can depend on the CT scanner, the ROI, and the patient itself.[31] Therefore, the selection of the threshold value is a subjective setting and can have a high influence on the accuracy of the resulting bone model. A threshold value that is selected too low results in an increased thickness of the cortex and artifacts in the resulting bone model. On the other hand, if the selected threshold value is too high, it can lead to voids in the bone model (Figure 41.1).[23] If translated to a patient-specific guide, a lower threshold leads to a guide that is too big and might sit loosely on the bone. Alternatively, a higher threshold leads to a smaller guide, which might not fit on the bone because the contact surface of the guide is a negative of the bone model. Manual segmentation allows the user to select or deselect pixels on each slice of the imaging data regardless of their gray value and can be very helpful to correct artifacts after automatic segmentation or to isolate specific bones. After segmentation, the software creates a 3D-mesh, which can then be exported as a Standard Tesselation Language (STL) file. The resulting file can then be imported into a Computer Aided Design (CAD) software to make further changes or design a patient-specific guide. The STL file can also be imported into a designated printing software to prepare it for 3D-printing.

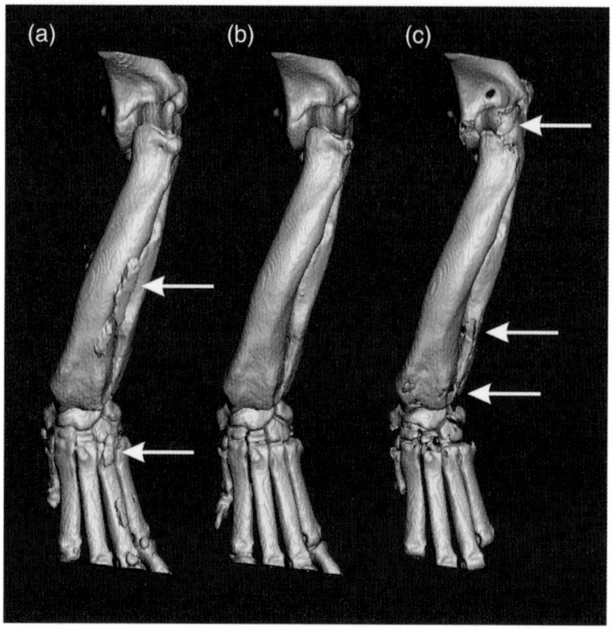

Figure 41.1 Different threshold settings and their influence on the resulting 3D model. The same imaging data was segmented with different threshold settings. In (a), the threshold was set too low, resulting in artifacts (arrows). In (b), the threshold was set correctly. In (c), the threshold was set too high, resulting in voids in the resulting bone model. *Source:* © Paul Schwarzmann.

Guide Design

The two most common applications of 3DP-PSGs are drill guides and saw guides. Drill guides are used to place screws or Kirschner Wires (K-wires) accurately in the bone for many different applications such as the stabilization of vertebrae,[9–18] the treatment of a humeral intracondylar fissure,[19] or fixation of an UAP.[20] Saw guides are used to make accurate cuts to create specific bone wedges; e.g., in the correction of angular and rotational deformities of the antebrachium[4–7] or the femur.[8]

Many different CAD-software programs can be used for pre-procedure planning and guide design. Since there is no clear tendency toward one specific software in the current literature, the decision of which software is used depends on the functions needed for a specific application, the costs of the software, the computing power of the PC, and personal preference. A commercial software program that is frequently used is 3-Matic (Materialise, Leuven, Belgium).[25,32,33] Free software programs that can be used are Meshmixer (Autodesk Inc., San Rafael, CA, USA)[5,20] or Tinkercad (Autodesk Inc., San Rafael, CA, USA).[27] Regardless of which software is used, the basic principles of designing a 3DP-PSG are the same. However, there are additional approaches on how to plan a surgery three dimensionally than the method described in the following paragraphs.

The principle for both, drill and saw guides, is a "press-fit" on the bone surface allowing the transfer of a surgical plan accurately to surgery. That means that there is only one possible location and orientation of the guide on the bone. After importing the STL file of the bone model in a CAD software, the first step of designing a guide is planning the surgery. This is done by defining either cuts for a saw guide or holes for a drill guide on the bone model.

When designing a drill guide, the first step is to digitally place one or several cylinders in the desired position where a hole should be drilled or a K-wire should be placed (Figure 41.2a). These cylinders stay in this position and are subtracted from the final guide (Figure 41.2b). The diameter of a cylinder should be selected slightly larger (0.1–0.2 mm) than the drill or the K-wire to avoid friction between the guide and the instrument and to counteract a slight shrinkage of the guide during the printing process. It is also possible to create a hole big enough to fit a standard

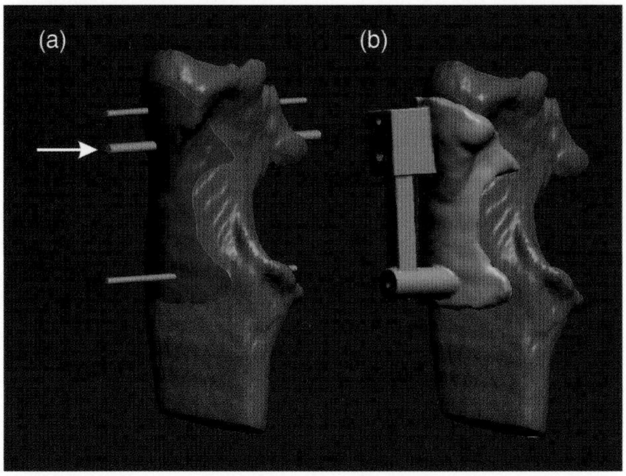

Figure 41.2 Design of a drill guide for the treatment of an ununited anconeal process (UAP). The cylinders in (a) represent two K-wires and the drill hole (arrow) for a screw to reattach the anconeal process. The cylinders are then subtracted from the final guide (b). *Source:* © Paul Schwarzmann.

drill sleeve.[34] In addition to the cylinder representing a drill hole, it can be favorable in many cases to add smaller cylinders representing K-wires to attach the guide to the bone while drilling. It is important that all cylinders are parallel to each other to allow the guide to be removed in surgery without removing the K-wires.

The design of a saw guide is more complex than the design of a drill guide and requires a good understanding of the principles of the performed surgery. When designing a saw guide for the correction of an angular limb deformity (ALD), it is essential to understand the Center of Rotation and Angulation (CORA) principles.[35]

In cases where a contralateral bone with a physiological conformation is present, this bone can be mirrored and used as a reference.[4] To define the cuts for a closing wedge ostectomy, the proximal joint surfaces of the affected and the unaffected, mirrored bone model are superimposed. A rectangular cuboid, which is generated in the software, is placed parallel to the proximal joint surfaces representing the guide for the proximal cut (Figure 41.3a). Additionally, a plane can be placed temporarily on the distal aspect of this cuboid to visualize the cut. For a closing wedge osteotomy, this plane should cut through a closing CORA. The cuboid and the affected bone are then combined and duplicated before the distal joint surfaces of the duplicated bone, and the mirrored, unaffected bone are aligned in all planes (Figure 41.3b). When the cuboid of the original affected bone is now separated and combined with the duplicated bone, this results in two cuboids representing the guides for a closing wedge osteotomy. If not previously done, two planes should be placed on the inner side of those cuboids. The cuboids are moved proximally and distally with the respective planes until the planes intersect at the closing CORA (Figure 41.3c). During this movement, the angle and the rotation of the cuboid must not be changed. If the wedge between those planes is now cut out and the cuboids are superimposed digitally, the ALD should be corrected in all planes (Figure 41.3d,e). However, some translation without altering any angle might be necessary to allow enough contact between the cortices. By simulating the osteotomy digitally, it is possible to assess the result, make corrections to the guide, and print the corrected bone for pre-bending a plate.

Other approaches to the design of a saw guide for the correction of an ALD include slots for the saw blade and a reduction guide. However, if a reduction guide is used, this compromises the flexibility of the reduction with regard to rotation and translation. A reduction guide is also needed if an open wedge osteotomy is performed. Therefore, the correction must be performed digitally and K-wires for the reduction guide need to be defined on the corrected bone. Afterwards, the bone with the K-wires in place is brought back to its original conformation, and a cutting guide is designed around the previously placed K-wires.

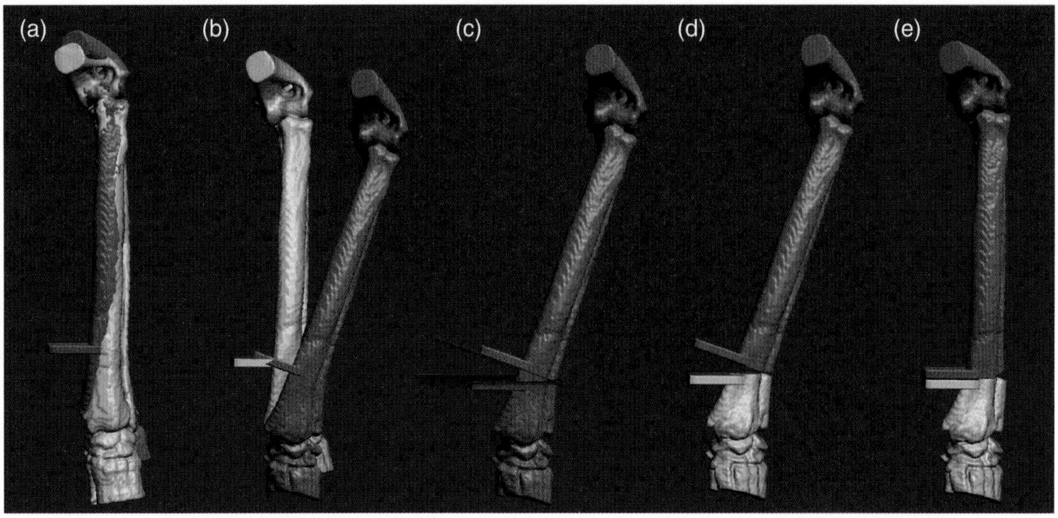

Figure 41.3 Defining the cuts for the correction of an ALD with a closing wedge osteotomy: (a) the proximal joint surfaces of the mirrored, physiological bone (gray) and the deformed bone (red) are superimposed and the proximal cut (cuboid) is placed parallel to the proximal joint surface; (b) the original deformed bone (gray) is combined with the proximal cut, duplicated and the distal joint surface of the copy (red) is aligned with the physiological bone resulting in one deformed bone aligned in the proximal joint surface and one deformed bone aligned in the distal joint surface. (c) Two planes are placed on the inner side of the cuboids representing the cuts. The cuboid of the original deformed bone that was proximally aligned with the physiological bone is separated and moved until the two planes cut on the opposite side of the bone. The guide can now be designed or a digital cut is made to evaluate the correction. (d) Two cuts are made digitally along the inner side of the cuboid. (e) The two cuboids are aligned together with the respective bone part resulting in a corrected bone. *Source:* © Paul Schwarzmann.

The surface, on which the guide should fit can either be selected with a "paint brush" tool (Figure 41.4a) (e.g., in Meshmixer) or a 3D object (e.g., a cuboid), is placed on the area of which the bone is later subtracted (e.g., Tinkercad).[27] In the first case, the area needs to be extruded and separated from the bone afterwards (Figure 41.4b). Areas, where soft tissues cannot be removed during surgery (e.g., joint capsule), should be spared because insufficient soft tissue removal compromises the accuracy of the guide significantly.[8] However, it is favorable to include significant landmarks of the bone that can easily be freed from soft tissue to allow a better press-fit and precise placement of the guide. While designing a saw guide, special attention needs to be paid to leave enough space for the implant to fit onto the desired area of the bone. The next step after creating the contact surface is to add support structures, such as bigger cylinders around the smaller cylinders for a drill guide or cuboids to make the guide less fragile. When designing a saw guide, cylinders representing K-wires are placed on the guide and subtracted from it. Those K-wires are used during surgery to attach the guide securely onto the bone while the cut is made. Additional K-wires can be planned and angled in a cross-pinning fashion to allow temporary fixation of the osteotomy. The different parts of the guide are combined and exported as an STL file for 3D-printing.

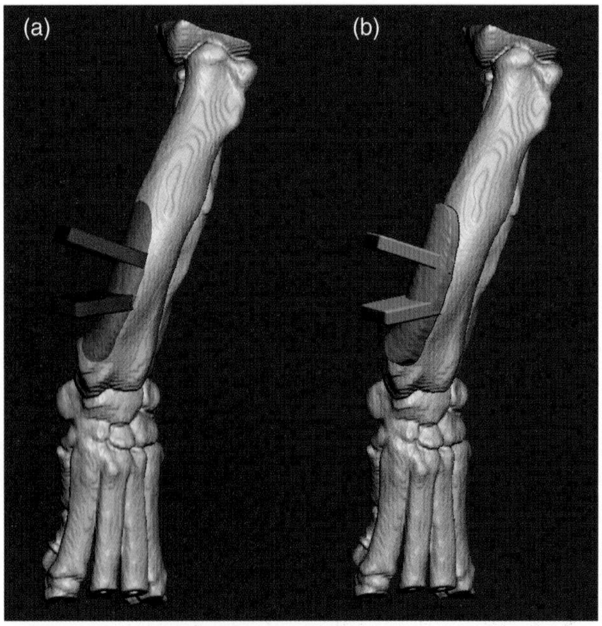

Figure 41.4 The surface on which the guide should fit is selected with a "paint brush" tool (a), extruded and combined with the cuts (b). *Source:* © Paul Schwarzmann.

3D-Printing Techniques

There are a variety of 3D-printing techniques that are all based on adding material layer by layer. The most commonly used techniques for producing 3DP-PSG are fused deposition modeling (FDM), stereolithography (SLA), and LCD resin printing. Other techniques used in veterinary medicine

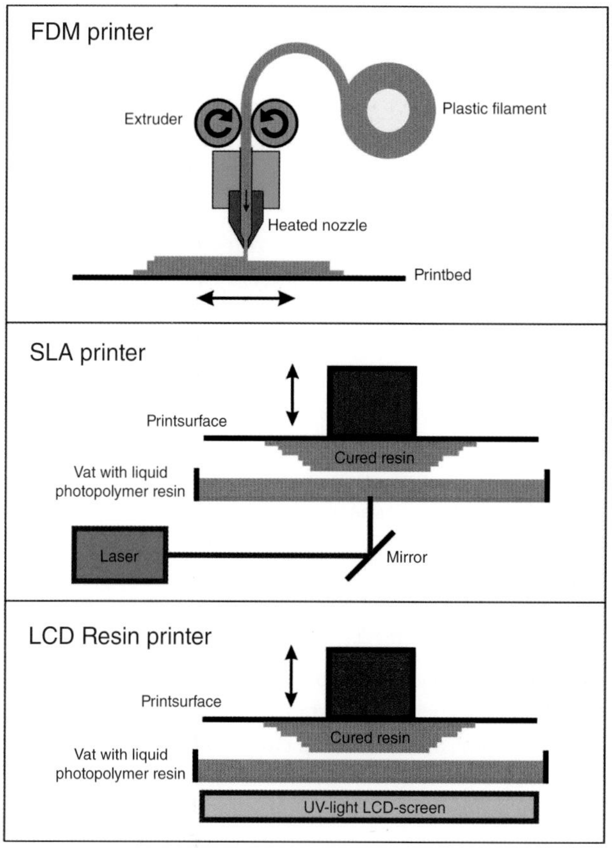

Figure 41.5 Schematic illustration of FDM, SLA, and LCD resin printers. *Source:* © Paul Schwarzmann.

are among other things metal printing technologies (electric beam melting and selective laser sintering), which are used for the production of patient-specific implants[7] and inkjet/polyjet (IJ/PJ) printers.[10,16,25]

FDM is based on melting and extruding thermoplastic through a nozzle (Figure 41.5). It is affordable and easy to use. However, support structures are needed in most cases[36] and it is not possible to steam sterilize most materials[21] which is one reason why SLA and LCD resin printing is more often used for surgical guides. There is a wide range of thermoplastics used for printing surgical guides, such as polylactic acid (PLA), acrylonitrile butadiene styrene (ABS), and several other materials with different mechanical and thermal properties.[37] While PLA and ABS deform significantly after steam sterilization, there are some materials, such as GreenTEC Pro (Extrudr, Lauterach, Austria), which show a relatively low deviation when steam sterilized.[37] In veterinary orthopedics, FDM is mostly used for printing bone models to visualize deformities, for pre-procedure training, or for pre-bending implants.[21] The author uses the FDM printer Prusa Mini+ (Prusa Research a.s., Prague, Czech Republic), which is very easy to use, can print with various materials, and has a layer thickness of 0.05–0.25 mm (https://www.prusa3d.com). A disadvantage of this printer is the relatively small print volume, which is sufficient for most applications but can be too small for printing larger models.

SLA and LCD resin printing are both based on the polymerization of a liquid resin in a vat using UV light emitted either from a laser (SLA) or a screen (LCD resin printer) under the vat (Figure 41.5). One advantage of SLA and LCD resin printers is the higher quality of the print compared to FDM printing.[36] It is also possible to use a large variety of materials, such as autoclavable, biocompatible, and transparent materials, like the Dental SG Resin (Formlabs, Sommerville, MA, USA), that are frequently used for surgical guides.[8,11,13–15,19,32] A disadvantage of SLA and LCD resin printing is the time-consuming but necessary cleanup and curing of the model.[36] The author uses the LCD resin printer, Phrozen Sonic Mighty 4K (Phrozen Technology, Hsinchu City, Taiwan), which offers a large build volume. It has a layer thickness of 0.01–0.3 mm and an xy resolution of 0.05 mm (https://phrozen3d.com).

In general, it can be said that it is beneficial to have both an SLA or LCD resin printer and an FDM printer. This allows to print accurate surgical guides with a resin printer and bone models for pre-procedure training with an FDM printer.

To print an STL file, it needs to be prepared with a print software and converted into the respective print format. Therefore, various commercial and free software programs are available, and most printers either come with a designated software or recommend a software to be used. Free software available for FDM printing is Ultimaker Cura (Ultimaker B.V., Utrecht, Netherlands). Free software for SLA or LCD resin printing is Chitubox (Chitubox, Shenzhen, China). With this software, the position of the model in the printer and the resolution can be defined, supports can be added manually or automatically, and the information for the printer is exported in the respective print format.

Surgical Procedure

When performing a surgical procedure with a 3DP-PSG, a standard approach to the desired area of the bone is performed. The approach should already be considered when designing the guide. One of the most important steps is to remove all soft tissues from the bone in the area where the guide will be placed because insufficient soft tissue removal is considered one of the main factors for inaccuracy.[8,13,19,25] When placing the guide on the bone, special attention should be paid to a correct "press-fit." When the position and orientation of the guide is considered satisfactory, it can be secured to the bone using K-wires through the designated holes, which are then shortened, to allow drilling or sawing (Figures 41.6, 41.7, and 41.8a).

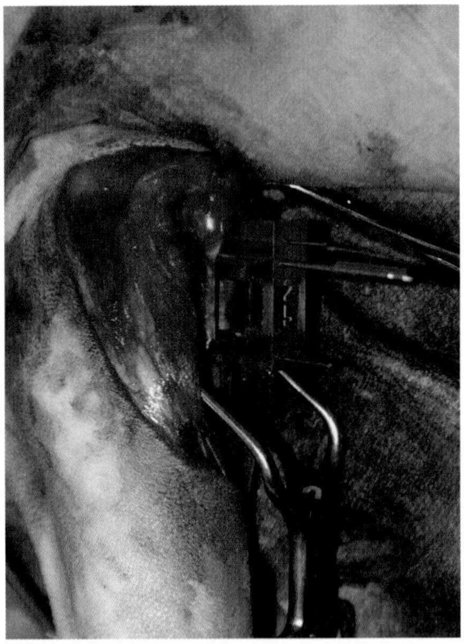

Figure 41.6 Application of a drill guide on the caudal aspect of the ulna for the reattachment of an ununited anconeal process. *Source:* © Paul Schwarzmann.

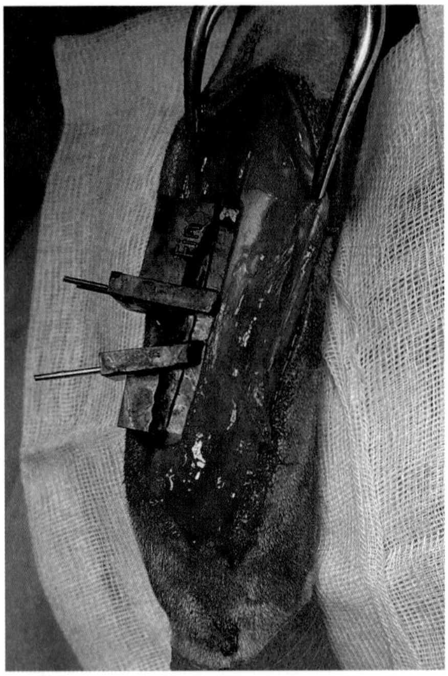

Figure 41.7 Application of a saw guide on the radius for the correction of an ALD. *Source:* © Paul Schwarzmann.

In the case of a drill guide, the drill can now be inserted into the designated hole. Once the drill is inserted in the guide, it is possible to review the trajectory of the drill bit with fluoroscopy. While drilling, special attention needs to be paid on any movement of the guide. After drilling, the guide can be removed, and a screw can be inserted in the drill hole.

When using a saw guide for a closing wedge osteotomy, the cuts are made with an oscillating saw along the given planes and the guide is cut before cutting the bone (Figure 41.8b,c). During this step, it is important to flush and suction to avoid too much debris from the guide remaining in the surgical site. After both cuts are made, the osteotomy is reduced by superimposing both cuboids. To get accurate anatomical reduction, translational movement is possible, but the axial and rotational alignment should be maintained. As soon as the reduction of the osteotomy is satisfactory, point-to-point bone reduction forceps can be applied to the guide to avoid movement (Figure 41.8d). Care should be taken not to apply too much pressure to avoid fracturing the guide. If holes are created for temporary fixation, K-wires can be used to cross-pin the osteotomy (Figure 41.8e). The osteotomy is now secured with an implant following the AO principles of fracture management.[38] Since an osteotomy equals a transverse or short oblique fracture, axial compression can be applied to increase stability and allow primary bone healing.[38] However, in some cases, the end-to-end contact of the cortices can be too small for applying compression. This is mainly the case in the correction of antebrachial ALDs due to the oval shape of the radius, and rotational correction is often necessary. After fixating the osteotomy, the guide is removed, and routine closure of the wound is performed. If a correction of the radius is performed, an osteotomy or ostectomy of the ulna should be performed[7] to facilitate movement of the fragments of the radius and to allow restoration of congruence in the elbow joint in cases where incongruence is present.[39]

If an open wedge osteotomy is performed, the guide is applied, and a single cut is made the same way as described for a closing wedge osteotomy. The guide is then removed while the K-wires remain in the bone. By inserting the K-wires in the designated holes of the reduction guide, the bone segments are aligned. The osteotomy can now be secured in this position using a bone plate.

Advantages and Disadvantages of 3D-Printing in Veterinary Orthopedics

A large review in human medicine showed several advantages of 3D-printing in orthopedics[40]: the possibility to print 3D-anatomical models allows the surgeon to better understand the pathology, to train the procedure on an accurate model, and to pre-contour implants before surgery, which results in a shorter time in the operating room. The accuracy of 3D-printed guides is generally considered to be high. This is especially favorable to prevent iatrogenic trauma, such as in spinal surgery,[27] and when placing a screw close to a joint, such as in the treatment of a humeral intracondylar fissure.[19] High accuracy also allows the surgeon to perform limb alignment correction in complex antebrachial angular limb deformities.[3–7] Assessing radial

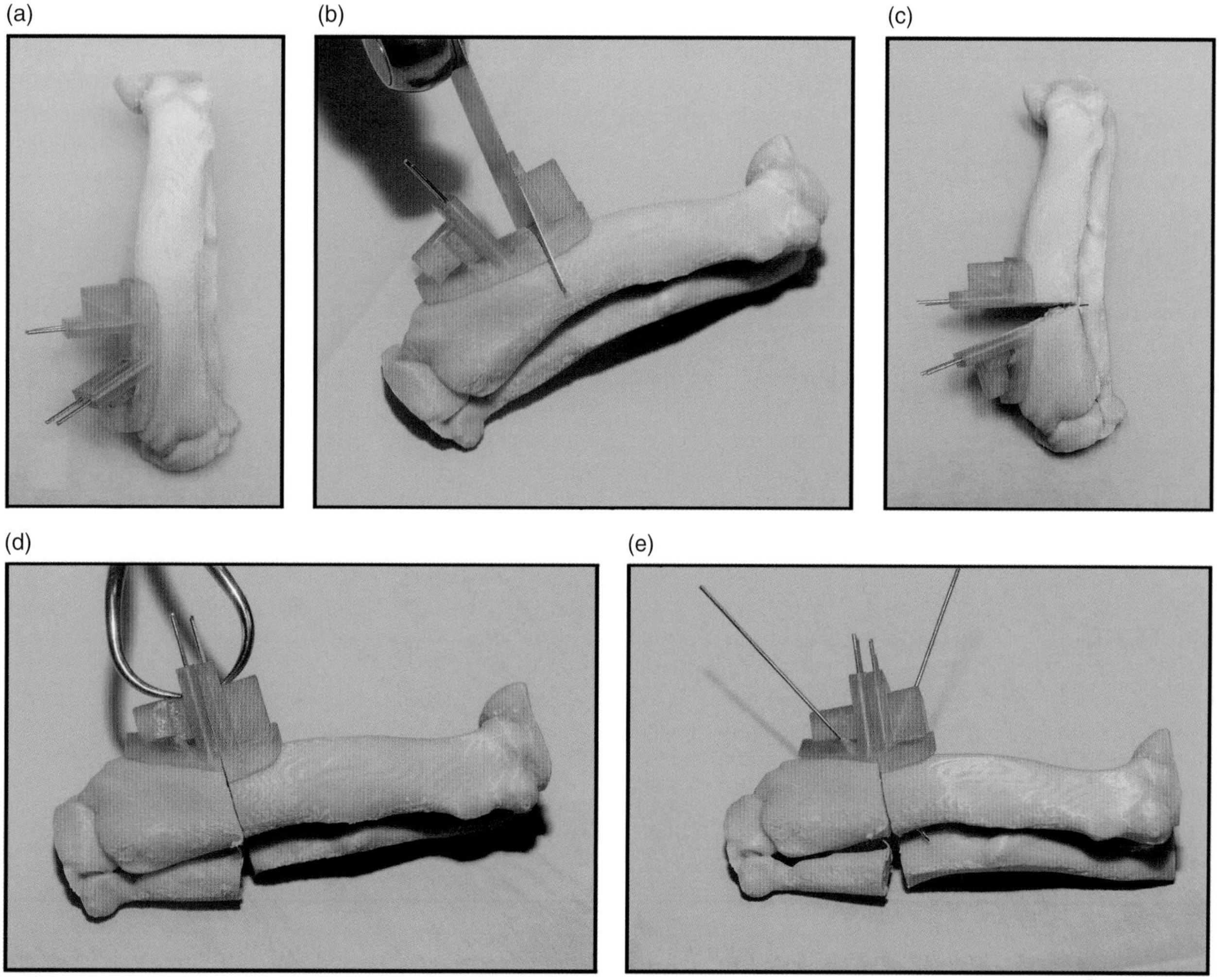

Figure 41.8 Surgical procedure of correcting an ALD with a 3D-printed saw guide simulated on a plastic bone: (a) the guide is placed "press-fit" on the bone and attached with K-wires through the designated holes; (b) the guide and the bone are cut with an oscillating saw along the given planes; (c) the wedge is removed; (d) the osteotomy is reduced by superimposing the planes of the guide. Thereby, translation is possible as long as the angles and the rotation are maintained, as given by the guide. The guide is then temporarily locked in place with point-to-point bone reduction forceps; (e) two K-wires are inserted into the designated holes of the guide to keep the osteotomy reduced while an implant is applied. The bone is printed with PLA with an FDM printer, and the guide is printed with an LCD resin printer. *Source:* © Paul Schwarzmann.

valgus in cases of an antebrachial ALD with two-dimensional radiographical measurements is highly inaccurate when significant radial torsion is present.[4] In these cases, it is possible to accurately assess all planes of a deformity when using 3D-imaging.[4]

One main disadvantage of 3DP-PSG is the time needed for the design and the production of the guide.[41] The time needed to design a 3DP-PSG is highly dependent on the complexity of the case, whether it is outsourced or designed in-house, the experience of the person designing the guide, and the type of the 3D-printer.[21] The time needed to produce the guide should always be weighted with the urgency of the procedure. While guides can be helpful for elective procedures or for stable patients, the time needed to produce the guides is too long for emergency situations. In the author's experience, the time needed to design a guide takes around three to four hours and up to eight hours in complex cases. The printing time varies with the size of the guide and whether an anatomical model is printed additionally or not. It varies between 2 and 4 hours for a smaller guide and up to 15–20 hours for a complete print of a medium to large bone model.

To allow accurate fit of a patient-specific guide, adequate soft tissue dissection is necessary in the area where the guide should be placed,[21] which causes additional trauma. This is especially relevant when designing the guide and selecting the surface where it should be placed during surgery. Easy positioning of the guide should be weighed against too much soft tissue trauma. Inadequate soft tissue dissection or a wrong selection of the contact area of the guide could lead to a higher inaccuracy of the guide. An important rule with the use of 3D-printed surgical guides is that the surgeon should have enough experience to recognize defective guides[40] and should be able to continue the surgery in the traditional way if the guide breaks or is defective.

Another big advantage of 3D-printing in veterinary orthopedics, in addition to 3DP-PSGs, is the possibility to practice specific procedures on plastic bones. Since training on cadavers is often limited by the number and availability of precisely-sized cadavers, 3D-printing allows the printing of plastic bones for surgical training. In contrast to commercially available plastic bones, 3D-printed bones are cheap and easily accessible. It is either possible to practice procedures on generic physiological bones (e.g., femoral head ostectomy, tibial plateau leveling osteotomy, and vertebral stabilization) or to train on bones with pathologic conformations (e.g., distal femoral osteotomy for varus deformity, and ALD correction) generated from a specific patient's limb CT scan. Thereby, it is possible to print bones from an actual patient allowing the surgeon to rehearse a complex procedure repeatedly in advance of the surgical procedure. The 3D-printing technique mostly used for simulating surgical procedures is FDM-printing since it provides a realistic bone model. When printing with an FDM printer, an interior structure is automatically created in most cases, which represents the medullary canal. Most filament materials also provide enough flexibility to withstand the forces applied by drilling, sawing, or inserting a K-wire without fracturing the model, which happens frequently with most materials used in a resin printer. However, especially when a saw is used on the model, specific materials with a higher heat resistance should be used to avoid melting of the material.

References

1 Hespel, A.M. (2018). Three-dimensional printing role in neurologic disease. *Vet. Clin. North Am. Small Anim. Pract.* 48 (1): 221–229.

2 Harrysson, O.L.A., Cormier, D.R., Marcellin-Little, D.J. et al. (2003). Rapid prototyping for treatment of canine limb deformities. *Rapid Prototyp. J.* 9 (1): 37–42.

3 Roh, Y., Cho, C., Ryu, C. et al. (2021). Comparison between novice and experienced surgeons performing corrective osteotomy with patient-specific guides in dogs based on resulting position accuracy. *Vet. Sci.* 8 (3): 40, 1–9.

4 Worth, A., Crosse, K., and Kersley, A. (2019). Computer-assisted surgery using 3D printed saw guides for acute correction of antebrachial angular limb deformities in dogs. *Vet. Comp. Orthop. Traumatol.* 32 (3): 241–249.

5 Kim, J., Song, J., Kim, S.Y. et al. (2020). Single oblique osteotomy for correction of congenital radial head luxation with concurrent complex angular limb deformity in a dog: a case report. *J. Vet. Sci.* 21 (4): e62, 1–7.

6 Longo, F., Penelas, A., Gutbrod, A. et al. (2019). Three-dimensional computer-assisted corrective osteotomy with a patient-specific surgical guide for an antebrachial limb deformity in two dogs. *Schweiz Arch. Tierheilkd* 161 (7): 473–479.

7 Carwardine, D.R., Gosling, M.J., Burton, N.J. et al. (2021). Three-dimensional-printed patient-specific osteotomy guides, repositioning guides and titanium plates for acute correction of antebrachial limb deformities in dogs. *Vet. Comp. Orthop. Traumatol.* 34 (1): 43–52.

8 Hall, E.L., Baines, S., Bilmont, A. et al. (2019). Accuracy of patient-specific three-dimensional-printed osteotomy and reduction guides for distal femoral osteotomy in dogs with medial patella luxation. *Vet. Surg.* 48 (4): 584–591.

9 Fujioka, T., Nakata, K., Nishida, H. et al. (2019). A novel patient-specific drill guide template for stabilization of thoracolumbar vertebrae of dogs: cadaveric study and clinical cases. *Vet. Surg.* 48 (3): 336–342.

10 Fujioka, T., Nakata, K., Nakano, Y. et al. (2020). Accuracy and efficacy of a patient-specific drill guide template system for lumbosacral junction fixation in medium and small dogs: cadaveric study and clinical cases. *Front. Vet. Sci.* 6: 494.

11 Hamilton-Bennett, S.E., Oxley, B., and Behr, S. (2018). Accuracy of a patient-specific 3D printed drill guide for placement of cervical transpedicular screws. *Vet. Surg.* 47 (2): 236–242.

12 Yu, Y., Kang, J., Kim, N. et al. (2022). Accuracy of a patient-specific 3D-printed drill guide for placement of bicortical screws in atlantoaxial ventral stabilization in dogs. *PLoS One* 17 (8): e0272336.

13 Toni, C., Oxley, B., Clarke, S. et al. (2021). Accuracy of placement of pedicle screws in the lumbosacral region of dogs using 3D-printed patient-specific drill guides. *Vet. Comp. Orthop. Traumatol.* 34 (1): 53–58.

14 Elford, J.H., Oxley, B., and Behr, S. (2020). Accuracy of placement of pedicle screws in the thoracolumbar spine of dogs with spinal deformities with three-dimensionally printed patient-specific drill guides. *Vet. Surg.* 49 (2): 347–353.

15 Toni, C., Oxley, B., and Behr, S. (2020). Atlanto-axial ventral stabilisation using 3D-printed patient-specific drill guides for placement of bicortical screws in dogs. *J. Small Anim. Pract.* 61 (10): 609–616.

16 Kamishina, H., Sugawara, T., Nakata, K. et al. (2019). Clinical application of 3D printing technology to the

surgical treatment of atlantoaxial subluxation in small breed dogs. *PLoS One* 14 (5): e0216445.

17 Gilman, O., Escauriaza, L., Ogden, D. et al. (2022). Thoracolumbar spinal stabilization with three dimensional-printed drill guides and pre-contoured polyaxial bone plates. *Vet. Comp. Orthop. Traumatol.* 36 (1): 46–52.

18 Mathiesen, C.B., de la Puerta, B., Groth, A.M. et al. (2018). Ventral stabilization of thoracic kyphosis through bilateral intercostal thoracotomies using SOP (String of Pearls) plates contoured after a 3-dimensional print of the spine. *Vet. Surg.* 47 (6): 843–851.

19 Easter, T.G., Bilmont, A., Pink, J. et al. (2020). Accuracy of three-dimensional printed patient-specific drill guides for treatment of canine humeral intracondylar fissure. *Vet. Surg.* 49 (2): 363–372.

20 Schwarzmann, P. and Haimel, G. (2021). Chirurgische Stabilisierung eines isolierten Processus anconaeus (IPA) mithilfe einer patientenspezifischen, 3D-gedruckten Bohrführung – zwei Fallberichte. *Wiener Tierärztliche Monatsschrift Vet. Med. Austr.* 108: 303.

21 Altwal, J., Wilson, C.H., and Griffon, D.J. (2022). Applications of 3-dimensional printing in small-animal surgery: a review of current practices. *Vet. Surg.* 51 (1): 34–51.

22 White, D., Chelule, K.L., and Seedhom, B.B. (2008). Accuracy of MRI vs CT imaging with particular reference to patient specific templates for total knee replacement surgery. *Int. J. Med. Robot. Comput. Assist. Surg.* 4 (3): 224–231.

23 Fitzwater, K.L., Marcellin-Little, D.J., Harrysson, O.L.A. et al. (2011). Evaluation of the effect of computed tomography scan protocols and freeform fabrication methods on bone biomodel accuracy. *Am. J. Vet. Res.* 72 (9): 1178–1185.

24 Beer, P., Park, B.H., Steffen, F. et al. (2020). Influence of a customized three-dimensionally printed drill guide on the accuracy of pedicle screw placement in lumbosacral vertebrae: an ex vivo study. *Vet. Surg.* 49 (5): 977–988.

25 Mariani, C.L., Zlotnick, J.A., Harrysson, O. et al. (2021). Accuracy of three-dimensionally printed animal-specific drill guides for implant placement in canine thoracic vertebrae: a cadaveric study. *Vet. Surg.* 50 (2): 294–302.

26 Oxley, B. (2017). Bilateral shoulder arthrodesis in a Pekinese using three-dimensional printed patient-specific osteotomy and reduction guides. *Vet. Comp. Orthop. Traumatol.* 30 (3): 230–236.

27 McCarthy, D.A., Granger, L.A., Aulakh, K.S. et al. (2022). Accuracy of a drilling with a custom 3D printed guide or free-hand technique in canine experimental sacroiliac luxations. *Vet. Surg.* 51 (1): 182–190.

28 Kang, J., Lee, S., Kim, N. et al. (2022). Minimally invasive mini-hemilaminectomy-corpectomy in cadaveric dogs: evaluation of the accuracy and safety of a three-dimensionally printed patient-specific surgical guide. *BMC Vet. Res.* 18 (1): 271.

29 Yushkevich, P.A., Piven, J., Hazlett, H.C. et al. (2006). User-guided 3D active contour segmentation of anatomical structures: significantly improved efficiency and reliability. *NeuroImage* 31 (3): 1116–1128.

30 Hespel, A.M., Wilhite, R., and Hudson, J. (2014). Invited review-applications for 3D printers in veterinary medicine: 3D printing in veterinary medicine. *Vet. Radiol. Ultrasound* 55 (4): 347–358.

31 Choi, J.Y., Choi, J.H., Kim, N.K. et al. (2002). Analysis of errors in medical rapid prototyping models. *Int. J. Oral Maxillofacial Surg.* 31 (1): 23–32.

32 Guevar, J., Bleedorn, J., Cullum, T. et al. (2021). Accuracy and safety of three-dimensionally printed animal-specific drill guides for thoracolumbar vertebral column instrumentation in dogs: bilateral and unilateral designs. *Vet. Surg.* 50 (2): 336–344.

33 Darrow, B.G., Snowdon, K.A., and Hespel, A. (2021). Accuracy of patient-specific 3D printed drill guides in the placement of a canine coxofemoral toggle pin through a minimally invasive approach. *Vet. Comp. Orthop. Traumatol.* 34 (1): 1–8.

34 Bongers, J.J., Wilkinson, N., Kurihara, M. et al. (2022). Accuracy of lumbosacral pedicle screw placement in dogs: a novel 3D printed patient-specific drill guide versus freehand technique in novice and expert surgeons. *Vet. Comp. Orthop. Traumatol.* 35 (6): 381–389.

35 Fox, D.B., Tomlinson, J.L., Cook, J.L. et al. (2006). Principles of uniapical and biapical radial deformity correction using dome osteotomies and the Center of Rotation of Angulation Methodology in dogs. *Vet. Surg.* 35 (1): 67–77.

36 Wilhite, R. and Wölfel, I. (2019). 3D printing for veterinary anatomy: an overview. *Anatom. Histol. Embryol.* 48 (6): 609–620.

37 Dautzenberg, P., Volk, H.A., Huels, N. et al. (2021). The effect of steam sterilization on different 3D printable materials for surgical use in veterinary medicine. *BMC Vet. Res.* 17 (1): 389.

38 Johnson, A.L., Houlton, J.E.F., and Vannini, R. (2005). *AO Principles of Fracture Management in the Dog and Cat*, 529 S. Davos Platz; Stuttgart: AO Publishing; Distribution by Thieme.

39 Vezzoni, A. and Benjamino, K. (2021). Canine elbow dysplasia. *Vet. Clin. North Am. Small Anim. Pract.* 51 (2): 439–474.

40 Tack, P., Victor, J., Gemmel, P. et al. (2016). 3D-printing techniques in a medical setting: a systematic literature review. *Biomed. Eng. Online* 15 (1): 115.

41 Martelli, N., Serrano, C., van den Brink, H. et al. (2016). Advantages and disadvantages of 3-dimensional printing in surgery: a systematic review. *Surgery* 159 (6): 1485–1500.

42

Mandibular Fractures

Caleb Hudson[1] *and Stephen C. Jones*[2]

[1] *Nexus Veterinary Specialists, Victoria, TX, USA*
[2] *Bark City Veterinary Specialists, Park City, UT, USA*

Key Points

- Restoration of proper dental occlusion is one of the main goals of mandibular fracture repair.
- Preoperative planning prior to mandibular fracture repair is vital to a successful outcome.
- A ventral approach to the mandible is typically recommended for stabilization of mandibular fractures using internal fixation.
- Circumferential wiring, interdental wiring combined with intraoral composite splinting, bone plate and screws, external skeletal fixation and temporary maxillomandibular fixation are common stabilization techniques utilized to treat mandibular fractures.
- Implants utilized for mandibular fracture fixation should be positioned to avoid tooth root impingement.
- Mandibular fractures have a high incidence of complications after surgical stabilization; however, most of these complications are avoidable with appropriate stabilization technique selection and excecution.

Introduction

Mandibular fractures are a common traumatic injury in dogs and cats and are often associated with hit by car accidents as well as gunshot injuries, animal attack/bite wounds, and falls from a height.[1–6] Patients diagnosed with mandibular fractures should be carefully assessed for evidence of additional injuries, as these fractures often occur in association with more widespread maxillofacial trauma (such as maxillary or orbital fractures). Mandibular fractures are usually open fractures in communication with the oral cavity due to the relatively thin oral mucosal tissue layer that covers the mandible and the firm attachment of the oral mucosal tissue to the underlying periosteum of the mandible.[2,3] Untreated mandibular fractures typically do not heal or they heal as poorly functional malunions. Various options exist for treatment of mandibular fractures, including both non-surgical (such as maxillomandibular splinting) and surgical stabilization options. Regardless of the method of fracture stabilization selected, one of the main considerations during mandibular fracture repair is restoration of normal dental occlusion.[3] Failure to restore proper dental occlusion may lead to long-term patient morbidity, including oral mucosal erosions, tooth damage, and/or persistent patient discomfort.[3]

The teeth occupy approximately 50% of the volume of the mandible, and consequently, fractures of the mandible often involve one or more teeth or tooth roots. Preservation of teeth involved in mandibular fractures should be attempted if possible. Stable teeth with an exposed root in a mandibular fracture site can typically be preserved.[5,7] A diseased or loose tooth in a mandibular fracture line or a tooth with a fractured root in association with a mandibular fracture may require extraction during mandibular fracture repair.[8]

Feeding tubes may be inserted intraoperatively at the time of mandibular fracture stabilization for use in the postoperative period at the discretion of the surgeon. Esophagostomy tubes are the feeding tube most commonly utilized after mandibular fracture repair, but gastrostomy tubes may also be utilized. The authors find that feeding

Techniques in Small Animal Soft Tissue, Orthopedic, and Ophthalmic Surgery, First Edition. Edited by Kristin A. Coleman.

Companion website: www.wiley.com/go/coleman/surgeries

tubes are rarely necessary for patient management after mandibular fracture repair in dogs, as most dogs will use their tongue to ingest a liquid diet soon after mandibular fracture stabilization. Cats are sometimes slow to eat in the postoperative period after mandibular fracture repair, particularly with maxillomandibular fracture stabilization techniques, so feeding tubes are more commonly placed in cats at the time of mandibular fracture repair.[9] If a feeding tube is placed at the time of surgery, it can be removed once the patient starts to eat orally in the postoperative period.

Biomechanical Considerations

The primary forces acting on mandibular fractures after repair are bending forces, and these forces can be quite large due to the strong masticatory musculature that attaches to the mandibles.[3,10] Following a mandibular fracture, the bending forces exerted on the mandible primarily cause the rostral segment of the mandible to displace in a ventral and caudal direction. This means that the alveolar (upper) surface of the mandible is the tension surface of the bone and the aboral or lower surface of the mandible is the compression surface.[3,10] In order for mandibular fractures to heal appropriately, the fixation technique selected must appropriately counteract the forces acting on the mandible in order to achieve a fracture site environment in which bone healing can occur. Optimally, mandibular fracture fixation technique should result in rigid stabilization of the mandibular bone segments, as this provides the optimal environment for healing. Most implants used in mandibular fracture repair are strongest when subjected to tensile forces, and therefore, from a biomechanical perspective, should optimally be placed on or close to the tension (alveolar) surface of the mandible.[3,10] With the exception of interdental wire with an intraoral composite splint, it is unfortunately not feasible to place most orthopedic implants on the tension surface of the mandible without damaging the teeth. This means that most implants (bone plates and screws or external fixator pins) utilized to stabilize mandibular fractures must be applied in a biomechanically suboptimal location on the mandible. Due to the suboptimal location in which these implants are often applied and due to the significant bending forces acting on the mandible, implant constructs utilized for mandibular fracture repair need to be quite strong to minimize the risk of implant failure or delayed union/malunion.

Anatomy

A good working knowledge of regional mandibular anatomy is required to streamline mandibular fracture stabilization and minimize the risk of iatrogenic complications. The reader is encouraged to review the excellent overview of mandibular anatomy, including the supporting neurovascular anatomy, in Chapter 12 prior to attempting mandibular fracture repair. The main muscles commonly encountered during the surgical approach to the mandible include the digastricus, the masseter, the medial and lateral pterygoids, the mylohyoideus, and in some cases, the genioglossus. The digastricus, which functions to open the mouth, originates on the occipital bone and attaches to the caudoventral aspect of the mandibular body. The medial and lateral pterygoid muscles attach to the medial aspect of both the ramus of the mandible and the angular process. The masseter muscle attaches to the ventrolateral portion of the mandibular ramus and the angular process. The pterygoid muscles and the masseter all function to close the mouth. The mylohyoideus is a thin muscle sheet that runs transversely between the mandibles and attaches to the medial aspect of the mandibular body bilaterally. The mylohyoideus functions to support the tongue ventrally. The geniohyoideus, which is rarely encountered during mandibular fracture repair, attaches to the medial aspect of the mandibular body bilaterally at the caudal edge of the mandibular symphysis and is positioned dorsal to the mylohyoideus. An understanding of dental anatomy is also important to optimize implant positioning for mandibular fracture stabilization and minimize the risk of damage to tooth roots during implant application, which might ultimately result in tooth loss or persistent patient discomfort in the future. Mandibular dental anatomy of the dog and cat is summarized in Figure 42.1. Permanent mandibular dentition in the dog consists of 3 incisors, 1 canine, 4 premolars, and 3 molars for a total of 11 teeth per mandible and 22 total mandibular teeth.[8] The incisors, canines, first premolar, and third molar of the dog all have one root while the second to fourth premolars and the first and second molars each have two roots.[8] Permanent mandibular dentition in the cat consists of 3 incisors, 1 canine, 2 mandibular premolars, and 1 mandibular molar for a total of 7 teeth per mandible and 14 total mandibular teeth.[8] The feline incisors and canine each have a single root while the premolars and molar each have two roots.[8]

Diagnostic Imaging

Mandibular fractures can usually be diagnosed based on physical examination due to the paucity of soft tissue structures around the mandibles and the significant mandibular instability that typically develops after even a simple unilateral mandibular fracture. Confirmation of diagnosis and determination of mandibular fracture configuration is achieved using diagnostic imaging. Traditionally, orthogonal skull radiographs, including oblique lateral projections, have been used to characterize mandibular fractures (Figure 42.2). Intraoral

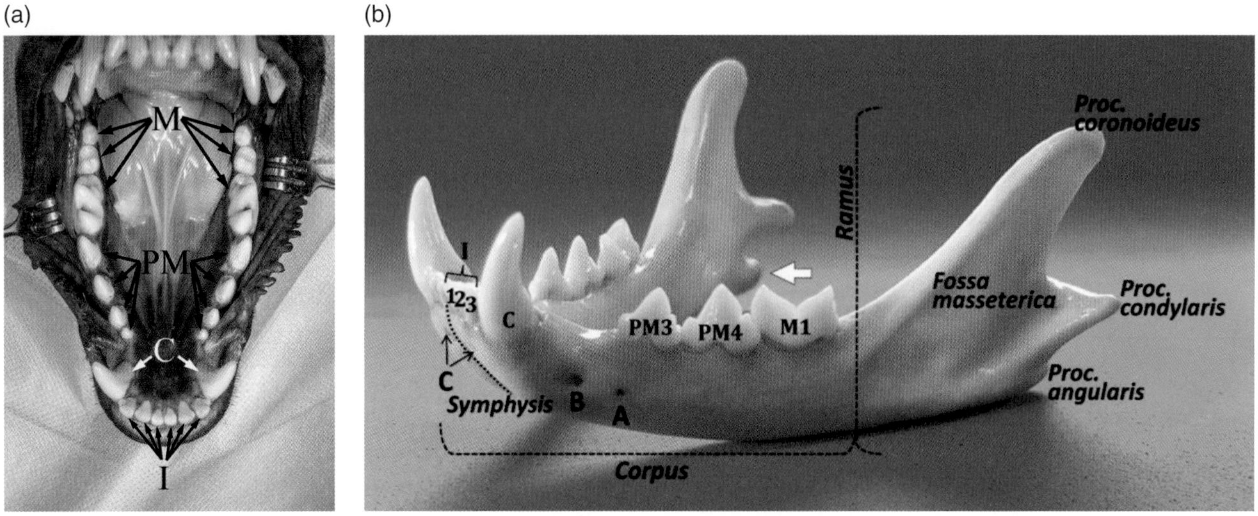

Figure 42.1 (a) Dorsal aspect of the canine lower jaw demonstrating normal dental anatomy. (b) Normal feline lower jaw demonstrating normal dental anatomy. Labeled structures include Molars (M), Premolars (PM), Canines (C), and Incisors (I). *Source:* (a) © Caleb Hudson. (b) Lombardero et al.[11] / MDPI / CC BY 4.0.

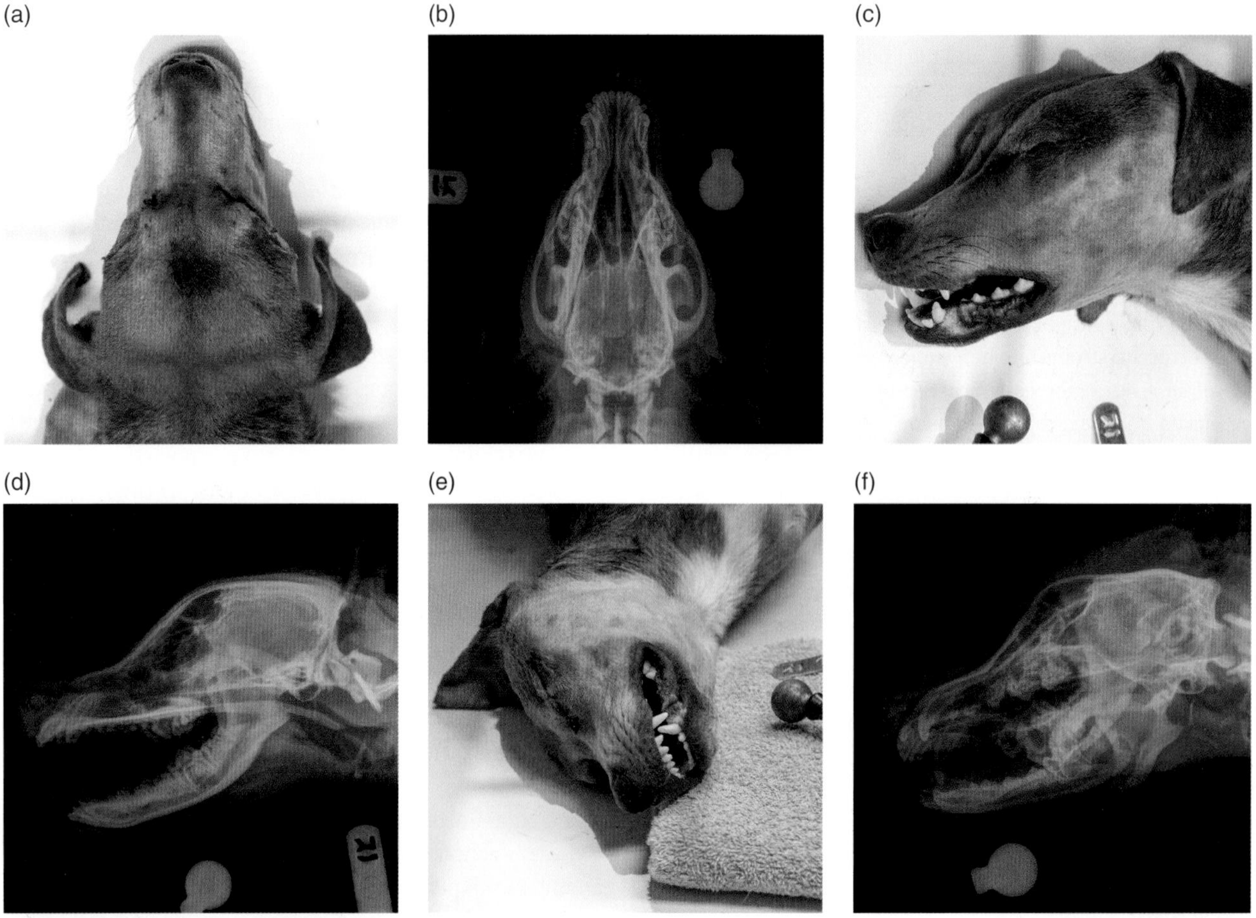

Figure 42.2 Paired photographs of a dog head positioned for skull radiographs with the radiographic image obtained in each position. (a) Head positioned for a DV radiographic projection. (b) DV radiographic projection of the skull. (c) Head positioned for a lateral radiographic projection. (d) Lateral radiographic projection of the skull – note the mandibular superimposition. (e) Head positioned for an oblique lateral projection isolating the ventral aspect of the right mandible. (f) Oblique lateral radiographic projection of the skull – note that the ventral aspect of the right mandible is visible without superimposition ventral to the left mandible. This position allows identification and assessment of a simple, right caudal mandibular body fracture. *Source:* © Caleb Hudson.

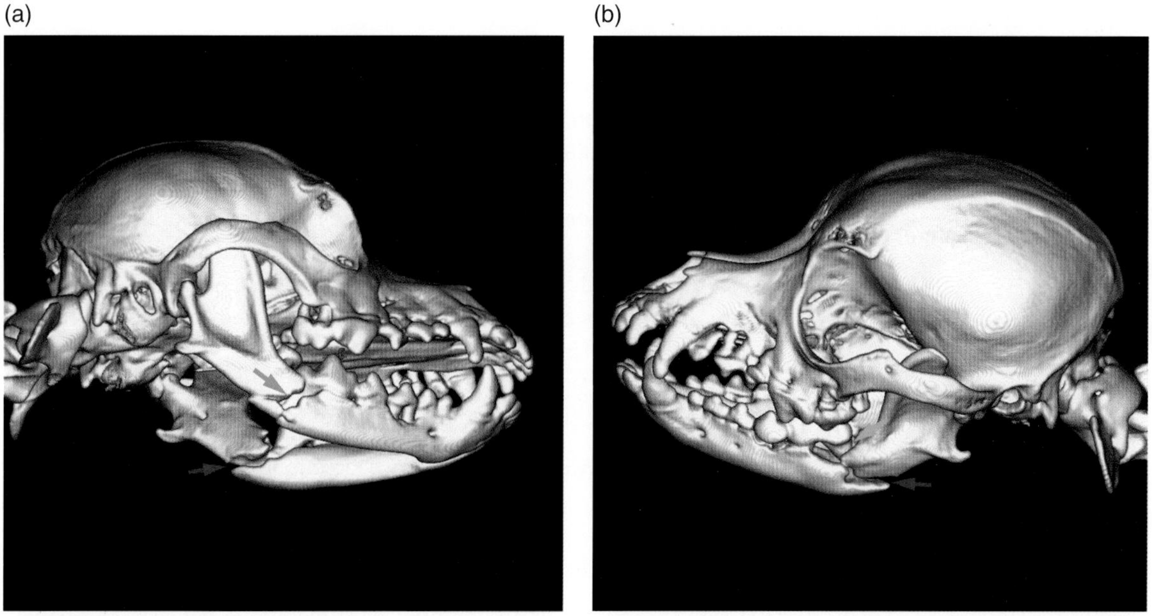

Figure 42.3 3D volume rendering of a skull CT scan from a dog with a bilateral mandibular fracture. Soft tissue structures have been subtracted to enhance assessment of fracture configuration. The right mandibular fracture (green arrow) is comminuted and best appreciated in image a. The left mandibular fracture (red arrow) is simple and is visible in images a and b. The caudal root of the first mandibular premolar is exposed in the fracture site on the left side (blue arrow). *Source:* © Caleb Hudson.

radiographs may also be utilized to gain more focused insight regarding mandibular fracture configuration. Due to the difficulty associated with interpretation of skull radiographs, particularly in the presence of multifocal maxillofacial injury, computed tomography (CT) scan is now commonly utilized to assess and characterize mandibular fractures. Mandibular fractures are more easily identified and more accurately characterized on CT images as compared to skull radiographs.[12] To simplify assessment of mandible fractures using CT scans and to guide surgical decision making, the CT images are often reconstructed into a virtual 3D image from which the surrounding soft tissue structures can be subtracted to facilitate assessment of the fractured bone (Figure 42.3).

Stabilization Options for Mandibular Fractures

Stabilization options for mandibular fractures may be divided into two major categories, those that are non-surgical versus those that involve surgery. Some guidelines for selection of mandibular fracture stabilization technique based on fracture location and configuration are summarized in Table 42.1. Non-surgical management of mandibular fractures is typically achieved via external maxillomandibular stabilization using a muzzle.[5,8] Muzzle stabilization of mandibular fractures does not result in rigid fracture site stabilization and is best utilized in young patients with

Table 42.1 Decision-making guidelines for selection of mandibular fracture stabilization method based on location, stability, and complexity of the mandibular fracture.

	Maxillomandibular stabilization	Interdental wire with intraoral composite splint	Bone plate(s) and screws	External skeletal fixation
Fracture location	Mid-body or caudal	Rostral to mid-body	Mid-body to caudal	Mid-body to caudal
Fracture site stability	Mildly unstable	Mild to moderate instability	Mild to severe instability	Mild to moderate instability
Fracture complexity	Simple to mildly comminuted	Simple or comminuted	Simple or comminuted	Simple or comminuted

simple, unilateral mandibular fractures that are only mildly unstable. Most mandibular fractures are best treated with surgical stabilization.

Surgical stabilization options for mandibular fractures may be subdivided into four major categories, including the following[3,8,10,13–15]:

- Maxillomandibular stabilization
- Wiring techniques
- Bone plates and screws
- External skeletal fixation

Surgical maxillomandibular stabilization has been described using a bi-gnathic encircling and retaining device (also known by the acronym BEARD).[9] The BEARD consists of a loop of nylon leader line that is tunneled subcutaneously circumferentially around the maxilla and both mandibles just caudal to the canine teeth and is secured ventral to the mandibles with a metal crimp or via a knot in the suture (Figure 42.4). The BEARD significantly restricts mandibular movement thereby facilitating fracture healing. It should be secured tight enough to allow the dog or cat sufficient jaw movement to eat soft/wet food and no more. The BEARD also helps maintain dental occlusion but, similar to muzzle stabilization of mandible fractures, the BEARD does not result in rigid fracture site stabilization. It is best suited for stabilization of caudal mandibular fractures that are not amenable to other forms of fracture stabilization, but can also be utilized in younger patients with simple, relatively stable mandible fractures.[9] The BEARD is commonly used in lieu of muzzle stabilization and is attractive in that it is mainly internal, thereby avoiding many of the challenges of muzzle stabilization such as muzzle dislodgement, moist dermatitis under the muzzle, and soiling of the tape muzzle. Although placing the BEARD is technically considered a surgery, it is very simple to perform, requires no specialized instrumentation, and does not need to be performed in a sterile OR setting.

Wiring techniques for mandibular fracture fixation may be subdivided into three groups[3,13,16]:

- Circumferential wire technique
- Intraosseous wire techniques
- Interdental wiring with intraoral composite splint techniques

The circumferential wire technique consists of a single strand of orthopedic wire, which is tunneled subcutaneously around both mandibles at the symphysis region just caudal to the canine teeth.[8,16] The wire is tensioned and secured ventrally using a twist knot. The circumferential wire technique is used to stabilize mandibular symphysis separation fractures. Intraosseous wire techniques involve the use of multiple interfragmentary wires inserted through tunnels drilled in each bone segment and used to

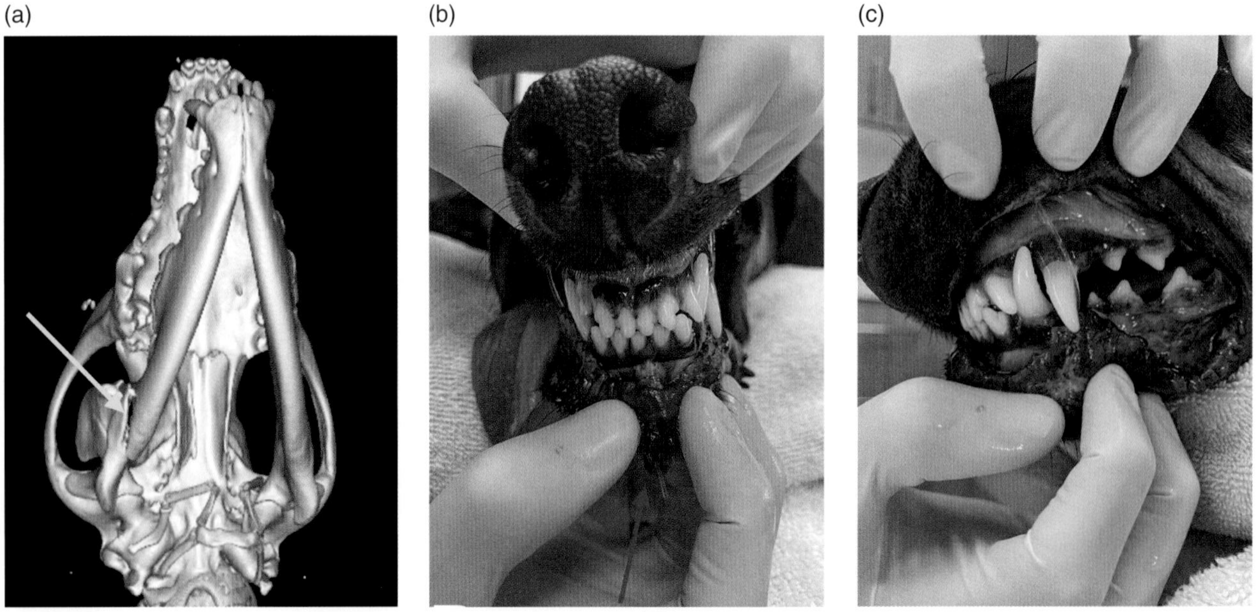

Figure 42.4 A three-year-old Doberman Pinscher dog with a mandibular fracture treated with a BEARD. (a) Three-dimensional volume rendering of a skull CT showing a minimally displaced caudal right mandibular fracture (yellow arrow). Note the considerable dental malocclusion despite the minor fracture displacement. (b) Rostral and (c) lateral photographs post-BEARD placement. Note the improvement in dental occlusion after the BEARD was placed. The nylon leader line was knotted ventral to the mandible (red arrow), allowing enough slack so that the dog could open his mouth enough to lap soft food/water. *Source:* © Stephen C. Jones.

reduce and compress mandibular bone segments together at the fracture site. Intraosseous wire techniques have historically been commonly utilized to stabilize mandibular fractures but are associated with a relatively high complication rate, as interfragmentary wires commonly loosen in the postoperative period and are not the optimal implant type to counteract bending forces.[3,10] The use of intraosseous wire techniques has decreased with the development of intraoral splinting and bone plate fixation techniques. Interdental wiring with intraoral composite splinting consists of a combination of one or multiple strands of orthopedic wire interwoven and twisted around the base of the crowns of multiple teeth spanning a mandibular fracture site over which a layer of dental acrylic is applied to create an intraoral splint.[8,13] Interdental wiring combined with an intraoral splint is an excellent technique for treating more rostral simple to mildly comminuted mandibular fractures.

Bone plate and screw fixation techniques are commonly utilized for mandibular fracture fixation as bone plate stabilization typically results in very rigid fracture site stabilization that can effectively resist strong bending forces.[3,10] Small locking bone plates are preferred for mandibular fracture fixation over non-locking plates, as locking plates provide angular stability and are very resistant to screw pullout even in the poor quality or thin bone that is often encountered in the mandible.[17] Reconstruction-style bone plates that allow plate-contouring to be performed in multiple planes are often utilized due to the non-linear shape of the majority of the mandible.[3,10] Bone plate stabilization is most applicable to fractures in the mid-body or ramus regions of the mandible. In the rostral portion of the mandible, bone plate fixation is difficult to utilize, as it is typically challenging or impossible to insert screws in the rostral mandible without tooth root impingement.

External skeletal fixator (ESF) techniques utilize end-threaded (recommended) or smooth (not recommended) pins percutaneously inserted into mandibular fracture segments and connected outside the body by an acrylic column or connecting bar to stabilize mandibular fractures. ESF techniques were commonly utilized for mandibular fracture stabilization prior to the development of small locking bone plating systems. Due to the limited and often relatively thin bone stock available for implant insertion in the mandible, ESF fixation typically does not result in rigid stabilization of mandibular fractures, and pin loosening or back-out is a common occurrence in the postoperative period.[3] For these reasons, ESF fixation is typically not the best choice for mandibular fracture fixation if a bone plate(s) construct could be utilized instead. When ESF fixation is selected, it is best applied to mid-body or rostral, unilateral mandibular fractures.

Preoperative Planning

Preoperative planning should always be performed prior to fracture stabilization surgery using preoperative radiographs and/or CT scan images. Appropriate preoperative planning starts with fracture assessment and categorization. The mandible can be divided into different regions for the purposes of preoperative planning (Figure 42.5). The region of the mandible affected by the fracture affects selection of stabilization technique. Mandibular fractures can also be classified as unilateral versus bilateral and as simple versus comminuted. Preoperative planning should also include determination of the desired stabilization technique, selection of implant type and size, and determination of where implants will be positioned on and inserted into the mandible (Figure 42.6). Measurements can be performed on the radiographs from identifiable bone landmarks to guide estimation of the location of tooth roots intraoperatively, which helps ensure that screws or pins will not impinge on tooth roots. If using bone plate fixation, the selected plate size will vary tremendously based on patient size and fracture location and configuration. In toy dogs and cats, 1.0 or 1.5 mm plates are often utilized, while in larger dogs, plates as large as 2.7 mm may sometimes be utilized. Preoperative contouring of the bone plate can also be performed using radiographs, a bone model, or a 3D-printed model of the mandible to guide contouring. Preoperative planning is optimally performed using orthopedic planning software. The authors prefer a software program called VPOP® Pro (VetSOS Education Ltd., Shrewsbury, England), which is cloud-based, affordable, and has an easy learning curve. When radiographs are used for preoperative planning, it is important to include a magnification correction marker of known size in the image

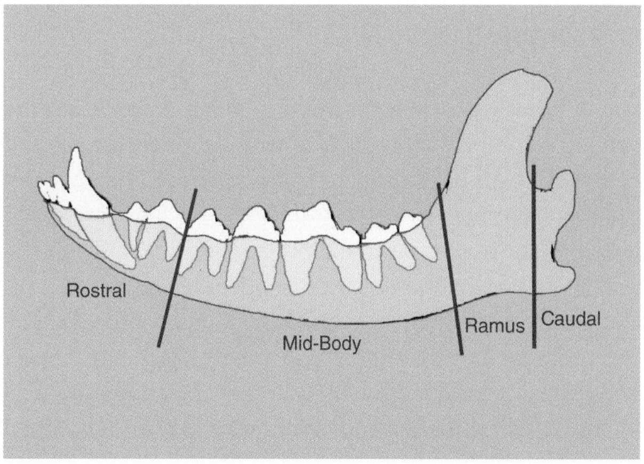

Figure 42.5 Illustration of the lateral aspect of the canine mandible with superimposition of the tooth roots over the bone of the mandible. The mandible can be divided into rostral, mid-body, ramus, and caudal regions to assist in decision making for fracture stabilization surgery. *Source:* © Caleb Hudson.

(a) (b)

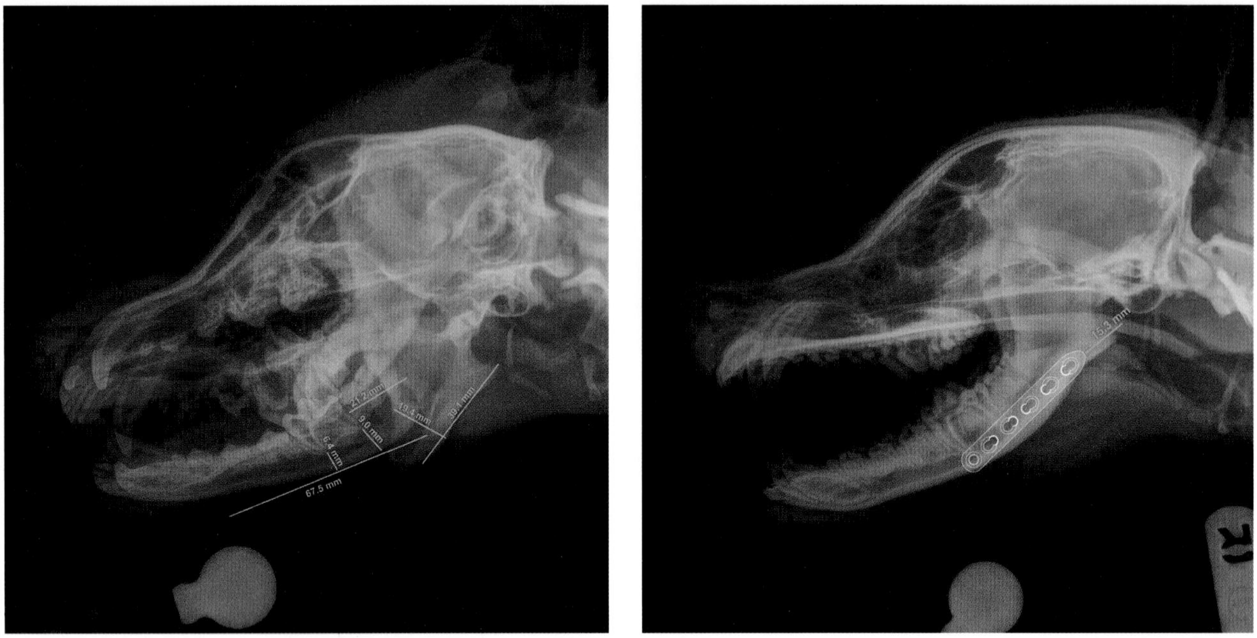

Figure 42.6 Preoperative planning performed on skull radiograph images from a dog with a simple mandibular body fracture using digital orthopedic planning software. (a) Lateral oblique radiographic projection with measurements performed to determine the dimensions of the cranial and caudal mandibular segments that are available for implant placement. The distance from the ventral aspect of the mandible to the ventral tip of several of the tooth roots has also been determined along with the distance from the fracture margin to the caudal tooth root of M1. (b) The template for a 2.7 mm locking bone plate has been positioned over the lateral aspect of the mandible, and the distance from the angular process to the caudal aspect of the plate has been measured. *Source:* © Caleb Hudson.

that is positioned an equivalent distance away from the radiographic plate as the mandible of interest. This magnification correction marker is used to size calibrate the image in the templating software so that measurements made using the software program will be accurate.

Patient Positioning, Airway Management, and Draping

Mandibular fracture repair is typically performed with the patient in dorsal recumbency when a bone plate and screws, an external fixator, or a circumferential wire stabilization technique is being utilized.[3] The hair is clipped over the entire ventral mandible region bilaterally to the level of the oral commissure dorsolaterally and with a caudal margin several cm caudal to the angular process. The clip margins can be abbreviated for isolated mandibular symphyseal separation fractures or very rostral mandibular fractures. For BEARD and interdental wiring combined with intraoral composite splinting stabilization techniques, the patient is typically positioned in sternal recumbency. For BEARD application, the hair should be clipped circumferentially over the rostral 3–5 cm of the muzzle.[9] For interdental wiring with intraoral splinting, clipping of hair may not be necessary, as the entire stabilization technique is intraoral; however, hair should be clipped from any portion of the mandible or maxilla that will be draped into the surgical field.

For simple mandibular fractures in which anatomic reduction can be achieved, standard oral endotracheal intubation is appropriate, as intraoperative assessment of occlusion is not critical. For comminuted mandibular fractures or any fracture in which anatomic reduction is not expected to be achieved, endotracheal intubation through a pharyngostomy approach should be considered to allow intraoperative assessment of occlusion to be used to guide mandibular bone segment alignment.[3] Endotracheal tube insertion through a pharyngostomy approach is recommended for BEARD stabilization of mandibular fractures to allow appropriate mouth closure and occlusion assessment intraoperatively.[9]

An inferior alveolar nerve block is recommended prior to mandibular fracture stabilization surgery. This block can be performed using standard bupivacaine or using a combination of standard bupivacaine and liposomal encapsulated bupivacaine (Nocita®, Elanco Animal Health, Greenfield, IN).

Standard aseptic skin preparation should be performed on all skin that will be draped into the sterile surgical field.

If the oral cavity will be included in the surgical field, aseptic preparation of the oral cavity should also be performed.[3,9] The tongue may be reflected into the pharyngeal region, and if any portion of the surgery will be intraoral, the pharynx may also be packed with gauze to protect the airway from hemorrhage intraoperatively.[3] Patient draping technique varies depending on the surgical approach and stabilization method being utilized. For bone plate application to a simple mandibular fracture, the draping may include only the ventral aspect of the mandible(s) and exclude the oral cavity from the surgical field. The oral cavity is draped into the surgical field during treatment of the majority of mandibular fractures to allow occlusion to be assessed intraoperatively as necessary.

Surgical Approach

For mandibular fractures treated with internal fixation, a ventral approach to the body and/or ramus of the mandible is typically performed (Figure 42.7).[18] With the patient in dorsal recumbency, the shaft of the mandible to be approached should be palpated. A skin incision is created over the ventral midline of the mandible, which extends parallel to the long axis of the mandible (Figure 42.7a). The incision should be centered over the mandibular fracture site, and the length of the incision should be about 1–2 cm longer than the length of the bone plate that is going to be applied to the fractured mandible. The subcutaneous tissue and platysma muscle are incised along the same line as the

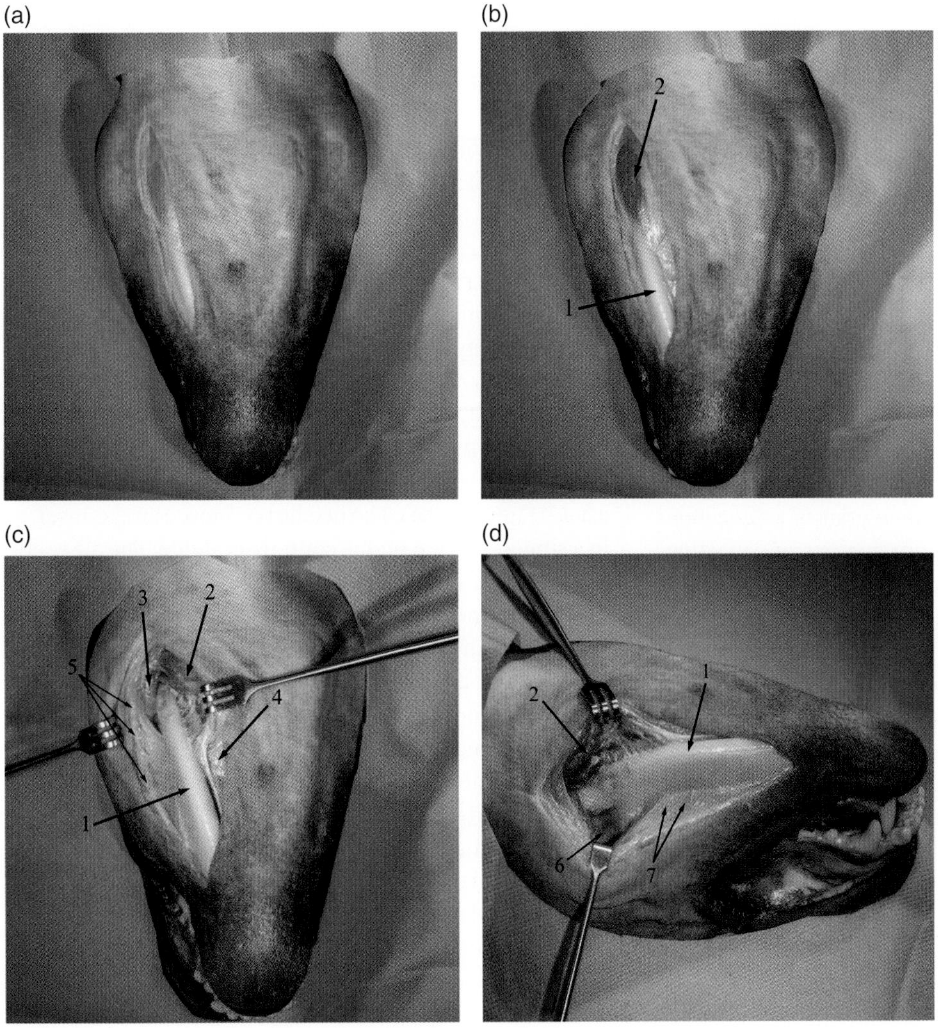

Figure 42.7 Ventral surgical approach to the body and ramus of the mandible. (a) The skin is incised over the ventral mandibular midline. (b) Subcutaneous tissue and platysma are incised to expose the body of the mandible and the digastricus muscle. (c) An incision is created at the junction between the digastricus and masseter to expose the caudal body of the mandible. (d) To expose the mandibular ramus, the digastricus is elevated off the ventral aspect of the mandible and retracted medially (ventral Senn retractor) while the masseter is elevated off of the lateral aspect of the ramus and retracted laterally (dorsal Senn retractor). Labeled structures include 1. Mandibular body. 2. Digastricus muscle. 3. Masseter muscle. 4. Mylohyoideus muscle. 5. Branches of facial vein and nerve. 6. Lateral aspect of mandibular ramus. 7. Oral mucosa. *Source:* © Caleb Hudson.

skin incision. The ventral aspect of the body of the mandible is now exposed in the surgical field (Figure 42.7b). To expose the caudal aspect of the mandibular body and lateral aspect of the ramus, the digastricus muscle is incised or separated from the masseter along the caudolateral aspect of the mandible (Figure 42.7c). The digastricus can be elevated off the ventral aspect of the mandibular body while the masseter is elevated off of the lateral aspect of the mandibular ramus to expose the ventral to middle regions of the mandibular ramus (Figure 42.7d). Care should be exercised to avoid damaging the branch of the facial vein, which runs just lateral to the mandibular body along with some smaller branches of the facial nerve (Figure 42.7c). If more medial exposure of the mandibular body is needed, the mylohyoideus can be elevated off of the medial aspect of the mandible. Bilateral mandibular fractures may be approached with two separate surgical approaches, each one centered over one of the mandibles. Alternatively, a single ventral midline skin incision may be created, and the skin edges at the incision site may be retracted laterally in either direction to provide access to each mandible in an alternating fashion.

Bone Graft Use in Mandibular Fracture Stabilization

Due to the relatively high risk of delayed healing or nonunion associated with mandibular fracture stabilization, the use of a bone graft is recommended during surgical stabilization of mandibular fractures. The most biologically active and inexpensive type of bone graft is a cancellous autograft. The cancellous autograft consists of cancellous bone collected from another bone in the patient's body that is packed in and around a fracture site to stimulate bone formation. The greater tubercle of the humerus is the most popular site for autogenous bone graft collection in dogs and cats and is easy to drape into the surgical field for mandibular fracture stabilization surgery if a ventral approach to the mandible is being performed.

Muzzle Stabilization Technique

Muzzle stabilization is best performed with the patient under light to moderate sedation and after administration of an injectable opioid analgesic drug, so that the mandibles can be digitally manipulated without patient resistance. Appropriate mandibular realignment should be performed such that normal dental occlusion is restored. A muzzle should be applied to the patient. The muzzle may be custom made from medical tape or may be a well-fitting commercially produced muzzle. The muzzle should be sized to allow a maximal gap of 0.5–1 cm between the incisors in small dogs and cats and 1–1.5 cm in larger dogs.[8] This limited ability to open the mouth will allow the patient to lap water and a liquid diet but will still preserve enough interdigitation of the canine teeth for proper dental occlusion to be maintained. Maintenance of partial interdigitation of the canine teeth also helps minimize movement at the fracture site, thereby facilitating bone healing. The patient should wear the muzzle until radiographic evidence of fracture healing is documented. Unilateral simple mandibular fractures in healthy patients without underlying bone pathology are expected to heal in 6–12 weeks after muzzle stabilization.[5] Muzzle stabilization of mandibular fractures commonly results in the development of moist dermatitis under the muzzle. The dermatitis typically resolves once the muzzle is removed.[8]

BEARD Stabilization Technique

A stab incision is created in the skin over the dorsal midline of the maxilla at the level of the base of the maxillary canine teeth. A 1.5″ 14- or 16-gauge hypodermic needle, which has been bent into a gentle curve, is inserted through the oral mucosa just caudal to the base of one maxillary canine and tunneled subcutaneously until the tip of the needle exits through the stab incision over the dorsal maxilla. One end of a strand of nylon leader line (50 lb test in cats or small dogs and 80–100 lb test in larger dogs) is inserted into the tip of the hypodermic needle and advanced until the leader line exits the hub of the needle in the oral cavity (Figure 42.8a). The needle is removed and re-inserted in a similar fashion on the contralateral side. The other end of the strand of leader line is inserted into the tip of the hypodermic needle and advanced until the tip of the suture strand exits the hub of the needle (Figure 42.8b). The needle is removed, and both ends of the suture are tensioned so that the dorsal loop of leader line is pulled through the dorsal stab incision in the skin with the strand of leader line sitting snuggly against the dorsal and lateral aspects of the maxilla in the subcutaneous tunnel. The muzzle is now elevated, and a 1–1.5 cm skin incision is created ventral to the mandibular symphysis region at the level of the base of the mandibular canine teeth. The curved hypodermic needle is inserted through this stab incision and advanced dorsally and laterally until the tip of the needle exits through the oral mucosa just caudal to the base of one of the mandibular canine teeth. The end of the nylon leader line on the same side as the hypodermic needle is inserted into the tip of the hypodermic needle and advanced until the leader line exits the hub of the needle ventral to the mandibular symphysis (Figure 42.8c). The needle is removed, and this same procedure is repeated on the contralateral side so that

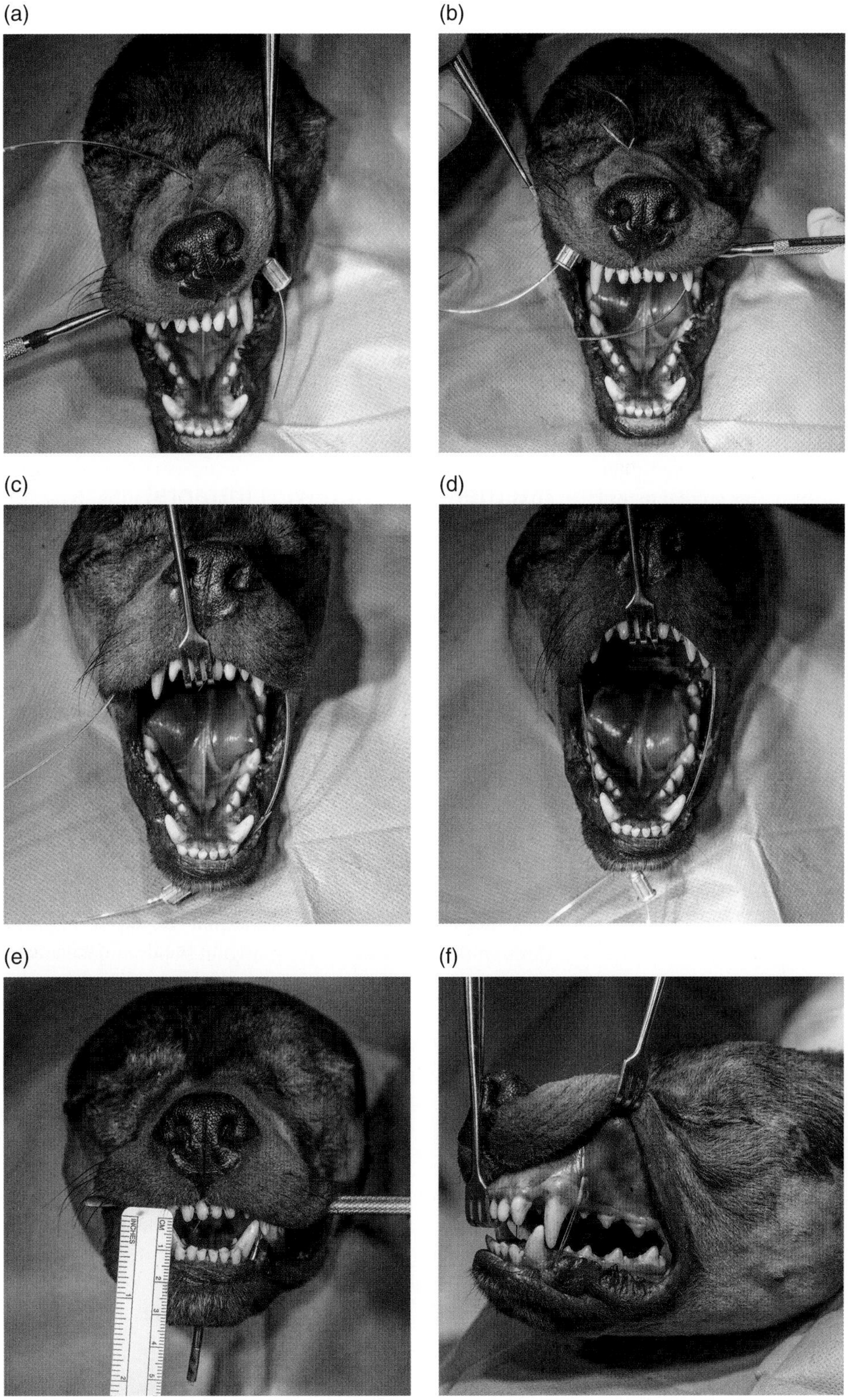

Figure 42.8 BEARD stabilization technique for mandibular fractures. (a) A 16-gauge, 1.5″ hypodermic needle has been bent into a curve and then inserted through the oral mucosa just caudal to the base of the maxillary canine and tunneled subcutaneously to exit at a stab incision on dorsal midline. One end of a strand of nylon leader line has been inserted through the needle from dorsal to ventral, exiting in the oral cavity. (b) The procedure from image a has been repeated on the contralateral side with the opposite end of the strand of nylon leader line. (c) The previously used hypodermic needle has been tunneled subcutaneously from a ventral stab incision over the mandibular symphysis to exit through the oral mucosa just caudal to the root of the mandibular canine. The ipsilateral end of the strand of nylon leader line is passed from dorsal to ventral through the hypodermic needle, exiting ventral to the mandibular symphysis. (d) The same procedure from image c has been repeated on the contralateral side with the opposite end of the strand of nylon leader line. (e) Both ends of the nylon leader line have been tensioned and crimp clamped ventral to the mandibular symphysis, resulting in partial closure of the mouth with an approximately 1–1.5 cm gap remaining between the incisors of the mandible and maxilla. (f) After completion of BEARD application, the nylon leader line crosses between the maxilla and mandible just caudal to the canine teeth. *Source:* © Caleb Hudson.

both ends of the strand of nylon leader line exit through the ventral stab incision (Figure 42.8d). Two or three metallic crimp clamps should be slid over both ends of the strand of nylon leader line. The mandible is manually reduced such that proper dental occlusion is restored. The crimps are slid dorsally against the undersurface of the mandibular symphysis, tensioning the loop of nylon leader line until the mouth is closed with approximately 0.5 cm of space between the incisors for a small dog or cat and 1–1.5 cm of space between the incisors in a larger dog. The most distal crimp clamp is crimped to maintain the mandible in the stabilized position while still allowing the oral cavity to open a small amount (Figure 42.8e,f). The crimp clamps may be left protruding from the ventral stab incision or may be pushed caudally into the subcutaneous space and the skin edges closed over the crimps. As an alternative to the crimp clamps, the nylon leader line ends can be tied together, with appropriate slack left in the nylon leader line to limit limited mouth opening, as above (Figure 42.4). The BEARD device is typically removed after three to four weeks but may remain in place for longer if necessary.[9] To remove the BEARD, the nylon leader line is cut, and the leader line and crimp clamps are removed through the ventral stab incision over the mandibular symphysis. An esophagostomy tube may be placed prior to BEARD stabilization of a mandibular fracture if desired at the discretion of the surgeon.

Circumferential Wire Stabilization Technique

A 1 cm stab incision is created in the skin ventral to the mandibular symphysis. A 1 or 1.5″ 16- or 18-gauge hypodermic needle, which has been bent into a gentle curve, is inserted through the stab incision at a level just caudal to the base of one mandibular canine and tunneled subcutaneously until the tip of the needle exits through the oral mucosa just caudal and lateral to the base of the mandibular canine. One end of a strand of 22-gauge (cats and small dogs) or 20-gauge (larger dogs) orthopedic wire is inserted into the tip of the hypodermic needle protruding into the oral cavity and advanced until the end of the wire exits through the hub of the needle (Figure 42.9a). The needle is removed and inserted in a similar fashion on the contralateral side of the mandible. The other end of the strand of orthopedic wire is inserted through the hypodermic needle in a similar fashion to the first side (Figure 42.9b), and the hypodermic needle is then removed. Both ends of the strand of orthopedic wire should be pulled ventrally to remove slack from the orthopedic wire and tensioned so that the wire strand is against the oral mucosa over the upper surface of the mandibles just caudal to the base of the canines. Mandibular symphysis reduction is performed manually, and the orthopedic wire is then tensioned and secured with a twist knot ventral to the mandibular symphysis (Figure 42.9c,d). Once the symphysis is palpably stable, the wire knot is bent over caudally into the subcutaneous tissues and then cut with at least three twists remaining. The skin incision can be closed to cover the wire twist knot or left open. The circumferential wire is typically removed about four weeks postoperatively by cutting the wire in the oral cavity and pulling the wire and associated wire knot out from the ventral aspect of the symphysis through a stab incision in the skin.

Interdental Wiring with Intraoral Composite Splint

The teeth should be assessed and cleaned prior to performing an interdental wiring technique. The mandibular bone segments should be aligned and dental occlusion assessed prior to wire application. Multiple acceptable techniques for interdental wiring have been described. The technique described here is based on the Stout multiple loop wiring technique.[19–21] A relatively long length of orthopedic wire should be selected with a gauge size of 22–24 in dogs and 24–26 in cats.[8,13,22] Interdental wiring utilizes the base of the tooth crown as an anchor point, and typically, two to three teeth should be incorporated on each side of the fracture site. One end of the wire strand should be inserted through the oral mucosa from lingual to buccal just caudal to the base of the most caudal tooth, which is going to be included in the fixation. Wire passage may be facilitated by the use of a hypodermic needle as a guide or by use of a small K-wire in an orthopedic drill to create a wire tract near the base of the crown. The wire is advanced around the buccal aspect of the tooth crown and then reinserted through the oral mucosa at the cranial base of the crown from buccal to lingual. The tip of the wire is then reversed, and the wire is reinserted through the mucosa just caudal to the base of the crown of the next most rostral tooth in a lingual to buccal direction. A small loop of wire is maintained on the lingual aspect of the mandible as the wire is advanced. This technique is repeated until a sufficient number of teeth have been looped with wire (Figure 42.10a). The opposite end of the strand of wire is passed from caudal to rostral along the lingual aspect of the mandible such that the end of the wire passes through each of the wire loops on the lingual aspect of the mandible. The two free ends of the wire are then twisted together to make a twist wire knot (Figure 42.10b). Each of the wire loops on the lingual aspect of the mandible is sequentially twisted to tension the wire around the base of the crowns of the teeth included in the fixation (Figure 42.10c). The twisted loops and the twisted

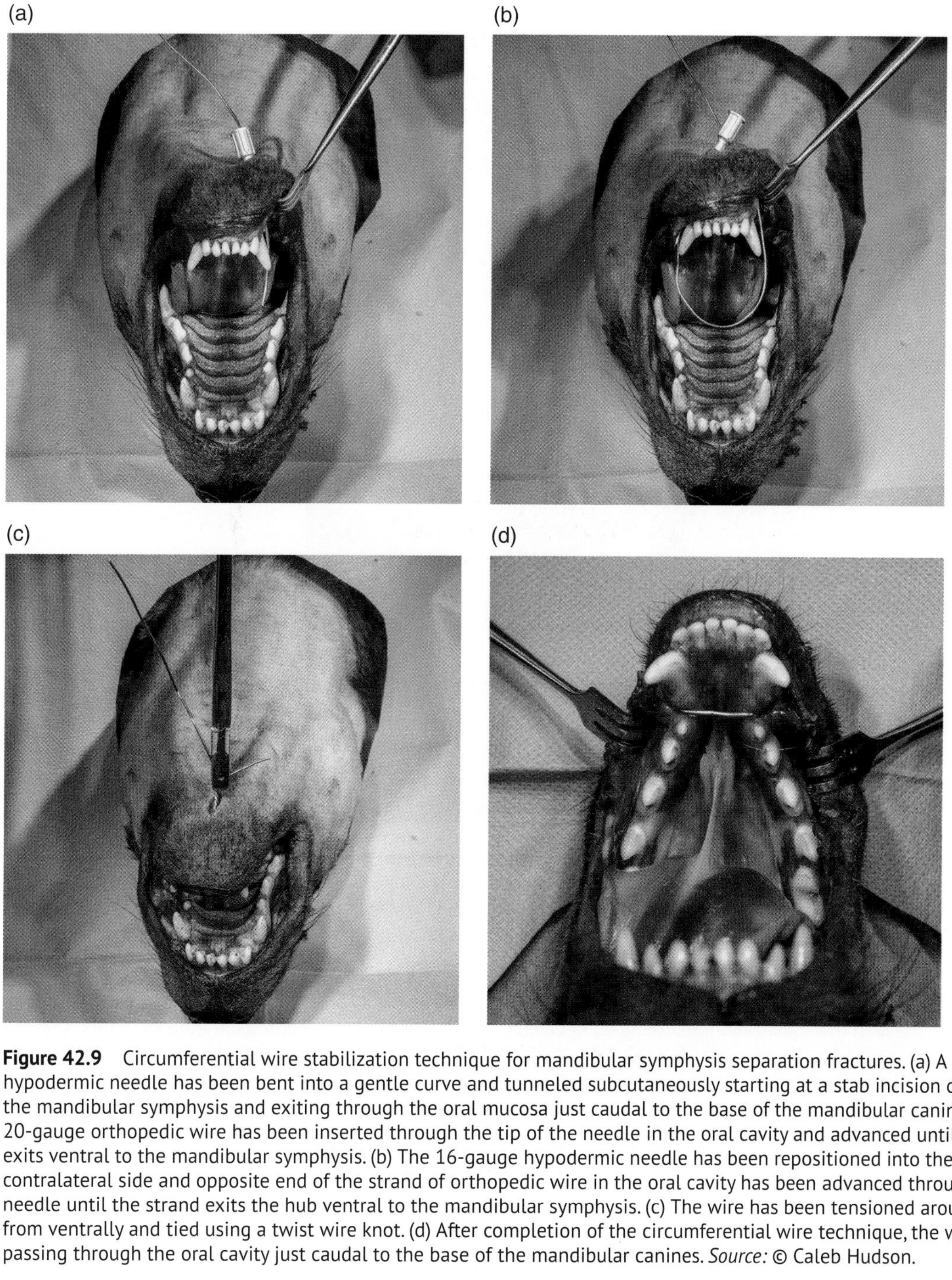

Figure 42.9 Circumferential wire stabilization technique for mandibular symphysis separation fractures. (a) A 16-gauge, 1.5″ hypodermic needle has been bent into a gentle curve and tunneled subcutaneously starting at a stab incision on ventral midline over the mandibular symphysis and exiting through the oral mucosa just caudal to the base of the mandibular canine tooth. A strand of 20-gauge orthopedic wire has been inserted through the tip of the needle in the oral cavity and advanced until the end of the wire exits ventral to the mandibular symphysis. (b) The 16-gauge hypodermic needle has been repositioned into the same position on the contralateral side and opposite end of the strand of orthopedic wire in the oral cavity has been advanced through the tip of the needle until the strand exits the hub ventral to the mandibular symphysis. (c) The wire has been tensioned around the mandibles from ventrally and tied using a twist wire knot. (d) After completion of the circumferential wire technique, the wire can be observed passing through the oral cavity just caudal to the base of the mandibular canines. *Source:* © Caleb Hudson.

ends of the wire strand are bent over close to the lingual surface of the mandible. The teeth included in the fixation should be etched with a phosphoric acid gel and dried prior to application of the intraoral composite splint.[8,13] Dental composite should be applied directly to the crowns of the teeth incorporated in the repair and on/around the interdental wire. The majority of the composite material should be kept on the lingual side of the mandible to minimize interference with normal dental occlusion (Figure 42.10d).[8] Once the composite has hardened, the splint can be smoothed and shaped using a burr.[8,13] A self-curing bis-acryl composite, such as MaxiTemp® (Henry Schein, Melville, NY), is the preferred material for the composite splint, as the lower cure temperature decreases the likelihood of thermal injury to the teeth or intraoral soft tissues.[24] Oral rinses with a chlorhexidine solution are an important component of the home care for patients treated with intraoral splints, as the splint tends to trap food particles.

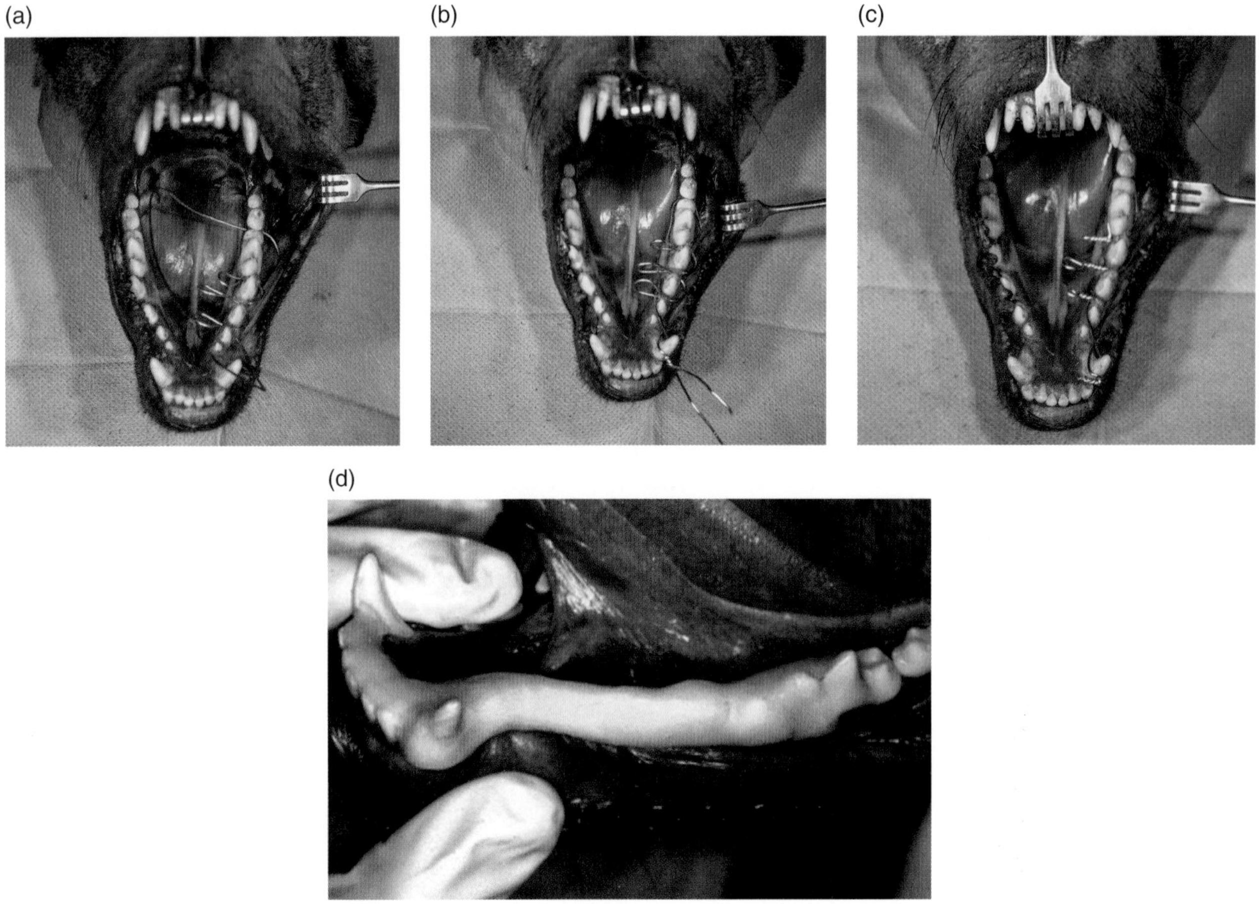

Figure 42.10 Interdental wiring (Stout multiple loop technique) with intraoral composite splint stabilization technique. (a) A length of orthopedic wire has been tunneled through the oral mucosa and passed around the base of multiple mandibular molars, premolars, and the canine tooth ipsilaterally, leaving multiple open loops of wire on the lingual side of the mandible. (b) The free end of the strand of orthopedic wire has been passed through the open loops and secured to the other end of the strand of orthopedic wire around the canine tooth using a twist wire knot. (c) Each of the free loops of orthopedic wire on the lingual aspect of the mandible has been sequentially tensioned using a twist knot, tightening the strand of orthopedic wire around the base of the crowns of the teeth included in the stabilization. (d) A completed intraoral splint after application of dental composite over the interdental wire and the crowns of the teeth included in the stabilization. *Source:* (a–c) © Caleb Hudson. (d) Cote[23] with permission from ELSEVIER.

Once radiographic evidence of bone healing is documented, the splint is removed by sectioning the composite and using extraction forceps or an elevator for removal.

Bone Plate(s) and Screws Stabilization Technique

A ventral surgical approach (Figure 42.11a) is typically performed to access the mandibular fracture site, and the mandibular fracture should be reduced. For simple fractures, anatomic reduction should be achieved. This is typically accomplished by grasping the rostral and caudal mandibular fracture segments with bone-holding forceps and manipulating the segments until the fracture segments are reduced (Figure 42.11b). A pointed bone-holding forceps can be applied to both mandibular fracture segments across the fracture site to maintain reduction (Figure 42.11c), or a temporary K-wire inserted perpendicularly across the fracture site may be used to temporarily maintain reduction. For comminuted fractures, the rostral and caudal mandibular segments should be aligned such that normal dental occlusion is re-established, but the comminuted fracture segments should not be anatomically reduced. The bone plate previously selected during preoperative planning should be positioned on the mandible in the desired position, and implant size, fit, and length should be assessed (Figure 42.11c,d). If a locking bone plate is being utilized, a minimum of two bicortical screws need to be applied on each side of the fracture site; however, as much of the mandible consists of relatively thin bone, three or four bicortical screws in each bone segment are preferred (Figure 42.11e). More screws are also required per segment if screws are inserted in a monocortical fashion. Preoperative planning

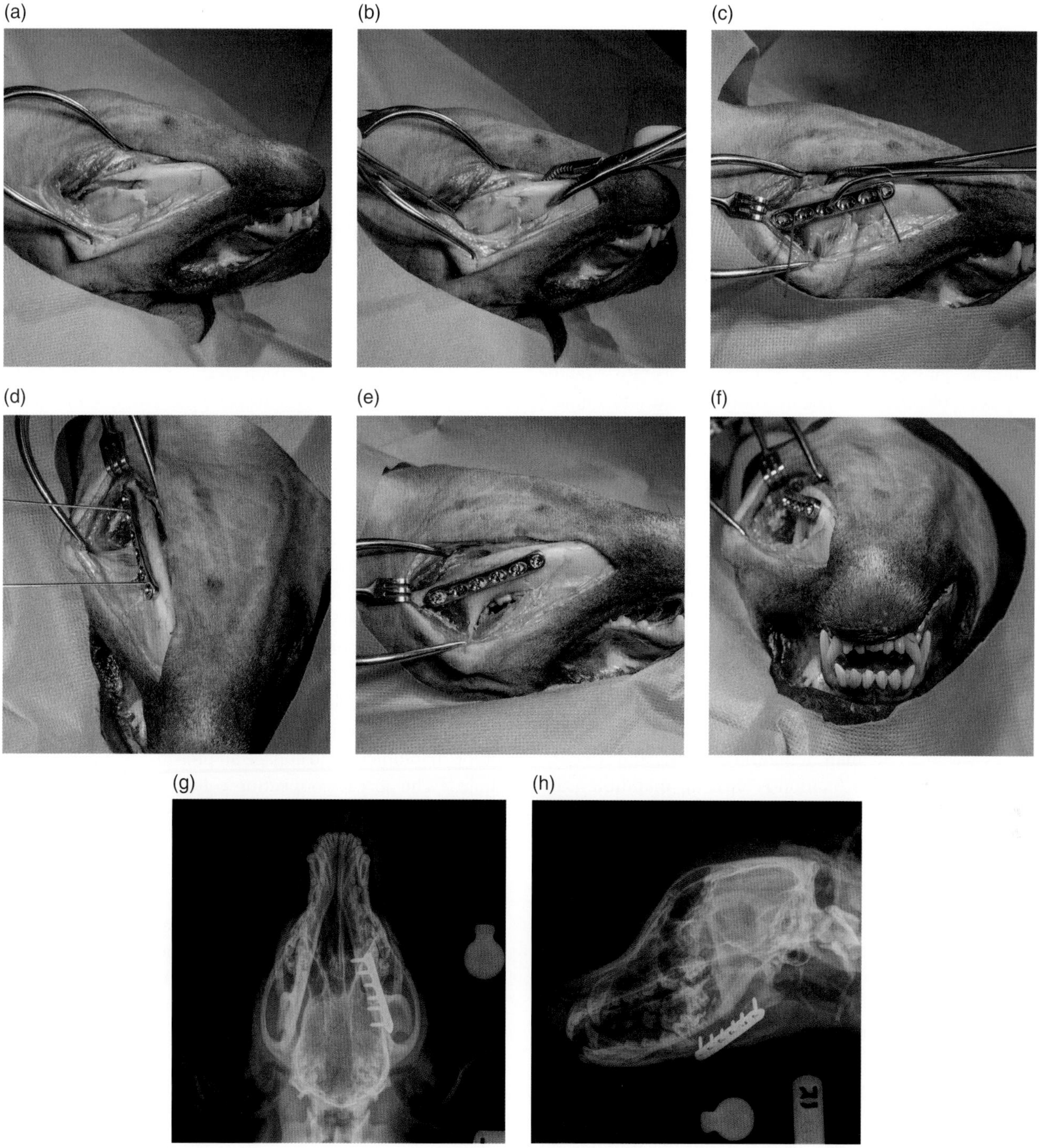

Figure 42.11 Bone plate and screws fixation of a simple, unilateral mandibular body fracture. (a) Exposure of the mandibular fracture site through a ventral approach. (b) Bone-holding forceps have been used to mobilize the mandibular segments and anatomically reduce the fracture site. (c) A precontoured bone plate has been applied to the lateral aspect of the mandibular body, bridging the fracture site, and temporarily fixed in position with two K-wires. Pointed bone-holding forceps are used to maintain anatomic reduction at the fracture site. (d) The bone plate has been both bent and twisted to match the contour of the mandibular body at the site of application. (e) Six locking screws have been inserted into the mandibular body through the bone plate, completing mandibular fracture stabilization. (f) Normal dental occlusion has been re-established by anatomic reduction of this simple, unilateral mandibular fracture. (g) Postoperative DV skull radiograph. (h) Postoperative lateral oblique skull radiograph. *Source:* © Caleb Hudson.

measurements should be assessed to ensure that screws inserted through the plate will not result in tooth root impingement. Use of intraoperative fluoroscopy, if available, is useful to guide screw insertion and minimize the risk of tooth root damage. Typically, screws should be inserted in the two end holes in the plate first. If both of the end holes are well-positioned over bone, all of the intervening plate holes are usually lined up such that all screws will engage the bone appropriately. A depth gauge should be used to determine the appropriate screw length for each hole, as excessively long screws may result in postoperative morbidity. Visual confirmation of the restoration of normal dental occlusion should be obtained once bone plate stabilization is completed (Figure 42.11f). Postoperative radiographs are obtained to assess fracture reduction and implant position (Figure 42.11g,h).

Long plates that span more of the mandibular body are preferred from a biomechanical perspective, but due to the non-linear shape of much of the mandible, application of longer plates without tooth root impingement may be challenging. If the use of a longer plate is desired, a reconstruction-style plate that allows contouring in multiple planes is often selected.[3,10] Use of two or more bone plates spanning the same mandibular fracture site is another strategy that can be utilized to increase the number of screws per bone segment and to achieve more rigid fixation that can more effectively counteract the forces acting on the mandibular fracture site after repair.[3] When multiple plate fixation is used for mandible fractures, the plates may both be applied to the lateral surface of the mandible (one plate closer to the alveolar margin and one closer to the ventral margin) or may be applied on different surfaces of the bone oriented at ~90° (such as the lateral surface and the ventral surface of the mandible), which is referred to as orthogonal plate fixation. Orthogonal plate fixation allows the implants to effectively counteract bending forces acting on the fractured mandible from multiple directions (Figure 42.12). When a plate is applied to the ventral aspect of the mandible, the screws are typically all inserted as monocortical screws that engage only the ventral cortex of the mandible to ensure that the screws do not impinge on tooth roots.

Surgical site closure is routine after mandibular fracture stabilization using bone plate fixation. Caudally, any elevated portions of the digastricus and/or masseter should be reapposed and sutured over the mandible and any portion of the bone plates located on the mandible in this region. Closure over the more rostral portion of the mandibular body consists of a two-layer closure of the subcutaneous layer and then the skin.

Bone plates typically are not removed after mandibular fracture healing unless an oral mucosal erosion exposes a portion of the plate in the oral cavity (more common if plates are applied to the medial aspect of the mandible or if excessively long screws are utilized). In rare cases, persistent patient discomfort or the development of an implant-associated infection may result in the need for implant removal.

External Fixator Stabilization Technique

External fixator stabilization may be performed as a minimally invasive procedure following the closed reduction of a mandibular fracture, or the fixator may be applied following an open ventral approach to the mandible, similar to the approach utilized for bone plate fixation. End threaded, positive profile pins (often called acrylic pins in smaller diameter sizes) are recommended for ESF application to mandibular fractures, and a minimum of three threaded pins should be applied to each major fracture segment (more are better). Pin insertion at slightly divergent angles is also recommended in the mandible. Pins may be inserted in a single mandible if a unilateral mandibular fracture is present or pins may be inserted into both mandibles (for bilateral fractures or to improve the strength of fixation for unilateral fractures). The connecting bar for ESF used to stabilize mandibular fractures is usually a column made of acrylic resin, as the resin can be molded to match the shape of the mandible and to engage all pins inserted in the mandible.[25] The acrylic connecting column should be applied leaving a 0.5–1 cm gap between the acrylic column and the skin to prevent impingement of the acrylic with the skin and to allow pin tract cleaning to be performed in the recovery period. Mandibular fracture healing after stabilization with an ESF construct is expected to occur over 6–12 weeks. Once radiographic evidence of fracture healing is obtained, the fixator should be removed by sectioning the acrylic column and unscrewing the threaded pins from the mandible.

Postoperative Management/Follow-up

Defects in the oral mucosa over the fracture site should be sutured closed following copious lavage to limit contamination of the fracture site from the oral cavity postoperatively.[3] In some cases, local flap techniques may be necessary to achieve oral mucosal closure if the fracture site has not been anatomically reduced or if oral mucosal tissue loss has occurred around the fracture site.

Analgesic therapy after mandibular fracture surgery typically consists of intermittent boluses of an injectable opioid drug for the first 12 hours postoperatively combined with an injectable non-steroidal anti-inflammatory drug.

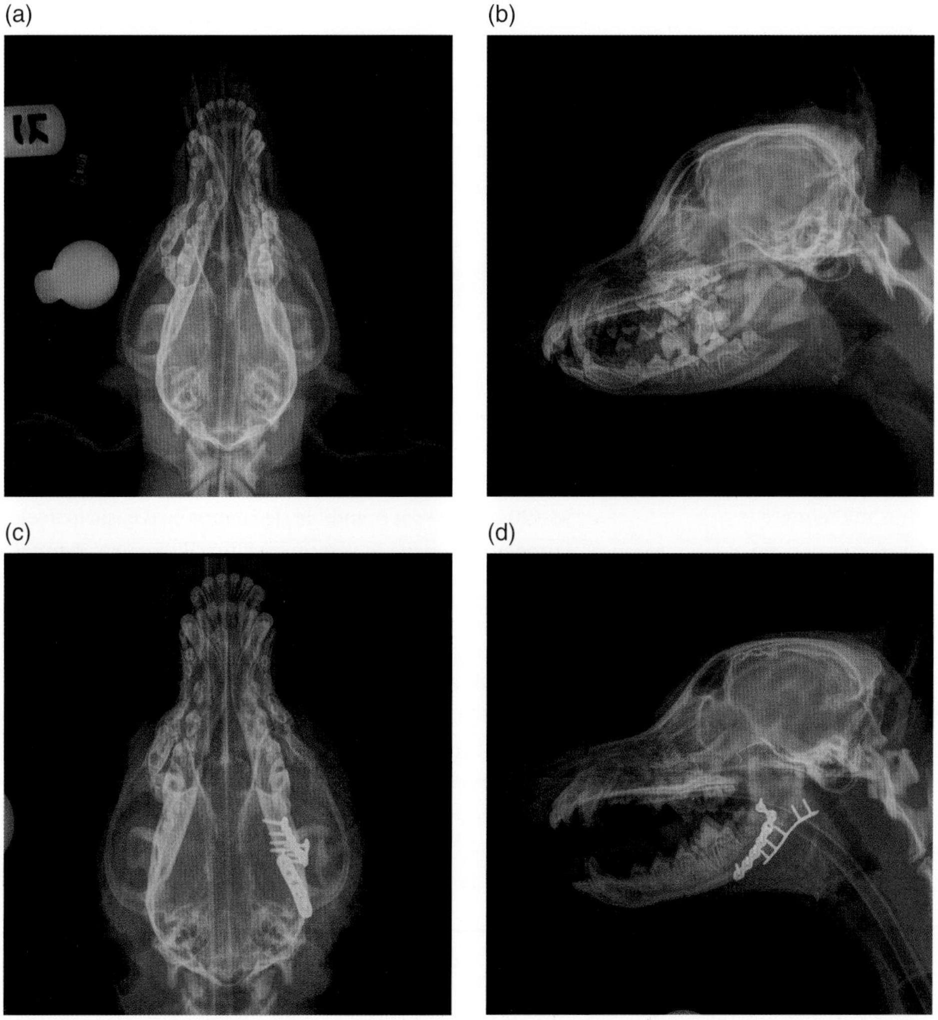

Figure 42.12 Preoperative and postoperative radiographs of a one-year-old, 6 kg mixed breed dog with a simple oblique caudal mandibular body fracture. The fracture was anatomically reduced and surgically stabilized using orthogonally positioned bone plates and screws. A 1.5 mm locking reconstruction-style, L-shaped plate was positioned on the lateral aspect of the mandibular body and ramus. A second 1.5 mm locking straight plate was positioned on the ventral aspect of the caudal mandibular body and angular process. All screws inserted through the ventrally positioned plate were monocortical. (a) Preoperative DV skull radiograph. (b) Preoperative lateral oblique skull radiograph. (c) Postoperative DV skull radiograph. (d) Postoperative lateral oblique skull radiograph. *Source:* © Caleb Hudson.

The day following surgery, patients are typically started on oral gabapentin and oral NSAID therapy, which is continued for 10–14 days postoperatively.

Antibiotic therapy is recommended after mandibular fracture stabilization surgery.[5,6] Postoperative antibiotic therapy has been shown to reduce the risk of osteomyelitis development in dogs after mandibular fracture stabilization surgery.[5] Empirical antibiotic therapy with a broad spectrum agent, such as amoxicillin with clavulanic acid or clindamycin, is often instituted for the first 7–10 days post-surgery. A bacterial culture sample should be obtained from the mandibular fracture site intraoperatively, and once culture and sensitivity results are available, antibiotic therapy can be altered as indicated by the test results.

Patients with mandibular fractures treated using maxillomandibular fixation techniques should be encouraged to lap a liquid diet but may initially have to be fed through a feeding tube. Patients in which rigid internal fixation of mandibular fractures has been achieved may be encouraged to take food orally starting the day following surgery. Convalescent patients should be fed soft food and not allowed access to chew toys until the mandibular fractures have healed.[3]

Follow-up radiographs are typically performed four weeks after surgery and then repeated every four weeks until bone healing is documented. Recheck skull radiographs or dental radiographs may be obtained depending on clinician preference and the location of the fracture.

Complications

Complications are common after mandibular fracture stabilization surgery, with reported complication rates ranging from 20% to >50% of cases.[5,6,9,13,15,25] Lower complication rates are typically reported after plate stabilization as compared to other forms of mandibular fracture stabilization. Most complications are minor, such as postoperative patient discomfort or drooling, mild malocclusion, or implant exposure in the oral cavity, but more severe complications requiring revision surgery, such as implant loosening, implant breakage, implant-associated infection, and non-union, are also reported after mandibular fracture stabilization surgery. Following the principles outlined in this chapter, including appropriately performed preoperative planning and implant selection, along with restoration of normal dental occlusion and provision of rigid fracture site stability, will help to minimize the development of postoperative complications.

References

1 Mulherin, B.L., Snyder, C.J., Soukup, J.W. et al. (2014). Retrospective evaluation of canine and feline maxillomandibular trauma cases. A comparison of signalment with non-maxillomandibular traumatic injuries (2003–2012). *Vet. Comp. Orthop. Traumatol.* 27 (3): 192–197.

2 Kitshoff, A.M., de Rooster, H., Ferreira, S.M. et al. (2013). A retrospective study of 109 dogs with mandibular fractures. *Vet. Comp. Orthop. Traumatol.* 26 (1): 1–5.

3 Boudrieau, R.J. (2018). Mandibular and maxillofacial fractures. In: *Veterinary Surgery: Small Animal*, 2e (ed. S.A. Johnston and K.M. Tobias), 1240–1265. St. Louis, MO: Elsevier.

4 Lefman, S. and Prittie, J.E. (2022). High-rise syndrome in cats and dogs. *J. Vet. Emerg. Crit. Care (San Antonio)* 32 (5): 571–581.

5 Umphlet, R.C. and Johnson, A.L. (1990). Mandibular fractures in the dog. A retrospective study of 157 cases. *Vet. Surg.* 19 (4): 272–275.

6 Umphlet, R.C. and Johnson, A.L. (1988). Mandibular fractures in the cat. A retrospective study. *Vet. Surg.* 17 (6): 333–337.

7 Freitag, V. and Landau, H. (1997). Histological findings in the alveolar sockets and tooth roots after experimental mandibular fractures in dogs. *J. Craniomaxillofac. Surg.* 25 (4): 203–211.

8 Reiter, A.M. and Soltero-Rivera, M.M. (2018). Dentistry for the surgeon. In: *Veterinary Surgery: Small Animal*, 2e (ed. S.A. Johnston and K.M. Tobias), 1224–1240. St. Louis, MO: Elsevier.

9 Nicholson, I., Wyatt, J., Radke, H. et al. (2010). Treatment of caudal mandibular fracture and temporomandibular joint fracture-luxation using a bi-gnathic encircling and retaining device. *Vet. Comp. Orthop. Traumatol.* 23 (2): 102–108.

10 Boudrieau, R.J. (2005). Fractures of the mandible. In: *AO Principles of Fracture Management in the Dog and Cat* (ed. A.L. Johnson, J.E. Houlton, and R. Vannini), 98–115. Davos, Switzerland: AO Publishing.

11 Lombardero, M., Alonso-Penarando, D., and Yllera, M. (2021). The cat mandible (I): anatomical basis to avoid iatrogenic damage in veterinary clinical practice. *Animals* 11: 405.

12 Bar-Am, Y., Pollard, R.E., Kass, P.H. et al. (2008). The diagnostic yield of conventional radiographs and computed tomography in dogs and cats with maxillofacial trauma. *Vet. Surg.* 37 (3): 294–299.

13 Guzu, M. and Hennet, P.R. (2017). Mandibular body fracture repair with wire-reinforced interdental composite splint in small dogs. *Vet. Surg.* 46 (8): 1068–1077.

14 Harasen, G. (2008). Maxillary and mandibular fractures. *Can. Vet. J.* 49 (8): 819–820.

15 Boudrieau, R.J. and Kudisch, M. (1996). Miniplate fixation for repair of mandibular and maxillary fractures in 15 dogs and 3 cats. *Vet. Surg.* 25 (4): 277–291.

16 Freeman, A. and Southerden, P. (2023). Mandibular fracture repair techniques in cats: a dentist's perspective. *J. Feline Med. Surg.* 25 (2): 1098612X231152521.

17 Miller, E.I., Acquaviva, A.E., Eisenmann, D.J. et al. (2011). Perpendicular pull-out force of locking versus non-locking plates in thin cortical bone using a canine mandibular ramus model. *Vet. Surg.* 40 (7): 870–874.

18 Piermattei, D.L. and Johnson, K.A. (2004). *Piermattei's Atlas of Surgical Approaches to the Bones and Joints of the Dog and Cat*, 4e, 33–45. Philadelphia, PA: Saunders.

19 Kern, D.A., Smith, M.M., Grant, J.W. et al. (1993). Evaluation of bending strength of five interdental fixation apparatuses applied to canine mandibles. *Am. J. Vet. Res.* 54 (7): 1177–1182.

20 Holmstrom, S.E., Frost, P.F., and Eisner, E.R. (1998). *Veterinary Dental Techniques: for the Small Animal Practitioner*, 2e. Philadelphia: WB Saunders.

21 Verstraete, F.J. (2003). Maxillofacial fractures. In: *Textbook of Small Animal Surgery*, 3e (ed. D. Slatter), 2190–2207. Philadelphia, PA: Saunders.

22 Muir, P. and Gengler, W.R. (1999). Interdental acrylic stabilisation of canine tooth root and mandibular fractures in a dog. *Vet. Rec.* 145 (2): 43–45.

23 Cote, E. (ed.) (2011). *Clinical Veterinary Advisor, ed 2.* St. Louis: Mosby.

24 Rice, C.A., Riehl, J., Broman, K. et al. (2012). Comparing the degree of exothermic polymerization in commonly used acrylic and provisional composite resins for intraoral appliances. *J. Vet. Dent.* 29 (2): 78–83.

25 Owen, M.R., Hobbs, S.J., Moores, A.P. et al. (2004). Mandibular fracture repair in dogs and cats using epoxy resin and acrylic external skeletal fixation. *Vet. Comp. Orthop. Traumatol.* 17 (04): 189–197.

43

Metacarpal and Metatarsal Fractures

Rebecca J. Webb

VetSurg, Ventura, CA, USA

Key Points

- Metacarpal and metatarsal fractures are common injuries encountered in dogs and cats.
- Factors such as which bones and how many are fractured, the location of the fractures, the displacement of the fracture segments, and patient factors are all carefully considered before the decision to pursue surgical intervention is chosen.
- Even if surgical stabilization is chosen for metacarpal or metatarsal fractures, the surgical fixation will need to be supported with external coaptation for a few weeks. The time spent in coaptation (e.g., a splint or soft-padded bandage) will depend on factors such as the patient's age and temperament, type of fracture, method of repair, and owner compliance.

Introduction

Metatarsal and metacarpal bone fractures can occur secondary to a range of injuries. Injuries can either be low impact, such as jumping off furniture, or high impact, such as being hit by a car. As there is very little soft tissue surrounding these bones, in cases with severe trauma, open fractures in this region are not uncommon. Fractures can range from simple transverse to comminuted, depending on the level of trauma sustained. The metacarpal and metatarsal bones are numbered 1–5 starting medially. Each metacarpal and metatarsal bone is divided into three regions, the proximal base, the middle body, and the distal head. The first metacarpal and metatarsal are non-weight-bearing, as they are significantly shorter than the other four (Figure 43.1).

Indications/Pre-op Considerations

Both conservative and surgical management of metatarsal and metacarpal fractures have been successfully employed for different fracture configurations in veterinary medicine. Several "rules" as to when surgical management should be pursued have been described over time. However, the accuracy of these recommendations is debated among surgeons, with some surgeons preferring a conservative approach for most, if not all, metacarpal and metatarsal fractures. Conservative management is typically recommended in the literature for minimally displaced fractures or fractures where at least one of the primary weight-bearing bones (metacarpal/metatarsal III or IV) is still intact.[1–4] Surgery is traditionally recommended in the following scenarios:

- If more than two metacarpals or metatarsals are fractured in the same limb;
- If the fractures involve both the primary weight-bearing metacarpals or metatarsals (III and IV);
- If the fractures involve the articular surface, as failure to restore joint congruity will lead to osteoarthritis;
- If the fracture fragments are displaced >50% and cannot be reduced manually under general anesthesia;
- If the fracture involves the base of metacarpal/metatarsal II or V, as this is where the collateral ligaments insert;
- In large breed, athletic, or working dogs.[3–6]

Techniques in Small Animal Soft Tissue, Orthopedic, and Ophthalmic Surgery, First Edition. Edited by Kristin A. Coleman.

Companion website: www.wiley.com/go/coleman/surgeries

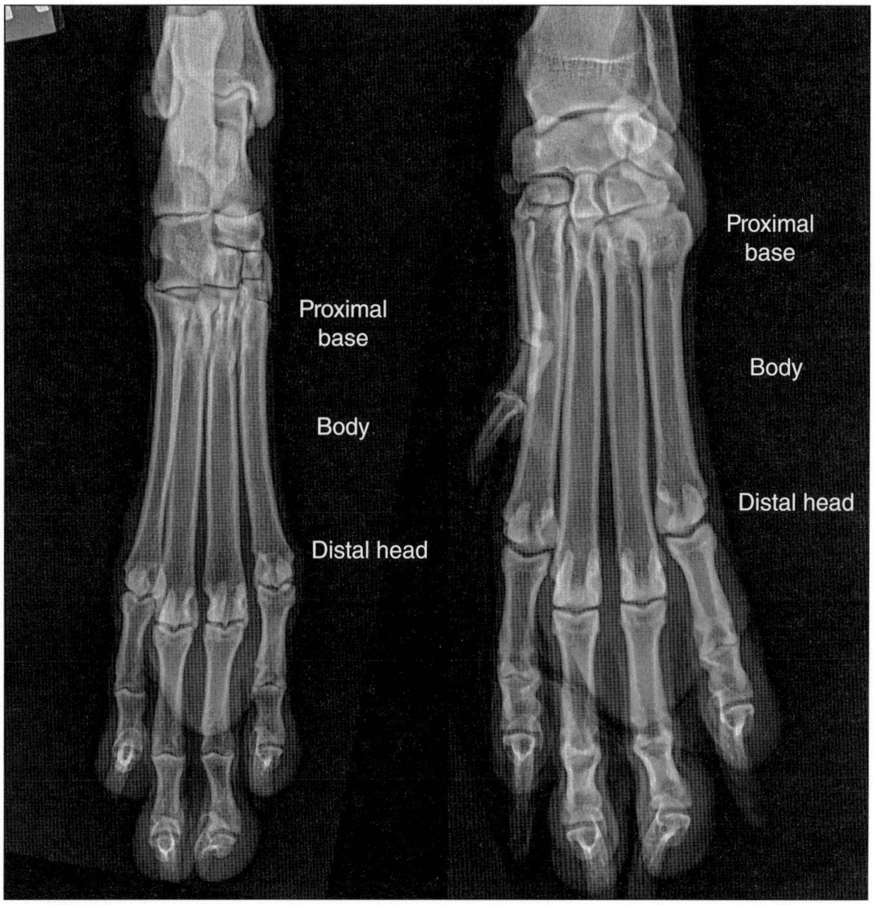

Figure 43.1 Craniocaudal radiographs of the canine metatarsals (left image) and metacarpals (right image) showing the proximal base, middle body, and distal head of the bones. The bones are numbered 1–5 from medial to lateral. *Source:* © Rebecca Webb.

Diagnostic Imaging

Orthogonal radiographs (dorsopalmar/dorsoplantar [DP] and lateral views) are standard for evaluation of fractures in this region. Additional radiographic views can be considered if needed, including (1) 45° lateral oblique views to evaluate fractures from the lateral aspect without superimposition of the metacarpals/metatarsals, (2) medial/lateral stressed views of the carpus/tarsus to evaluate for collateral laxity, and (3) DP and lateral views with the toes spread to evaluate the digits more thoroughly. The digits can be spread by applying tape to each of the digits and adhering the other end of the tape to the radiology table to spread them. A computed tomography (CT) scan can also be performed to evaluate these fractures but typically is not required prior to surgery.

Cases that are presented secondary to serious trauma should be fully evaluated and stabilized prior to surgical repair being considered. During systemic stabilization, support of the fractures with a splinted bandage to improve patient comfort and wound care, if applicable to the case, are recommended until definitive repair can be pursued. Open wounds associated with fracture fragments should be evaluated and given wound management prior to surgical fixation. These wounds can range from pinpoint dermal defects secondary to puncture from the underlying sharp bony fragments, which are still likely to be successfully addressed with surgical stabilization of the fracture(s), to large shearing wounds with loss of the overlying soft tissue. Extensive tissue loss, as is seen in shearing injuries, is challenging when considering surgical fixation of this region, as there is minimal neighboring loose skin to close defects in this area. Due to this, these defects often must be healed by second intention. Recognizing this is important, as any implants applied to the metatarsal or metacarpal bone fractures are likely to be exposed while the overlying tissue heals, increasing the risk of infection. A plan to remove implants once healed is often required. This should be taken into consideration when making the initial surgical plan, as some implants and fixation methods used in this area are especially challenging to remove, such as dowel pinning. As such, implants that may result in high morbidity to the patient with attempted explantation should be avoided in these cases.

Patients who present with wounds (either small or large) should be given basic wound care and started on a broad-spectrum antibiotic (such as amoxicillin–clavulanic acid or cefpodoxime) prior to surgery to help reduce the risk of infection. Generally, fractures that are simple in nature will have more load-sharing between the fracture fragments and the implants when reconstructed. In cases like these, simpler constructs can be successful. In cases with heavy comminution and minimal load-sharing between the bone fragments and the construct and in larger patients, stronger constructs, such as bone plating, are typically indicated.

Surgical Procedure

Patient Preparation

Clipping of the entire foot and interdigital region is recommended to give the surgeon access to the distal aspect of the metatarsals/metacarpals. Due to the interdigital skin folds and ungual regions surrounding the nails, sterile preparation of the digits can be challenging. Following diligent clipping of hair in the region, performing a foot soak can be helpful prior to performing a final sterile preparation. To perform a foot soak, the digits and foot should be soaked in 4% chlorhexidine or 10% povidone-iodine solution. This can be performed by filling an examination glove with the solution and placing the foot within it for three to five minutes. Porous tape or an elastic adhesive bandage (such as Vetap™) is used to secure the top of the glove around the metacarpals/metatarsals during soaking time to prevent spillage of scrub solution from the glove (Figure 43.2). Following this foot soak, the foot is hung in the operating room for ease of

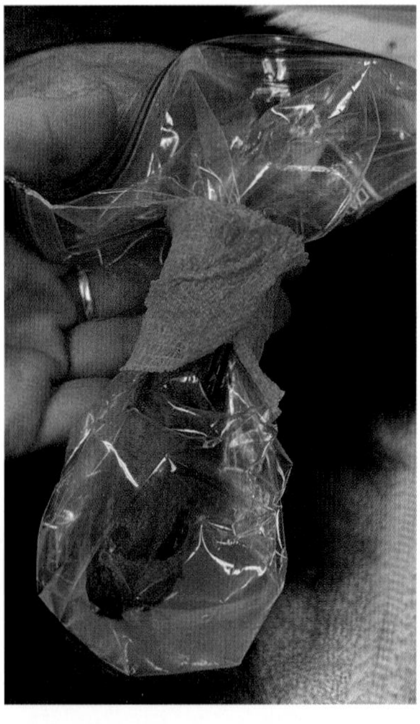

Figure 43.2 Paw soak. Following clipping of the fur of the digits, the paw is soaked in a surgical preparation solution while the patient is moved into the operating room. *Source:* © Rebecca Webb.

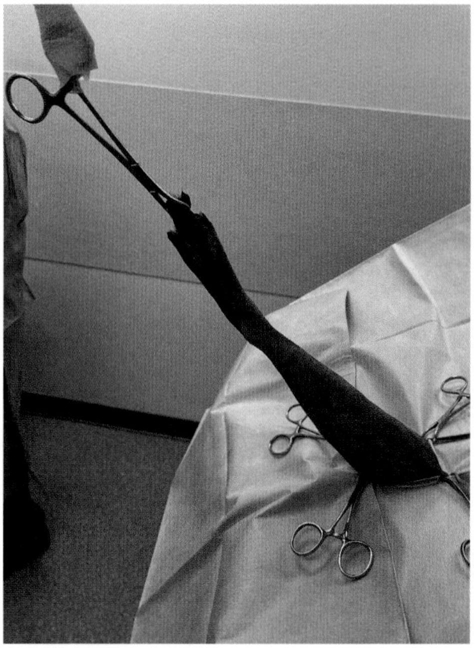

Figure 43.3 The paw is suspended to allow final surgical preparation of the paw and limb using a sterile towel clamp placed in the interdigital space. The towel clamp is then used to suspend the limb using tape around the handle to secure the limb to an overhead light or IV pole. *Source:* © Rebecca Webb.

draping, and a final surgical preparation of the limb is performed. To hang the foot, a sterile Backhaus towel clamp can be placed in the interdigital space and then secured to tape to suspend the foot and distal limb from an IV pole or similar structure for the preparation and draping to be performed (Figure 43.3). Once the patient has been draped, the sterile surgeon or surgical assistant grasps the foot, and a non-sterile surgical assistant can remove the towel clamp from the digits to release the foot to the surgical team.

Approach and General Considerations

Fracture Types

Fractures of the Base These fractures are typically avulsions of ligamentous insertions. Given the pull of the ligamentous structures, these fractures are susceptible to displacement, malunion, and potential secondary joint instability. Surgical fixation is the treatment of choice for these fractures. Options for isolated fracture (and not joint instability) include interfragmentary lag screw placement or a buttress plate.

Fractures of the Body Fractures of the shaft can be managed either conservatively or surgically. The decision between the two depends on multiple factors described above, including the number of bones involved, the level of displacement of the fragments, the inherent stability of the fracture, and the configuration of the fracture. Common methods for fixation include bone plating, dowel pinning, intramedullary pinning, and external fixator placement.

Fractures of the Head Fractures in this region are commonly intraarticular owing to their location. Given their small distal segment, they are often unstable and require surgical fixation. Commonly these fractures are repaired with interfragmentary lag screws.

Surgical Approach and Instrumentation

Depending upon the metatarsal or metacarpal bones that are fractured, the surgical approach will differ. If access to a single metatarsal or metacarpal bone is required, an incision over the dorsal aspect of that specific bone is made to access the fracture. If two neighboring bones need to be accessed, the dorsal incision can be centered between the two. If access to all four metatarsals or metacarpals is required, options include one central dorsal incision (in small patients where the overlying soft tissues can easily be shifted to gain access to all four bones), two separate incisions centered between M2+3 and M3+4 (in larger patients where there is less mobility of the overlying soft tissues), or one elongated S-shape incision to span all four meta-bones. Some clinicians prefer a medial or lateral approach when dealing with fractures of M2 and M5, respectively.

Given the small nature of these bones and their fragility, fine instrumentation for manipulation is recommended. The use of hemostats to manipulate the bone fragments can be helpful, and small Hohmann retractors and/or Gelpi retractors are important for holding back the dorsally-located extensor tendons while manipulating, reducing, and stabilizing the fracture fragments. In addition, the use of a small hand chuck can be helpful when using Kirshner wires or pins.

Fixation Methods

Dowel Pinning Dowel pins are intramedullary Kirshner wires, which are placed retrograde from the fracture site to align the bone. A K-wire that almost fills the medullary canal of the bone is selected, and the wire is advanced into the longer of the two bone fragments until it is seated. The wire is then cut to leave approximately 5–15 mm of the wire protruding from the fracture site. Using gentle manipulation, the fracture is distracted, and the protruding end of the wire is seated into the intramedullary canal of the shorter fragment. Gentle twisting of the two fragments along the wire is helpful to complete the reduction. The placement of the intramedullary pins will restrict bending motions at the fracture site, which means dowel pinning and intramedullary pinning are best suited for simple fracture stabilization in which load-sharing between the implant and bone is present. In addition, dowel and intramedullary pinning is often only appropriate for midbody non-comminuted fractures, as proximal or distal fractures lack substantial bone for seating of the implant (Figure 43.4).[7]

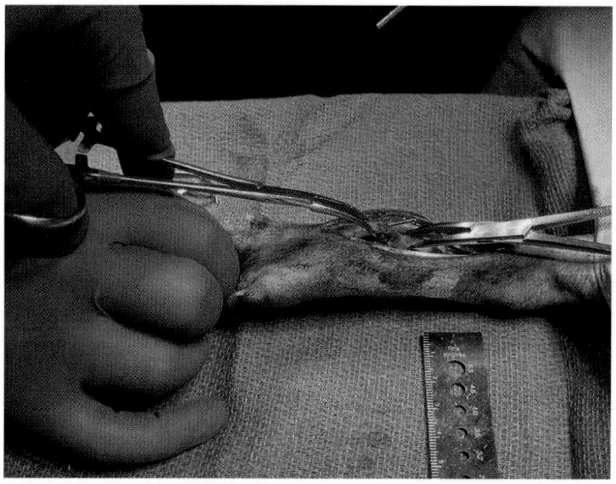

Figure 43.4 Dowel pinning. The pin has been placed into the longer distal metatarsal and cut short. In the image, the fracture is being distracted to allow insertion of the exposed pin into the medullary cavity of the proximal fragment. *Source:* © Rebecca Webb.

Intramedullary Pinning Intramedullary Kirshner wires are placed normograde from either the proximal or distal metacarpal metatarsal bone fragment. The K-wires are started at the dorsal aspect of the bone to avoid impingement of the neighboring joint and then advanced into the intramedullary canal. Once the pin is advanced to the level of the fracture site, the fracture is held in reduction while the pin is advanced into the other fragment of the fracture. Once the pin has been advanced appropriately, it is bent close to the dorsal entry point on the metacarpal or metatarsal bone and cut short. Compared to dowel pinning (above), this technique has the advantage of ease of retrieval of the pin if explanation is required. The disadvantages of this technique are the potential for impingement of the overlying extensor tendons, potential for damage to the joint surfaces by the pin (leading to osteoarthritis), and implant exposure due to the small amount of overlying soft tissues in this region.

Bone Plating Small bone plates (typically 1.5 and 2.0 mm plates) can be used in appropriately-sized patients (Figure 43.5). These plates are typically placed on the dorsal surface; however, some clinicians prefer to plate metacarpal/metatarsal II medially and V laterally. This medial or lateral placement avoids any impingement of the plate and screws with the extensor tendons, and due to the scarcity of soft tissues in this region, the approach is simplified. Clinicians should ensure when plating on the medial or lateral surface that their plate is adequately

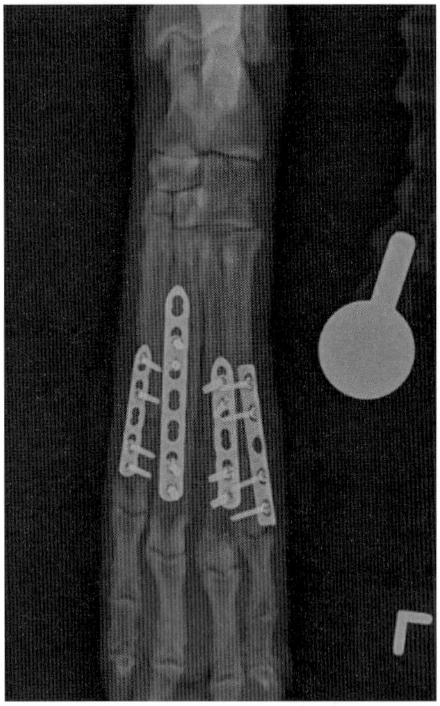

Figure 43.5 Bone plating. This patient had plating of left MT II-V fractures. *Source:* © Rebecca Webb.

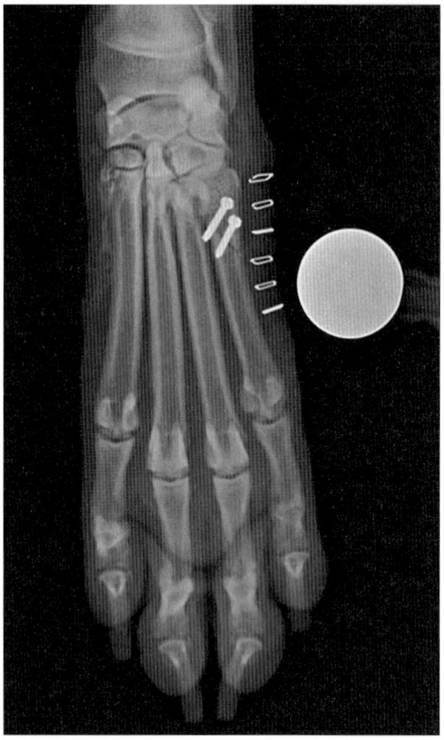

Figure 43.6 Interfragmentary screw placement in a short oblique fracture of proximal metacarpal V. *Source:* Courtesy of Dr. Desmond Tan.

contoured, as the bone is more curved on these surfaces than it is dorsally.[8]

External Fixator External skeletal fixation can be employed in appropriate cases. Typically, a combination of small pins and epoxy putty is most common with small connecting bars being used in larger patients (due to their increased weight). Pins can be placed transversely across the fragments or in combination with an intramedullary tie-in.[1] The placement of external fixators is beneficial in cases with open fractures, as the ESF implants are eventually removed. However, clinicians should be cautious during case selection, as accurate placement of fixator pins into the small metacarpal and metatarsal bones can be challenging. The use of fluoroscopy is helpful to allow these procedures to be performed in a closed manner, and therefore, improve the biology of the fracture site.

Interfragmentary Screw Placement of an interfragmentary screw is recommended in cases with oblique fractures. This method is most commonly utilized in fractures of the proximal base of metacarpal/metatarsal II and V (Figure 43.6). Fixation of fractures to the proximal base of these bones is important, as they are the areas of insertion of the collateral ligaments. Untreated fractures in this area can lead to instability of the joints, leading to osteoarthritis long term. Placement of an interfragmentary screw is helpful in these proximal fractures, as the small proximal fragment often precludes the placement of a bone plate in these cases. These screws are ideally placed for stabilizing long oblique fractures (where the fracture length is at least twice the diameter of the bone). A minimum of two screws are placed to prevent the bony fragments from rotating on a single screw. The screw is typically placed in lag fashion, although in small bones where the clinician is concerned about fragmentation of the bone with placement, the fracture is anatomically reduced and placed in a standard fashion. Typically, cortical screws are used for this, and screw size should be determined based on the patient's bone width at the level of the fracture.

Potential Complications

Due to the small size of these bones, implant size is often limited. For this reason, bandages are often used in addition to internal fixation, and bandage-associated disease is common in these patients. Other complications include delayed or non-union of the fractures. This is not uncommon in these patients due to the poor soft tissue surroundings of the metatarsals and metacarpal bones. Often, despite a failure of bony union, a fibrous union occurring in small patients can still be quite functional. Non-union is likely of higher consequences in sporting and large breed dogs, and in these cases, the use of bone grafts can be considered at the time of the surgery to assist healing. Other complications include osteomyelitis, implant loosening/infection, synostoses, and osteoarthritis.

Post-op Care/Prognosis

Limited leashed activity and strict confinement at home are recommended until a bridging callus forms, which may be four to eight weeks depending on patient signalment and other individual factors.

External Coaptation

Bandaging is used following surgery in most cases. Casts should technically stabilize "the joint above" and should extend to the proximal antebrachium or crus for patient comfort and to reduce the risk of bandage morbidity. They are typically used when the repair has minimal strength (typically in cases with intramedullary pinning or dowel pinning). The length of time to use a cast in these cases is debatable, but in the author's practice is commonly two to three weeks, after which it is reduced to a splint (caudal for the metacarpals and caudolateral for the metatarsals) for three to four weeks followed by a soft-padded bandage for one to two weeks. In cases where plating is performed, a splint (caudal for the metacarpals and caudolateral for the metatarsals) is commonly used for the first three to four weeks given the large weight of these patients and the small size of the implants used. When external coaptation is used without surgical stabilization, a cast is typically used for four to six weeks followed by a caudal or caudolateral splint for three to four weeks. Patients in external coaptation should have their bandage changed weekly.

Radiographs

Radiographs should be performed at regular intervals to monitor healing of the fractures and to monitor the implants. The first radiographs are typically performed at four to six weeks and then performed every four weeks until healing is complete.

Many of these fractures heal uneventfully. However, factors that may impact healing include open fractures, the degree of comminution, articular fractures, and fractures with a high degree of displacement.[9,10]

References

1. Fitzpatrick, N., Riordan, J.O., Smith, T.J. et al. (2011). Combined intramedullary and external skeletal fixation of metatarsal and metacarpal fractures in 12 dogs and 19 cats. *Vet. Surg.* 40 (8): 1015–1022.
2. Piras, A. and Bruecker, K.A. (2021). Common pathology associated with the digits and metacarpal region. *Vet. Clin. Small Anim.* 51: 263–284.
3. Muir, P. and Norris, J.L. (1997). Metacarpal and metatarsal fractures in dogs. *J. Small Anim. Pract.* 38 (8): 344–348.
4. Johnson, A.L. (2013). Management of specific fractures - metacarpal, metatarsal, phalangeal and sesamoid fractures and luxations. In: *Small Animal Surgery*, 4e (ed. S.A. Johnston and K.M. Tobias), 1163–1168. Missouri, USA: Elsevier.
5. Wernham, B.G.J. and Roush, J.K. (2010). Metacarpal and metatarsal fractures in dogs. *Compend. Contin. Educ. Vet.* 32 (3): E1–E7.
6. Kapatkin, A.S., Garcia-Nolen, T., and Hayashi, K. (2018). Carpus, metacarpus and digits. In: *Veterinary Surgery Small Animal*, 2e, 920–938. Johnston, S.A., Tobias, K.M. Missouri, USA: Elsevier.
7. Zahn, K., Kornmayer, M., and Matis, U. (2007). 'Dowel' pinning for feline metacarpal and metatarsal fractures. *Vet. Comp. Orthop. Traumatol.* 20 (4): 256–263.
8. Piras, A. and Guerrero, T. (2012). Minimally invasive repair of metabones. *Vet. Clin. North Am. Small Anim. Pract.* 42 (5): 1045–1050.
9. Manley, P.A. (1981). Distal extremity fractures in small animals. *J. Vet. Orthop.* 2 (2): 38–48.
10. Kornmayer, M., Failing, K., and Matis, U. (2014). Long-term prognosis of metacarpal and metatarsal fractures in dogs. A retrospective analysis of medical histories in 100 re-evaluated patients. *Vet. Comp. Orthop. Traumatol.* 27 (1): 45–53.

44

Humeral Condylar Fractures

Nathan T. Squire[1] and David Dycus[2]

[1] *Gulf Coast Veterinary Specialists, Houston, TX, USA*
[2] *Ortho Vet Consulting, Severn, MD, USA*

Key Points

- Humeral condylar fractures are common, making up approximately 41–44% of all humeral fractures in the dog.
- Most humeral condylar fractures involve the lateral aspect and occur in skeletally immature dogs.
- Humeral condylar fractures can occur in the medial aspect, and, if they occur, they are usually in skeletally mature dogs.
- Complex T-Y humeral condylar fractures (also termed "bicondylar" fractures) account for about 20% of all humeral condylar fractures.
- Given the articular nature of humeral condylar fractures, anatomical reconstruction with avoidance of steps or gaps at the articular surface is the key to fixation.
- Transcondylar screw placement is key for articular reconstruction.
- Ancillary fixation should be robust with anti-rotational Kirschner wires or epicondylar plates.
- With appropriate fixation, outcomes are expected to be good, though the development of elbow osteoarthritis is possible.

Introduction

The canine and feline humerus is a complex bone, having an "S-shape" from the lateral perspective and terminating distally with the humeral condyle, which is divided into medial and lateral components. It should be noted that there is only one humeral condyle with medial and lateral portions; there are no separate medial and lateral humeral condyles. The medial part of the humeral condyle is termed the *trochlea* and articulates with the ulna, while the lateral part of the humeral condyle is termed the *capitulum* and articulates mainly with the radial head. Caudally, the olecranon fossa articulates with the anconeal process of the ulna and provides important medial-lateral stability when the elbow is extended. Two prominent bony landmarks, the medial and lateral epicondyles, are present on the medial and lateral aspects of the humeral condyle and serve as the origin for the flexor and extensor muscle groups, respectively, along with the medial and lateral collateral ligaments of the elbow. The distal metaphysis, proximal to the condyle, is divided by the supratrochlear foramen.[1] It should be noted that, in cats, the supratrochlear foramen is not perforated as it is in the dog. Therefore, condylar fractures in the cat are less common. However, in cats, there is a supracondylar (i.e., epicondylar) foramen just proximal to the medial epicondyle, through which the median nerve and brachial artery pass. Caution should be taken when making surgical approaches and when placing implants for fracture fixation in this region.

The maturation of the distal part of the humerus entails the formation of both the trochlea and the capitulum, which arise from separate centers of ossification. These centers typically fuse by roughly 85 days (3 months), followed by fusion of the entire condyle to the metaphysis by

Techniques in Small Animal Soft Tissue, Orthopedic, and Ophthalmic Surgery, First Edition. Edited by Kristin A. Coleman.

Companion website: www.wiley.com/go/coleman/surgeries

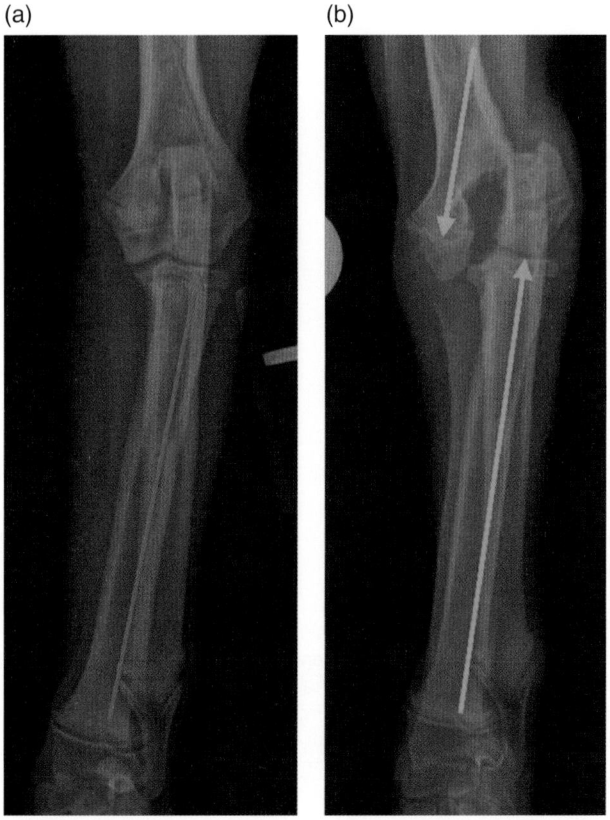

Figure 44.1 Cranio-caudal radiographs displaying an intact (left) humeral condyle and a Salter–Harris type IV fracture (right). (a) Note how as the load transfers through the antebrachium (orange arrows) it is passed through the elbow with the majority of the load through the humeral capitulum and the lateral epicondylar crest. (b) Because of the load transfer and the natural shearing force through (green arrows) the humeral capitulum and weaker lateral epicondylar crest, there is a predisposition for fracture through the lateral humeral condyle, extending through the lateral epicondylar crest. When this occurs, there is proximal displacement. *Source:* © Dr. David Dycus.

5.5–6 months of age.[2] Weight-bearing of the antebrachium is directed from the radial head through the capitulum and lateral epicondylar crest. The lateral epicondylar crest is smaller and weaker than the medial epicondylar crest. In the skeletally immature dog, prior to the fusion of these centers and the metaphysis, the softness of the bone in the lateral epicondyle in conjunction with the forces applied through the radial head during weight-bearing to the humeral capitulum predispose dogs to Salter–Harris type IV fractures that involve the articular surface of the condyle (Figure 44.1). In dogs, lateral condylar fractures are the most common (~70%), with complex T/Y fractures involving both components of the condyle (~20%) and medial condylar fractures (10%) being significantly less common (Figure 44.2).[2,3] Patient signalment is an important consideration when evaluating fusion of the humeral condyle. Humeral intracondylar fissure (HIF), previously referred to as incomplete ossification of the humeral condyle (IOHC), is characterized by a fissure in the sagittal plane bisecting the humeral condyle that persists past the normal age of ossification (Figure 44.3). English Springer Spaniels, French Bulldogs, and other breeds have been reported to be at a higher risk for this condition.[4,5]

The neurovascular structures surrounding the distal aspect of the humerus are robust and intricate, and they must be accounted for when considering the surgical approach and implantation for fracture repair. Laterally, the radial nerve traverses the humerus from caudoproximal to craniodistal approximately 2/3 of the way distally along the diaphysis, superficial to the brachialis muscle. This nerve crosses the elbow joint cranial to the lateral epicondyle before sending a deep branch to the extensor carpi radialis and terminates by innervating the underside of the supinator muscle on the radius and continuing distally in the interosseous space. This nerve innervates muscles that control both elbow and carpal extension. The median nerve lies on the craniomedial surface of the humerus, while the ulnar nerve courses caudomedially prior to crossing the elbow joint. The median nerve runs adjacent to the brachial artery and vein cranially, while the collateral ulnar artery and vein follow the course of the ulnar nerve caudally.[6]

Indications and Preoperative Considerations

As with all fracture patients, a comprehensive evaluation is crucial to rule out concurrent effects of trauma on the body as a whole. Patients presenting with a history of significant trauma should have a complete physical exam (including both orthopedic and neurologic evaluation), baseline bloodwork (typically, a complete blood count and serum chemistry panel), three-view chest radiographs, and evaluation of the abdominal cavity, usually either via abdominal-focused assessment of ultrasonographic trauma (AFAST) or abdominal radiographs. This evaluation is important for patients who have sustained significant trauma, such as from vehicular trauma, or who have a complex T-Y condylar fracture. For skeletally immature patients that suffer lower velocity trauma, such as a fall from an elevated surface, and have a Salter–Harris type IV lateral condylar fracture, a complete physical examination and baseline bloodwork are typically sufficient. Following the establishment of patient stability, two-view radiographs of the affected limb are performed. It is often useful to obtain contralateral humeral radiographs both for interpretation of the fracture site and for surgical planning. Patients who present with a lack of significant trauma with a humeral condylar fracture should be carefully evaluated for the

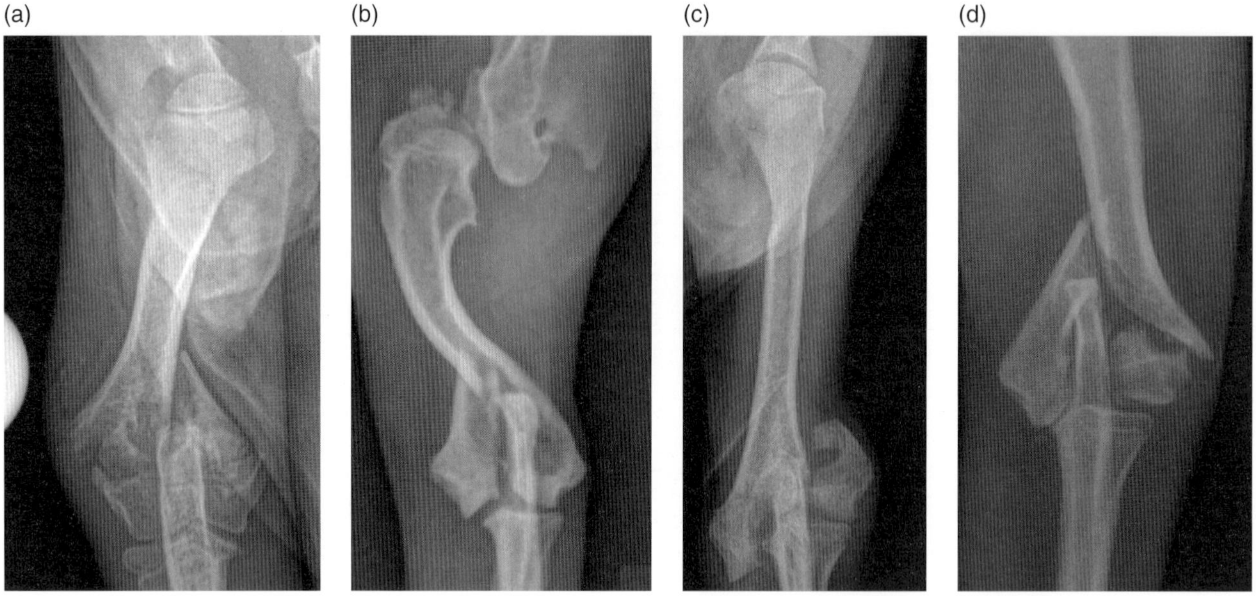

Figure 44.2 Cranio-caudal radiographs of various distal humeral fractures. (a) A supracondylar distal humeral fracture in a skeletally immature dog. Note how there is the fracturing of the humerus just proximal to the supratrochlear foramen involving both epicondylar crests. The fracture, however, does not extend into the articular surface. (b) A medial humeral condylar fracture in a skeletally mature dog. The fracture is articular in nature and extends through the medial epicondylar crest. In addition, this patient has glenoid dysplasia and a resultant angular deformity of the humerus. (c) A lateral humeral condylar fracture (Salter–Harris type IV) in a skeletally immature dog. The fracture is articular in nature and extends through the lateral epicondylar crest. (d) A complex "T-Y" humeral condylar fracture. The fracture is articular in nature and involves both the lateral and medial epicondylar crest. *Source:* © Dr. David Dycus.

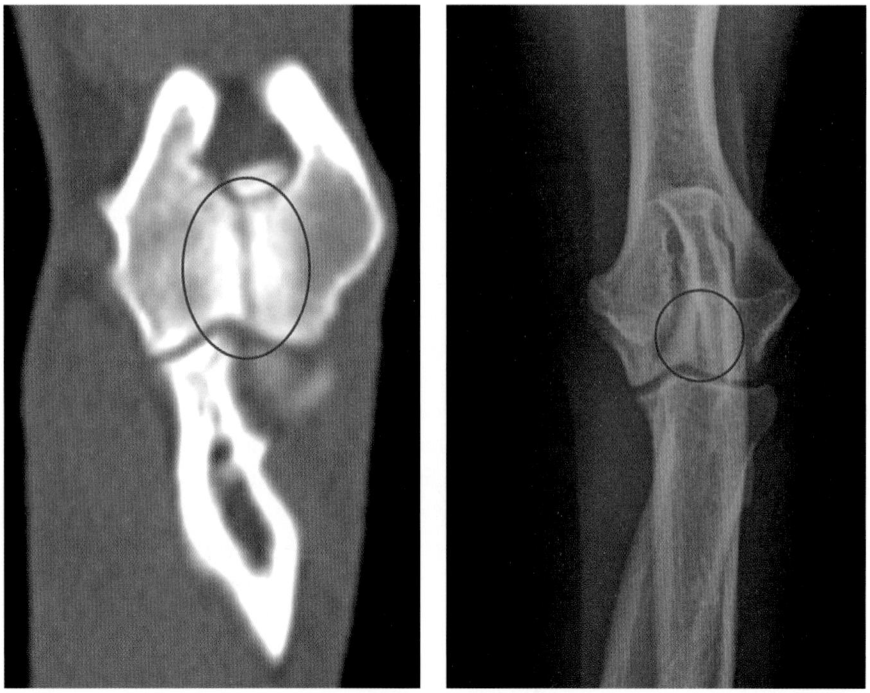

Figure 44.3 Images of humeral intracondylar fissure (HIF) in a three-year-old English Springer Spaniel. On the left is an axial CT image depicting the fissure (red oval). The image on the right is a cranio-caudal radiograph with the fissure evident (red circle). In some cases, a $10–15^{0}$ craniolateral-caudomedial oblique view is required to identify the fissure on plain radiographs. *Source:* © Dr. David Dycus.

presence of underlying HIF, particularly in predisposed breeds. This screening involves two-view radiographs of the affected and contralateral humerus, and/or 10° obliqued craniolateral-caudomedial radiographs, and/or a CT scan (Figure 44.3).[7] Neurologic evaluation of the affected limb(s) should involve careful evaluation of radial nerve function, as this nerve crosses the distolateral aspect of the humerus and is, at times, compromised by the initial trauma or by the fracture itself.

After orthopedic and neurologic evaluation, analgesics should be administered. Most commonly, this involves a full mu opioid, such as fentanyl, hydromorphone, or methadone, if the patient is to remain hospitalized. Nonsteroidal anti-inflammatories (NSAIDs) may be administered judiciously, but caution should be used in patients with significant trauma, hypotension, renal compromise, or other preexisting conditions that increase the risk for side effects. In the absence of open wounds, antibiotics are not necessary to administer to fracture patients upon admission to the hospital. If a patient is confirmed or suspected to have an open fracture, broad-spectrum antibiotics should be administered as soon as possible, as this has been shown to improve outcomes in this population.[8]

Prior to the definitive correction, the limb may be temporarily stabilized in a Spica splint. It is crucial that external coaptation immobilizes both the elbow and the shoulder to appropriately protect the fracture site and the adjacent soft tissue structures. A common error is to place a soft-padded bandage that stops at the level of the axilla proximally. This will act as a fulcrum on the fracture site, increasing patient discomfort and the likelihood of additional trauma. Alternatively, the limb may be left without a bandage, as most patients will protect the fracture site by reducing or eliminating weight-bearing on the affected limb.

Treatment options for humeral condylar fractures are numerous and are based on multiple factors, including fracture configuration, fracture chronicity, patient age, presence of HIF, and others. As with any articular fracture, anatomical reconstruction of the joint surface is critical with the avoidance of any steps or gaps. In general, medial or lateral humeral condylar fractures are treated with a transcondylar screw placed either in a lag or positional fashion. Following articular reconstruction, adjunctive fixation is needed to achieve fracture stability. This can be completed with a bone plate on the ipsilateral epicondylar region of the distal humerus or with an anti-rotational K-wire placed from the humeral epicondyle and driven proximally through the epicondylar crest to exit the contralateral cortex. However, recent evidence suggests adjunctive K-wire fixation is more prone to complications compared to plating, as an epicondylar plate is biomechanically stronger than an adjunctive K-wire.[9,10] Repair solely with pins has been reported and may be feasible when other fixation methods are not readily available or in exceptionally small patients; however, the authors do not recommend this approach.[11] Complex "T-Y" fractures of the humeral condyle are significantly more unstable and, therefore, require more robust fixation. This typically involves the placement of a transcondylar screw or screws as mentioned above, in addition to medial and lateral bone plates. Plates placed for unicondylar or bicondylar fractures are typically placed in a bridging fashion, and locking implants are preferred to non-locking implants by the authors, particularly in juvenile patients with soft cancellous bone that increases the likelihood of screw pull-out with conventional cortical screws. In addition, the complex distal anatomy of the humerus makes the exact contouring that is required for non-locking implants challenging. Preoperative templating for appropriate implant selection can be performed with digital software or more conventional acrylic templating. It is imperative that radiographs are appropriately calibrated to ensure accurate templating.

Apart from Salter–Harris type I or type II fractures, both of which are uncommon, humeral condylar fractures are articular in nature and, therefore, require anatomic reconstruction and rigid fixation. Because of the articular nature of the fracture and damage to the joint, it is imperative to consult with owners that articular fractures initiate the process of osteoarthritis, and this is expected to develop over time. However, many dogs with humeral condylar fractures have an excellent to good long-term prognosis if the joint surface is able to be reconstructed. Failure to achieve an anatomic reduction of the fracture may result in loss of elbow range of motion, ongoing lameness, and the development of more significant osteoarthritis during the recovery period and afterward.[12,13] Management of osteoarthritis falls outside the scope of this chapter but is nevertheless an important component of communicating a realistic prognosis to the owner.

Surgical Procedure

Due to the importance of anatomic reconstruction of the joint surface and the complex osseous anatomy involved in fracture fixation, intraoperative fluoroscopy can be helpful for humeral condylar fracture repair. Where fluoroscopy is not available, additional surgical exposure may be useful or even necessary to confirm appropriate fracture reduction and implant placement.

Complex T-Y humeral fractures and medial humeral condylar fractures, both of which occur considerably less commonly, will not be discussed in this chapter. Referral to a board-certified surgeon should be considered in these cases given their complexity and need for specialized equipment and techniques.

Lateral Humeral Condylar Fractures

The affected forequarter is clipped circumferentially from the dorsal midline or the level of the scapula distally to at least the level of the carpus, and a routine sterile preparation is performed. The animal may be placed either in dorsal or lateral recumbency with the affected limb up. Dorsal recumbency facilitates both the use of intraoperative fluoroscopy and performing a medial approach to the humeral condyle, if necessary.

A lateral approach to the humeral condyle is performed by making a curvilinear skin incision overlying the distal humerus and extending distally over the lateral humeral epicondyle and the proximal aspect of the radius. Electrosurgery is used for hemostasis as needed. The skin and subcutaneous tissue are incised on the same line. This will expose the lateral head of the triceps caudal to the humerus, and an incision is made in the fascia just cranial to this muscle belly, which is then extended distally over the extensor muscles of the antebrachium. While located further proximally than for most exposures to lateral condylar fractures, care must be taken to preserve the radial nerve, which courses distally underneath the brachialis muscle and is located cranial to the lateral head of the triceps. An incision is then made between the extensor carpi radialis and the common digital extensor and extended proximally to elevate the distal aspect of the origin of the extensor carpi radialis. This will expose the lateral humeral epicondyle and epicondylar crest. The underlying joint capsule is incised with an "L"- shaped incision to access the joint and to visualize the cranial aspect of the humeral condyle.[6]

Fracture reduction can be achieved in a variety of ways, using Vulsellum forceps, AO point-to-point forceps, or a humeral condylar clamp applied to both the medial and lateral aspects of the condyle. Frequently, the trochlea is subluxated medially away from the semilunar notch of the ulna and must be reduced prior to attempting fracture reduction to ensure appropriate congruity of the elbow joint. Reduction of the trochlea can be achieved in some cases by either flexion or extension of the elbow followed by a cranially directed force to move the trochlea back into the semilunar notch of the ulna. The fracture site can be challenging or impossible to visualize directly with a lateral approach to the joint, and fracture reduction is often assessed indirectly via gentle palpation of the cranial aspect of the condyle with a Freer periosteal elevator. Step defects in the articular surface must be avoided as part of anatomic reconstruction. In simple, reconstructable fractures, anatomic reduction of the epicondylar crest can often be used as an indirect representation of fracture reduction at the articular surface. If intraoperative fluoroscopy is available, orthogonal views of the elbow joint can be obtained to ensure anatomic reduction of the fracture prior to implant placement. For a fracture where anatomic reduction cannot be achieved or confirmed, procedures such as an olecranon osteotomy or a triceps tenotomy can be performed to improve visualization of the axial aspect of the condyle. It should be noted that these procedures result in increased morbidity and additional risk for complications.

When appropriate fracture reduction is confirmed, the condyle is stabilized with the placement of a transcondylar screw. In most cases, this is a cortical screw placed either in a positional or lag fashion. In very young patients with soft metaphyseal bone, a positional screw may be desirable, as this increases the thread purchase of the screw, reducing the likelihood of screw pull-out or loosening, but comes at the cost of sacrificing a degree of compression. The use of a washer positioned under the head of the screw helps to distribute the load placed on the lateral cortex when the screw is tightened and is frequently used in young patients. Placement of screws exceeding 40% of the height of the condyle distal to the supracondylar foramen as measured on preoperative radiographs has been shown to cause an increased risk of medial epicondylar fissure fractures.[14] The ideal entry point for this screw is just cranial and distal to the lateral humeral epicondyle, with the exit point located in a similar location on the medial side with respect to the medial humeral epicondyle (Figure 44.4). Angulation distally may result in penetration of the articular surface of the condyle, whereas angulation too proximally may result in penetration of the supracondylar foramen and interference with the anconeal process during elbow extension.

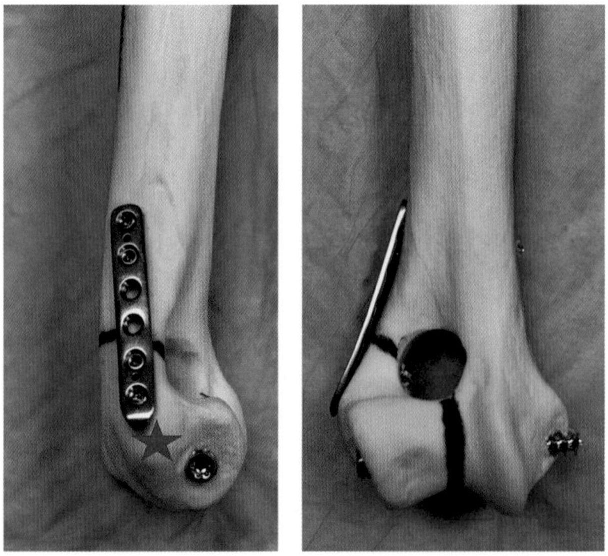

Figure 44.4 Saw bone model demonstrating the ideal placement locations for a transcondylar screw and a lateral epicondylar plate on the distal humerus. The lateral epicondyle is demonstrated by the star in the image on the left. Note that the transcondylar screw is placed just distal and cranial to this readily identifiable landmark. *Source:* © Dr. David Dycus.

While ideal to avoid the distal humeral physis with the transcondylar screw, there is no evidence that this affects the likelihood of a successful repair. In addition, with the contouring of a lateral epicondylar plate, it is common for the distal-most screw in the plate to cross the physis anyway. C-shaped aiming guides are available to facilitate accurate passage of a K-wire or drill-bit across the condyle. Intraoperative fluoroscopy can be used to confirm the appropriate path for screw placement, if available.

An alternative to conventional cortical screws involves the use of headless compression screws. These are screws with two threaded portions separated by a central smooth shaft that allows for compression to be generated across a fracture line without the need for drilling of separate glide and thread holes. In addition, headless compression screws are available as cannulated screws starting with 2.4 mm diameter screws and larger, which facilitates placement over a pre-placed K-wire. Another advantage of these screws is their ability to be countersunk below the level of the cortical bone at the insertion point, reducing the risk of soft tissue irritation or impingement postoperatively. These screws may be more desirable than conventional cortical screws placed in lag fashion in juvenile patients with soft bone due to the purchase of screw threads in both the cis and trans fragments, though this has not been evaluated specifically for humeral condylar fractures.

Positional screw placement is achieved by completely drilling across the condyle with one size drill bit appropriately selected for the chosen size of screw. To place a screw in lag fashion, a glide hole is first drilled in the cis cortex, followed by a threaded hole in the trans cortex. For an in-depth description of lag screw placement, the reader is directed to AO Principles of Fracture Management in the Dog and Cat, AO Publishing, Switzerland, 2005. In young patients with softer bones, it is important not to over-tighten the lag or positional screw. In such cases, a washer can be used. As the screw is being tightened, it is important to prevent rotation of the fracture fragment about the axis of the screw. Therefore, it is important that some form of bone-holding forceps are used to aid in reduction.

Following placement of the transcondylar screw, the epicondylar crest is secured either with an anti-rotational K-wire or with an epicondylar bone plate. If placing a K-wire, the starting point is just caudal to the head of the transcondylar screw. The K-wire is directed up the epicondylar crest and exits through the medial cortex of the distal diaphysis (Figure 44.5a). Since this method of fixation is usually reserved for smaller patients, the size of the K-wire ranges from a 0.9 mm (0.035″) to a 1.6 mm (0.062″) K-wire. The anti-rotational pin width cannot exceed the width of the humeral epicondyle as measured on pre-operative radiographs.

Recent literature suggests that the placement of an epicondylar bone plate is biomechanically superior to the placement of an anti-rotational K-wire for stability at the fracture site.[9] In dogs where an appropriately-sized plate is available, this is the preferred method of fixation for lateral humeral condylar fractures. As discussed previously, locking implants are preferred by the authors. When placing the plate, a thorough knowledge of regional anatomy is crucial to avoid screw placement into the joint space. Distal screws must be angled in such a way as to avoid the articular surface of the condyle (either cranially, distally, or caudally), as well as the supracondylar foramen. Because the main function of this plate is to provide anti-rotational support, it is often sufficient to engage the distal fracture fragment with two monocortical locking screws. The proximal segment can be secured with either two or three locking screws (Figures 44.4 and 44.5b).

The surgery site is thoroughly lavaged prior to closure. The extensor carpi radialis is sutured to its origin on the lateral epicondyle using a long-acting monofilament absorbable suture, such as polydioxanone or polyglyconate, along with the deep fascia of the extensors of the antebrachium. The brachialis muscle is closed to the cranial border of the lateral head of the triceps. The subcutaneous tissues and skin are closed routinely.

Potential Complications

There are several potential complications of lateral humeral condylar fracture repair, most of which are nonspecific to the procedure and are consistent with complications observed with other fracture repairs. Figure 44.6 demonstrates a few examples of potential complications observed following repair of this fracture configuration.

Surgical site infection (SSI) is a known risk of fracture repair.[15] Minor SSIs involve the skin and/or subcutaneous tissue and are most commonly managed with broad-spectrum antibiotic therapy with or without minor wound care, if required. Typical clinical signs associated with superficial SSI include swelling, redness, discharge, and/or dehiscence of the skin incision. These findings are most commonly noted within the first two weeks following surgery. Deep SSI entails an infection involving the implants that were placed at the time of surgery or progression of an untreated/unrecognized superficial SSI. Deep SSI is complicated by the potential development of a biofilm, often rendering systemic oral antibiotic therapy ineffective at completely clearing the infection. Clinical signs of deep SSI may appear similar to superficial SSI or may include worsening lameness, pain at the surgical site on palpation, or, uncommonly, systemic signs, such as lethargy, fever, or poor appetite. Performing radiographs of the surgical site along with sampling of joint fluid are indicated in these cases given the potential for involvement of the elbow

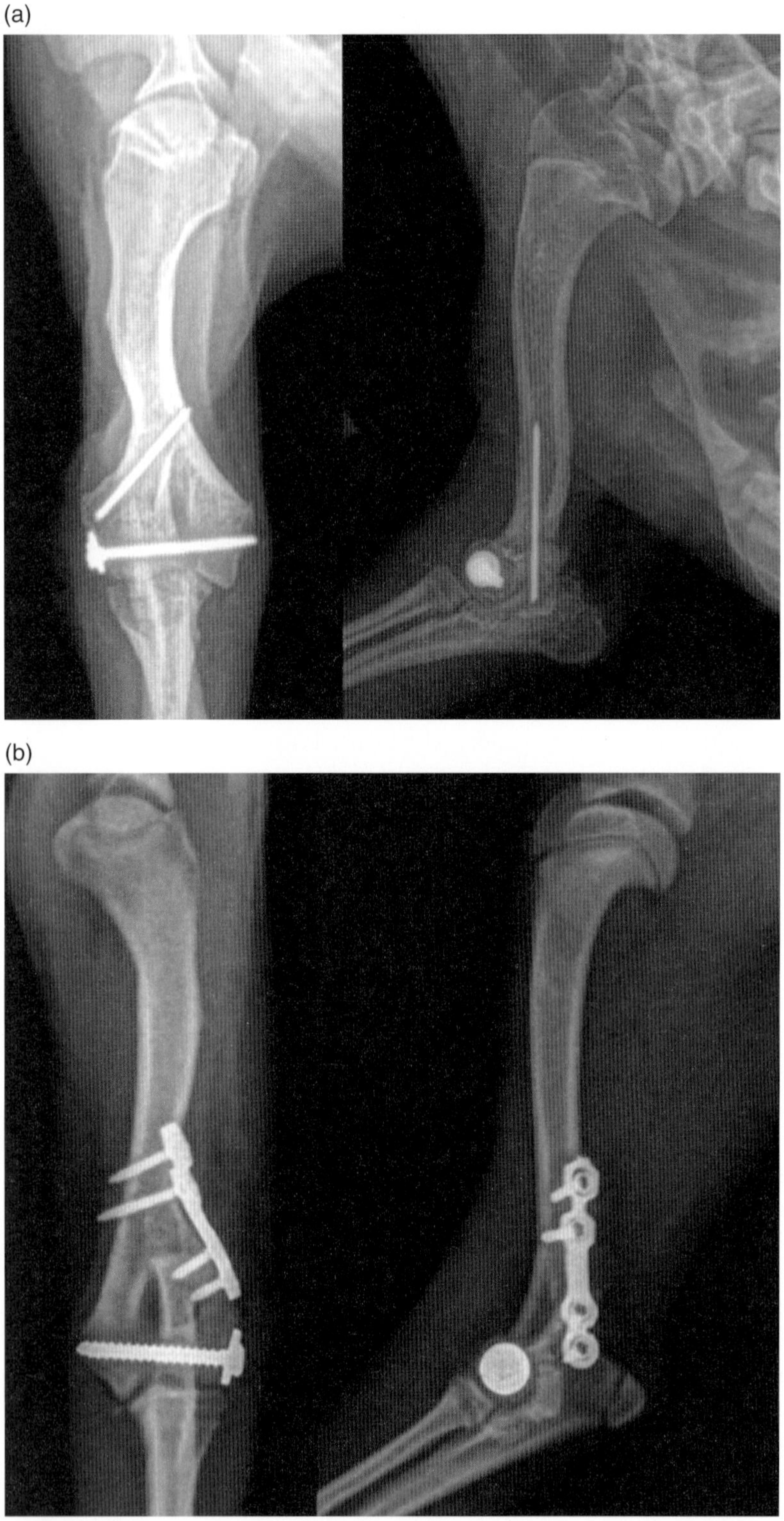

Figure 44.5 Cranio-caudal and medial-lateral postoperative radiographs of surgical repair of a lateral humeral condylar fracture using a transcondylar screw and washer and an anti-rotational pin (a) and a transcondylar screw and washer with an epicondylar bone plate and screws (b). Close inspection of the articular surface reveals a small step in image a, and appropriate anatomic reconstruction in image b. Both patients had a good clinical outcome. *Source:* © Dr. David Dycus.

joint. If deep SSI develops, implant removal after complete healing of the fracture site may be necessary.

Implant loosening, implant failure, nonunion, delayed union, and malunion are all potential complications that can occur.[2] The risk of implant-associated complications is mitigated by appropriate postoperative activity restriction. Recent literature suggests that the use of a lateral epicondylar plate reduces the likelihood of postoperative implant complications as compared to the more traditional anti-rotational K-wire.[12,16] Owners should be instructed to monitor for clinical signs such as a sudden decrease in weight-bearing, signs of pain, or swelling of the affected

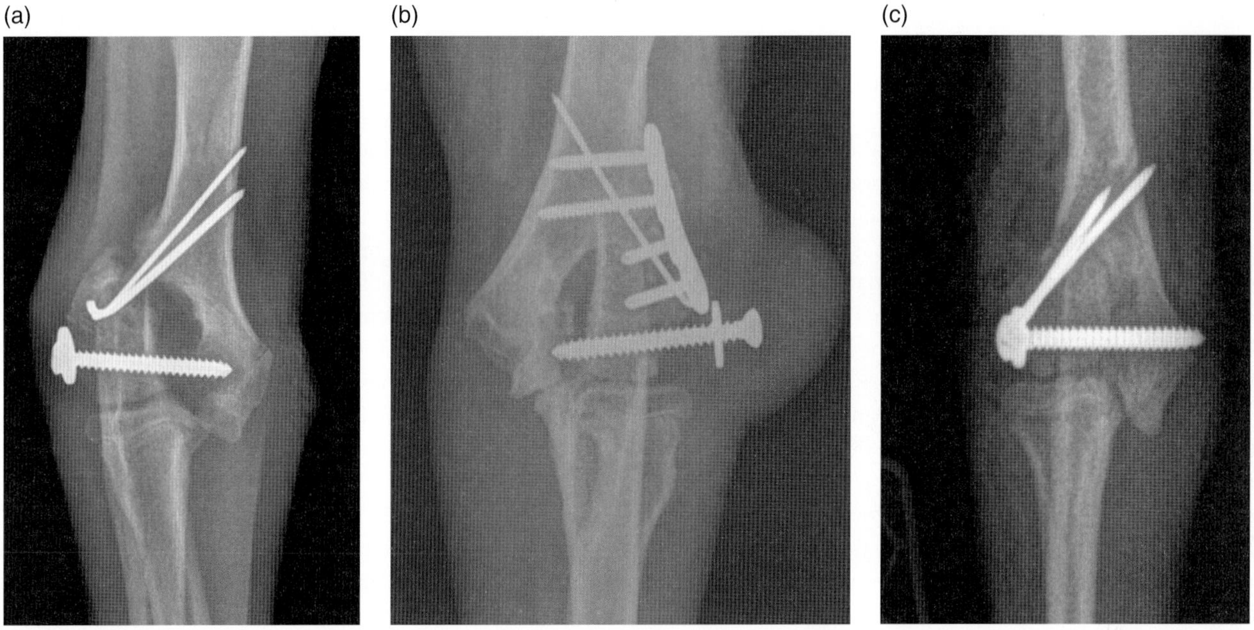

Figure 44.6 (a) A cranio-caudal radiograph showing catastrophic failure of a previously surgically repaired Salter–Harris IV lateral condylar fracture that was repaired with a transcondylar screw and washer and two anti-rotational K-wires. There is poor bony purchase of the K-wires in the distal fragment, resulting in a loss of K-wire engagement. In addition, the transcondylar screw has backed out slightly. Upon further inspection, it does not appear the transcortex of the humeral condyle was engaged with the screw initially, further weakening the construct. The displacement of the fracture following implant breakdown has resulted in a large gap and step of the articular surface. Surgical revision would be required and would entail implant removal along with fracture reduction and placement of new implants. (b) A cranio-caudal radiograph showing implant breakdown of a previously surgically repaired Salter–Harris IV lateral humeral condylar fracture that was repaired with a transcondylar screw and washer, K-wire, and lateral epicondylar plate. There is poor bony purchase of the K-wire in the distal fragment, resulting in a loss of K-wire engagement. The transcondylar screw has backed out, resulting in significant soft tissue swelling. However, the improved biomechanical strength with the addition of the lateral epicondylar plate prevented catastrophic failure (as noted in Figure 44.6a). Surgical revision would be required and would entail the removal of the screw and replacement with a longer screw. (c) A cranio-caudal radiograph showing a previously surgically repaired Salter–Harris type IV lateral condylar fracture that was repaired with a transcondylar screw and washer and two anti-rotational K-wires. While there appears to be good compression of the intra-articular fracture and good reduction of the lateral epicondylar crest, there is poor reduction of the articular component with a large step of the articular surface. This degree of step would be considered unacceptable. Once noted on immediate postoperative radiographs, the patient should return to the operating room for implant removal, improved reconstruction of the articular surface, and placement of implants. Failure to recognize the step defect would likely result in continued pain and lameness for the patient. *Source:* © Dr. David Dycus.

elbow. Development of these signs should prompt urgent reexamination by a veterinarian or the surgeon who performed the surgery.

Postoperative osteoarthritis is to be expected with articular fractures and has been shown to occur independently of how well-reduced the fracture is at the time of surgery.[17] Despite this, most studies show that the majority of patients have good to excellent outcomes following surgical repair, which is consistent with the authors' experience.[12,18] Regardless, owners should be counseled prior to surgery regarding this expectation, and appropriate guidelines should be established for ongoing osteoarthritis management monitoring and therapy.

Despite the involvement of the distal humeral physis, limb length discrepancy, and angular limb deformities are both rarely observed following surgery even if a transcondylar screw, or a screw placed through an epicondylar plate, violates the distal humeral physis.[2]

Postoperative Care

Following surgery, patients are hospitalized for analgesic and anesthetic recovery purposes. In the absence of a preoperative nerve block (radian, ulnar, median, and musculocutaneous [RUMM] block or brachial plexus block), most patients require the use of a full mu opioid and other injectable analgesics during the first 12–24 hours. In addition, injectable and/or oral NSAIDs are continued or started provided that the patient is a good candidate to receive this class of medication. Upon discharge, appropriate oral analgesics such as NSAIDs, opioids, and gabapentin/pregabalin can be used. In addition, the authors routinely use oral sedatives, such as trazodone or acepromazine, for the first two to four weeks after surgery in patients who are likely to be active or difficult to confine. Controversy surrounds the need to send home postoperative antibiotics. In cases where there is a break in sterility or there is any concern for contamination of the surgical site, antibiotics should be sent home. Outside of this, it is up to the veterinarian to determine the need for postoperative antibiotics.

The incision site is covered with an adhesive bandage that can be removed upon discharge or a few days following surgery. The authors do not routinely use a bandage or splint following a humeral condylar fracture. However, if a bandage or splint is placed to protect the surgery site or as part of the treatment of concurrent wounds, it is *imperative* that the bandage extends above the shoulder, such as with a "cross-your-heart" bandage or a Spica splint. Bandages that do not fully immobilize the shoulder will act as a fulcrum on the fracture site and will increase the risk of complications and/or pain.

Recovery following a humeral condylar fracture can take as little as 4 weeks in a skeletally immature animal to as long as 8–12 weeks in a skeletally mature animal. During recovery, activity restriction is paramount. High-impact activities, such as running, jumping, or playing, must be prohibited to reduce strain on the implants and fracture site until fracture healing has been radiographically confirmed. Patients should be maintained on a leash at all times while not in an enclosure at home. The first two weeks consist of short elimination walks only. Pending the recheck orthopedic exam two weeks after surgery, leash walks may be increased by five minutes' duration weekly thereafter. A second recheck appointment, with radiographs, is scheduled four to six weeks postoperatively to ensure appropriate fracture healing and static orthopedic implants. If radiographic healing is complete at that time, normal activity may be gradually resumed over the course of the following three to four weeks.

Formal physical rehabilitation is a highly useful addition to the postoperative care protocol for patients with humeral condylar fractures. It is aimed at achieving early return to function, maintaining and improving elbow range of motion, improving patient comfort level, and may be beneficial to earlier detection of complications.

References

1 Evans, H.E. and deLahunta, A. (2013). The skeleton. In: *Miller's Anatomy of the Dog*, 4e, 129–132. St. Louis: Elsevier.

2 Tobias, K.M. and Johnston, S.A. (2017). Fractures of the humerus. In: *Veterinary Surgery: Small Animal Expert Consult*, 2e, 820–836. St. Louis: Elsevier.

3 Smith, M.A.J., Jenkins, G., Dean, B.L. et al. (2020). Effect of breed as a risk factor for humeral condylar fracture in skeletally immature dogs. *J. Small Anim. Pract.* 61 (6): 374–380.

4 Moores, A.P. and Moores, A.L. (2017). The natural history of humeral intracondylar fissure: an observational study of 30 dogs. *J. Small Anim. Pract.* 58 (6): 337–341.

5 Moores, A. (2006). Humeral condylar fractures and incomplete ossification of the humeral condyle in dogs. *In Practice* 28 (7): 391–397.

6 Johnson, K.A. and Peermattei, D.L. (2014). Approach to the lateral aspect of the humeral condyle and epicondyle in the dog. In: *Piermattei's Atlas of Surgical Approaches to the Bones and Joints of the Dog and Cat*, 5e, 202–205. St. Louis: Elsevier.

7 Meyer-Lindenberg, A., Heinen, V., Fehr, M. et al. (2002). Incomplete ossification of the humeral condyle as the cause of lameness in dogs. *Vet. Comp. Orthop. Traumatol.* 15 (03): 187–194.

8 Tillson, D.M. (1995). Open fracture management. *Vet. Clin. North Am. Small Anim. Pract.* 25 (5): 1093–1110.

9 Coggeshall, J.D., Lewis, D.D., Iorgulescu, A. et al. (2017). Adjunct fixation with a Kirschner wire or a plate for lateral unicondylar humeral fracture stabilization. *Vet. Surg.* 46 (7): 933–941.

10 Eayrs, M.K., Guerin, V., Grierson, J. et al. (2021). Repair of fractures of the lateral aspect of the humeral condyle in skeletally mature dogs with locking and non-locking plates. *Vet. Comp. Orthop. Traumatol.* 34 (6): 419–426.

11 Cinti, F., Pisani, G., Vezzoni, L. et al. (2017). Kirschner wire fixation of Salter–Harris type IV fracture of the lateral aspect of the humeral condyle in growing dogs. A retrospective study of 35 fractures. *Vet. Comp. Orthop. Traumatol.* 30 (1): 62–68.

12 Sanchez Villamil, C., Phillips, A.S.J., Pegram, C.L. et al. (2020). Impact of breed on canine humeral condylar fracture configuration, surgical management, and outcome. *Vet. Surg.* 49 (4): 639–647.

13 Kvale, E., Kalmukov, I., Grassato, L. et al. (2022). Epicondylar plate fixation of humeral condylar fractures in immature French bulldogs: 45 cases (2014–2020). *J. Small Anim. Pract.* 63 (7): 532–541.

14 Jenkins, G. and Moores, A.P. (2022). Medial epicondylar fissure fracture as a complication of transcondylar screw

placement for the treatment of humeral intracondylar fissure. *Vet. Surg.* 51 (4): 600–610.

15 Pratesi, A., Moores, A.P., Downes, C. et al. (2015). Efficacy of postoperative antimicrobial use for clean orthopedic implant surgery in dogs: a prospective randomized study in 100 consecutive cases. *Vet. Surg.* 44 (5): 653–660.

16 Perry, K.L., Bruce, M., Woods, S. et al. (2015). Effect of fixation method on postoperative complication rates after surgical stabilization of lateral humeral condylar fractures in dogs. *Vet. Surg.* 44 (2): 246–255.

17 Gordon, W.J., Besancon, M.F., Conzemius, M.G. et al. (2003). Frequency of post-traumatic osteoarthritis in dogs after repair of a humeral condylar fracture. *Vet. Comp. Orthop. Traumatol.* 16 (01): 01–05.

18 Gluding, D., Häußler, T.C., Büttner, K. et al. (2022). Retrospective evaluation of surgical technique, complications and long-term outcome of lateral and medial humeral condylar fractures in 80 dogs. *New Zealand Vet. J.* 70 (6): 349–356.

45

Canine Elbow Dysplasia

Joey A. Sapora

Department of Clinical Sciences, Colorado State University, Fort Collins, CO, USA

Key Points

- Having a fundamental understanding of the components of Canine Elbow Dysplasia is important for formulating a diagnostic and treatment plan.
- Early identification of CED allows for prompt owner education, allows for the institution of a lifelong joint health plan early in life, and can identify cases that maybenefit from surgical intervention.
- Developing comfort with an orthopedic examination of the elbow relies on the palpation of both normal and abnormal patients. Common locations of joint effusion, the feel of normal bony prominences, and certain maneuvers that may elicit pain in clinically affected patients are all required for a thorough evaluation.
- Radiographs of the elbow are the most important screening diagnostic for patients with CED and radiographic changes occur in predictable locations.
- Various surgical procedures may be recommended in dogs with CED, and an awareness of these surgical procedures is required for appropriate owner education and case management.

Introduction

Canine Elbow Dysplasia (CED) is a commonly encountered orthopedic condition in veterinary general practice that causes lameness in juvenile, medium to large breed dogs. The use of the term dysplasia to explain the complex syndrome that leads to osteoarthritis and pain of the canine elbow may be an oversimplification, particularly to pet owners. The term Developmental Elbow Disease[1] has been proposed to better capture the complexity of a condition where the relationship between genetics, biology, and biomechanics has not been fully elucidated. For clarity, the traditional term of CED will be applied in this chapter. Semantics aside, it is important to acknowledge the intricate and often frustrating condition of CED to optimize client education and patient care. This chapter will review the etiopathogenesis of CED, discuss common physical exam findings, diagnostic radiographic technique, and management strategies for various stages and components of the disease.

Etiopathogenesis of Canine Elbow Dysplasia

Ununited anconeal process (UAP) in the dog was first recorded in the 1950's,[2,3] and medial coronoid disease, osteochondritis dissecans, and humeroradioulnar incongruity were first described in the 1970's.[4–6] The International Elbow Working Group (IEWG) defined Elbow Dysplasia almost 15 years later to consist of four entities: fragmented medial coronoid process (FCP), osteochondrosis (OC) of the medial humeral condyle, UAP, and elbow joint incongruity.[6]

The hereditary nature of CED is well-established with multiple genes and environmental factors playing a role in the end-stage manifestation of elbow osteoarthritis.[7–11] The prevalence of cases of "elbow joint disease" presenting to primary care veterinary practices is around 0.56%,[12] while the incidence of CED ranges from 0% to 55% depending upon the patient's breed, the population evaluated, and the screening protocols applied.[10] Some of the breed prevalence and odds ratios for UAP, medial coronoid disease, OC of the medial humeral condyle, and elbow joint incongruity

Techniques in Small Animal Soft Tissue, Orthopedic, and Ophthalmic Surgery, First Edition. Edited by Kristin A. Coleman.

Companion website: www.wiley.com/go/coleman/surgeries

	Elbow dysplasia	FCP	Elbow incongruity	OCD	UAP
Bernese Mountain Dog	0.260[g], 0.234[a], 0.200[e], 0.153[d]	0.966[d] OR 140.1[i]	0.503[d]	0.270[d]	OR 50.5[i]
Rottweiler	0.542[f], 0.381[g], 0.345[a], 0.330[e]	OR 36.1[i]		OR 174[j]	OR 27.4[j]
Chow Chow	0.486[g], 0.472[a]	OR 16.6[i]		OR 108.8[i]	OR 13.3[i]
Chinese Shar Pei	0.310[e], 0.240[g]				OR 4.6[i]
Newfoundland	0.260[e], 0.227[g] 0.214[a]	OR 10.9[i]		OR 261[i]	OR 13.8[i]
German Shepherd Dog	0.178[g], 0.165[a], 0.120[e]	OR 43.7[i]		OR 14.9[i]	OR 8.2[i]
English Setter	0.144[a], 0.142[g]				OR 3.7[i]
Bullmastiff	0.145[a], 0.142[g]	OR 38.9[i]			
English Springer Spaniel	0.159[a], 0.125[g]				
Labrador Retriever	0.178[c], 0.130[e], 0.091[a], 0.056[d]	0.980[d] OR 20.5[i]	0.060[d]	0.132[d] OR 109.4[10]	OR 8.5[i]
Golden Retriever	0.180[e], 0.087[a], 0.052[d]	0.968[d] OR 5.5[i]	0.063[d]	0.254[d] OR 42.4[i]	OR 4.9[i]
Greater Swiss Mountain Dog	0.180[e], 0.088[a]				
Estrela Mountain Dog	0.165[b]				
American Staffordshire Terrier	0.161[g]				
Irish Water Spaniel	0.156[g]				
Tibetan Mastiff	0.138[g]				
Bloodhound	0.131[g]				
Mastiff	0.131[g], 0.128[a]	OR 48.4[i]			OR 20.2[i]
Gordon Setter	0.126[g]	OR 19.8[i]			
Bouvier Des Flanders	0.089[a]	OR 19.5[i]			
Australian Cattle Dog	0.085[a]				
Rhodesian Ridgeback	0.080[e], 0.050[a]				
Leonberger	0.040[e]				
Australian Shepherd	0.027[a]				
Bassett Hound		OR 19.5[i]			OR 2.7[i]
Irish Wolfhound		OR 93.4[i]			
Saint Bernard		OR 53.4[i]			OR 14.2[i]
Great Dane				OR 87.0[i]	
Skye Terrier			0.490[h]		
Pomeranian					OR 3.7[i]

Figure 45.1 Published prevalence rates of Elbow Dysplasia based upon breed noted in the current small animal literature, in addition to prevalence and odds ratios for FCP, Elbow Incongruity, OCD, and UAP. Prevalence is the proportion of a population that has the condition over a set period of time and can be more easily interpreted as a percent. Odds ratio can be thought of as the odds the condition will occur in that breed compared to it not occurring. [a]Baers et al. (2019). [b]Alves-Pimenta, S., Colaco, B., Silvestre, A.M., et al. (2013). Prevalence and breeding values of elbow dysplasia in the Estrela mountain dog. *Veterinarni Medicina* 58, 2013 (9): 484–490. [c]Morgan, J.,P., Wind A., Davidson A.P. (1999). Bone dysplasias in the labrador retriever: a radiographic study. *Journal of the American Animal Hospital Association* 35(4):332–340. [d]Lavrijsen, I., Heuven, H., Voorhout, G., et al. (2012). Phenotypic and genetic evaluation of elbow dysplasia in Dutch Labrador Retrievers, Golden Retrievers, and Bernese Mountain dogs. *The Veterinary Journal* 193(2):486–492. [e]Coopman, F., Verhoeven, G., Saunders, J., et al. (2008). Prevalence of hip dysplasia, elbow dysplasia and humeral head osteochondrosis in dog breeds in Belgium. *The Veterinary Record* 163(22):654–658. [f]Beuing, R., Mues, C.H., Tellhelm, B., et al. (2000). Prevalence and inheritance of canine elbow dysplasia in German Rottweiler. *Journal of Animal Breeding and Genetics* 117(6):375–383. [g]Oberbauer, A., Keller, G., Famula, T. (2017). Long-term genetic selection reduced prevalence of hip and elbow dysplasia in 60 dog breeds. *PloS one* 12(2):e0172918. [h]Lappalainen, A., Hyvärinen T., Junnila J., et al. (2016). Radiographic evaluation of elbow incongruity in Skye terriers. *Journal of Small Animal Practice* 57(2):96–99. [i]LaFond, E., Breur, G.J., Austin, C.C. (2002). Breed susceptibility for developmental orthopedic diseases in dogs. *Journal of the American Animal Hospital Association* 1;38(5):467–477.

currently published in the literature are listed in Figure 45.1. For example, a Gordon Setter has a CED prevalence of 0.126[g], meaning 12.6% of the population is suspected to have CED (or 126 out of every 1,000). The odds ratio for Gordon Setters being diagnosed specifically with FCP is an OR of 19.8[i], meaning that the odds of FCP occurring in this breed are 19.8 times more likely than other breeds.

CED is not limited to medium and large breed dogs, with chondrodystrophic and toy breed dogs being affected as well.[13,14] Male dogs, specifically male German Shepherd Dogs and Labrador Retrievers, may be at a higher risk of CED than female dogs.[11,15] Identified environmental risk factors that *may* contribute to the disease include increased body weight, increased food intake, higher proportional intake of fat, and exercise involving chasing after balls and sticks thrown by the owner.[16,17] It is also important to note that long-term reduced food intake has been shown to decrease the severity of osteoarthritis over time, an expected sequela of CED.[16]

As there are no curative medical or surgical interventions available to treat CED, prevention of the disease through judicious breeding strategies is required. This starts with early identification and client education. Given the polygenic nature of the condition, the development of a single genetic test to screen for CED is unlikely for quite some time. Screening based on Estimated Breeding Values (EBV) is recommended and has been shown to be superior to screening based on phenotype. EBVs have been used for decades in livestock populations and involve tracking and measuring heritable traits using statistical models. This industry-tested process is superior to phenotypic selection and provides faster genetic progression when attempting to decrease the prevalence of CED in various canine populations.[8,9,18–20] These tools are already being employed by certain universities and the Orthopedic Foundation for Animals (OFA) to combat hip and elbow dysplasia.

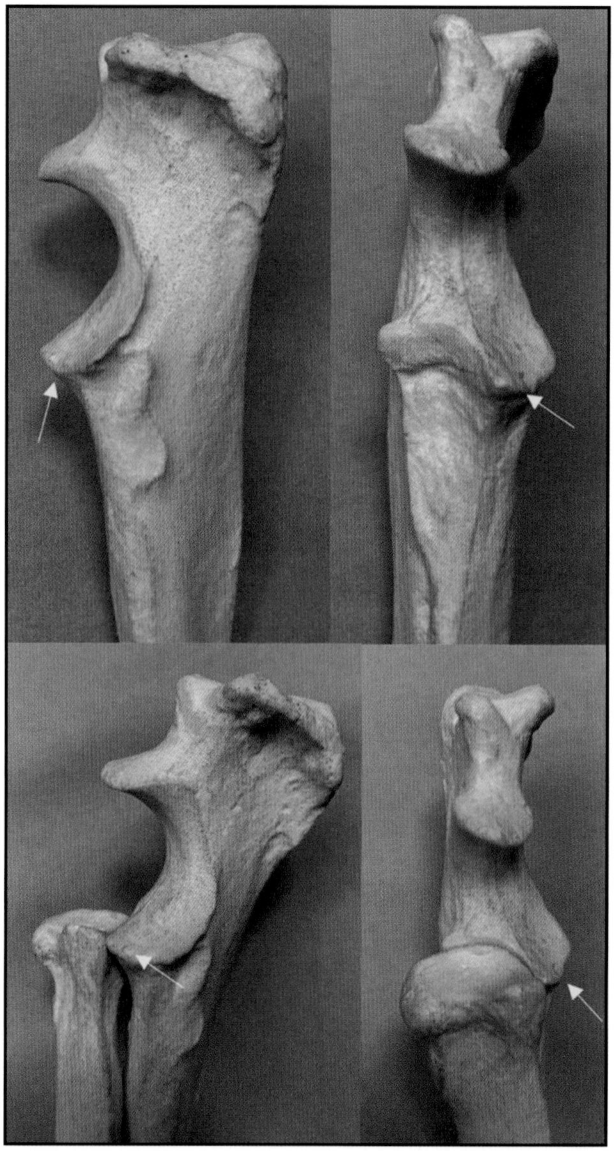

Figure 45.2 Anatomic specimens of the canine ulna showing the medial coronoid process (yellow arrow) from a medial (top left) and cranial (top right) view of the proximal ulna. Bottom images are similar views with the addition of the radius. Note the size of the medial coronoid and its intimate association with the radial head. *Source:* Image courtesy of Joey Sapora.

Components of Canine Elbow Dysplasia

Fragmented Medial Coronoid Process (FCP) and Medial Compartment Disease (MCD)

The medial coronoid process forms the most distomedial aspect of the trochlear notch and increases the contact area of the ulna with the humerus[21] (Figure 45.2). The medial coronoid process is cartilaginous at birth, and complete ossification, occurring from base to apex, has been shown to occur in small dogs by 16 weeks of age and in larger dogs by 20 weeks of age.[22] Changes to the medial coronoid process can include fissuring, fragmentation, and subchondral bone fatigue that commonly involve either the coronoid apex or base.[23] Studies have demonstrated that histologic changes to the coronoid originate in deeper layers of the articular cartilage, mainly in the calcifying zone, prior to any changes at the level of the articular surface. Retained hyaline cartilage and excessive amounts of Type X collagen have been identified in affected coronoids.[24–26] FCP is the most common form of CED (>96%), and the disturbance in ossification is thought to also give rise to cleft formation as a result of either normal physiologic or abnormal biomechanical forces.[10,24] These biomechanical forces are the premise behind elbow joint incongruity and its contribution to FCP development. For example, a patient with a "short radius" leading to an "elevated" medial coronoid at the level of the elbow joint may have an increased load placed over the medial coronoid, leading to fragmentation. Approximately 24% of FCP cases have computed tomographic (CT) signs of joint incongruity. FCP can occur as a single entity or in conjunction with OC or, less commonly, with UAP.[27]

With computed tomography and arthroscopy now commonplace in small animal specialty hospitals, we are better able to characterize FCP pathology and its relationship with arthroscopic cartilage change. These cartilage changes mainly affect the humeroulnar articulation along the medial aspect of the joint with the degree of joint incongruity and the presence of an FCP correlating with the degree of cartilage injury present.[28] The descriptive term Medial Compartment Disease (MCD) is now preferred over "medial coronoid disease," to describe the severe and sometimes widespread cartilage wear that may be present with or without the presence of coronoid pathology or joint incongruity.[29,30] These changes include chondromalacia, full-thickness cartilage erosions, and "kissing lesions" believed to be secondary to humeroulnar conflict. Although there is currently controversy about which terms should be used with inconclusive verbiage used in the published texts, that debate is beyond the scope of this chapter.

While asynchronous bone growth can lead to humeroulnar conflict, a musculotendinous contribution from the biceps brachii and brachialis muscle complex has also been proposed.[31] The biceps brachii and brachialis muscle complex inserts along the radial tuberosity in addition to the ulna along the medial aspect of the joint, and contraction causes both flexion of the elbow in addition to supination. This leads to rotation of the radial head along the radial incisure of the ulna, essentially squeezing the medial coronoid into the radial head.[31,32] This focal pressure over time is theorized to contribute to FCP and is the rationale for the Biceps Ulnar Release Procedure (BURP).

Osteochondrosis of the Medial Humeral Condyle

OC refers to the failure of the normal process of endochondral ossification, in which hyaline cartilage is replaced with bone.[33] This normal endochondral ossification is required for the developing medial coronoid, anconeal process, and humeral condyle. In 1976, Olsson was one of the first to consider that all three of these conditions (FCP, UAP, OCD) could, in fact, be manifestations of OC,[33] and it is still proposed that FCP, UAP, and asynchronous growth between the radius and ulna may be clinical manifestations of this disease.[34]

The underlying etiology of OC of the medial humeral condyle is believed to be a combination of genetic and environmental factors, including nutritional imbalance, rapid growth, physical activity, and microtrauma.[23] The role that elbow incongruity plays in the development of elbow OC is unclear. Diets high in calcium and phosphorus, as well as excessive vitamin D intake, have been associated with the development of OC.[35–37] It is reported more commonly in males than females.[23]

Ununited Anconeal Process

The anconeal process of the ulna does not have a separate center of ossification in small breed dogs,[2,38] but the failure of appropriate fusion of this process is well-documented in many large and giant breeds,[39] with the German Shepherd Dog overrepresented.[27]

Mineralization of the process begins by around 10–16 weeks of age with complete fusion occurring at approximately 20 weeks.[40,41] The process is termed "ununited" if ossification is not completed by 20 weeks of age, and it was the first described component of CED initially reported in the 1950's.[2,3] The currently accepted pathogenesis for UAP involves asynchronous growth of the radial head relative to the ulna, leading to a "longer radius" generating increased pressure across the anconeal process.[23] This likely occurs in the early phase of radial growth (ages four to five months). As some patients can have both UAP and FCP concomitantly with a short radius, a subsequent stunted radial growth phase (five to six months of age) has also been proposed.[23,27]

Joint Incongruity

The role of elbow incongruity in the proposed manifestations of FCP and UAP has been well-established[42–44] with up to 60% of dogs with FCP having underlying joint incongruity.[45] Three forms of elbow incongruity are proposed and these include radioulnar incongruity (RUI), humeroulnar incongruity, and radial incisure incongruity.[29] RUI is further broken down into positive RUI (short radius) and negative RUI (short ulna). A "short radius" is suspected to place supra-physiologic loads on the medial coronoid leading to FCP, while a "short ulna" is suspected to place supra-physiologic loads on the anconeal process leading to UAP.[46] Humeroulnar incongruity has more recently been investigated[47–49] and refers to the congruency of the trochlear notch with the humeral articulation. Some patients may have an abnormal "C-shape" to their trochlear notch, appearing to have a more shallow, or in other cases, a more acute curve to the notch, which is suspected to alter the biomechanics of the joint.[46,50] Assessment of radial incisure and humeroulnar incongruity is complex and requires advanced diagnostic imaging, and its role in the progression of disease is yet to be fully understood.

When considering elbow incongruity in general practice, a routine radiographic elbow series will aid in the detection of severe RUI (step ≥3 mm). More subtle RUI, in addition to a detailed assessment of humeroulnar and radial incisure incongruity, is better evaluated with a CT scan, however, the estimation of incongruity can be affected by patient positioning. In models of experimentally induced RUI, arthroscopic assessment has been shown to be a more sensitive and reproducible technique when compared to radiographic and CT analysis.[51]

Physical Exam Findings

Characteristic gait changes in patients with CED include lifting up of the head as the painful limb strikes the ground during the stance phase (i.e., "head bob") and decreased stride length during the swing phase of the gait cycle. In bilaterally affected patients, weight is often shifted caudally onto the pelvic limbs. At a stand, patients with medial compartment disease may shift their weight to the lateral compartment and tend to stand with slight external rotation of the distal extremity (pseudovalgus, Figure 45.3) or may have a bow-legged stance (elbow abduction) when more severely affected.[23]

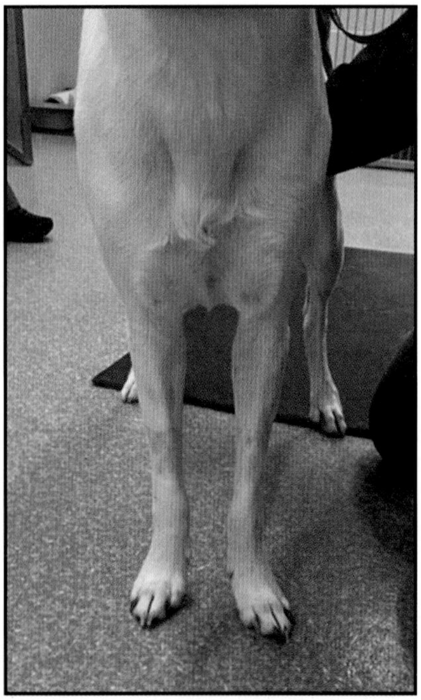

Figure 45.3 A one-year-old spayed female mixed breed dog with elbow dysplasia characterized by medial coronoid process fragmentation and 3 mm of positive RUI (left > right). Note the external rotation of the left forepaw, a conformational change thought to improve comfort related to medial compartment pain. *Source:* Image courtesy of Joey Sapora.

Palpation of joint effusion during the standing exam can improve the detection of subtle effusion as the joint is loaded. The effusion may or may not be present and is most commonly identified along the lateral aspect of the joint between the lateral epicondyle and olecranon, underneath the anconeus muscle (Figure 45.4). With chronicity, remodeling of the joint occurs, and normal bone prominences become less identifiable, particularly along the lateral compartment. Discomfort may be elicited when placing the joint through a range of motion depending upon the degree of effusion and capsulitis present. The diagnosis of medial compartment disease based on a pain response is challenging, and patients can be asymptomatic. It is also important to note that the degree of synovial inflammation is directly related to exposure to subchondral bone, which may be present in varying degrees based on the stage of OC or medial compartment disease.[23]

Various maneuvers that should be performed include a complete range of motion assessment, full elbow flexion, pronated flexion, elbow hyperextension, and the "Campbell's test."

Elbow Range of Motion

Subjective assessment for the normal range of motion of the canine elbow includes full elbow extension to approximately 180°, and flexion of the elbow with the dorsal aspect of the carpus reaching the level of the shoulder (Figure 45.4). This degree of normal elbow flexion may not be normal for well-muscled breeds (i.e., French Bulldogs, English Bulldogs, Pit Bulls, etc.).

Elbow Flexion

With the patient standing, the antebrachium and caudal aspect of the elbow can be supported to perform isolated elbow flexion (Figure 45.4). A pain response may be elicited in patients with medial compartment disease, which can include yelping, the patient pulling up and away from the maneuver, or hopping toward the contralateral limb. Pain upon full flexion is one of the more reliable indicators of diseases of the medial compartment of the elbow (FCP, medial compartment disease, OCD). Holding the elbow in moderate flexion followed by supination of the antebrachium may elicit pain, in addition to pronation followed by full elbow flexion.

Elbow Hyperextension

To perform isolated elbow extension, the antebrachium is supported and a cranially directed force is applied to just proximal to the elbow (Figure 45.4). The shoulder should remain immobilized. Pain upon elbow hyperextension is a more common abnormality associated with UAP.

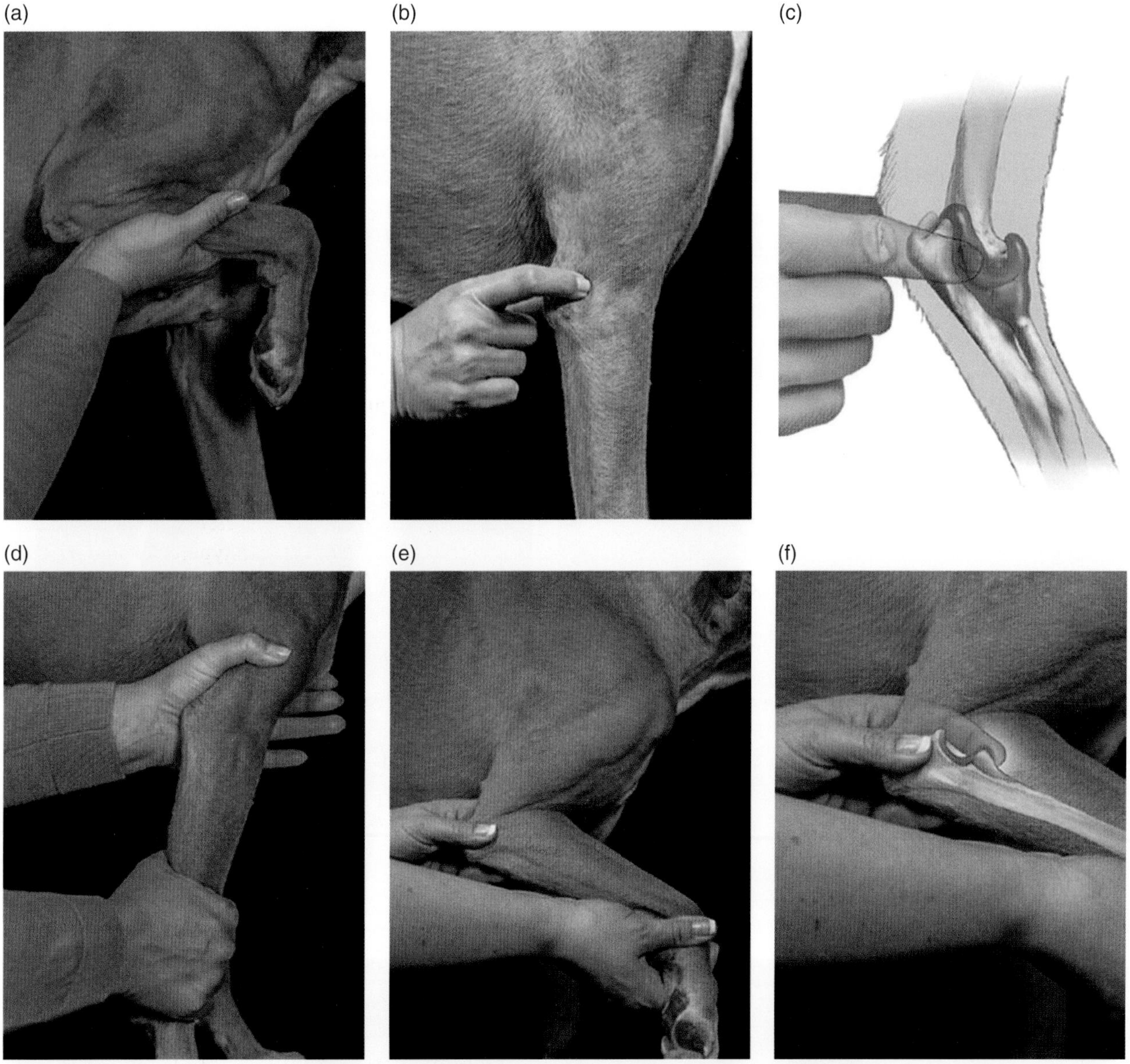

Figure 45.4 (a) Full flexion of the elbow is performed by placing the examiner's hand along the caudal aspect of the antebrachium and applying an upward pressure. (d) Hyperextension of the elbow is performed by stabilizing the humerus just proximal to the elbow and drawing the antebrachium caudally. Note how the shoulder is not extended simultaneously. (b,c) Palpation of joint effusion caudal to the humeral epicondyles. (e,f) The "Campbell's test" can be performed by pronating and supinating the limb while holding the elbow and carpus at 90° of flexion and applying gentle pressure over the medial coronoid process. *Source:* Felix Duerr, 2019 / with permission from JOHN WILEY & SONS, INC.

The "Campbell's Test"

Initially developed to assess collateral ligament instability,[52] this maneuver can be helpful when assessing young dogs in which joint remodeling and decreased range of motion have not yet developed. This test involves first holding the elbow and carpus at 90° of flexion. A moderate amount of pressure is then applied over the region of the medial coronoid (approximately 1 cm distal to medial epicondyle in a large-breed dog), and the elbow is then fully supinated and pronated. Discomfort may be elicited in some patients with CED (Figure 45.4).

Diagnostic Imaging

Radiographs are the mainstay for early identification of CED in juvenile patients and can aid in tracking the progression of the disease. Comfort with normal radiographic anatomy of the canine elbow is required for early identification of disease. The following radiographic elbow series is recommended for screening patients with suspected CED.[6,23,53]

Neutral (120°) Mediolateral Projection

Patient Positioning: With the patient in lateral recumbency, the desired elbow to be imaged is placed against the table, closest to the image detector (i.e., affected side down) (Figure 45.5). The elbow is positioned at a neutral angle, approximately 120°, with slight flexion of the carpus to avoid supination. The beam is centered just distal to the medial epicondyle.

Common abnormalities:

- Blunting or irregularities to the silhouette of the medial coronoid process (Figure 45.6).
- Increased sclerosis of the subtrochlear notch of the ulna with a loss of trabecular pattern. This subtrochlear sclerosis may also obscure the margins of the lateral coronoid (Figure 45.7).
- Osteophyte formation on the dorsal aspect of the anconeal process, cranial aspect of the radial head, and profiles of the medial and lateral humeral condyles.
- Joint incongruity – most commonly noted between the radial head and lateral coronoid process, generating a "short radius" or a "short ulna" (Figure 45.8). It is important to note that while severely incongruent joints can be

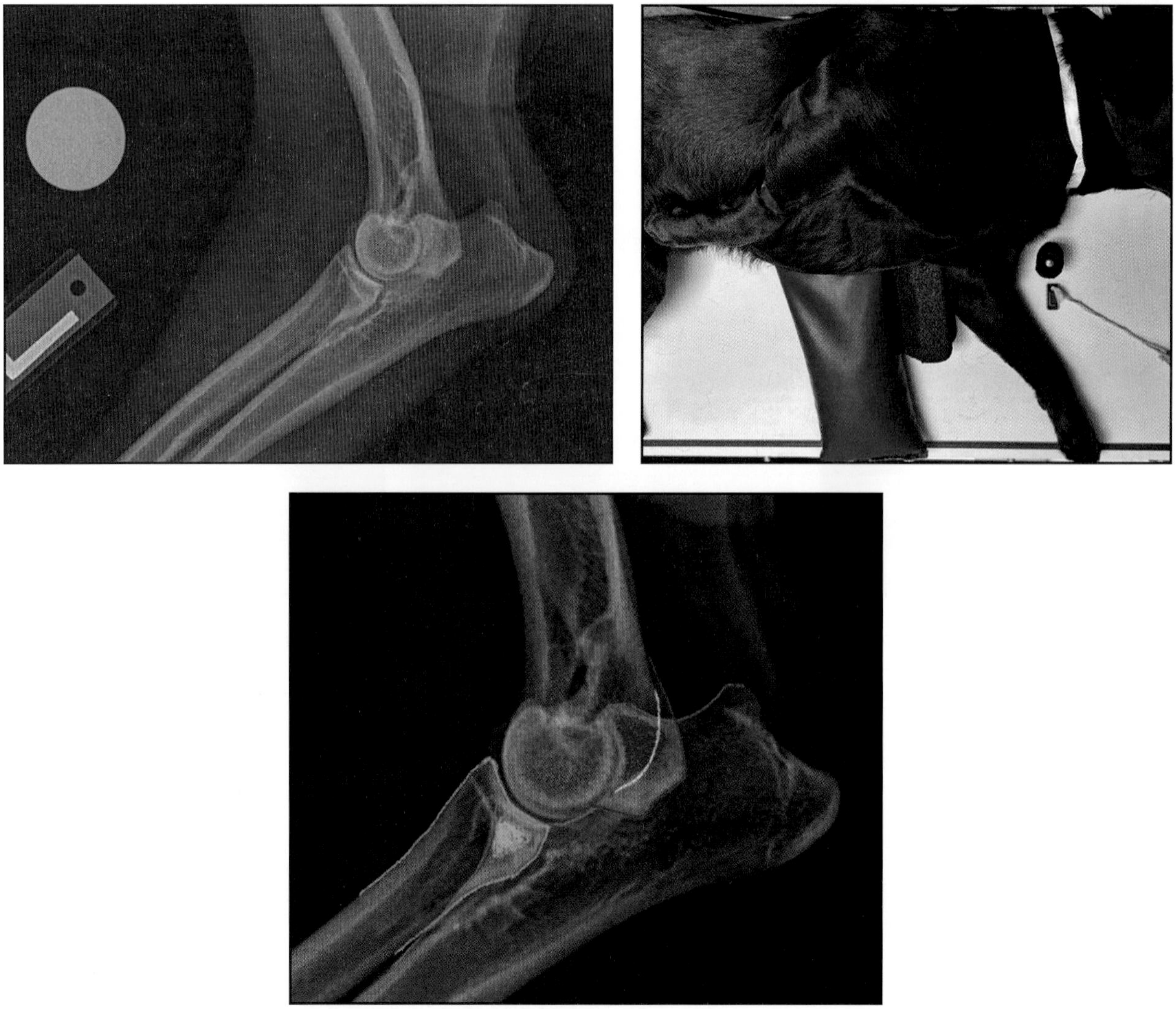

Figure 45.5 Neutral (120°) mediolateral projection of a normal elbow in a 1-year-old castrated male Labrador Retriever (top left). Appropriate positioning for the neutral mediolateral projection with calibration ball, limb marker, and use of hands-free radiographic technique (top right). Normal radiographic anatomy of the canine elbow, lateral projection (bottom): green line – radius; blue line – ulna; yellow shade – medial coronoid process; red shade – lateral coronoid process; purple shade – anconeal process; white line – lateral humeral epicondyle; pink line – medial humeral epicondyle. *Source:* Image courtesy of Joey Sapora.

identified radiographically, accurate quantification or grading is unreliable using radiographs alone. For diagnosing RUI, arthroscopy has been shown to be superior to both CT and radiography.[51]

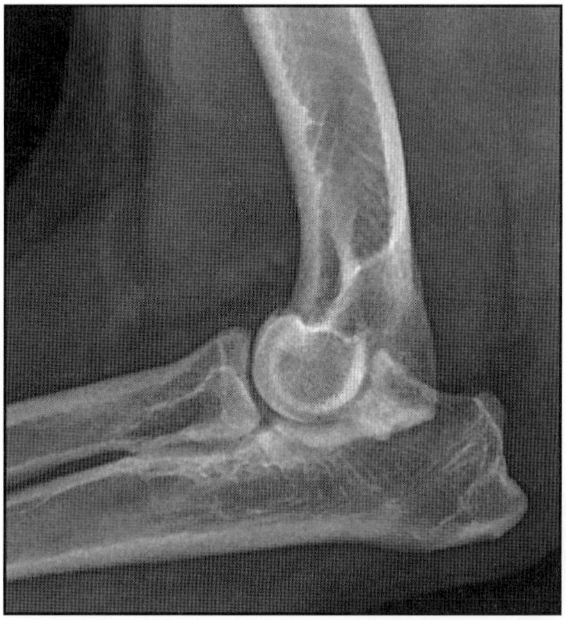

Figure 45.6 A six-year-old spayed female Labrador Retriever with advanced Canine Elbow Dysplasia (CED). Note the severe blunting of the medial coronoid process. *Source:* Image courtesy of Joey Sapora.

Flexed (45°) Mediolateral Projection

(Figure 45.9)

Patient Positioning: The patient remains in lateral recumbency with the desired elbow to be imaged resting against the table. The elbow is positioned at a flexed angle, approximately 45°, with slight flexion of the carpus to avoid supination. The beam is centered just distal to the medial epicondyle.

Common abnormalities: This view is most useful for the assessment of the anconeal process for abnormalities including osteophytosis (Figure 45.10) and UAPs (Figure 45.11).

Craniocaudal Projection with 15° Pronation

(Figure 45.12)

Patient Positioning: The patient is rotated into sternal recumbency with the pelvic limbs in lateral recumbency, away from the limb to be imaged. The head and neck are gently flexed away from the leg to be imaged (same direction as pelvic limbs), and the carpus is rotated inwards (pronated approximately 15°). The beam is centered over the crease in the skin overlying the cranial aspect of the joint.

Common abnormalities:

- Osteophyte formation over the medial and lateral humeral condyles, as well as the medial coronoid process (Figures 45.13 and 45.14).

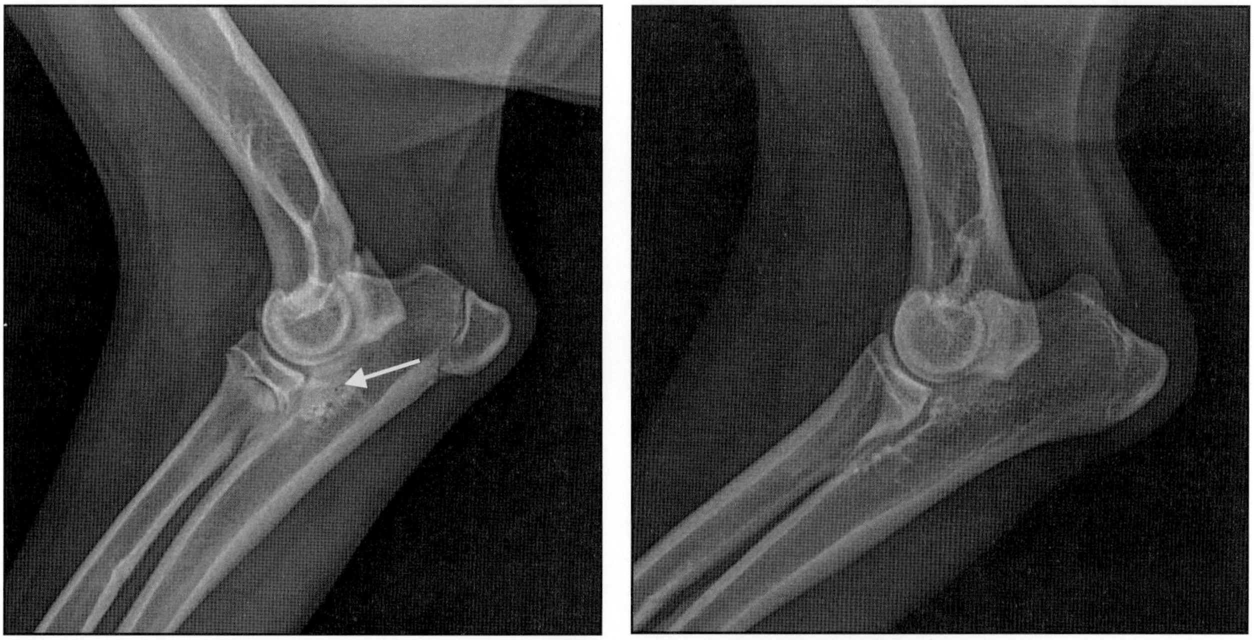

Figure 45.7 On the left is a lateral radiograph of the left elbow of a five-month-old male intact Golden Retriever with evidence of subtrochlear sclerosis (STS) denoted by the yellow arrow. Compare this STS to the image on the right of a one year old Retriever with a normal left elbow. Note the lack of sclerosis and visible trabecular pattern of the ulna adjacent to the medial coronoid (right image). *Source:* Image courtesy of Joey Sapora.

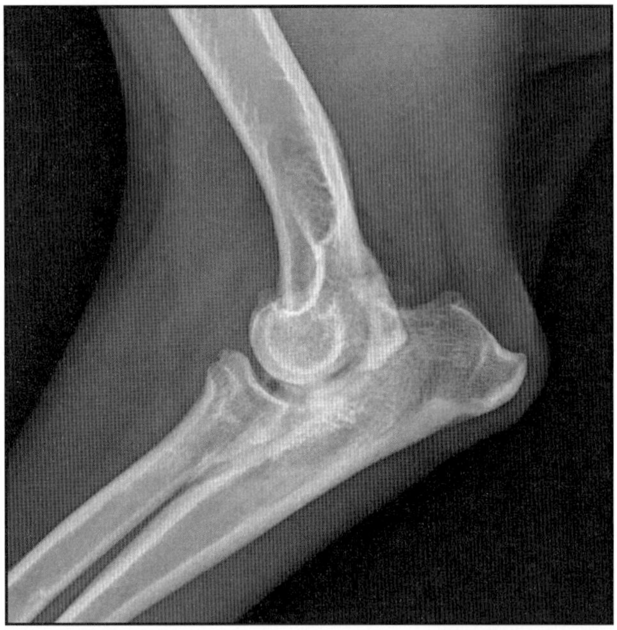

Figure 45.8 Neutral (120°) mediolateral projection of the elbow of a one-year-old castrated male Australian Cattle Dog. Note the "short radius" when compared to the ulna, generating positive radioulnar incongruence (RUI) at the level of the elbow. This degree of radiographic RUI is severe. *Source:* Image courtesy of Joey Sapora.

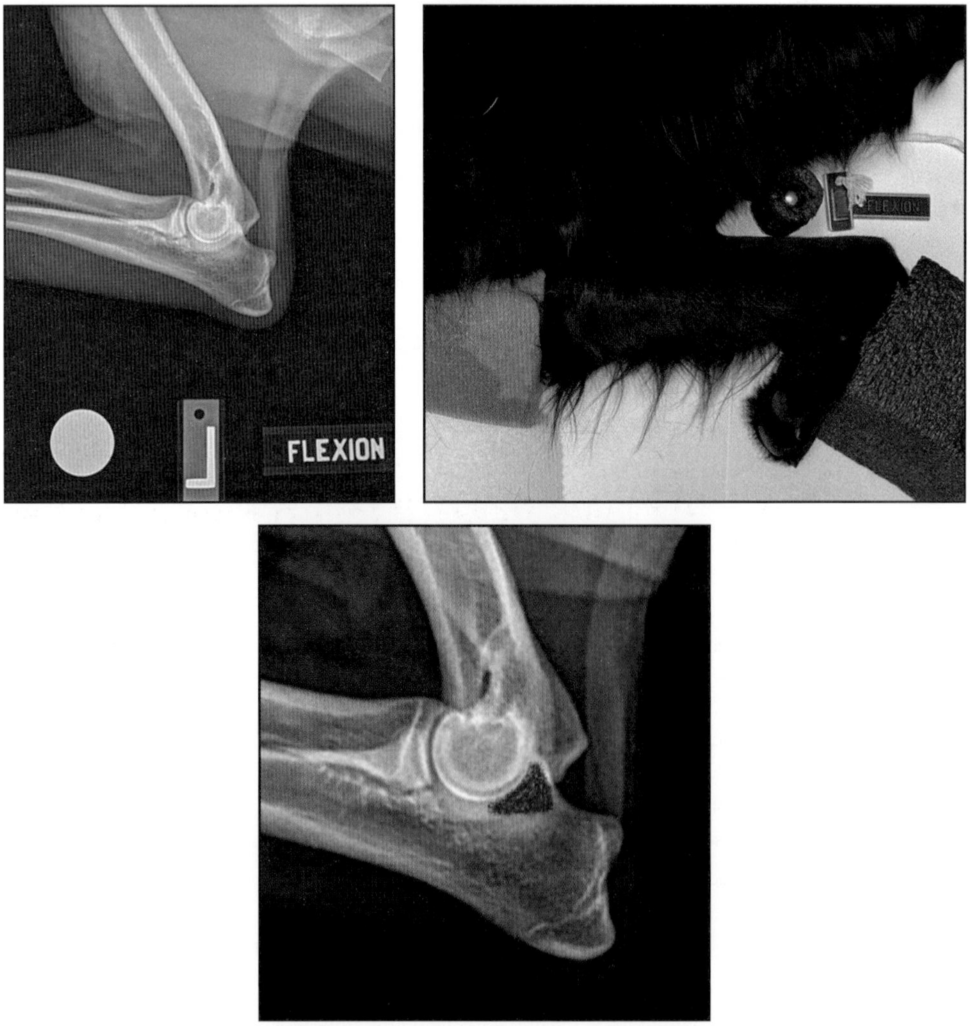

Figure 45.9 Flexed (45°) mediolateral projection of a normal elbow in a one-year-old castrated male Flat-Coated Retriever (top left). Appropriate patient positioning (top right). Note how the anconeal process (purple shade) is better visualized with less superimposition of the humeral epicondyles when flexed to this degree (bottom). *Source:* Image courtesy of Joey Sapora.

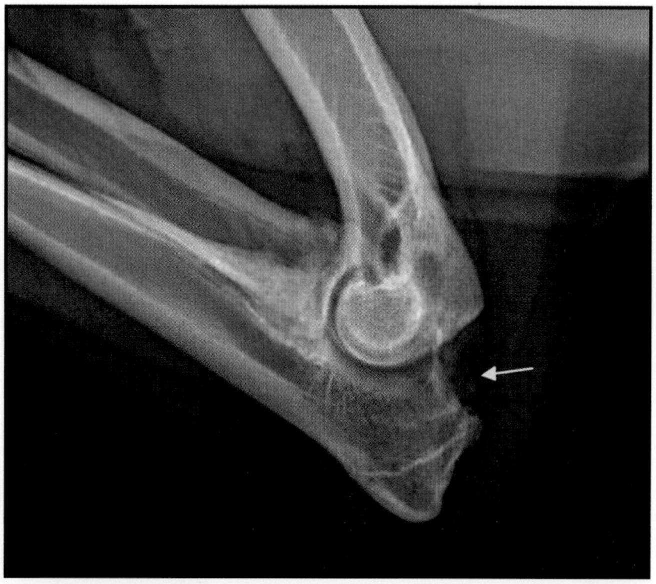

Figure 45.10 A five-year-old castrated male Australian Shepherd with CED. Note the osteophytosis present along the dorsal aspect of the anconeal process (yellow arrow). *Source:* Image courtesy of Joey Sapora.

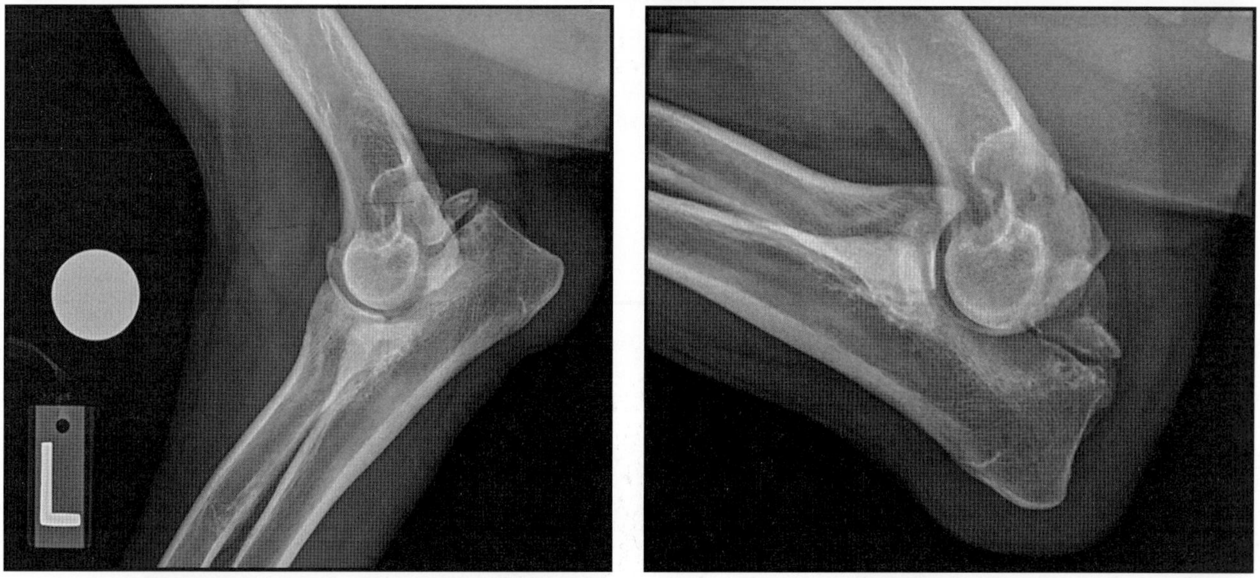

Figure 45.11 A two-year-old castrated male German Shepherd Dog with an ununited anconeal process (UAP). Note the improved visualization of the UAP on the flexed (45°) view (right image) with narrowing of the radiolucent fissure, suggestive for UAP instability. This patient also has evidence of a "short ulna." *Source:* Image courtesy of Joey Sapora.

- Decreased medial coronoid density with possible fragmentation. Do not mistake the sesamoid in the supinator muscle for a medial coronoid fragment.
- OC of the medial humeral condyle.

Multiple grading schemes have been developed for the radiographic scoring of CED. The IEWG guidelines (Figure 45.15) for scoring CED are based upon the identification of osteoarthrosis and signs of a primary lesion. Again, radiographic interpretation of joint incongruity can be unreliable and radiographic assessment of osteophytosis has been shown to be a poor predictor of the severity of arthroscopic pathology for CED.[54]

Subtrochlear sclerosis (STS) is a very reliable indicator of the presence of medial coronoid pathology, and increasing the severity of STS increases the sensitivity in detecting medial coronoid pathology and correlates with disease severity (Figure 45.7).[55] Ulnar STS has also been shown to be the most common radiographic finding in dogs <12 months of age with medial coronoid disease, while blurring of the cranial aspect of the medial coronoid was the most common radiographic finding in dogs >12 months of age.[56] While attempts at quantifying STS as a percentage or by using digital methods may provide a means for objective assessment, subjective evaluation by an experienced

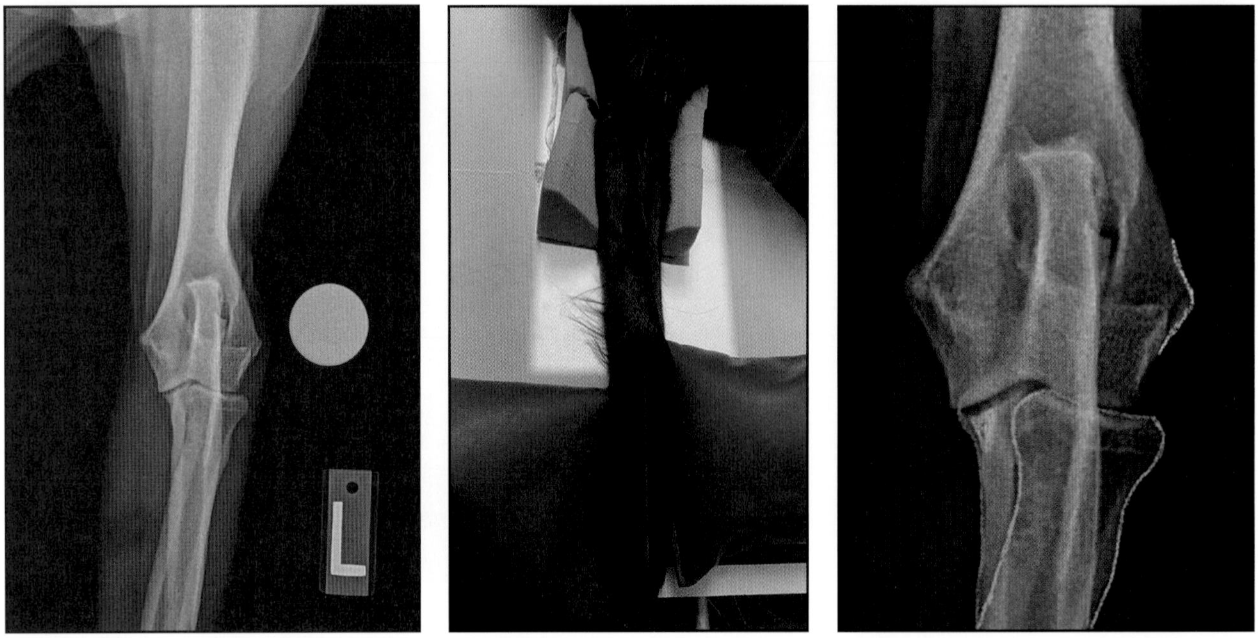

Figure 45.12 Craniocaudal projection with 15° of pronation of a normal elbow in a one-year-old castrated male Flat-Coated Retriever (left). Appropriate craniocaudal positioning (center). Normal radiographic anatomy of the canine elbow, Cr-Cd projection: green line – radius; blue line – ulna; yellow shade – medial coronoid process; pink line – medial humeral epicondyle; white line – lateral humeral epicondyle (right). *Source:* Image courtesy of Joey Sapora.

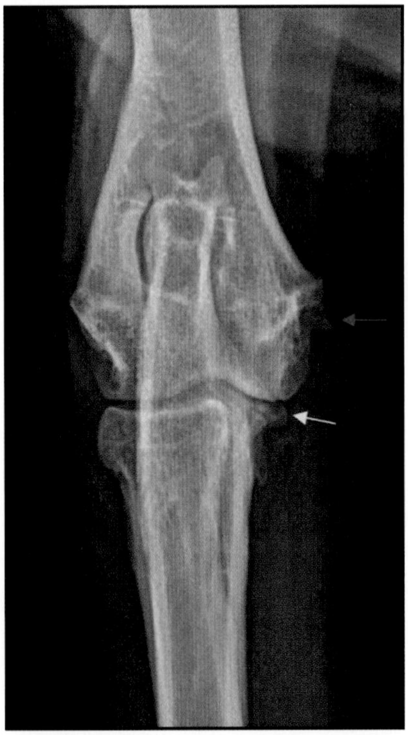

Figure 45.13 A two-year-old castrated male Labrador Retriever with medial coronoid osteophytosis (yellow arrow) and medial humeral condylar osteophytosis (blue arrow). *Source:* Image courtesy of Joey Sapora.

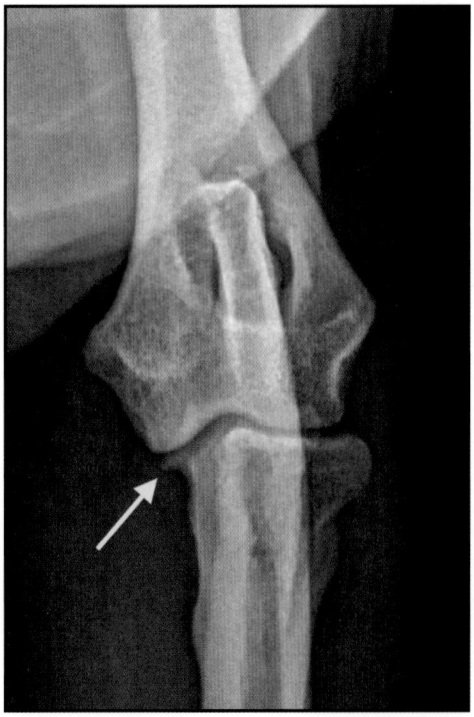

Figure 45.14 A three-year-old spayed female Rottweiler with evidence of early osteophytosis of the medial coronoid process (yellow arrow). CT identified a large FCP. *Source:* Image courtesy of Joey Sapora.

Elbow dysplasia scoring		Radiographic findings
0	Normal elbow joint	Normal elbow joint, No evidence of incongruity, sclerosis or arthrosis
1	Mild arthrosis	Presence of osteophytes < 2 mm, sclerosis of the base of the coronoid processes - trabecular pattern still visible Step =/> 2 mm between radius and ulna
2	Moderate arthrosis or suspect primary lesion	Presence of osteophytes 2 – 5 mm Obvious sclerosis (no trabecular pattern) of the base of the coronoid processes Step of 3–5 mm between radius and ulna (INCONGRUITY) Indirect signs for other primary lesion (UAP, FCP/Coronoid disease, OCD)
3	Severe arthrosis or evident primary lesion	Presence of osteophytes > 5 mm Step of > 5 mm between radius and ulna (obvious INCONGRUITY) Obvious presence of a primary lesion (UAP, FCP, OCD)

Figure 45.15 International Elbow Working Group guidelines for radiographic scoring of Elbow Dysplasia.

practitioner may be the most helpful diagnostic tool readily available for early identification of disease, as even mild STS is a cause for concern in the juvenile patient.

Computed Tomography (CT) provides a more detailed and three-dimensional assessment of the canine elbow compared to radiography and can aid in early diagnosis. The value of a CT scan in the decision-making process for surgical treatment of elbow dysplasia is predominantly surgeon-dependent. Benefits include accurate characterization of the components of CED prior to surgery, multiplanar assessment of the humeroradioulnar articulations, more accurate detection of concomitant lesions (i.e., focal OC lesions, radial incisure pathology, panosteitis, etc.), and post-operative evaluation of patients experiencing a suboptimal recovery (coronoid re-fragmentation can rarely occur). In addition, it can provide more accurate prognostic information to clients regarding joint health prior to surgery (Figure 45.16).

Ultimately, arthroscopic examination of the joint remains the ideal diagnostic test for assessing articular cartilage for potential pathology and radioulnar incongruence (Figure 45.17).[51,56] Additional diagnostic modalities that can be utilized for CED include nuclear scintigraphy,[57] ultrasonography,[53] PET-CT scans, and MRI. Despite the availability of advanced cross-sectional imaging, the importance of pain with elbow manipulation, most notably flexion, remains the mainstay for early identification of disease.

Surgical Treatment Options

Fragmented Medial Coronoid Process (FCP) and Advanced Medial Compartment Disease (MCD)

No definitive treatment option exists for the many clinical manifestations of CED. The preferred local treatment for FCP is a subtotal coronoidectomy (SCO), a procedure in which the abnormal portion of the medial coronoid process is removed.[58] This is most commonly performed at the time of an arthroscopic exam of the joint utilizing an osteotome or arthroscopic shaver. Arthroscopic subtotal coronoidectomy (Figure 45.18) has been shown to provide a shorter convalescent period for patients, however, when compared to open arthrotomy, the development of future osteoarthritis cannot be avoided.[59] Despite this progression of arthritis, long-term improvement and, in some cases, resolution of lameness can be achieved in dogs following SCO.[54]

While dogs with isolated FCP and only mild changes to their joint cartilage have a more favorable prognosis following SCO, fragment removal alone will not palliate clinical signs in patients with more global cartilage wear. This can be the case in older patients with advanced medial compartment disease (Figure 45.19), and in those with changes affecting predominantly the medial aspect of the humeroulnar joint additional advanced osteotomies and

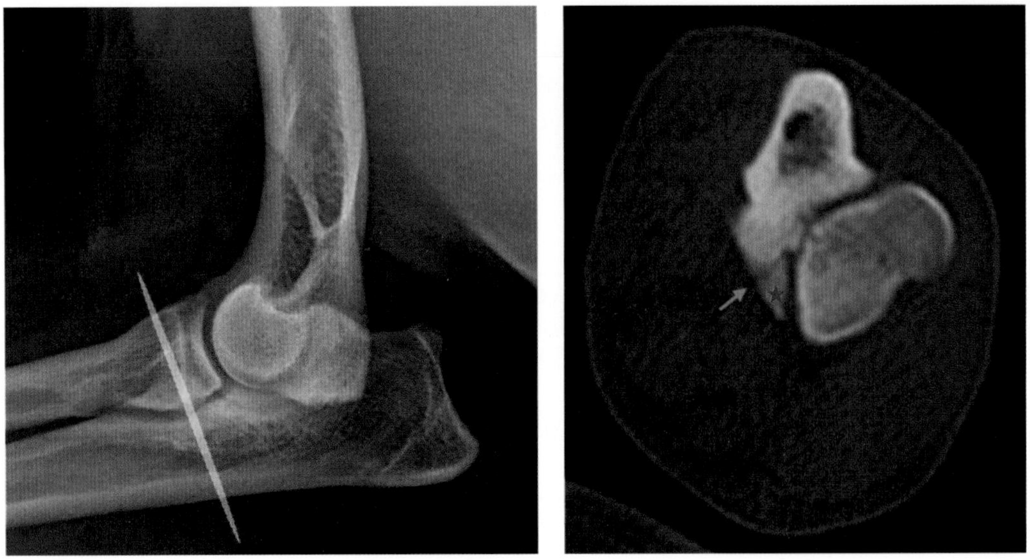

Figure 45.16 The image on the left is a lateral radiograph of a canine elbow. The yellow disc is the radius and ulna in cross-section (transverse plane) with the corresponding CT image on the right. On the CT image, the red star denotes the medial coronoid process, with the green arrow identifying clear fragmentation. This fragmentation was not noticeable radiographically. *Source:* Image courtesy of Joey Sapora.

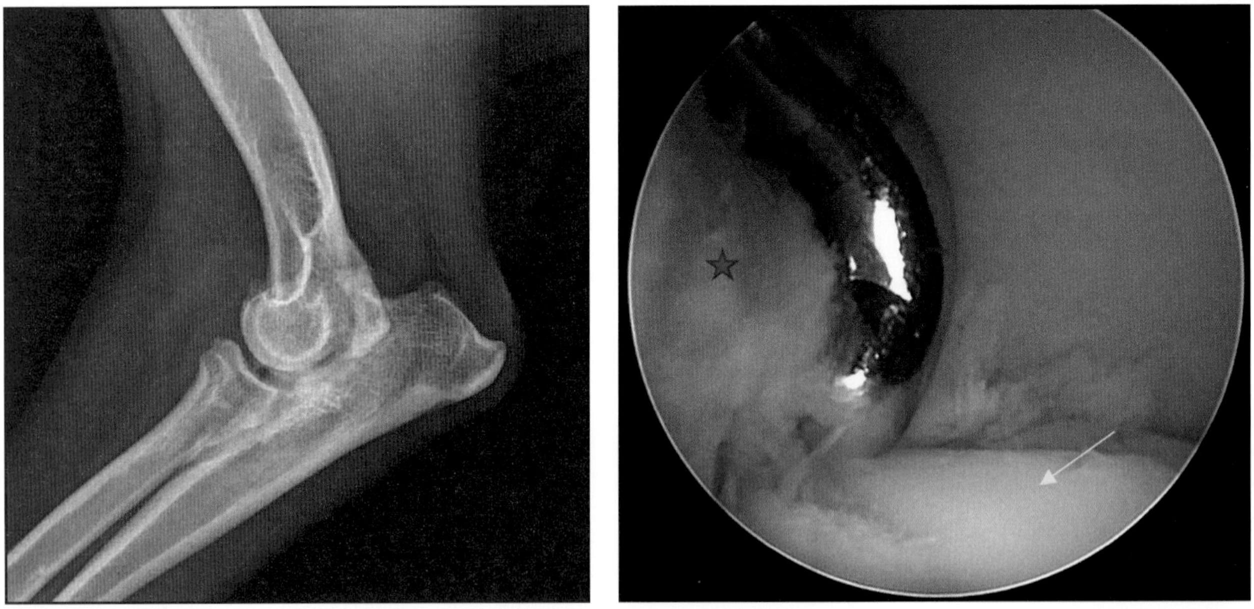

Figure 45.17 An 11-month-old spayed female Australian Cattle Dog. Note the radiographic evidence of positive RUI (short radius) in the image on the left, and the corresponding arthroscopic exam showing a large step defect between the radial head (yellow arrow) and ulna (blue star) in the image on the right. *Source:* Image courtesy of Joey Sapora.

synthetic implants have been developed. These include the sliding humeral osteotomy (SHO), proximal abducting ulnar osteotomy (PAUL), canine unicompartmental elbow (CUE), and elbow replacement systems (KYON BANC, TATE, Iowa State).[60] Careful case selection and ample client communication are required prior to pursuing these interventions.

Osteochondrosis (OC) of the Medial Humeral Condyle

Treatment for medial humeral condylar OC involves arthroscopic identification and removal of the diseased cartilaginous flap followed by agitation of the sclerotic subchondral bone. This is most commonly performed through

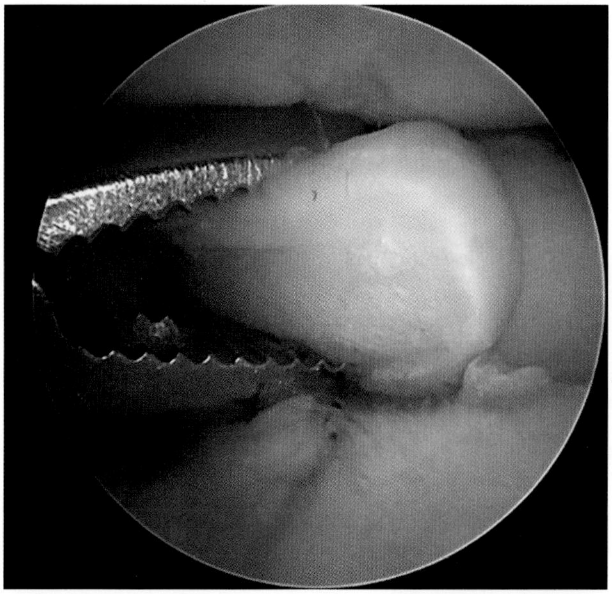

Figure 45.18 Arthroscopic subtotal coronoidectomy with retrieval of a fragmented medial coronoid process. *Source:* Image courtesy of Joey Sapora.

micropicking or osteostixis (microdrilling), which involves creating subchondral bone tunnels approximately 3–5 mm deep and spaced 2–3 mm apart. Bleeding should be observed, and the generation of these vascular channels promotes the formation of a more stable fibrocartilaginous defect (Figure 45.20).

Radioulnar Elbow Incongruence

For treatment of elbow incongruence (Figure 45.8), ulnar ostectomies are considered when cross-sectional imaging reveals moderate incongruence with a cutoff of >4 mm proposed.[58] Ostectomies that may be considered include distal dynamic ulnar ostectomies for patients 4–5 months of age and bi-oblique dynamic proximal ulnar osteotomies for patients 5–12 months of age.[23] Case selection and surgical technique are critical when performing an ulnar ostectomy on a juvenile patient, as complications may arise including radioulnar synostosis resulting in the development of an angular limb deformity, delayed unions, varus deformities, and worsening elbow incongruity. When rotational instability with excessive loading of the biceps

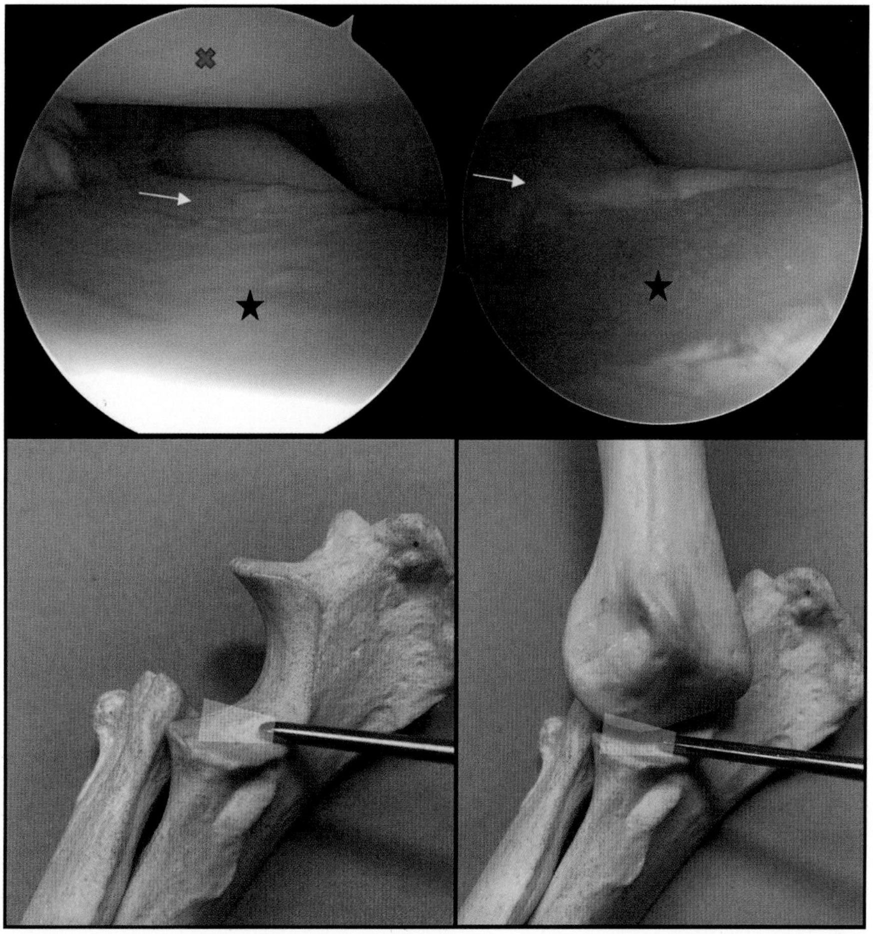

Figure 45.19 Top – Two juvenile patients with CED with evidence of medial coronoid fragmentation (yellow arrow). The patient on the top left has only mild cartilage wear to the humeral trochlea (blue cross) and the base of the medial coronoid (black star). Despite being similar in age, the patient on the top right has more severe cartilage eburnation with exposure of subchondral bone, classic for "medial compartment disease." Bottom – anatomic specimens showing the viewing angle of the scope, replicated by placement of a probe, with and without the humerus for clarity. Source: Image courtesy of Joey Sapora.

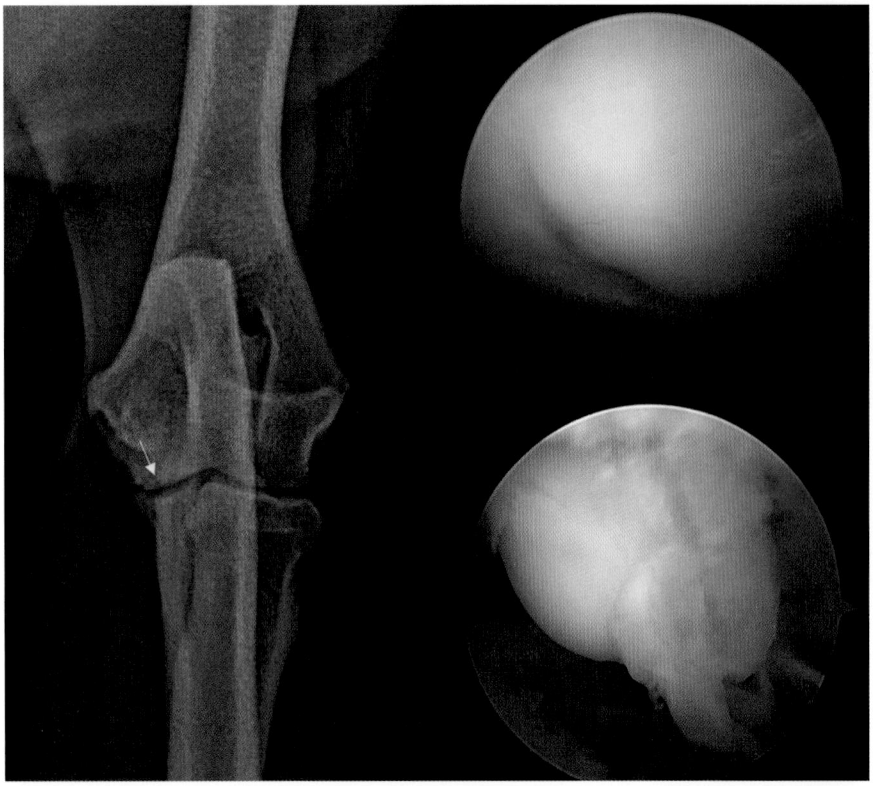

Figure 45.20 A one-year-old intact male Labrador Retriever with radiographic evidence of medial humeral trochlear sclerosis and a focal concavity consistent with osteochondrosis (left). The same patient's arthroscopy revealed a very large, 5 mm × 6 mm OCD flap (top right) that was easily elevated with blunt probing and removed (bottom right). *Source:* Image courtesy of Joey Sapora.

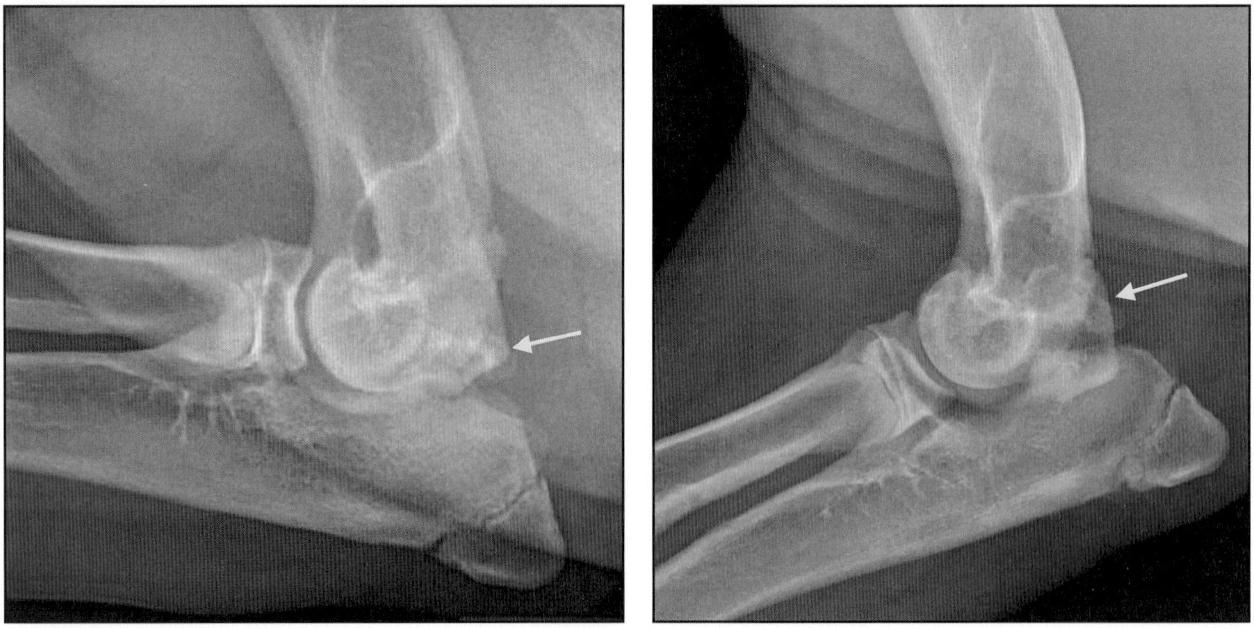

Figure 45.21 A five-month-old intact male Pitbull with radiographic evidence of a suspected unstable UAP (yellow arrows). *Source:* Image courtesy of Joey Sapora.

brachii/brachialis muscle complex is suspected, the biceps ulnar release procedure (BURP) may be considered. These are often recommended in juvenile patients with cartilage or subchondral bone pathology affecting the radial incisure based upon arthroscopic exam or cross-sectional imaging.[58]

United Anconeal Process (UAP)

For the treatment of UAP, early identification is paramount (Figure 45.21). Surgical treatment with screw fixation and release of the ulna can allow for the fusion of the anconeal process and the avoidance of elbow osteoarthritis. This is most effective in large breed dogs between four to six months of age and giant breed dogs up to nine months of age.[61] Fusion of the process is preferred over the removal of the fragment, as UAP removal leads to a significantly reduced range of motion and accelerated osteoarthritis. In adult dogs, UAP removal is the only treatment and is reserved for cases where the UAP has detached from its fibrocartilaginous attachment and is unstable. Otherwise, medical management is recommended. Determination of whether or not the UAP is stable is based on radiographs and arthroscopic examination.

Medical Management of Canine Elbow Dysplasia

Despite the age of diagnosis and if surgical intervention is pursued, long-term osteoarthritis management is recommended for all dogs with CED. Management strategies that have the greatest body of evidence for efficacy include weight management, exercise, and dietary optimization with the addition of omega-3 fatty acid supplementation, nonsteroidal anti-inflammatory drug (NSAID), and anti-nerve growth factor monoclonal antibody medications.[62] A lean body weight targeting a BCS of 4–5/9 is recommended. Regular but moderate daily activity that does not precipitate lameness should be encouraged. Nerve pain medications (gabapentin and amantadine) can be considered for adjunct pain management. Further therapy can include the addition of disease-modifying agents like polysulfated glycosaminoglycans, physical therapy with a certified canine rehabilitationist, and, for advanced disease, intraarticular biologic injections (platelet-rich plasma, hyaluronic acid, triamcinolone, etc.). Radiocolloid intraarticular products (Synovetin OA®) are a newer addition to the repertoire of managing canine osteoarthritis with promising early results. Treatment involves the injection of radioactive isotopes that have limited tissue penetration (<0.3 mm for Synovetin OA®), ensuring only local treatment effects. These isotopes undergo phagocytosis by inflammatory macrophages, causing cell destruction of these inflammatory macrophages over a sustained period of time.[63] Radiation isolation following treatment is required according to state and local ordinances. Additional prospective clinical trials are needed to optimize case selection and identify the part intraarticular radiocolloids play in the complex treatment of CED.

References

1 Fitzpatrick, N. ed. (2013). New insights into the etiopathogenesis, scoring & treatment algorithm for developmental elbow disease. *Proceedings American College of Veterinary Surgeons Symposium, San Antonio, Texas*, 285–289.

2 Cawley, A.J. and Archibald, J. (1959). Ununited anconal processes of the dog. *J. Am. Vet. Med. Assoc.* 134 (10): 454–458.

3 Stiern, R.A. (1956). Ectopic sesamoid bones at the elbow (patella cubiti) of the dog. *J. Am. Vet. Med. Assoc.* 128 (10): 498–501.

4 Tirgari, M. (1974). Clinical radiographical and pathological aspects of arthritis of the elbow joint in dogs. *J. Small Anim. Pract.* 15 (11): 671–679.

5 Olsson, S.E. (1971). Degenerative joint disease (osteoarthrosis): a review with special reference to the dog. *J. Small Anim. Pract.* 12 (6): 333–342.

6 Hazewinkel, H.A.W. ed. (2022). Pathogenesis of fragmentation of coronoid process. *Proceedings 34th annual meeting of the International Elbow Working Group*, Nice, France, 7–12.

7 Mäki, K., Groen, A., Liinamo, A.E. et al. (2002). Genetic variances, trends and mode of inheritance for hip and elbow dysplasia in Finnish dog populations. *Anim. Sci.* 75 (2): 197–207.

8 Malm, S., Fikse, W., Danell, B. et al. (2008). Genetic variation and genetic trends in hip and elbow dysplasia in Swedish Rottweiler and Bernese Mountain Dog. *J. Anim. Breed. Genet.* 125 (6): 403–412.

9 Lewis, T.W., Blott, S.C., and Woolliams, J.A. (2013). Comparative analyses of genetic trends and prospects for selection against hip and elbow dysplasia in 15 UK dog breeds. *BMC Genet.* 14 (1): 1–12.

10 Lavrijsen, I., Heuven, H., Voorhout, G. et al. (2012). Phenotypic and genetic evaluation of elbow dysplasia in Dutch Labrador Retrievers, Golden Retrievers, and Bernese Mountain dogs. *Vet. J.* 193 (2): 486–492.

11 Janutta, V., Hamann, H., Klein, S. et al. (2006). Genetic analysis of three different classification protocols for the evaluation of elbow dysplasia in German shepherd dogs. *J. Small Anim. Pract.* 47 (2): 75–82.

12 O'Neill, D.G., Brodbelt, D.C., Hodge, R. et al. (2020). Epidemiology and clinical management of elbow joint disease in dogs under primary veterinary care in the UK. *Canine Med. Genet.* 7: 1–15.

13 Hans, E.C., Saunders, W.B., Beale, B.S. et al. (2016). Fragmentation of the medial coronoid process in toy and small breed dogs: 13 elbows (2000–2012). *J. Am. Anim. Hosp. Assoc.* 52 (4): 234–241.

14 Lappalainen, A., Hyvärinen, T., Junnila, J. et al. (2016). Radiographic evaluation of elbow incongruity in Skye terriers. *J. Small Anim. Pract.* 57 (2): 96–99.

15 Morgan, J.P., Wind, A., and Davidson, A.P. (1999). Bone dysplasias in the labrador retriever: a radiographic study. *J. Am. Anim. Hosp. Assoc.* 35 (4): 332–340.

16 Kealy, R.D., Lawler, D.F., Ballam, J.M. et al. (2000). Evaluation of the effect of limited food consumption on radiographic evidence of osteoarthritis in dogs. *J. Am. Vet. Med. Assoc.* 217 (11): 1678–1680.

17 Sallander, M.H., Hedhammar, A., and Trogen, M.E.H. (2006). Diet, exercise, and weight as risk factors in hip dysplasia and elbow arthrosis in Labrador retrievers. *J. Nutr.* 136 (7): 2050S–2052S.

18 Woolliams, J.A., Lewis, T.W., and Blott, S.C. (2011). Canine hip and elbow dysplasia in UK Labrador retrievers. *Vet. J.* 189 (2): 169–176.

19 Oberbauer, A., Keller, G., and Famula, T. (2017). Long-term genetic selection reduced prevalence of hip and elbow dysplasia in 60 dog breeds. *PLoS One* 12 (2): e0172918.

20 Baers, G., Keller, G.G., Famula, T.R. et al. (2019). Heritability of unilateral elbow dysplasia in the dog: a retrospective study of sire and dam influence. *Front. Vet. Sci.* 6: 422.

21 Fox, S., Bloomberg, M., and Bright, R. (1983). Developmental anomalies of the canine elbow. *J. Am. Anim. Hosp. Assoc.* 19: 605–615.

22 Breit, S., Künzel, W., and Seiler, S. (2004). Variation in the ossification process of the anconeal and medial coronoid processes of the canine ulna. *Res. Vet. Sci.* 77 (1): 9–16.

23 Vezzoni, A. and Benjamino, K. (2021). Canine elbow dysplasia: ununited anconeal process, osteochondritis dissecans, and medial coronoid process disease. *Vet. Clin. North Am. Small Anim. Pract.* 51 (2): 439–474.

24 Lau, S.F., Hazewinkel, H.A.W., Grinwis, G.C.M. et al. (2013). Delayed endochondral ossification in early medial coronoid disease (MCD): a morphological and immunohistochemical evaluation in growing Labrador retrievers. *Vet. J.* 197 (3): 731–738.

25 Crouch, D.T., Cook, J.L., Lewis, D.D. et al. (2000). The presence of collagen types II and X in medial coronoid processes of 21 dogs. *Vet. Comp. Orthop. Traumatol.* 13 (04): 178–184.

26 Danielson, K.C., Fitzpatrick, N., Muir, P. et al. (2006). Histomorphometry of fragmented medial coronoid process in dogs: a comparison of affected and normal coronoid processes. *Vet. Surg.* 35 (6): 501–509.

27 Meyer-Lindenberg, A., Fehr, M., and Nolte, I. (2006). Co-existence of ununited anconeal process and fragmented medial coronoid process of the ulna in the dog. *J. Small Anim. Pract.* 47 (2): 61–65.

28 Samoy, Y., Van Vynckt, D., Gielen, I. et al. (2012). Arthroscopic findings in 32 joints affected by severe elbow incongruity with concomitant fragmented medial coronoid process. *Vet. Surg.* 41 (3): 355–361.

29 Michelsen, J. (2013). Canine elbow dysplasia: aetiopathogenesis and current treatment recommendations. *Vet. J.* 196 (1): 12–19.

30 Duerr, F.M. (2020). Elbow Region. In: *Canine Lameness*, 195–221. Wiley.

31 Hulse, D., Young, B., Beale, B. et al. (2010). Relationship of the biceps-brachialis complex to the medial coronoid process of the canine ulna. *Vet. Comp. Orthop. Traumatol.* 23 (03): 173–176.

32 Wilson, D.M., Goh, C.S., and Palmer, R.H. (2014). Arthroscopic biceps ulnar release procedure (BURP): technique description and in vitro assessment of the association of visual control and surgeon experience to regional damage and tenotomy completeness. *Vet. Surg.* 43 (6): 734–740.

33 Mason, T., Lavelle, R., Skipper, S. et al. (1980). Osteochondrosis of the elbow joint in young dogs. *J. Small Anim. Pract.* 21 (12): 641–656.

34 Johnston, S.A. and Tobias, K.M. (2017). Osteochondrosis. In: *Veterinary Surgery Small Animal Second Edition* (ed. G. Breur and N. Lambrechts), 1372. Elsevier.

35 Schoenmakers, I., Hazewinkel, H.A., Voorhout, G. et al. (2000). Effects of diets with different calcium and phosphorus contents on the skeletal development and blood chemistry of growing great danes. *Vet. Rec.* 147 (23): 652–660.

36 Hedhammar, A., Wu, F.M., Krook, L. et al. (1974). Overnutrition and skeletal disease. An experimental study in growing Great Dane dogs. *Cornell Vet.* 64 (2): Suppl 5:-160.

37 Lavelle, R. (1989). The effects of the overfeeding. *Nutrition of the Dog and Cat: Waltham Symposium* Number 7, Cambridge University Press.

38 Frazho, J.K., Graham, J., Peck, J.N. et al. (2010). Radiographic evaluation of the anconeal process in skeletally immature dogs. *Vet. Surg.* 39 (7): 829–832.

39 LaFond, E., Breur, G.J., and Austin, C.C. (2002). Breed susceptibility for developmental orthopedic diseases in dogs. *J. Am. Anim. Hosp. Assoc.* 38 (5): 467–477.

40 Gustafsson, P.O., Olsson, S.E., Kasström, H. et al. (1975). Skeletal Development of Greyhounds, German Shepherd Dogs and Their Crossbreed Offspring: An Investigation with Special Reference to Hip Dysplasia. *Acta Radiol. Diag.* 16 (344_suppl): 81–107.

41 Hanlon, G. and Spurrel, F. (1967). Elbow dysplasia with reference to the maturation of the procesus anconeous in the German shepherd dogs. *Minn. Vet.* 7: 11–15.

42 Corley, E., Sutherland, T., and Carlson, W. (1968). Genetic aspects of canine elbow dysplasia. *J. Am. Vet. Med. Assoc.* 153 (5): 543–547.

43 Kirberger, R. and Fourie, S. (1998). Elbow dysplasia in the dog: pathophysiology, diagnosis and control. *J. S. Afr. Vet. Assoc.* 69 (2): 43–54.

44 Sjöström, L. (1998). Ununited anconeal process in th dog. *Vet. Clin. North Am. Small Anim. Pract.* 28 (1): 75–86.

45 Eljack, H. and Böttcher, P. (2015). Relationship between axial radioulnar incongruence with cartilage damage in dogs with medial coronoid disease. *Vet. Surg.* 44 (2): 174–179.

46 Alves-Pimenta, S., Ginja, M.M., and Colaço, B. (2019). Role of elbow incongruity in canine elbow dysplasia: advances in diagnostics and biomechanics. *Vet. Comp. Orthop. Traumatol.* 32 (02): 087–096.

47 Alves-Pimenta, S., Ginja, M.M., Colaço, J. et al. (2015). Curvature radius measurements from the ulnar trochlear notch in large dogs. *Anat. Rec.* 298 (10): 1748–1753.

48 Alves-Pimenta, S., Ginja, M., Fernandes, A.M. et al. (2016). Curvature radius measurements from the humeral trochlea in large dogs. *Anat. Rec.* 299 (8): 1012–1014.

49 Alves-Pimenta, S., Colaço, B., Fernandes, A.M. et al. (2017). Radiographic assessment of humeroulnar congruity in a medium and a large breed of dog. *Vet. Radiol. Ultrasound* 58 (6): 627–633.

50 Wind, A.P. and Packard, M. (1986). Elbow incongruity and developmental elbow diseases in the dog: Part II. *J. Am. Anim. Hosp. Assoc.* 22: 725–730.

51 Wagner, K., Griffon, D.J., Thomas, M.W. et al. (2007). Radiographic, computed tomographic, and arthroscopic evaluation of experimental radio-ulnar incongruence in the dog. *Vet. Surg.* 36 (7): 691–698.

52 Farrell, M., Draffan, D., Gemmill, T. et al. (2007). In vitro validation of a technique for assessment of canine and feline elbow joint collateral ligament integrity and description of a new method for collateral ligament prosthetic replacement. *Vet. Surg.* 36 (6): 548–556.

53 Cook, C.R. and Cook, J.L. (2009). Diagnostic imaging of canine elbow dysplasia: a review. *Vet. Surg.* 38 (2): 144–153.

54 Fitzpatrick, N., Smith, T.J., Evans, R.B. et al. (2009). Radiographic and arthroscopic findings in the elbow joints of 263 dogs with medial coronoid disease. *Vet. Surg.* 38 (2): 213–223.

55 Draffan, D., Carrera, I., Carmichael, S. et al. (2009). Radiographic analysis of trochlear notch sclerosis in the diagnosis of osteoarthritis secondary to medial coronoid disease. *Vet. Comp. Orthop. Traumatol.* 22 (01): 7–15.

56 Lau, S.F., Theyse, L.F., Voorhout, G. et al. (2015). Radiographic, computed tomographic, and arthroscopic findings in Labrador retrievers with medial coronoid disease. *Vet. Surg.* 44 (4): 511–520.

57 Van Bruggen, L.W., Hazewinkel, H.A., Wolschrijn, C.F. et al. (2010). Bone scintigraphy for the diagnosis of an abnormal medial coronoid process in dogs. *Vet. Radiol. Ultrasound* 51 (3): 344–348.

58 Fitzpatrick, N. and Yeadon, R. (2009). Working algorithm for treatment decision making for developmental disease of the medial compartment of the elbow in dogs. *Vet. Surg.* 38 (2): 285.

59 Meyer-Lindenberg, A., Langhann, A., Fehr, M. et al. (2003). Arthrotomy versus arthroscopy in the treatment of the fragmented medial coronoid process of the ulna (FCP) in 421 dogs. *Vet. Comp. Orthop. Traumatol.* 16 (04): 204–210.

60 Bruecker, K.A., Benjamino, K., Vezzoni, A. et al. (2021). Canine elbow dysplasia: medial compartment disease and osteoarthritis. *Vet. Clin. Small Anim. Pract.* 51 (2): 475–515.

61 Boiocchi, S. (2022). Elbow Ostechondritis Dissecans (OCD): diagnosis and results from surgical treatment. *Proceedings 34th annual meeting of the International Elbow Working Group* Nice, France: 24-30.

62 Monteiro, B.P., Lascelles, B.D.X., Murrell, J. et al. (2022). 2022 WSAVA guidelines for the recognition, assessment and treatment of pain. *J. Small Anim. Pract.* 64 (4): 177–254.

63 Lattimer, J., Fabiani, M., Gaschen, L. et al. (2023). Clinical effectiveness and safety of intraarticular administration of a ^{117m}Tin radiocolloid (Synovetin OA^{TM}) for treatment of early and intermediate grade osteoarthritis of the elbow in a dose finding study conducted in 44 dogs. *Vet. Radiol. Ultrasound* 64 (2): 351–359.

46

Femoral Head and Neck Ostectomy (FHO)

Kristin A. Coleman

Gulf Coast Veterinary Specialists, Houston, TX, USA

Key Points

- The goal of a femoral head and neck ostectomy (FHO) is to reduce or eliminate pain in the hip joint compared to pre-operative status. This procedure has the best chance of success with aggressive postoperative physical therapy.
- Osteoarthritis of the hip can be quite painful and debilitating, and, in small animals for whom total hip replacement (THR) is not an option or is not pursued, FHO should be considered when medical management is not sufficient to control pain.
- There are pros and cons to the craniolateral and ventral approaches to the FHO, and these should be considered prior to surgery for each patient.
- Tips for FHO procedural success: know the anatomy, always find palpably identifiable structures to aid in dissection, don't try to make a mini-approach, RETRACT, double-check the femur angle prior to osteotomy, take the hip through range of motion prior to closing, and obtain radiographs postoperatively.

Introduction

Femoral head and neck ostectomy (FHO) is a procedure with many different names and acronyms, including, but not limited to, femoral head and neck excision (FHNE), femoral head and neck osteotomy, and excision arthroplasty. FHO is performed to address the diseased, injured, or luxated coxofemoral joint.[1–7] FHO was first developed in 1928 for human septic tuberculosis of the coxofemoral joint as the *Girdlestone excision arthroplasty*, and it has since been adopted in veterinary medicine as a "salvage procedure" treatment option for severe hip joint osteoarthritis secondary to hip dysplasia or other causes (Figure 46.1), fractures of the femoral head or neck, Legg-Calve-Perthes disease or other forms of avascular necrosis of the femoral head or neck, neoplasia, and acute or chronic hip luxation. Other indications include capital physeal fractures, acetabular fractures, and metaphyseal osteopathy of the femoral neck.[7–14] The basic goal of the procedure is to remove the femoral head and neck to alleviate the pain from bone-on-bone contact between the femur and pelvis by allowing a "pseudo-joint" to form, which is composed of dense fibrous tissue over the cut edge of femur, with the remaining hip musculature to provide support.

FHO may be performed via one of two approaches: the traditional craniolateral approach and the more recently described ventral approach. Ventral FHO (vFHO) was originally reported in 1968 for addressing femoral neck fractures, but it is now used as a treatment for many other orthopedic diseases and conditions in small animals.[15] While there are no long-term studies evaluating objective outcome measures for animals undergoing ventral FHO, the perceived benefits include better visualization of the lesser trochanter compared to the craniolateral approach

Techniques in Small Animal Soft Tissue, Orthopedic, and Ophthalmic Surgery, First Edition. Edited by Kristin A. Coleman.

Companion website: www.wiley.com/go/coleman/surgeries

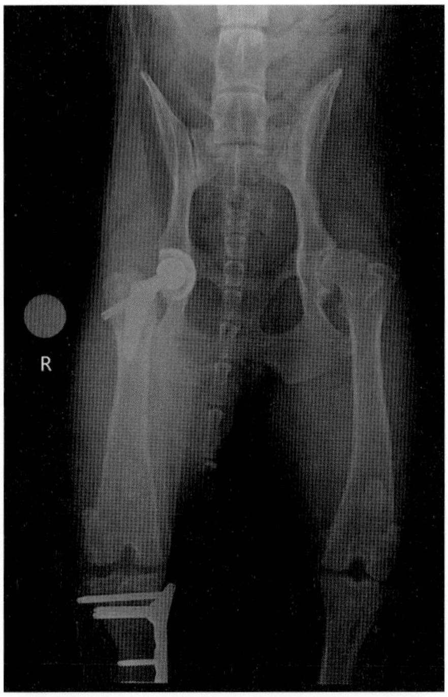

Figure 46.1 Craniocaudal radiograph of the pelvis of a large breed dog with significant degenerative joint disease, characterized by marked osteophytosis, of the left coxofemoral joint. A non-cemented total hip replacement has previously been performed on the right hip in this patient, and a tibial plateau leveling osteotomy (TPLO) plate is present on the medial aspect of the right tibia. *Source:* © Kristin Coleman.

and the ability to perform the procedure bilaterally without having to re-position the patient. The main benefit of the ventral approach over the more traditional craniolateral approach includes preservation of the cranial-dorsal musculature and soft tissue support structures that need to take over the function of the hip post-FHO, including the dorsal joint capsule and deep gluteal muscle tendon. Additionally, the only muscle transection that is needed in the ventral approach is the pectineus muscle. As pectineal myotomy has been described previously as a treatment option for hip dysplasia,[9] the ventral approach offers a potential inherent advantage if the pectineus is not re-apposed at the conclusion of surgery.

Sparing the dorsal support structures with the ventral approach could potentially minimize the craniodorsal malposition of the femur and "limb-shortening" postoperatively that is reported following the traditional craniolateral approach.[8,16] Subjectively, return to comfortable function in the limb is faster with the ventral approach versus the craniolateral approach. The cases when craniolateral approach is beneficial compared to the ventral approach are in patients with craniodorsal hip luxation or patients that have excessive inguinal fat that may hinder clear identification of surgical landmarks. Potential disadvantages of the ventral approach include proximity of the surgical dissection to the medial circumflex femoral artery and vein, that it is a subjectively more tedious procedure than that of the craniolateral approach (per the lack of visualization of the medial aspect of the greater trochanter), the challenge of removing additional bone after initial ostectomy, and the need to retract the iliopsoas muscle to begin the osteotomy.[16] Overall, choice of approach is dependent upon the surgeon's preference and comfort level, the patient, and the disease process being treated.

Indications/Pre-operative Considerations

A thorough conversation with the client is an important step prior to surgery to educate them about their pet's disease process and the treatment options available. They should be counseled on other potential options for their pet depending on the animal's age and presenting complaint. Such options include continued medical management, primary fracture repair (if an acute fracture is present), or other hip dysplasia surgical interventions such as juvenile pubic symphysiodesis (JPS), double or triple pelvic osteotomy, or total hip replacement (THR).[17] As previously mentioned, while the goal of surgery is to make the patient more comfortable, a residual lameness may remain, and the kinematics of the limb are permanently altered. Owners should also be reminded that the success of surgery relies heavily upon their willingness to pursue physical therapy postoperatively, either with a professional rehabilitation therapist or with at-home stretching and exercising.

Anatomy

Even before surgery, the surgeon should palpate the various bony prominences in the proximal hindlimb area to ensure accuracy in surgical approach and execution. The triad of prominences of the craniolateral approach is the iliac crest, the ischiatic tuberosity, and the greater trochanter, with the latter representing the landmark around which the FHO incision is based. There are a few important structures to avoid during this surgical approach, particularly the sciatic nerve. This nerve runs just caudodorsal to the coxofemoral joint and is the main reason for externally rotating the femur while retracting prior to femoral neck transection. During the ventral approach, there is less risk of encountering the sciatic nerve.

During the vFHO, care should be taken to identify and protect the femoral artery, femoral vein, and saphenous nerve, all of which lie on the cranial aspect of the pectineus muscle. After the pectineus muscle is transected and reflected distally, the medial circumflex femoral artery and vein are visualized tracking caudally and medially to the acetabulum with small branches that may be possibly disturbed during retraction. The majority of the muscles that are encountered are separated from their neighboring muscles and not transected. The only muscle to be potentially partially transected in the craniolateral approach is the deep gluteal muscle tendon, which is re-apposed at the end of the procedure, and the only muscle to be transected in the ventral approach is the pectineus muscle, which is not re-apposed. When the deep gluteal tendon is transected, this is typically performed in an "L"-shaped incision, ensuring that enough tendon of insertion is preserved for closure at the end of the procedure. In the author's experience, this transection is not always necessary as part of FHO.

It is advisable to frequently palpate the coxofemoral joint to not lose sight of the target located deep within the surgical site. This is easily done by grasping the hindlimb at the distal femur and manipulating the femur through a range of motion, including adduction and abduction, to identify the joint or even just the luxated femoral head if this is the disease process being treated.

Instruments for FHO

Having the proper instrumentation is essential to any surgical procedure, and this is especially true of orthopedic surgeries. A general surgery pack should, at minimum, include a Bard blade handle, Brown-Adson forceps, Metzenbaum scissors, curved Mayo scissors, a variety of hemostats, needle-holders, and suture-cutting scissors. An FHO surgery pack also includes a Gelpi perineal retractors (minimum of 2), Senn and/or Army-Navy retractor, (optional) Hat spoon or round ligament cutter, Freer periosteal elevator (or other elevator), Hohmann retractors (minimum of 2), sagittal saw or an osteotome and mallet, and a bone rasp. The ability to lavage the surgical site, particularly during the osteotomy to cool the saw blade, and suction are recommended for this procedure. The additional instrument needed for the ventral approach is the right angle forceps (Figure 46.2).

Surgical Procedure

Craniolateral Approach

The patient is positioned in lateral recumbency with the affected side facing up.[18] The affected hindlimb is clipped and prepped circumferentially from the stifle and proximally to the inguinal region medially and to the dorsal midline laterally. This allows the entire limb to be in the sterile field and manipulated throughout the procedure, which is important for confirming the completeness of the cut at the end of surgery. Self-adhesive, such as white tape, may be used to cover the non-shaved portion of the limb, and an exam glove is convenient to place around the paw.

A "dirty prep" is performed using dilute chlorhexidine scrub and non-sterile saline until the gauze lacks visible dirt or surface debris prior to taking the patient into the operating theater. Once the patient is positioned at the end of the surgery table, a standard hanging limb preparation is performed with a sterile glove using dilute chlorhexidine and sterile saline for a minimum of three rounds. At this point, quarter-draping may commence, being sure to place

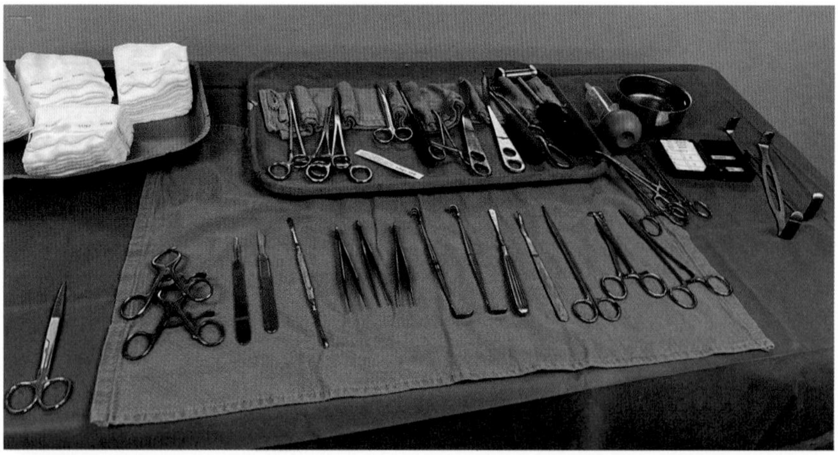

Figure 46.2 Standard instrument table for FHO. Counterclockwise from top left: gauze, sharp/sharp suture-cutting scissors, two small/pediatric Gelpi retractors, #15 Bard blade with handle, #10 Bard blade with handle, Freer periosteal elevator, three thumb forceps (Brown-Adson, two types of rat-tooth), two Senn retractors (one sharp, one blunt), Adson periosteal elevator, Hohmann retractor, curved Metzenbaum scissors, point-to-point bone reduction forceps, Mayo-Hegar needle holders, two Army-Navy retractors, sharps container, bowl with sterile saline, bulb syringe, several curved hemostats, and tray of instruments that are not commonly used (other than the two Hohmann retractors) in this procedure. If power equipment is not available, it is important to include a sharp osteotomes of various sizes and a mallet for performing FHO. Not pictured: monopolar electrosurgery pen and sagittal saw, which are on the patient table that is draped separately in some cases. *Source:* © Kristin Coleman.

the sticky drape or sterile Huck towel at least 1 cm in the sterile field from the hair to reduce the risk of hair contamination during the procedure. A water-impermeable segment of drape or sterilized aluminum foil is used to grasp the distal aspect of the hindlimb. A non-sterile assistant may "cut down" the limb from its hanging position (commonly, an IV pole), and after covering the paw with the water-impermeable material, a sterile self-adhesive bandaging material (e.g., 3M™ Vetrap™) is used to secure the drape or foil to the limb until no bandage material is visualized. A patient drape (with a small fenestration through which the sterilely prepped hindlimb is passed) is then used to cover both the patient and the caudally-located instrument table (Figure 46.3a). One of the keys to this procedure is remaining aware of the location of the palpably identifiable greater trochanter. While performing this procedure in the early stages, it may help to mark the skin with a sterile marker on the proposed incision prior to cutting.

An incision through the skin and subcutaneous layers may either be straight or curvilinear (with the curved portion oriented cranially at the dorsal aspect). The incision is started dorsally just craniodorsal to the palpable greater trochanter and extends distally to approximately 1/3–1/2 of the femoral length parallel to and along the cranial aspect (Figure 46.3b). The incision should essentially be centered on and cranial to the greater trochanter (Figure 46.3c), which allows for the incision to be directed over the coxofemoral joint in most animals. This will also permit visualization of the caudally-located biceps femoris, and an incision should be made through the superficial leaf of the fascia lata on the cranial edge of the biceps femoris to separate it from the cranially-located tensor fascia latae (Figure 46.4). The division between these muscles is not always obvious; the change in fiber directions of one muscle compared to the other aids in identifying the partition. Once these two muscles are separated and the superficial and deep leaves of the fascia lata have been incised, a Gelpi perineal retractor is placed to aid in identifying the dorsally-located gluteal muscles (Figure 46.5). Care should be taken caudally to not place the Gelpi retractor too deeply, as the sciatic nerve courses distally along the caudolateral aspect of the femur deep to the biceps femoris. The shiny fascia of the vastus lateralis muscle will be seen at this point, and the incision is continued proximally between the tensor fascia latae muscle (cranial) and superficial gluteal muscle (caudal).

Note: Cats have a muscle that is derived from the biceps femoris that is part of the "hamstring" muscle group called the *caudofemoralis*. This muscle is located just caudal to the superficial gluteal muscle. The caudofemoralis muscle is absent in the dog and should not be confused with the gluteal muscles in the cat.[18]

Using a Senn retractor and an assistant, retract the middle gluteal muscle dorsally to reveal the characteristic deep gluteal muscle tendon with its insertion onto the greater

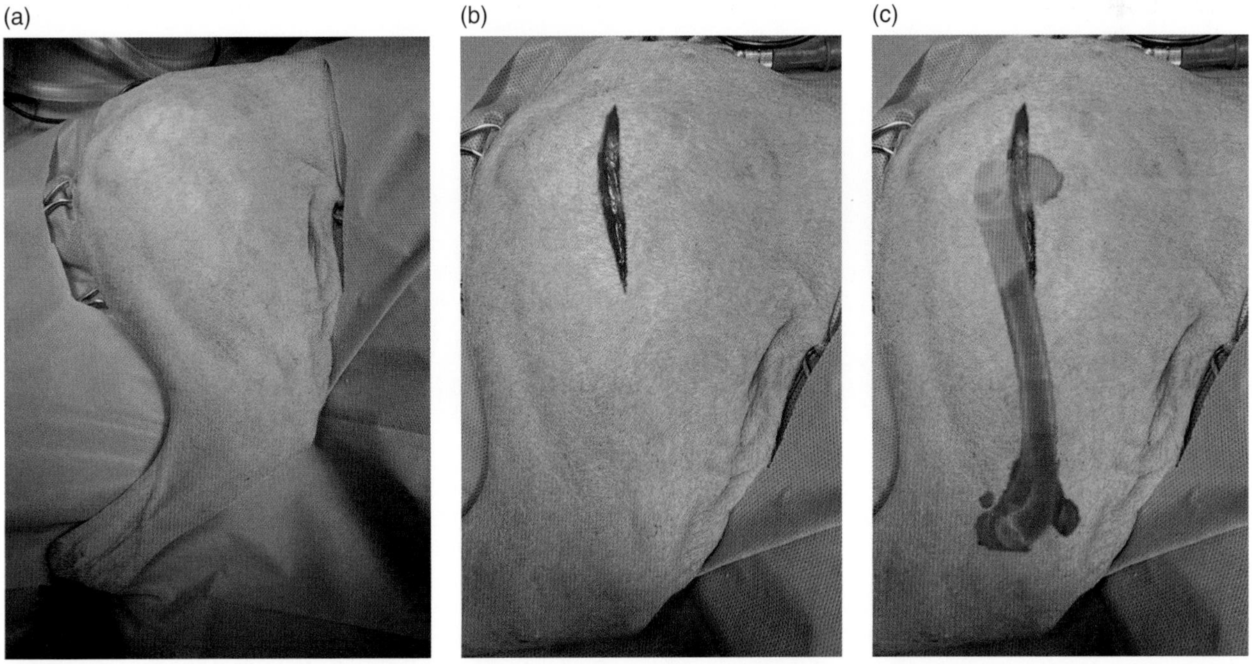

Figure 46.3 Canine patient undergoing right FHO via craniolateral approach: *initial incision*. Cranial is to the right of each image. (a) Patient is positioned in left lateral recumbency. (b) A straight or curvilinear incision is made through the skin and subcutaneous tissue just cranial to the palpable greater trochanter to ensure that the surgical site is positioned over the coxofemoral joint. (c) Image B with femur overlay to demonstrate the proper placement of the incision to approach the hip. *Source:* © Kristin Coleman.

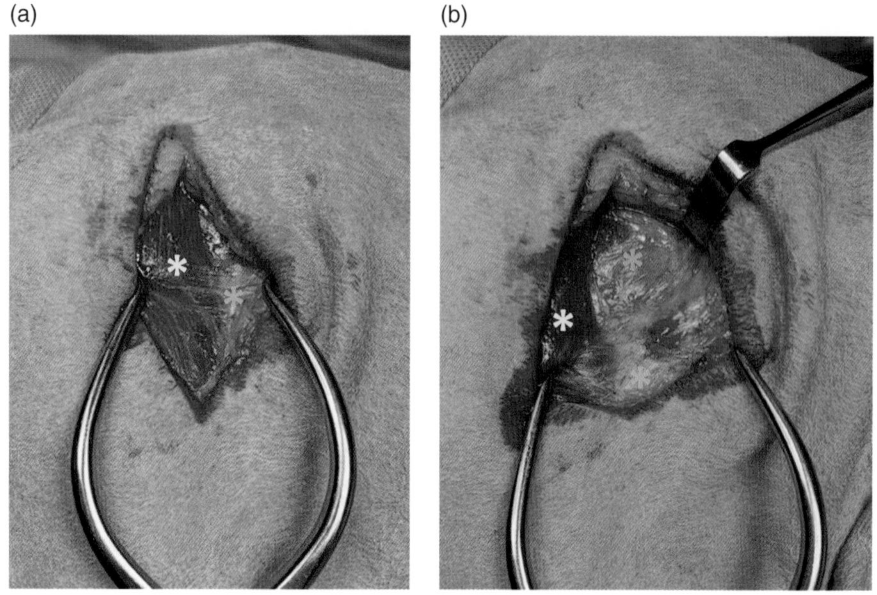

Figure 46.4 Craniolateral approach to the right hip of a canine patient: *incising the fascia lata*. Cranial is to the right in each image. (a) Incision is made through the skin and subcutaneous layers, and Gelpi retractors are placed to visualize the proper position of the next structures to separate: the biceps femoris (yellow *) and superficial leaf of the fascia lata (blue *). (b) After the superficial leaf of the fascia lata is incised, Gelpi retractors may be placed deeper into the surgical site to further retract the biceps femoris caudally and allow visualization of the deep leaf of the fascia lata and underlying tensor fascia latae (lime green *). Alternatively, to avoid inadvertent trauma to the sciatic nerve, a sterile assistant may retract the biceps femoris with Army-Navy retractors. *Source:* © Kristin Coleman.

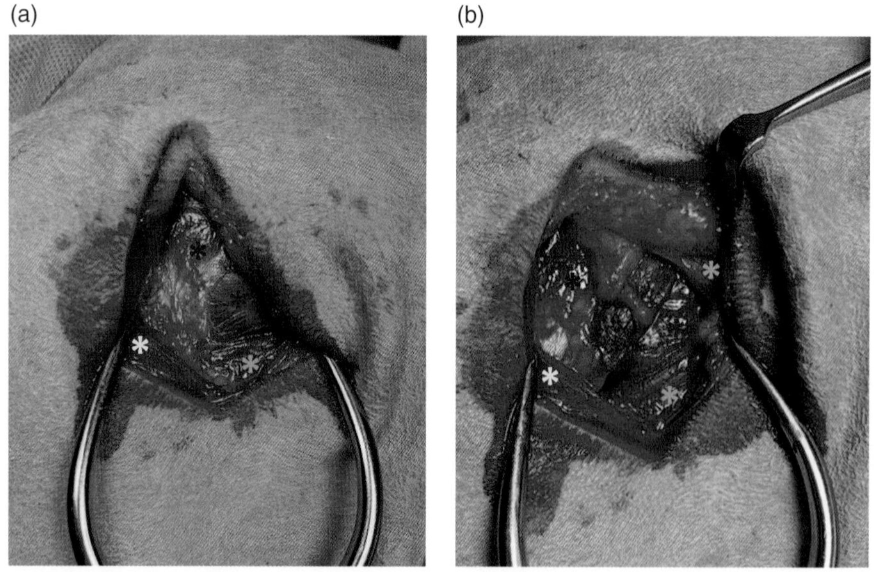

Figure 46.5 Craniolateral approach to the right hip of a canine patient: *dissection*. Cranial is to the right in each image. (a) After incising through both leaves of the fascia lata to separate the TFL (lime green *) from the biceps femoris (yellow *), the superficial gluteal muscle (violet *) is visualized. (b) Dissection is performed at the cranial aspect of the superficial gluteal muscle to separate it from the cranioventrally-located TFL and retract it caudodorsally to expose the underlying middle gluteal muscle (dark blue *). *Source:* © Kristin Coleman.

trochanter (Figure 46.6). In larger patients, an Army-Navy retractor may provide better visualization of this landmark. The deep gluteal tendon may be partially transected (~50% from the ventral aspect in the transverse direction) to aid in the exposure of the coxofemoral joint, but the author does not always find this necessary for adequate exposure of the femoral head and neck. If a tenotomy is performed, a stay suture should be placed onto the tendon for later re-apposition to the remaining tendon fibers onto the greater trochanter. Directly beneath the deep gluteal

(a) (b)

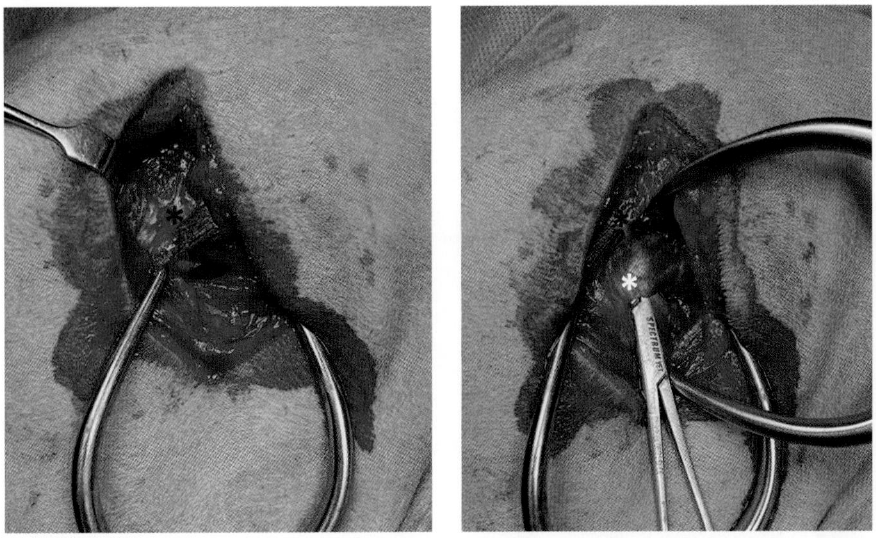

Figure 46.6 Craniolateral approach to the right hip of a canine patient: *the gluteal muscles*. Cranial is to the right in each image. (a) Gelpi retractors are re-positioned to retract the TFL cranially and the superficial gluteal muscle (violet *) caudally, and a Senn retractor is retracting the biceps femoris muscle caudally. (b) A second pair of Gelpi retractors is placed perpendicular to the first pair to retract the middle gluteal muscle dorsally (dark blue *) and allow exposure of the deep gluteal muscle tendon (white *), under which a curved mosquito hemostat is placed. A partial deep gluteal tenotomy may be performed at this point; if this is performed, the recommendation is to place a stay suture on the cranial side of the tendon to allow easy identification at the time of closure. *Source:* © Kristin Coleman.

tendon is the coxofemoral joint capsule, which may or may not be intact depending on the underlying reason for performing the FHO (e.g., chronic craniodorsal hip luxation may not have an appreciable joint capsule remaining on the dorsolateral aspect). If it is intact, an incision should be made through the capsule along the dorsal acetabular rim with a blade (#10, 11, or 15), then the round ligament (i.e., ligament of the head of the femur) should be transected (if intact) with a Hat spoon, round ligament cutter, or curved Mayo scissors. This step is most readily achieved with external rotation and adduction of the femur.

*Note: Cats, unlike dogs, have a muscle covering the lateral aspect of the coxofemoral joint capsule at this level called the *articularis coxae*. This must be transected in the cat to access the joint.[18]

As the femur is rotated, the lesser trochanter should be palpable as it moves from a medial to a cranial location with external rotation. This is important, as the lesser trochanter is the distal landmark for the osteotomy. In the cases when a lesser trochanter is not readily palpable, it can be identified by the hip flexor muscle (i.e., the iliopsoas), which becomes taut in hip extension or external rotation.

In preparation for the femoral neck osteotomy, the femoral head is ideally luxated from the acetabulum and held in a more superficial location with Hohmann retractors on the cranial and caudal aspects. To improve the reproducibility of orientation, the hindlimb is externally rotated until the patella is facing directly upwards. Soft tissues (notably, the origin of the vastus lateralis muscle) should be elevated and pushed distally from the femoral neck. Gelpi retractors should be introduced in the surgical site to improve exposure at 90° angles to each other (Figure 46.7a). Once the femoral neck is exposed, a line (created with either electrosurgery or a blade) is drawn or etched on the femoral neck for the proposed cut, which extends proximally (between the femoral head and greater trochanter) in either a straight line or slightly concave line to end immediately proximal to the lesser trochanter (Figure 46.7b). The author recommends having a radiograph of the patient's pelvis in the operating room prior to completing the ostectomy. Observation of a craniocaudal radiograph of the pelvis, in which the patellae are ideally facing cranially, allows the surgeon to more accurately gauge the location of the osteotomy in the space between the femoral head and greater trochanter to completely remove the femoral neck. This is accomplished with an osteotomy that ends proximally just medial to the medial border of the greater trochanter and ends distally just proximal to the lesser trochanter. As mentioned previously, the femur should be externally rotated by grasping the distal femur (do not grasp the crus to rotate, which could strain ligaments of the stifle) to the point of the patella "facing the ceiling," which allows the osteotomy to be a bit farther from the sciatic nerve than if it was left in a neutral position.

The osteotomy may be performed in a variety of ways with osteotome or sagittal saw being described.[25] If an

(a) (b)

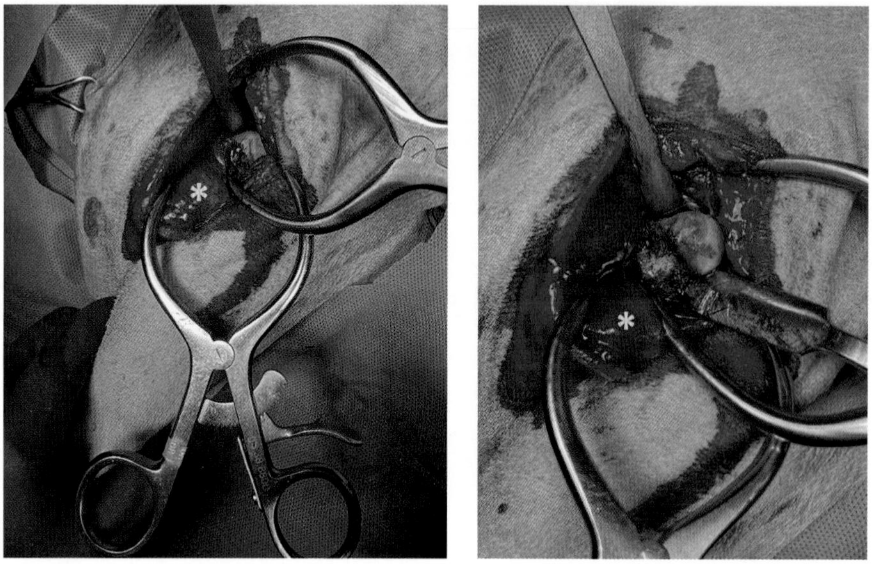

Figure 46.7 Craniolateral approach to the right hip of a canine patient: *isolating the femoral head and neck.* Cranial is to the right in each image. (a) Following either partial deep gluteal tenotomy or retracting it dorsally, the coxofemoral joint capsule is incised, the round ligament is transected (if still intact), and the femoral head is luxated to allow for improved visualization. Dissection may commence on the femoral neck to elevate the vastus lateralis muscle (light gray *) and retract it distally to the point of the less trochanter and caudally to the point of the greater trochanter. To aid in ideal positioning, the femur should be externally rotated by an assistant holding the distal femur to result in the patella "facing the ceiling." (b) Retractors are placed to keep soft tissues away from the sagittal saw blade or osteotome's path to prevent iatrogenic damage. The author prefers to use perpendicular Gelpi retractors and a Hohmann retractor at each side of the bone near the osteotomy "entrance" and "exit." Care should be taken when placing the caudal/dorsal Hohmann retractor and ensure that it is directly between the deep gluteal muscle and femoral neck to avoid sciatic nerve impingement. Finally, after palpating the lesser trochanter and ensuring adequate dissection, monopolar electrosurgery is used on the bone to mark the trajectory of the osteotomy prior to cutting. *Source:* © Kristin Coleman.

osteotome is chosen, it should be perpendicular to the bone (if correctly externally rotated), and it should rest on the ridge of bone cranial to the trochanteric fossa just medial to the greater trochanter and point toward the lesser trochanter, which allows the cut to be made in a direction away from the sciatic nerve. It is preferable to err on the side of taking too small a segment of bone, as more can always be removed with either Rongeurs or a bone rasp. An osteotomy cut made with an osteotome that is directed too far distally carries the risks of inadvertent removal of the lesser trochanter or fracture of the femur. The author prefers to use a sagittal saw, while an assistant lavages and suctions intermittently throughout the cut. Proper placement of the Hohmann retractors is essential during the ostectomy to protect the surrounding tissues.

After either type of ostectomy, palpate the femoral neck region for sharp edges or remnants, which may be rasped or grasped with rongeurs. The limb may then be taken through a range of motion to ensure there is no remaining femoral neck to impinge upon the pelvis. If the extension is limited or if a "click" is appreciated, that may mean that bone-on-bone impingement from a remnant of the femoral neck is occurring. After lavage and instilling local anesthetic into the surrounding tissues, closure may commence. If there is a joint capsule remaining to close, 1 or 2 cruciate mattress ligatures of a long-term absorbable monofilament suture may be placed; if there is no appreciable capsule, skip this step. If a deep gluteal tenotomy was performed, re-appose the tendon with a long-term absorbable monofilament suture in a proper tendon apposition pattern (e.g., cruciate mattress, locking loop, 3-loop pulley). After the deep and superficial leaves of the tensor fascia are apposed with long-term absorbable monofilament suture in a simple continuous pattern, the subcutaneous and skin layers are closed routinely.

Following surgery, POST-OPERATIVE RADIOGRAPHS MUST BE TAKEN. This should always be performed both to assess the completion and success of the FHO, as well as to establish, from a legal perspective, that the procedure has been appropriately performed. If there is a femoral neck remaining on the postoperative craniocaudal view, the patient should be taken back to surgery to remove more of the femoral neck, since this has the potential to cause discomfort due to impingement with the acetabulum.

Ventral Approach

The patient is positioned in dorsal recumbency with the limbs abducted to allow access to the femoral triangle of the affected side or sides (Figure 46.8).[18] The entire limb and caudoventral abdomen should be clipped, prepped, and draped in the surgery field, which allows for manipulation of the limb during surgery and would allow for conversion to the craniolateral approach if needed. The paw should be wrapped as described for the craniolateral approach. To start the procedure, the lateral aspect of the limb should be relatively flat on the table.

The femoral arterial pulse and adjacent pectineus muscle (which lies just caudal to the femoral artery and vein and saphenous nerve) are palpated, and a skin incision is made centered over the origin of the pectineus muscle and is made parallel to the femur (Figure 46.9). Resist the urge to incise too distally on the limb, since the origin of the pectineus muscle should be the midway point of the incision. Careful blunt dissection with right angle forceps is then carried out to isolate the origin of the pectineus muscle along the cranial, caudal, and lateral (deep) aspects, which is then transected at the musculotendinous junction on the iliopubic eminence with either a #15 blade or monopolar electrosurgery (Figure 46.10). If transected at this junction and not in the center of the muscle, hemorrhage will be minimal. The joint capsule is easily visualized once the pectineus muscle is released, and Gelpi retractors may be carefully placed to avoid the surrounding vasculature.

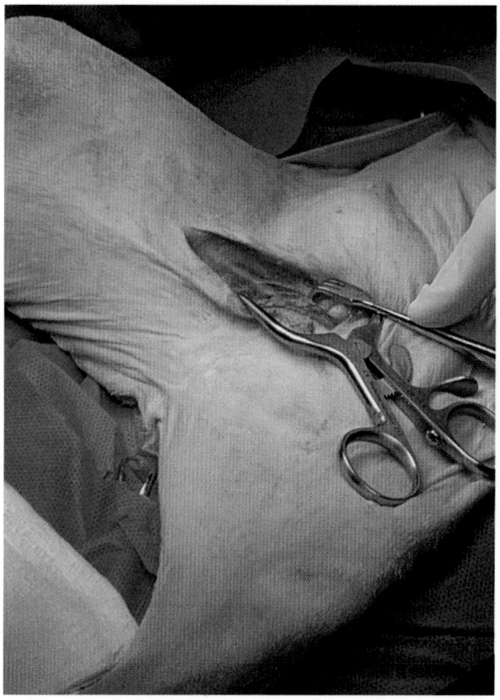

Figure 46.9 Ventral approach to the right hip of a feline patient: *initial incision*. Cranial is to the right. Using the palpable pulse of the femoral artery, the taut pectineus muscle is identified just caudally. An incision is then made directly over or immediately cranial to this muscle belly. The origin of the pectineus muscle on the iliopubic eminence is the center of the incision, which should extend from the inguinal region to distally, parallel to the femoral shaft. After incising through skin and subcutaneous layers, Gelpi retractors are placed, and blunt Senn retractors may be used to hold back the inguinal fat from the surgical site. *Source:* © Kristin Coleman.

(a)

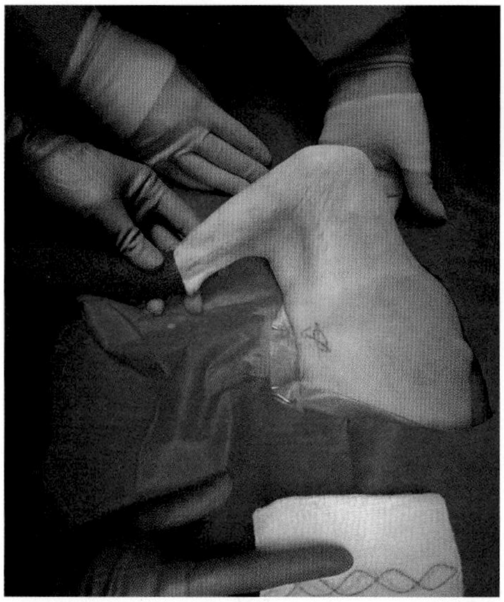

(b)

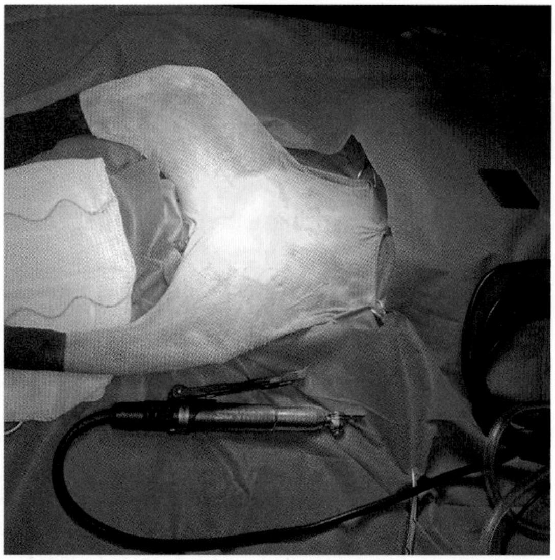

Figure 46.8 Ventral approach to the hip(s) of feline patients: *positioning*. Cranial is to the right in each image. Both patients are in dorsal recumbency. (a) With surgeon standing at the caudal aspect of the patient, the assistant stands on the lateral aspect, which allows for retraction of the tissues and manipulating the angle of the femur. The instrument table is draped separately from the patient. (b) If single-stage bilateral vFHO is being performed, both hindlimbs may be draped in at the same time as shown. These limbs are draped proximally enough to allow for conversion to a craniolateral approach if needed. *Source:* © Kristin Coleman.

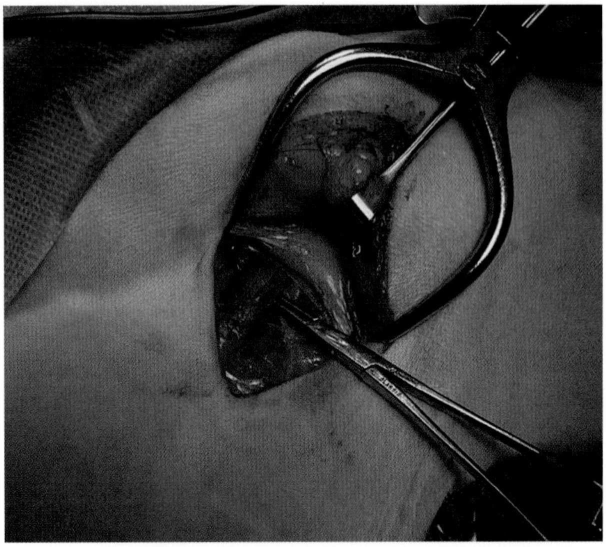

Figure 46.10 Ventral approach to the right hip of a feline patient: *dissection and isolation of pectineus muscle.* Cranial is to the left and up in the image. Right angle forceps are used to dissect parallel to the pectineus muscle on the cranial and caudal aspects until the forceps may be passed completely around the lateral (deep) aspect of the muscle. At this point, the origin of the muscle is transected along the iliopubic eminence. *Source:* © Kristin Coleman.

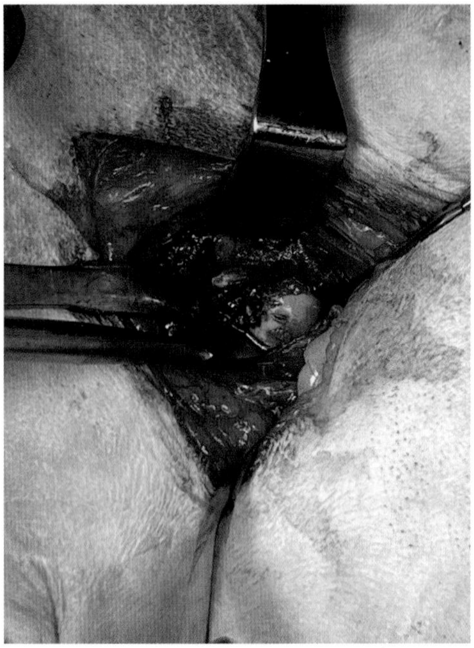

Figure 46.11 Ventral approach to the right hip of a feline patient: *dissection and isolation of femoral neck.* Cranial is to the top, the inguinal/medial region is to the right, and the remainder of the right hindlimb is mostly to the left of the image. The joint capsule has been incised over this caudoventrally luxated femoral head, and while the osteotomy may be easier with the hip reduced, it is typically easier to perform dissection with the femoral head and neck elevated superficially within the surgical site (i.e., transect the round ligament and luxate medially). In this image, two elevators are being used to elevate the femoral head out of the acetabulum, a Hohmann retractor is protecting the soft tissues caudal to the femoral neck, and an Army-Navy retractor is retracting the iliopsoas muscle distally to allow placement of the osteotome or sagittal saw blade just proximal to the lesser trochanter. *Source:* © Kristin Coleman.

After transecting the pectineus muscle from the origin and reflecting distally, the medial circumflex femoral artery and vein, which are branches of the cranially-located femoral artery and vein, will be seen coursing transversely in a cranial to caudal direction over the femoral neck region. These vessels should be elevated and retracted proximally during further dissection. The next structure to note is the iliopsoas muscle, which is palpated on its lesser trochanter insertion during the ventral approach; note that it is not seen in the craniolateral approach. Visualizing this muscle will help in identifying the lesser trochanter, which is important for making the proper osteotomy.

The joint capsule is then sharply incised using a scalpel blade or electrosurgery pen to reveal the femoral head. The author prefers not to luxate the hip out of the acetabulum at this point but leaves it in situ to help with stabilization during the osteotomy. Time and care should be taken to ensure sufficient joint capsule has been removed from the femoral neck to allow accurate removal of both the femoral head and neck. The best exposure of the neck of the femur can be developed by placing Hohmann retractors cranial and caudal to the femoral neck (Figure 46.11).

The author recommends having a bone model of a pelvis and femur in the operating theater for reference to help guide the correct orientation of the FHO cut, which should begin at the lesser trochanter and be directed in a way to remove all of the femoral head and neck. The surgeon MUST have an assistant to support and hold the affected hind leg in proper orientation during the execution of the FHO cut from either approach. This assistant is positioned on the lateral aspect holding the Hohmann retractor and the limb, and the surgeon is positioned at the caudal aspect of the leg and table with the osteotome or sagittal saw. There are other techniques that have been described to aid the surgeon in a more accurate osteotomy angle.[19]

As the pelvic limb is typically abducted in a frog-legged position, the orientation of the cut is typically directed toward the pelvis by the assistant elevating the limb to ~40° to the osteotome or saw blade. The insertion of the iliopsoas muscle on the lesser trochanter can readily be palpated; however, the greater trochanter will not be visualized due to the limited exposure of this approach and its dorsal-lateral location. If the orientation of the FHO cut is too perpendicular to the shaft of the femur, it may risk inadvertent damage to the greater trochanter.

When performing the osteotomy, this author likes to mark the start of the osteotomy just proximal (~2 mm) to the lesser trochanter (which is easier to palpate via this approach) with an osteotome (even if a sagittal saw will eventually be the tool to make the cut), and the osteotome or saw blade should remain vertical the entire time. The angle of the osteotomy is approximately 25–45° parallel with the shaft of the femur. When performing the osteotomy, it is essential to have an assistant scrubbed into the surgery to help hold the retractors and limb to allow for accurate orientation of the cut. Soft tissues are protected on either side of the femoral neck with Hohmann and Gelpi retractors (Figure 46.12).

*Note: It is very important not to be too perpendicular to the bone with the femoral osteotomy, as inadvertent fracture of the greater trochanter may occur. Osteotomy should be carried out with either a sharp osteotome and mallet or a power-driven sagittal saw. This part of the procedure should not be rushed, such that the osteotomy is performed at the correct angle resulting in removal of the entire femoral head and neck without iatrogenic damage to the greater trochanter.

The osteotomy site should be carefully palpated following completion to confirm the appropriate configuration of the FHO osteotomy (lifting the leg can facilitate palpation of the dorsal aspect of the cut), and the hip should be taken through a range of motion to assess for any roughened edges or areas of impingement. If there are rough edges and adequate bone has been removed, rasping is sufficient for smoothing. After assessing the excised femoral head and neck, the surgeon may carefully replace the osteotome or sagittal saw with retractors still in place to excise the remaining femoral neck if not all of the intended neck was removed. Lavage is performed, hemostasis is confirmed, and closure is performed.

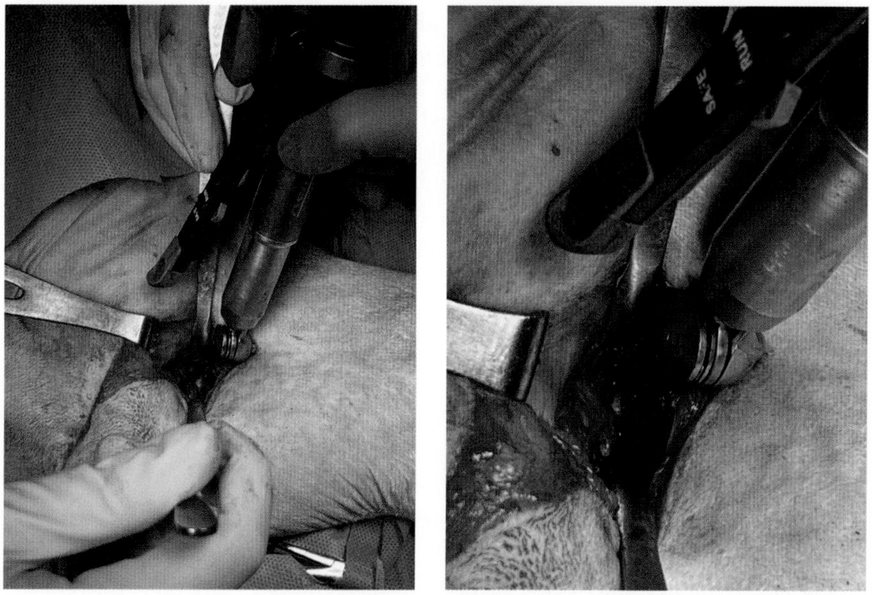

Figure 46.12 Ventral approach to the left hip of a feline patient: *femoral neck osteotomy*. Cranial is to the top of the image. Hohmann retractors are placed on either side of the femoral neck, and Army-Navy retractors are used to keep the inguinal fat out of the way for visualizing the femoral head and neck. Even if using a sagittal saw to perform the osteotomy, it is helpful to at least score the cortical bone just proximal to the lesser trochanter with an osteotome initially to prevent the saw blade from slipping. *Source:* © Kristin Coleman.

While reapposition of the pectineus has been described elsewhere, the author does not recommend this step during closure due to perceived associated tension and postoperative discomfort. Subcutaneous tissue (3-0 or 4-0 short-term absorbable monofilament suture in a simple continuous pattern) and skin are closed routinely (Figure 46.13).

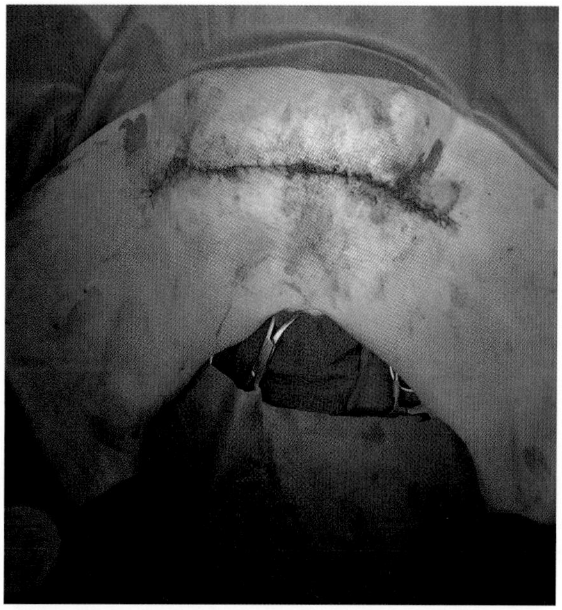

Figure 46.13 Ventral approach to the bilateral hips of a feline patient: *closure following bilateral single-stage FHOs*. Cranial is to the top of the image. After lavaging the surgical site, closure is routine with apposition of the (optional) deep subcutaneous layer (3-0 or 4-0 short-term absorbable monofilament suture in a buried simple interrupted pattern), superficial subcutaneous layer (3-0 or 4-0 short-term absorbable monofilament suture in a simple continuous pattern), and skin (4-0 non-absorbable monofilament suture in a simple continuous pattern [in this image]). *Source:* © Kristin Coleman.

Before the patient is recovered from anesthesia, postoperative hip-extended craniocaudal pelvic radiographs should be performed to confirm the appropriate orientation and completeness of the ostectomy.

Leaving too much of the femoral neck can be a technical pitfall of limb and saw positioning intra-operatively and should be corrected when found on palpation or on the postoperative radiographs while the patient is still anesthetized.

Potential Complications

An intra-operative complication commonly encountered by those performing an FHO for the first few times is that their initial craniolateral approach is not over the aponeurosis between the tensor fascia lata and the biceps femoris. This may be addressed by shifting the skin incision either cranially or caudally to find this muscular division, since it is not recommended to simply start dissecting onto the femur. A major intra-operative complication is sciatic nerve transection, which may be avoided by using proper retraction (especially at the time of osteotomy) and by externally rotating the limb to point the "patella to the ceiling."

An additional commonly noted complication is incomplete removal of the femoral neck at the time of surgery, which can be seen on radiographs taken while the patient is still anesthetized.[20] Inadequate removal of the femoral neck may cause pain and limb dysfunction due to continued bone-on-bone contact between the remaining femoral neck and acetabular rim, sciatic nerve damage, or sciatic nerve entrapment.[2,5,21,22] This frustrating complication may be avoided by utilizing a bone rasp after the ostectomy in surgery, by ensuring that the cut goes from the medial aspect of the greater trochanter to the lesser trochanter, by removing more femoral neck if a "click" is palpated when taking the limb through range of motion prior to closure, and by returning to the operating room if needed to remove additional bone after postoperative radiographs are obtained. A recent cadaveric study in cats was performed to evaluate the ideal positioning of the feline femur for radiographs to most accurately evaluate the completeness of an FHO, and it was found that craniocaudal views of the femur in external rotation (30° and 45°) had the highest sensitivity, specificity, and accuracy for assessing the adequacy of the FHO in cats.[7] Performing these radiographs may improve postoperative recognition of an insufficient ostectomy.

There are technical challenges to the vFHO approach, including the relatively blind nature of the osteotomy, the limited exposure of the coxofemoral joint in comparison to the craniolateral approach, the need to retract the iliopsoas muscle, the difficulty associated with the removal of additional bone following the initial osteotomy, and the proximity of the femoral artery and vein. The recommendation for mitigating these risks is to practice the vFHO approach on one or more cadavers prior to performing it in a client-owned patient. When performing the osteotomy, the angulation of the femur being held by the assistant must be confirmed prior to cutting. It is more difficult to remove additional bone following the initial osteotomy than to ensure appropriate positioning the first time. One unique, but major, potential complication with the vFHO is accidental osteotomy of the greater trochanter (Figure 46.14). The risk of this major complication can be decreased by having a bone model in the O.R. to increase the likelihood that the trajectory of the osteotomy is accurate and by having an assistant in the O.R. to hold the limb at the appropriate angle for osteotomy.

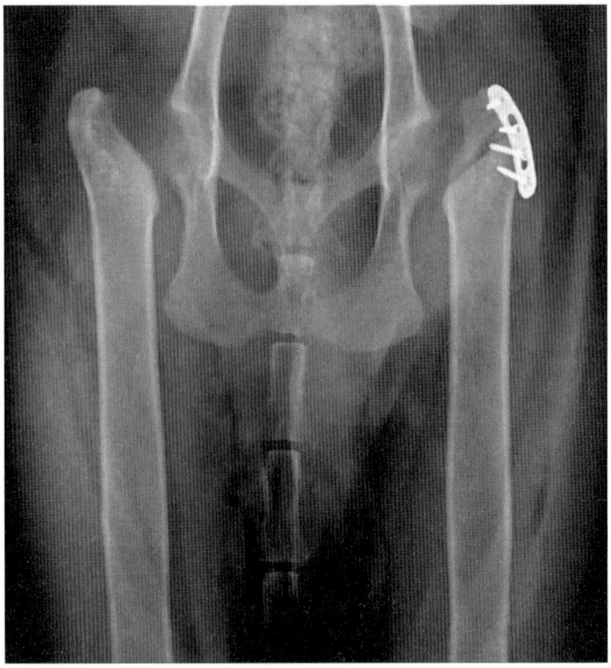

Figure 46.14 Craniocaudal radiograph of feline pelvis after bilateral vFHO. Following accidental osteotomy of the greater trochanter, a four-hole 2.4 mm LCP was applied to stabilize the fracture via a craniolateral approach to the hip.

Postoperative Care/Prognosis

Following surgery and postoperative radiographs (Figure 46.15), the patient is usually kept overnight in the hospital for a gradual transition from injectable to oral pain medications. A hard cone collar and sling are sent home with the patient the day after surgery with sedatives, usually trazodone (3–10 mg/kg PO up to every 8 hours PRN), and pain medications, typically including gabapentin (10 mg/kg PO every 8–12 hours), a NSAID (if appropriate for the patient),[23] and sometimes amantadine (1–5 mg/kg PO every 12–24 hours). While the postoperative discomfort may not warrant use of all three analgesics, encouraging

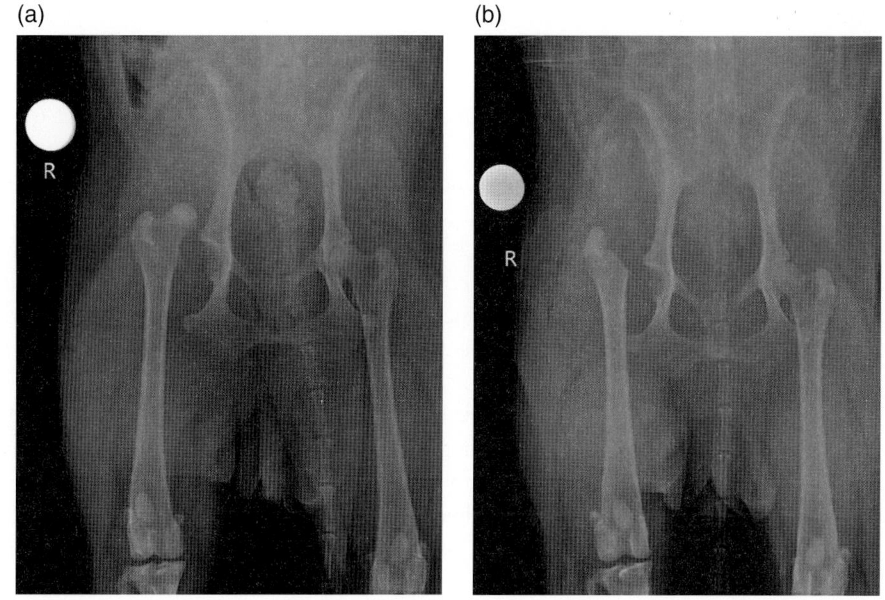

Figure 46.15 Craniocaudal pelvic radiographs of a dog after hit-by-golfcart trauma. (a) The pre-operative radiograph (along with the orthogonal lateral view) revealed craniodorsal luxation of the right hip. (b) The postoperative image revealed that the appropriate amount of femoral neck was removed via FHO. This particular patient also sustained severe muscle trauma that required months of professional physical therapy, which eventually led to a positive outcome and nearly-absent right hindlimb lameness. *Source:* © Kristin Coleman.

the patient to use the affected hindlimb is of utmost importance for a successful outcome following FHO. For two weeks, the patient should be prevented from licking their incision(s) by use of the cone collar to reduce the risk of infection or dehiscence. Confinement should consist of a crate, pen, or small room with several leashed walks of 5–10 minute duration per day for the first two weeks. From weeks three to eight postoperatively, the patient should be prevented from running, jumping, and playing but should be confined only to a small room to allow more movement than typical orthopedic postoperative recoveries. Physical therapy is encouraged during this time, especially passive range of motion of the affected coxofemoral joint(s) by the owners at home.

Reported outcomes following FHO vary widely,[7,24] though in many cases an inconsistent or poor outcome is noted when comparing this salvage procedure to those that restore a normally functioning joint, such as THR.[17,22] Despite these findings, the majority of the studies investigating clinical function, gait analysis, and owner satisfaction following FHO in cats revealed a successful and good to excellent outcome, especially compared to their pre-operative status.[3,8,9,12] In a 2010 study evaluating dogs and cats a few years following their FHO procedure via physical examination and recheck radiographs, functional results were good in 38%, satisfactory in 20%, and poor in 42%, despite 96% owner satisfaction.[8] However, these outcomes may not be an accurate representation of an appropriately performed FHO, given that six out of the 15 cats in the study had incomplete resection of the femoral neck noted on their immediate postoperative radiographs.[7,8]

In a recent study,[26] 90% of owners considered the outcome of FHO surgery to be good to excellent with their dogs returning to normal physical activity postoperatively. However, when evaluated at recheck, the dogs had less muscle mass, less hip extension, and less weight-bearing on the operated limb when standing. Despite these findings, the trot gait was unaffected, and there were no differences between the limbs regarding stance or swing phase or weight-bearing during step.[26] Because many of the conditions for which an FHO is recommended could also be treated with THR, clients should be informed that a THR is not typically an option if FHO fails to deliver the desired outcome. FHO is often chosen as the more economical surgical alternative compared to THR, in addition to a reduced likelihood of major complications requiring revision surgery.

References

1 Spreull, J. (1961). Excision arthroplasty as a method of treatment of hip joint diseases in the dog. *Vet. Rec.* 73: 573–576.

2 Harper, T.A.M. (2017). Femoral head and neck excision. *Vet. Clin. North Am. Small Anim. Pract.* 47 (4): 885–897.

3 Yap, F.W., Dunn, A.L., Garcia-Fernandez, P.M. et al. (2015). Femoral head and neck excision in cats: medium- to long-term functional outcome in 18 cats. *J. Feline Med. Surg.* 17 (08): 704–710.

4 Johnson, K.A. (2010). Outcome of femoral head ostectomy in dogs and cats. *Vet. Comp. Orthop. Traumatol.* 23 (5): III–IV.

5 Harasen, G. (2004). The femoral head and neck ostectomy. *Can. Vet. J.* 45 (2): 163–164.

6 Lippincott, C.L. (1992). Femoral head and neck excision in the management of canine hip dysplasia. *Vet. Clin. North Am. Small Anim. Pract.* 22 (3): 721–737.

7 Howser, A.L., Vinayak, A., Ward, M.P. et al. (2020). Effects of femur position on radiographic assessment of femoral head and neck excision completeness in cats. *Vet. Comp. Orthop. Traumatol.* 33: 130–136.

8 Off, W. and Matis, U. (2010). Excision arthroplasty of the hip joint in dogs and cats. Clinical, radiographic, and gait analysis findings from the Department of Surgery, Veterinary Faculty of the Ludwig-Maximilians-University of Munich, Germany. 1997. *Vet. Comp. Orthop. Traumatol.* 23 (5): 297–305.

9 Berzon, J.L., Covell, S.J., Trotter, E.J. et al. (1980). A retrospective study of the efficacy of femoral head and neck excisions in 94 dogs and cats. *Vet. Surg.* 9: 88–92.

10 Basher, A.W.P., Walter, M.C., and Newton, C.D. (1986). Coxofemoral luxation in the dog and cat. *Vet. Surg.* 15 (5): 356–362.

11 Daly, W. (1978). Femoral head and neck fractures in the dog and cat: a review of 115 cases. *Vet. Surg.* 7 (2): 29–38.

12 Queen, J., Bennett, D., Carmichael, S. et al. (1998). Femoral neck metaphyseal osteopathy in the cat. *Vet. Rec.* 142 (7): 159–162.

13 Perry, K. (2016). Feline hip dysplasia: a challenge to recognise and treat. *J. Feline Med. Surg.* 18 (3): 203–218.

14 Keller, G.G., Reed, A.L., Lattimer, J.C. et al. (1999). Hip dysplasia: a feline population study. *Vet. Radiol. Ultrasound* 40 (5): 460–464.

15 DeAngelis, M. and Hohn, R.B. (1968). The ventral approach to excision arthroplasty of the femoral head. *J. Am. Vet. Med. Assoc.* 152 (2): 135–138.

16 Winders, C.L.B., Vaughn, W.L., Birdwhistell, K.E. et al. (2018). Accuracy of femoral head and neck excision via a craniolateral approach or a ventral approach. *Vet. Comp. Orthop. Traumatol.* 31 (2): 102–107.

17 Liska, W.D., Doyle, N., Marcellin-Little, D.J. et al. (2009). Total hip replacement in three cats: surgical technique, short-term outcome and comparison to femoral head ostectomy. *Vet. Comp. Orthop. Traumatol.* 22 (6): 505–510.

18 Johnson, K.A. (2014). *Piermattei's Atlas of Surgical Approaches to the Bones and Joints of the Dog and Cat*, 5e. Philadelphia, PA: Saunders.

19 O'Donnell, M.D., Warnock, J.J., Bobe, G. et al. (2015). Use of computed tomography to compare two femoral head and neck excision ostectomy techniques as performed by two novice veterinarians. *Vet. Comp. Orthop. Traumatol.* 28 (5): 295–300.

20 Sapora, J.A., Palmer, R.H., and Goh, C.S.S. (2021). Ventral femoral head and neck ostectomy: standard versus novel K-wire guided technique using a premeasured ostectomy angle in canine cadavers. *Vet. Surg.* 50 (6): 1201–1208.

21 Vinayak, A., Kerwin, S.C., Ward, M.P. et al. (2006). Effects of femur position on radiographic assessment of completeness of femoral head and neck excision in medium- to largebreed dogs. *Am. J. Vet. Res.* 67 (1): 64–69.

22 Fitzpatrick, N., Pratola, L., Yeadon, R. et al. (2012). Total hip replacement after failed femoral head and neck excision in two dogs and two cats. *Vet. Surg.* 41 (1): 136–142.

23 Liska, W.D., Doyle, N.D., and Schwartz, Z. (2010). Successful revision of a femoral head ostectomy (complicated by postoperative sciatic neurapraxia) to a total hip replacement in a cat. *Vet. Comp. Orthop. Traumatol.* 23 (2): 119–123.

24 Grisneaux, E., Dupuis, J., Pibarot, P. et al. (2003). Effects of postoperative administration of ketoprofen or carprofen on short- and long-term results of femoral head and neck excision in dogs. *J. Am. Vet. Med. Assoc.* 223 (7): 1006–1012.

25 Penwick, R.C. (1992). The variables that influence the success of femoral head and neck excision in dogs. *Vet. Med.* 87 (4): 325–333.

26 Engstig, M., Vesterinen, S., Morelius, M. et al. (2022). Effect of femoral head and neck osteotomy on canines' functional pelvic position and locomotion. *Animals* 12 (13): 1631.

47

Lumbosacral Steroid Epidural

Rebecca S. Salazar

Gulf Coast Veterinary Specialists, Houston, TX, USA

Key Points

- Lumbosacral (LS) steroid injections are an alternative to surgical intervention in dogs with lumbosacral disease.
- LS disease often requires advanced imaging for definitive diagnosis.
- LS disease is often very painful and can lead to end-of-life discussions.
- Surgery may not be an option for some patients; therefore, medical management is a must.
- With the appropriate training, epidurals are straightforward and can be performed with patients under heavy sedation.
- Patients often find such relief from LS injections, and they are subsequently able to live at their full potential.

Introduction

Lumbosacral (LS) degenerative disease, canine degenerative lumbosacral stenosis (DLSS), or lumbosacral stenosis, is lower back pain that can be associated with neurologic dysfunction.[1] DLSS often occurs in middle-aged to older medium- to large-breed dogs with an over-representation of German Shepherd dogs and working-type breed dogs.[1–3] There is likely a correlation between work-related stress and breed predisposition that plays a role in DLSS.[1,2]

The vertebral canal and intervertebral foramina at disk spaces L7-S1 can become narrowed due to disk degeneration, protrusion, or congenital stenosis.[1] In addition, bone and soft tissue proliferation can lead to compression of the *cauda equina*.[1] The pain associated with DLSS is attributed to direct nerve compression and/or damage to the neighboring soft tissue structures.[1] In humans, this discomfort is known as lower back pain. The direct nerve compression, whether congenital or acquired, causes significant discomfort, which is often exacerbated by certain types of movements.[1,2] Most clinical signs are consistent with lower motor neuron paresis, significant pain on tail manipulation, and owner-perceived pain.[1–3] However, other clinical signs include intermittent or persistent lameness, reluctance to jump, climb, or stand, spontaneous vocalization for no apparent reason, excessive reaction to manual manipulation and certain movements, and/or worsening lameness induced by exercise.[1–3] If not managed appropriately, DLSS can lead to severe neuropathic pain by overexpression of calcium channels, substance P, and calcitonin gene-related peptide leading to a chronic pain condition.[1,2,4–6]

Diagnosis of DLSS is based on a combination of clinical signs, imaging, and ruling out other differentials.[1] The minimal diagnosis database must include thoracolumbar radiographs to rule out bone-associated neoplasia, discospondylitis, trauma, or other vertebral anomalies.[1] Contraindications for lumbosacral steroid injections include some bleeding disorders and active skin disease or infection.[7] In addition, abnormal pelvic anatomy, from congenital or trauma, can make epidurals difficult, however, can be accomplished.[7]

Techniques in Small Animal Soft Tissue, Orthopedic, and Ophthalmic Surgery, First Edition. Edited by Kristin A. Coleman.

Companion website: www.wiley.com/go/coleman/surgeries

Regarding DLSS within the current veterinary literature, there is no consensus on definitive treatment and no evidence that surgical intervention is better than medical management.[1,2] The current conclusion in human medicine regarding the role of surgical management of humans with lower back pain due to lumbosacral disease is the same as veterinary medicine.[8,9] Options for managing DLSS include oral pain medications, weight loss, physical therapy, lumbosacral steroid injections, and surgical intervention.[10] Some dogs cannot tolerate certain classes of oral medications given daily, with the most commonly given drug class being the non-steroidal anti-inflammatories (NSAIDs). NSAIDs can have unfortunate side effects with devastating consequences.[11] Further discussion of NSAIDs and other oral pain medications is beyond the scope of this chapter. Strengthening core muscles in dogs with DLSS has been reported as an effective treatment, however, physical rehabilitation alone warrants more investigation.[1,10] In the author's experience, physical rehabilitation does play an important role in conjunction with lumbosacral steroid injections.

Lumbosacral steroid injections are minimally invasive, fairly easy to perform, and have little to no side effects. Surgical intervention may be considered if the dog does not respond favorably to the series of injections or if the injections become more frequently indicated over time.[1,12,13] A retrospective study, including a client questionnaire, found 79% of dogs had improved clinical signs and 53% had no clinical signs after a series of lumbosacral steroid injections,[13] and this conclusion was that lumbosacral steroid injections between the seventh lumbar vertebra and the sacrum are safe, effective, and should be considered prior to acute surgical intervention.[12,13]

Methylprednisolone acetate (MPA) is a particulate steroid and due to the long duration of action (half-life of 139 hours) is preferred.[14] Particulate steroids offer a longer duration of action due to the local depot effect, resulting in the continuous release of drugs over a long period of time.[14–17] Other particulate steroids include betamethasone and triamcinolone.[16] MPA should not be given intrathecally, as subarachnoid administration can cause severe meningeal inflammation; therefore, care needs to be taken to ensure the drug is given epidurally.[14] MPA dose for lumbosacral steroid epidural is 1 mg/kg, with a minimum drug volume of 0.5 mL. In addition, 0.1–0.3 mL of saline flush is needed to compensate for volume dose loss within the needle shaft and line.[13]

All steroids can have side effects, and Salmelin et al. reported polyuria, polydipsia, polyphagia, temperament changes, urinary incontinence, and diarrhea in dogs given steroid epidurals. All reported side effects resolved in a few days and required no medical intervention.[15] The author chronicles minimal side effects, and all reported side effects subsided within days of initial discovery and required no medical intervention. Human literature reports up to 33% of inadvertent systemic administration of steroid injectate, causing side effects that are highly variable.[14,16]

Lumbosacral steroid injections can be done under general anesthesia or heavy sedation, and the author prefers the latter. Whether utilizing heavy sedation or anesthesia, multiparameter monitoring should be performed, along with an intravenous catheter being placed. Other drugs can be utilized in the LS (lumbosacral) epidural space for pain management; however the author recommends veterinary anesthesia and pain management literature for LS epidural drug specifics as the specifics are beyond the compass of this chapter. Post-procedure, the author usually administers gabapentin and an NSAID (if not contraindicated) for one to three days post-injection. This is due to the pain of patient manipulation during the procedure, inflammation caused by the epidural process, and decreased overall inflammation from DLSS. It is not advised to keep dogs on long-term NSAIDs when receiving steroid epidurals due to cumulative adverse gastrointestinal side effects.[18]

Initial treatment interval protocols vary considerably from a single injection to three injections given over two-week intervals to four injections over a one-year period.[13] The author follows an initial treatment protocol extrapolated from the veterinary and human literature. The initial treatment schedule is as follows: preliminary injection (day 1), second injection 14–16 days following the day 1 injection, and third injection 40–50 days following the day 1 injection. The author has several patients who require maintenance injections every 6–12 months. The maintenance injections are administered based on the patient's response to the initial three-injection treatment, reoccurrence of clinical signs, and owner-perceived pain. Along with clinical assessment, the author utilizes a clinical questionnaire for owners to gauge the efficacy of the initial series of injections and subsequent injections that may be required.

Epidural Supplies

- Clippers
- Skin preparation solution(s)
- Lumbosacral injection needle
  - Tuohy needle or spinal needle with loss-of-resistance syringe (Figure 47.1)
  - Nerve-stimulator needle and nerve stimulator (Author preference) (Figure 47.2)
- Syringes and needles for sedation drugs
- Steroid medication and flush (Figure 47.3)
- Lidocaine for initial infiltrate (Figure 47.3)
- Sterile gloves
- +/− Fenestrated drape (Figure 47.4)

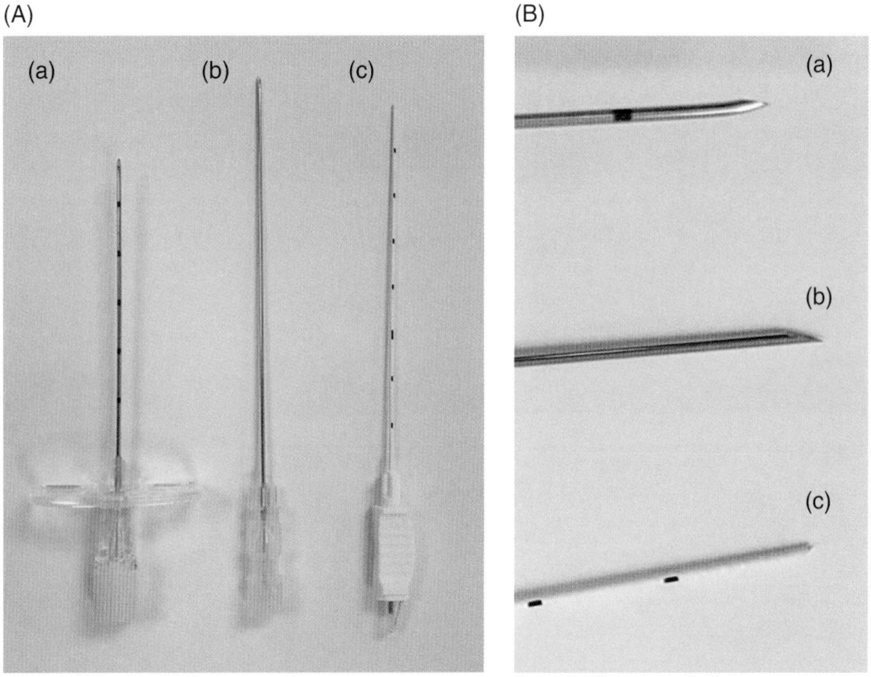

Figure 47.1 (A) Tuohy needle with wings (a), spinal needle (b), and nerve-stimulation needle (c) with the cords removed. Note the Tuohy and the spinal needle have stylets that are to be removed, and the (B) bevels of the needles are shaped differently. The different bevel shapes create a different tissue drag with each needle when advancing through tissues, thus, creating a different feeling for the user when placing the needle into the lumbosacral epidural space. *Source:* © Rebecca Salazar.

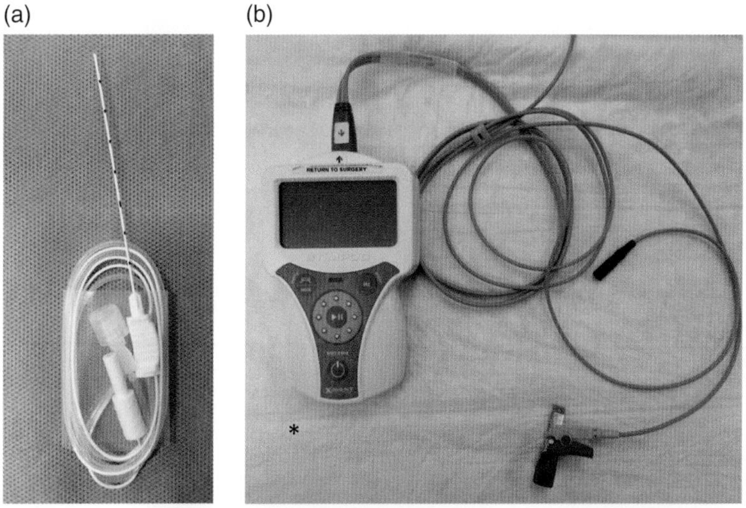

Figure 47.2 Nerve stimulator (b) and stimulating echogenic needle (a). The nerve stimulator has a clip that is to be applied to the patient's skin (*). The black male end attaches to the white female end of the needle. The drug goes through the clear line attached to the needle. The black dots along the shaft of the needle correlate with centimeters. *Source:* © Rebecca Salazar.

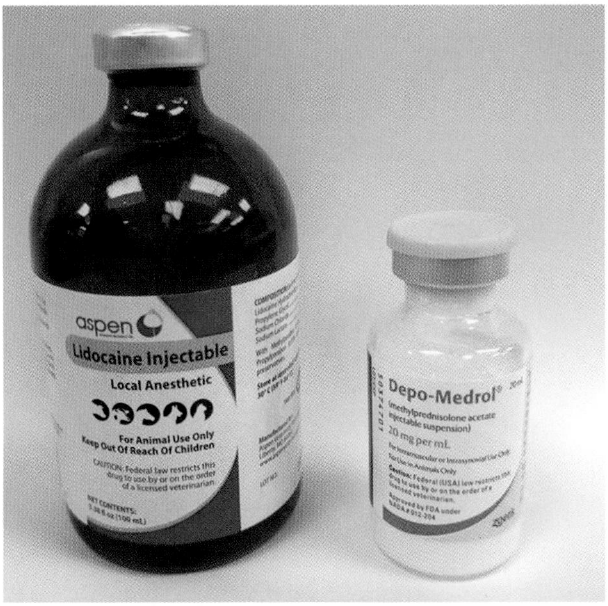

Figure 47.3 Drugs used for steroid epidural injection: lidocaine as an infiltrative block, methylprednisolone acetate (one-time use only) placed in the LS space. *Source:* © Rebecca Salazar.

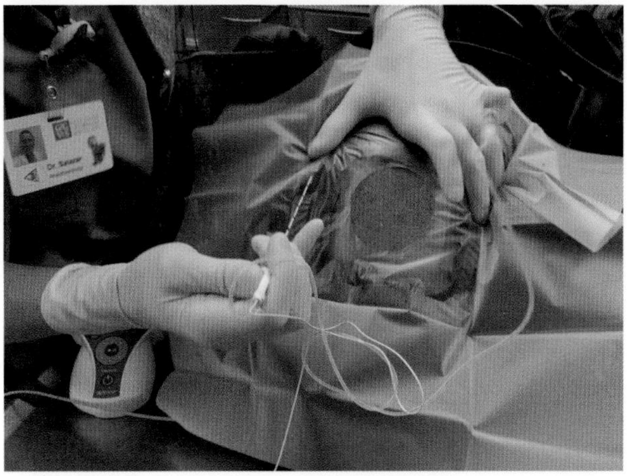

Figure 47.4 Example of procedure and fenestrated drape used in steroid epidural injections. The dominant hand is holding the nerve-stimulating needle and the non-dominant hand is palpating the anatomical structures associated with finding the LS space. *Source:* © Rebecca Salazar.

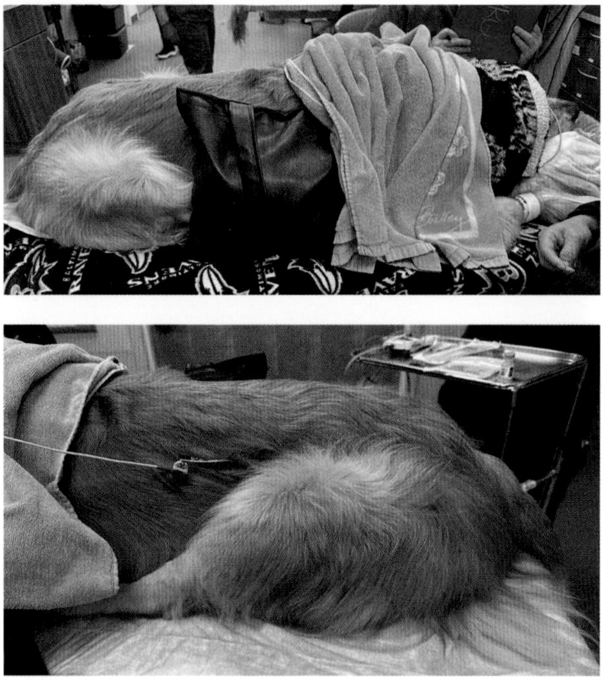

Figure 47.5 Dogs should be placed in sternal recumbency for LS steroid injection. The animal is placed sternally with the hips flexed, and legs are pulled into a cranial position. There are bean bags stabilizing the lateral aspects of the body, so the animal is not tilting too far to either side. *Source:* © Rebecca Salazar.

Procedure:

- Sedate the patient and place an intravenous catheter.
- Connect multiparameter monitoring equipment.
- Place the patient in sternal recumbency with coxofemoral joints in a completely flexed position allowing the legs to be tucked under patient. This is done to "open" the lumbosacral space (Figure 47.5).
- Locate the puncture site, which is between the spinous processes of L7 and S1 on dorsal midline (Figures 47.6 and 47.7).
- Clip hair over the injection site and perform rough preparation.
  - Deem that skin is acceptable and that there are no appreciable skin infections.
- Inject 1–2 mL of 20% lidocaine within the subcutaneous tissue layers over the injection site, taking care not to inject into the LS epidural space (Figure 47.8).
- Aseptically prepare the LS injection site.
- The needle is to be inserted perpendicular to the skin on the dorsal midline caudal to the spinous process of L7 (Figure 47.9).
- Wingless needles are to be handled with the index finger and thumb of the dominant hand. The non-dominant hand can be used to palpate the anatomical landmarks or to provide additional stabilization of the needle (Figure 47.10).
- As the needle is advanced through the skin and subcutaneous tissues, usually no resistance is felt. The needle is to be advanced through the interspinous ligament where initial resistance will be felt.
- ***There are several ways to confirm the correct epidural placement of the needle***. The author prefers electrolocation. Loss of resistance and hanging drop technique are options; however, these methods can be more challenging to ensure proper placement of the needle in the LS space. Often time radiographs or fluoroscopy are required to ensure exact needle placement in the LS location.

(a) (b)

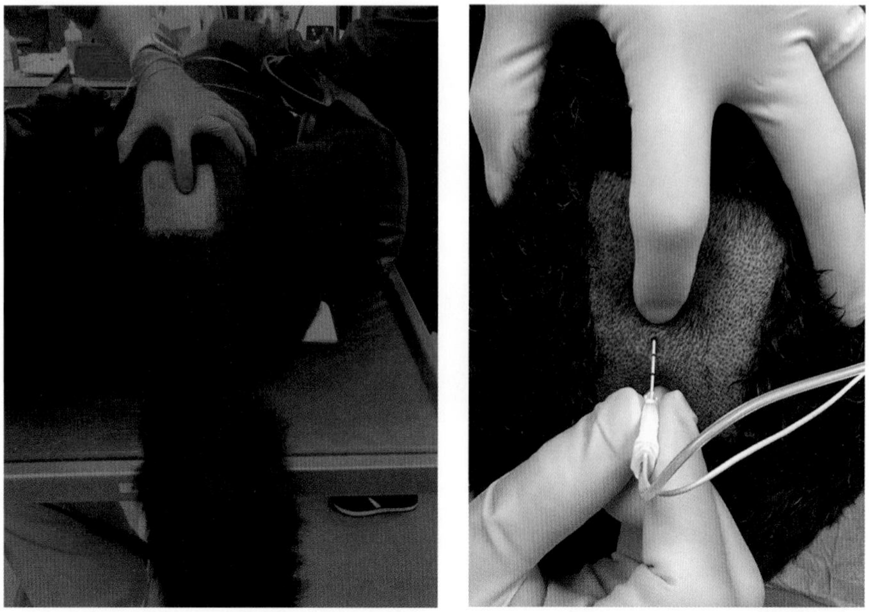

Figure 47.6 Location of needle placement for LS steroid epidural. The non-dominant hand is used to maintain contact with the correct anatomy (a). The middle finger and the thumb are placed on the iliac wings while the index finger is currently in the space between the dorsal spinous process of lumbar vertebra 7 and the most cranial aspect of the sacrum. The dominant hand is used to insert the needle perpendicular and maintain contact with the needle (b). *Source:* © Rebecca Salazar.

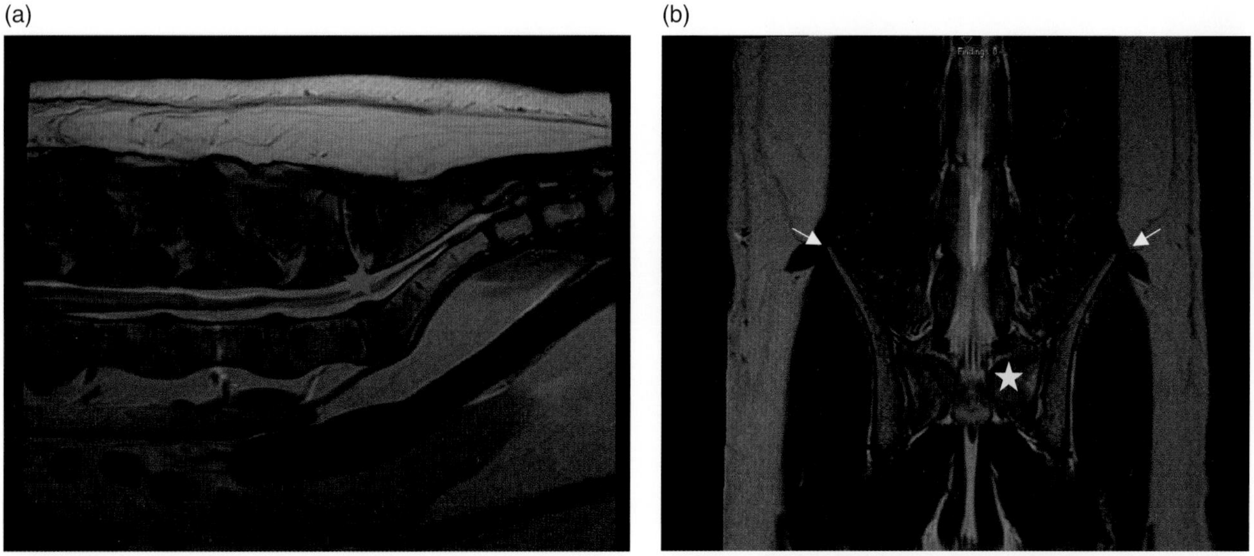

Figure 47.7 T2-weighted sagittal MRI (3T) image through the caudal lumbar region (a). The red star indicates a healthy lumbosacral spinal canal. Cranial to the red star is the lumbar vertebra seven (L7) and directly caudal is the sacrum. Below the star is the intervertebral disk between L7 and S1. The image provides a visual for needle placement and the importance of angling the needle perpendicular to the skin. The LS space is not "open" in this patient due to the coxofemoral joints in complete extension. T2-weighted dorsal MRI (3T) image through the caudal lumbar region (b). The white arrows indicate the iliac wings and adjacent to the yellow star is the *cauda equina*. *Source:* Courtesy of Dr. Cisco Guevara.

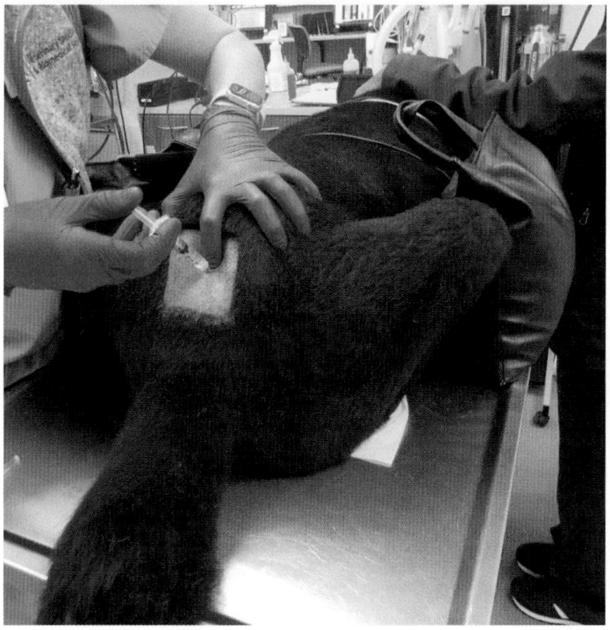

Figure 47.8 Position of lidocaine injection within the tissues surrounding the epidural space. *Source:* © Rebecca Salazar.

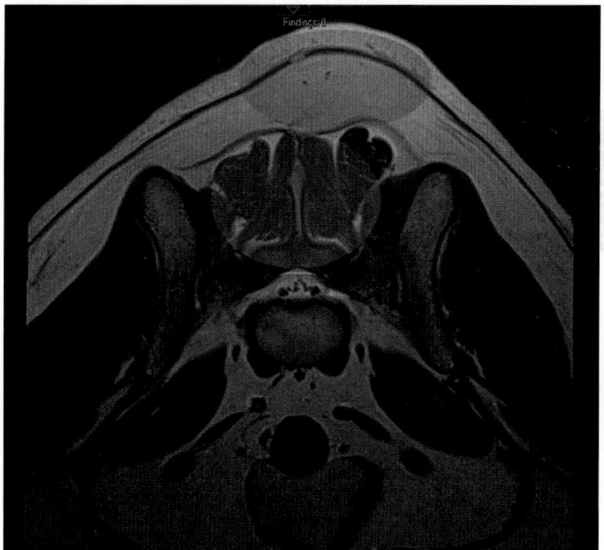

Figure 47.9 T2-weighted transverse MRI image through the lumbosacral space. Red-shaded oval correlates with the skin, fat, and subcutaneous tissues. Orange-shaded oval represents the muscles and the caudal aspect of the transverse process of L7, yellow thin line is the ligamentum flavum, green-shaded oval is the epidural space, and blue-shaded oval is the bone of the sacrum. *Source:* Courtesy of Dr. Cisco Guevara.

- **Electrolocation** (Figure 47.11)
  - Each layer of the spinal cord requires a different threshold current to elicit a motor response.[19,20] The electrical threshold to elicit limb and or tail twitches is around 0.3 mA/0.1 ms. Twitches are not usually seen until the needle has penetrated the epidural space. The nerve stimulator needs to be engaged during needle advancement prior to penetration of the epidural space.[19,20] The author does not go over 0.8 mA/0.1 ms when utilizing electrolocation. Once

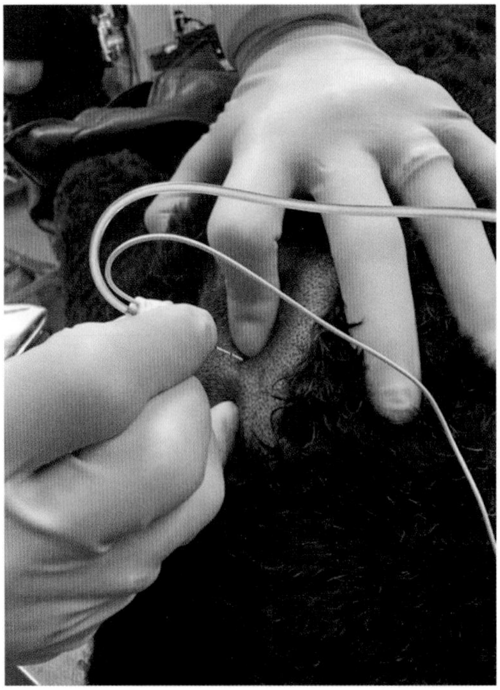

Figure 47.10 The non-dominant hand is used to palpate the anatomical landmarks, and the dominant hand is used to stabilize and place the needle into the epidural space. The pinky of the dominant hand is used to balance against the skin of the animal, while the thumb and index finger secure the shaft of the needle. *Source:* © Rebecca Salazar.

in the correct LS epidural location, the tail will twitch, indicating correct placement. The nerve stimulator can then be paused.

- **Loss of Resistance** (Figure 47.12)
  - Prior to entering the lumbosacral space, the stylet is removed from the needle, and a syringe with air or fluid is connected. Very slight pressure is applied to the syringe as the needle is advanced, until there is a sudden loss of resistance. This indicates entrance into the epidural space. If multiple attempts are made, there can be air-pocketing, thus, a false positive for LS epidural location can occur. The drug should flow smoothly without resistance and glide into the space as the syringe plunger is pushed with light pressure. If this smooth flow of the drug is not occurring, the author advises to take out the needle and start again.
- **Hanging Drop**
  - Prior to entering the lumbosacral space, the stylet is removed from the needle, and a drop of saline is placed in the hub of the needle. As the needle penetrates the epidural space, the fluid will be aspirated and pulled into the epidural space due to subatmospheric pressure within the vertebral canal.

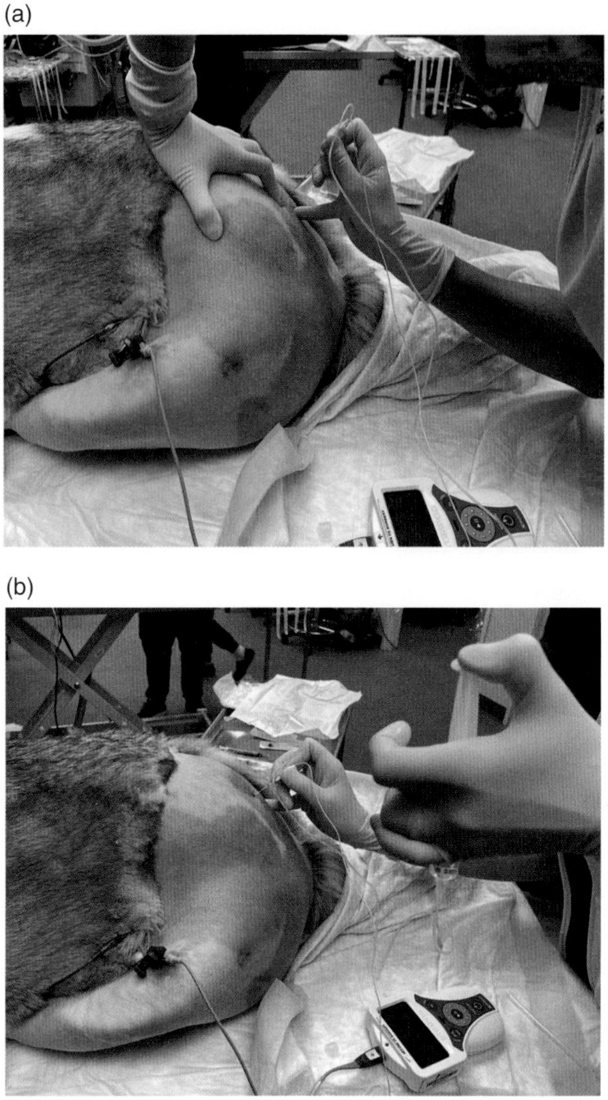

Figure 47.11 Anatomical location is felt with the non-dominant hand while the dominant hand inserts the needle into the epidural space in the top images (a). The grounding clip is attached to the shaved skin, and the needle is attached to the nerve stimulator via a cord. The dominant hand is stabilizing and holding the needle in the correct space while the non-dominant hand is pushing the drug into the epidural space in the bottom image (b). *Source:* © Rebecca Salazar.

This type of technique is useful in large-breed dogs. If the epidural space has previously been penetrated, the aspiration of fluid may be slow or not occur at all.

- If the needle comes into contact with bone, it should be withdrawn slightly and redirected. Movements need to be controlled to minimize the risk of surrounding tissue iatrogenic trauma with the needle.

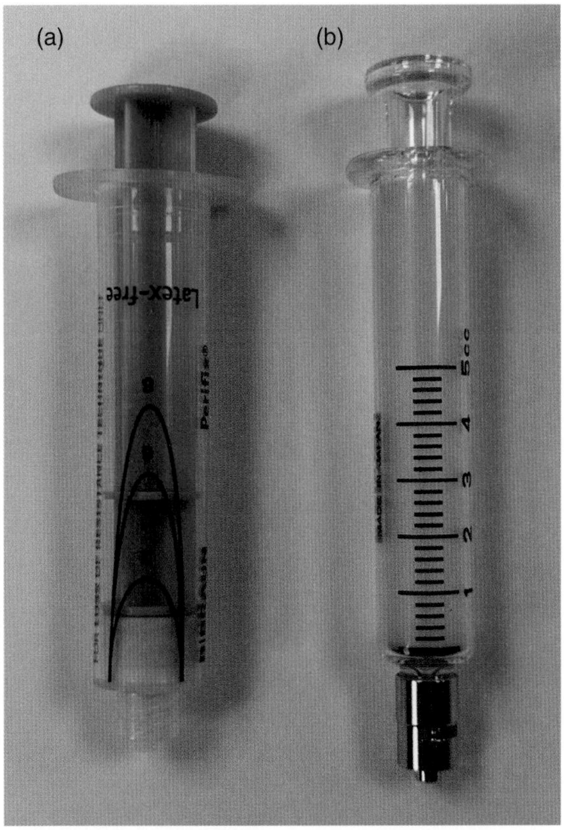

Figure 47.12 Loss of resistance (LOR) syringe plastic (a) and glass (b). The glass LOR syringe can be re-sterilized while it is not advised to re-sterilize the plastic syringe. LOR syringes are used to confirm correct needle placement in the epidural space. *Source:* © Rebecca Salazar.

- Once the epidural space is correctly identified, assess the needle hub for blood or cerebral spinal fluid. If either of the two is observed, the needle is removed, and the procedure is to start over from the beginning.
- Once it has been determined safe to inject the steroids, verbally confirm the injectate on the syringe and administer slowly over one to two minutes. There should be no resistance when administering drugs into the epidural space.
- During and after epidural injection, monitor for pain, tachycardia, hypotension, arrythmias, muscle twitches, tremors, and seizures. In the author's experience, dogs can be sore the day after the injection and can appear somewhat worse per the owners. By day three post-injection, improvement of clinical signs should be apparent and should continue to improve over the course of the injectate series.

Overall, lumbosacral corticosteroid injections can provide amelioration of clinical signs secondary to DLSS, and in most patients, they can offer a long-term recovery rate of up to 70%.[13] The procedure is efficient, cost-effective, can be done on an outpatient basis, and requires minimal supplies. Correct diagnosis is key, and adjuvant physical therapy is highly encouraged. Per the author, if the dog requires injections with increased frequency and the steroid is exhibiting a shorter duration of action via alleviation of clinical signs, surgical intervention with possible additional imaging should be discussed.

References

1 Worth, A., Meij, B., and Jeffery, N. (2019). Canine degenerative lumbosacral stenosis: prevalence, impact and management strategies [published correction appears in Vet Med (Auckl). 2020 Feb 04;11:15]. *Vet. Med.* 10: 169–183. https://doi.org/10.2147/VMRR.S180448.

2 Worth, A.J., Thompson, D.J., and Hartman, A.C. (2009). Degenerative lumbosacral stenosis in working dogs: current concepts and review. *N. Z. Vet. J.* 57 (6): 319–330. https://doi.org/10.1080/00480169.2009.64719.

3 Harcourt-Brown, T.R., Granger, N.P., Fitzpatrick, N. et al. (2019). Electrodiagnostic findings in dogs with apparently painful lumbosacral foraminal stenosis. *J. Vet. Intern. Med.* 33 (5): 2167–2174. https://doi.org/10.1111/jvim.15589.

4 Matiasek, K., Steffen, F., and Gödde, T. (2011). Entrapped L7 dorsal root ganglia show an increased expression of calcium channel subunit alpha-2-delta (poster presentation). Selected research communications of the 23rd symposium of the ESVN-ECVN Cambridge. *J. Vet. Int. Med.* 26 (1): 218–219.

5 Kobayashi, S., Kokubo, Y., Uchida, K. et al. (2005). Effect of lumbar nerve root compression on primary sensory neurons and their central branches - changes in the nociceptive neuropeptides substance P and somatostatin. *Spine* 30 (3): 276–282. https://doi.org/10.1097/01.brs.0000152377.72468.f4.

6 Kobayashi, S., Sasaki, S., Shimada, S. et al. (2005). Changes of calcitonin gene-related peptide in primary sensory neurons and their central branch after nerve root compression of the dog. *Arch. Phys. Med. Rehabil.* 86 (3): 527–533. https://doi.org/10.1016/j.apmr.2004.03.037.

7 Grubb, T. and Lobprise, H. (2020). Local and regional anaesthesia in dogs and cats: descriptions of specific local and regional techniques (part 2). *Vet. Med. Sci.* 6 (2): 218–234. https://doi.org/10.1002/vms3.218.

8 Horváth, G., Koroknai, G., Acs, B. et al. (2010). Prevalence of low back pain and lumbar spine degenerative disorders. Questionnaire survey and clinical-radiological analysis of a representative Hungarian population. *Int. Orthop.* 34 (8): 1245–1249. https://doi.org/10.1007/s00264-009-0920-0.

9 Zaina, F., Tomkins-Lane, C., Carragee, E. et al. (2016). Surgical versus non-surgical treatment for lumbar spinal stenosis. *Cochrane Database Syst. Rev.* 2016 (1): CD010264. https://doi.org/10.1002/14651858.CD010264.pub2.

10 Spinella, G., Bettella, P., Riccio, B. et al. (2022). Overview of the current literature on the most common neurological diseases in dogs with a particular focus on rehabilitation. *Vet. Sci.* 9 (8): 429. https://doi.org/10.3390/vetsci9080429.

11 Narita, T., Sato, R., Matoishi, K. et al. (2007). The interaction between orally administered non-steroidal anti-inflammatory drugs and prednisone in healthy dogs. *J. Vet. Med. Sci.* 69 (4): 353–363. https://doi.org/10.1292/jvms.69.353.

12 Gomes, S.A., Lowrie, M., and Targett, M. (2020). Single dose epidural methylprednisolone as a treatment and predictor of outcome following subsequent decompressive surgery in degenerative lumbosacral stenosis with foraminal stenosis. *Vet. J.* 257: 105451. https://doi.org/10.1016/j.tvjl.2020.105451.

13 Janssens, L., Beosier, Y., and Daems, R. (2009). Lumbosacral degenerative stenosis in the dog. The results of epidural infiltration with methylprednisolone acetate: a retrospective study. *Vet. Comp. Orthop. Traumatol.* 22 (6): 486–491. https://doi.org/10.3415/VCOT-08-07-0055.

14 Mienke, R., Van Wijck, A.J.M., Kalkman, C.J. et al. (2012). Safety assessment and pharmacokinetics of intrathecal methylprednisolone acetate in dogs. *Anesthesiology* 116: 170–181.

15 Salmelin, B., Fitzpatrick, N., Rose, J., et al. (2019). Safety profile of methylprednisolone acetate epidural injection in dogs treated for lumbosacral disease. *BSAVA Congress Proceedings*. p. 546.

16 Pountos, I., Panteli, M., Walters, G. et al. (2016). Safety of epidural corticosteroid injections. *Drugs R D* 16 (1): 19–34. https://doi.org/10.1007/s40268-015-0119-3.

17 Mehta, P., Syrop, I., Singh, J.R. et al. (2017). Systematic review of the efficacy of particulate versus nonparticulate corticosteroids in epidural injections. *PM R* 9 (5): 502–512. https://doi.org/10.1016/j.pmrj.2016.

18 Campoy, L. and Read, M.R. (2013). Chapter 14, Epidural and spinal anesthesia. In: *Loco-Regional Anesthetic Blocks for Small Animal Patients*, 227–259. Ames, IA: Wiley-Blackwell.

19 Riviere, J.E. and Papich, M.G. (2009). Chapter 30: Glucocorticoids, mineralocorticoids, and adrenolytic drugs. In: *Veterinary Pharmacology and Therapeutics*, 9e. Ames, IA: Blackwell Publishing.

20 Garcia-Pereira, F.L., Hauptman, J., Shih, A.C. et al. (2010). Evaluation of electric neurostimulation to confirm correct placement of lumbosacral epidural injections in dogs. *Am. J. Vet. Res.* 71 (2): 157–160.

48

Pelvic Fractures

Rebecca J. Webb

VetSurg, Ventura, CA, USA

Key Points

- Pelvic fractures are a common orthopedic problem in dogs that require prompt diagnosis and appropriate medical or surgical intervention for a successful outcome.
- A thorough orthopedic and neurological examination, thoracic radiographs, urinary tract evaluation, and systemic patient stabilization are necessary before considering surgical intervention.
- Luxation of the sacroiliac joint is a common concurrent injury with fractures of the pelvis and can lead to neurologic deficits, which should be identified and assessed prior to surgical intervention.
- Sacroiliac luxations can be managed either conservatively, when minimally displaced and/or chronic and stable, or surgically.
- Postoperative care, including adequate nursing care and urinary tract care, is critical for a successful outcome in these patients.

Introduction

Pelvic fractures in dogs are a common orthopedic injury that can result from trauma, such as being hit by a vehicle or falling from a height. Due to the "box-like structure" of the pelvis, for displacement of fragments to occur, there must be two, but often three, separate fractures or "disruptions to the box of the pelvis" present. The most common fracture configuration is the trio of fractures to the ilium, ischium, and pubis. Sacroiliac luxation (+/− concurrent sacral fracture) is a common concomitant injury that when present, can constitute one of these three "fractures" and allow displacement of the pelvis. Bilateral sacroiliac luxation alone can also lead to significant displacement of the pelvis without additional fractures.

Due to the level of trauma required to cause these fractures, they are often associated with significant injuries to other body systems, such as urinary tract avulsions or ruptures resulting in uroabdomen, hernias, and neurological injury. While some of these injuries are obvious at the time of presentation (such as wounds or other fractures), other injuries, such as urinary tract trauma and neurological injury, may only be apparent following thorough physical exam, patient stabilization, and diagnostic imaging. It is important that the clinician performs a detailed clinical and neurological examination prior to making a surgical plan for the patient, as these patients often present acutely following trauma and need to be systemically stabilized prior to surgical intervention for their fractures.

Indications/Pre-op Considerations

Indications

The decision of whether to treat a patient with pelvic fractures medically or surgically is based on a multitude of factors, including the location, orientation, and displacement of the fractures, degree of pelvic canal narrowing, concurrent injury to other organ systems, fractures of the forelimbs, and client/patient factors. The goals of surgical management are to restore weight-bearing, accurately reduce articular fractures, restore pelvic canal width, and

Techniques in Small Animal Soft Tissue, Orthopedic, and Ophthalmic Surgery, First Edition. Edited by Kristin A. Coleman.

Companion website: www.wiley.com/go/coleman/surgeries

improve patient comfort and early mobility. The weight-bearing segments of the pelvis include the acetabulum, ilium, sacroiliac joint, and sacrum. Typically, fractures of these areas are candidates for surgical repair. Rarely, fractures of the pubic bone may occur in combination with a ventral abdominal hernia. While these fractures may be considered for surgical repair, other fractures of the pubis and ischium are typically managed conservatively since they are not part of the weight-bearing axis when an animal ambulates.

Conservative management typically consists of strict crate restriction, nursing care, and physical therapy when the fragments have become stable enough to allow some activity. Typical candidates for this therapy include stable, minimally displaced fractures of the ilium, minimally displaced luxation of the sacroiliac joint, and most pubic or ischial fractures. Clinicians should pay particular attention to medial displacement of the fragments causing pelvic canal narrowing, as this can lead to long-term problems for the animal, such as obstipation and difficulty during parturition in intact females. It is important to recognize that following diagnosis, further shifting of the fragments may occur, especially if the client and patient are noncompliant with activity restrictions. When the conservative route is chosen, frequent follow-up with the patient is of vital importance within the first 7–10 days to monitor for this. During this time, the patient should be reassessed with radiographs, rectal examination, and complete orthopedic and neurological examination to determine if conservative management is still appropriate. If shifting has occurred leading to narrowing of the pelvic canal by 50% or more, surgery should be reconsidered. The pursuit of surgery after this window of time is of questionable benefit, as significant callus formation and muscle contraction make surgical reduction more challenging and may lead to a higher rate of iatrogenic trauma. Cases presenting after this window should be evaluated on a case-by-case basis to determine the risk versus benefit of pursuing surgical repair.

Preoperative Considerations

Patients will typically present with a severe or non-weight-bearing lameness. If there are additional injuries to the forelimbs or concurrent neurological injury, the patient may be nonambulatory.

Concurrent injuries to the urinary tract, respiratory system, body wall, skin (traumatic wounds), and neurological systems are common, and each of these systems should be thoroughly evaluated prior to surgery. In addition, baseline CBC and chemistry are recommended to evaluate the patient's systemic stability prior to surgery. Due to blood loss from the fractures and trauma, some patients may require blood products for stabilization prior to anesthesia.

Urinary Tract

Evaluation of the urinary tract is important in trauma patients. A palpable bladder at the time of presentation and a visible bladder on radiographs do not rule out injury to the urinary tract. In patients presenting with pelvic fractures, over 1/3 of these patients will have trauma to the urinary tract diagnosed, of which 16% required surgery to repair the injury. Most of these injuries are to the bladder, but a small proportion occur in the urethra or ureters.[1] Repeated evaluation for free abdominal fluid during hospitalization of these patients is important to diagnose these injuries, and if they are suspected, a positive contrast cystourethrogram or ultrasound should be performed. In patients who are nonambulatory and require extended stabilization prior to surgery, a urinary catheter is often placed. However, it is important to note that the placement of a urinary catheter will limit the clinician's ability to evaluate neurological control of the bladder until the catheter is removed.

Respiratory System

Thoracic radiographs should be performed as part of the initial diagnostic evaluation of any patient presenting with trauma. Injuries to the respiratory system are commonly diagnosed, including pulmonary contusions, diaphragmatic hernia, and rib fractures among others. When present, repair of a diaphragmatic hernia should precede surgical intervention for the fractures. Pulmonary contusions can vary in significance; while patients with mild contusions may be comfortable breathing room air, patients with significant contusions may require supplemental oxygen therapy until they improve. Respiratory stabilization of these patients should be prioritized prior to considering surgical repair, which may take around 72 hours to resolve, and repeat thoracic radiographs should be performed to re-evaluate the patient prior to considering an anesthetic event.

Neurological System

Injury to the spinal cord or the peripheral nerves (commonly, the lumbosacral trunk and sciatic nerve) can occur secondary to polytrauma. In cases with pelvic fractures, trauma to the lumbosacral trunk is most frequently seen and is commonly associated with craniomedial displacement of ilial wing fractures.[2] Luxation of the sacroiliac joint can lead to trauma to the neighboring lumbosacral trunk and sacral nerves. Trauma to these nerves can lead to deficits in innervation of the anal sphincter and urinary bladder, as well as to the sciatic nerve and all of its innervations. Of those patients with neurological deficits, approximately 80% had good functional recovery within 16 weeks following initial trauma.[2] However, the absence of deep pain to the limb, loss of perineal sensation, and absence of anal tone are concerning physical exam findings, and the severity of this injury should be conveyed to the client at diagnosis. A tip is to perform the patient's neurological exam either prior to pain medication administration or if opioids or gabapentin have been administered, wait until the effects have abated; ataxia secondary to gabapentin or sedation secondary to opioids may be confused with a neurologic deficit.

Abdominal Wall

Avulsion of the insertion of the rectus abdominus muscle on the pubis or fracture to the pubis can lead to concurrent ventral abdominal herniation of the viscera. This herniation can lead to entrapment and necrosis of the herniated viscera if not recognized early. Repair of the hernia is typically expedited and performed when the patient is stable.

Surgical Procedures

Ilial Fracture

Ilial fractures most commonly occur in the midbody of the ilium and are typically oblique (Figure 48.1). The location of the fracture may vary but typically is located immediately caudal to the sacroiliac joint. The caudal fragment typically displaces medially and cranially. This may lead to significant pelvic canal narrowing or damage to the nearby lumbosacral trunk.

General Preparation

The hind limb and hemipelvis should be clipped of fur from one inch past the dorsal midline (onto the other side of the pelvis) to the midline of the ventral abdomen. The clip should extend caudally to include the perineum on the surgical side and an inch or two cranial to the palpable wing of the ilium. Along the limb, the clip should extend to just past the tarsus, as the proximal limb will be included in the field. Placement of an anal purse string suture is recommended to help prevent contamination of the sterile field. A hanging limb prep of the clipped field should be performed, this allows the surgeon to have access to the limb for manipulation during surgery, which is helpful for reduction.

Approach

The approach for ilial fractures is primarily through a lateral incision followed by a "gluteal roll-up". During this approach, a lateral incision is made over the ilium, and the gluteal muscles are released from their origin on the ilium ventrally and cranially then retracted or "rolled up" dorsally to access the underlying ilium and cranial aspect of the acetabulum.[3] The use of multiple Gelpi (or other) retractors is recommended to adequately expose the ilium.

Reduction of the fracture can be achieved through multiple routes. Initially, manipulation of the caudal fragment with bone-holding forceps to distract it caudally and laterally from its medial position is attempted. During

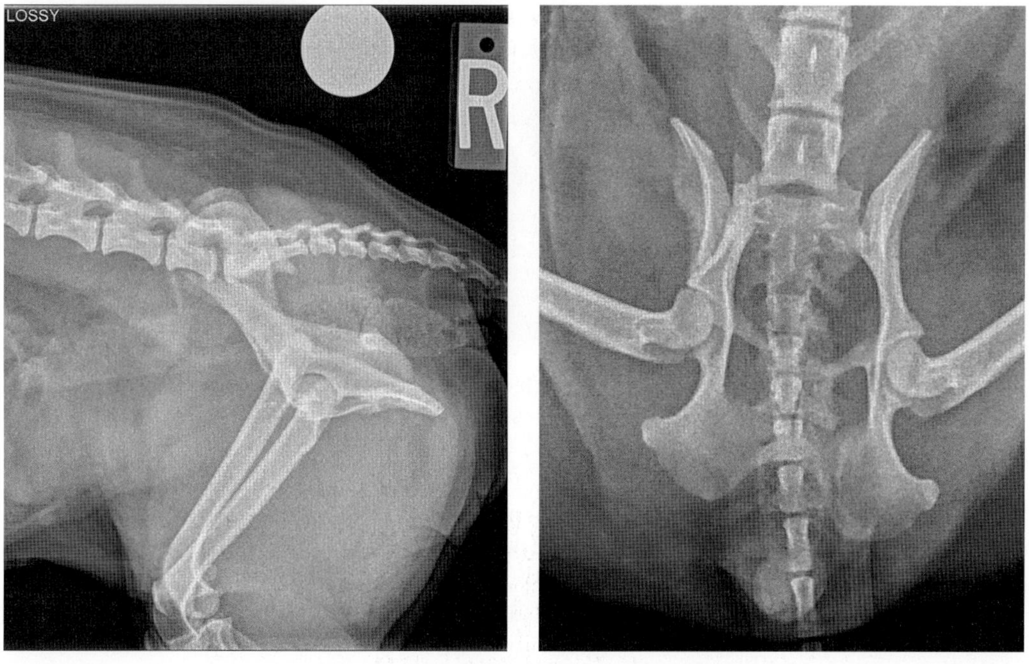

Figure 48.1 Pre-operative radiographs of a closed long oblique ventromedially displaced right ilial wing fracture in a small breed dog. *Source:* © Rebecca Webb.

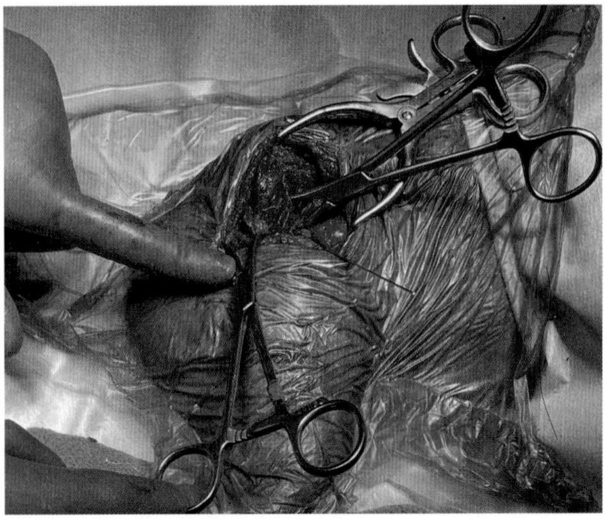

Figure 48.2 Right long oblique ilial fracture in the process of reduction. The towel clamp being held in the image is around the greater trochanter to aid in the manipulation of the fragments for reduction. The cranial clamp is placed across the long oblique fracture in this case to complete the reduction. Patient's head is to the right of the image. *Source:* © Rebecca Webb.

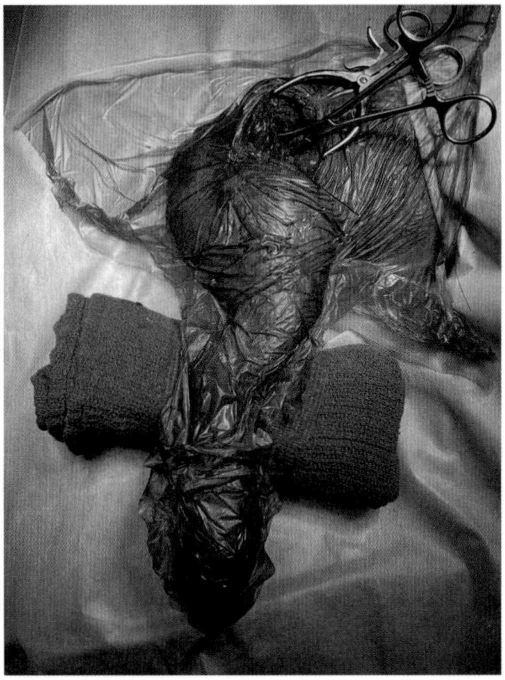

Figure 48.3 A rolled sterile towel is placed underneath the limb to prevent adduction of the limb and assist with the reduction of the long oblique right ilial fracture. Patient's head is to the right of the image. *Source:* © Rebecca Webb.

placement of the forceps and manipulation of the fragment, the surgeon should pay particular care to avoid damage to the lumbosacral trunk on the dorsal and medial aspect of the ilium. The greater trochanter can be used as a secondary point of manipulation of the fragment. The placement of a large towel clamp around the greater trochanter can give the clinician more power to distract and manipulate the caudal segment (Figure 48.2). During the reduction of the fracture, it can be helpful to place a rolled towel underneath the limb to prevent adduction of the limb toward the body, which will aid further in reduction (Figure 48.3).

These methods of manipulation are often sufficient for cats and small dogs. However, in large dogs or in patients with chronic fractures, further manipulation may be required. Manipulation of the ischium, provided it is intact, can be helpful in these cases by grasping the palpable ischiatic tuberosity. To access the area, a small approach over the palpable tuber ischii is made, and bone-holding forceps are placed around the ischium. The caudal segment can then be distracted caudally and manipulated into the desired position more easily than with the previously mentioned methods. This method should be used with care in young patients with open physes and soft bone, as damage to the physis or fracture of the bone can occur in these patients. Once the fragments are mostly reduced, pointed reduction forceps are placed across oblique fractures to complete the reduction (Figure 48.4). A tip is to use reduction forceps with a blunted tip (e.g., clamshell bone reduction forceps) in young animals or those with soft bones to reduce the risk of iatrogenic trauma. To secure the reduction, a small Kirshner wire (K-wire) can be placed across an oblique fracture to maintain the reduction (Figure 48.4). This K-wire is helpful, as it often allows the clinician to

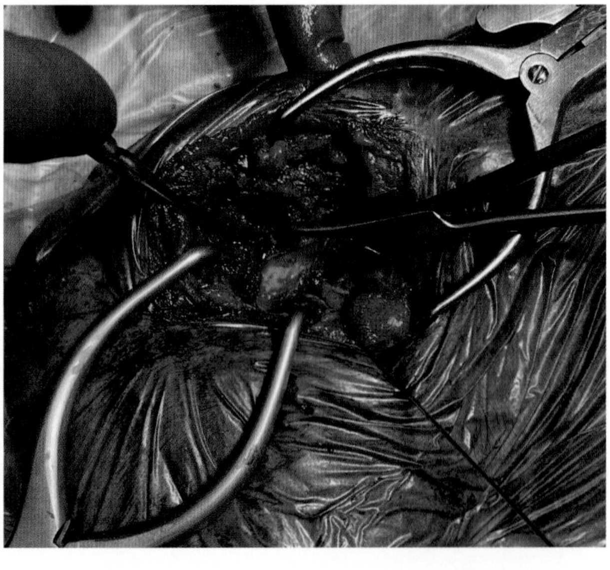

Figure 48.4 The central pointed reduction forceps are placed across a long oblique right ilial fracture, and visualization is improved with two Gelpi retractors. Following the placement of the forceps, a small Kirshner wire has been placed across the oblique fracture in a cranioventral to caudodorsal direction to maintain the reduction during the application of the implant. Patient's head is to the right of the image. *Source:* © Rebecca Webb.

remove the pointed reduction forceps and allow easier access to the bone for bone plate and screw placement. Placement of the wire can be challenging due to the narrow width of the ilial wing; it is helpful to place a finger from the clinician's nondominant hand in the region where the clinician wants the wire to exit, as this will help improve the clinician's accuracy with the placement of the K-wire. If this is done, be careful to not drill the pin into the finger positioned at the exit site.

Descriptions of using the plate to help reduce challenging ilial fractures have been described.[4] It is important to recognize that accurate contouring of the plate based on radiographs of the opposite ilial wing prior to placement is required for this technique to provide consistent results. In addition, the clinician should be aware that the ilial wing is narrow, and the purchase of the screws within the bone is only over a short segment. Due to this, the clinician should take care that only a small amount of reduction is expected from this method of utilizing the plate for reduction, as larger shifts of the ilial fragments may overpower the implant and lead to screw loosening or screw pull-out.

Implantation

Final fixation of the fracture is most commonly achieved using plates and screws (Figure 48.5). Lag screws placed across a long oblique fracture can be used either as a secondary component of stabilization in addition to a plate or as the primary fixation method. Although the use of lag screws as a primary fixation seems simple in concept, placement of these screws can be challenging. For the lag screw to function appropriately, they should be placed at a 90° angle to the fracture, but this can be a challenging angle to achieve given the large overlying muscle mass of the pelvis. In addition, the width of the ilial wing in this location is slim, which makes the placement of the screws across the wing challenging, often limiting the size of the screw that can be used, and therefore, limits the strength of the final construct. For the lag screws to be used as the primary stabilization method, a minimum of two are placed to prevent rotation of the fragments along a single screw.

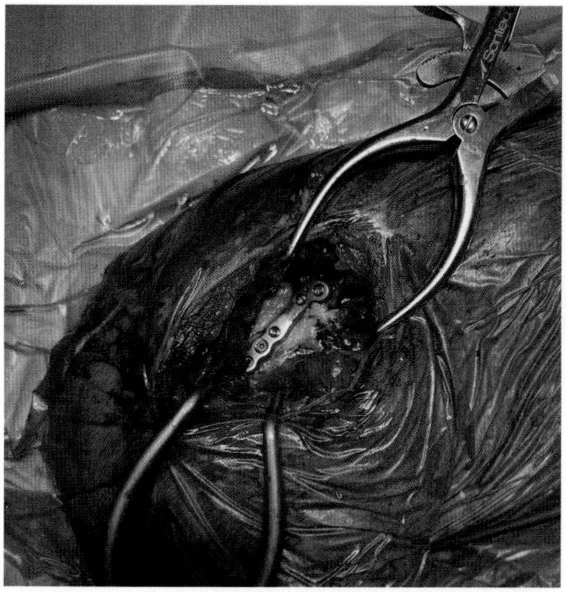

Figure 48.5 Placement of an Arthrex OrthoLine™ 2.0 mm locking T-plate across a long oblique fracture of the right ilium. Patient's head is to the right of the image. *Source:* © Rebecca Webb.

Plate placement is commonly performed on the lateral surface, however, ventral and dorsal plating have also been described.[5–7] Once the fracture is adequately reduced, an appropriately sized plate is selected. Generally, a 2.7 mm plate is selected for cats and small dogs, and 3.5 mm plates are used for large breed dogs.[8] When performing ventral or dorsal plating of the ilium, the size of the plate will typically decrease due to the thin profile of the ilium in these locations. Ideally, locking plates are recommended, as they have a significantly lower reported risk of screw loosening.[9] In cases with a short bone segment either cranially or caudally, a T-plate can be used to increase the number of screws able to be placed in the small fragment. In addition, the use of TPLO-LCP plates has been reported for the fixation of ilial fractures, as the plate has a cluster of locking screws that can be helpful with short fragments that cannot accommodate the length necessary for screw purchase of a straight plate.[10]

The bone of the ilial wing is thin and soft cranially, and screws placed in this region are typically weaker and subject to loosening. Due to this, it is recommended to place a minimum of three screws (at least two of which should be bicortical) in the cranial segment and, ideally, plan for a longer plate span in this region. In the thicker caudal ilial bone, a minimum of two bicortical screws should be placed, however, three is optimum (Figure 48.6). Once the appropriately sized implant is selected, the plate should be contoured to the ilial wing. During screw placement, the clinician should be aware of the approximate width of the ilial wing (measured on preoperative calibrated radiographs), since there is potential for the screw to be drilled directly into the vertebrae or spinal canal on the medial aspect. Although the engagement of a screw within the sacral body appears to provide good initial stability, the long-term effect on stability is unknown, and clinicians should be aware of the potential to place the implant into the spinal canal inadvertently. External fixators have been used historically for the treatment of ilial fractures but have largely fallen out of favor due to the morbidity of pin tracts through the highly muscled pelvis.

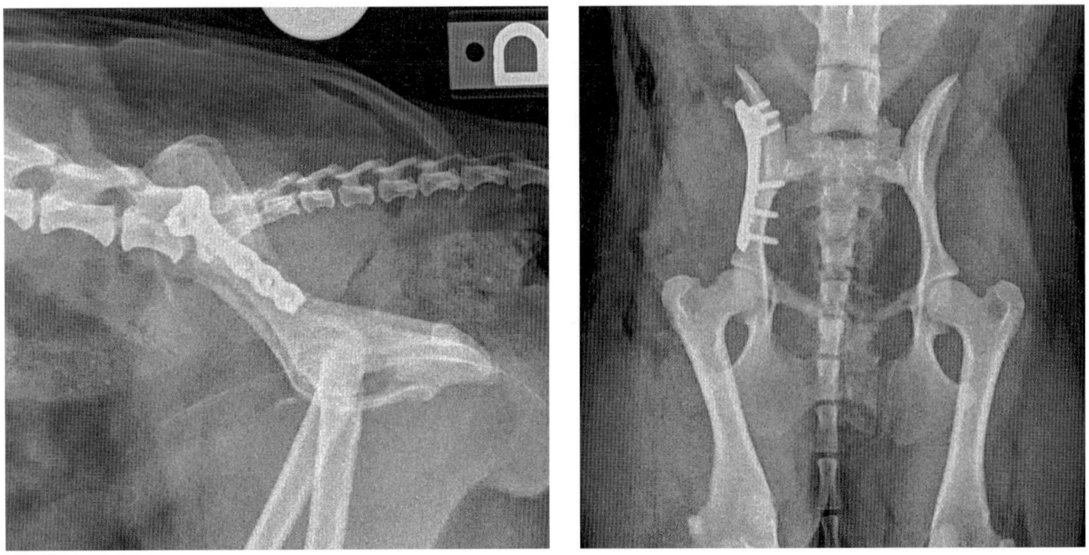

Figure 48.6 Post-operative radiographs of the long oblique right ilial wing fracture from Figure 48.1 post-repair with an Arthrex OrthoLine™ locking T-plate. *Source:* © Rebecca Webb.

Acetabular Fractures

Acetabular fractures pose a significant challenge to surgeons. These fractures are challenging to visualize, and even with a large approach, accurate apposition of the fragments is of paramount importance to reduce long-term osteoarthritis within the joint. Fractures of the acetabulum are classified as simple transverse, oblique, or comminuted and are classified according to their location within the acetabulum (cranial, dorsal, central, or caudal portions) (Figure 48.7). Conservative management for fractures within the caudal segment of the acetabulum used to be recommended. This segment of the acetabulum was historically suggested to be non-weight-bearing, likely because patients with these fractures typically will present with a

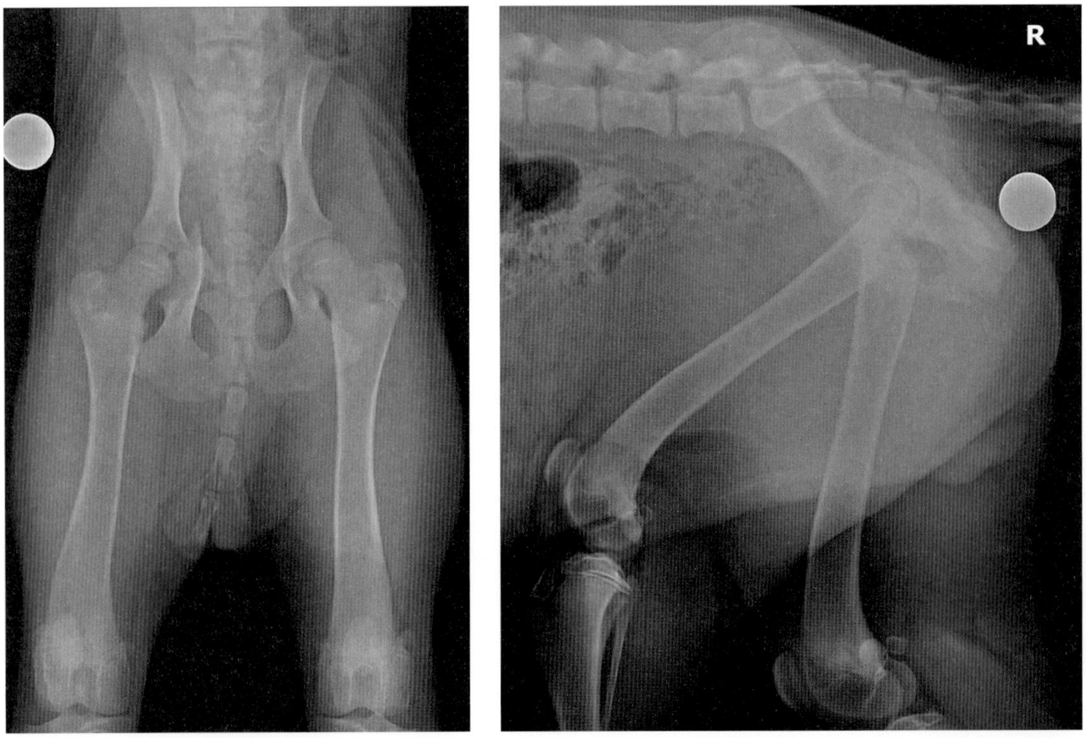

Figure 48.7 Pre-operative radiographs of an immature mid-sized dog with an acetabular fracture in the cranial portion of the right acetabulum. *Source:* Courtesy of Dr. Desmond Tan.

weight-bearing lameness at diagnosis. However, research has shown this segment appears to be fully weight-bearing during ambulation, and long-term follow-up of cases managed with conservative management showed lameness secondary to moderate to severe degenerative joint disease.[11,12] Due to this, the location of the fracture should not be the only factor when deciding whether to pursue surgical repair of an acetabular fracture. However, the difficulty in reducing and stabilizing caudal acetabular fractures should be considered when determining treatment options.

When involvement of the acetabulum is suspected, accurate imaging of the area is of vital importance to prepare the clinician for surgery. In addition to the standard ventrodorsal and lateral radiographs of the pelvis, oblique views can be helpful to further evaluate the fracture conformation. An oblique view is typically taken with the patient in lateral recumbency with the fractured side of the pelvis on the radiology table. The nonaffected limb is then abducted to rotate the pelvis and expose the acetabulum. Ideally, computed tomography (CT) is utilized in these cases to provide accurate information about the fracture. CT has the added benefit of 3-D reconstruction to allow the clinician to understand the fracture and plan the surgery more precisely.

In patients with comminuted, nonreconstructable fractures of the acetabulum or with clients who are unable to pursue surgical correction, salvage surgical options are typically recommended. Femoral head and neck ostectomy (FHO) is typically recommended for these cases. Bridging and stabilization of the acetabulum has been recommended in these patients to improve comfort and improve early limb function, however, this is not imperative in most cases. Clinicians should be cautious recommending FHO for acetabular fractures in young, rapidly growing patients, as fusion of the femoral neck osteotomy site to the acetabulum could occur if the patient is not using the limb consistently following surgery. Depending on the patient's comfort, FHO may be delayed a week or two in these patients, or alternatively, the client should be invested in aggressive physical therapy to prevent this from occurring.

General Preparation

General preparation of the patient for an acetabular fracture repair is the same as for ilial fracture repair described previously.

Approach

A dorsal approach to the coxofemoral joint with greater trochanteric osteotomy is typically recommended for central, dorsal, and cranial fractures with a caudal approach used for caudal fractures.[13,14] The clinician should take particular care to avoid damage to the nearby sciatic nerve in dissection and especially during retraction for these approaches.

Reduction

Reduction is typically challenging for acetabular fractures, as manipulation of the individual fragments is limited by the small approach and overlying musculature. Grasping the greater trochanter of the femur with reduction forceps can be helpful to manipulate the acetabular fragment if the round ligament remains intact (Figure 48.2), and grasping the ischium as discussed previously can be helpful to manipulate the caudal segment for reduction. An incision in the dorsal joint capsule to visualize the joint surface is imperative to ensure accurate reduction of the fracture. A slender instrument, such as a Freer periosteal elevator, may be inserted into the joint to palpate the joint surface and help evaluate adequate reduction. The previously mentioned towel clamp on the greater trochanter can also be used to gently distract the femoral head from the acetabulum and increase visualization. Once reduced, small K-wires or pointed reduction forceps can be placed to stabilize the fracture fragments during implantation, although the placement of either can be challenging due to the muscle mass and proximity of the joint surface. Continued manual reduction of the fracture may be required to maintain reduction during contouring and plating.

Implantation

Fixation of acetabular fractures is typically performed with plates and screws. It is important with the placement of a bone plate in this location that the plate is accurately contoured to the bone surface, since this is an articular fracture that requires anatomic reduction, and tightening of cortical screws on either side of the fracture could lead to shifting of the bone fragments with a loss of reduction. Given the heavy need for contouring, standard straight plates are challenging to use for this location. Acetabular reconstruction plates are made for this purpose but are traditionally nonlocking implants. Surgeons should take care with the nonlocking acetabular plates; although they come precontoured, they typically still require significant additional contouring to prevent a loss of reduction during plate placement. Newer acetabular plates are locking and can simplify the implantation process by preventing the shifting of the fragments during plate placement (Figure 48.8). String of Pearls (SOP) plates are locking plates that are more easily contoured than a straight plate and can be helpful in this location. Straight locking plates can also be used, but they require heavy contouring to place appropriately to ensure the absence of screws within the acetabular fossa post-operatively (Figure 48.9). Clinicians should also be aware of the direction the locked screws are being directed, as this can be significantly altered post-contouring.

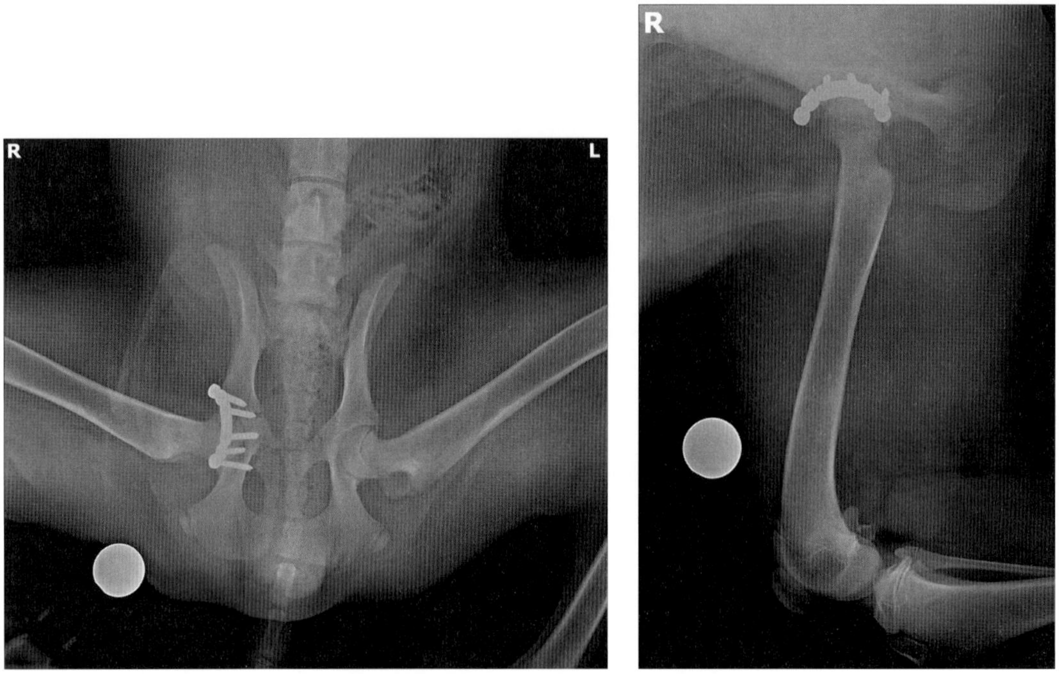

Figure 48.8 Post-operative radiographs of the patient from Figure 48.7. The right acetabular fracture has been reduced and repaired with a 2.7 mm locking acetabular plate. *Source:* Courtesy of Dr. Desmond Tan.

There is a described technique using a combination of screws, orthopedic wire, and poly(methyl methacrylate) (PMMA) to stabilize the fractures.[15] This repair method has been used in different fracture configurations and has the advantage of not requiring perfect plate-contouring.

Sacroiliac Luxation

Introduction

Sacroiliac luxation refers to the dislocation of the joint between the sacrum and the ilium (Figure 48.10). The dislocation can cause pain, lameness, and an inability to ambulate. Sacral fractures may also accompany sacroiliac luxations, so the clinician should pay close attention to the imaging performed to evaluate for this, in addition to performing a thorough neurological assessment of the patient. Following sacroiliac luxation, the wing of the ilium is usually displaced dorsally and cranially, and the caudal hemipelvis often displaces medially to narrow the pelvic canal. This pelvic canal narrowing is important to evaluate, since if it is not corrected, long-term issues, such as obstipation (particularly in cats), can result.

Diagnostic Imaging

Accurate diagnostic imaging is important to diagnose a sacroiliac luxation. Ventrodorsal and lateral radiographs are performed, but diagnosis is typically made on the ventrodorsal view in which a step defect can be seen between the sacrum and the ilium (Figure 48.11). While luxations with significant displacement are more straightforward to diagnose, patients with mild displacement may only be diagnosed on appropriately positioned radiographs. Due to patient comfort, accurate positioning can be challenging, so heavy sedation or anesthesia may be required to position the patient appropriately to get a straight ventrodorsal view. The clinician should carefully evaluate the radiographs for evidence of concurrent sacral fractures. These can be sometimes challenging to diagnose on radiographs alone, so if there is any consideration of a sacral fracture being present, a CT should be pursued to evaluate the area in more detail prior to surgical repair.

Conservative Versus Surgical Management

Several factors determine whether surgical or conservative management of a sacroiliac luxation is most appropriate, including the severity of displacement and instability, the presence or absence of neurological defects, the presence of other fractures or co-morbidities, and the client's financial resources. Conservative management is typically indicated when there is minimal displacement and no or minimal palpable instability, when the patient is showing minimal discomfort, or if finances prevent surgical intervention. Surgical intervention leads to a quicker return to function, whereas the return to function with medical management is highly variable with a possible period of extended (three to four weeks) nursing care required. Historically, most sacroiliac luxations were managed conservatively. This is likely due to the challenge of accurate

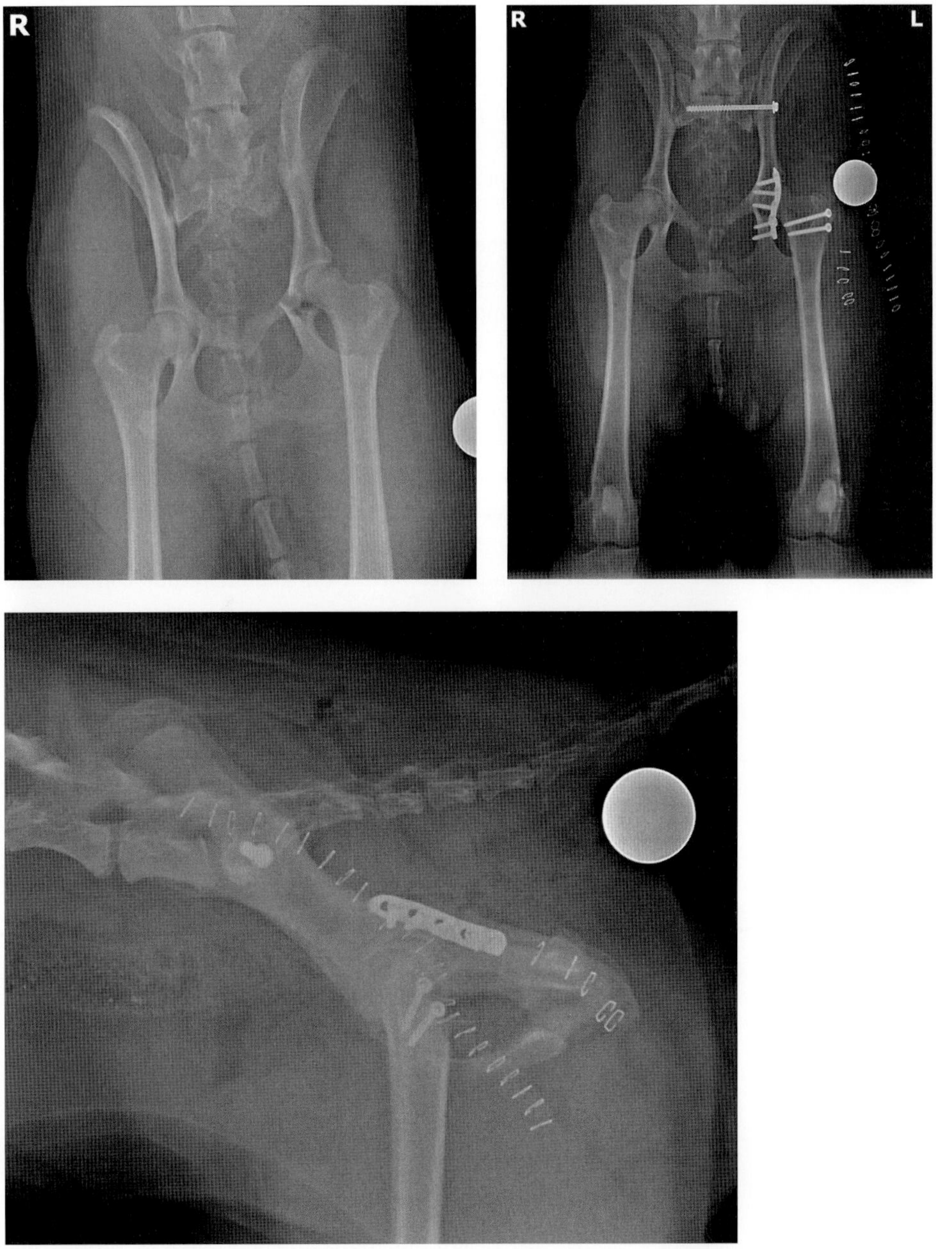

Figure 48.9 Pre- and post-operative radiographs of a mid-sized dog with a unilateral left sacroiliac luxation, a central to caudal short oblique acetabular fracture on the same side, as well as pubic and ischial fractures. A greater trochanteric osteotomy was performed to allow access to the acetabular fracture, and the fracture repaired with a 2.7 mm straight locking compression plate. The osteotomy of the greater trochanter was repaired using two 2.7 mm cortical lag screws. In addition, the left sacroiliac luxation was fixed using a single sacroiliac lag screw. *Source:* Courtesy of Dr. Desmond Tan.

implant placement through an open technique and the risks of nerve injury if the implant placed penetrates the sacral canal or damages the nerve roots. However, with the introduction of minimally invasive techniques using intra-operative fluoroscopy, the surgical procedure has been simplified and the risks of surgery reduced, which makes surgical stabilization and its more rapid return to function a more attractive option.[16] If medical management is pursued, it is important for clinicians to recognize that, just as with ilial fractures managed conservatively, further displacement of the ilial wing can occur in the first few weeks following injury, especially if instructions for strict confinement and activity restrictions aren't adhered to by the client. Therefore, a similar schedule as described above for medical management of ilial fractures of early, frequent rechecks is recommended to reassess for potential displacement and pelvic canal narrowing and ensure medical management is still the recommended therapy.

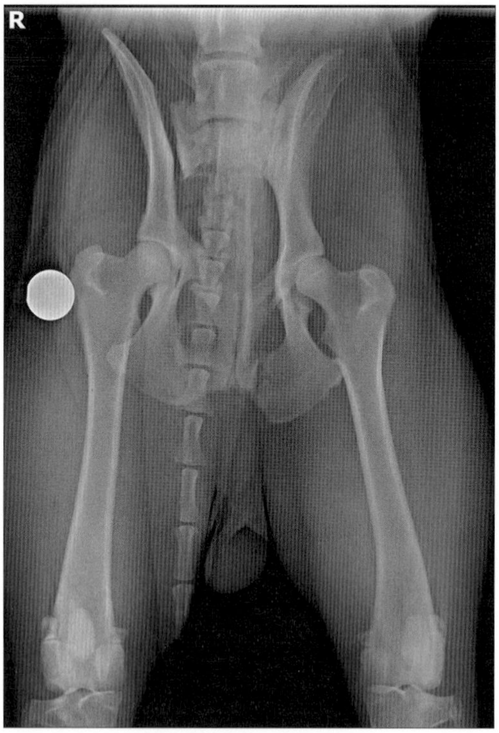

Figure 48.10 Pre-operative ventrodorsal radiograph showing a unilateral right sacroiliac luxation with concurrent pubic and ischial fractures. *Source:* Courtesy of Dr. Desmond Tan.

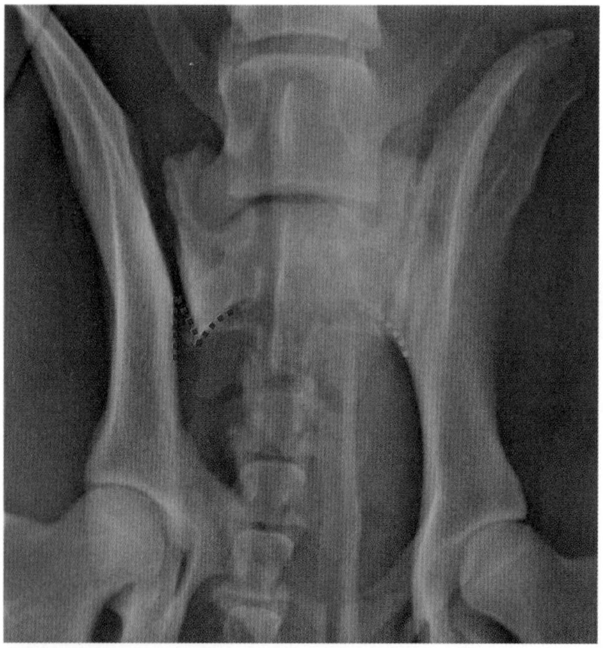

Figure 48.11 Ventrodorsal radiograph showing the characteristic step defect between the caudal aspect of the sacrum and the ilial wing. The joint marked with the green line shows a smooth transition between the sacrum and the ilium and is normal. The joint marked with the red line shows the step defect consistent with a sacroiliac luxation. *Source:* Courtesy of Dr. Desmond Tan.

Surgical Procedures

Multiple techniques for surgical stabilization of sacroiliac luxation have been described. The most common procedure is the placement of a sacroiliac lag screw, but other techniques include transilial bolt, trans-sacral screw and nut placement, and transiliosacral pinning among others.[17–19] A number of approaches have been proposed for sacroiliac luxation repair, including both open surgical approaches and minimally invasive approaches. The more common approaches for open stabilization include the dorsolateral and ventrolateral approaches, although in regions where intra-operative imaging is widely available, the minimally invasive approach is prevalent (Figure 48.12).[20,21] When comparing the two open approaches, the dorsolateral approach will typically provide superior visualization of the sacral body compared to the ventral approach. When comparing them retrospectively, the reduction of the luxation was improved for the dorsolateral group compared to the ventral group, however, there was no significant difference in the screw placement or clinical complications for either group.[22]

Accurate placement of the sacroiliac lag screw within the body of the sacrum is important for successful fixation. Initial mechanical studies found that the length of the screw should traverse at least 60% of the sacral body width to prevent post-operative loosening.[23] Another study showed that the placement of two screws was mechanically superior to one (each screw of approximately 60% of sacral width).[24] A recent mechanical study evaluated the placement of two shorter (average 23% sacral body width) screws and found the combination of two shorter screws to be mechanically stronger when compared to a singular screw of 60% sacral width. The use of shorter screws may be advantageous to reduce the risk of iatrogenic injury during placement.[25] In addition, the authors found no mechanical difference between the placement of the sacroilial screw in lag or positional fashion.[25]

The use of intra-operative imaging, such as fluoroscopy, is of significant benefit to avoiding inadvertent screw placement into the spinal canal and to improve the stability of the construct. In one study, the use of intra-operative imaging to guide screw placement was found to result in fewer screws exiting the sacrum and a greater sacral screw engagement length.[26] Improvements in the placement of sacroilial screws lead to a more stable construct. When comparing open with minimally invasive approaches, the minimally invasive approach with fluoroscopy was found to consistently lead to better screw placement and had a lower incidence of post-surgical screw loosening.[27]

The open placement of sacroilial lag screws is well-described in multiple textbooks, including safe corridors for screw placement in both dogs and cats.[4,28] Surgeons should be very comfortable with the regional anatomy and

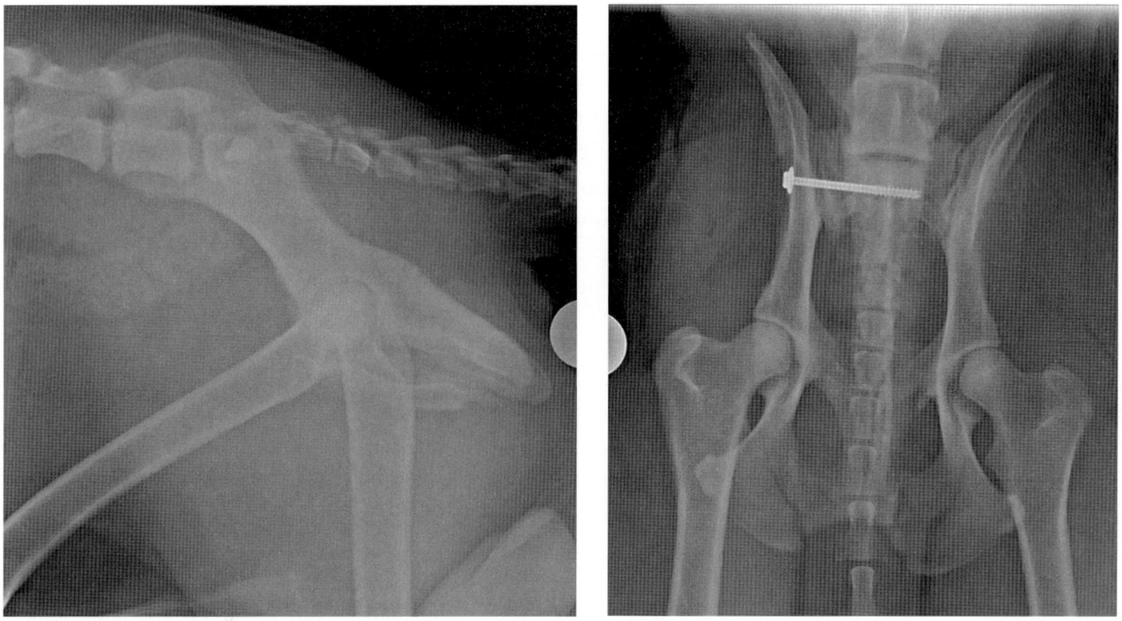

Figure 48.12 Post-operative radiographs of a minimally invasive sacroiliac 4.5 mm lag screw for right SI stabilization. *Source:* Courtesy of Dr. Desmond Tan.

have experience with the repair of more straightforward pelvic trauma prior to considering the pursuit of sacroiliac luxation repair.

Potential Complications

The potential complications of the above surgeries include nerve damage, implant failure/loosening, fracture malunion, and degenerative joint disease (particularly for acetabular fractures). Nerve damage is a severe complication, which can range in severity from mild neuropraxia to complete loss of function. These injuries typically lead to weakness or loss of sensation of the hind limbs (typically, sciatic nerve injury), loss of function and sensation to the tail, loss of function of the bladder, or fecal incontinence (sacral nerves). Knowing the patient's neurological status prior to surgery will help the clinician evaluate if the neurologic dysfunction is secondary to the original injury or iatrogenic after the surgical intervention. Careful retraction during surgery and a thorough knowledge of anatomy are essential to prevent this from occurring. Neurological function improves in most cases following surgical stabilization of a pelvic fracture; however, a lack of improvement after three to four months gives a poor prognosis for return to function, and amputation should be considered.[2]

Degenerative joint disease of some description is expected following acetabular fracture repair due to the level of trauma this joint has sustained. Careful reconstruction of the joint surface and adequate stabilization are key factors to reduce its severity post-surgery. Implant failure (typically, screw loosening) is seen with some frequency, particularly in the cranial aspect of the ilium and in the placement of sacroiliac lag screws. This may lead to a range of consequences ranging from mild pelvic canal narrowing, which is likely of minimal significance, to complete fixation failure requiring revision surgery. This particular complication may be mitigated by the use of locking screws instead of cortical screws for fracture fixation.

Post-op Care/Prognosis

The level of nursing care required by these patients following surgery is typically substantial. Post-surgery considerations include adequate pain control, bladder care, and mobility support.

Patients with pelvic fractures can have significant pain and discomfort. This discomfort is typically intensified when the patient is manipulated and moved as required for cleaning and physical therapy. Patients who cannot move on their own should be rotated every few hours to improve circulation and prevent the formation of ulcers. The patient's comfort should be controlled using analgesics (oral and injectable as needed), nonsteroidal anti-inflammatories (as tolerated by the patient), and local anesthetics infiltrated at the time of surgery (e.g., epidural, Nocita® at surgical site). Patients may need additional pain management to allow for nursing care (frequent changing of bedding/bathing, etc.) depending on their level of comfort.

The patient should be assisted to stand multiple times a day; this helps to regain muscular function, encourages the recovery of normal urination and defecation, reduces the risk of "bed sores" over bony prominences, and reduces the potential for blood-pooling, which in humans can lead to blood clots. This assistance can be provided with either a commercially designed sling or a towel used as a sling for support. Harnesses that provide mobility support for the front and hind limbs (such as the Help-Em-Up Harness® [Blue Dog Designs, LLC]) are very helpful for manipulation of the patient both in the hospital and at home, as the clients will have a handle on the harness (both on front end and back end) for easier control and handling.

Urinary care is of vital importance during the post-operative period. Patients can have difficulty urinating due to the inability to stand or inability to posture to urinate, due to concurrent urinary tract trauma, or due to neurological deficits. Urinary care is typically performed either with an indwelling urinary catheter or frequent bladder expression.

Post-surgical activity restriction is typically 8–10 weeks and consists of slow leashed walks until the fractures show signs of adequate healing radiographically. Once this occurs, a gradual reintroduction of activity over another four to six weeks is typically recommended. The patient's progression back to normal activity can be variable depending on the injuries sustained, but typically, most patients are fully recovered at four to six months post-surgery. Physical therapy can help increase the speed of this recovery and is helpful for these patients. Radiographs are performed at regular intervals to monitor healing and monitor for implant complications. The first radiographs are typically taken at six to eight weeks and repeated in another month in cases with incomplete healing on the first set of post-operative radiographs.

References

1 Selcer, B.A. (1982). Urinary tract trauma associated with pelvic trauma. *J. Am. Anim. Hosp. Assoc.* 18 (5): 785–793.

2 Jacobson, A. and Schrader, S.C. (1987). Peripheral nerve injury associated with fracture or fracture dislocation of the pelvis in dogs and cats: 34 cases (1978–1982). *J. Am. Vet. Med. Assoc.* 190 (5): 569–572.

3 Johnson, K.A. (2014). Approach to the ilium through a lateral incision. In: *Piermattei's Atlas of Surgical Approaches to the Bones and Joints of the Dog and Cat*, 5e (ed. K.A. Johnson), 316–319. Missouri, USA: Elsevier.

4 Moens, N.M. and DeCamp, C.E. (2018). Fractures of the pelvis. In: *Veterinary Surgery Small Animal*, 2e (ed. S.A. Johnston and K.M. Tobias), 938–956. Missouri, USA: Elsevier.

5 Breshears, L.A., Fitch, R.B., Wallace, L.J. et al. (2004). The radiographic evaluation of repaired canine ilial fractures (69 cases). *Vet. Comp. Orthop. Traumatol.* 17 (2): 64–72.

6 Langley-Hobbs, S.J., Meeson, R.L., Hamilton, M.H. et al. (2009). Feline ilial fractures: a prospective study of dorsal plating and comparison with lateral plating. *Vet. Surg.* 38 (3): 334–342.

7 Hamilton, M.H., Evans, D.A., and Langley-Hobbs, S.J. (2009). Feline ilial fractures: assessment of screw loosening and pelvic canal narrowing after lateral plating. *Vet. Surg.* 38 (3): 326–333.

8 Koch, D. (2005). Implants: description and application; screws and plates. In: *AO Principles of Fracture Management in the Dog and Cat* (ed. A.L. Johnson, J.E.F. Houlton, and R. Vannini), 27–52. Stuttgart, Germany: AO Publishing.

9 Schmierer, P.A. (2015). Screw loosening and pelvic canal narrowing after lateral plating of feline ilial fractures with locking and nonlocking plates. *Vet. Surg.* 44 (7): 900–904.

10 Guthrie, J.W. and Kalff, S. (2018). Tibial plateau levelling osteotomy locking-compression plates for stabilization of canine and feline ilial body fractures. *J. Small Anim. Pract.* 59 (4): 232–237.

11 Moores, A.L., Moores, A.P., Brodbelt, D.C. et al. (2007). Regional load bearing of the canine acetabulum. *J. Biomech.* 40 (16): 3732–3737.

12 Boudrieau, R.J. and Kleine, L.J. (1988). Nonsurgically managed caudal acetabular fractures in dogs: 15 cases (1979–1984). *J. Am. Vet. Med. Assoc.* 193 (6): 701–705.

13 Johnson, K.A. (2014). Approach to the caudal aspect of the hip joint and body of the ischium. In: *Piermattei's Atlas of Surgical Approaches to the Bones and Joints of the Dog and Cat*, 5e (ed. K.A. Johnson), 350–354. Missouri, USA: Elsevier.

14 Johnson, K.A. (2014). Approach to the craniodorsal and caudodorsal aspects of the hip joint by osteotomy of the greater trochanter. In: *Piermattei's Atlas of Surgical Approaches to the Bones and Joints of the Dog and Cat*, 5e (ed. K.A. Johnson), 340–345. Missouri, USA: Elsevier.

15 Lewis, D.D., Stubbs, W.P., Neuwirth, L. et al. (1997). Results of screw/wire/polymethylmethacrylate composite fixation for acetabular fracture repair in 14 dogs. *Vet. Surg.* 26 (3): 223–234.

16 Tomlinson, J. (2012). Minimally invasive repair of sacroiliac luxation in small animals. *Vet. Clin. North Am. Small Anim. Pract.* 42 (5): 1069–1077.

17 Pratesi, A., Grierson, J.M., and Moores, A.P. (2018). Single transsacral screw and nut stabilization of bilateral sacroiliac luxation in 20 cats. *Vet. Comp. Orthop. Traumatol.* 31 (1): 44–52.

18 Parslow, A. and Simpson, D.J. (2017). Bilateral sacroiliac luxation fixation using a single transiliosacral pin: surgical technique and clinical outcomes in eight cats. *J. Small Anim. Pract.* 58 (6): 330–336.

19 Tonks, C.A., Tomlinson, J.L., and Cook, J.L. (2008). Evaluation of closed reduction and screw fixation in lag fashion of sacroiliac fracture-luxations. *Vet. Surg.* 37 (7): 603–607.

20 Johnson, K.A. (2014). Approach to the wing of the ilium and dorsal aspect of the sacrum. In: *Piermattei's Atlas of Surgical Approaches to the Bones and Joints of the Dog and Cat*, 5e (ed. K.A. Johnson), 312–315. Missouri, USA: Elsevier.

21 Johnson, K.A. (2014). Approach to the ventral aspect of the sacrum. In: *Piermattei's Atlas of Surgical Approaches to the Bones and Joints of the Dog and Cat*, 5e (ed. K.A. Johnson), 320–322. Missouri, USA: Elsevier.

22 Singh, H., Kowaleski, M.P., McCarthy, R.J. et al. (2016). A comparative study of the dorsolateral and ventrolateral approaches for the repair of canine sacroiliac luxation. *Vet. Comp. Orthop. Traumatol.* 29 (1): 53–60.

23 DeCamp, C.E. and Braden, T.D. (1985). Sacroiliac fracture-separation in the dog: a study of 92 cases. *Vet. Surg.* 14: 127–130.

24 Radasch, R.M., Merkley, D.F., Hoefle, W.D. et al. (1990). Static strength evaluation of sacroiliac fracture-separation repairs. *Vet. Surg.* 19 (2): 155–161.

25 Hanlon, J., Hudson, C.C., Litsky, A.S. et al. (2022). Mechanical evaluation of canine sacroiliac joint stabilization using two short screws. *Vet. Surg.* 51 (7): 1061–1069.

26 Silveira, F., Quinn, R.J., Adrian, A.M. et al. (2017). Evaluation of the use of intraoperative radiology for open placement of lag screws for stabilization of sacroiliac luxation. *Vet. Comp. Orthop. Traumatol.* 30 (1): 69–74.

27 Rollins, A., Balfour, R., Szabo, D. et al. (2019). Evaluation of fluoroscopic-guided closed reduction versus open reduction of sacroiliac fracture-luxations stabilized with a lag screw. *Vet. Comp. Orthop. Traumatol.* 32 (6): 467–474.

28 Johnson, A.L. (2013). Management of specific fractures – sacroiliac luxations and fractures. In: *Small Animal Surgery*, 4e (ed. S.A. Johnston and K.M. Tobias), 1168–1173. Missouri, USA: Elsevier.

49

Medial Patellar Luxation Repair

Ross H. Palmer

Department of Clinical Sciences, Colorado State University, Fort Collins, CO, USA

Key Points

- Patellar luxation is the product of insufficient static patellar constraints combined with variable degrees of mal-alignment of the skeleton with overlying quadriceps-patellar mechanism (QPM).
- More severe grades of patellar luxation (III–IV) are commonly associated with profound soft tissue distortions and skeletal deformities even in small breeds of dogs and often require more advanced diagnostics (computed tomography) and complex surgical techniques (corrective osteotomies) for effective treatment.
- Thorough patient examination including accurate luxation grading and detection of skeletal deformities is key to appropriate patient selection.
- The 50/50 Rule is used to determine the necessity for and dimensions of the various trochleoplasty techniques described herein.
- The Line A-B Rule is used to determine the necessity for and the direction and magnitude of tibial tuberosity transposition described herein.
- Balancing of soft tissue tension is an important aspect of surgical treatment of MPL; the complexity of which is reduced in less severe grades of luxation (II).

Introduction

Patellar luxation is a common cause of lameness in dogs and less commonly in cats and can be either medial or lateral. This chapter will focus on medial patellar luxation (MPL), as it is more common overall. Canine MPL is graded I-IV according to severity.[1]

- Grade I – patella can be manually luxated but returns to normal position when released.
- Grade II – patella luxates during stifle flexion or ambulation and remains luxated until stifle extension or manual reduction. The frequency of spontaneous luxation/reduction is variable.
- Grade III – patella is continually luxated and can be manually replaced but will reluxate spontaneously when manual pressure is removed.
- Grade IV – patella is luxated continually and cannot be manually reduced.

Etiopathogenesis of Medial Patellar Luxation

Healthy static and dynamic patellofemoral joint constraints support normal patellar tracking. *Static constraints* include normal patellofemoral joint conformation in which the patella glides through a deep femoral sulcus bounded by medial and lateral trochlear ridges throughout a full range of stifle joint motion. Static constraints also include balanced tension within the joint capsule, retinaculum, and medial/lateral femoropatellar ligaments. *Dynamic constraint* is provided by proper alignment of the quadriceps-patellar

Techniques in Small Animal Soft Tissue, Orthopedic, and Ophthalmic Surgery, First Edition. Edited by Kristin A. Coleman.

Companion website: www.wiley.com/go/coleman/surgeries

mechanism (QPM) with the underlying skeleton and is necessary for normal patellar tracking.

MPL may be congenital, developmental, or traumatic, but the majority are developmental in nature. While not fully understood, malalignment of the QPM with the underlying skeleton plays a key role in MPL development and condition severity, and it is key to understanding the relationship between MPL grade and the surgical treatments necessary.

The patella is a sesamoid bone within the active quadriceps muscle group. Tensile forces within the quadriceps group may either pull the patella firmly into the femoral trochlear sulcus or generate forces favoring medial or lateral patellar luxation, depending upon the skeletal malalignment relative to the overlying QPM (Figure 49.1). When QPM forces favoring patellar luxation are relatively small, the static constraints of the patellofemoral joint are able to maintain normal patellar tracking. When these static constraints are incapable of overcoming strong active QPM forces, spontaneous patellar luxation occurs. There is a profound difference between lesser MPL grades (I–II) and more severe grades (III–IV) upon skeletal development and soft tissue distortions. Sustained displacement of QPM relative to the skeleton (i.e., grade III–IV patellar luxation) during skeletal development can lead to anatomical changes in the femur and tibia. The absence of sustained normal retro-patellar compression on the femur can lead to trochlear hypoplasia, as well as the development of a misplaced pseudo-sulcus. The bowstring effect of sustained medial QPM displacement can contribute to coxa vara, femoral varus, and external torsion, as well as medialization of the tibial tuberosity and external tibial torsion.[2–4] MPL causes internal rotation of the stifle joint and, when sustained, can lead to profound soft tissue distortions, such as medial capsular/fascial contracture, lateral capsular/fascial stretching, and likely alterations to meniscal shape/structure.

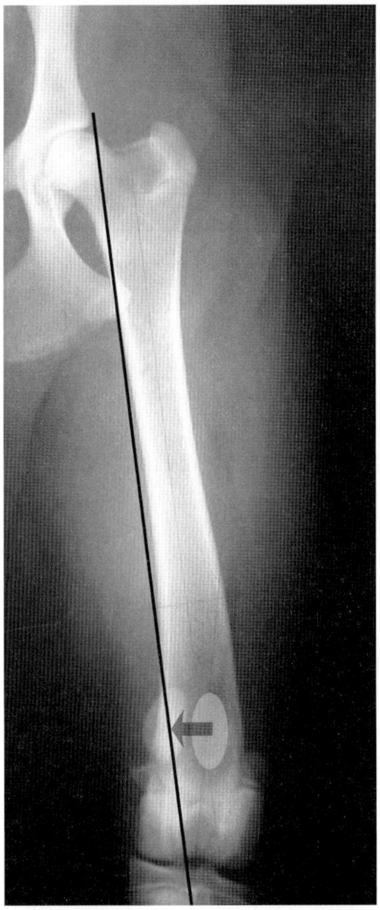

Figure 49.1 Dynamic patellofemoral joint constraint. The patella is a sesamoid within the powerful quadriceps muscle group. When there is skeletal malalignment with the overlying quadriceps patellar mechanism (QPM), quadriceps tonus may exert a force favoring patellar luxation (medial in this example).

Gait Observation and Physical Examination

Careful observation of gait is essential and must be correlated with limb palpation findings to fully assess the luxation grade and associated skeletal deformities that may result. In brief, lesser grades of patellar luxation (I–II) are much less likely to be associated with major soft tissue distortions and skeletal deformities, because the QPM is properly aligned with the underlying skeleton most of the time in these cases (i.e., the patella is reduced more often than it is luxated). In contrast, more severe grades of patellar luxation (III–IV; especially grade IV) are commonly associated with profound soft tissue distortions and skeletal deformities even in small breeds of dogs.[2,3]

Gait observation includes classifying the gait as normal or lame, grading the lameness, and describing any lameness as sustained versus episodic. The degree of lameness may vary according to gait: stance, walk, trot, run, and ascending versus descending stairs. Grade II MPL is often characterized by an episodic skipping gait in which the gait may be normal one moment and non-weight-bearing the next. It is also important to note that some dogs, especially terrier breeds, can display such a skipping gait but do not have patellar luxation. Gait observation also includes noting pelvic limb conformation. Dogs with MPL often appear to be "bowlegged" (i.e., genu varum), and this may be a true skeletal deformity or may merely be a postural change that resolves when the patella is reduced.[5] Finally, it is important to note the foot position during stance and correlate it with the luxation grade; for instance, internal rotation of the foot (i.e., "pigeon-toed posture") with grade III luxation is likely the result of internal stifle rotation. In contrast, the normal orientation of the foot in association with grade IV MPL is strongly suggestive of an external tibial torsional deformity; this is because grade IV MPL means the stifle (proximal tibia relative to the femur) is internally rotated, yet the foot remains in the normal orientation rather than being aligned with the proximal tibia.

When lameness is detected, it is important to correlate the patellar position (normal versus medial versus lateral). The direction of spontaneous patellar luxation must be determined before performing surgical correction. It may be preferable to palpate the patellar position with the patient in a standing position for several reasons: (1) it can be correlated with the gait that was observed immediately prior, (2) stance keeps the quadriceps active and, therefore, more reflective of the dynamic QPM, and (3) it is relatively easy to simultaneously extend the hip such that the rectus femoris is placed under tension. (Note: the rectus femoris is the only of the four quadriceps muscles to span the hip as well as the stifle joint). Standing exam may also be helpful in detecting joint effusion / periarticular fibrosis that is particularly common when there is concomitant cranial cruciate ligament disease (CrCLD). If the patella is difficult to palpate, it can be helpful to follow the tibial tuberosity and patellar ligament proximally. Once detected, the patella is held between the thumb and forefinger as the hip is extended and the stifle joint is rotated internally (to assess for MPL) and externally (to assess for LPL). When luxation is detected, it should be graded, and any patellofemoral crepitus is noted, which is an indicator of cartilage erosion of the patella and/or trochlear ridge. While tibial tuberosity position may be noted, it is ideal to reduce the patella before doing so, because medial luxation rotates the entire tibia internally such that apparent medialization of the tibial tuberosity may be postural rather than anatomic. To that end, in most instances, final decisions about the patient need for tibial tuberosity transposition (and trochleoplasty) are typically made intra-operatively, as will be discussed. It is important to evaluate for cranial drawer and/or cranial tibial thrust instability, as concurrent treatment of MPL and CrCLD, while advisable, is a more complex surgical procedure that is associated with higher rates of surgical complication; referral to a surgical specialist may be advised.

Diagnostic Imaging

Stifle radiographs help to confirm luxation (though grade II MPL may appear normal), detect degenerative changes, and identify occult co-morbidities. Radiographs of the femur and tibia are often required to detect complicating skeletal deformities, but caution should be exercised because subtle shifts of a three-dimensional object (such as a bone) can create the artifactual appearance of a deformity on a two-dimensional radiographic image.[6,7]

Mediolateral (M-L) positioning is often simpler than latero-medial position when seeking to obtain a sagittal plane image of the stifle, femur, or tibia. An M-L stifle view is helpful for detecting joint effusion and caudal superimposition of the patella upon the femoral condyle, which may suggest patellar luxation.

Caudo-cranial (Cd-Cr) position is often simpler than the cranio-caudal position when seeking to obtain a frontal plane image of the stifle, femur, or tibia. The direction of patellar luxation, when present, can be detected on properly positioned Cd-Cr views.

Properly positioned sagittal- and frontal-plane radiographs can be used as a screening tool to rule out significant skeletal deformities, but computed tomography (CT) is advised to definitively diagnose and quantify deformity.[7] Failure to detect and treat skeletal deformities contributing to grade III and IV MPL is a common cause of postoperative re-luxation.

Surgical Treatment

It must be noted that patellar luxation corrective surgery is "part art and part science"; as such, the following is reflective of that current reality. Surgery is generally indicated for those cases of symptomatic MPL, particularly if the symptoms are progressing in frequency and/or severity. Grade II and some early/mild grade III MPLs can typically be managed by some combination of trochleoplasty, tibial tuberosity transposition, and soft tissue tension balancing. The final decision regarding the necessity of these procedures is typically performed intra-operatively. The necessity of and planning for femoral and tibial corrective osteotomies, most common with grade III and grade IV MPLs, is typically performed pre-operatively from CT images and emphasizes the importance of deformity detection and luxation grading through correlation of gait, stifle examination, and imaging.

It is important to note that surgical treatment of MPL is not performed identically in each patient or even within defined grades of luxation; instead, it is important to make pre- and intra-operative assessments to identify the factors contributing to luxation in the individual patient such that surgical treatment can be customized accordingly. Bony contributors to MPL, such as trochlear hypoplasia and medial displacement of the tibial tuberosity, cannot be corrected with soft tissue treatments, and soft tissue contributors to MPL, such as medial joint capsular contracture and lateral capsular stretching, cannot be corrected with bony treatments.

The typical sequence of surgical assessments and treatments is as follows:

1) **Reduce the patella.** It is easiest to make a surgical approach to an anatomically correct joint. This is, of

course, not possible with grade IV MPL and emphasizes the importance of luxation grading, so that the surgery being performed is commensurate with the training, skills, and experience of the surgical team.

2) **Surgical approach.** While arguments can be made for either medial or lateral parapatellar arthrotomy, medial parapatellar arthrotomy may be preferred in most MPL cases for reasons of cosmesis and to serve as a capsular release when needed for grade III and IV MPLs. Medial parapatellar arthrotomy does not negate the possibility of lateral capsular/fascial imbrication when needed.
3) **Assess the need for and, if necessary, the dimensions of trochleoplasty using the 50/50 Rule.** Abrasion, wedge recession, block recession, or semi-cylindrical recession trochleoplasty is performed as indicated.
4) **Assess the need for and, if necessary, the magnitude of tibial tuberosity transposition (TTT) using the Line A-B rule.** TTT is performed as indicated.
5) **Soft tissue tension balancing as indicated.** A combination of medial soft tissue release and/or lateral imbrication (tightening) is performed according to the degree of soft tissue distortion that correlates with luxation grade.

The patient is typically positioned in dorsal recumbency with the pelvic limbs toward the end of the table and, when the hip is abducted, the tibia can lie flat with its lateral surface on the surgical table and oriented in the perfect M-L orientation (sagittal plane). Once the proper patient position on the table is confirmed, the limb is suspended per usual so that an aseptic hanging limb preparation and draping can be performed.

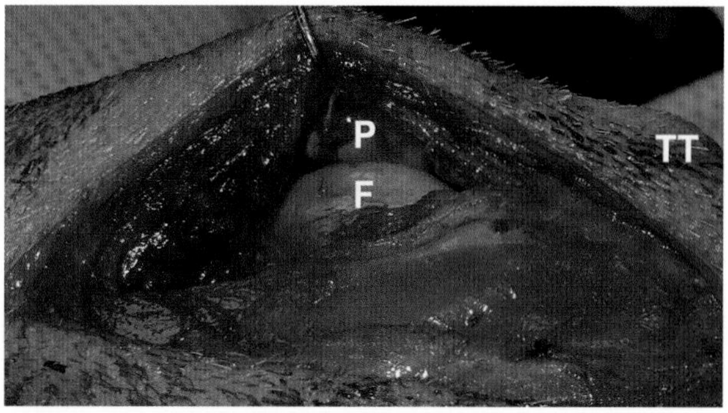

Figure 49.2 Medial stifle arthrotomy (P = patella; F = femoral medial trochlear ridge; TT = tibial tuberosity). The 50/50 Rule is a subjective visual assessment used to determine if the patient requires a trochleoplasty and, if so, what the length and depth dimensions of the trochleoplasty should be. The patellofemoral joint is viewed through the full extension/flexion stifle range of motion to assess if at least 50% of its length and depth is always within the trochlear sulcus.

Trochleoplasty

The need for trochleoplasty is assessed via the 50/50 rule (Figure 49.2). This is a subjective visual assessment in which, following arthrotomy, the patellofemoral joint is visualized from full stifle joint extension to full flexion while asking the question, *"Is 50% of the depth and length of the patella contained within the trochlear sulcus?"*. If the answer is YES, the patient does not need a trochleoplasty. If the answer is NO, trochleoplasty is indicated, and the dimensions of which should satisfy the 50/50 rule. For instance, it is relatively common to discover "relative patella alta" in which only the distal 30%–40% of the patella is within the trochlear sulcus during full stifle extension. In this instance, the trochleoplasty is extended proximal to the native trochlear sulcus, such that the 50/50 rule is satisfied. Often erosion of the proximal extent of the medial trochlear ridge (and mirrored erosion of the disto-lateral patellar articular surface) is noted to support this conclusion. One could certainly argue that the stifle is not typically held in full extension during the gait cycle, but a slight exaggeration of the proximal trochleoplasty dimension in an effort to reduce the reported incidence of postoperative re-luxation is the rationale.[8] As to the abaxial dimensions of the trochleoplasty, it is essential that the trochleoplasty be able to receive the full width of the patella; thus, these are typically "just within guardrails" represented by the peaks of the medial and lateral trochlear ridges. While making too narrow of a trochleoplasty is a common surgical error, it is also important that the trochleoplasty not be so wide as to excise the trochlear ridges. The dimensions of the selected trochleoplasty, per the 50/50 rule assessment, are typically outlined with a scalpel blade prior to performing either wedge or block trochleoplasty.

Generally, techniques that preserve the healthy hyaline cartilage of the trochleoplasty are indicated. These include wedge recession, block recession, and semi-cylindrical recession trochleoplasty techniques; while there are theoretic advantages and disadvantages of each of these relative to one another, each can be effectively used. Abrasion trochleoplasty removes the existing cartilage from the trochlear sulcus and is replaced by less congruent and resilient fibrocartilage. Abrasion trochleoplasty is, therefore, only indicated when preservation of healthy hyaline cartilage is not feasible (e.g., revision of previous abrasion trochleoplasty, intra-operative complication with recession trochleoplasty, etc.).

Wedge Recession Trochleoplasty (WRT)

The dimensions of WRT, as for all trochleoplasties, are determined by the 50/50 rule and are outlined with a scalpel blade into the articular cartilage. The abaxial cuts are typically made with a handheld, manual patellar saw; these saws typically have a fine/thin kerf (such that little bone is removed) and fine teeth (such that they cut smoothly). It is important to start the cut at the apex of each trochlear ridge and apply minimal pressure to each smooth to/fro motion of the angled cut toward the proximal and distal apexes of the wedge. This is truly an acquired skill and art that takes some practice. Power reciprocating saws may be used, but the principles of a fine saw kerf and teeth, as well as practiced training, are still relevant. Power oscillating saws are not ideal for this procedure in the hands of most surgeons.

Once the osteochondral (OC) wedge is liberated, it is preserved in a blood-soaked sponge. If the wedge were immediately returned to the recipient bed, little recession would be accomplished. Instead, the walls of the recipient bed are slightly widened and deepened. While classical descriptions of this technique call for a third abaxial saw cut, the author utilizes a scalpel blade to precisely shave cancellous bone from the walls and deep apex of the recipient bed (Figure 49.3a). It is also often advisable to use a rongeur or scalpel blade to excise the apical tip of the OC wedge segment (Figure 49.3b). The wedge is returned to the recipient bed to assess the satisfaction of the 50/50 rule, as well as the ability to accomplish a satisfactory press fit that will resist postoperative migration (Figure 49.3c). It is relevant to note that the wedge can be inverted, such that what was originally proximal is now distal, if that accomplishes a more satisfactory press fit and 50/50 rule compliance. In fact, an asymmetric inverted wedge recession trochleoplasty has been described, whereby intentional

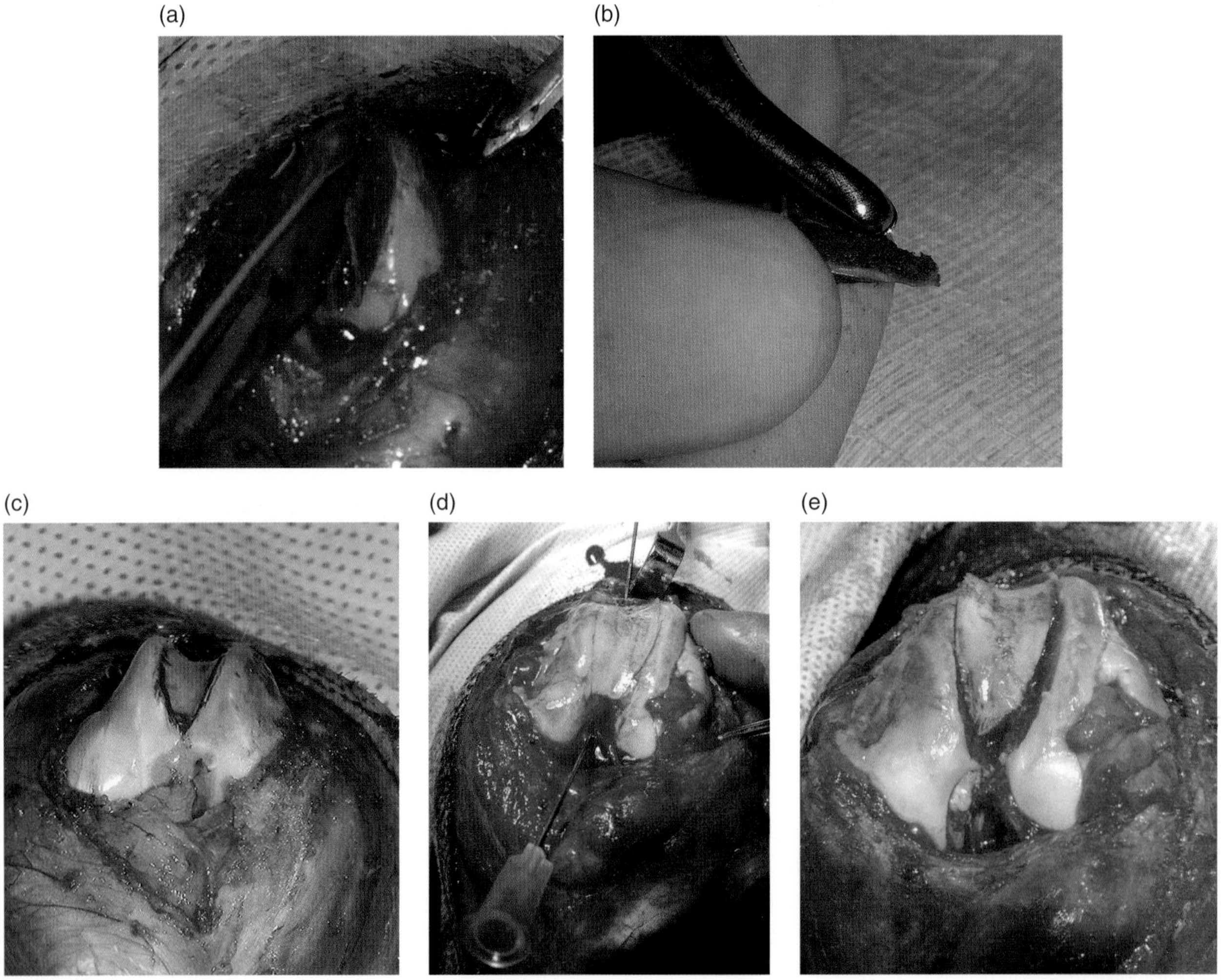

Figure 49.3 Wedge recession trochleoplasty (WRT). (a) Using a scalpel blade to precisely deepen and widen the recipient bed. (b) Rongeur or a scalpel blade can be used to excise the cancellous tip of the apex of the wedge to allow its recession into the recipient bed. (c) Properly performed, WRT should preserve the hyaline cartilage surface, produce firm press-fit fixation in the recipient bed, and satisfy the 50/50 Rule. (d) Asymmetric inverted wedge trochleoplasty is indicated for hypoplasia of the medial trochlear ridge. The procedure uses a steep, nearly vertical cut on the medial side and a shallow cut on the lateral side of the wedge. The needles are marking the planned proximal and distal apices of the asymmetric wedge. (e) When the wedge is inverted, it produces a more prominent medial ridge. Because firm press-fit is not always achievable with this method, a fine transverse K-wire may be required for the fixation of the wedge.

proximo-distal inversion of an asymmetrically harvested wedge is used to correct medial trochlear ridge hypoplasia (Figure 49.3d,e).[9] In this situation, secure press-fit fixation may not be achievable, and the use of a fine transverse K-wire may be required for fixation of the wedge to the medial and lateral trochlear ridges.

Block Recession Trochleoplasty (BRT)

The dimensions of BRT, as for all trochleoplasties, are determined by the 50/50 rule, and the abaxial boundaries are outlined with a scalpel blade into the articular cartilage. The proximal and distal transverse boundaries can be marked with firm pressure applied to an osteotome. Since the basilar cuts will progress from distal to proximal and the thickness between the superficial and deep basilar cuts determine the amount of recession, it is often helpful to pre-mark both levels of cuts at the distal transverse margin.

Once the boundaries have been marked, the abaxial cuts are typically made with a handheld, manual patellar saw. The saw and the surgical technique are like that described for the WRT except that these cuts are angled only 10°–15° toward the midline of the sulcus rather than to the center of the sulcus as with WRT. A common technical error is a failure to angle the abaxial cuts sufficiently, which ultimately results in the inability to achieve a press fit of the OC block into the recipient bed. Power reciprocating saws may be used, and the principles of a fine saw kerf and teeth remain relevant. Regardless of the saw used, the abaxial cuts are carried to the depth of the planned deep basilar cut.

The superficial basilar cut is made with a sharp, thin profile osteotome (Figure 49.4a). It is important to visualize

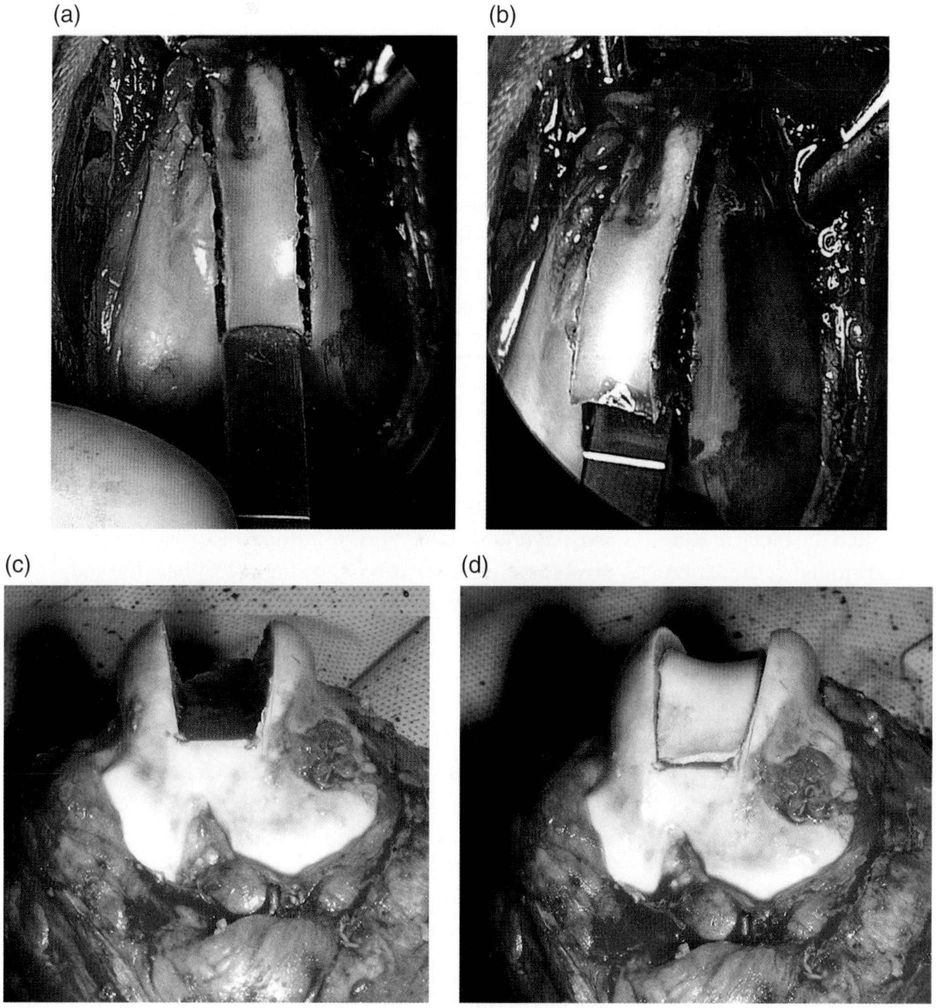

Figure 49.4 Block recession trochleoplasty (BRT). (a) An appropriately sized, thin-profile, osteotome is used to make the superficial basilar cut. (b) The OC block will begin to rise from the bed as the basilar cut progresses, but the surgeon must complete the cut to its proximal terminus and avoid the urge to lever the block upward. (c) The deep basilar cut has been made, the depth of which will determine the amount of recession achieved. The base of the recipient bed and OC block are rasped if necessary to create congruent surfaces. (d) Properly performed, BRT should preserve the hyaline cartilage surface, produce firm press-fit fixation in the recipient bed, and satisfy the 50/50 Rule.

the desired depth of the cut at its proximal-most terminus. One common error is to orient the osteotome too tangential to the distal femoral articular surface when starting the cut; this can result in the hyaline cartilage being sheared from the subchondral bone, whereas the goal is to create an OC block. As the superficial basilar cut progresses from distal to proximal, the surgeon must guide the osteotome down the center of the sulcus (protecting the medial and lateral trochlear ridges). The surgeon must also complete the superficial basilar cut from its distal origin to its proximal terminus and resist the urge to lift the osteotome in hopes of "popping" the block from its base (this will fracture the OC block) (Figure 49.4b). Once the intact OC block is liberated, any undulations of its osseous base are smoothed with a rongeur or rasp, and the block is temporarily stored in a blood-soaked sponge.

The deep basilar cut is performed like the superficial cut, but a narrower width of osteotome is often needed, owing to the angulation of the abaxial walls. The cancellous bone "matchstick" that is liberated is saved in a blood-soaked sponge, as it can be used as a bone graft for TTT or as a shim to help secure the OC block if the abaxial walls were insufficiently angulated. Any undulations in the basilar cut are smoothed with an osteotome or rasp so that there will be a congruence of the OC block's base when it is press-fit into the recipient bed (Figure 49.4c,d). The block is returned to the recipient bed to assess the satisfaction of the 50/50 rule as well as the ability to accomplish a satisfactory press fit that will resist postoperative migration. Once satisfaction with the 50/50 rule is confirmed, poor press-fit fixation owing to insufficient angulation of the abaxial walls can be managed with either of two escape strategies. First, the bony matchstick can be trimmed to create one or more shims along one wall, against which the block is compressed and the excess matchstick is trimmed at the articular surface. Alternatively, a fine K-wire can be placed to capture the subchondral bone of the block as the wire passes from one trochlear ridge to the other. This fine wire is typically bent firmly against the abaxial margin of each trochlear ridge to prevent migration.

Semi-Cylindrical Recession Trochleoplasty (SCRT)

The SCRT is a recently introduced technique performed using a commercially available instrument set.[10,11] The system allows for a two-step cutting process in which the thickness of bone excised between the first superficial cut and the second deeper cut (in addition to the kerf of the saw blade) corresponds to the degree of recession achieved, similar to the BRT. The dimensions of SCRT, as for all trochleoplasties, are determined by the 50/50 rule. Next, the diameter of the hole saw is determined by the width of the trochlear sulcus; this can be accomplished intraoperatively by matching the variously-sized blades to the patient's trochlea. The goal, as with other trochleoplasties, is to have the blade cut from the center of the medial and lateral trochlear ridges and ensures that the cut does not extend abaxially beyond the apex of the trochlear ridges. When the perfect saw blade diameter is not available, it is preferable to err toward a smaller hole saw diameter. A 0.045″ (1.1 mm) K-wire is placed from distal to proximal beneath the center of the trochlear sulcus with the aid of an aiming guide; this K-wire will serve as a guide wire for positioning the SCRT cutting guide. The K-wire is inserted through an aiming guide starting just proximal to the intercondylar fossa of the distal femur and is aimed to exit proximal to the femoral trochlear articular cartilage; the proximal target for pin exit is such that any noted trochlear ridge erosion is centered between the proximal-most and distal-most boundaries of the planned trochleoplasty (Figure 49.5a). The SCRT cutting guide that corresponds to the selected SCRT hole saw diameter is threaded onto the K-wire using the guide cannulation that best corresponds to the desired depth of the first, superficial-most cut (Figure 49.5b). The depth of the first cut is deep enough to generate an OC autograft (rather than only a chondral flap) yet superficial enough to allow adequate deepening with the second, deeper cut. It is important to maintain alignment of the first, superficial cut with the K-wire and to keep it centered between the trochlear ridges while copious saline lavage is used for cooling. This is particularly important given the inherent flexibility of the K-wire, which can easily be bent, resulting in altered alignment of the saw blade and cut. The harvested OC graft is temporarily stored in a blood-soaked sponge. While the first cut is being performed, it is important to apply copious lavage and to intermittently cease drilling to minimize thermal damage to the cartilage and bone. In the author's experience, it is relatively common for the OC autograft to become lodged in the center of the saw blade. A Freer periosteal elevator wrapped in moistened gauze can be used to atraumatically lever the OC graft free in these cases. The depth of the guide is adjusted in preparation for the second, deeper cut by sliding it off the current guide wire cannulation (note which hole it is in) and shifting it to a guide wire cannulation closer to the large center SCRT saw cannulation (Figure 49.5c). The spacing between each guide wire cannulation is 1.5 mm, such that shifting the guide two holes closer to the SCRT saw cannulation will result in 3 mm of deepening with the sulcoplasty. Once the guide is adjusted, the second, deeper cut is made to produce a thin semicylindrical cancellous bone wafer that can be saved and later used for grafting of a tibial tuberosity transposition if indicated (Figure 49.5d). While not part of the originally published technique, some surgeons prefer to make the second deeper cut using the next smaller diameter SCRT saw in order to accomplish a tighter press fit of the OC autograft

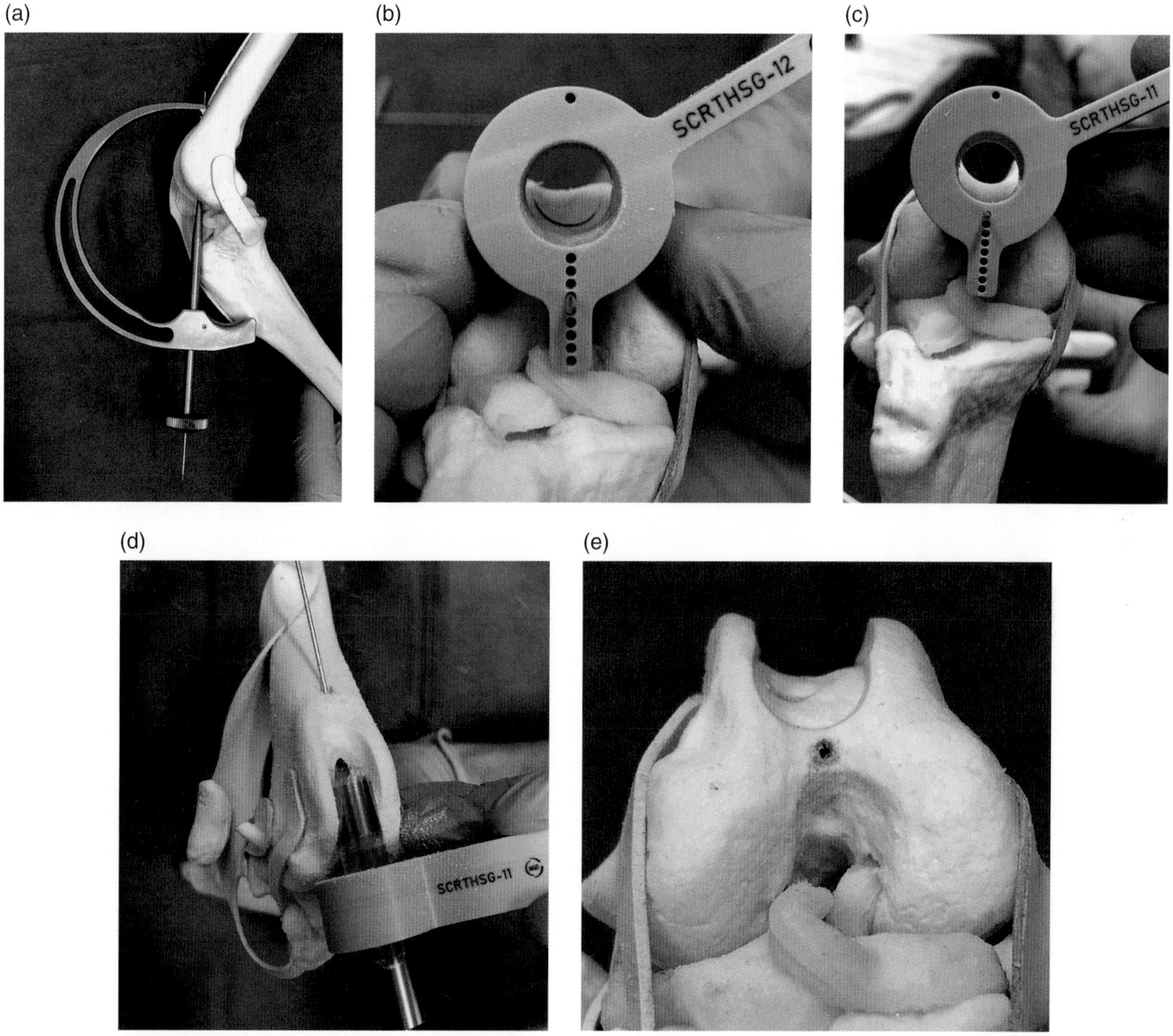

Figure 49.5 Semi-cylindrical recession trochleoplasty (SCRT). (a) An aiming guide is used to properly place a guide wire for the SCRT saw guide. (b) An SCRT saw guide that corresponds to the proper saw blade diameter is placed upon the guide wire at the appropriate depth to yield a semi-cylindrical OC graft. (c) The saw guide is repositioned on the guide wire in preparation for the second, deeper cut. (d) The cancellous thickness of the second, deeper cut will determine the degree of sulcus depth created. Some surgeons prefer to step down one size in saw blade diameter for this deeper cut as shown here. (e) Properly performed, SCRT should preserve the hyaline cartilage surface, produce firm press-fit fixation in the recipient bed, and satisfy the 50/50 Rule.

into the recipient bed.[11] The SCRT trochleoplasty is evaluated and adjusted until satisfaction of the 50/50 rule and press fit of the OC graft is achieved (Figure 49.5e).

Tibial Tuberosity Transposition (TTT)

A sterilizable power drill is needed for proper TTT fixation. A sterilizable power oscillating saw, as will be discussed later, is preferable to an osteotome and other instruments for creating the osteotomy. There are several cost-effective options for sterilizable power equipment, including the purchase of refurbished units from a reputable orthopedic equipment reseller. It is not advisable to perform MPL corrective surgery if the surgeon and facility are not properly equipped to perform TTT.

The need for TTT is assessed using the Line A-B rule (Figure 49.6). This is a subjective visual assessment in which the patella is reduced, and the stifle is extended. In the absence of tibial torsion, the patient's toes will point in the same direction as the reduced patella. When the patient's toes are not pointed in the same direction as the patella, they are usually pointing laterally, and this is an indication of external tibial torsion that was hopefully detected pre-operatively. Assuming the absence of tibial torsion, the reduced patella is identified as Point A and the center of the metatarsus as Point B. An imaginary line A-B

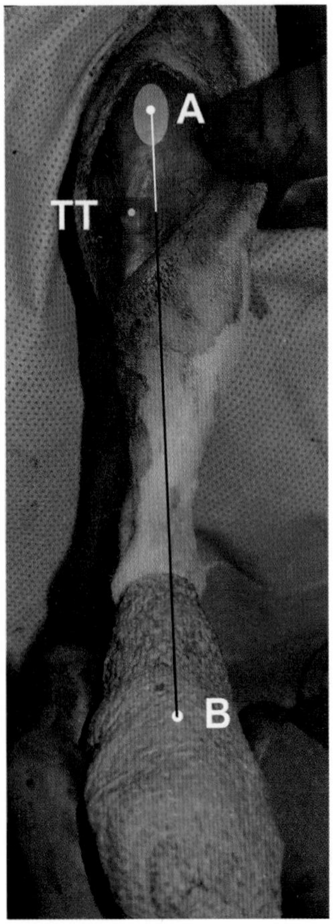

Figure 49.6 The Line A-B Rule is a subjective visual assessment used to determine if the patient requires a tibial crest transposition and, if so, the magnitude of the transposition. The patella is reduced, and the stifle joint is extended. Provided that there is no tibial torsion present, the foot will be pointing in the same direction as the patella. The reduced patella defines Point A and the center of the metatarsus defines Point B. The tibial tuberosity (TT) is viewed to determine if it falls on Line A-B. If not, it is transposed in the direction and magnitude required to position it upon that line.

is drawn while asking the question, *"Is the tibial tuberosity on Line A-B?"*. If the answer is YES, the patient does not need a TTT. If the answer is NO, TTT is indicated, and the direction and magnitude of the TTT is such that it will satisfy the Line A-B rule. In the case of MPL, when TTT is indicated, it is typically in the lateral direction.

Next, the surgeon should plan and mark the position of the planned tibial crest osteotomy that will permit safe and effective TTT. The tibial osteotomy courses from the tubercle of Gerdy proximally in a disto-cranial direction toward the distal terminus of the tibial crest, usually leaving a 2–3 mm intact bony bridge distally (Figure 49.7a). Because the cut is usually made from the medial side of the tibia, it is important to extrapolate a line from the tubercle of Gerdy, which is on the lateral tibial surface, to the medial side of the proximal tibia. The tubercle of Gerdy is the small bony prominence that marks the cranial border of the tibial extensor sulcus through which the long digital extensor (LDE) tendon passes. It is important to distinguish Gerdy's tubercle from the caudal border of the LDE extensor sulcus (sometimes referred to as "Gerdy's big sister"), which may be more prominent and easily palpable in some dogs. The line extrapolated medially from Gerdy's tubercle can be done visually or by passing a K-wire from lateral to medial through the joint capsule and fat pad.

Monopolar cautery is then used to draw the line on the medial surface of the tibia from the proximal-most origin of the planned osteotomy to its distal terminus. This will allow the surgeon to focus on making an accurate cut while performing the osteotomy. Retraction of the patellar tendon with a Hohmann retractor or placement of a towel clamp around the tendon to distract cranially can be used to protect it from injury while performing the osteotomy.

Regardless of the instrument used to make the tibial crest osteotomy, it is important that the cut remains in the frontal plane. This can be difficult to do, especially for the novice surgeon, because the proximal tibia has a triangular shape in cross-section. The author advises that the tibia be held by an assistant in the perfect M-L (sagittal plane) orientation with the lateral surface of the crus firmly against the draped surgical table. With the limb held in this sagittal plane position, orienting the osteotomy perpendicular to the surgical table will ensure it is in the frontal plane (Figure 49.7b). An adjustable osteotomy guide and associated patient-specific planning service, originally designed for tibial tuberosity advancement (TTA), are commercially available for TTT planning and execution (www.ossability.com).

Many cutting instruments have been used to make the tibial crest osteotomy. Having trained thousands of veterinarians and veterinary students to perform TTT, the author has noted that the use of a sagittal saw seems to be associated with the best precision, the least number of intra-operative complications, and the fastest learning curve. Osteotomes can be used effectively but must be sharp and can be difficult, especially for the novice, to maintain in the frontal plane while also following the planned osteotomy trajectory. Power reciprocating saws can be very precise but are not uniformly available, even in some specialty practices. When cutting from the medial surface with an oscillating saw, a line is initially scored along the cautery-drawn line. The osteotomy is progressively deepened as the cut works from proximal to distal. When gentle pressure is applied to the saw blade, it will cut more effectively (versus firm pressure), and it is possible to feel when the lateral cortex is penetrated, such that the blade minimally disrupts the cranial tibial musculature on the lateral tibial surface and these tissues do not need to be elevated laterally.

(a) (b)

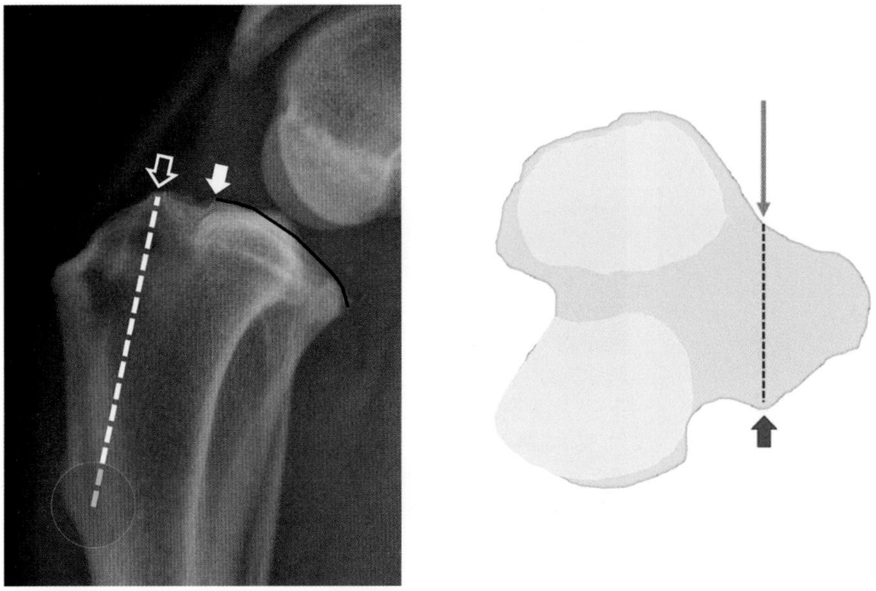

Figure 49.7 Tibial crest osteotomy landmarks. (a) The osteotomy passes from the level of Gerdy's tubercle (open white arrow) proximally in a disto-cranial direction to terminate 2–3 mm from the distal termination of the tibial crest (orange-shaded circle); thus, protecting the long digital extensor tendon as it passes through the extensor sulcus (orange curved line) and the cranial-most (closed white arrow) margin of the tibial articular surface (black line). (b) It is important to keep the osteotomy oriented in the frontal plane (red dotted line). To do so, a line from Gerdy's tubercle (blue arrow) can be extrapolated from the lateral to the medial side of the tibia (red dotted line). The tibia can be held by an assistant flat upon the draped surgical table as a power sagittal saw is oriented perpendicular to the table surface (gray arrow) to create a frontal plane osteotomy from medial to lateral across the tibial crest.

Once the TTT cut is completed (leaving the intact 2–3 mm distal bony bridge), the stifle joint is extended to allow for easier lateral transposition of the tibial crest segment. Transposition should be performed slowly over approximately one minute to reduce the chances of fracture of the bony bridge. If it is overly difficult to transpose, confirm that the stifle is extended, the osteotomy extends through the lateral cortex, and that the distal bony bridge is not too large. Maintain slow, sustained lateral pressure on the tibial tuberosity until the transposition appears to satisfy the Line A-B rule. At this point, pass a hypodermic needle or fine K-wire firmly along the medial cortical surface of the transposed tuberosity and deeply into the freshly exposed osteotomy bed of the tibia; this "door-stopper needle" prevents the tibial crest segment from slamming shut to its original position without damaging the small tibial crest segment (Figure 49.8a). If the Line A-B rule is not truly satisfied, the TTT can be readjusted, and a new door-stopper needle placed for temporary fixation. Once the Line A-B rule is satisfied, the door stopper needle maintains proper TTT orientation until definitive fixation with K-wires can be achieved.

Numerous methods to secure the TTT have been described. For the sake of training the novice surgeon, the author prefers two K-wires (one proximal to the other); a figure-of-eight tension band wire can be applied to this K-wire fixation in selected instances. The proximal-most K-wire is placed through the fibers of the patellar tendon as it inserts on the tibial tuberosity (Figure 49.8b). The K-wire is ~20–25% the diameter of the bone in this location and is directed from the tibial tuberosity in a caudo-medial direction to fully penetrate the cortical bone at the caudo-medial margin of the proximal tibia. While it is mechanically desirable to have K-wires oriented perpendicular to the tibial long axis, it may not be possible to do so in this location, as it may risk iatrogenic penetration of the stifle joint. It is often helpful for the surgeon to grasp the proximal tibia in their non-dominant hand with their thumb on the tibial tuberosity/crest region and their fingers at the caudo-medial tibial margin; this hand is compressing the osteotomy while the fingers serve as a target for aiming the K-wire. The dominant hand is used to drill the K-wire through the insertional Sharpey's fibers of the patellar tendon toward the "target fingers" on the caudo-medial tibial margin. As the far-cortex is approached, the surgeon moves their fingers slightly to allow for safe, full penetration of the far-cortex in this location (Figure 49.8c). The second K-wire is typically placed distal to the tibial tuberosity, through the narrower tibial crest segment, and this may require a slightly smaller diameter K-wire to be used. Once again, this K-wire is aimed to exit the caudo-medial margin of the tibia, but remote to the exit point of the more

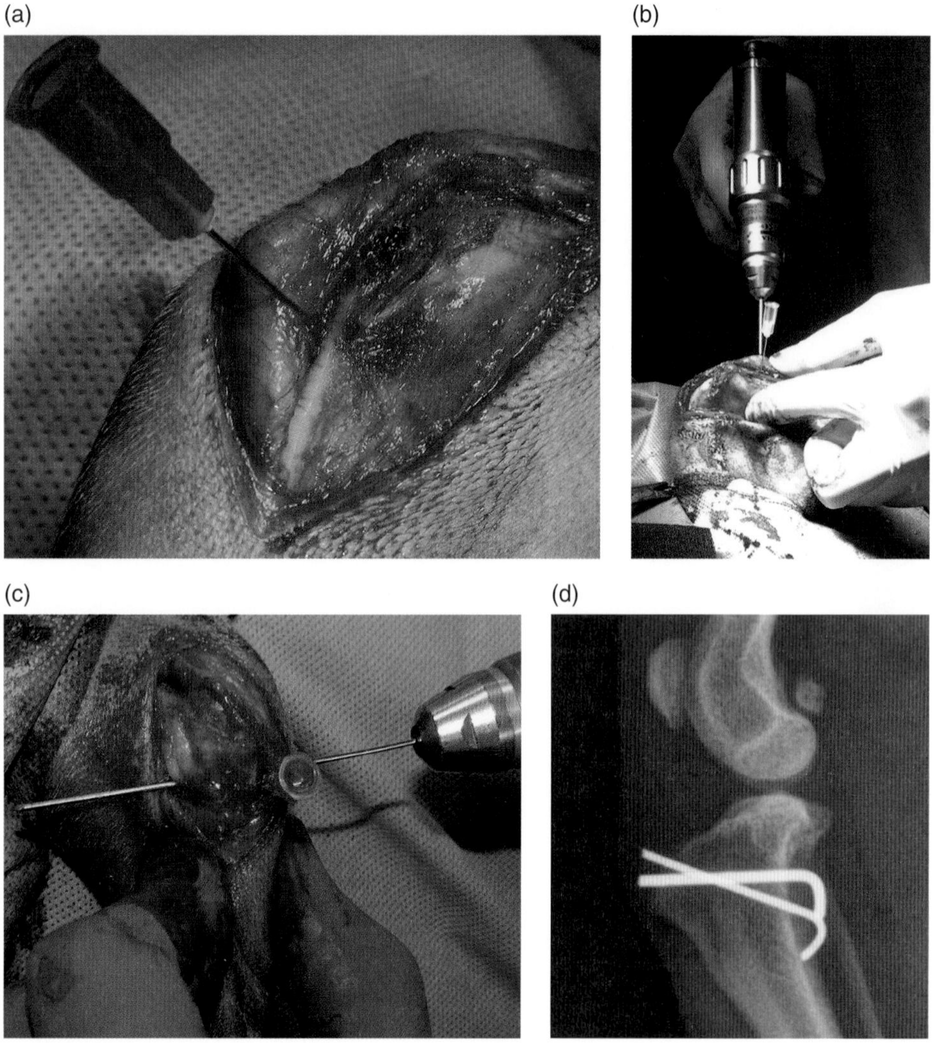

Figure 49.8 Tibial tuberosity transposition fixation. (a) Temporary "door stopper needle" holding the transposed tibial tuberosity in position until definitive fixation is applied. (b) The surgeon compresses the tibial crest osteotomy by placing the fingers of their non-dominant hand at the caudo-medial margin of the tibia and directs the first K-wire through the insertional fibers of the patellar ligament to exit adjacent to their fingers at the caudo-medial margin. (c) If properly directed, the K-wire can exit the caudo-medial tibial margin and be withdrawn until flush with the tibial tuberosity if desired (it is generally left protruding at the tibial tuberosity if a figure-of-eight tension band wire is planned). (d) The wire can be twisted over at the caudal margin of the tibia so that it will be retrievable in the future if desired, as shown in this postoperative radiograph.

proximal K-wire (to reduce a stress concentrator effect that may predispose to fracture).

Countersinking Versus Bending the K-Wires

When a figure-of-eight tension band is applied, it is preferable to bend the more proximal wire to serve as a hook to retain the tension band wire (Figure 49.9). Otherwise, K-wires bent at the cranial margin of the tibia can predispose to skin irritation and draining wounds since there is sparse soft tissue coverage in this area. Some surgeons may opt to countersink the K-wires flush with the cranial cortex, but this makes the K-wires difficult to retrieve in the future if necessary. Either way, bending or countersinking of the K-wire at the cranial margin should be done carefully to avoid iatrogenic fracture of this relatively small tibial crest segment.

One solution that allows for cranial surface countersinking plus future retrievability has been dubbed "the Danish Twist" by the author. This technique is possible when K-wires are properly directed to exit the caudo-medial margin of the tibia (Figure 49.8c). In this instance, the K-wire is advanced through the caudo-medial exit point as the tibia is externally rotated, and the caudal tibial musculature is retracted from the exiting wires. The caudo-medially protruding ends of the K-wires can then be grasped and retrieved until the cranial tip is flush with the cranial cortex. The long, caudo-medially protruding ends of the K-wires can then be bent flush with the medial tibial

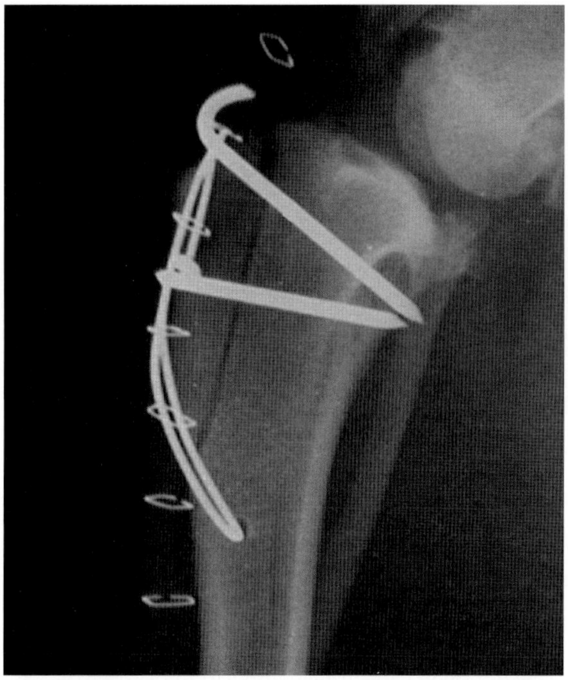

Figure 49.9 Tibial crest tension band fixation. Note that the proximal-most K-wire is bent at the tibial tuberosity to serve as a hook to secure the figure-of-eight wire. Note also that the transverse bone tunnel for the distal anchorage of the figure-of-eight wire is distal to the osteotomy and ~30% of the distance from the cranial cortex to the caudal cortex.

surface and cut (Figure 49.8d). This Danish Twist technique is not relevant for the proximal-most K-wire used in a figure-of-eight tension band, as it is desired to have the bent hook at the tibial tuberosity in this instance to retain the tension band wire (Figure 49.9).

Tension Band Fixation of the TTT

A figure-of-eight tension band wire is relatively easy to add to the described K-wire fixation, adds considerable resistance to the strong tensile forces of the QPM, and reduces the risk of postoperative avulsion fracture of the TTT. Tension band fixation may be indicated in several instances:

- When the tibial osteotomy is complete, and no intact distal bony bridge remains
- When questionable postoperative patient/owner compliance is anticipated
- When bilateral simultaneous TTT procedures are performed
- When TTT is performed in a cat, because cats are prone to jumping to high elevations via explosive QPM contractile forces, making TTT complications relatively common in this species[12]

To place a figure-of-eight tension band wire (Figure 49.9), a transverse tibial tunnel is drilled in the frontal plane distal to the TTT osteotomy and ~30% of the bone diameter caudal to the cranial tibial cortex (the goal is to feel a near- and far-cortex as this tunnel is drilled). Cranial tibial musculature is elevated slightly at the level of the transverse tibial tunnel to create a small, lateral soft tissue window. Spool wire (22 g for cats and small dogs; 20 g for medium dogs; 18 g for large dogs) is passed from medial to lateral, and the tip of the wire is retrieved through the lateral soft window as it emerges from the lateral cortex. The ends of the wire are then passed upward (proximally) and criss-crossed to form the bottom of the "8." Next, the end of the wire that was retrieved from the lateral soft tissue window and has now crossed to the medial side of the tibial tuberosity is passed around the proximal-most K-wire. The question is raised as to whether this wire end should pass from medial to lateral UNDER or OVER the patellar tendon? It is the author's opinion that the wire should pass such that it least distorts the pathway of the patellar tendon. Thus, the wire should pass under the tendon in some patients and over the tendon in others; this will depend upon the tibial tuberosity morphology and position of the proximal-most K-wire in it. If the tightening of a wire passes over the tendon and squeezes into the tendon during tightening, it should be repositioned under the tendon and vice versa. As the top loop of the figure-of-eight is formed, the twist will be on the lateral side. The wire is initially pulled snug by hand as the first twist or two is formed. Then, a wire twister is applied, and the twist is pulled straight back as the twist is tightened. The twist knot is made until the figure-of-eight tension band is taut, but excessive tightening is avoided, as it will deform the proximal K-wire. A gentle twisting motion is made as the wire is folded over into a small lateral soft tissue window and is cut with ~3 twists remaining with the patient.

Bending K-Wires

Whether bending the K-wire at the tibial tuberosity or at the caudo-medial tibial margin (as with the Danish Twist technique), the goal is to attain an acute bend of the K-wire at the level of the bone without permitting the K-wire to cut through the bone in the process. It is easiest to achieve this acute bend if the wire is left long until the bend is complete. Special K-wire benders are commercially available and can prove helpful. The K-wire bender is, first, passed down to the base of the wire at the bony surface to create the acute bend and a properly designed instrument takes some of the load off the bony wall. Next, the instrument is withdrawn ~8 cm on the K-wire before making a counter-bend. The length of the wire between the acute bend and the counter-bend serves as a lever arm to maximize the acute bend at the bony surface. At times, regional anatomy may dictate that the acute bend is initially directed disto-medially, but the wire can be cut with a 3–5 mm bent tip in

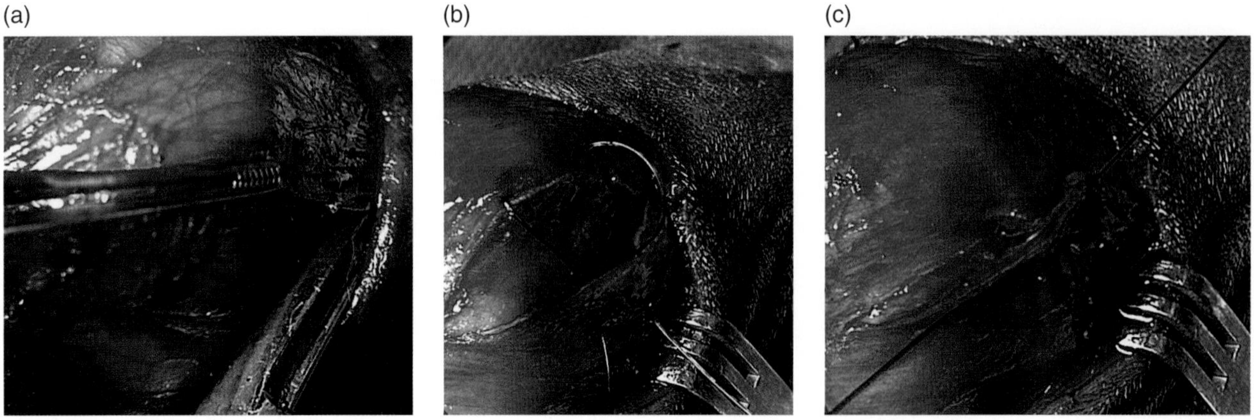

Figure 49.10 Lateral fascial imbrication. (a) A lateral fascial incision is made. (b) Vest-over-pants imbricating suture pattern is placed in the fascia. (c) Suture tightening results in imbrication via fascial overlap.

most instances that is then rotated into a position that is flush with the regional tissues.

Soft Tissue Tension Balancing

After completing the necessary bony procedures, it is important to assess the need for soft tissue tension balancing. Even this portion of the correction can be challenging in grade III and IV MPLs, owing to the marked soft tissue distortions that are often present. In milder grades of MPL, soft tissue tension balancing is typically less daunting.

In general, there may be soft tissues (joint capsule and fascia) that require release on the medial side of the stifle with MPL while tissues on the lateral side may require tightening in the form of imbrication. In the instance of medial arthrotomy as described herein, lateral imbrication can often be achieved by, first, incising the lateral parapatellar fascia (Figure 49.10a). This incised fascia can then be imbricated by using an overlapping (vest-over-pants), everting (horizontal mattress), or inverting (Lembert) suture pattern (Figure 49.10b,c). Alternatively, some surgeons may opt to excise a margin of fascia and directly reappose it (the more tissue that is excised, the more tightening that is achieved). The patella is closely observed during lateral imbrication to make sure that the lateral tightening does not create a lateral luxation. In some instances, the lateral imbrication may need to be decreased or counter-opposed with medial stifle reconstruction. In other instances, lateral imbrication may not be necessary at all. In some instances, the medial capsular and fascial release is left open (no surgical apposition of these layers), and surgical site closure commences with the closure of the deep subcutaneous tissues. In most instances of grade II MPL, either medial release or re-apposition of the medial arthrotomy with gentle lateral fascial imbrication will suffice, but the procedures performed are customized to the needs of the individual patient.

Postoperative Care

Postoperative care consists of a short-term continuation of peri-operative antimicrobial therapy (at surgeon discretion), analgesia for 10–14 days, convalescent activity restriction, and trained physical rehabilitation if available. Recheck examinations are typically scheduled at 10–14 days for suture removal and at 45 and 90 days for progress assessment. Radiographs are made on day 45 when a TTT has been performed to assess healing and implant stability. Duration and intensity of leash walks are progressively increased on a weekly basis after day 45 if TTT is healed or healing routinely. Return to full activity is not permitted before day 90 and may be delayed further in complex cases, including corrective osteotomies.

References

1 Roush, J.K. (1993). Canine patellar luxation. *Vet. Clin. North Am. Small Anim. Pract.* 23 (4): 855–868.

2 Yasukawa, S., Edamura, K., Tanegashima, K. et al. (2016). Evaluation of bone deformities of the femur, tibia, and patella in Toy Poodles with medial patellar luxation using computed tomography. *Vet. Comp. Orthop. Traumatol.* 29 (1): 29–38.

3 Yasukawa, S., Edamura, K., Tanegashima, K. et al. (2021). Morphological analysis of bone deformities of the distal femur in Toy Poodles with medial patellar

luxation. *Vet. Comp. Orthop. Traumatol.* 34 (5): 303–311.

4 Hulse, D.A. (1981). Pathophysiology and management of medial patellar luxation in the dog. *Vet. Med. Small Anim. Clin.* 76 (1): 43–51.

5 Tomo, Y., Edamura, K., Yamazaki, A. et al. (2022). Evaluation of hindlimb deformity and posture in dogs with grade 2 medial patellar luxation during awake computed tomography imaging while standing. *Vet. Comp. Orthop. Traumatol.* 35 (3): 143–151.

6 Swiderski, J.K., Radecki, S.V., Park, R.D. et al. (2008). Comparison of radiographic and anatomic femoral varus angle measurements in normal dogs. *Vet. Surg.* 37 (1): 43–48.

7 Palmer, R.H., Ikuta, C.L., and Cadmus, J.M. (2011). Comparison of femoral angulation measurement between radiographs and anatomic specimens across a broad range of varus conformations. *Vet. Surg.* 40 (8): 1023–1028.

8 Wangdee, C., Hazewinkel, H.A.W., Temwichitr, J. et al. (2015). Extended proximal trochleoplasty for the correction of bidirectional patellar luxation in seven Pomeranian dogs. *J. Small Anim. Pract.* 56 (2): 130–133.

9 Fujii, K., Watanabe, T., Kobayashi, T. et al. (2013). Medial ridge elevation wedge trochleoplasty for medial patellar luxation: a clinical study in 5 dogs. *Vet. Surg.* 42 (6): 721–726.

10 Blackford-Winders, C.L., Daubert, M., Rendahl, A.K. et al. (2021). Comparison of semi-cylindrical recession trochleoplasty and trochlear block recession for the treatment of canine medial patellar luxation: a pilot study. *Vet. Comp. Orthop. Traumatol.* 34 (3): 183–190.

11 Conzemius, M. Semi-cylindrical recession trochleoplasty (SCRT) technique. https://www.ngdvet.com/product_details.php?cid=110#:~:text=Semi%2DCylindrical%20Recession%20Trochleoplasty%20or,wedge%20recession%20or%20abrasion%20sulcoplasty (accessed 26 December 2023); https://www.youtube.com/watch?v=lELMsHHN1Lc (accessed 26 December 2023).

12 Rutherford, L., Langley-Hobbs, S.J., Whitelock, R.J. et al. (2015). Complications associated with corrective surgery for patellar luxation in 85 feline surgical cases. *J. Feline Med. Surg.* 17 (4): 312–317.

50

Extracapsular Stabilization for the Cranial Cruciate Ligament-Deficient Stifle

Trent T. Gall

Gall Mobile Veterinary Surgery, Longmont, CO, USA

Key Points

- Good knowledge of the stifle anatomy is key to surgical success.
- Understanding stifle anatomy and potential variances in that anatomy is key to recognizing the ideal surgical patients.
- Finding the proper isometric anchor points on the femur and tibia for extracapsular suture placement is essential for a good outcome and stifle range of motion postoperatively.
- Postoperative confinement, activity restrictions, and rehabilitation are extremely important for overall success of this surgery.

Introduction

Extracapsular stabilization (ECS) of the stifle joint encompasses many surgical techniques that all have similar principles and objectives. The fundamental strategy is mimicking the stabilizing properties of the cranial cruciate ligament (CrCL). This is accomplished by placing a synthetic material outside the joint capsule (extracapsular), spanning from the femur to the tibia in a caudal to cranial direction on the lateral aspect of the stifle joint. Ultimately, these techniques rely on the body to create periarticular fibrosis around the synthetic material for long-term stability, while short-term stability is provided by the synthetic material. The two main forces ECS controls are cranial tibial translation (cranial tibial drawer motion or tibial thrust) and excessive internal rotation. ECS is safe, relatively inexpensive (depending on the synthetic material of choice), and is a relatively easy procedure that has good results. This procedure can easily be performed by general practitioners with some practice and appropriate patient selection.

Anatomy

Knowing the anatomy of the stifle joint is important for surgical success. It is imperative to understand that the stifle joint is not a pure hinge joint; the stifle joint moves in three planes. The author likes to simplistically think of these three planes as the following: (1) Hinge, which is flexion and extension of the tibia in relation to the femur. (2) Glide, as there is a small amount of gliding motion of the femur on the tibia. (3) Rotation, the third plane is a small amount of normal internal rotation of the tibia. The term "screw-home" mechanism has been used to describe the human knee joint and has been adopted in veterinary literature. In brief, this term is to describe the different constraints present through a normal range of motion. Since the stifle joint normally moves in three planes, it is important to keep that in mind during surgical stabilization. This is so the surgeon does not overtighten the ECS and eliminate one or more of the natural movement planes, which could result in excessive patient discomfort, cartilage

Techniques in Small Animal Soft Tissue, Orthopedic, and Ophthalmic Surgery, First Edition. Edited by Kristin A. Coleman.

Companion website: www.wiley.com/go/coleman/surgeries

damage leading to progression of osteoarthritis,[1,2] or premature ECS synthetic material failure.

The bones that make up the stifle joint are the femur, tibia, and patella. The patella is a sesamoid bone (the largest sesamoid in the body) of the quadriceps muscles. There are three other sesamoid bones (fabellae) in the stifle joint, but these can be variable on which ones are present in any given stifle joint (Figure 50.1). Two of these sesamoids are the lateral and medial sesamoids of the gastrocnemius muscle (lateral and medial fabellae), and the attachment of the lateral femoral fabellae is often called the fabello-femoral ligament. This is not actually a ligament but is the tendon of origin of the gastrocnemius muscle to the femur. For descriptive purposes, this attachment will be called the fabello-femoral ligament in this chapter and is also called this term in other textbooks. The third sesamoid of the stifle other than the patella is the sesamoid of the popliteus muscle. In the author's experience, not all dogs have a lateral or medial fabella or a popliteal sesamoid. These differences can even be present in the same dog being different between the two hind limbs. This is a very good reminder and one of the reasons to perform pre-operative radiographs to determine the specific anatomy of the limb being operated. If there is no lateral fabella, a traditional extracapsular suture stabilization will not work, since there is no lateral fabella to anchor the synthetic material. In these patients, a bone anchor or femoral bone tunnel will be needed. It is much better to be prepared for that scenario prior to surgery via radiographs than to discover the lack of a lateral fabella during surgery and not have the appropriate hardware or backup surgical plan.

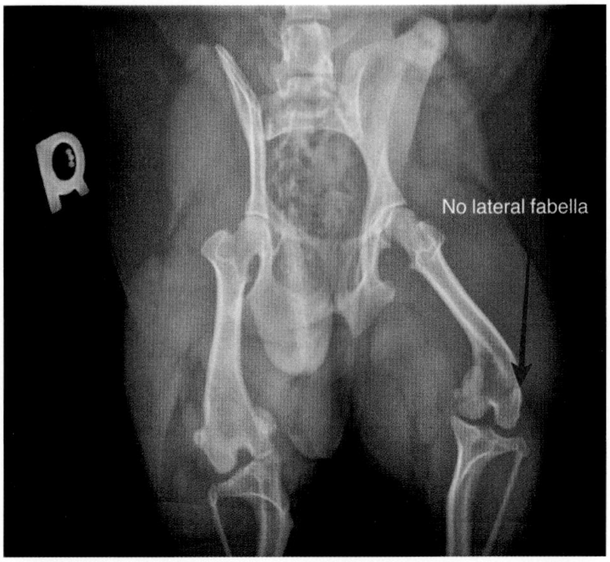

Figure 50.1 Radiograph of a small breed dog that is missing the left lateral fabella. Blue arrow is pointing to the absence of a lateral fabella. *Source:* © Trent Gall.

The popliteal sesamoid is also variable, both in its position (which can change on radiographs based on joint/limb position) and if it is present or not (Figures 50.2 and 50.3). This normal sesamoid can be mistaken for an intraarticular osseous body (joint mouse) on radiographs if the surgeon is not familiar with the normal anatomy.

The ligament stabilizers in the stifle are the medial collateral ligament (MCL), lateral collateral ligament, CrCL,

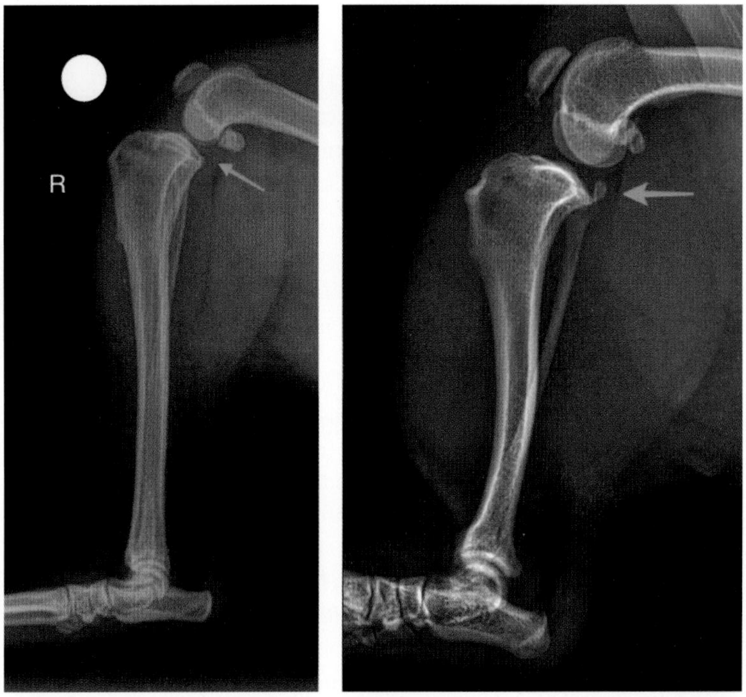

Figure 50.2 Radiograph of a dog with no right popliteal sesamoid (left image) and a radiograph of a dog with a popliteal sesamoid (right image). The green arrows point to the area of the popliteal sesamoid bone. On a cranial-caudal view of the dog with a popliteal sesamoid, the sesamoid can appear to be in the joint space. This is not an abnormal osseous body (joint mouse) but is a normal, but variable, anatomy. *Source:* © Trent Gall.

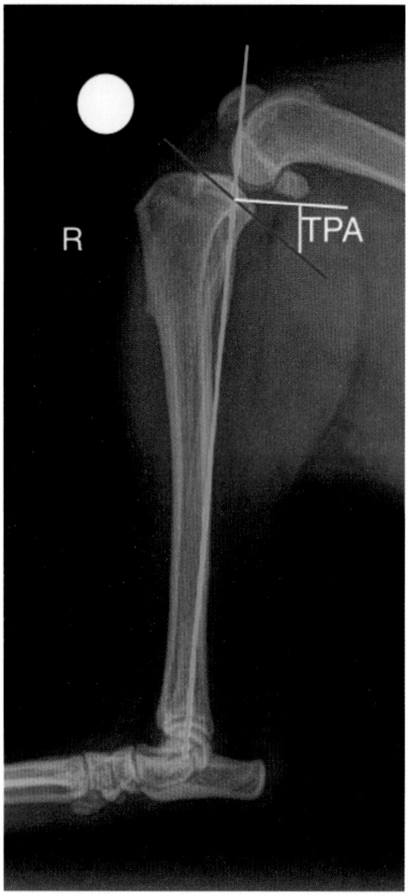

Figure 50.3 The TPA can be measured by drawing one vertical line from the center of the tarsus through the center of the intercondylar eminence (tibial long axis – green line). The second line is the top of the tibial plateau (tibial plateau axis – blue line), the reference line perpendicular to the tibial long axis line (white line). *Source:* © Trent Gall.

and caudal cruciate ligament (CdCL). The CrCL has two bands, the craniomedial band and the caudolateral band. There are also the two menisci, the medial and lateral menisci, and the patellar tendon that also provide stability to the stifle joint.

Pathophysiology

CrCL pathology is the leading cause of canine hind limb dysfunction. CrCL pathology can simplistically be broken down into three categories: (1) juvenile traumatic injuries, (2) mature/adult traumatic injuries, and (3) degenerative CrCL disease. Juvenile CrCL injuries are somewhat rare. These typically occur in skeletally immature animals that sustain a traumatic event. The Sharpey's fibers of the CrCL attaching to the bone are often stronger than the bone, which results in an avulsion fracture of either the insertion or origin of the CrCL with excess pressure. These injuries can be treated with re-attachment of the avulsed piece of bone if that osseous segment is large enough for surgical re-attachment, but since juvenile injuries also can result in a mid-body rupture of the CrCL itself, other treatment options are available.

Other treatment options for juvenile patients with CrCL tears include epiphysiodesis, CBLO, and a staged approach with eventual ECS placement. Performing an epiphysiodesis involves placing a transphyseal screw in a particular position to utilize the remaining growth of the proximal tibial physis. This technique closes the cranial aspect of the proximal tibial growth plate with the screw, and as the animal grows, the caudal aspect of the growth plate continues to grow while the cranial aspect is stopped from growing by the transphyseal screw. With this ideally controlled variation in growth across the proximal tibial physis, the tibial plateau angle (TPA) decreases, which effectively levels the TPA and creates stability, consistent with the theory behind a tibial plateau osteotomy (TPLO). This technique requires precise placement of the transphyseal screw and a relatively narrow age window to effectively level the tibial plateau.[3] Another technique is a corrective osteotomy that spares the growth plates, such as a CORA-based leveling osteotomy (CBLO). The final treatment option is conservative management until the animal is skeletally mature, followed by performing an ECS technique. An ECS should not be performed in young growing animals, since the ECS could constrain the joint too much, resulting in abnormal bone growth (causing an angular limb malformation) and/or excessive cartilage strain, which, as stated before, can lead to early progression of osteoarthritis.

Pure traumatic injuries are less common in veterinary medicine as compared to human medicine. These are the result of an acute excessive force being applied to the stifle joint. Traumatic CrCL injuries can happen in any age of animal, and if there is an isolated CrCL tear (i.e., not a deranged stifle with multiple ligamentous injuries), an ECS is an appropriate surgical stabilization for this type of injury. When exploring the stifle joint, it is usually noted that the torn ends of the CrCL have a frayed, mop-head appearance or even a hematoma on the CrCL. Once under general anesthesia, these animals should be closely evaluated for damage to the other ligaments and stabilizers of the stifle, such as the collateral ligaments and caudal cruciate ligament. It is recommended to assess for medial and lateral instability (i.e., valgus and varus, respectively) and the presence of caudal drawer (i.e., proximal tibial subluxation caudally in relation to the distal femur). When three or more stabilizing ligaments in the stifle are damaged, this is referred to as a deranged stifle. In the author's experience, this is more common in cats than in dogs. The repair for a deranged stifle diagnosis is beyond the scope of this chapter.

The most common type of stifle pathology is a degenerative process of the CrCL. Despite years of study and countless publications, the exact mechanism is yet to be understood on why the CrCL can undergo this disease process. Most likely, there are both genetic and environmental factors that contribute to this disease process, which is seemingly why the contralateral CrCL can become affected in approximately 22–54% of patients.[4–9] Given the high predilection to the contralateral limb being affected, it is highly advisable to pass this information to the owners to prepare them for the possibility of the contralateral limb experiencing a CrCL injury at some point in the future. To date, there have been three studies looking at the heritability of CrCL rupture in purebred dogs in three high-risk breeds for CrCL injuries: the Newfoundland, the Labrador Retriever, and the Boxer. Looking at these three studies together, the heritability is in the range of 0.3–0.5 (approximately 30–50% chance that the disease risk is genetic), and one can extrapolate that the general canine population with CrCL disease has a genetic component as well. For further information on the proposed cause of CrCL disease, an in depth description of the pathophysiology of CrCL disease can be found in the two following text books: *Advances In The Canine Cranial Cruciate Ligament*, second edition, ed. Peter Muir. *Veterinary Surgery Small Animal*, second edition, eds. Spencer A. Johnston and Karen M. Tobias.

Pre-operative Considerations/Indications

Patient Selection

To optimize surgical success, it is key to carefully select patients for any surgical procedure. ECS stabilization is one of these procedures in which case selection has a direct impact on surgical success. Increased body weight and younger age have been associated with increased risk of postoperative complications.[10] The authors of this study found that younger dogs have an increased risk of complications, and they speculated that this is due to increased activity of the young dogs with more challenging post-op exercise restrictions. They also noted that heavier dogs had an increased risk of complications. While the authors didn't give specific guidelines on what age or weight would be optimal in performing ECS surgery, many surgeons, including this author, have some "loose" guidelines for this recommendation.

In this author's experience, dogs weighing over 40 lb are not ideal candidates for ECS surgery, and young and/or active dogs are not ideal ECS candidates, presumably due to increased activity and difficulty in successfully limiting their activity postoperatively. Middle age to older dogs and those that lead a more sedentary lifestyle seem to be better ECS surgical candidates, but, as stated above, these are "loose" guidelines. The patient's activity, ability to be appropriately restricted postoperatively, owners' expectations, patient co-morbidities, and finances all play a role in selecting patients for ECS stabilization. Another factor to consider is the patient's TPA. Many surgeons express concern that with a higher TPA, there is a higher ECS failure rate or decreased long-term successful clinical outcome. A study that specifically looked at small breed dogs (<20 kg) with a TPA above 30° found that those who had a TPLO performed had better long-term clinical outcomes and were less likely to require NSAID administration than those dogs that underwent a lateral fabello-tibial suture procedure.[11] In this author's experience, this general rule seems to apply. Measurement of the TPA on pre-surgical radiographs is another reason to perform high quality radiographs prior to surgical decision-making (Figure 50.3).

Patients with suspected partial CrCL injuries also are not considered ideal candidates for ECS stabilization, since these patients lack substantial laxity in the stifle to begin with. Knowing the limitations of a surgical technique is imperative to surgical success and how to direct clients in decision-making.

Diagnosis

The diagnosis of a CrCL injury is based on the signalment and history of the patient, the physical examination, and radiographic signs. The history of the lameness can be variable but typically for an acute tear of the CrCL, the patient often presents for a non-weight-bearing to minimally weight-bearing lameness of the hind limb. Another typical presentation is a waxing and waning lameness that is worse after exercise and worse after getting up from a lying position. The physical exam often finds a hind limb lameness at a walk and trot. Often, these patients will "kick out" the affected limb while sitting to avoid full flexion of the stifle joint; this is referred to as a positive "sit test." Patients with a CrCL injury are typically painful on full flexion and extension of the stifle, and dogs with suspected partial tears are often painful on full extension of the stifle. Stifle effusion is often palpated by feeling over the medial and lateral aspects of the patellar tendon and appreciating the loss of the sharp edge of this tendon. Medial periarticular fibrosis can be felt on the proximal part of the tibia; this is termed medial buttress.

The cranial drawer test is a good test for determining the degree of laxity from a torn CrCL. The cranial drawer test is performed by first placing the dog in lateral recumbency with the affected leg facing up. One hand is placed on the femur with the pointer finger on the patella and the thumb on the lateral fabella, ensuring that the thumb gradually slides into position from cranial to caudal to avoid pinching the peroneal nerve when grasping the fabella. This hand is simply stabilizing the femur to prevent movement when the other hand is manipulating the tibia. The second hand is placed on the tibia with the pointer finger on the tibial tuberosity and the thumb on the fibular head. The hand on the tibia is then moved cranially while the hand on the femur is kept still and stabilizing the femur from moving. This cranial translation is the “cranial drawer sign.” Dogs with partial tears usually don’t have cranial drawer unless the knee is in flexion and only the craniomedial band of the CrCL is torn. It is advised to perform the cranial drawer test in flexion, extension, and a standing angle.

A cranial tibial compression test can be performed as well. This is performed by placing a hand on the femur with the thumb on the fabella, and the pointer finger spans the joint and places caudal pressure on the tibial tuberosity, which is somewhat mimicking the position and pressure of a fabello-tibial suture. The limb is positioned at a standing angle, and the second hand is placed on the foot and then flexes the hock joint. A positive cranial tibial compression test is if the proximal tibia subluxates cranially relative to the femur when the hock is flexed. This maneuver takes more practice to effectively utilize, but if the patient is very tense, large, or heavily muscled, a tibial compression test is often easier to perform successfully in diagnosing stifle instability than eliciting cranial drawer motion. Sedation may be needed to help confirm the diagnosis and can be very helpful when performing radiographs to get ideal positioning.

Radiographs are highly recommended to help confirm the tentative diagnosis of a CrCL injury, rule out other differentials, such as neoplasia or infection, and to assess the patient’s anatomy for surgical planning. As mentioned above, the patient’s anatomy can play a key role in what procedure to advise (e.g., higher TPA or lack of lateral fabella may negate the ECS option). Another benefit of preoperative radiographs is that it gives a baseline of the presence of osteoarthritis. Well-positioned radiographs are essential to accurately evaluating the patient’s anatomy, as well as identifying subtle changes that are consistent with a CrCL injury. The best positioning for a diagnostic stifle radiograph is a perfectly lateral view with the stifle in the center of the beam. The femoral condyles are directly, or as close as possible to directly, superimposed. The stifle and hock joint are at 90° (a “90/90 view”). The X-ray beam is centered on the stifle joint, and the radiograph incorporates the hock in the field of view. Collimation is important to achieve as detailed radiographs as possible (Figures 50.4–50.6).

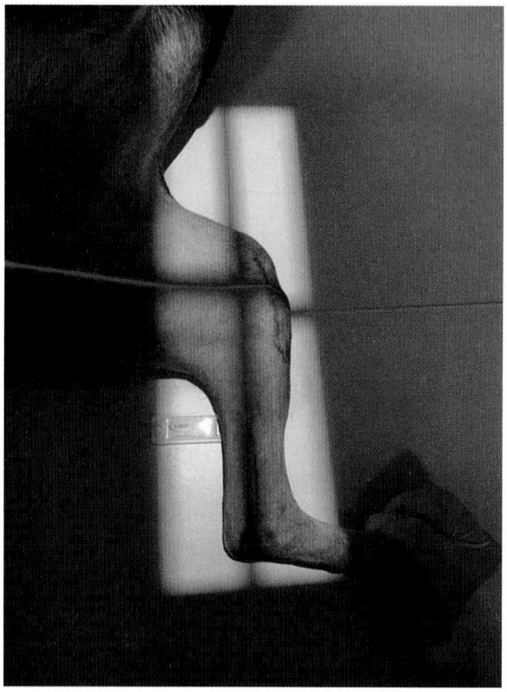

Figure 50.4 The patient is in lateral recumbency with the stifle and hock positioned at 90° angles. The X-ray beam is centered on the stifle joint, and the hock joint is in the field of view. While this image shows an unprotected hand holding the hind paw in position for demonstration purposes, there are commercially-available blocks to assist in positioning the patient’s limb without exposing staff to unnecessary radiation. *Source:* © Trent Gall.

Suture Material Selection

There are many ECS materials on the market. The two broad categories of suture used for ECS are nylon leader line and braided material, and there are multiple brands of each on the market. Each material type has its own pros and cons to the use and application of ECS material. Nylon leader line has been in use in veterinary medicine for many years and is still a very tried and true material to use. The benefits of nylon leader line are the ease of application, affordable instrumentation for placement, inexpensive material, and has been studied extensively over the years. The downside of nylon leader line is that it has a lower tensile strength compared to braided material. Also, when tying knots in the leader line, there is considerable knot “bulk,” but this can be mitigated by using leader line size-specific crimp clamps on certain sizes of leader line. Currently, the nylon leader line sizes come in 20-, 40-, 60-, 80-, and 100-lb test weights. However, only 40-, 80-, and 100-lb test weights come with crimp clamps of the same sizes.

The advantage of using crimp clamps is their low profile nature, which decreases soft tissue irritation compared to a bulky knot, and the crimp clamps are stronger than using knots.[12] A rough guideline for which suture size to use is to use the patient’s weight. For example, if the patient is 15 lb then the appropriate choice would be 20-lb test weight. If the patient was 41 lb the appropriate weight would be either 60- or 80-lb test weight. The author prefers to use nylon leader line with crimp clamps and avoids 60-lb test

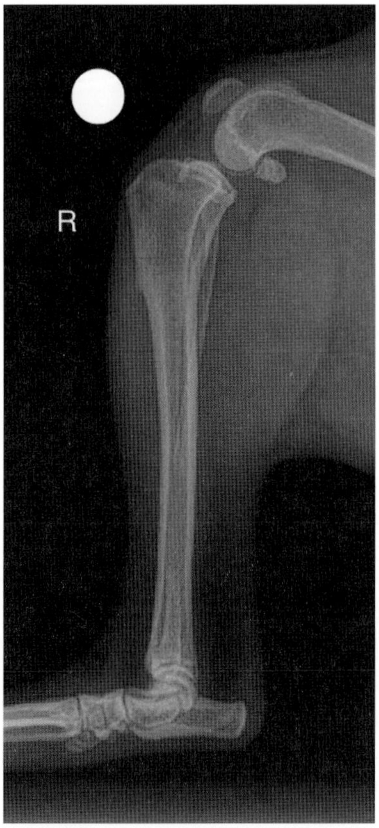

Figure 50.5 The femoral condyles are directly superimposed over each other. Note in this radiograph there is stifle effusion (cranial displacement of the fat pad and caudal out-pouching of the caudal joint pouch). The tibia is also in slight cranial drawer, as the intercondylar imminence should be more directly below the femoral condyle. These are all signs consistent with a CrCL injury. *Source:* © Trent Gall.

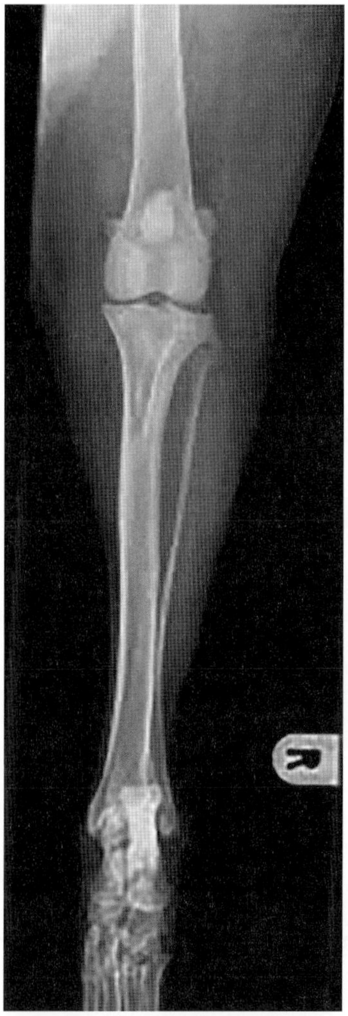

Figure 50.6 A straight anterior/posterior (AP), cranial/caudal view, or a caudal/cranial view. Note the patella is centered, the fabellae are symmetrically bisected by the femoral cortices, and the hock joint is straight. *Source:* © Trent Gall.

weight, since this would be a very large suture knot and impossible to get a secure knot. The 20-lb test weight is small enough that the suture knot is usually not an issue with smaller patients. That being said, the author has had several small patients with very little muscle mass and thin skin where the 20-lb knot caused a persistent seroma. In one case, the nylon leader line and knot was removed and replaced with a softer braided material, which successfully resolved the underlying soft tissue irritation due to the knot and secondary seroma.

When using crimp tubes (Figure 50.7), which are placed around the leader line and then crimped to hold it in position, a crimping tool is needed. It is important to note that the surgeon should not mix and match materials and instrumentation from different manufacturers. Each crimping tool is calibrated to the specific manufacturer's crimp clamp or tube. By mixing and matching systems, it is possible to either overcrimp, which could transect the leader line or tube, or under-crimp the crimp tube, which could lead to suture slippage and implant failure. For example,

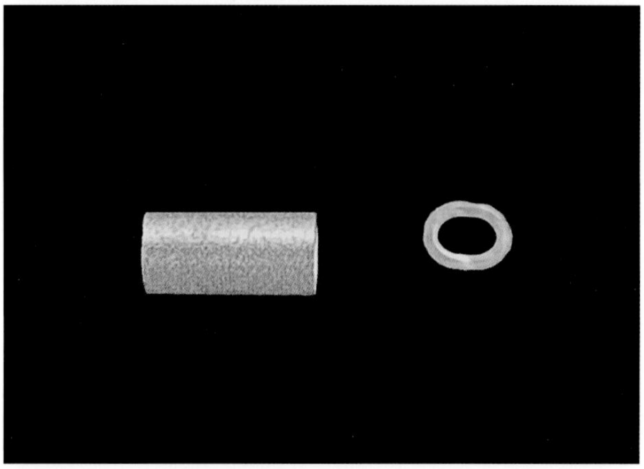

Figure 50.7 Example of a 40-lb stainless steel crimp tube. Some companies also add special coatings, such as titanium-nitride, to their crimp tubes. *Source:* © Trent Gall.

do not use Securos leader line with an Everost crimping tool. Stay with the same manufacturer for whichever system you choose. Some manufacturer's crimping tools have a "stopper" to know when the crimp tube is adequately compressed enough to securely hold the suture or leader line. This is useful to prevent under- or overcrimping of the crimp tube (Figures 50.8 and 50.9).

There are multiple options for obtaining suture to use for ECS placement. The first option is an individually-wrapped suture with the swaged-on needle of particular sizes (Figure 50.10), which is very convenient, since it uses a one-time use a sharp swaged-on needle (Figure 50.11), is of appropriate suture length for ECS placement in CrCL injuries, and is sterile in the pack. The second option is to purchase a roll of nonsterilized nylon leader line (e.g., essentially, fishing line), cut anticipated lengths of suture that are needed for the procedure, and then sterilize the strands individually. With this second option, a variety of cruciate needles would be needed to have on hand, since these will be non-swaged-on sutures that require threading at the time of surgery. When sterilizing the length of suture material, be sure to cut off enough suture material to easily work with. The author prefers approximately 14–18 in. (35.56–45.72 cm). Another tip is to sterilize the nylon leader line strand in a double peel pouch. This way, the surgeon can take the inner pouch when the outer pouch is opened over the surgical field since the line likes to "spring" out. According to the company, it is not recommended to steam-sterilize nylon leader line more than once, since multiple steam sterilization cycles can weaken the nylon leader line.

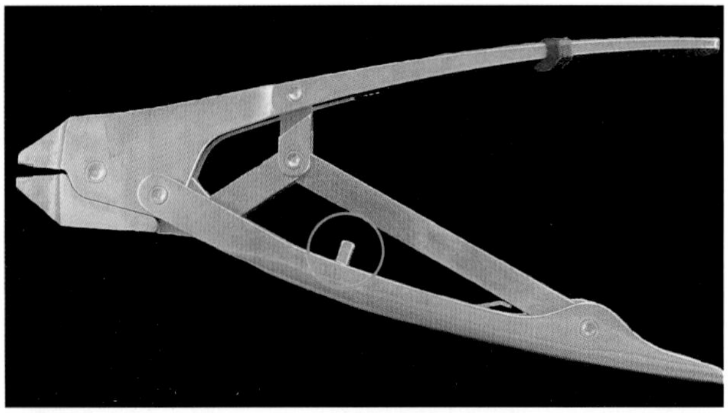

Figure 50.8 The stopper on a Securos® "Power X" crimping tool to prevent under- or overtensioning of the crimp tube. This picture is of the crimping tool in the open position. *Source:* © Trent Gall.

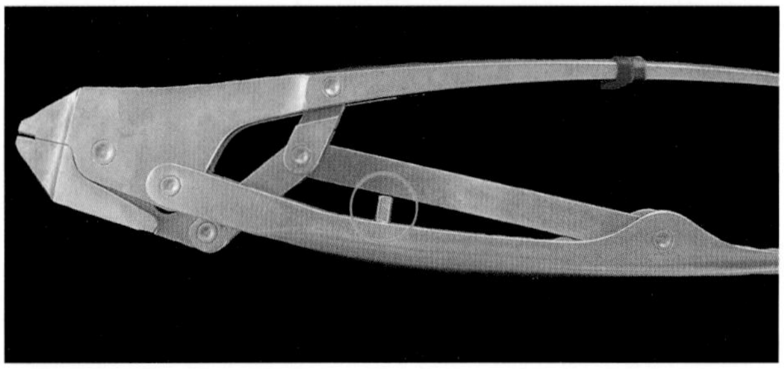

Figure 50.9 The stopper is in the closed position. With this Securos® "Power X" crimping tool, it is impossible to overcrimp a crimp tube. If the crimping tool is fully compressed, the surgeon knows the crimp tube is fully crimped. *Source:* © Trent Gall.

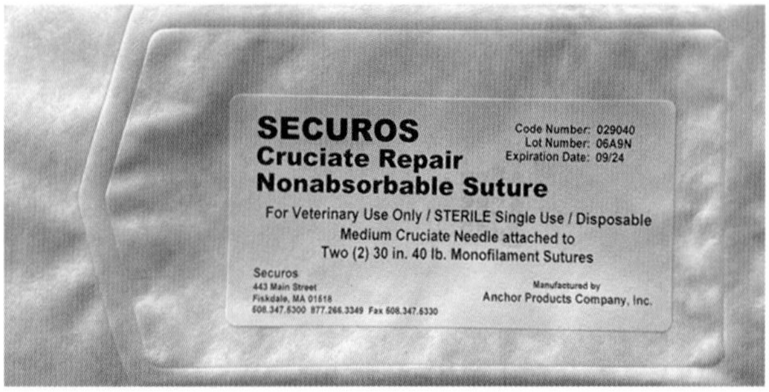

Figure 50.10 Example of a pre-made suture "kit," which includes a double-stranded swaged-on needle with two lines of suture material. *Source:* © Trent Gall.

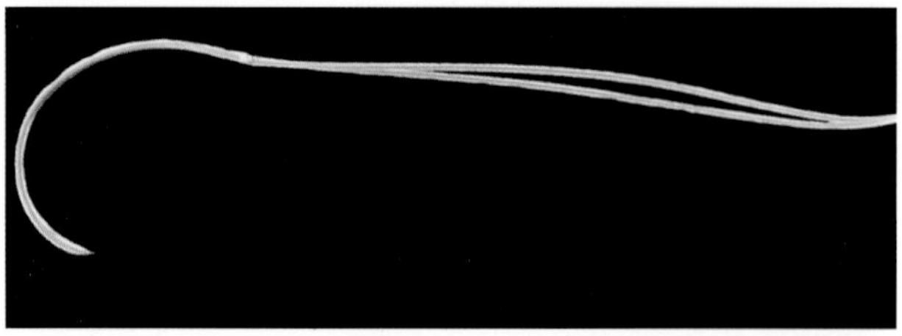

Figure 50.11 Example of a swaged-on needle with double strands of leader line. *Source:* © Trent Gall.

Tools that are helpful in the surgeon's armamentarium for performing an ECS placement with nylon leader line are the following: a crimping tool (specific to the crimp tubes and the leader line, use the same manufacturer), a tensioning device (helps tension the leader line with precision by allowing for various suture tension assessments during stifle range of motion prior to final clamp crimping), and a Jacobs chuck and key for drilling the proximal tibial bone tunnel(s) with a Steinmann pin (Figure 50.12).

In surgery, the extracapsular fabello-tibial leader line can be placed as either a single strand or a double strand. The author prefers using a double strand with two crimp clamps (one crimp tube on each nylon line). The double-strand technique is stronger than a single-strand technique.[13] Once the material is passed around the lateral fabella and through a tibial tunnel(s), the material is tensioned and then either tied or crimp-clamped to secure its position (Figure 50.13).

There are multiple braided suture options for performing an ECS procedure (Figure 50.14). The pros to using a braided suture material are that these materials have a higher tensile strength compared to nylon leader line and are made of a softer material, which perceivably could

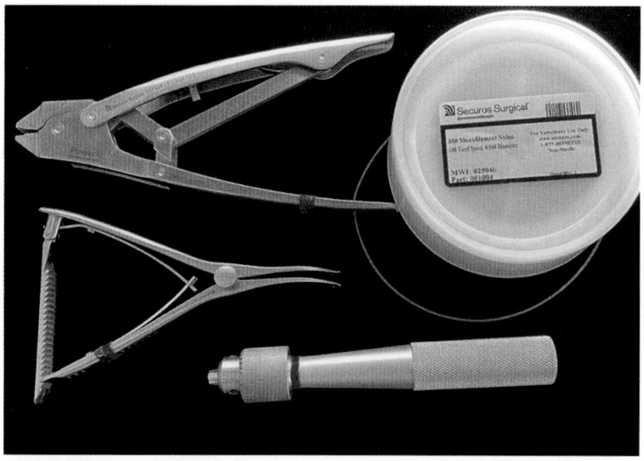

Figure 50.12 Instrumentation for performing an ECS stabilization using nylon leader line. Crimping tool (Securos® Power X), tensioner, Jacobs chuck, spool of unsterilized nylon 80# leader line. *Source:* © Trent Gall.

result in less potential tissue irritation at the level of the cut suture ends compared to firm leader line edges. The cons to using a braided suture is that there is a potential for a higher infection rate compared to monofilament given that braided material can harbor bacteria. Other contraindications include that braided material can "saw" through

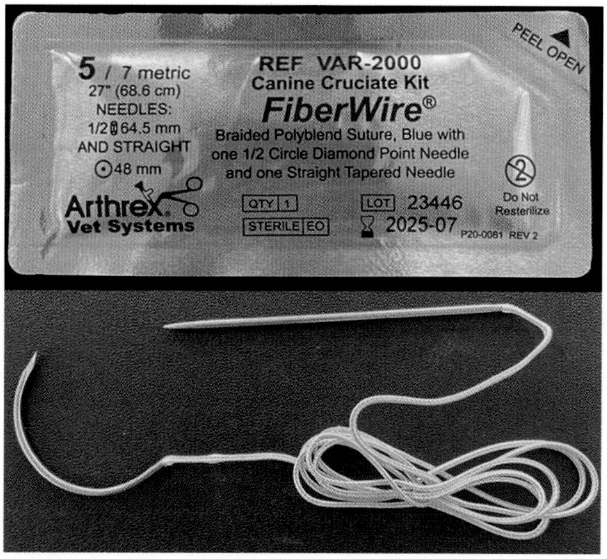

Figure 50.14 Example of a braided material (FiberWire™ by Arthrex®) and the cruciate ligament "kit." *Source:* © Trent Gall.

the fabello-femoral ligament, and since the material is sometimes stronger than the fabello-femoral ligament, it can avulse the fabella with excessive force. The braided material is also often much more expensive than the nylon

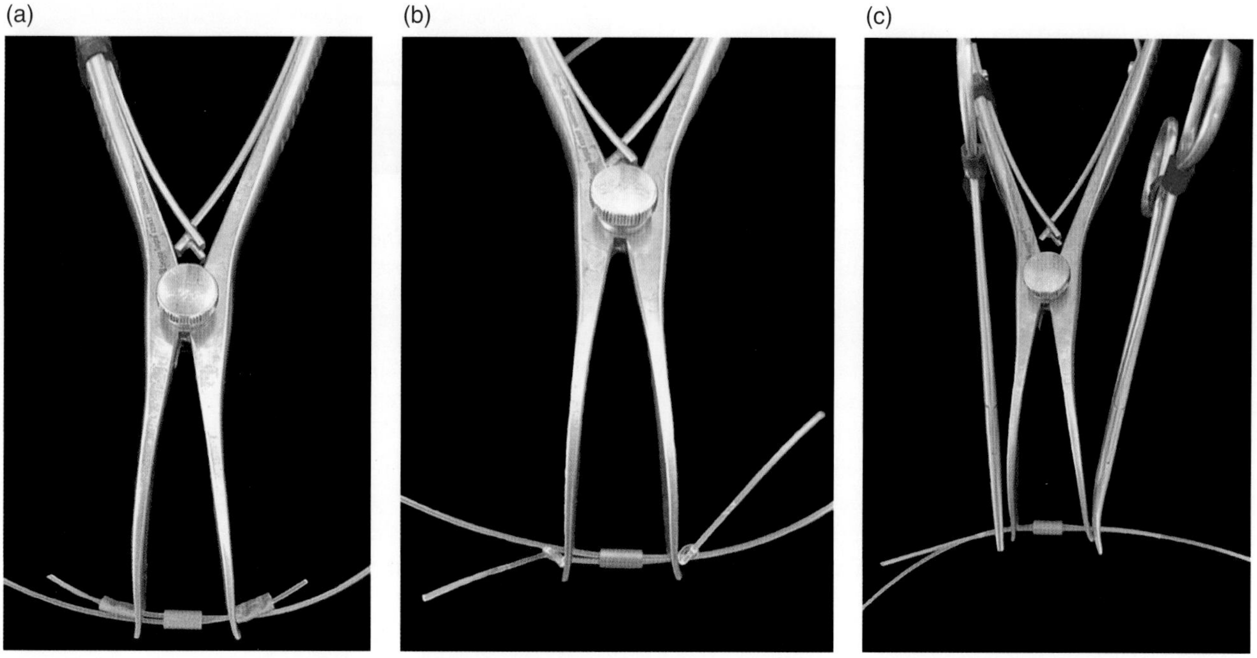

Figure 50.13 Three examples of ways to tension the ECS nylon leader line. (a) Using a three crimp clamp technique. One central crimp clamp has the two ends of the nylon running through it in opposite directions. Two additional crimp clamps are placed on the free ends of the nylon (one strand each) then crimped. The tensioner is then placed between the two free end clamps and tensioned; finally, the central crimp clamp is then crimped once appropriate tension is achieved. (b) Using a knot technique. A central crimp clamp is placed as described in (a), and a knot is placed on each free end of the suture material to give the tensioner something to press against. The tensioner is then placed between the two knots until tensioned as desired, and the central clamp is then crimped (three crimps are recommended per tube). (c) Using a hemostat technique. A central crimp clamp is placed as described in (a), and the tensioner is placed between two hemostats that are placed on the free ends of the nylon (one strand only in each hemostat). The tensioner is then tensioned as desired, and the central crimp clamp is then crimped in place. *Source:* © Trent Gall.

leader line. Strict asepsis is needed for any surgery in which an implant is being used, but an even higher standard of asepsis is needed when using a braided material. When using a braided material, the author performs a "dirty" scrub in the induction area with chlorhexidine scrub followed by alcohol rinse, performed three times. The patient is then transported to the operating room. Typically, once the patient is connected to the anesthesia machine and gas inhalant, positioned, and connected to monitoring equipment, the limb is dry and ready for a hanging leg surgical scrub. For this aseptic OR preparation, the author performs a second chlorhexidine scrub with sterile saline using sterile gloves, followed by an iodine-based solution (DuraPrep™ by 3M™). This is allowed to air dry for three to five minutes, then an iodine-impregnated sticky drape is placed over the limb once the patient is draped in (Ioban™ by 3M™). This extra scrub protocol seems to help decrease the chance of both the braided material and the surgeon from coming into contact with the skin, which can never be fully sterilized; just aseptically prepared.

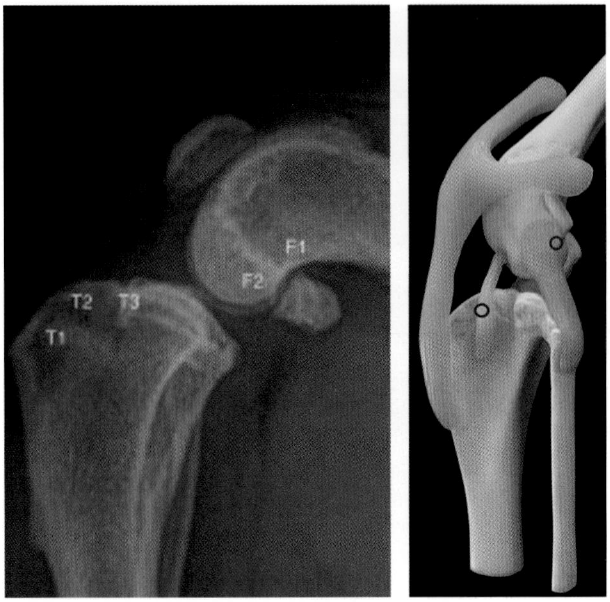

Figure 50.15 Femoral and tibial anchor sites. Based on experimental data, F2 and T3 are the most desirable of the quasi-isometric points.[14] *Source:* © Trent Gall.

Locations and Methods for Securing ECS Material to the Femur and Tibia

The goal of any ECS is to eliminate excessive internal rotation and cranial tibial drawer motion in flexion and extension. This is achieved by a strong material that is anchored onto the femur and the tibia in perfect isometric locations (i.e., the material is in the same amount of tension through stifle range of motion). Unfortunately, in the clinical setting, there is no perfect isometric location on the femur and tibia. The closest that we can get is "quasi-isometric" due to the cam-shaped femur and individual differences in anatomy. For this reason, there are multiple variations of anchor points. The classic femoral anchor point loops the suture around the lateral fabella (if it is present) through the fabello-femoral ligament, and an alternative anchor point on the femur uses a bone anchor, for which, there are many bone anchors on the market at various price points. This femoral anchor site is often called the F2 location, which is derived from a cadaveric study attempting to identify isometric points for ECS placement (Figure 50.15).[14]

If using a bone anchor, it is recommended to predrill the hole using a power drill with a drill bit of the appropriate size corresponding to the size of the bone anchor (Figure 50.16). The anchor must be angled slightly proximal and cranial to avoid coming out the backside of the femur and to avoid the femoral notch, which could damage cartilage, damage the origin of the caudal cruciate ligament, or be a source of continued pain or discomfort (Figure 50.17).

Landmarks on the tibia that are helpful for ECS placement are the *tubercle of Gerdy* and *Gerdy's "sister."* Gerdy's "sister" point does not have a formal name. The *tubercle of Gerdy* is often easily palpated as the protuberance just cranial to the long digital extensor (LDE) tendon groove, and *Gerdy's "sister"* is the smaller protuberance on the caudal aspect of the LDE groove. According to one study, the ideal location for the tibial anchor point is the T3 site (Figure 50.15).[14,15] This site is quite proximal on the tibia, just below the joint (approximately 2–3 mm), just cranial to Gerdy's "sister" in the LDE groove but under the LDE, and on the angled portion of the proximomedial tibia. Another site that is slightly less quasi-isometric but is easier to access is the T2 site. This T2 site can be easier to visualize by elevating the cranial tibial muscle.

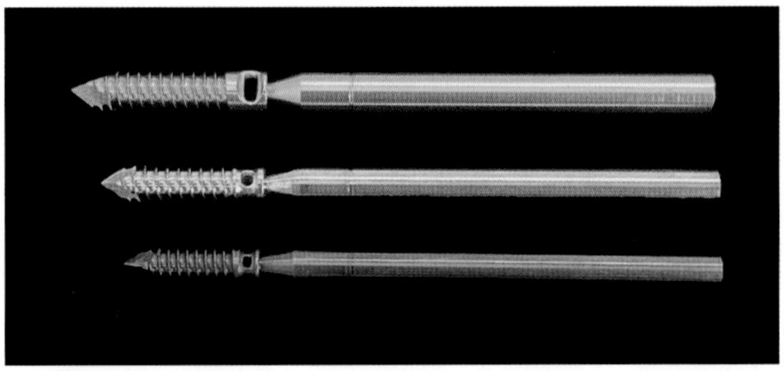

Figure 50.16 Examples of titanium bone anchors (Securos®) with a break-away insertion shaft. It is recommended that a hole is predrilled with the appropriate drill bit, then after the bone anchor is screwed into place and appropriately seated in the bone, the shaft is snapped off. Technically, it is possible to insert bone anchors with cutting threads, such as these in the above image, without pre-drilling a hole. There are many other bone anchors on the market; this is only one example. *Source:* © Trent Gall.

The tibial anchor point can either be via one or two bone tunnels. The first of the methods utilizing one bone tunnel

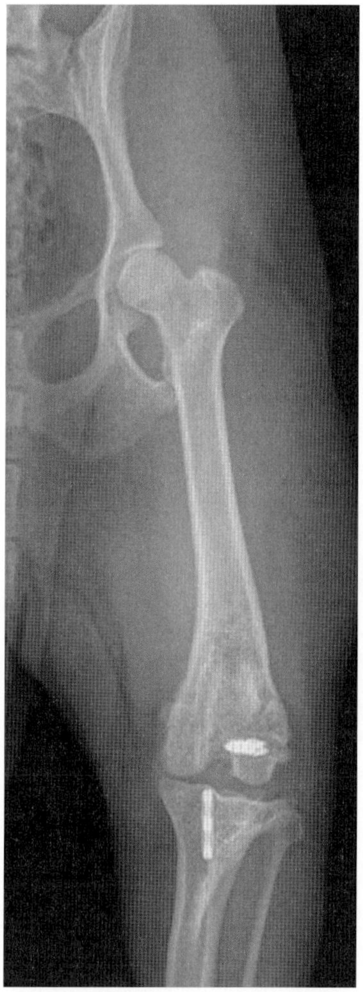

Figure 50.17 Bone anchor placement. Note the bone anchor is not intruding into the trochlear notch, although the bone anchor could have ideally been angled slightly more proximally (towards the hip). This patient also has a suture button on the tibia for anchoring the suture material to the tibia. *Source:* © Trent Gall.

involves the suture passing through the single bone tunnel, through a suture button, and back through the same bone tunnel (Figure 50.18), followed by the suture being tensioned and then tied or crimped.

The tibia anchor point can also be two bone tunnels. The second bone tunnel is placed roughly 5–10 mm distal and slightly cranial to the first bone tunnel or directly distal to the first tunnel. The second bone tunnel should not be below the level of the insertion of the patellar tendon. Since this distance between the two bone tunnels is a sort of "bone bridge," care must be taken to make sure this is not too narrow; otherwise, with tension (by the surgeon or by the patient during or after recovery), this "bone bridge" can break away and lose stabilization of the stifle joint (Figure 50.19).

A third way (second method utilizing one bone tunnel) to anchor to the tibia in ECS placement is through one proximal tibial bone tunnel as previously described, exiting

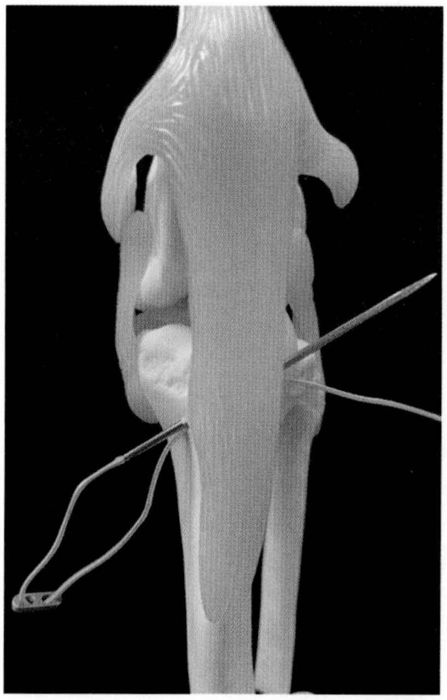

Figure 50.18 Placement of one proximal tibial bone tunnel using a suture button. Note the angle of the tunnel trajectory to match the forces being placed on the suture going to the lateral fabella or corresponding femoral bone anchor.
Source: © Trent Gall.

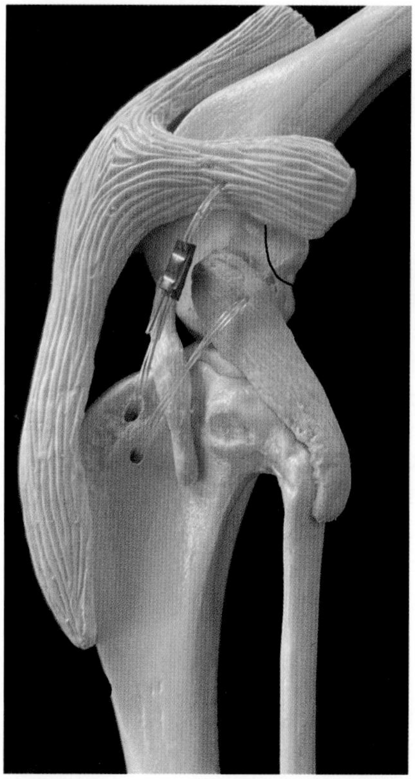

Figure 50.19 Tibial bone tunnel placement for using a two bone tunnel technique utilizing the T2 tibial anchor point and a second tunnel directly distal to T2. *Source:* © Trent Gall.

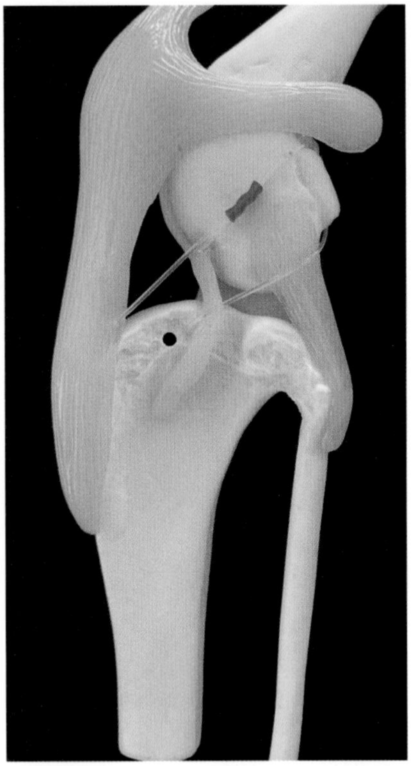

Figure 50.20 One proximal tibial bone tunnel technique, in which the suture is passed through the tunnel then under the patellar tendon, as close to the tendon as possible to try to avoid entering the joint. *Source:* © Trent Gall.

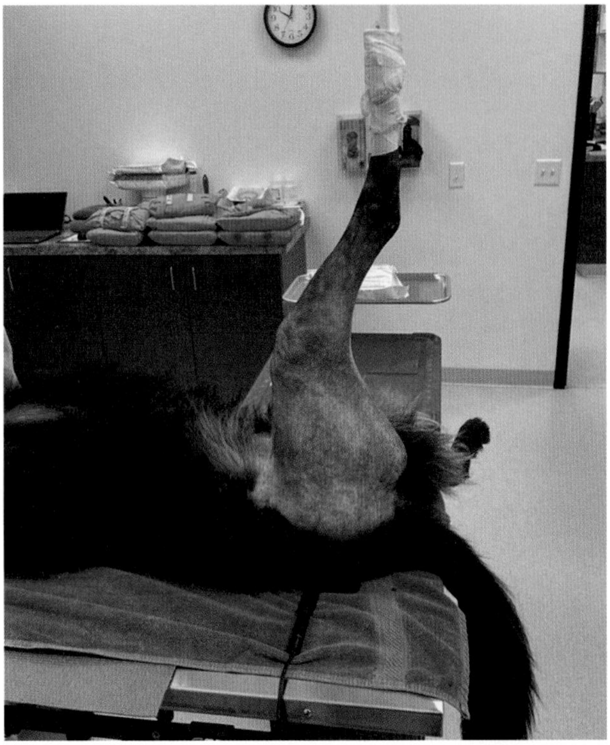

Figure 50.21 Example of a patient being positioned at the end of the surgical table and the limb being prepared for a "hanging limb" surgical scrub. *Source:* © Trent Gall.

medially on the tibia, then passing the suture under the patellar tendon in the space between the joint capsule and patellar tendon (Figure 50.20).

The author has had to remove several extracapsular sutures that have been passed under the patellar tendon but unfortunately into the stifle joint, and due to the presumed intra-articular irritation from this suture, these were converted to a one tibial bone tunnel with a suture button technique. Care must be taken not to place the bone tunnel(s) too cranial or distal on the tibia. The tibial tuberosity is very easy to approach in this area, and it is tempting to place the bone tunnel(s) in this location; however, this is a terrible location due to lack of isometry. If the tibial anchor point is placed in the tibial tuberosity, the stifle will be stable in flexion and extension, but this anchor point will put undue stress on the suture material through normal stifle movements due to being overly taut in certain positions and then overly loose in other positions during a range of motion.

Surgical Technique

Positioning

The patient is positioned with the hind limbs close to the end of the table, and the surgeon stands at the "foot" of the surgical table (Figure 50.21). The patient is positioned in dorsal recumbency, slightly obliqued away from the surgery limb (i.e., obliqued toward the contralateral laterality). The patient is positioned in this way for easy access to the lateral aspect of the limb. The other three limbs are tied to the table to minimize patient movement. A "V" trough, towels, or "V'ed" surgical table can be used to help keep the patient in the dorsal obliqued position.

Sterile Preparation

A standard surgical "hanging limb" surgical scrub is performed. This is performed by first placing an exam glove over the hind paw and then wrapping the paw with porous white tape. This tape is then hung from a surgical lamp, an IV pole, or from a ceiling-mounted system. Once the surgical scrub is performed, the surgeon is scrubbed in and the limb has been sterilely quarter-draped as far proximally as possible, a waterproof wrap (sterilized aluminum foil, sterilized drape material, etc.) is placed over the foot by the surgeon. Sterile self-adherent bandaging material (e.g., 3M™ Vetrap™) is then wrapped around the waterproof material. This allows the surgeon to manipulate the whole limb while staying sterile by not touching the distal limb/foot. This material can be purchased in sterile form, such as 3M™ Coban™, or this bandaging material can be

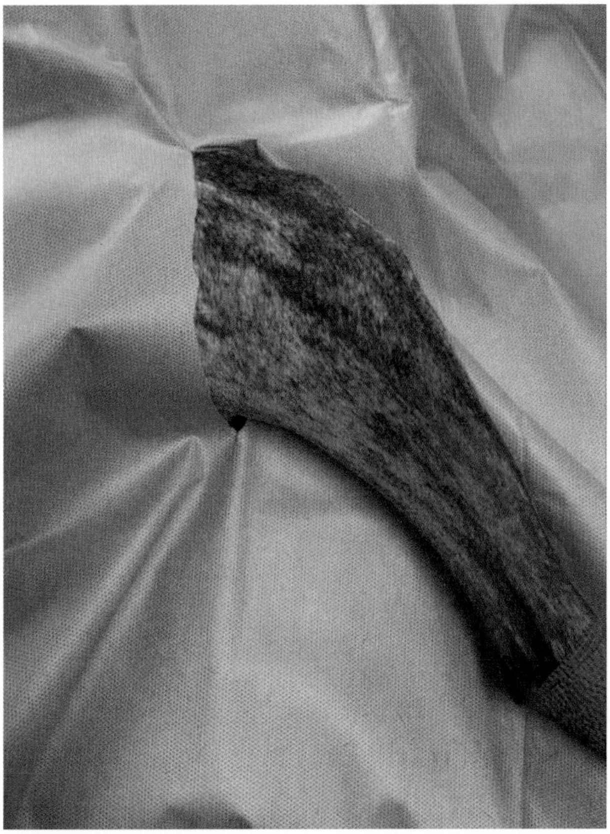

Figure 50.22 Patient positioned in obliqued dorsal recumbency. This is a lateral view of the right hind limb. The patient's head is towards the top of the picture, and the tail is towards the bottom of the picture. *Source:* © Trent Gall.

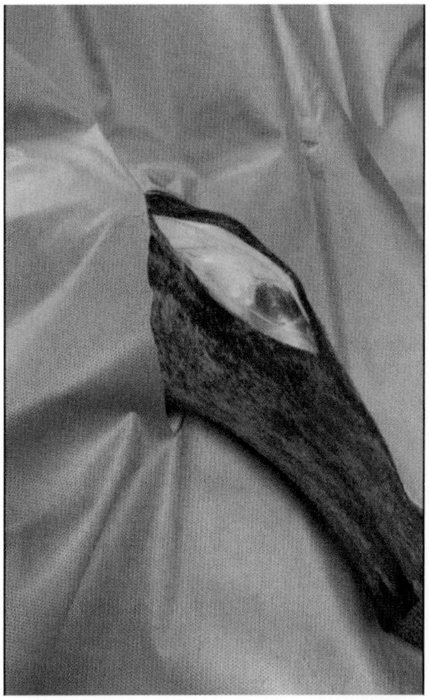

Figure 50.23 Craniolateral skin incision is made from proximal to the patella to distal to the tibial tuberosity. *Source:* © Trent Gall.

sterilized via steam autoclave, which is the most common and economical practice. Another sterilization practice is either plasma sterilization or ethylene oxide gas sterilization (EtO). The patient is then draped with a sterile surgical drape (Figure 50.22).

Approach

A craniolateral skin incision is performed from proximal to the patella to just distal to the tibial tuberosity (Figure 50.23). The subcutaneous tissues are gently dissected to the point of the lateral biceps fascia. Either a lateral parapatellar arthrotomy or a medial parapatellar arthrotomy is performed (by reflecting the skin incision over the medial aspect of the stifle joint) (Figure 50.24). The author prefers to perform a medial parapatellar arthrotomy for several reasons. A medial parapatellar arthrotomy makes visualization of the medial joint compartment easier than the lateral approach, especially since the medial meniscus has a much higher incidence of damage requiring intervention than the lateral meniscus. Also, by performing a medial parapatellar arthrotomy, the lateral joint capsule is left untouched which makes the placement of the ECS material easier.

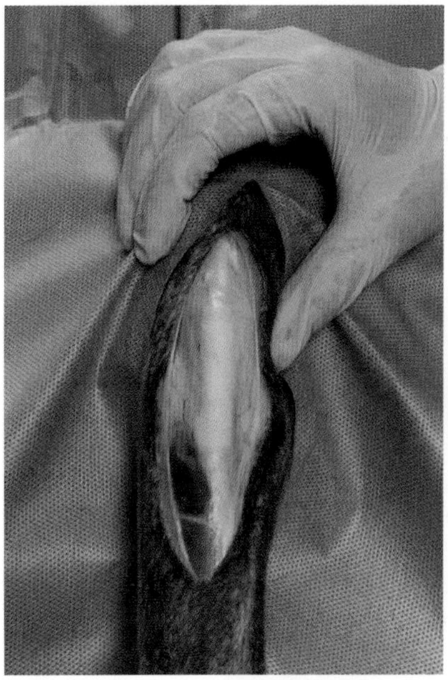

Figure 50.24 After the craniolateral incision is made through the skin and subcutaneous layers, the incision is reflected medially to perform a medial parapatellar arthrotomy. If performing a lateral parapatellar arthrotomy, this step is not needed. *Source:* © Trent Gall.

When performing a lateral parapatellar arthrotomy, the surgeon must be very careful not to cut the long digital extensor tendon. This is completely avoided by performing a medial parapatellar arthrotomy.

Arthrotomy

An arthrotomy is performed mid-way between the patella and tibial tuberosity with a #11 blade (see Figures 50.25–50.27 for details). The CrCL is visualized, and the torn portion

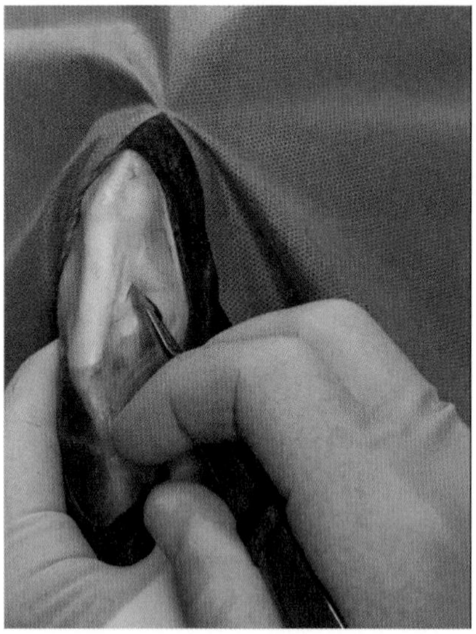

Figure 50.25 Stab incision with a #11 blade is made into the medial parapatellar space, approximately 1/3 (between proximal 1/3 and distal 2/3) to 1/2 distance between the patella and tibial tuberosity. Aim the blade proximally towards the patella. A tip is to make a stab incision 3–4 mm medial to the patellar tendon, which leaves enough tissue to be able to place suture for closure. Do not aim distally with the blade. The cranial pole of the meniscus is immediately distal to this location and care must be taken to avoid cutting the cranial pole of the meniscus. *Source:* © Trent Gall.

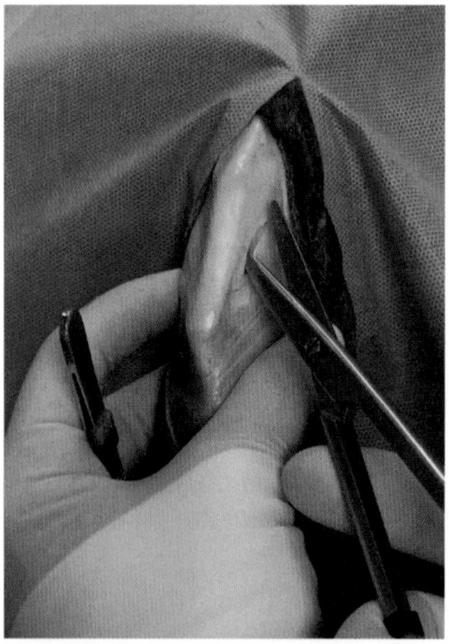

Figure 50.26 The medial parapatellar arthrotomy is extended proximally with Mayo (ideally, curved) scissors. As the incision is continued proximally, aim away from the patella. *Source:* © Trent Gall.

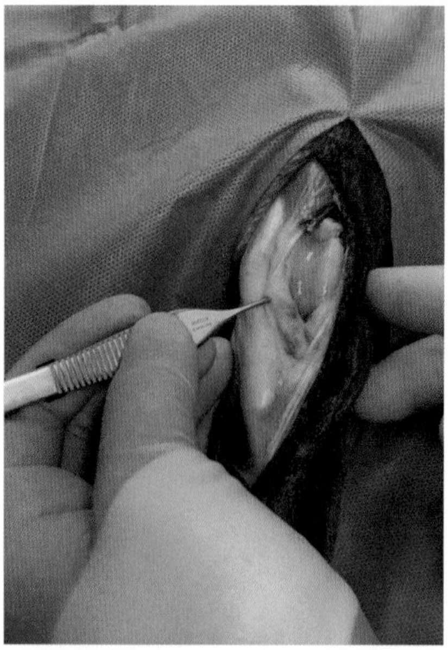

Figure 50.27 The patella is luxated laterally to give full exposure to the joint. Note that sometimes on larger dogs and more heavily-muscled dogs, some muscle fibers will need to be split proximal and medial to the patella to get this exposure. As the surgeon gains experience with stifle explores, a "mini" arthrotomy can be performed, where the patella is not fully luxated. However, the full stifle arthrotomy with luxation of the patella gives the best exposure for thorough stifle explore. *Source:* © Trent Gall.

can be debrided with single-action rongeurs for better visualization of the menisci. The caudal cruciate ligament is palpated with a meniscal probe to confirm that it is intact. The medial meniscus is then probed with a meniscal probe to assess for any tears, particularly in the caudal pole. If the medial meniscus is damaged, the damaged portion is removed. This is not an easy procedure, especially in very small dogs or dogs with a lot of periarticular fibrosis. Instruments that are very helpful for a thorough joint exploration are small Gelpi retractors (either 3.5″ or 5.5″), a stifle distractor (being held by an assistant is ideal and makes this portion of the procedure much quicker, since it allows the surgeon to use both hands and still have the stifle distracted to provide optimal visualization), a meniscus probe, a small pair of mosquito hemostats or meniscus hemostats, a sharp dura hook can be helpful in small spaces, a sharp 3-prong Senn retractor or sharp two-prong rake retractor, and suction (Figures 50.28–50.30).

Torn portions of the meniscus are very difficult to "grab," so a small sharp dura hook can be very helpful for "grabbing" the meniscus. Debriding a torn meniscus can be a very frustrating procedure due to the small working space and need to protect the axially-located CdCL, the abaxially-located MCL (in cases of medial meniscal tears), and the surrounding cartilaginous surfaces, so the surgeon must remember that this portion of the procedure can be difficult for even the most skilled and experienced surgeon.

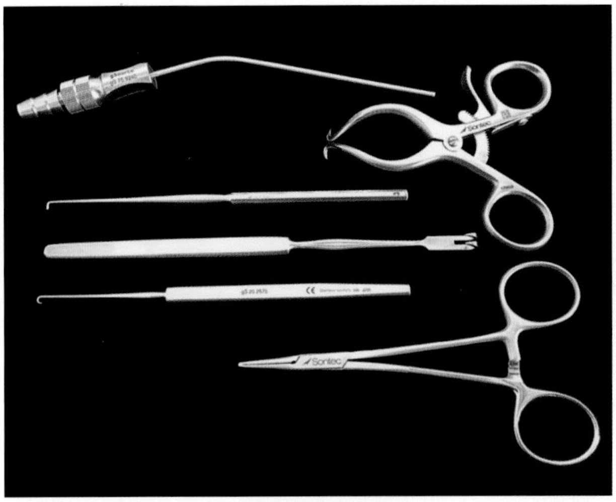

Figure 50.28 Instruments that are helpful for exploring the stifle joint. From top to bottom of the image: a 7-French Frazier suction tip, a 3.5″ Gelpi perineal retractor, a meniscal probe, a sharp two-prong rake retractor (or sharp 3-prong Senn retractor), a dura nerve hook, a small straight mosquito hemostat. *Source:* © Trent Gall.

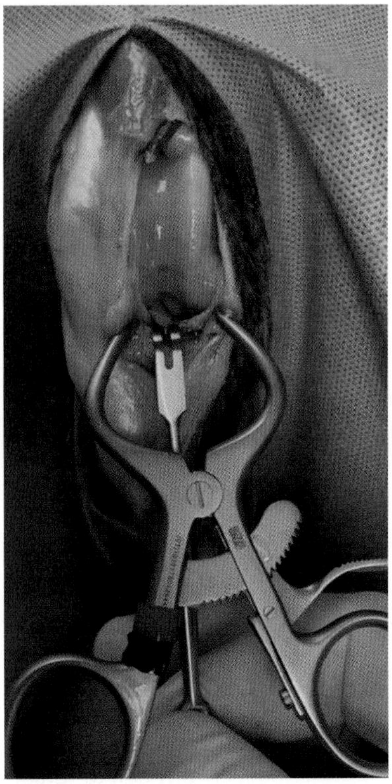

Figure 50.29 Gelpi retractors and a sharp two-prong rake (or sharp Senn retractor) are placed to help visualize the joint. *Source:* © Trent Gall.

Once the meniscus is determined to be normal, or damaged portions removed to be best of one's abilities while not causing more cartilage damage, the lateral meniscus is quickly evaluated. Damage to the lateral meniscus is extremely rare, but this author believes it is worthwhile to at least visualize the lateral meniscus for damage.

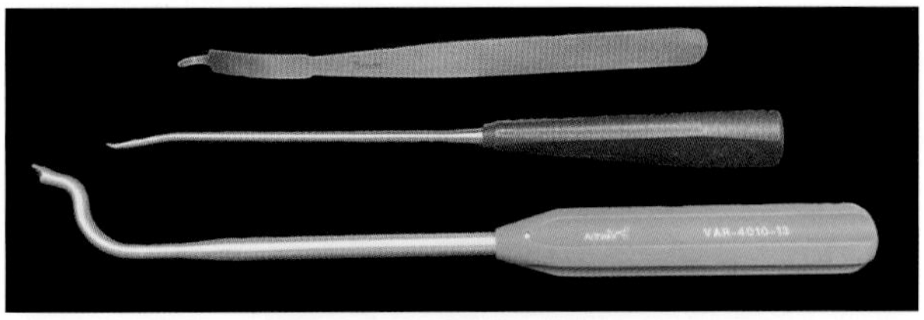

Figure 50.30 Examples of stifle distractors. From top to bottom of the image: a small Hohmann retractor, a Ventura stifle thrust lever / distractor (IMEX®), an Arthrex® stifle distractor. *Source:* © Trent Gall.

Once inspection of the stifle joint and any debridement is finished (Figures 50.31 and 50.32), the joint is lavaged with sterile saline or sterile LRS. The joint capsule is then closed either with simple interrupted sutures, cruciate sutures, or a simple continuous pattern. Some surgeons prefer to close the joint capsule separately from the overlying tissue, this author prefers one single simple continuous suture pattern for both joint capsule and overlying fascia. Depending on the patient size, 3-0, 2-0, or 0 are typical sizes using an absorbable long-term monofilament suture to close the joint. The author prefers to use a longer-lasting suture, such as PDS™ (polydioxanone, or Maxon™ polyglyconate).

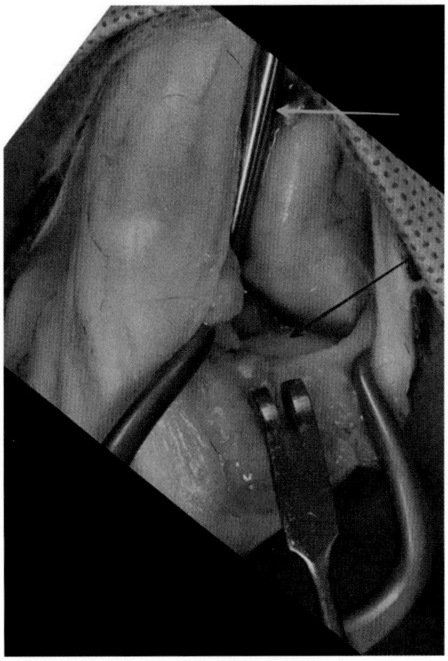

Figure 50.31 A stifle distractor is placed (green arrow). The assistant holds the stifle distractor to put cranial pressure on the proximal tibia by pressing from the caudal tibial notch and a sharp two-prong rake (or sharp Senn retractor) to pull distally on the soft tissues. The assistant and small Gelpi retractors distracting the joint capsule medially and laterally allow the surgeon to probe the medial meniscus (blue arrow) and explore the joint with improved visualization. *Source:* © Trent Gall.

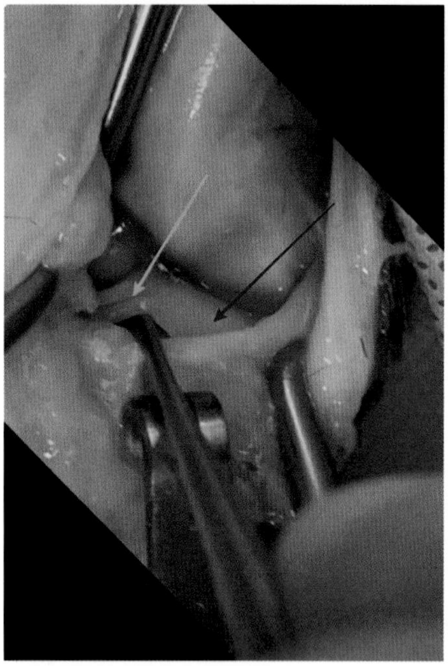

Figure 50.32 A meniscal probe is probing under the axial aspect of the medial meniscus looking for any tears or defects. The green arrow is the caudal menisco-tibial ligament. If a meniscal release was to be performed, this is the location for a medial meniscal release. The blue arrow is the caudal horn of the medial meniscus. *Source:* © Trent Gall.

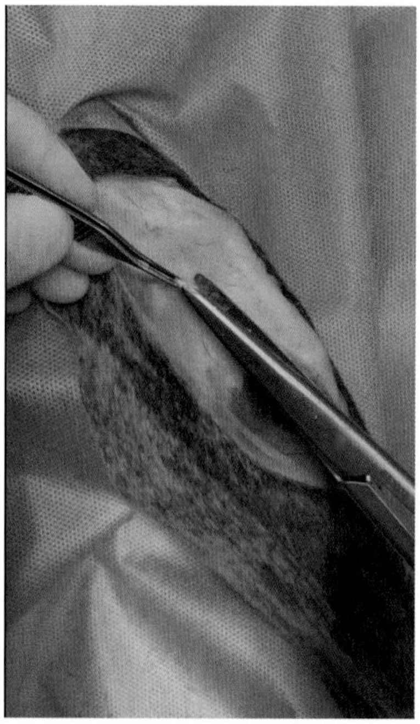

Figure 50.33 Approach to lateral fabella after medial arthrotomy closure. The skin is allowed to roll back to the lateral position. The biceps fascia is tented with thumb forceps, and a "nick" is made in the fascia. This small incision needs to be in the fascia only and not through the joint capsule. This will be an extracapsular incision in the fascia only. *Source:* © Trent Gall.

If using a medial parapatellar arthrotomy, the skin is allowed to roll back over to the lateral aspect where the initial incision was performed.

Approach to Lateral Fabella

The biceps fascia is tented, and either a stab incision is performed with a #11 or 15 blade or Mayo scissors are used the "nick" the fascia, being careful to not incise the joint capsule (Figure 50.33). Mayo scissors are used to extend the incision proximally in a caudal lateral direction (away from the patella), stopping once muscle fibers are identified. In the author's experience with larger and more heavily-muscled dogs, the incision needs to split some muscle fibers to get to the level of the lateral fabella. The incision is extended distally to the level of the joint (Figure 50.34).

At this level, the incision can be directed caudally to help with exposure (basically making a flap of fascia in the shape of an "L"), but the incision must NOT go past the level of the fibular head (Figure 50.35). The peroneal nerve runs in this area, and extreme care must be taken to avoid damaging the peroneal nerve! Once the fascial incision is made, the lateral fabella can be identified (Figure 50.36). Take time to observe the broad attachment of the gastrocnemius muscle with its sesamoid, the lateral fabella, onto the caudal femur (fabello-femoral ligament). The fibers of this attachment are more robust at the proximal portion of the lateral fabella. This is an important landmark for placing the suture material, and these fibers are very important to engage when passing the suture/cruciate needle.

Approach to the Proximal Tibia

At this point, the surgeon can either pass the suture material around the fabella or, as this author prefers to do, prepare the proximal tibia. One must decide if they will be using one bone tunnel and passing the material under the patellar tendon, through two bone tunnels, or one bone tunnel and utilizing a suture button. The T3 or T2 site for tibial anchor point can be found via several ways. The first option is to create a small approach directly parallel to the long digital extensor (LDE) tendon, and using Gelpi retractors to retract the small incision open, drill the bone tunnel 2–3 mm distal from the joint surface. The second option is to excise the fascia of the cranial tibial muscle attachment to the tibial crest then elevate the muscle away from the proximal tibia using a periosteal elevator or monopolar electrosurgery right along the bone (Figure 50.37). The bone tunnel is 2–3 mm distal from the joint surface and caudal towards the T3 site, care being taken not to damage the LDE (Figures 50.38 and 50.39a). If a second bone tunnel is performed, it is ~5–10 mm (patient size-dependent) distal and either slightly cranial to the first bone tunnel or

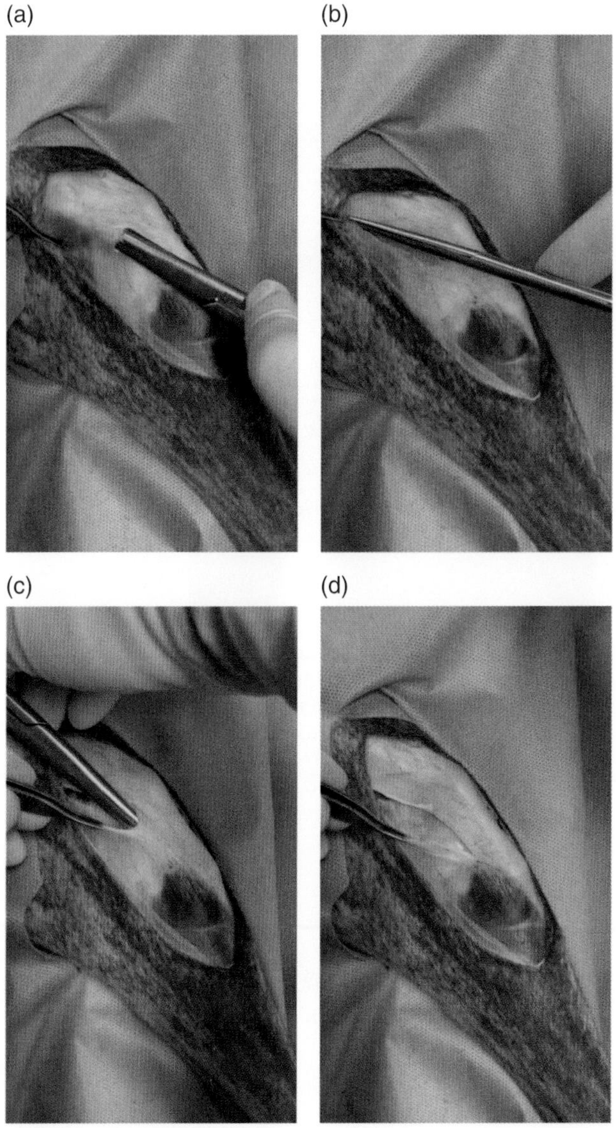

Figure 50.34 (a) The Mayo scissors can be tunneled proximally, still outside of the joint capsule and below the fascia. (b) The incision is continued proximally between muscle bellies. Sometimes, the muscle fibers need to be split to obtain adequate exposure of the lateral fabella. (c) The fascial incision is continued distally. (d) The distal extent of the fascial incision should reach the proximal aspect of the cranial tibial muscle. *Source:* © Trent Gall.

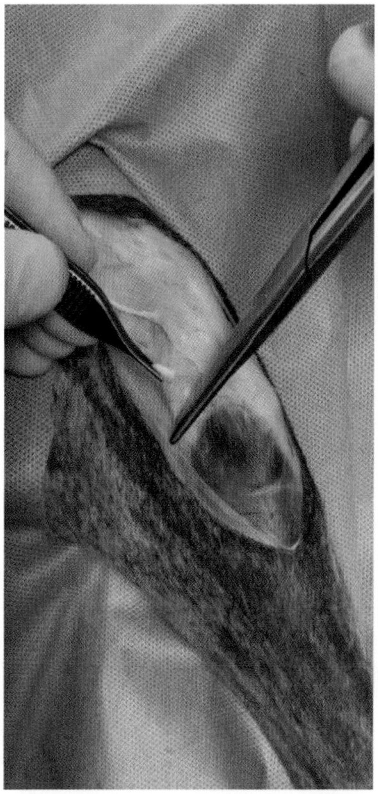

Figure 50.35 If the exposure is not adequate to reach the lateral fabella, a perpendicular incision in the fascia leaf can be performed to make a fascial L-shaped "flap." Care must be taken NOT to extend this incision caudally past the fibular head. The peroneal nerve is directly next to the fibular head and can be damaged if this incision is carried too far caudally. *Source:* © Trent Gall.

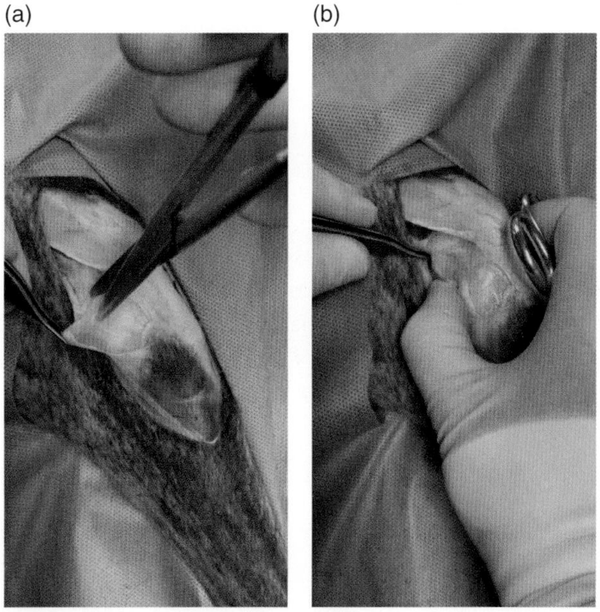

Figure 50.36 (a) The underlying fascial attachments can be gently dissected away to gain exposure to the lateral fabella. (b) Exposure and palpation of the lateral fabella. *Source:* © Trent Gall.

directly distal to the first bone tunnel (Figure 50.39b). Care must be taken to preserve this "bone bridge" and avoid suture pull-out and breaking of this bone bridge.

The size of the bone tunnel(s) is determined by the size of the material being used. The surgeon must consider if one or two strands will be occupying the same hole. Use a Steinman pin or K-wire just big enough to easily pass the material or needle, but not too big to compromise the bone bridge or tibial integrity.

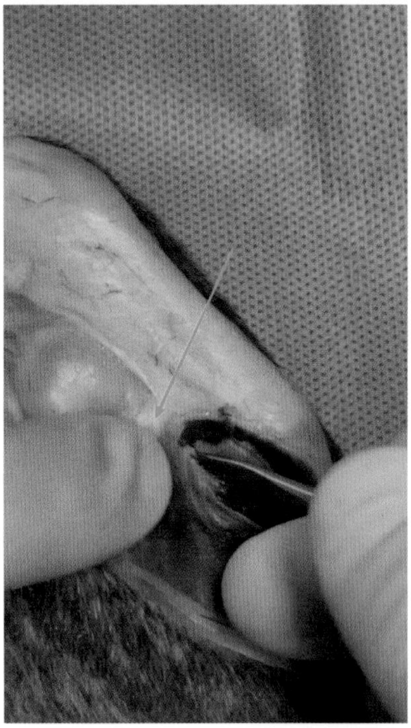

Figure 50.37 Elevation of the cranial tibial muscle using a periosteal elevator from the proximolateral tibia to expose the T2 or T3 site. Green arrow is indicating the location of the long digital extensor (LDE) tendon. *Source:* © Trent Gall.

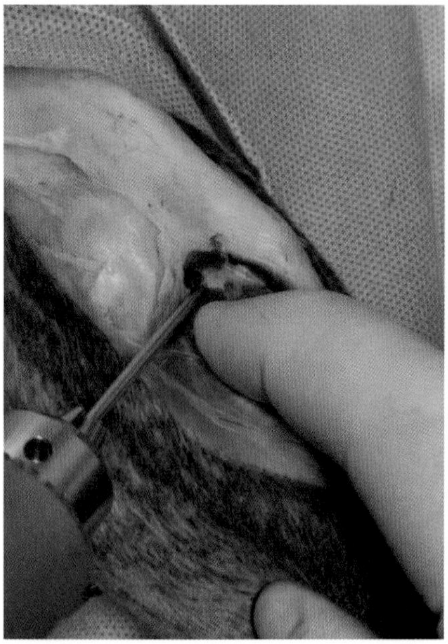

Figure 50.38 A Jacobs chuck with a Steinman pin starting the proximal bone tunnel approximately 3 mm from top of the tibia. Due to the flair at the top of the tibia, a small pilot hole is started by angling the pin towards the joint (~90° to the bone surface). Once there is a "divot" (so the pin doesn't slide down the tibial flair), the pin is leveled and aimed slightly distal and cranial on the tibia. *Source:* © Trent Gall.

Passage of the Suture Material: Femoral Anchor Point

Anchoring the suture material to the femur may be accomplished by passing the material around the lateral fabella. The author tends to prefer passing the needle from a distal to proximal direction to visualize the needle coming through the tough fibers (fabello-femoral ligament, or more anatomically correct, the fibers of origin of the gastrocnemius muscle), which is essentially the "holding layer" of the suture for ECS placement (Figure 50.40a,b). This is another portion of the surgery that can be difficult and frustrating. If the surgeon is having a hard time passing the needle around the lateral fabella and exiting in those fibers of attachment of the gastrocnemius muscle, a small pair of curved mosquito or Kelly hemostats can be first used to "make a tunnel" for the needle to follow. This can

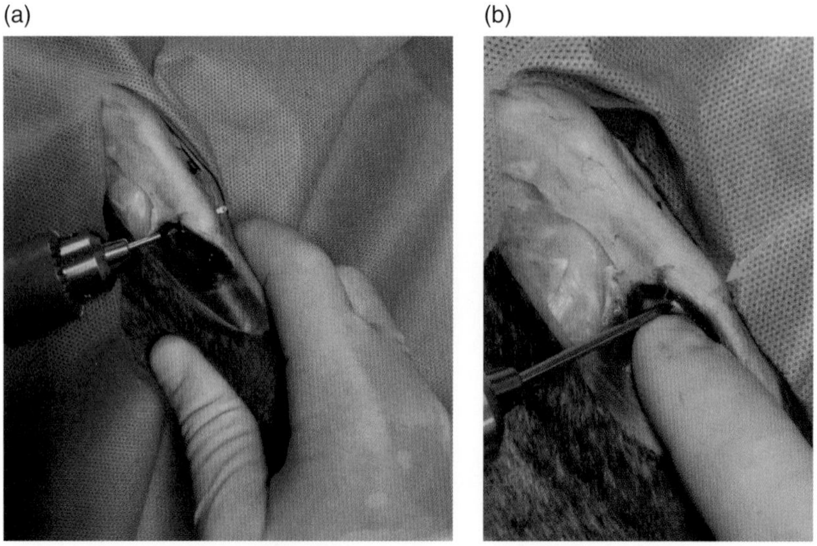

Figure 50.39 (a) The bone tunnel aimed slightly distal and cranial on the proximal tibia and exiting the medial side. (b) If performing a two-bone tunnel technique, the second bone tunnel is distal to the first bone tunnel and possibly a little cranial. Do not go past the distal end of the patellar tendon fibers (green arrow). *Source:* © Trent Gall.

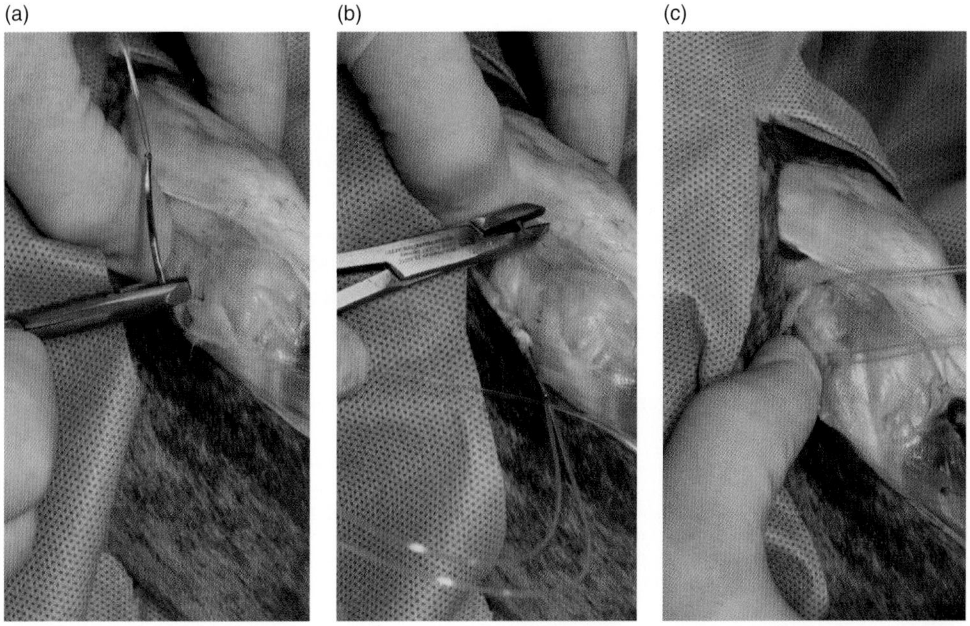

Figure 50.40 (a) The cruciate needle with double-stranded swaged-on nylon leader line is being passed around the lateral fabella using wire-twister needle-holders. (b) The cruciate needle is continued around the lateral fabella. Be sure to follow the curve of the needle when pulling the needle through. (c) The two strands are now passed around the lateral fabella, the strands are pulled to make sure they feel secure and don't feel like they will slip off the fabella. *Source:* © Trent Gall.

also help identify if the path is truly behind the fabella by using the hemostats to move the fabella. Once the needle is passed along with the suture material, grasp both ends of the material and firmly pull to make sure the suture is secure and not wanting to slip off the back side or proximal aspect of the lateral fabella (Figure 50.40c). One of the author's mentors would say it should feel "as if you could lift the dog off the table and throw it over your shoulder," if placed correctly. If there is no lateral fabella, a bone anchor can be used for securing the suture material to the femur. The bone anchor is placed in the femoral condyle approximately 2–3 mm from the femoral fabella joint space, and as mentioned previously, it is recommended that the anchor hole be predrilled with the appropriately-sized drill bit angling cranial and proximal. The bone anchor needs to be seated well in the femur but angled away from the femoral notch from which the caudal cruciate ligament originates.

Passage of the Suture Material: Tibial Anchor Point

The suture material now can be passed through the bone tunnel(s). If using a two-bone tunnel technique, the suture material that exits distal to the fabella is passed through the distal bone tunnel, exits the medial side, and back through the more proximal bone tunnel. Make sure when placing the suture material in the tibia to not place the material on top of the attached cranial tibial muscle; tunnel under the muscle (Figure 50.41). Placing the suture material on

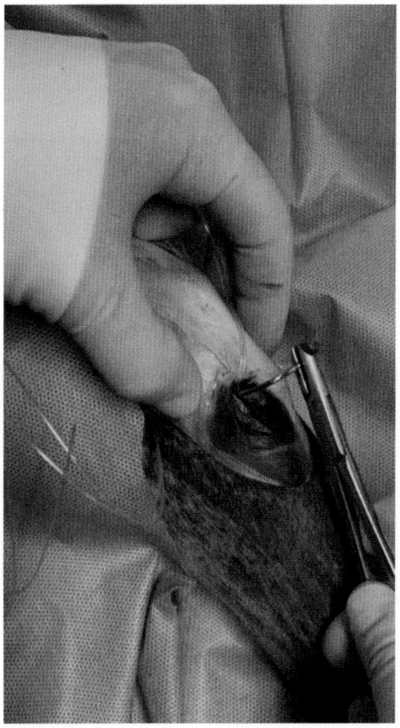

Figure 50.41 The nylon suture is passed under the remaining attachment of the cranial tibial muscle and then through the proximal tibial bone tunnel. If the tibia isn't too wide (as on small breed dogs), the cruciate needle can be passed directly through the bone tunnel. At this point, the needle can be removed, and the nylon suture passed by itself through the bone tunnel. Another option to help guide the suture through the bone tunnel is using a large gauge hypodermic needle (12-gauge to 18-gauge, depending on suture size). *Source:* © Trent Gall.

top of the muscle will cause pain and premature loosening of the material if the muscle atrophies. If using a one-bone tunnel technique and a suture button, run one end of the suture material through the bone tunnel, through the suture button on the medial aspect, and then back through the same bone tunnel. If using the one bone tunnel technique and under the patellar tendon, pass the suture material through the bone tunnel and then under the patellar tendon, trying not to breach the joint capsule (Figures 50.42 and 50.43).

Tensioning the Suture Material

The author recommends "flossing" the suture material back and forth to work out any slack in the system by hand prior to using a tensioning device, which is also a convenient time to match the strands and ensure the free ends match each other (Figure 50.44). The stifle is placed in approximately 100° of flexion during tensioning. If using a crimping system, there are several ways to use the tensioning device by placing different obstructions on the free ends of the suture on which the tensioner can grasp

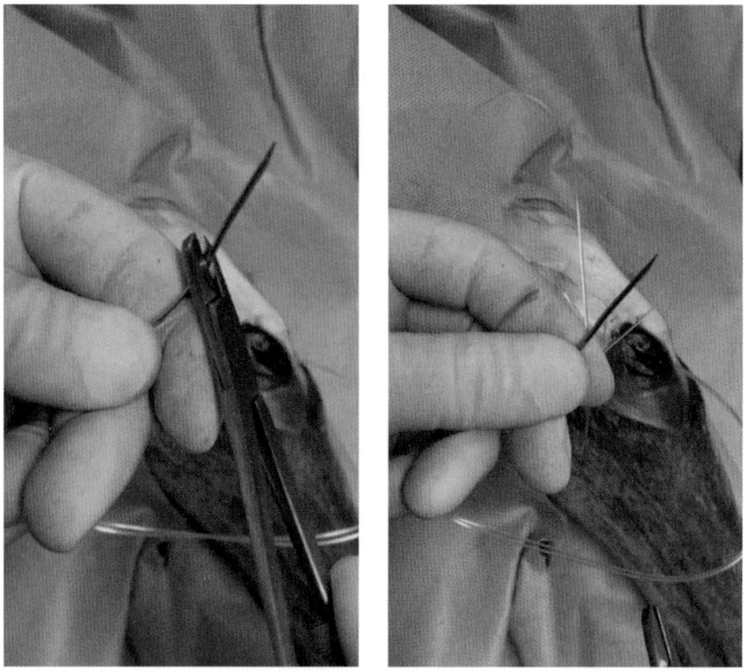

Figure 50.42 If the tibia is too wide and the cruciate needle cannot be passed through, the needle can be straightened with heavy needle-holders or wire-twisters to help aid in passing through the bone tunnels. *Source:* © Trent Gall.

(a) (b)

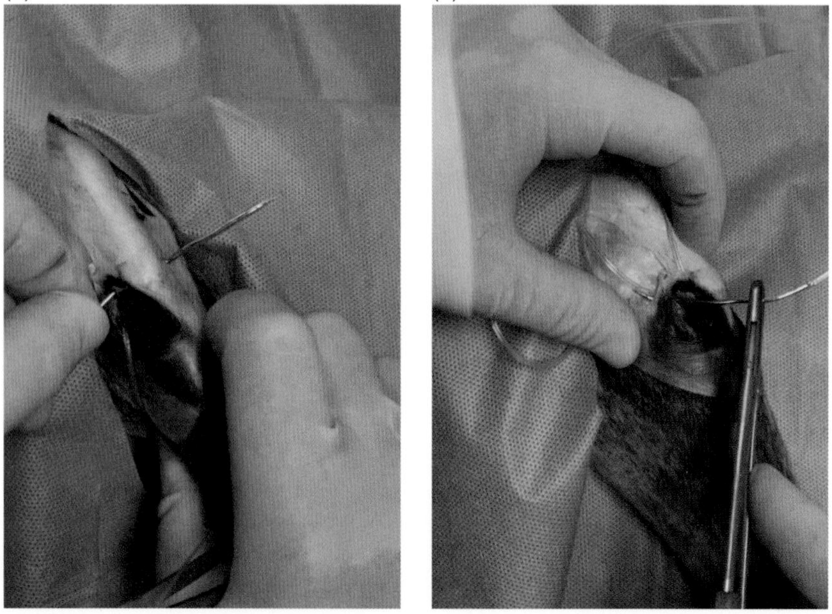

Figure 50.43 (a) The suture material is being passed through the proximal bone tunnel and then through the distal bone tunnel on the medial side of the tibia. (b) The suture is passed under the cranial tibial muscle. *Source:* © Trent Gall.

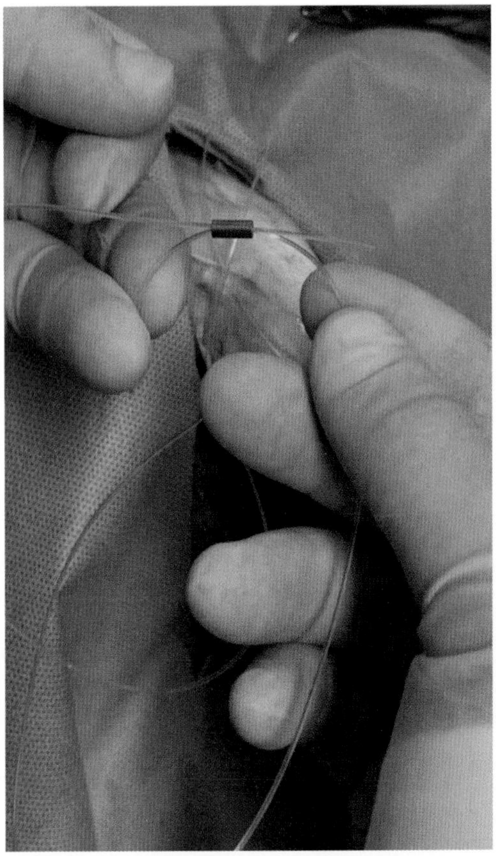

Figure 50.44 The needle is cut off the suture material. The two ends of the corresponding suture line are passed in opposing directions through the crimp clamp. *Source:* © Trent Gall.

(see Figure 50.13 for the three main methods). The first method is by using multiple crimp clamps. First, place the crimp clamp that is going to be used for securing the two strands by passing the strands opposite of each other through the ends of the crimp clamp. Next, use a second crimp clamp on one of the free ends of the suture, crimp it in place. Slide a third crimp clamp on the other free end of suture material and crimp in place. Place the tensioning device between the two compressed crimp clamps and start to tension. A tip with this method is to place the crimp clamps on the free ends close to the center crimp tube, since the tensioner will not reach the proper tension if the clamps are placed far on the suture ends. A second method for using the tensioner is to tie a knot on each free suture end. A third method is to use two hemostats on the free ends (Figure 50.45).

For all three methods, the tensioner is ratcheted one click at a time. Squeeze to get a click, test for cranial drawer motion, squeeze the tensioner to get a click to tighten or "tension" the suture ends, test for cranial drawer motion, and continue this process until there is only 1–2 mm of drawer motion. Be careful not to overtension the suture material and completely eliminate cranial drawer. This could cause external rotation of the foot, which can both cause a lameness and prematurely loosen the suture material. Once the surgeon is pleased with the tension, the crimper tool is used to make the crimps on the crimp tube. Depending on the manufacturer, this will either be one clamping motion or three clamping motions to make a total of three indentations in the crimp tube. Make sure the

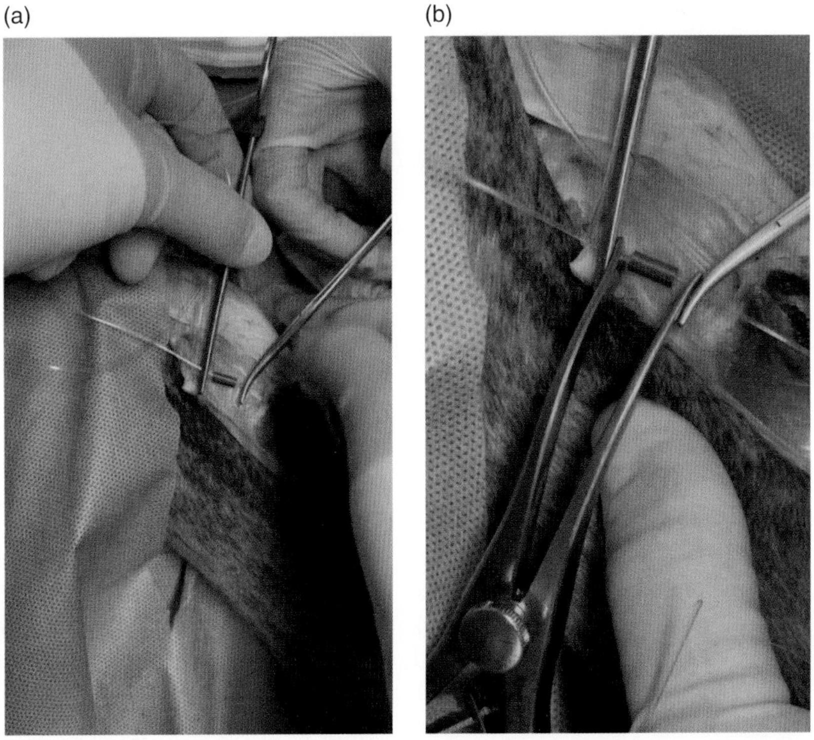

Figure 50.45 (a) The two hemostat technique for tensioning is being demonstrated. The hemostats are only on one suture line each, so the tensioning device can slide the suture lines to tension them. (b) The tension device in place and tensioned to eliminate *most* of the instability to cranial drawer. Only 1–2 mm of cranial drawer should be present, since overtensioning will result in external rotation of the foot. *Source:* © Trent Gall.

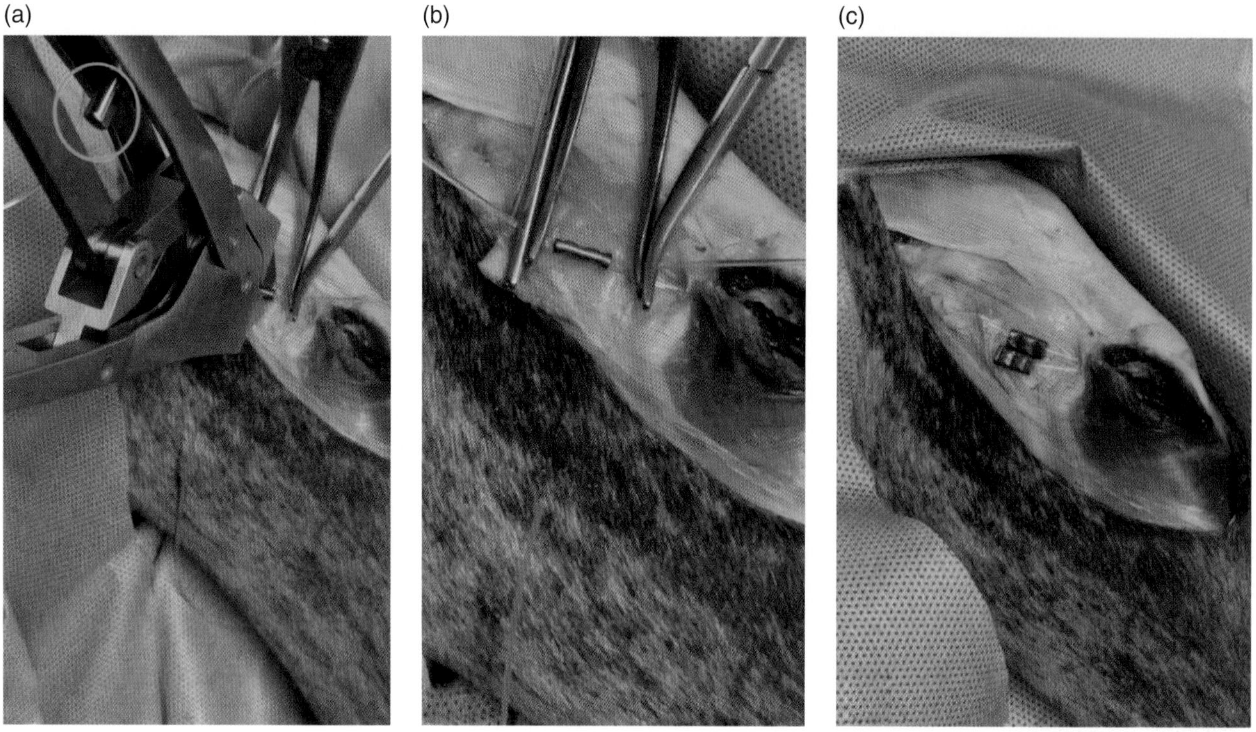

Figure 50.46 (a) The crimping tool is being placed. Note the peg stopper circled in green on this Securos Power X crimper. This peg should touch the metal bar under it to get the proper crimp compression. (b) Fully compressed crimp clamp in place. (c) Example of two-strand technique with the second crimp clamp in place. Note the crimps are beside each other. If the clamps were offset, it is possible the crimp clamp could cut through the adjacent suture line. *Source:* © Trent Gall.

two outside crimp indentations are not too close to the edge of the crimp clamp, which could cut the suture material when the crimper tool is fully clamped down. Most crimper tools have a stopper that must be compressed by the handles to achieve the appropriate crimp in the crimp tube (Figure 50.46).

This is a good opportunity to note that the surgeon must use the same manufacturer for all the crimp tubes, suture material, and crimping tools. These are all calibrated to achieve the most secure crimp with materials from the same company. Do not mix and match systems, which can lead to suture failure due to an inadequate crimp. If placing a second suture line (as part of the recommended double-strand), this is tensioned in the exact same manner as the first. Be careful when tensioning the second line, as it is very easy to overtension and create slack in the first suture line.

If using a suture material that doesn't have an associated crimp clamp, a slip knot is tied at first and tensioned by hand to assess for cranial drawer motion. Once the surgeon is happy with the tension, the slip knot is locked, and square knots are placed. A total of three to four square knots (six to eight throws) is sufficient. The downside of using square knots is that the knots create a large knot bulk (especially with nylon leader line suture) that can sometimes be felt through the skin and become a source of inflammation and seroma formation. The author has had to remove several lateral sutures on very small thin skin dogs due to constant irritation from the nylon/fishing line knot. These were subsequently replaced with a softer material, such as FiberWire™ from Arthrex®.

Closure

Flush the surgical site with sterile saline. Close the fascia of the biceps with either a simple continuous pattern or an imbricating pattern. Some people believe that slightly imbricating the fascia will help facilitate the fibrosis process. Depending on the patient size, 3-0, 2-0, or 0 are typical sizes using an absorbable long-term monofilament suture to close the biceps fascia. The author prefers to use a longer-lasting suture, such as PDS™ (polydioxanone) or Maxon™ (polyglyconate). The author also likes to flush the surgical site once again with sterile saline prior to closing the subcutaneous tissue with an absorbable short-term monofilament suture, such as Monocryl™ (poliglecaprone 25) or Biosyn™ (Glycomer 631). The skin is then routinely closed Figure 50.47.

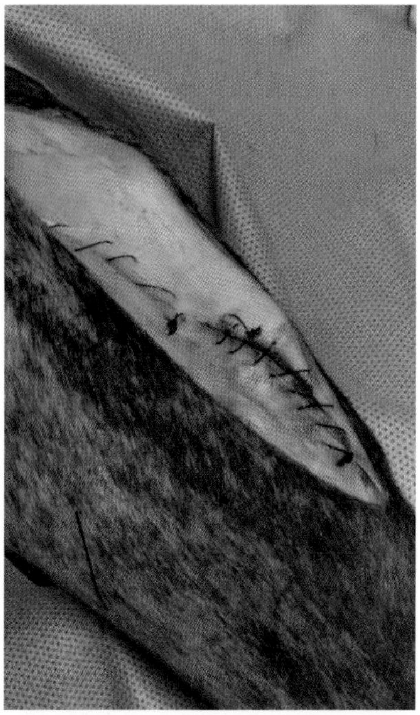

Figure 50.47 Closure of the fascia and fascia over the cranial tibial muscle. Then routine subcutaneous closure and skin closure. *Source:* © Trent Gall.

Postoperative Considerations

The patient must be kept from overactivity, otherwise, complications can occur. The author prefers the following restrictions:

- The first two weeks are the strictest. Leash walks outside for bathroom purposes only and then back inside, which results in walks that are no longer than five minutes in duration.
- No running, jumping, or rough play for the entirety of 12 weeks.
- At two weeks postsurgery, the author likes to re-examine the patient to make sure the incision has healed. At this point, the patient can start ~10-minute leash walks two to four times a day. This continues until 8–10 weeks postsurgery, then the patient can start with a leash walk or stretches to "warm" the patient up prior to allowing short amounts of off-leash time. This starts with five minutes off-leash, and every three to five days, the client may increase the duration of off-leash time.
- By 12–14 weeks after surgery, the patient can be back to normal activity. The author likes to start the patient in a professional canine rehabilitation program two weeks postsurgery if possible. Recheck exams at 2-, 8- and 16-weeks postsurgery are recommended. The patient should have minimal to no lameness by 8–10 weeks postsurgery.

Potential Complications

ECS material can stretch, break, break the bone tunnel, avulse the lateral fabella, pull out the bone anchor, or "saw" through the fabello-femoral ligament, all resulting in failure of the ECS material. Incisional complications, such as dehiscence or infection, either superficial skin infection or deeper infection around the ECS material, may occur. Peroneal nerve deficits can occur if the ECS material is passed too close to or entraps the peroneal nerve or if too aggressive of a surgical approach is performed. Postsurgical or late meniscal injuries can happen as well. If there is persistent lameness due to one of the complications, it is advisable to perform a revision surgery. At the revision surgery, a thorough exploration of the stifle should be performed to look for a late meniscal injury (i.e., postliminary meniscal tear if it occurs postoperatively, latent meniscal tear if it was missed during the original surgery) or other intra-articular pathology. If there is persistent instability, another ECS should be placed or consider a different procedure, such as a TPLO.

References

1 Chailleaux, N., Lussier, B., De Guise, J. et al. (2007). In vitro 3-dimensional kinematic evaluation of 2 corrective operations for cranial cruciate ligament-deficient stifle. *Can. J. Vet. Res.* 71 (3): 175–180.

2 Kim, S.E., Pozzi, A., Kowaleski, M.P. et al. (2008). Tibial osteotomies for cranial cruciate ligament insufficiency in dogs. *Vet. Surg.* 37 (2): 111–125.

3 Vezzoni, A., Bohorquez Vanelli, A., Modenato, M. et al. (2008). Proximal tibial epiphysiodesis to reduce tibial plateau slope in young dogs with cranial cruciate ligament deficient stifle. *Vet. Comp. Orthop. Traumatol.* 21 (4): 343–348.

4 Buote, N., Fusco, J., and Radasch, R. (2009). Age, tibial plateau angle, sex, and weight as risk factors for contralateral rupture of the cranial cruciate ligament in Labradors. *Vet. Surg.* 38 (4): 481–489.

5 Cabrera, S.Y., Owen, T.J., Mueller, M.G. et al. (2008). Comparison of tibial plateau angles in dogs with unilateral versus bilateral cranial cruciate ligament rupture: 150 cases (2000–2006). *J. Am. Vet. Med. Assoc.* 232 (6): 889–892.

6 Chuang, C., Ramaker, M.A., Kaur, S. et al. (2014). Radiographic risk factors for contralateral rupture in dogs

with unilateral cranial cruciate ligament rupture. *PLoS One* 9 (9): e106389.

7 de Bruin, T., de Rooster, H., Bosmans, T. et al. (2007). Radiographic assessment of the progression of osteoarthrosis in the contralateral stifle joint of dogs with a ruptured cranial cruciate ligament. *Vet. Rec.* 161 (22): 745–750.

8 Doverspike, M., Vasseur, P.B., Harb, M.F. et al. (1993). Contralateral cranial cruciate ligament rupture: incidence in 114 dogs. *J. Am. Anim. Hosp. Assoc.* 29: 167–170.

9 Muir, P., Schwartz, Z., Malek, S. et al. (2011). Contralateral cruciate survival in dogs with unilateral non-contact cranial cruciate ligament rupture. *PLoS One* 6 (10): e25331.

10 Casale, S.A. and McCarthy, R.J. (2009). Complications associated with lateral fabellotibial suture surgery for cranial cruciate ligament injury in dogs: 363 cases (1997–2005). *J. Am. Vet. Med. Assoc.* 234 (2): 229–235.

11 Tikekar, A., De Vicente, F., McCormack, A. et al. (2022). Retrospective comparison of outcomes following tibial plateau levelling osteotomy and lateral fabello-tibial suture stabilisation of cranial cruciate ligament disease in small dogs with high tibial plateau angles. *N. Z. Vet. J.* 70 (4): 218–227.

12 Anderson, C.C., Tomlinson, J.L., Daly, W.R. et al. (1998). Biomechanical evaluation of a crimp clamp system for loop fixation of monofilament nylon leader material used for stabilization of the canine stifle joint. *Vet. Surg.* 27 (6): 533–539.

13 Aisa, J., Calvo, I., Buckley, C.T. et al. (2015). Mechanical comparison of loop and crimp configurations for extracapsular stabilization of the cranial cruciate ligament-deficient stifle. *Vet. Surg.* 44 (1): 50–58.

14 Roe, S.C., Kue, J., and Gemma, J. (2008). Isometry of potential suture attachment sites for the cranial cruciate ligament deficient canine stifle. *Vet. Comp. Orthop. Traumatol.* 21 (3): 215–220.

15 Hulse, D., Hyman, W., Beale, B. et al. (2010). Determination of isometric points for placement of a lateral suture in treatment of the cranial cruciate ligament deficient stifle. *Vet. Comp. Orthop. Traumatol.* 23 (3): 163–167.

51

Osteochondrosis

Stephen C. Jones[1] *and Caleb Hudson*[2]

[1] *Bark City Veterinary Specialists, Park City, UT, USA*
[2] *Nexus Veterinary Specialists, Victoria, TX, USA*

Key Points

- Osteochondrosis represents a developmental disorder of articular cartilage that leads to the formation of a cartilage flap within the joint.
- This condition usually affects young large and giant breed dogs.
- Although many different joints can be affected, caudal humeral head lesions represent the vast majority of osteochondrosis lesions seen.
- Radiographs are typically sufficient to make a diagnosis, but in some cases, advanced imaging modalities, such as computed tomography (CT), are required for definitive diagnosis.
- The goals of treatment are to remove the painful cartilage flap and to reestablish a congruent joint surface.
- The prognosis following surgical treatment depends on the joint affected, the method of treatment chosen, and the patient's age at the time of treatment.

Introduction

Osteochondrosis (OC) is a developmental orthopedic disease that affects the differentiation of physeal chondrocytes leading to the development of a focal necrotic articular cartilage lesion.[1] Physiologic loading of the OC lesion can result in cracks, fissures, and the formation of a cartilaginous flap. Once a flap has developed, the condition becomes known as osteochondritis dissecans (OCD). OCD usually affects young, rapidly-growing large and giant breed dogs with affected dogs often exhibiting clinical signs in the first 6–12 months of life.[1,2] Great Danes, Newfoundlands, German Shepherds, Mastiffs, Rottweilers, Irish Wolfhounds, Labrador Retrievers, and Golden Retrievers are known to be at-risk breeds for the development of OCD.[1–3]

OCD can affect many joints in dogs and cats. OCD has been reported in the caudal humeral head,[3] elbow joint,[3] stifle joint,[4] tibio-tarsal joint,[5] glenoid cavity,[6] vertebra,[7–10] patella,[11] tibial tuberosity,[12] distal radius,[13] acetabulum,[13] and femoral head.[1] OCD of the caudal humeral head accounts for the majority of cases in dogs (76%), followed by the stifle joint (16%), the tarsus (4.5%), and the distal humerus (3.5%).[3] This book chapter will discuss only these four most common locations. OCD in other locations is very rare and accounts for a very small percentage of the overall number of OCD cases seen in dogs.

Etiology

The exact etiology and underlying pathogenesis of OC is still not fully understood. Even the name of the condition itself lends itself to confusion. The word "osteochondritis" suggests an inflammatory etiology, but histological studies of bone removed during surgical OC lesion debridement fail to show any signs of osteonecrosis. In fact, histological findings strongly support a pathogenesis characterized by failure of endochondral ossification secondary to localized avascular necrosis of the epiphyseal cartilage.[14] A range of environmental and genetic risk factors have been proposed.

Techniques in Small Animal Soft Tissue, Orthopedic, and Ophthalmic Surgery, First Edition. Edited by Kristin A. Coleman.

Companion website: www.wiley.com/go/coleman/surgeries

Historically, trauma was considered a primary causative factor for OC in people. In most cases, however, no single traumatic event is reported. Repetitive cartilage stress may play a more important role as a precipitating factor for the onset of clinical signs and lameness. Dietary factors, such as copper deficiency, excess phosphorus, and excess dietary energy, have also been implicated in the development of OC.[14] Genetics seem to play an important role in the development of OC. In horses, for example, offspring from affected sires are more than twice as likely to develop OC as those from normal sires.[15] Despite well-documented evidence suggesting that genetics play an important role in the etiopathogenesis of OC in multiple species, specific genes and alleles related to OC have not yet been identified. Ultimately, the development and clinical expression of OC are likely the result of a combination of etiological risk factors, both genetic and nongenetic in nature.

Indications and Pre-op Considerations

History and Physical Examination

Dogs with OCD most commonly present with signs of thoracic or pelvic limb lameness anywhere between 5 and 10 months of age.[13] The magnitude of lameness can vary from dog to dog, but it often starts insidiously and eventually becomes an obvious toe-touching lameness with non-weight-bearing lameness occasionally seen. Some dogs can present much later in life, and in some patients, OCD may be found incidentally on radiographic examination.[3] As the OCD disease process progresses, joint inflammation causes effusion, decreased range of motion, and pain on joint manipulation. Crepitus is occasionally palpable in more chronic cases.

Diagnostics

Plain Radiography

Radiographs performed in the early stages of stifle OCD often demonstrate a faint radiolucent defect beneath the articular margin. The surgeon should closely scrutinize the radiographs, as this finding can be subtle and easy to miss (Figure 51.1). Soft tissue opacity in the joint space secondary to joint effusion is usually appreciated in stifle and tarsal joints with OCD. Given the summation of other bones and/or dense overlying soft tissue, joint effusion is more difficult to see in the elbow and shoulder joints. If clinical suspicion of OCD exists and regular orthogonal radiographs are not confirmatory, oblique projection radiographs should be acquired (Figure 51.2). As the disease progresses, a more distinct round-to-oval-shaped radiolucent defect at the articular surface is seen. Typically, a ring of sclerotic bone surrounds this radiolucent defect (Figure 51.1). In some instances, the cartilaginous flap mineralizes and can be seen overlying the radiolucent defect, or it can become detached and is seen as a mineralized joint mouse elsewhere in the joint (Figure 51.1).

Computed Tomography

Computed tomography (CT) can help better delineate the osseous anatomy at the level of the articular surface and results in increased detection of OCD lesions as compared to radiographs.[16] Furthermore, it has been shown that radiographs consistently underestimated the size of OCD lesions in the caudal humeral head when compared with CT.[17] CT, therefore, is considered the preferred diagnostic modality when articular defect reconstruction is to be attempted. In addition to improving the accuracy of lesion size determination, CT permits the surgeon to develop a better understanding of the exact location and topography of the lesion. Some surgeons find it helpful to create a 3D surface rendering (digital and/or printed) of the affected joint, to better appreciate the lesion location and size. It is important, however, to realize that surface reconstructions do not account for cartilaginous defects and/or subchondral bone pathology and, thus, may underestimate the true size of the articular cartilage lesion.

Additional Diagnostics

Early in the formation of a cartilaginous OCD flap and prior to the development of trabecular bone sclerosis, an OCD lesion may not be radiographically identifiable. In the shoulder joint, the use of positive contrast arthrography was found to be 88% accurate in the detection of discontinuity of the cartilage associated with nonmineralized flaps.[18] However, in the same study, CT accuracy at detecting thickened cartilage covering a subchondral defect where no surface cartilage defect existed was only 55%.[18] Ultrasonography (US) has been shown to be a useful imaging modality for detecting nonmineralized cartilage flaps in the canine shoulder joint. In one study of 29 joints with OC/OCD lesions, 21 joints were fully visualized and 8 were partially visualized using US.[19] Magnetic resonance imaging (MRI) has also been shown to be a valuable diagnostic modality in the detection of canine shoulder OC/OCD lesions (Figure 51.3).[20] A recent study found that the odds of detecting an OC lesion were 3.2 times higher with MRI than US.[21] Interestingly, in that same study, diagnostic accuracy of OC/OCD was highest for MRI (94.4%), followed by radiography (88.9%), with US having the lowest accuracy of the modalities compared (82.6%).[21] While MRI is a theoretically appealing imaging modality in cases of OC/OCD, limited availability, the necessity of general

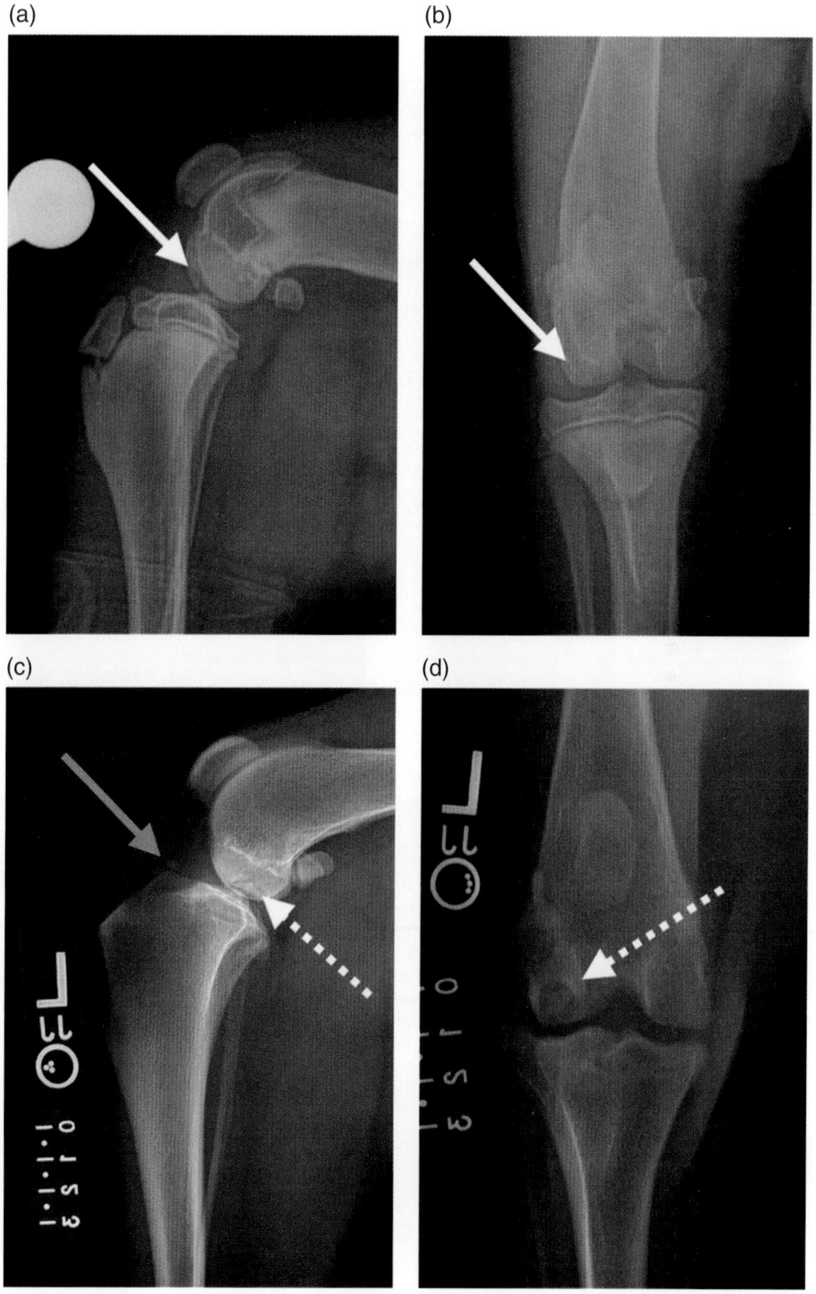

Figure 51.1 Lateral (a,c) and craniocaudal (b,d) radiographs of a 4-month-old Labrador (a,b) and an 18-month-old German Shepherd (c,d). Note how discernible the radiolucent defect and the surrounding trabecular sclerosis are in the older (dotted white lines) versus the younger (solid white line) dog. The surgeon should pay close attention to the joint contour and opacities in the younger patients where the OCD lesion can easily be missed. Note also the mineralized body in the cranial joint pouch of the older dog (orange arrow, c). This presumably represents a detached mineralized OCD flap. *Source:* © Stephen C. Jones.

anesthesia, and high procedural costs along with a lack of comparative studies assessing the diagnostic accuracy of MRI for OCD in joints other than the shoulder are limitations to the widespread use of MRI as a diagnostic imaging modality for OC/OCD in dogs.

Considerations

OC is commonly found in the affected joint bilaterally, even if the dog or cat is not displaying clinical signs in the contralateral limb. OCD is reported to be present bilaterally in 16%, 41%, 75%, and 40% of humeral head, distal humerus, stifle, and tarsus cases, respectively.[4,5,22,23] The veterinarian is advised to perform diagnostic imaging on the affected and the contralateral joints, even if clinical signs are only present unilaterally. The presence of a radiographically identifiable lesion, in the absence of clinical signs, however, presents a conundrum. While radiographically identifiable OC lesions in younger patients (<6 months) may be clinically silent, these lesions often progress to a flap (OCD) over time and ultimately result in clinical lameness. Conversely, some patients with clinically asymptomatic OC lesions go on to heal by bone infilling of the subchondral

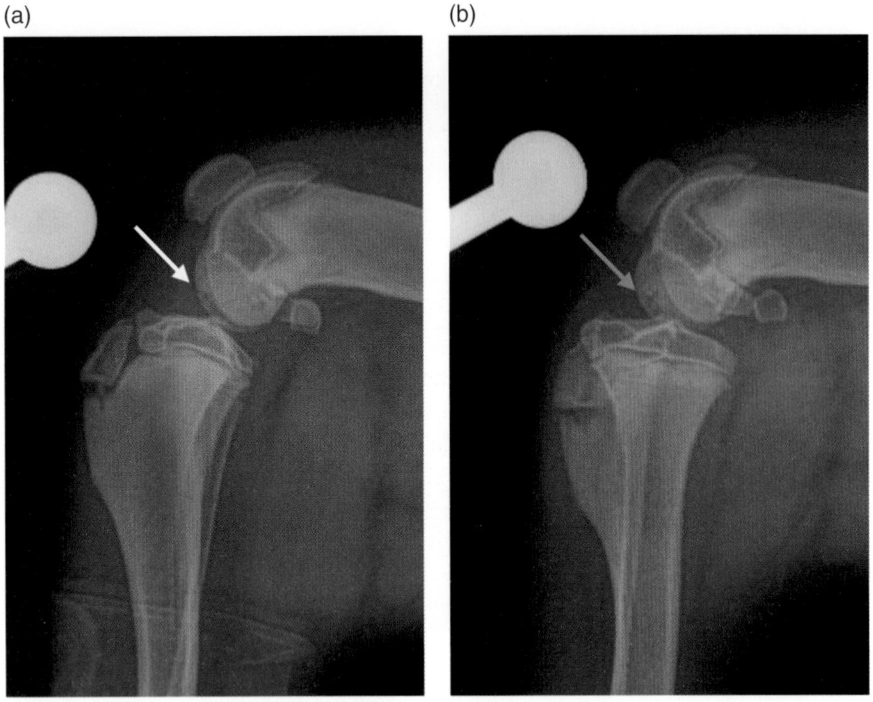

Figure 51.2 Lateral stifle radiographs of a dog with OCD of the lateral femoral condyle. Note that the lesion is not easily appreciated on the straight lateral (a) view (white arrow) but becomes more obvious when an oblique (b) view is acquired (orange arrow). *Source:* © Stephen C. Jones.

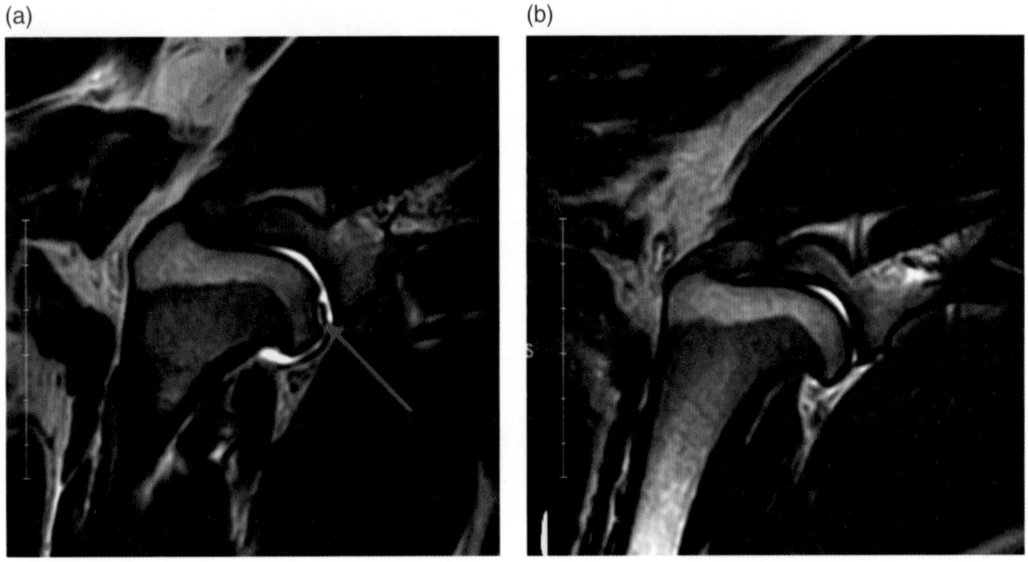

Figure 51.3 T2-weighted 3-Tesla sagittal MRI images of the left (a) and right (b) shoulder joints in a 12-month-old Dutch Shepherd with a left-sided OCD lesion. The hyperintense (bright) joint fluid can be seen surrounding the hypointense (dark) flap (red arrow). *Source:* © Stephen C. Jones.

OC defect and do not progress to flap formation with the associated pain and lameness. The decision of whether to perform surgery on the clinically unaffected side is, therefore, challenging with no clearly correct answer. Ultimately, the decision to operate unilaterally or bilaterally should be made in concert with the owner. Ideally, it is best to adopt a wait-and-see approach on the nonclinical side. The owner, however, must be aware of the potential necessity for second-side surgery at a later date. The joint affected should be considered in the decision-making process for unilateral versus bilateral surgery. Debridement of a nonclinical OC lesion in the shoulder, where OC/OCD lesion debridement is expected to have a very good prognosis for functional outcome post-operatively, is more justifiable than debridement of a nonclinical lesion in other joints, where the prognosis after surgery is less favorable. Another option is to visually assess the nonclinical side at the time of the initial surgery. This is especially appealing when using arthroscopy, which is minimally invasive and, therefore, is expected to result in minimal patient morbidity on the nonclinical side. When deciding on whether to make an open surgical approach on a clinically silent side, the veterinarian should take into account the size of the lesion radiographically, the presence of other radiographic factors that may indicate ongoing joint pathology (joint effusion, for example), and owner factors (economics, logistics, etc.). If diagnostic arthroscopy/arthrotomy is performed, the presence of a visible cartilage defect and/or visible evidence of joint synovitis would warrant cartilage lesion debridement.

If the surgeon is planning to perform a joint resurfacing procedure, careful scrutiny of the patient's skin for evidence of dermatitis or pyoderma should be performed. Any pre-existing skin disease should be treated aggressively until completely resolved before attempting a joint resurfacing procedure, where a surgical site infection would be likely to result in a catastrophic outcome.

In some patients with large OCD lesions affecting the medial aspect of the humeral condyle, the femoral condyle, or the trochlea of the talus, or in patients with advanced degenerative joint disease (DJD) present at the time of OCD diagnosis, the prognosis associated with surgical debridement or partial joint resurfacing procedures may be guarded. In this group of patients, joint replacement surgery may be considered as a first-line treatment option for OCD. Even if OCD lesion debridement is ultimately selected over joint replacement surgery, it is important to educate owners prior to OCD debridement surgery on the expected outcome for the affected joint to ensure that reasonable expectations exist.

Treatment Options

The goals of any OCD treatment are to reestablish a congruent joint surface, to provide an improved long-term functional outcome, and to minimize OA progression. OCD treatment options consist of conservative management, open/arthroscopic removal of the cartilage fragment with debridement/stimulation of the subchondral bed, osteochondral autograft transplantation, osteochondral allograft transplantation, synthetic osteochondral resurfacing, and total joint replacement. Treatment decisions should be based on patient considerations such as the joint affected, patient age, degree of lameness, underlying OA, patient temperament, and comorbidities, OCD lesion type (location and topography), and owner factors such as economic considerations, compliance, and post-operative management/outcome expectations. While this chapter will focus primarily on the treatment of OCD lesions with an arthrotomy approach, it should be noted that arthroscopy presents a much less invasive option for the treatment of most cases of OCD and, where possible, is the preferred treatment approach over arthrotomy.

Specialized Surgical Instrumentation

OCD flap removal and subchondral bone debridement are facilitated with the use of specialized instrumentation due to the limited working space available inside most joints and the need to treat the OCD lesion while minimizing iatrogenic damage to the surrounding articular cartilage. The optimal instrumentation for OCD debridement is arthroscopic hand instruments, which were designed for use during arthroscopic surgery but which can be utilized just as effectively during open surgery. Arthroscopic hand instruments have small tips and a long, thin shaft designed to fit into a small joint space. The most common arthroscopic hand instruments utilized for OCD lesion debridement include graspers, blunt probes (meniscal probes), and curettes. Graspers are used to grasp and remove the flap from the joint (Figure 51.4a). Blunt probes are used to manipulate the flap and assess the depth of the OCD defect (Figure 51.4b). A curette is used to conservatively debride the subchondral bone bed in the OCD defect until healthy, bleeding bone is observed (Figure 51.4c). An arthroscopic power shaver can also be utilized through an arthrotomy approach to debride the subchondral bone bed of the OCD lesion after flap removal. A micropick is also sometimes utilized to create focal microfractures in the subchondral bone bed and promote vascular ingrowth (Figure 51.4d). If an arthroscopic grasper is not available, a small mosquito hemostat can be used in most patients to grasp and remove the OCD flap.

Surgical Treatment of OCD

General principles of surgical technique utilized for OCD lesion treatment are similar between joints, regardless of the surgical treatment technique being utilized. General principles of each surgical treatment technique will be covered in this section, while variations from the standard technique that may be applicable to specific joints will be mentioned further in the sections pertaining to each individual joint.

Cartilage Fragment Removal with Debridement/Stimulation of the Subchondral Bed

After an arthrotomy (or arthroscopy) has been performed, the joint should be thoroughly evaluated by visual inspection and probing. The OCD lesion should be identified and thoroughly inspected. The cartilage flap should be grasped

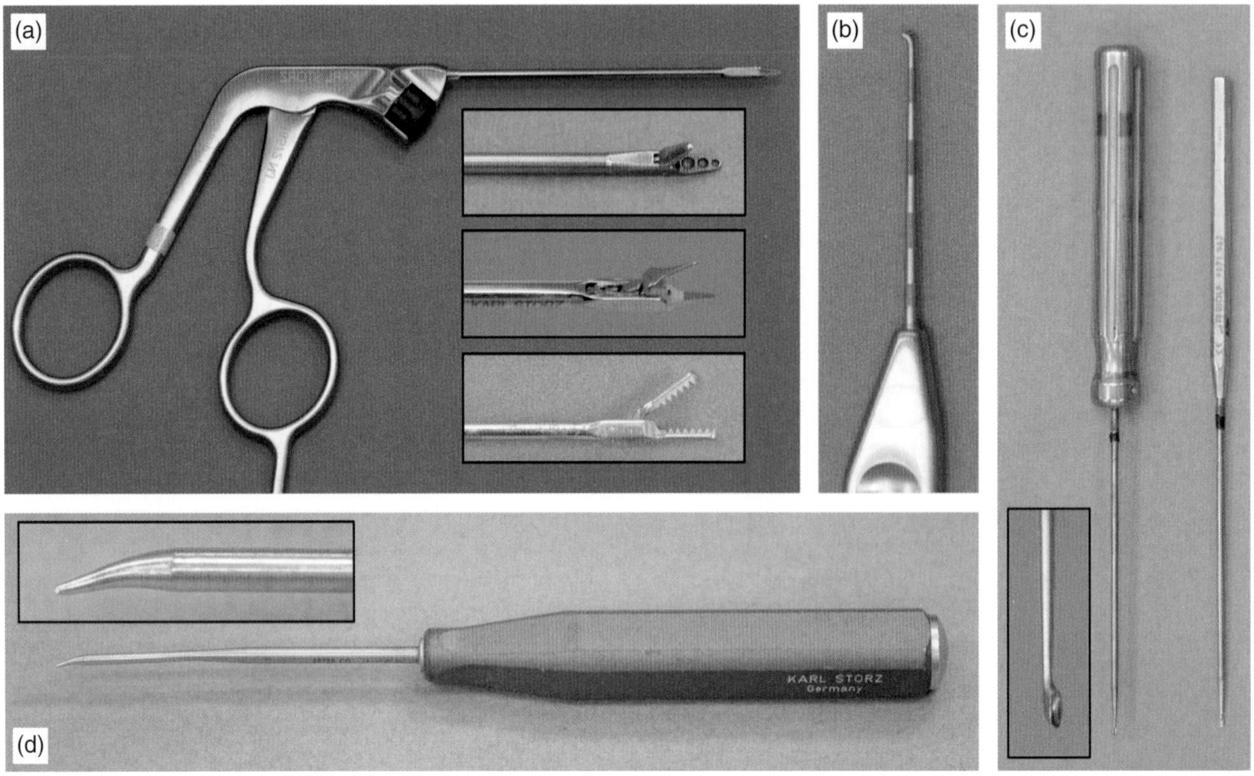

Figure 51.4 (a) Arthroscopic graspers are used to grasp and remove the flap from the joint. (b) Shown here is a meniscal probe. Blunt probes, such as the meniscal probe, are used to manipulate the flap and assess the depth of the OCD defect. (c) A curette is used to conservatively debride the subchondral bone bed in the OCD defect until healthy, bleeding bone is observed. (d) A micropick is occasionally utilized to create focal microfractures in the subchondral bone bed and promote vascular ingrowth from the subchondral metaphysis. *Source:* © Caleb Hudson.

and gently pulled and manipulated to remove it from the joint surface. Careful probing around the lesion often reveals additional cartilage that is not appropriately adhered to the subchondral bone; this cartilage should also be removed using a grasper or curette. Following flap removal, the subchondral bed is debrided down to a bleeding surface. This can be performed using a curette, high-speed burr, arthroscopic shaver, or some other instrument capable of removing the often-dense sclerotic subchondral bone of the OCD bed. The premise behind curettage of the subchondral bone is to create hemorrhage, which promotes infiltration of pluripotent mesenchymal stem cells from the subjacent metaphyseal bone into the lesion bed, thereby initiating repair and lining of the defect with fibrocartilage.[1,2] To encourage bleeding and blood vessel ingrowth in OCD lesions where the underlying bone bed is very sclerotic, a technique referred to as microfracture can be utilized. Microfracture consists of the creation of multiple small holes in the sclerotic surface of the subchondral bone so that the underlying, more normally vascularized bone can communicate with the bone surface. Microfracture is performed by impacting the tip of a micropick into the subchondral bone surface of the OCD defect. Typically, numerous small holes are created, separated from each other by approximately 1–2 mm. When performed correctly, hemorrhage should be observed from the defects created in the sclerotic subchondral bone.[24]

Joint Resurfacing Techniques

As an alternative to flap extirpation and curettage of the subchondral bed, the surgeon may opt to resurface the OCD lesion. A detailed description of the surgical techniques available for joint resurfacing is beyond the scope of this chapter but can be found in the pertinent literature cited herein. The OCD lesion can be resurfaced using an osteochondral autograft, harvested from the dog's own stifle joint.[25] While this technique offers the ability to resurface the lesion using the patient's own hyaline cartilage, thereby minimizing the chances of graft rejection, it does result in donor-site morbidity and the inability to match recipient site cartilage thickness or surface topography. Osteochondral allograft transplantation (graft obtained from a donor dog cadaver) negates the issues with donor site morbidity, but these grafts are more susceptible to graft rejection and, in theory, have the potential for disease transmission.[26] One significant advantage of an allograft over an autograft, however, is the

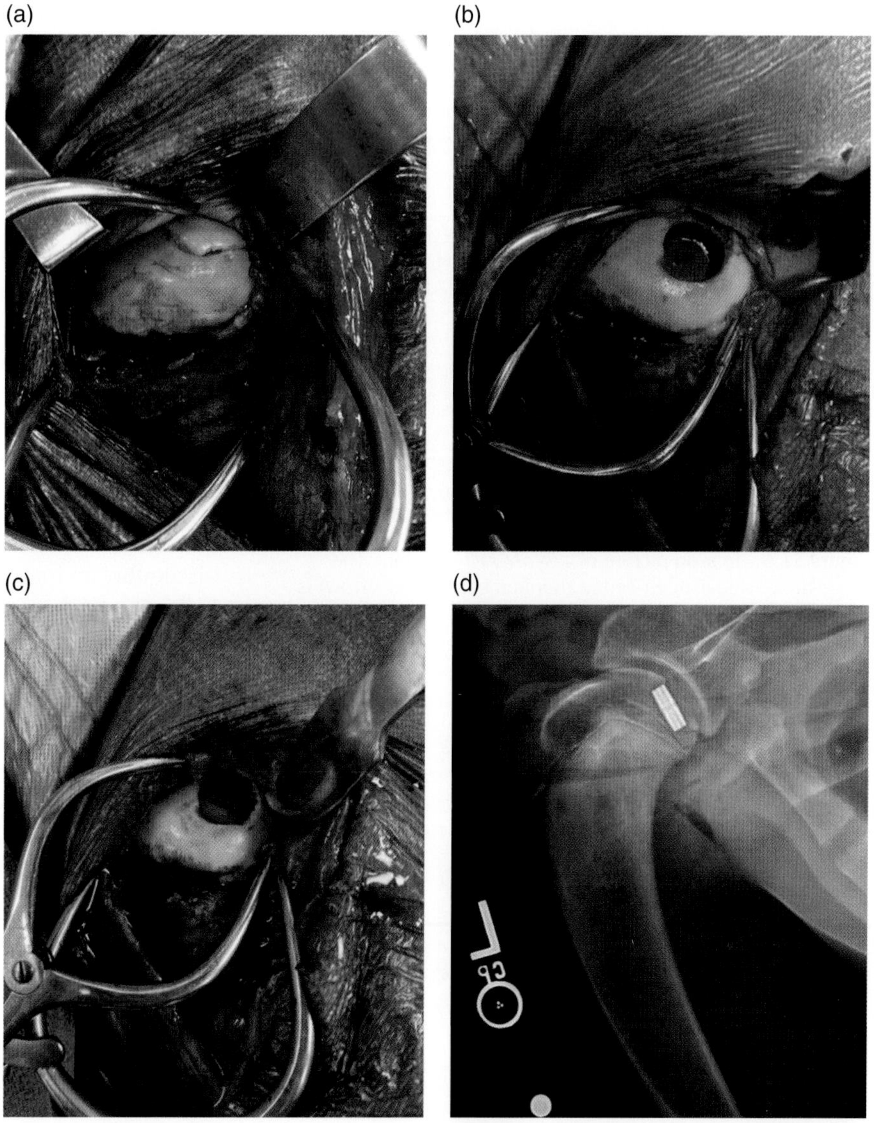

Figure 51.5 Intra-op (a–c) and post-op lateral radiographic image (d) of a dog with a caudal humeral head OCD lesion (a) repaired utilizing the SynACART® synthetic resurfacing implant. After flap removal, the recipient bed is prepared (b) using custom-designed instruments, and the implant is impacted into the final position (c). Note that the radiolucent polycarbonate urethane surface is not identified on the radiograph (d). *Source:* © Stephen C. Jones.

ability to match the cartilage thickness and topography of the OCD site. More recently, synthetic resurfacing has become another available treatment option for dogs with OCD (Figure 51.5).[27,28] SynACART® (Arthrex® Vet Systems, Naples, FL) is a commercially available synthetic implant designed for the resurfacing of osteochondral defects. It is biphasic with a three-dimensional, open-celled titanium scaffold base specifically designed to allow for bone ingrowth and overgrowth. The upper portion of the implant is made of polycarbonate urethane (PCU), which is fused to the titanium scaffold base by an injection-molding process (Figure 51.6).

While not utilized on a regular basis for OCD treatment, custom joint resurfacing implants can be manufactured to precisely match the contour of the affected region of the joint surface of an individual patient. Custom joint resurfacing implants are usually manufactured using 3D printing technology guided by a CT scan of the affected and contralateral joints. These custom joint resurfacing implants are considered somewhat experimental at the present time, as there is no standardization in the manufacturing process and no data available on long-term outcomes associated with the use of these implants. The use of a synthetic implant offers a number of advantages, including the immediate availability of implants with a long storage life, no risk of disease transmission, and no donor site morbidity. Conversely, however, available implants only come in a limited number of sizes, they have a flat surface, making it very difficult to match the contour of the surrounding joint surfaces, and they are circular in shape, making it difficult to match the often oval shape of OCD lesions (Figure 51.7). In addition, the long-term wear characteristics of these synthetic implants are unknown. The use of synthetic implants for joint resurfacing also introduces the risk of implant-associated complications, such as failure of osteointegration, biofilm formation, and/

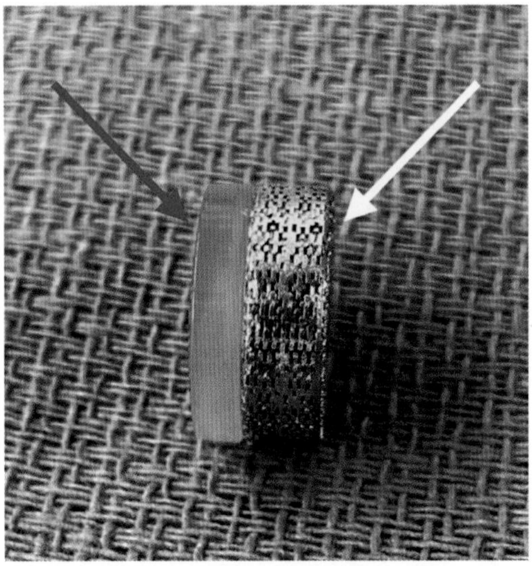

Figure 51.6 End-on picture of a SynACART® implant. The three-dimensional, open-celled titanium base (white arrow) is designed to allow for bone ingrowth. The upper part (red arrow) is made of polycarbonate urethane and is the portion of the implant at the joint surface. *Source:* © Stephen C. Jones.

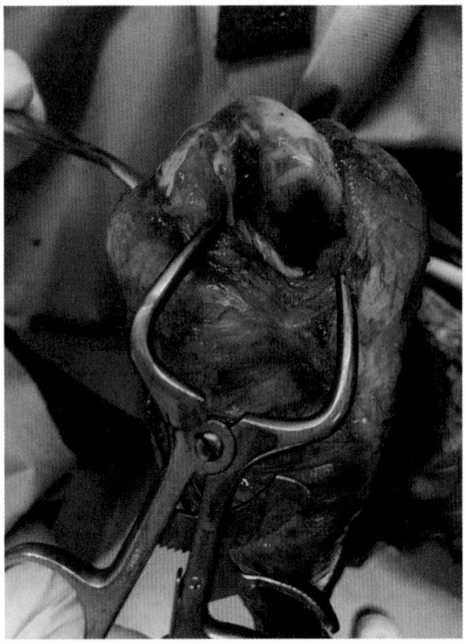

Figure 51.7 Intra-operative image following SynACART® resurfacing of a medial femoral condylar OCD lesion. Note the oval/elongated shape of the OCD lesion. Given the imperfect fit between the lesion and the circular SynACART® implant, it was chosen to resurface the more caudal portion of the condyle, as this region articulates more with the tibial plateau. *Source:* © Stephen C. Jones.

or implant failure. Despite the appeal of resurfacing OCD lesions, to date, no studies have demonstrated the superiority of any form of resurfacing when compared to the traditional technique of flap removal and subchondral bone stimulation.

Total Joint Replacement

Off-the-shelf joint replacement implants currently exist for the canine elbow, stifle, and tarsus. While not routinely performed by most surgeons at the present time, joint replacement of the stifle, elbow, and tarsus is routinely performed by a small group of surgeons who are considered specialists in joint replacement. Although joint replacement is not routinely needed in the treatment of OCD, total joint replacement can be an excellent option for patients with very large OCD lesions that are not amenable to partial joint resurfacing or for patients who have previously had OCD lesion debridement or partial joint resurfacing performed and are not responding well.

Humeral Head – Surgical Technique

Discomfort and lameness typically persist as long as the OCD flap remains attached to the humeral head. Conservative therapy, universally considered inferior to surgical intervention, involves vigorously exercising the dog until the flap becomes loose and detaches. While detachment of the flap may result in clinical relief, incomplete detachment may result in prolonged disability and pain. Furthermore, the detached flap can migrate into the bicipital bursa, causing inflammation and pain. For these reasons, when possible, surgical intervention is recommended over conservative therapy.

Multiple arthrotomy approaches to the shoulder have previously been described, several of which can be successfully utilized for debridement on an OCD lesion affecting the caudal humeral head. The shoulder can be approached via a craniolateral, caudolateral, or caudal approach.[29] Each approach has specific advantages and disadvantages. The challenge with all three of these approaches is the necessity for a large incision with significant soft tissue dissection (Figure 51.8). In addition, for most of these approaches, a tenotomy is required, resulting in more significant patient morbidity (Figure 51.8). More recently, a less invasive craniolateral approach to the shoulder, that does not require a tenotomy, has been described for the treatment of OCD in dogs.[22] This modified Cheli approach is the authors' preferred surgical approach when utilizing an arthrotomy for humeral head OCD debridement.

To perform an arthrotomy approach to the shoulder, the patient is placed in lateral recumbency with the affected leg up. It is helpful to have the dog close to the edge of the table with the affected leg hanging off the side (Figure 51.9). This allows the surgeon to easily manipulate the leg during the surgery. For example, with the Modified Cheli approach,[22] the shoulder joint must be hyper-flexed to gain access to the OCD lesion, and this is

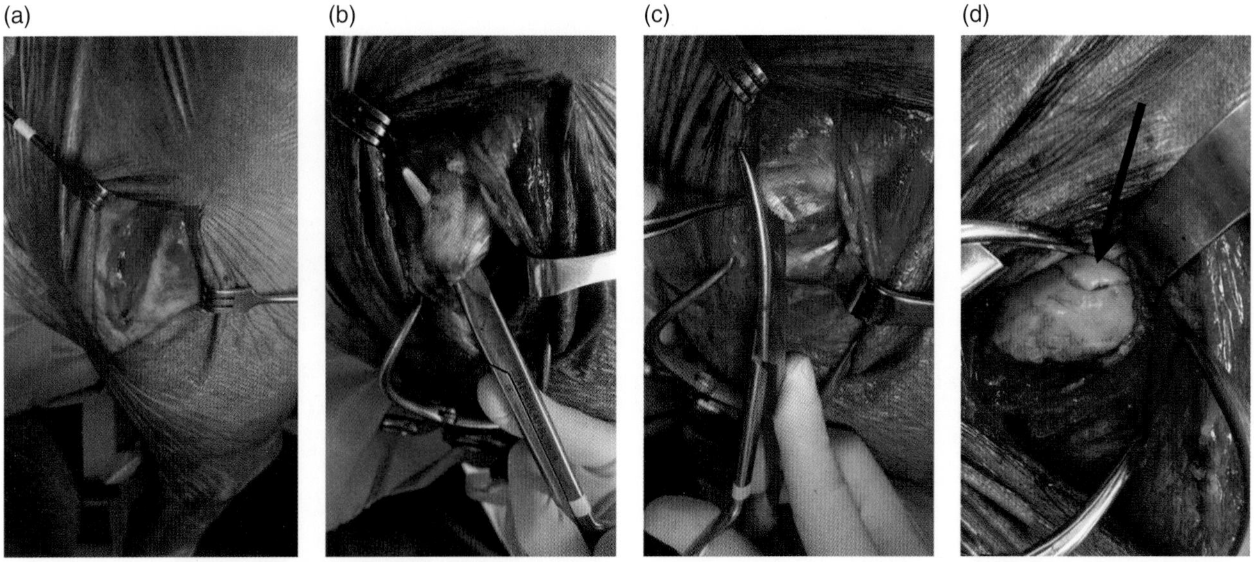

Figure 51.8 Craniolateral[29] approach to the left shoulder joint in a dog with a caudal humeral head OCD lesion. (a) A large soft tissue incision is required. (b) Shown here is the undermining of the infraspinatus tendon from the joint capsule and greater tubercle. (c) A tenotomy of the infraspinatus is utilized with this approach. (d) Significant soft tissue dissection and retraction are required with this approach. Note that the large OCD lesion (black arrow) is easily seen with this approach. *Source:* © Stephen C. Jones.

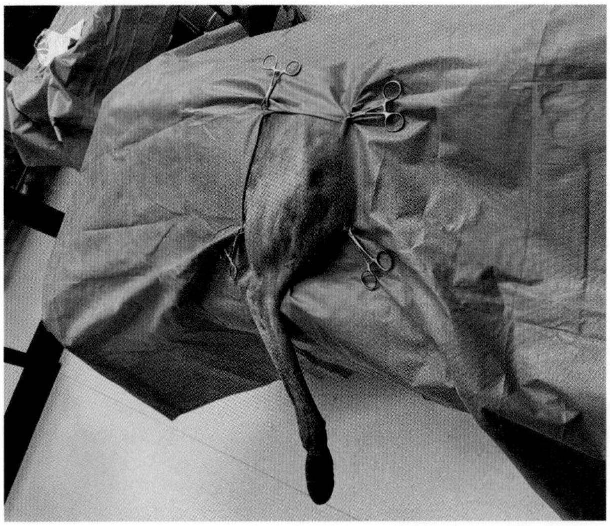

Figure 51.9 A patient is positioned on the surgery table prior to surgical debridement of a caudal humeral head OCD. Note that the patient is positioned close to the edge of the table with the shoulder, elbow, and carpal joints all draped in. This allows easy manipulation of the shoulder and elbow joints during surgery, to help improve access to the OCD lesion. *Source:* © Stephen C. Jones.

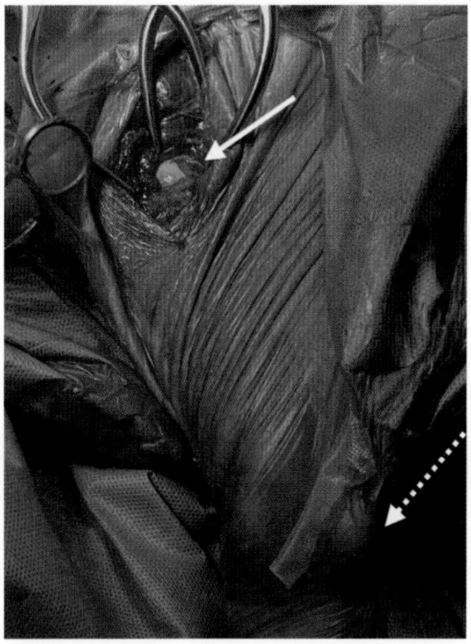

Figure 51.10 Caudo-lateral[29] approach for surgical debridement of a humeral head OCD lesion. The entire leg has been draped in to allow manipulation during surgery. Note that the elbow joint has been externally rotated (dotted arrow), resulting in internal shoulder rotation, thereby, providing greater access to the caudo-medially located OCD lesion (solid arrow) in this case. *Source:* © Stephen C. Jones.

greatly facilitated by appropriate patient positioning. In addition, with all surgical approaches, both internal and external rotation of the humerus can greatly aid in the exposure of the lesion during surgery (Figure 51.10). Surgical site preparation may be performed by clipping and draping a small region centered over the shoulder joint, in which case the limb is manipulated intra-operatively through the patient drape. Alternatively, the entire limb from the proximal scapula distally may be prepared and draped into the surgical field to improve the ease of intra-operative limb manipulation.

Humeral head OCD can be treated by lesion debridement and subchondral bone stimulation,[30] osteochondral autograft transfer,[25] osteochondral allograft transplantation,[26] synthetic osteochondral resurfacing,[28] and hemiarthroplasty.[31] The surgeon should have a clear idea of what the intended treatment will be and should be adequately prepared with appropriate instruments and any required implants ahead of time. Regardless of the intended treatment to be performed, surgical intervention should be performed as soon as possible after diagnosis. It has been shown that earlier diagnosis and treatment of humeral head OCD strongly influences the rate of recovery and can also reduce the amount of future osteoarthritis development.[32]

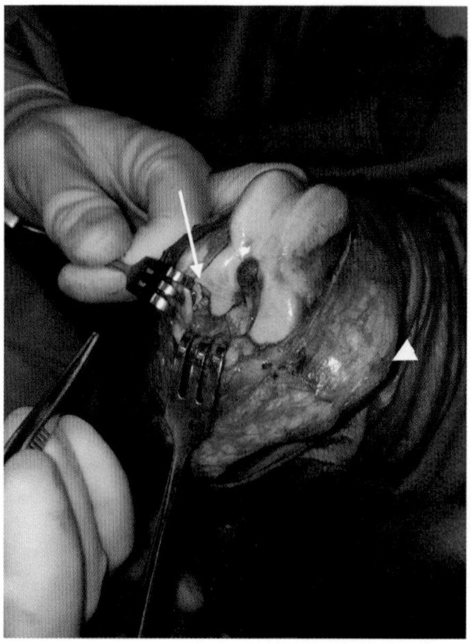

Figure 51.12 Intra-operative image of a dog being treated for an OCD lesion of the lateral femoral condyle (white arrow). A full lateral parapatellar arthrotomy has been performed. The patella (arrowhead) has been luxated medially and the stifle is flexed fully to optimize exposure. *Source:* © Stephen C. Jones.

Stifle – Surgical Technique

The stifle joint is commonly affected by OCD, representing 16% of all OCD cases in dogs in one report.[3] Although rare, OCD of the stifle joint has been described in cats (Figure 51.11).[33,34] The vast majority of stifle OCD lesions (96%) are reported to affect the lateral femoral condyle with 75% of patients having bilateral disease.[4] OCD of the medial femoral condyle is also reported,[27] and the incidence of medial femoral OCD appears to be increasing over time. Cases involving the intercondylar fossa have also been reported.[35]

The patient is typically positioned in dorsal recumbency with the limb to be operated on hanging off of the end of the table for either an arthrotomy or arthroscopy approach to the stifle joint. A medial or lateral parapatellar arthrotomy is performed ipsilateral to the side of the lesion (Figure 51.12).[36] For the majority of stifle OCD lesions, maximal stifle flexion is required to gain access to the caudal aspect of the lesion. Even with a full craniomedial/craniolateral arthrotomy, access to very caudal lesions can be inadequate (Figure 51.13), so intermeniscal desmotomy can be performed to help improve access to the most caudal aspect of the OC/OCD lesion. Performance of the desmotomy allows the cranial

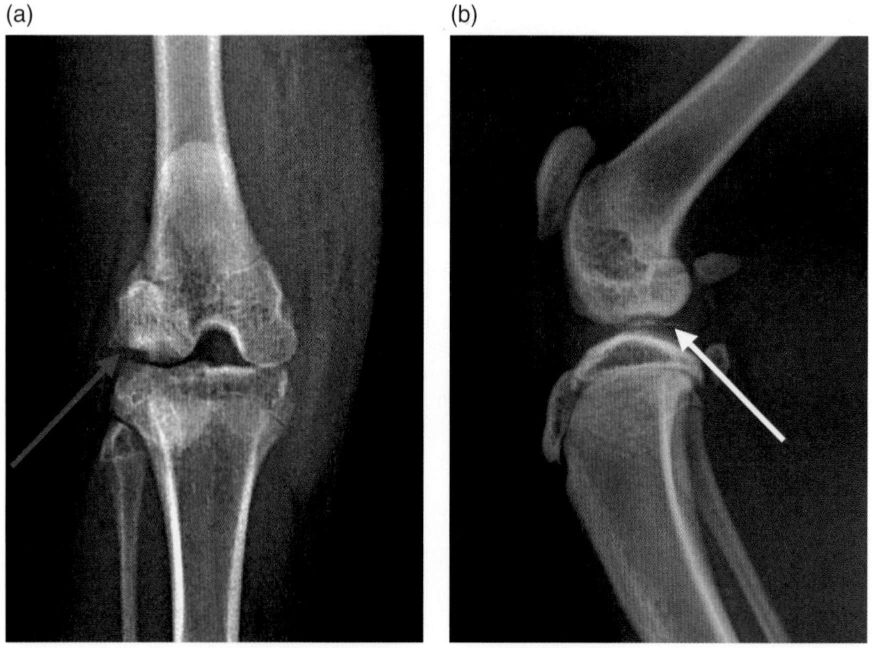

Figure 51.11 Craniocaudal (a) and lateral (b) stifle radiographs in a cat with an OCD lesion of the lateral femoral condyle. This can be seen as a radiolucent concave defect with subjacent trabecular bone sclerosis (red arrow). A mineralized flap is seen slightly distal and caudal to the concave defect on the lateral view (white arrow). *Source:* © Caleb Hudson.

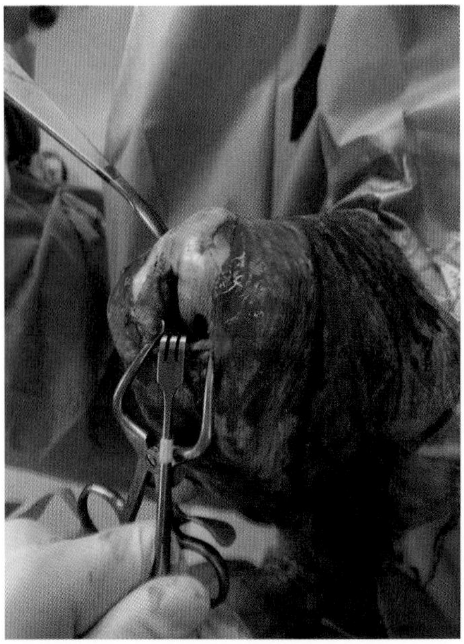

Figure 51.13 Intra-operative image of a dog being treated for an OCD lesion of the medial femoral condyle. Note that even with full stifle flexion, it is challenging to see/access the most caudal aspect of the OCD lesion. In this case, an intermeniscal desmotomy was performed to obtain adequate exposure of the lesion. *Source:* © Stephen C. Jones.

pole of the meniscus to be displaced abaxially, giving the surgeon increased working space to access the lesion. It should be noted that the long-term effects of the performance of an intermeniscal desmotomy are unknown and, thus, should only be employed when absolutely necessary.

Considering that joint surface incongruity likely leads to local and global joint inflammation, which tends to promote secondary osteoarthritis progression and likely increases the risk of additional joint lesions (meniscal damage, kissing lesions of the opposing joint surface, and cruciate ligament degeneration), surgical intervention is considered the optimal treatment approach for OCD lesions of the stifle joint. As with lesions of the humeral head, OCD of the stifle can be treated by flap excision and debridement of the subchondral bed,[37] osteochondral allografts,[26,38] osteochondral autografts,[38–40] or synthetic joint resurfacing.[27] As OCD lesions usually occur on a weight-bearing portion of the femoral condyle and typically affect a relatively large percentage of the surface area of the condyle, treatment with flap excision and debridement often results in unacceptable joint malarticulation and abnormal loading along with progressive meniscal wear, all of which tend to result in joint dysfunction and rapid osteoarthritis development. For these reasons, dogs with femoral condyle OCD often develop end-stage DJD at a relatively young age and may ultimately be candidates for total knee replacement surgery.

Distal Humerus – Surgical Technique

Osteochondritis dissecans lesions are considered one of the components of elbow dysplasia and are typically located medially on the humeral trochlea. Medial coronoid disease is concurrently present in the majority of cases of humeral trochlear OCD. The surgeon should closely assess the patient pre-operatively for evidence of medial coronoid disease or any of the other components of elbow dysplasia. Given the inherently low sensitivity of radiographs for the detection of elbow osteochondral pathology, CT is the preferred diagnostic modality when available (Figure 51.14).

The surgeon should be aware of the potential for cartilage wear lesions to develop on the humeral trochlea secondary to medial coronoid disease; a so-called "kissing lesion" (Figure 51.15). These cartilage wear lesions often result in subchondral bone sclerosis of the humeral trochlea, which can resemble the hyperattenuation seen on CT images in the subchondral bone around an OCD lesion (Figure 51.14). Kissing lesions may also vaguely resemble an OCD lesion during visual inspection in surgery but can be differentiated from an OCD lesion by the lack of a free cartilage flap. Failure to identify and treat coronoid disease and/or other components of elbow dysplasia at the time of OCD lesion treatment may result in suboptimal patient outcomes and persistent lameness and disability.

A medial intermuscular approach is used to access the elbow joint for assessment and treatment of both OCD and

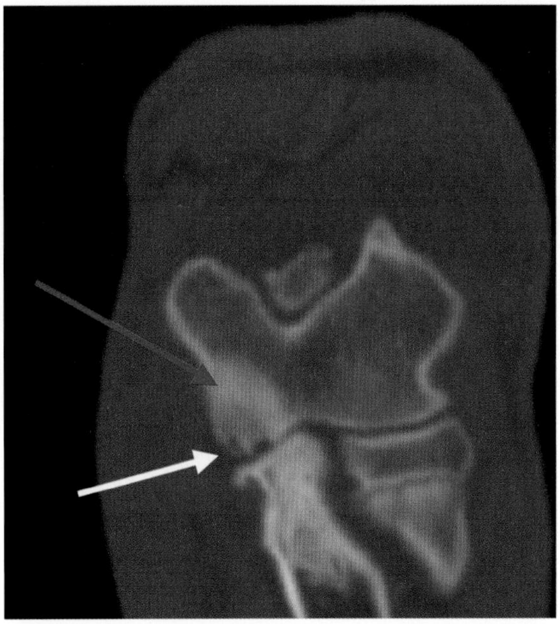

Figure 51.14 Frontal plane computed tomography reconstruction image of the elbow joint of a dog with an OCD lesion of the humeral trochlea. Note the hypoattenuating lesion associated with the OCD lesion (white arrow) and the subjacent hyperattenuation associated with sclerotic bone (red arrow). *Source:* © Stephen C. Jones.

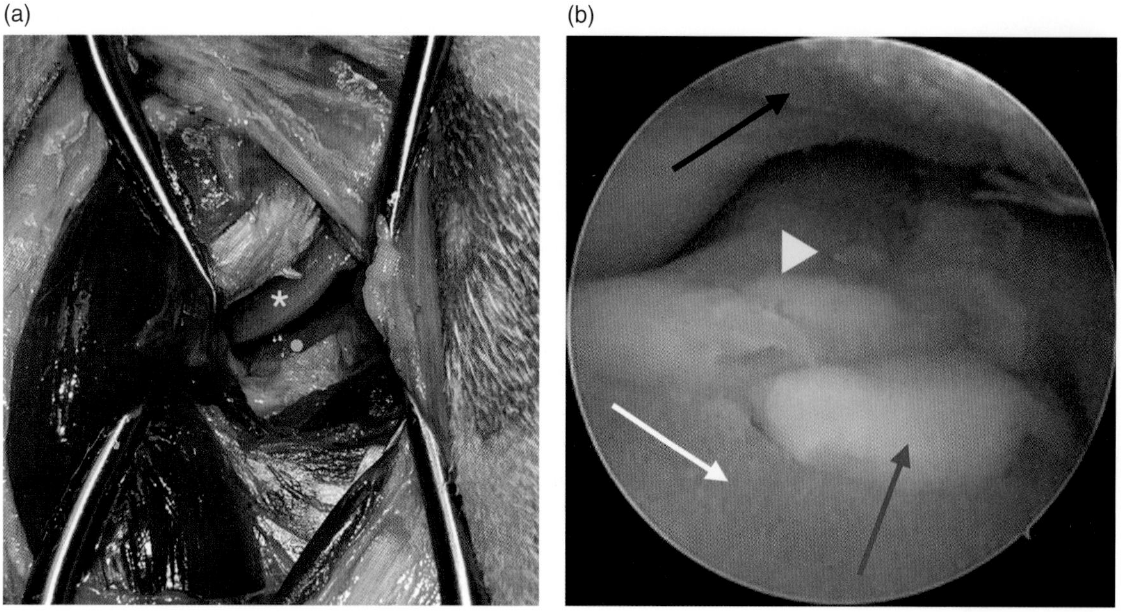

Figure 51.15 (a) Inter-muscular medial elbow arthrotomy[41] and (b) arthroscopic view of an elbow joint with medial coronoid disease. (a) Note the limited view of the trochlea (yellow star) and medial coronoid (blue dot) afforded by an arthrotomy. (b) Note the fragment at the apex of the medial coronoid (red arrow) with complete loss of cartilage of the medial coronoid (white arrow). Using arthroscopy also allows good visualization of the radial head (yellow arrowhead) and the articular margin of the humerus. Note also the kissing lesion of the humeral trochlea (black arrow). *Source:* © Stephen C. Jones.

medial coronoid disease.[41] It is worth noting the superiority of arthroscopy over an arthrotomy for assessment of the medial compartment of the elbow joint. The intermuscular approach provides a limited view of the medial joint compartment (Figure 51.15) and may lead to missed diagnoses (such as coronoid disease, for example) and, therefore, incomplete treatments rendered. Depending on the treatment selected for the OCD lesion, an alternative medial approach to the elbow joint, utilizing an osteotomy of the medial humeral epicondyle, has been described.[41] This approach does provide better access to the medial joint space but comes at the risk of more severe potential post-operative complications, including fixation failure of the medial epicondylar osteotomy, especially in younger dogs with softer bone.

Reported surgical options for OCD of the elbow include treatment by flap removal and subchondral bone stimulation,[42] osteochondral autografts,[23] osteochondral allografts,[26] and synthetic osteochondral implants. Partial or total elbow replacement is also a treatment option for dogs with end-stage DJD affecting the medial compartment or entire joint, respectively.

Tarsus – Surgical Technique

Tarsal OCD in the dog may affect the medial or lateral ridge of the talus, leading to pain, lameness, and progressive DJD. Approximately 79% of cases affect the medial ridge, with 21% reportedly affecting the lateral ridge.[5] Anatomic complexity of the tibio-tarsal joint can make radiographic diagnosis of talar OCD challenging. A craniocaudal projection of the tarsus with the joint in full extension is the most useful radiographic view to help detect OCD of the plantar aspect of the medial trochlear ridge, the most common location for talar OCD. Conversely, less than half of all OCD lesions of the lateral talar ridge are documented on joint-extended craniocaudal tarsal radiographs. A comprehensive overview of additional radiographic views that can be utilized to help diagnose tarsal OCD lesions is available.[5] Despite the utility of these different radiographic views, many cases of tarsal OCD go undiagnosed using conventional radiographs.[5] If available, CT, which affords the surgeon a three-dimensional assessment of this complex joint, allows more accurate determination of lesion presence, location, and size (Figure 51.16).[16,17] Although patient signalment (young, large breed dogs) should lead to clinical suspicion of OCD, the surgeon should thoroughly assess each patient for other sources of lameness attributable to the tarsal joint. Collateral ligament stability, for example, should be carefully assessed pre-operatively. Avulsion fractures of the talofibular portion of the short component of the lateral collateral ligament can create an osteochondral defect on the plantar aspect of the lateral talar ridge, and this can mimic an OCD lesion of that region. Isolated fragmentation of the medial malleolus can also be mistaken for an OCD lesion, given the

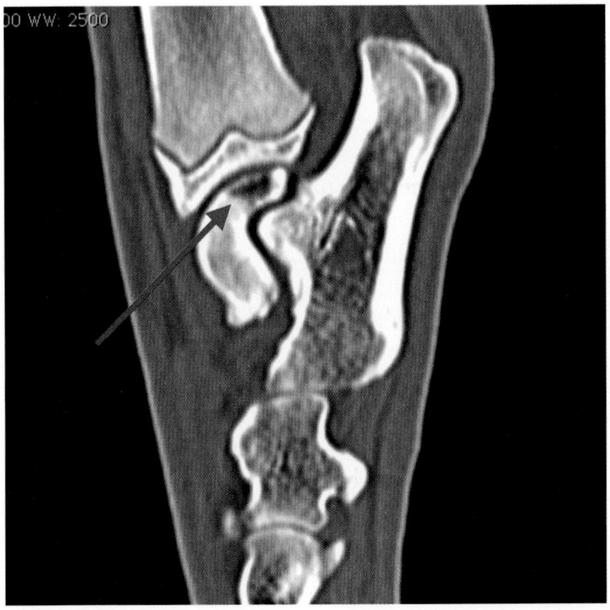

Figure 51.16 Sagittal computed tomographic image of a tarsus from an eight-month-old Labrador retriever. Note the easily identifiable hypoattenuating OCD lesion of the medial ridge of the talus (red arrow). This lesion was not identified on standard orthogonal radiographs of the tarsus. *Source:* Courtesy of Dr. Nina Kieves.

proximity to the medial trochlear ridge of the talus.[43] In the absence of an additional OCD lesion in the joint (present in 50% of fragmentation cases), fragmentation of the medial malleolus often does not warrant surgical intervention.[43]

Five different surgical approaches have been described for the tibio-tarsal joint, including: dorsolateral, dorsomedial, plantarolateral, plantaromedial, and caudal.[5] Depending on the approach, the dog is either positioned in dorsal or lateral recumbency, with the tarsus extended to permit access to more dorsal lesions and flexed to allow access to more plantar lesions. All five approaches have the benefit of being relatively minimally invasive with no osteotomies or desmotomies required.[5]

Scientific reports support the benefits of OCD flap removal with subchondral bone stimulation. Similar to OCD of the humeral head, research suggests that affected dogs benefit from earlier intervention and flap removal. The benefits associated with OCD flap removal and subchondral stimulation may be limited to the short term, as the findings of some clinical studies have suggested that the long-term outcome is no different between joints that did and did not undergo operative treatment.[44,45] Furthermore, lower success rates have been reported in dogs operated after 12 months of age.[44] The poorer longer-term outcomes associated with the tarsal OCD flap removal and debridement presumably are associated with the significant incongruity that results in this tight joint after flap removal and debridement, which tend to result in significant progression of osteoarthritis. The use of osteochondral allografts for tarsal OCD is scarcely reported in the literature.[26] To the author's knowledge, there are no published reports on the use of osteochondral autografts for the treatment of talar OCD in dogs. Recently, partial talar synthetic resurfacing to treat an extensive medial talar OCD lesion was reported in one dog with a good long-term outcome described.[46] This case was performed using a custom-designed prosthesis which was implanted using patient-specific, 3D-printed drill guides. Although custom joint resurfacing technology is in its infancy in the veterinary world, the authors expect custom-designed implants to become more popular in the coming years. Over time, reducing technology costs will likely allow patient-specific implants to become the gold standard for many types of resurfacing procedures in companion animals.

Potential Complications

Potential complications when performing arthroscopic debridement of OCD lesions tend to be infrequent and minor in nature. The most common complications post-assessment of any joint arthroscopically are extravasation of fluids used during arthroscopy and post-operative bruising (Figure 51.17). Extravasation of isotonic crystalloid fluids used during arthroscopy results in soft tissue swelling around the arthroscopy ports. This swelling is short-lived, much like giving a subcutaneous bolus of fluids, and will usually self-resolve within 24 hours.

Bruising is common after any surgical intervention. Once there is no active hemorrhage post-operatively, this is typically left alone and will self-resolve. In the case where a large dissection has been performed and significant bruising seems to be developing, the veterinarian may decide to place a compression bandage to reduce any ongoing oozing or bleeding, thereby, reducing the severity of the bruising.

Seroma formation is arguably the most common complication seen following an arthrotomy to treat OCD. This is especially true for an arthrotomy where a large intermuscular approach has been performed, for example, with the approaches to the shoulder joint. As is the case with any seroma, conservative therapy is highly recommended with warm compresses, massaging, and time considered the treatments of choice. Seroma formation can largely be avoided by meticulous closure of the soft tissues, particularly the subcutaneous layer, and strict exercise restriction in the early post-operative period. The use of a compression bandage can also be helpful in preventing and treating seromas. This, however, is often

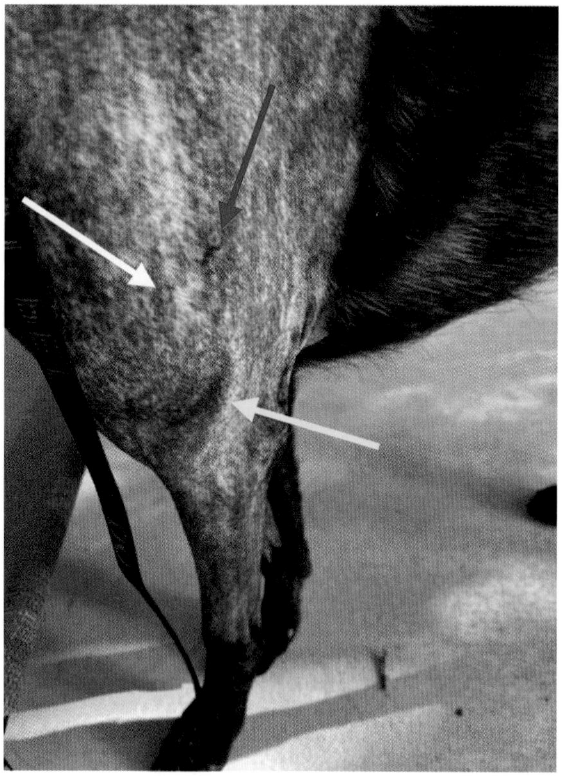

Figure 51.17 Picture of the shoulder and brachium area of a mixed-breed dog four days postarthroscopic debridement of a humeral head OCD lesion. The white and red arrows indicate the location of the scope and instrument portals, respectively. Note the minor, ventrally-dependent bruising as indicated by the yellow arrow. *Source:* © Stephen C. Jones.

difficult or impractical for the more proximal joints with a large peri-articular soft tissue mass (e.g., the shoulder and stifle joints).

Surgical site infection is an uncommon complication following OCD surgery. As mentioned earlier however, when performing a resurfacing procedure, be that an autograft, an allograft, or a synthetic resurfacing procedure, infection can be catastrophic and can result in failure of osseous integration of the graft and/or the necessity to remove the graft/implant completely.

The veterinarian needs to carefully assess the patient's skin pre-operatively for any evidence of dermatitis or pyoderma. Any evidence of skin disease should be treated and be completely resolved before attempting a resurfacing procedure. Arguably, the most important contributor to post-operative infection is incisional trauma by the patient. The patient should be sent home with an appropriately-sized Elizabethan collar and the owner strongly counseled about its importance.

Iatrogenic nerve injury is another rare but significant complication post-OCD surgery. The surgeon should familiarize themselves with the pertinent regional anatomy before attempting surgery to treat OCD.

Post-Operative Care

Patients can generally be discharged from the hospital within 24 hours following OCD surgery. In fact, with improvements in pain management protocols, many of these patients can now be treated as outpatients being discharged on the same day as surgery. Where possible, a lightweight soft-padded bandage is advised for three to four days post-operatively. As mentioned previously, it is imperative that the dog or cat cannot lick or bite at the incision post-operatively. Having a bandage in the early post-operative period helps prevent incisional self-trauma but should not be relied upon. In the authors' opinion, a hard-plastic E-collar is the only repeatably reliable deterrent to prevent licking and biting at the surgery site. If the placement of a bandage is impractical, cold compression of the surgery site daily for the first three to five days can greatly help with discomfort and swelling. Strict exercise restriction is required in the post-operative period. The main goal of any recovery program is to provide slowly increased and controlled loading. In cases with debridement, return to off-leash activity may be slowly introduced over the four to six week post-operative timeframe. Return to normal activity should be slower for allograft, autograft, or synthetic resurfacing, with full return to high-impact activity being closer to three to four months post-operatively (see below). During this time, the dog should not be allowed to run, jump, climb, or play. The patient should be kept in a confined area when inside the house and should be on a short leash whenever they are taken outside.

Sample Rehabilitation Protocol for Resurfacing Procedure

Phase I: 0–4 Weeks

Cage rest with sling support when outside the cage, to avoid excessive load on the lesion. Passive joint range of motion should be performed with controlled weight-bearing and light-controlled load-shifting.

Phase II: 5–8 Weeks

Slow, early load-bearing with controlled 10-minute leash walks twice daily beginning in week 5. Walk duration can be increased by 5 minutes each additional week; the dog can therefore walk 15 minutes twice daily in week 6 and 20 minutes twice daily in week 7, etc. If a complex grafting procedure is performed or the dog displays any discomfort during convalescence, the frequency and/or duration of the walking should be curtailed. Again, no running, jumping, or playing is permitted during this time.

Phase III: 9–12 Weeks

Continued progressive increase in the duration of daily leash walks, with the incorporation of on-leash jogging. Short durations of off-leash activity in a confined area, such as inside the house or in a small backyard, is permitted. Progressively increase the off-leash activity over this time with the goal of complete resumption of normal activity after 12-weeks of recovery.

Prognosis

The prognosis following surgical treatment of OCD depends largely on the joint affected, the method of treatment chosen, and the patient's age at the time of treatment. Conservative therapy tends to be most successful when employed in young dogs with minimal to no clinical signs, small radiographic lesions, and no joint mice.[47] Overall, however, surgical intervention carries a better prognosis than conservative therapy. Older dogs with more chronic lameness tend to have a more guarded prognosis after surgical treatment.[47]

Flap removal and debridement remain the most commonly employed surgical treatment for dogs with OCD. Treatment of the caudal humeral head via flap removal and subchondral bed stimulation carries the best prognosis of all joints affected by OCD in the dog with the prognosis reported to be good to excellent.[47] While no studies have compared long-term outcomes between arthroscopy and arthrotomy, OA development and subtle lameness are still expected long-term after arthroscopic flap removal and subchondral bone stimulation of the humeral head.[17] Prognosis after flap removal and subchondral bone stimulation is described as guarded to poor for the stifle, elbow, and tarsal joints.[1,39,47] The location of the lesion in the joint, the size of the lesion, and how aggressively the subchondral bone is debrided all seem to affect the prognosis. In most cases, surgery improves clinical signs and reduces lameness, but moderate to severe OA progression tends to cause long-term disability for cases of OCD in the stifle, elbow, and tarsal joints.

Studies comparing clinical outcomes of dogs treated with traditional OCD lesion debridement versus those treated with a resurfacing procedure are lacking. Clinical outcomes with lesion debridement and curettage, in locations other than the caudal humeral head, however, suggest that alternative treatments should be considered. Evidence in the human literature suggests resurfacing of knee OCD lesions provides a superior outcome to those with only debridement.[48,49] The poor outcomes with debridement only are attributed to the loss of articular cartilage architecture in the weight-bearing portions of the joint, with the resultant incongruity and abnormal cartilage loading leading to the rapid development of OA.[39] In a randomized clinical trial in people, autograft treatments had significantly better 10-year functional outcomes when compared to microfracture cases, but both groups were improved over presurgical outcome.[50] However, 75% of patients in the autograft group maintained the same physical activity level compared to only 37% in the microfracture group.[50]

In a recent retrospective study in dogs with OCD affecting all major joints, the use of osteochondral allograft transplantation was found to be a viable treatment for both focal and complex cartilage detects.[26] In total, 30 out of 35 cases had a successful outcome; conversely, 5 cases had an unsuccessful outcome, each with a major complication.[26] Osteochondral autografts were successfully employed in the caudal humeral head of 14 dogs (16 shoulders).[25] At long-term evaluation, only one of the 12 dogs examined had lameness in the treated limb.[25] Similar subjectively good outcomes were found when osteochondral autografts were used to treat stifle[39,40] and elbow[23] OCD lesions. Successful long-term outcomes following synthetic osteochondral resurfacing were reported in 24 dogs (28 shoulders) with OCD of the caudal humeral head.[28] In that study, only one dog had a major complication, an implant-associated infection, necessitating implant removal. Although no inference can be made about the superiority of one treatment modality over another, the aforementioned resurfacing studies offer hope that their use (be that an allograft, autograft, or synthetic resurfacing) will improve the historically guarded prognosis for dogs treated for OCD, particularly in the elbow, stifle, and tarsal joints.

References

1 Harari, J. (1998). Osteochondrosis of the femur. *Vet. Clin. North Am. Small Anim. Pract.* 28 (1): 87–94.

2 Cook, J.L., Hung, C.T., Kuroki, K. et al. (2014). Animal models of cartilage repair. *Bone Joint Res.* 3 (4): 89–94.

3 Nečas, A., Dvořák, M., and Zatloukal, J. (1999). Incidence of osteochondrosis in dogs and its late diagnosis. *Acta Vet. Brno* 68 (2): 131–139.

4 Montgomery, R.M., Milton, J.L., Henderson, R.A. et al. (1989). Osteochondritis dissecans of the canine stifle. *Compend. Cont. Educ. Pract. Vet.* 11 (10): 1199–1206.

5 Fitch, R.B. and Beale, B.S. (1998). Osteochondrosis of the canine tibiotarsal joint. *Vet. Clin. North Am. Small Anim. Pract.* 28 (1): 95–113.

6 Bilmont, A., Mathon, D., and Autefage, A. (2018). Arthroscopic management of osteochondrosis of the glenoid cavity in a dog. *J. Am. Anim. Hosp. Assoc.* 54 (5): e54503.
7 Bartels, J.E., Dorn, A.S., and Britt, A.L. (1970). Osteochondrosis of the vertebrae in a dog. *Can. Vet. J.* 11 (3): 47–51.
8 Alexander, J.E. and Pettit, G.D. (1967). Spinal osteochondrosis in a dog. *Can. Vet. J.* 8 (2): 47–49.
9 Mathis, K.R., Havlicek, M., Beck, J.B. et al. (2009). Sacral osteochondrosis in two German Shepherd dogs. *Aus. Vet. J.* 87 (6): 249–252.
10 Hanna, F.Y. (2001). Lumbosacral osteochondrosis: radiological features and surgical management in 34 dogs. *J. Small Anim. Pract.* 42 (6): 272–278.
11 Palierne, S., Palissier, F., Raymond-Letron, I. et al. (2010). A case of bilateral patellar osteochondrosis and fracture in a cat. *Vet. Comp. Orthop. Traumatol.* 23 (02): 128–133.
12 Skelly, C.M., McAllister, H., and Donnelly, W.J.C. (1997). Avulsion of the tibial tuberosity in a litter of greyhound puppies. *J. Small Anim. Pract.* 38 (10): 445–449.
13 Poulos, P.W. (1982). Canine osteochondrosis. *Vet. Clin. North Am. Small Anim. Pract.* 12 (2): 313–328.
14 McCoy, A.M., Toth, D., Dolvik, N.I. et al. (2013). Articular osteochondrosis: a comparison of naturally-occurring human and animal disease. *Osteoarthr. Cartil.* 21 (11): 1638–1647.
15 Lykkjen, S., Roed, K.H., and Dolvik, N.I. (2012). Osteochondrosis and osteochondral fragments in Standardbred trotters: prevalence and relationships. *Equine Vet. J.* 44 (3): 332–338.
16 Gielen, I., van Ryssen, H., and van Bree, H. (2005). Computerized tomography compared with radiography in the diagnosis of lateral trochlear ridge talar osteochondritis dissecans in dogs. *Vet. Comp. Orthop. Traumatol.* 18 (02): 77–82.
17 Zann, G.J., Jones, S.C., Selmic, L.S. et al. (2022). Long-term outcome of dogs treated by surgical debridement of proximal humeral osteochondrosis. *Vet. Surg.*.
18 van Bree, H. (1993). Comparison of the diagnostic accuracy of positive-contrast arthrography and arthrotomy in evaluation of osteochondrosis lesions in the scapulohumeral joint in dogs. *J. Am. Vet. Med. Assoc.* 203 (1): 84–88.
19 Vandevelde, B., Van Ryssen, B., Saunders, J.H. et al. (2006). Comparison of the ultrasonographic appearance of osteochondrosis lesions in the canine shoulder with radiography, arthrography, and arthroscopy. *Vet. Radiol. Ultrasound* 47 (2): 174–184.
20 van Bree, H., Degryse, H., Van Ryssen, B. et al. (1993). Pathologic correlations with magnetic resonance images of osteochondrosis lesions in canine shoulders. *J. Am. Vet. Med. Assoc.* 202 (7): 1099–1105.
21 Wall, C.R., Cook, C.R., and Cook, J.L. (2015). Diagnostic sensitivity of radiography, ultrasonography, and magnetic resonance imaging for detecting shoulder osteochondrosis/osteochondritis dissecans in dogs. *Vet. Radiol. Ultrasound* 56 (1): 3–11.
22 Vezzoni, A., Vezzoni, L., Boiocchi, S. et al. (2020). A modification of the Cheli craniolateral approach for minimally invasive treatment of osteochondritis dissecans of the shoulder in dogs: description of the technique and outcome in 164 cases. *Vet. Comp. Orthop. Traumatol.* 34 (02): 130–136.
23 Fitzpatrick, N., Yeadon, R., and Smith, T.J. (2009). Early clinical experience with osteochondral autograft transfer for treatment of osteochondritis dissecans of the medial humeral condyle in dogs. *Vet. Surg.* 38 (2): 246–260.
24 Steadman, J.R., Briggs, K.K., Rodrigo, J.J. et al. (2003). Outcomes of microfracture for traumatic chondral defects of the knee: average 11-year follow-up. *Arthroscopy* 19 (5): 477–484.
25 Fitzpatrick, N., Van Terheijden, C., Yeadon, R., and Smith, T.J. (2010). Osteochondral autograft transfer for treatment of osteochondritis dissecans of the caudocentral humeral head in dogs. *Vet. Surg.* 39 (8): 925–935.
26 Franklin, S.P., Stoker, A.M., Murphy, S.M. et al. (2021). Outcomes associated with osteochondral allograft transplantation in dogs. *Front. Vet. Sci.* 8: 759610.
27 Egan, P., Murphy, S., Jovanovik, J. et al. (2018). Treatment of osteochondrosis dissecans of the canine stifle using synthetic osteochondral resurfacing. *Vet. Comp. Orthop. Traumatol.* 31 (2): 144–152.
28 Murphy, S.C., Egan, P.M., and Fitzpatrick, N.M. (2019). Synthetic osteochondral resurfacing for treatment of large caudocentral osteochondritis dissecans lesions of the humeral head in 24 dogs. *Vet. Surg.* 48 (5): 858–868.
29 Piermattei, D.L. and Johnson, K.A. (2004). The scapula and shoulder joint. In: *Piermattei's Atlas of Surgical Approaches to the Bones and Joints of the Dog and Cat*, 4e, 126–141. Philadelphia, PA: Saunders.
30 Johnston, S.A. and Tobias, K.M. (2018). The shoulder. In: *Veterinary Surgery Small Animal*, 2e, 805–808. St. Louis, MO: Elsevier.
31 Sparrow, T., Fitzpatrick, M.J., and Blunn, G. (2014). Shoulder joint hemiarthroplasty for treatment of a severe osteo- chondritis dissecans lesion in a dog. *Vet. Comp. Orthop. Traumatol.* 27 (3): 243–248.
32 Biezyński, J., Skrzypczak, P., Piatek, A. et al. (2012). Assessment of treatment of Osteochondrosis dissecans (OCD) of shoulder joint in dogs – the results of two years of experience. *Pol. J. Vet. Sci.* 15 (2): 285–290.
33 Herrin, K.V., Allan, G., Black, A. et al. (2012). Stifle osteochondritis dissecans in snow leopards (Uncia uncia). *J. Zoo Wildl. Med.* 43 (2): 347–354.

34 Ralphs, S.C. (2005). Bilateral stifle osteochondritis dissecans in a cat. *J. Am. Anim. Hosp. Assoc.* 41 (1): 78–80.

35 Kulendra, E., Lee, K., Schoeniger, S., and Moores, A.P. (2008). Osteochondritis dissecans-like lesion of the intercondylar fossa of the femur in a dog. *Vet. Comp. Orthop. Traumatol.* 21 (2): 152–155.

36 Piermattei, D.L. and Johnson, K.A. (2004). The hindlimb. In: *Piermattei's Atlas of Surgical Approaches to the Bones and Joints of the Dog and Cat*, 4e, 392–399. Philadelphia, PA: Saunders.

37 Johnston, S.A. and Tobias, K.M. (2018). Stifle joint. In: *Veterinary Surgery Small Animal*, 2e, 1164–1165. St. Louis, MO: Elsevier.

38 Glenn, R.E. Jr., McCarty, E.C., Potter, H.G. et al. (2006). Comparison of fresh osteochondral autografts and allografts: a canine model. *Am. J. Sports Med.* 34 (7): 1084–1093.

39 Cook, J.L., Hudson, C.C., and Kuroki, K. (2008). Autogenous osteochondral grafting for treatment of stifle osteochondrosis in dogs. *Vet. Surg.* 37 (4): 311–321.

40 Fitzpatrick, N., Yeadon, R., van Terheijden, C., and Smith, T.J. (2012). Osteochondral autograft transfer for the treatment of osteochondritis dissecans of the medial femoral condyle in dogs. *Vet. Comp. Orthop. Traumatol.* 25 (2): 135–143.

41 Piermattei, D.L. and Johnson, K.A. (2004). The forelimb. In: *Piermattei's Atlas of Surgical Approaches to the Bones and Joints of the Dog and Cat*, 4e, 252–265. Philadelphia, PA: Saunders.

42 Johnston, S.A. and Tobias, K.M. (2018). Surgical diseases of the elbow. In: *Veterinary Surgery Small Animal*, 2e, 871–872. St. Louis, MO: Elsevier.

43 Newell, S.M., Mahaffey, M.B., and Aron, D.N. (1994). Fragmentation of the medial malleolus of dogs with and without tarsal osteochondrosis. *Vet. Radiol. Ultrasound* 35 (1): 5–9.

44 Breur VCOT 1989 Breur GJ, Spaulding KA, Braden TD. Osteochondritis dissecans of the medial trochlear ridge of the talus in the dog. *Vet. Comp. Orthop. Traumatol.* 1989;2(4):168–176.

45 Smith, M.M., Vasseur, P.B., and Morgan, J.P. (1985). Clinical evaluation of dogs after surgical and nonsurgical management of osteochondritis dissecans of the talus. *J. Am. Vet. Med. Assoc.* 187 (1): 31–35.

46 Schmierer, P.A. and Böttcher, P. (2023). Patient specific, synthetic, partial unipolar resurfacing of a large talar osteochondritis dissecans lesion in a dog. *Vet. Surg.* 52 (5): 731–738.

47 Demko, J. and McLaughlin, R. (2005). Developmental orthopedic disease. *Vet. Clin. North Am. Small Anim. Pract.* 35 (5): 1111–1135.

48 Murray, J.R.D., Chitnavis, J., Dixon, P. et al. (2007). Osteochondritis dissecans of the knee; long- term clinical outcome following arthroscopic debridement. *Knee* 14 (2): 94–98.

49 Sanders, T.L., Pareek, A., Johnson, N.R. et al. (2017). Nonoperative management of osteochondritis dissecans of the knee: progression to osteoarthritis and arthroplasty at mean 13-year follow-up. *Orthop. J. Sports Med.* 5 (7): 2325967117704644.

50 Gudas, R., Gudaite, A., Pocius, A. et al. (2012). Ten-year follow-up of a prospective, randomized clinical study of mosaic osteochondral autologous transplantation versus microfracture for the treatment of osteochondral defects in the knee joint of athletes. *Am. J. Sports Med.* 40 (11): 2499–2508.

52

Arthrocentesis

Carolyn L. Chen[1], Leah P. Hixon[2], and Emily C. Viani[3]

[1] *Department of Small Animal Medicine and Surgery, University of Georgia, Athens, GA, USA*
[2] *Colorado Canine Orthopedics, Colorado Springs, CO, USA*
[3] *Tufts Veterinary Emergency Treatment & Specialties, Walpole, MA, USA*

Key Points

- Arthrocentesis is a common technique utilized to diagnose diseases of the joints.
- Appropriate sampling technique and knowledge of local anatomy is required to obtain a useful sample and avoid iatrogenic damage to the affected joint.
- Given that no specialized equipment is required, any clinician can perform arthrocentesis with the appropriate training.

Introduction

Joints, or articulations, form when two or more bones are united by a combination of fibrous, elastic, or cartilaginous tissue. They are divided into three main groups: fibrous, cartilaginous, and synovial joints. Synovial joints permit the greatest degree of movement and are the most commonly involved when considering diagnostic sampling. All synovial joints are characterized by a joint cavity, a joint capsule, synovial fluid, and articular cartilage.[1] The shoulder, elbow, carpus, hip, stifle, and tarsus are all synovial joints.

Arthrocentesis is the aspiration of synovial fluid from a joint space. Synovial fluid analysis is recommended in diagnostic workup for joint disease. It is useful for categorizing types of diseases, such as immune-mediated, inflammatory, infectious, and occasionally, neoplastic. Synovial fluid analysis can be beneficial in diagnosing joint disease in a rapid manner based on cytology and cell count numbers. Osteoarthritis typically shows evidence of mild inflammatory change with mild to moderate increases in mononuclear cell numbers. Moderate to severe increases in mononuclear cell numbers and nondegenerative neutrophils is a more supportive cytology indicative of immune-mediated polyarthritis; whereas degenerative neutrophils with or without organisms is indicative of infective arthritis.[2–4] The reader is directed to other texts for further detail regarding specific diseases of the joint and associated cytology and culture findings.[2,4,5]

Arthrocentesis is a simple diagnostic procedure that carries minimal morbidity when performed appropriately. The procedure does not require extensive training or specialized equipment, lending itself to be a widely accessible diagnostic and therapeutic tool for the general veterinary clinician. Appropriate knowledge of pertinent anatomy and practice can quickly make arthrocentesis an invaluable tool for the diagnosis and treatment of a wide variety of joint diseases.[6] This chapter is meant to provide the clinician with tools and information to become successful at performing arthrocentesis of various joints in the dog and cat.

Indications/Pre-procedure Considerations

There are several indications for performing arthrocentesis and joint taps in veterinary patients, which can be categorized broadly into diagnostic and therapeutic reasons. Synovial fluid may be aspirated to obtain an initial diagnosis or to guide treatment for an ongoing disease process, such

Techniques in Small Animal Soft Tissue, Orthopedic, and Ophthalmic Surgery, First Edition. Edited by Kristin A. Coleman.

Companion website: www.wiley.com/go/coleman/surgeries

as septic arthritis or immune-mediated polyarthritis. Therapeutic indications for placing a needle into the joint may include injecting medications, such as platelet-rich plasma (PrP), or flushing joints to treat septic arthritis. Flushing the joint can also be utilized to check joint capsule integrity as part of a complete wound evaluation.

The clinician must remember to evaluate the patient as a whole prior to performing arthrocentesis. While most patients can tolerate arthrocentesis with sedation, the patient's cardiovascular status and anesthetic candidacy must be evaluated to allow for a safe sedation or anesthetic event should general anesthesia be necessary. Smaller dogs and cats may require more extensive sedation or anesthesia to prevent iatrogenic hemorrhage from trauma to the synovium secondary to movement during the procedure.

Steps should be taken to ensure efficiency and decrease patient morbidity, including appropriate patient positioning and preparation. The clinician should decide how many joints need to be sampled and accordingly position the patient such that the least amount of repositioning is needed to access all joints. In cases where clearly one joint is affected, the clinician may elect to only sample said joint. If trying to diagnose immune-mediated polyarthritis, multiple joints, preferably distal joints, such as a carpus and/or tarsus, should be sampled even if only one joint seems clinically affected.[5] Anticipated tools needed for the procedure should be laid out for easy access, including but not limited to sterile needles (22-gauge being the most commonly used), syringes, slides, gloves, culture tubes, and sample tubes (Figure 52.1).

Aseptic technique should be practiced when preparing the sites for arthrocentesis. The skin overlying the desired sample site should be evaluated for overt disease that would increase the chances of complication with this procedure. Although it has been demonstrated that effective aseptic skin preparation is possible without clipping short-haired dogs, the authors still recommend that the fur over the joint of interest is clipped to allow sterile preparation and decrease the chance of iatrogenic introduction of joint infection.[7]

Surgical Procedure

Once positioned appropriately, the fur over the joints of interest is clipped, and the skin is aseptically prepared. Sterile gloves should be worn to facilitate palpation of the joint. It has been shown that larger syringes can generate more vacuum but result in relatively less needle control.[8] Therefore, it is recommended to choose a syringe that is just large enough for a sample but not too small such that viscous joint fluid cannot be aspirated. This is most commonly a 3 mL syringe. Regular hypodermic needles have a relatively long bevel, which may preclude the lumen from entering the joint completely in smaller joints. In those cases, a spinal needle, which has a short bevel, may be of better yield.[9]

The clinician can decide whether or not to attach the needle to the syringe prior to or after the insertion of the needle into the joint. See below for techniques specific to each joint. Negative pressure is gently applied to the syringe, keeping in mind that normal joint fluid is viscous and requires more time to travel through the needle into the syringe. If no joint fluid is appreciated, sometimes

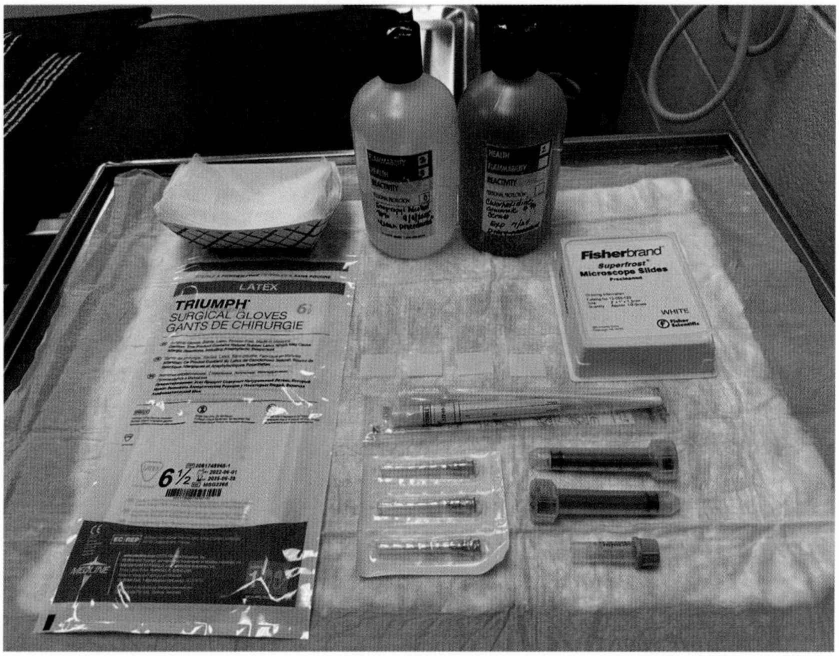

Figure 52.1 Common supplies used for arthrocentesis include (starting from the left in a clockwise direction): sterile gloves, gauze, aseptic scrub materials, microscope slides, culturette, syringes, collection tubes, and hypodermic needles. *Source:* © Carolyn Chen, Leah Hixon, Emily Viani.

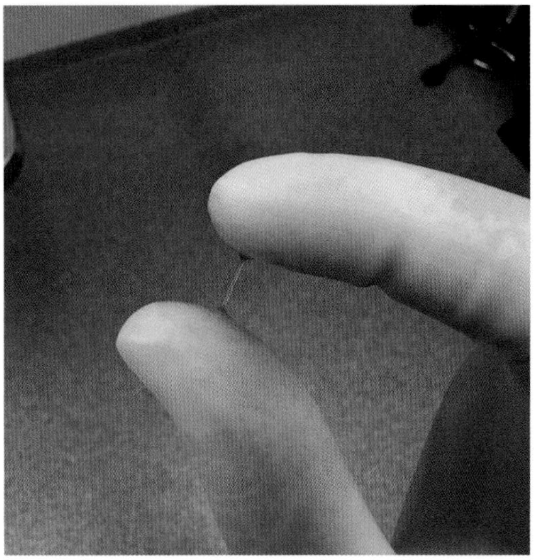

Figure 52.2 Normal joint fluid should be clear to straw-colored and quite viscous. A watery joint fluid that lacks the normal sticky consistency indicates an inflammatory component. *Source:* © Carolyn Chen, Leah Hixon, Emily Viani.

rotating the needle on its axis and re-aspirating may help dislodge any tissue that is blocking the lumen. Negative pressure should be released prior to redirecting and re-aspirating the joint. Oftentimes, only a small amount of fluid, such as only enough to fill the needle hub, is required to achieve a diagnosis; the quality of the fluid is prioritized over the quantity.[10] After synovial fluid has successfully been sampled, negative pressure is released, and the syringe and needle are removed from the joint. Alternatively, in efforts to prevent blood contamination, the clinician can firmly hold the needle hub in place while disconnecting the syringe. The needle is then removed.

The gross appearance of the synovial sample can often give the clinician a hint as to whether pathology is present or not in the joint. Normal joint fluid should be quite viscous, clear, and straw-colored (Figure 52.2). Synovial fluid is a thixotropic fluid; it is less viscous when shaken, and will return to the original viscosity at rest.[10] It should not be mistaken for a clot.

Samples from arthrocentesis should be immediately transferred to the medium of choice, whether it be for cytology or for culture. If there is blood contamination, the fluid may be placed in an EDTA tube to prevent clotting. However, EDTA will interfere with the mucin clot test[1] and culture results.[10] To preserve cell morphology, direct smear slides should be prepared right after obtaining the sample. The clinician should keep in mind that because of the viscous nature of the joint fluid, the spreader slide should be moved slowly and evenly.[11] If the clinician wishes to culture the synovial fluid, the sample should be kept in the sterile syringe, placed in an aerobic culturette, or placed in a blood culture tube. Aerobic culturette tubes should be placed in the refrigerator and shipped on ice packs.[12] It has been shown in human prosthetic joint infections that blood culture tubes have higher sensitivity, specificity, and positive and negative predictive values when compared with standard tissue and swab samples.[13] Additionally, blood cultures were shown to have improved detection rates in human septic arthritis as compared to traditional agar plates.[14] Although it has been shown that a slight delay in sample incubation is not detrimental to the results,[15,16] it is still strongly recommended to incubate the blood culture tubes as soon as possible. The blood culture tubes should never be refrigerated or frozen.[17]

Shoulder

The shoulder joint is a ball-and-socket, diarthrodial joint that involves the articulation of the glenoid cavity of the scapula with the head of the humerus.[18] It is a highly moveable joint, allowing flexion, extension, abduction, and adduction. The main movement of the shoulder is flexion and extension.[19] The bony anatomy of the joint consists of the distal extremity of the scapula and the proximal humerus. Along the lateral surface of the shoulder is the spine of the scapula, which starts from the middle of the dorsal border and extends distally to the glenoid end, which forms a pointed structure known as the acromion process. The lateral surface of the humerus is the deltoid tuberosity and the brachial groove. An important feature to note at the proximal humerus is the crest of the greater tubercle. The craniolateral bony projection on the lateral surface of the proximal humerus is the greater tubercle, whereas the smaller bony prominence at the medial aspect is the lesser tubercle.[18]

The primary ligaments of the glenohumeral joint are the joint capsule and the two glenohumeral ligaments. The joint capsule attaches proximally at the periphery of the labrum, which is the glenoid lip that surrounds the glenoid. The joint capsule attaches distally to the distal portion of the humeral head. The glenohumeral ligaments, both lateral and medial, arise from the supraglenoid tubercle and end caudal to the lesser tubercle of the humerus. These collateral ligaments bridge the joint on the lateral and medial aspects.[18,20–22]

There are multiple muscles, nerves, and vessels also comprising the anatomy of the shoulder joint. The tendon of the biceps brachii muscle, supraspinatus and infraspinatus muscles, subscapularis muscle, omotransversarius and deltoideus muscles, and tendons of the teres major and minor muscles are all involved in the shoulder joint anatomy. The biceps brachii muscle originates from the supraglenoid tubercle of the scapular bone, crosses the shoulder joint, and inserts on the cranial surface of the humerus to the joint capsule at the intertubercular groove.[18,21,23] It is at the intertubercular groove where the joint capsule surrounds the tendon of the biceps brachii muscle, and it is held in place by the transverse humeral retinaculum. The axillary, subscapularis, brachial and radial nerves, and arteries are located cranial to the shoulder joint, while the subscapularis artery and nerve are located caudally.[18,20,21]

Knowledge of the anatomy of the shoulder joint is vital prior to performing arthrocentesis to minimize complications and contamination. For arthrocentesis of the shoulder joint, it is necessary for the patient to be sedated. The sedated patient is placed in lateral recumbency. Important landmarks to palpate prior to arthrocentesis are the greater tubercle and acromion (Figure 52.3). In general, the joint is located distal to the acromion and proximal to the greater tubercle. Using sterile technique, a 22-gauge needle attached to a 3cc syringe, is inserted and directed craniolateral to caudomedial, entering the joint between the greater tubercle and the acromion, shown in Figure 52.4.[24–26] A longer needle may be required for large dogs. Once the needle is advanced into the joint, synovial fluid can be aspirated. Synovial fluid analysis is critical in diagnosing immune-mediated and septic disease of the shoulder joint; however, these diseases are less common in the shoulder joint. It is more common for shoulder joint disease to be consistent with degenerative joint disease, in which case synovial analysis can be normal despite intra-articular disease. If degenerative joint disease is suspected in the joint, further diagnostics, such as advanced imaging (radiographs, musculoskeletal ultrasound, or computed tomography) is recommended in addition to synovial analysis.[24,25]

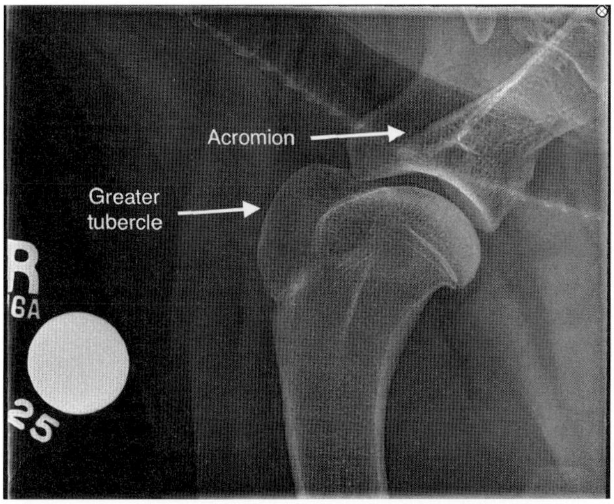

Figure 52.3 Lateral radiograph of the right canine shoulder. The acromion and the greater tubercle of the humerus are important landmarks for shoulder arthrocentesis and are labeled. *Source:* © Carolyn Chen, Leah Hixon, Emily Viani.

Elbow

The elbow is a hinge joint with a range of motion of 36° in flexion and 165° in extension. Motion in torsion and mediolateral plane is limited due to the anconeal process and collateral ligaments,[27,28] which make it a "ginglymus" joint. The medial collateral ligament attaches proximally to the medial epicondyle of the humerus and then divides into cranial and caudal crura. It attaches distally to the radius and ulna. The lateral collateral ligament is stronger than the medial, attaches proximally to the lateral epicondyle of the humerus, and divides in a similar manner to the medial collateral ligament. The annular ligament is located deep in the collateral ligaments and prevents cranial translation of the radius by its attachments on the

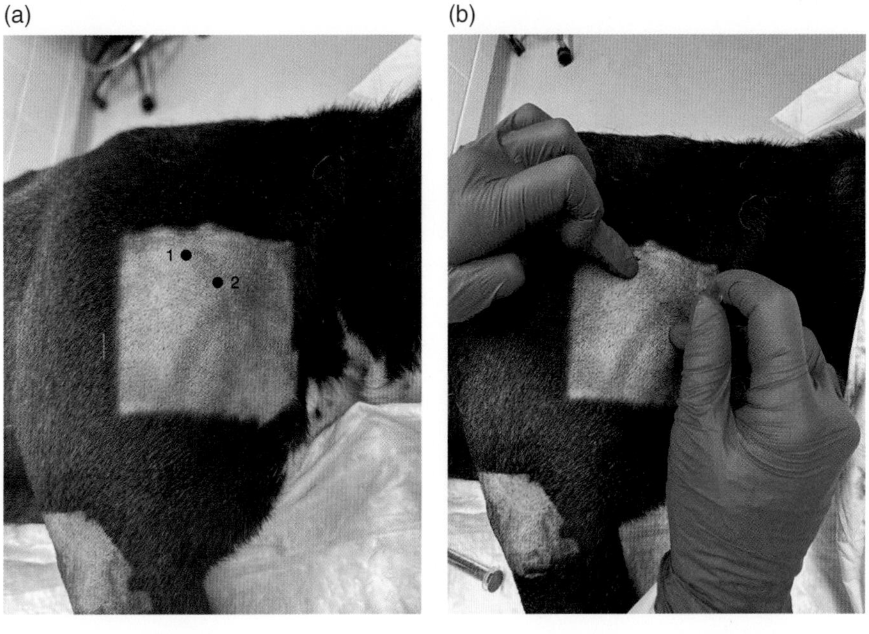

Figure 52.4 (a) The right shoulder joint, lateral aspect. The patient is in left lateral recumbency with cranial to the right and caudal to the left. 1, acromion; 2, greater tubercle. (b) The joint is located distal to the acromion and proximal to the greater tubercle. The needle is inserted and directed craniolateral to caudomedial, entering the joint. The fingertips are on the palpable landmarks immediately prior to sterile arthrocentesis. *Source:* © Carolyn Chen, Leah Hixon, Emily Viani.

proximal radius and ulna. The ligaments are external to the joint capsule. The joint capsule encloses the joint and forms two compartments: cranial and caudal. An inner synovial layer and an outer fibrous layer comprise the joint capsule.[27,29,30]

The extensor muscles of the elbow consist of the triceps brachii muscle, anconeus, and tensor fasciae antebrachii muscles. They are innervated by the radial nerve. Flexor muscles consist of the biceps brachii and brachialis muscles. Flexion of the elbow joint by these muscles is via innervation by the musculocutaneous nerve. In contrast to the canine, the supratrochlear foramen is usually absent in felines; however, a supracondylar foramen is present in the humerus. This serves as an opening for the median nerve and brachial artery. Another difference between the canine and feline anatomy is the presence of the epitrochlearis muscle in the cat. This muscle is present on the proximomedial surface of the elbow articulation, which arises from the medial epicondylar crest and inserts on the olecranon to function with the triceps musculature to extend the elbow. Lastly, while the brachioradialis muscle is a thin strip of muscle in the canine, it is well-developed in the feline.[31] The median nerve and artery runs along the medial aspect of the elbow. The ulnar nerve and collateral ulnar artery cross the caudomedial aspect of the joint and continue distally between the flexor carpi radialis and superficial digital flexor muscles. Lastly, the radial nerve crosses craniolateral to the joint, with the deep branch running under the proximocranial border of the extensor carpi radialis muscle.[32,33]

Elbow arthrocentesis is subjectively more difficult in comparison to other joints, and as such, there are several methods performed to obtain joint fluid. For the first of three methods, place the patient in lateral recumbency with the affected elbow facing up in a neutral position. Palpate two landmarks: the lateral epicondyle of the humerus and olecranon (Figures 52.5 and 52.6a). Using a 22-gauge, 1-in. needle and 3cc syringe, position the needle parallel to the long axis of the ulna, halfway between the two landmarks, in a distomedial direction (Figure 52.6b–d). The needle can be inserted just medial to the lateral epicondylar ridge, proximal to the olecranon process. Once in the joint, the needle should be between the lateral epicondylar crest of the humerus and the anconeal process of the ulna.[4] Alternatively, as the second method, the needle can be inserted into the joint space between the radial articular fovea and the ulnar lateral coronoid process. This location can be configured based on palpation of the lateral epicondyle first, then targeting distal to this anatomical location. This is similar to the third method, which is obtaining joint fluid from the medial aspect of the elbow, mirroring portal locations for arthroscopy. For this method, the patient is

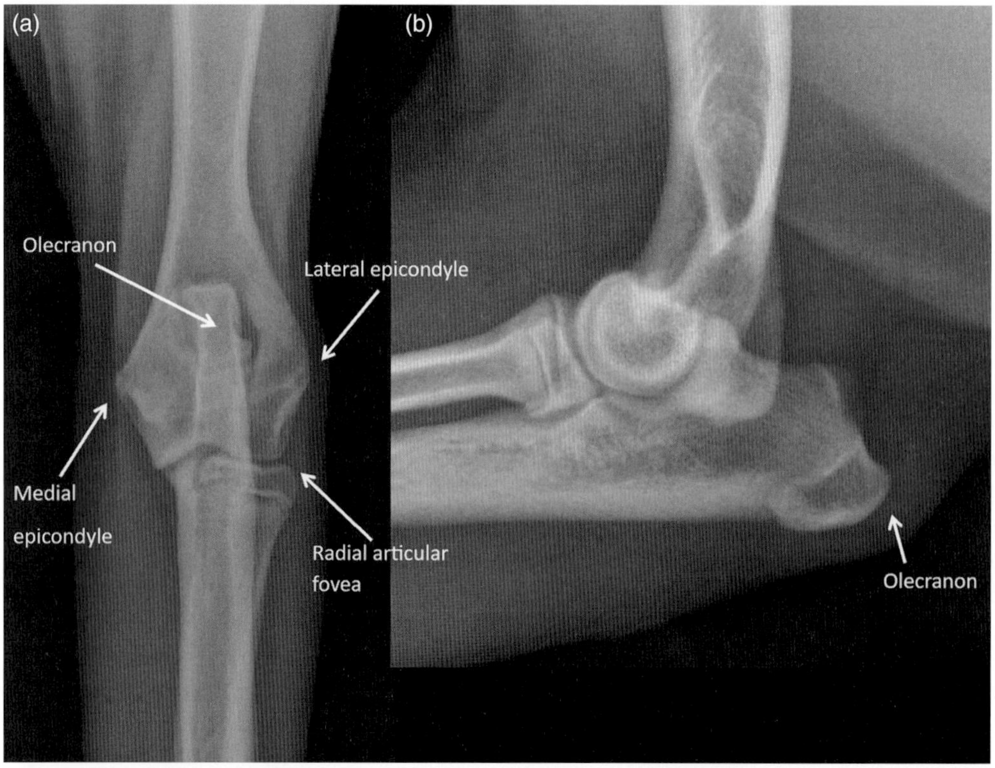

Figure 52.5 (a) Cranial-caudal radiograph of the canine elbow. (b) Lateral view of the canine elbow. *Source:* © Carolyn Chen, Leah Hixon, Emily Viani.

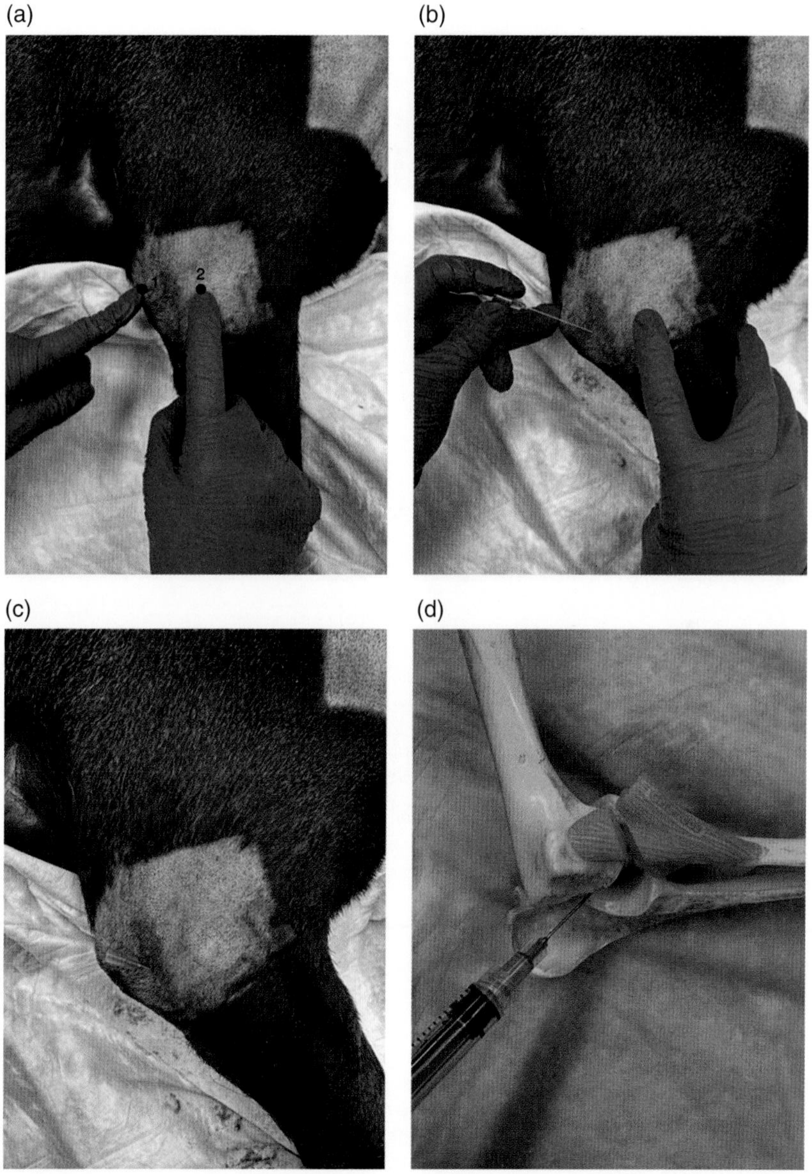

Figure 52.6 (a) The right elbow joint, lateral aspect. The patient is in left lateral recumbency with cranial to the right and caudal to the left. 1, olecranon; 2, lateral epicondyle of the humerus. (b) The needle is positioned parallel to the long axis of the ulna, halfway between the two landmarks in a distomedial direction. The needle is inserted into the joint just medial to the lateral epicondylar ridge, proximal to the olecranon process. (c) Once in the joint, the needle should be between the lateral epicondylar crest of the humerus and the anconeal process of the ulna. (d) A model of the right elbow showing the position of the needle in the joint. Cranial is to the right and caudal is to the left. *Source:* © Carolyn Chen, Leah Hixon, Emily Viani.

positioned in lateral recumbency with the affected elbow down. For easier entry into the joint, a rolled towel should be placed on the laterodistal aspect of the elbow, and a non-sterile assistant may gently abduct the elbow (toward the floor, as if pushing into valgus position) with the carpus flexed. After locating the palpable medial epicondyle, a line is imagined (or drawn) parallel to the radial diaphysis, and approximately 45° caudally and 6–10 mm in length (varies with patient size) from the medial epicondyle in a caudodistal direction is the joint space. Care must be taken to precisely identify this medial landmark prior to blindly attempting arthrocentesis due to the proximity of the caudally-located ulnar nerve, the cranially-located median nerve, and the even more cranially-located median artery on the medial aspect (Figure 52.7).[1,33,34]

Carpus

The carpus consists of multiple joints formed from the various bony articulations amongst the radius, ulna, and the seven carpal bones, which are arranged in two transverse rows plus a small medial sesamoid bone located in the tendon of insertion of the musculus abductor digiti I pollicis longus on the proximomedial aspect of the first metacarpal bone. The proximal row includes the radial carpal bone, ulnar carpal bone, and accessory carpal bone. The distal row includes the first through fourth carpal bones.[35] From proximal to distal, the three main joints are the antebrachiocarpal joint, the middle carpal joint, and the carpometacarpal joint. Of these, the antebrachiocarpal joint is the most commonly sampled space. This joint is located between the distal part of the radius, called the trochlea

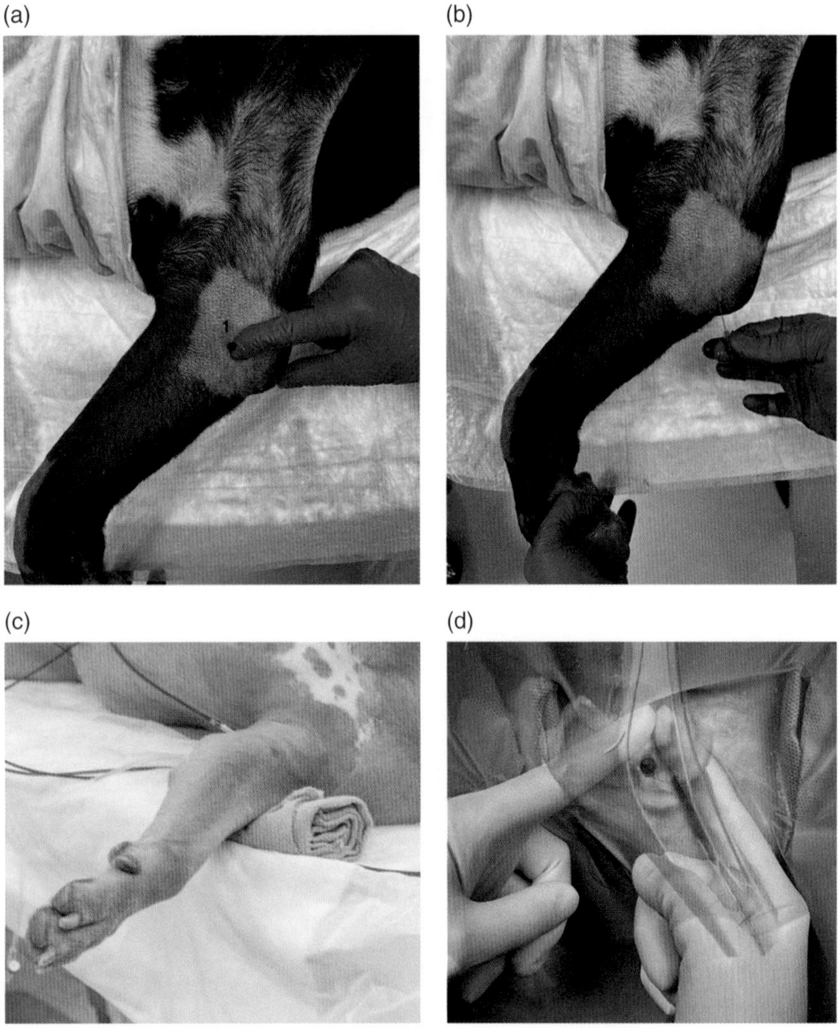

Figure 52.7 The elbow joint can also be approached medially. (a) The right elbow joint, medial aspect. The patient is in right lateral recumbency with the left forelimb held in abduction by an assistant with cranial to the left and caudal to the right. 1, medial epicondyle is palpated in this image. (b) The needle is inserted perpendicular to or angled slightly proximally to parallel the trochlear surface. (c) To aid in "breaking open" the joint, a rolled towel should be placed on the laterodistal aspect of the elbow, and a nonsterile assistant may gently abduct the elbow (toward the floor, somewhat pushing into valgus position) with the carpus flexed. (d) The left elbow joint, medial aspect, cranial to the right, and caudal to the left. The two fingertips in this image are converging on the palpable medial epicondyle, and the right pointer finger is kept parallel to the radial diaphysis. The left pointer finger is angled 90° from the right finger (i.e., perpendicular to the radius), and the hypodermic needle is easily inserted into the joint space, which is halfway between these two fingers (i.e., 45° from the radius) and approximately 6–10 mm in length from the medial epicondyle depending on the size of the patient. Care must be taken to precisely identify this medial landmark prior to blindly attempting arthrocentesis due to the proximity of the caudally-located ulnar nerve, the cranially-located median nerve, and the even more cranially-located median artery on this medial aspect. *Source:* (a) and (b) © Carolyn Chen, Leah Hixon, Emily Viani; (c) © Caleb Hudson; (d) © Kristin Coleman.

radii, and the ulna and the proximal row of carpal bones (Figure 52.8).

The dorsal aspect of the carpus should be shaved and aseptically prepared. To position for sampling, the carpus is flexed to 90° by the clinician or an assistant, and a depression just distal to the radius is palpated; this is the antebrachiocarpal joint space (Figure 52.9). The needle should be inserted within this area perpendicular or angled slightly proximally to the joint, just medial to the common digital extensor tendon and the cephalic vein, both of which pass over the center of the dorsal aspect of the joint space. If there is resistance, the angle of carpal flexion can be slowly adjusted along with careful needle redirection until the joint space is found. Alternatively, the middle or carpometacarpal joints can also be sampled with maximal flexion of the carpus and careful palpation of the spaces between the rows of bones. The distal two joints communicate, but not with the antebrachiocarpal joint.[1]

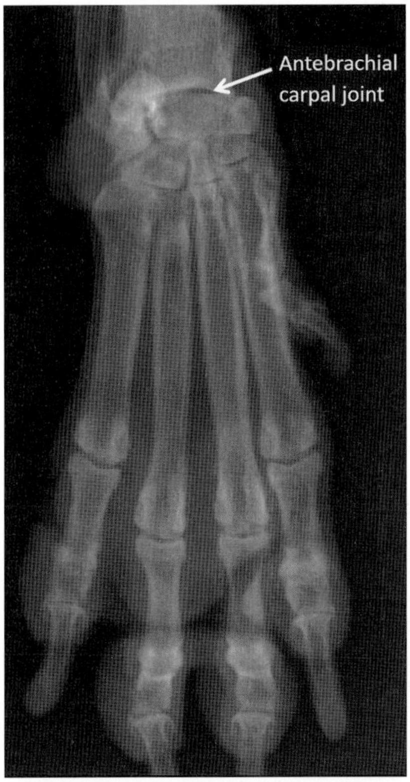

Figure 52.8 Craniocaudal view of the canine carpus. Antebrachiocarpal joint labeled with white arrow. The needle should be inserted within this depression perpendicular or angled slightly proximally to the joint. *Source:* © Carolyn Chen, Leah Hixon, Emily Viani.

Hip

As a diarthrodial, ball-and-socket articulation between the femoral head and acetabulum, the coxofemoral joint allows a wide range of joint motion. Stabilizers of the coxofemoral joint include primary and secondary stabilizers. The three primary stabilizers of the hip joint include the ligament of the head of the femur, the joint capsule, and the dorsal acetabular rim. The ligament of the head of the femur extends from the fovea capitis of the femoral head to the acetabular fossa. The joint capsule attaches near the acetabular rim on the medial aspect and laterally on the femoral neck. Secondary stabilizers of the joint include a fibrocartilaginous band that extends laterally from the dorsal acetabular rim, known as the acetabular labrum, and the transverse acetabular ligament, which is located ventrally and extends across the acetabular notch. Additional secondary stabilizers of the coxofemoral joint include the deep, middle, and superficial gluteal muscles that traverse the joint and lie dorsal and cranial to the femur.[36] The iliopsoas, quadratus femoris, internal and external obturators, and gemelli are additional muscles that traverse the hip joint. Due to the large amount of muscle coverage of this joint, arthrocentesis of the hip joint is considered the most challenging joint to obtain samples from.[1]

Arthrocentesis of the hip joint is uncommon to perform, as joint effusion cannot be palpated within this joint. The patient must be adequately sedated for hip arthrocentesis. Due to the depth of this joint, a 20 or 22-guage, 3-in. spinal needle may be required to reach the joint in a medium or large-breed dog (Figure 52.10). A 1.5-in. 20 or 22-gauge needle may be sufficient for smaller dogs and cats. The patient is placed in lateral recumbency with the affected joint up with the femur in slight abduction and slight external rotation (Figure 52.11). Traction can be placed by a nonsterile assistant to allow a slim opening of the joint space. Palpate the greater trochanter (Figures 52.11 and 52.12) then a nonsterile assistant should slightly abduct and distract the limb, opening up the coxofemoral joint space. Just cranial to the greater trochanter, insert the needle perpendicular to the long axis of the femur in a lateral to medial direction. If the dorsal acetabular rim is encountered, angle the needle slightly distal. If needed, ultrasound can be used to guide the needle. Arthrocentesis at the caudal aspect of the joint is avoided due to the presence of the sciatic nerve running dorsocranially to ventrocaudally in this location.[1]

Stifle

The stifle is one of the most common joints to perform arthrocentesis due to the ease of acquisition of joint fluid and to investigate the common causes of stifle effusion, such as septic arthritis, osteoarthritis, and IMPA. The patellar ligament, which runs on the cranial aspect of the joint from the patella to the tibial crest, palpates as a distinct, longitudinal structure in a normal stifle. On either side of the patellar ligament, the medial and lateral joint pouch should palpate as soft and concave, similar to an "apple bruise." With stifle effusion, the patellar ligament becomes less distinct as the joint pouch on either side distends and protrudes (Figure 52.13).

Due to the complex intra-articular nature, appropriate knowledge of anatomy is required. The articular surfaces of the stifle joint are separated by the menisci, leading to the classification of the stifle joint as a complex condylar synovial joint. The stifle is limited to flexion-extension and rotation. The lateral and medial femoral condyles and cranial surface of the femoral trochlea are considered to be the three major articular areas of articulation of the distal femur. The condyles are separated by the intercondyloid fossa, where the cruciate ligaments originate. At the cranial aspect of the femur, continuous with the articular surfaces of the condyles lies the femoral trochlea, where the patella articulates with the femur.[37]

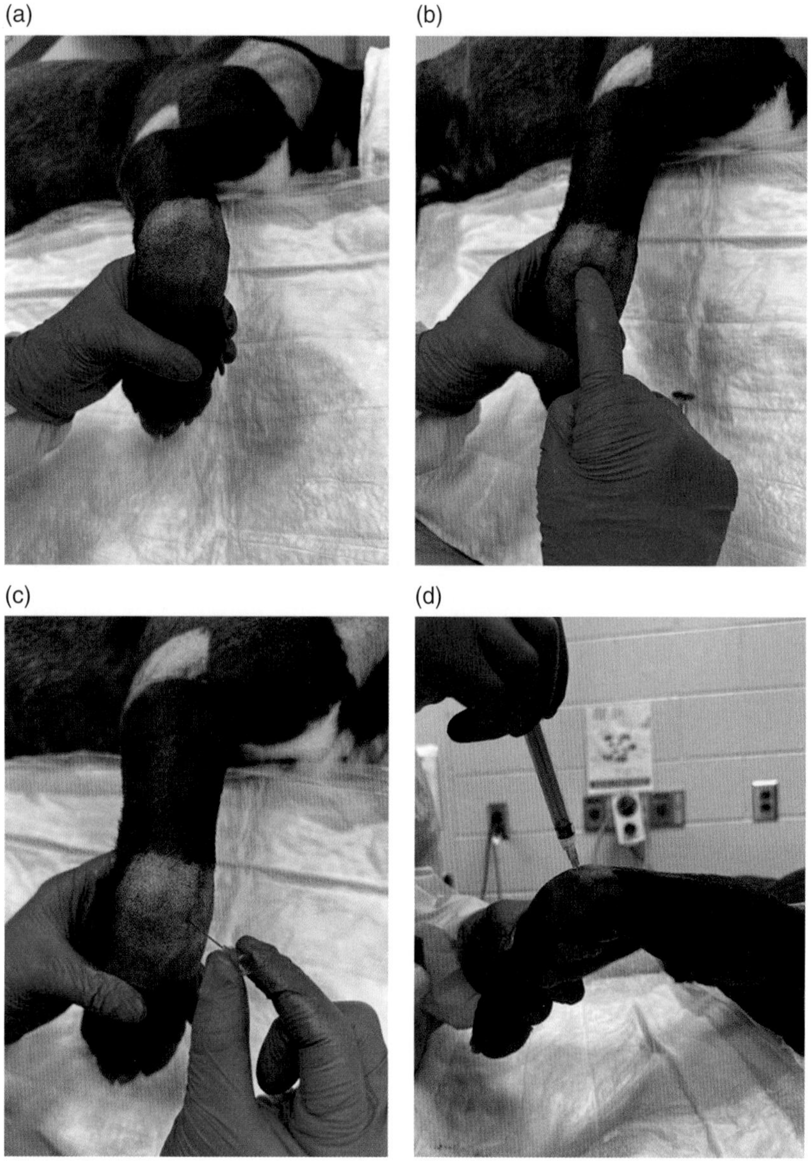

Figure 52.9 (a) Craniocaudal view of the right carpus. Cranial is to the right and caudal is to the left. The carpus is held in a 90° flexion. A tip is to keep a hand on the paw to gently extend and flex the carpus to find the palpable antebrachiocarpal joint depression. (b) A depression just distal to the radius is palpated, as shown here. This is the antebrachiocarpal joint space. (c) The needle should be inserted within this area perpendicular or angled slightly proximally to the joint, just medial to the common digital extensor tendon and the cephalic vein, both of which pass over the center of the dorsal aspect of the joint space. (d) An alternative view of carpal arthrocentesis. The syringe is attached to the needle and gentle aspiration should be performed to evacuate synovial fluid. *Source:* © Carolyn Chen, Leah Hixon, Emily Viani.

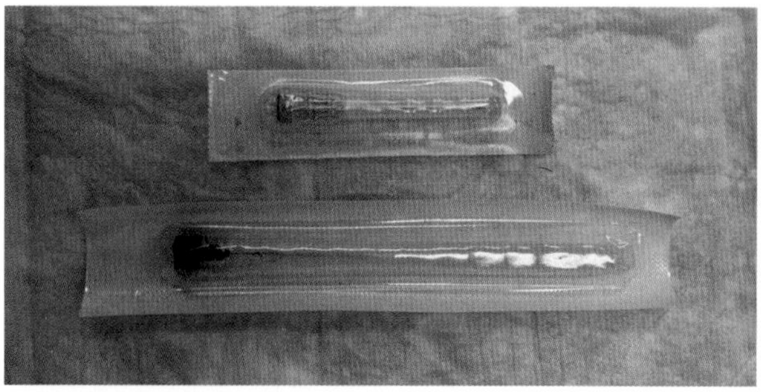

Figure 52.10 Common needle choices for hip arthrocentesis. For smaller dogs and cats, a 1.5-in. 22-gauge needle (above) may be sufficient. For larger dogs, a spinal needle may be needed (below) due to the depth of this joint. *Source:* © Carolyn Chen, Leah Hixon, Emily Viani.

The articular surface of the tibia is divided into medial and lateral condyles, with a nonarticular surface, the intercondylar eminence, separating these two regions. The two tubercles of the intercondylar eminences articulate with the femur on their abaxial surfaces. Cranial to the intercondylar eminence lies an oval depression for the insertion of the cranial cruciate ligament and cranial meniscus ligaments. The caudal intercondyloid area also consists of a depression that serves as the attachment to the caudal meniscus ligaments. The caudal cruciate ligament attaches to the lateral edge of the popliteal notch, which separates the tibial condyles. At the cranial margin of the lateral tibial condyle lies the long digital extensor (LDE) tendon, which runs in the extensor groove.

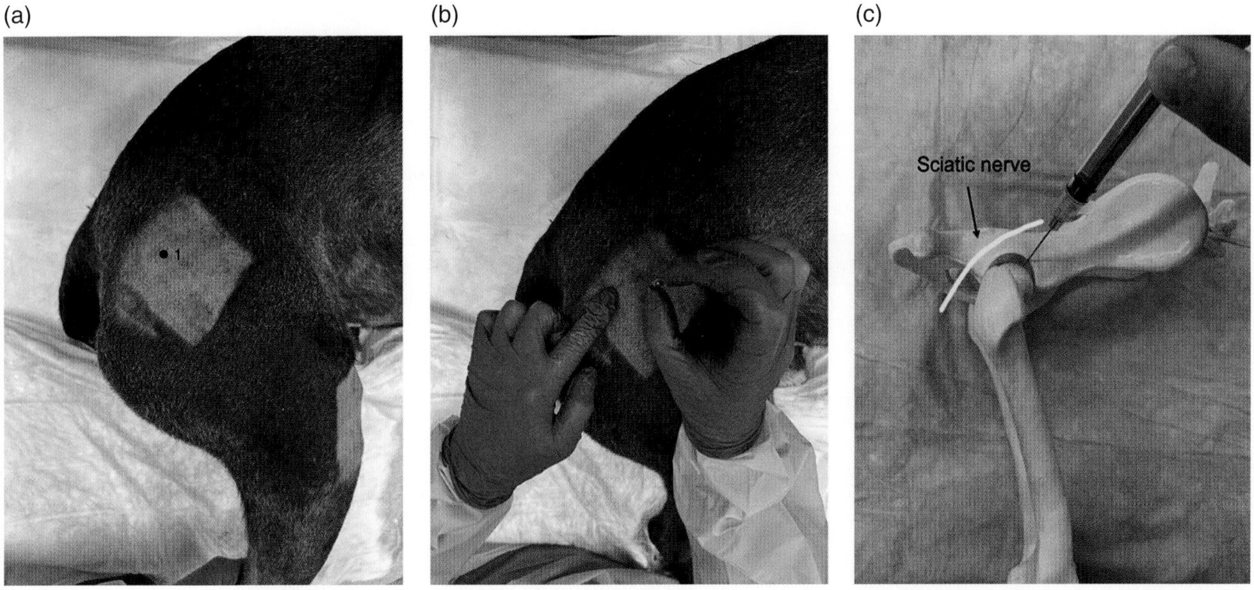

Figure 52.11 (a) Positioning for right hip arthrocentesis. The patient is in left lateral recumbency. Cranial is to the right, and caudal to the left. 1, greater trochanter of the femur. (b) Just cranial to the greater trochanter, insert the needle perpendicular to the long axis of the femur in a lateral to medial direction. If the dorsal acetabular rim is encountered, the needle can be angled slightly distally. The caudal aspect of the joint should be avoided due to the presence of the sciatic nerve. (c) A model demonstrating appropriate needle placement in the right coxofemoral joint. Cranial is to the right. *Source:* © Carolyn Chen, Leah Hixon, Emily Viani.

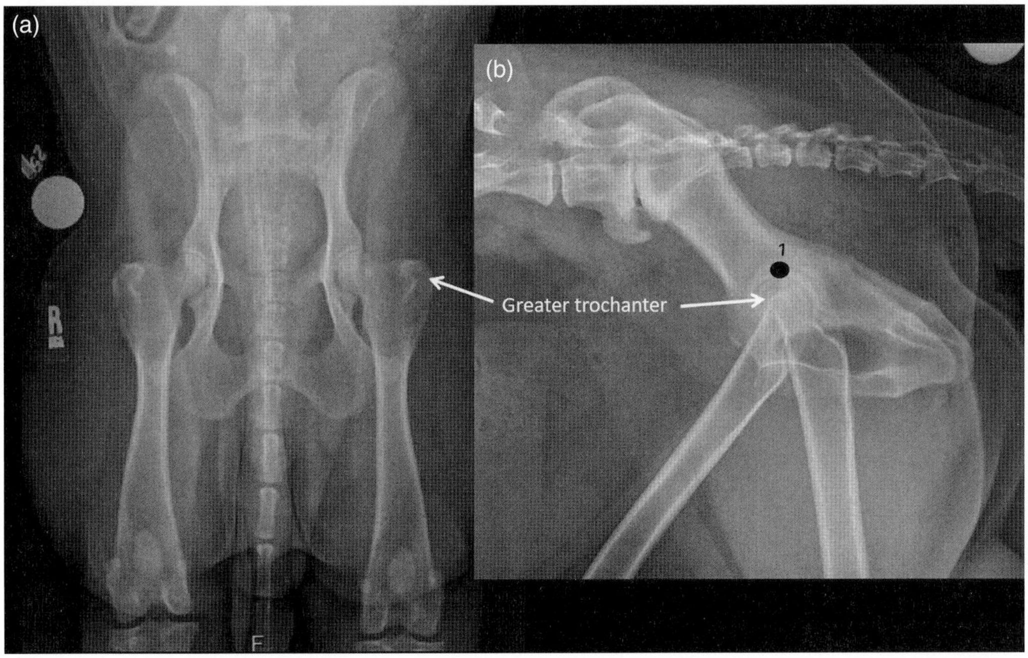

Figure 52.12 (a) Craniocaudal view of the canine pelvis. (b) Lateral view of the canine pelvis. Palpable greater trochanter labeled with white arrow. 1, location of insertion of the needle for coxofemoral arthrocentesis. *Source:* © Carolyn Chen, Leah Hixon, Emily Viani.

A palpable bony prominence, referred to as the *tubercle of Gerdy* in humans, is located at the proximal end of the tibia and corresponds to the cranial aspect of the extensor groove of the LDE in dogs.[37]

For stifle arthrocentesis, the patient is placed either in lateral recumbency with the affected limb externally rotated 90° or in dorsal recumbency (Figure 52.14). The stifle is flexed slightly, then the cranial aspect of the stifle is shaved and sterilely

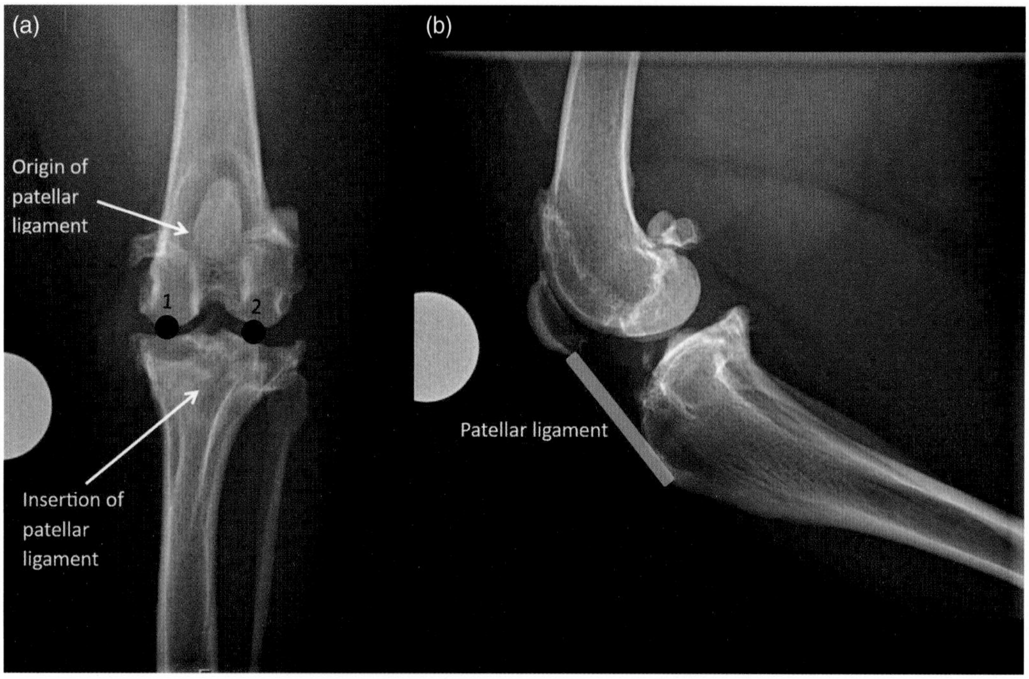

Figure 52.13 (a) Craniocaudal view of the canine stifle. (b) Lateral view of the canine stifle. Blue rectangle representing the patellar ligament, originating on the patella and inserting on the tibial crest. 1, insertion point of the needle in the medial joint pouch. 2, insertion point of the needle in the lateral joint pouch. *Source:* © Carolyn Chen, Leah Hixon, Emily Viani.

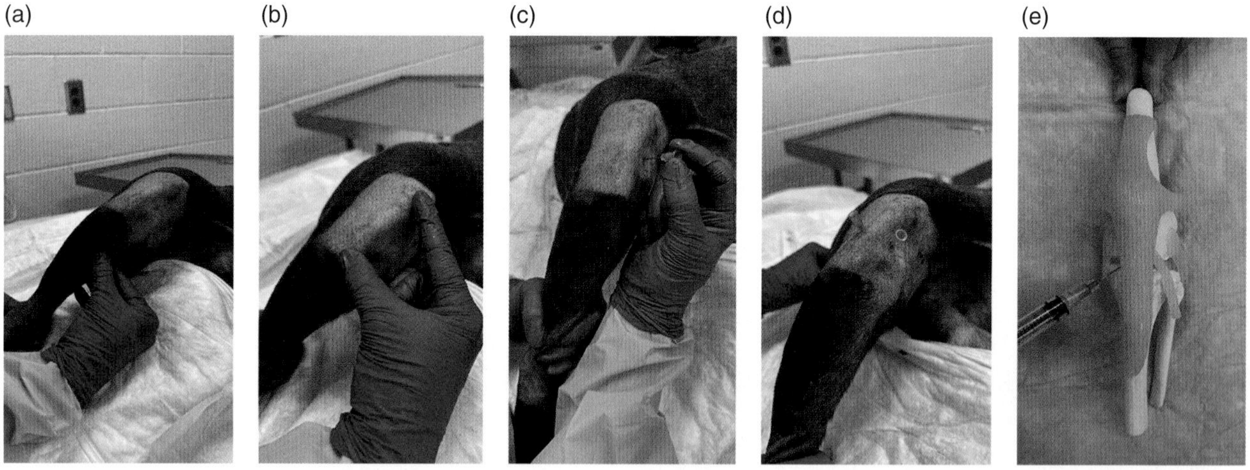

Figure 52.14 (a) Right stifle arthrocentesis. The dog is in left lateral recumbency. Cranial is to the right of the image. The stifle is held such that both the lateral and medial aspects of the joint can be accessed easily. (b) The patella (index finger) and the tibial tuberosity (thumb) are palpated. Running between these two structures is the patellar ligament. (c) The needle is inserted halfway between the medial condyle of the femur and the proximal tibia, aiming toward the intercondylar notch, or toward the opposite fabella (in this case, the lateral fabella). (d) Pictured are needle insertions for stifle arthrocentesis on either side of the patellar ligament. (e) A model demonstrating insertion of the needle medial to the patellar ligament. *Source:* © Carolyn Chen, Leah Hixon, Emily Viani.

prepped from the proximal patella to the tibial tuberosity. A 22-gauge, 1.5-in. needle is inserted just medial or lateral to the patellar ligament, midway between the patella and tibial crest (halfway between the proximal tibia and medial or lateral condyle), aiming toward the intercondylar notch. A tip is to aim for the opposite fabella with the needle in the joint (e.g., the needle inserted medial to the patellar tendon aims toward the lateral fabella). While some clinicians have success with the insertion of the needle through the center of the patellar ligament, the authors do not recommend performing this in lieu of a paratendon technique if possible to avoid traumatizing the patellar ligament and the intra-articular structures.

Tarsus

The tarsus, similar to the carpus, is also a composite of articulations of which the tarsocrural joint allows the greatest amount of movement and is the easiest to sample. This joint is formed by the articulations between the trochlea of the talus and the cochlea of the tibia (Figure 52.15). The bones of the tarsus line up into multiple rows, with the calcaneus and talus making up the proximal row, and the first, second, and third tarsal bones in the distal row. The fourth tarsal bone completes the distal row laterally, and extends proximally into the center row, sitting next to the central tarsal bone.[35]

With the patient in lateral recumbency and affected limb up, the tarsus is first put through a range of motion to best identify the tarsocrural joint. The joint is then placed in a neutral standing position (Figure 52.16a), which is about 115–125° in the cat, versus 135°–145° in the dog.[38] The skin centered over the lateral malleolus should be clipped and aseptically prepared, extending from the cranial aspect of the joint to the caudal aspect. The lateral malleolus of the fibula is palpated, and the needle is inserted just medial to it on the dorsolateral aspect of the joint, in a plantaromedial direction (Figure 52.16b). An alternative approach is to align the needle parallel to the calcaneus and insert it into the plantarolateral joint space just medial to the lateral malleolus (Figure 52.16c,d). If needed, arthrocentesis of the other tarsal joints is possible with careful palpation but is rarely indicated and difficult to achieve.

Potential Complications

The most common complication of arthrocentesis is failure to obtain an appropriate synovial fluid sample. Appropriate anatomical knowledge and experience improve the chances of obtaining a diagnostic sample. Iatrogenic blood contamination is another common complication and is indicated by blood "streaks" that are not mixed within the sample. This can be reduced when leaving the joint by releasing negative pressure from the syringe plunger prior to the removal of the needle from the joint. Alternatively, the affected portion may be expressed prior to submitting the "clean" sample. Some clinicians prefer to use a butterfly catheter in an appropriately-sized patient, as they can select which portions of the sample to save and which to remove. Submitting a sample of peripheral blood can often help a cytologist differentiate the blood cell counts of each sample.

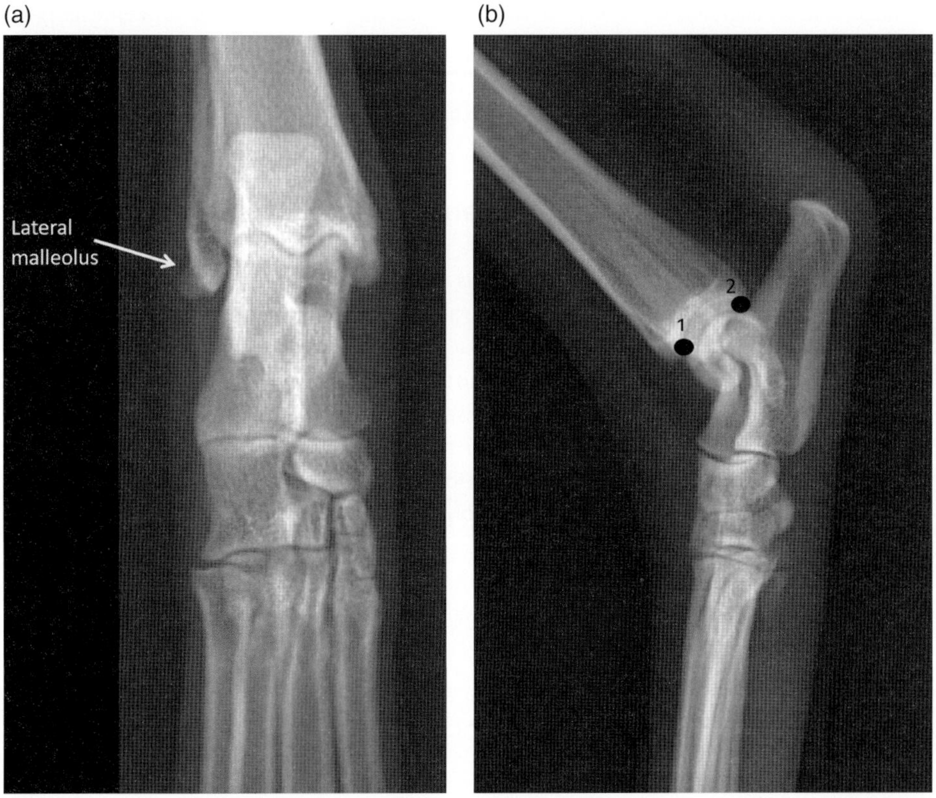

Figure 52.15 (a) Craniocaudal view of the canine tarsus. (b) Lateral view of the canine tarsus. 1, insertion location on the dorsolateral aspect of the joint, cranial to the medial malleolus; 2, alternative approach with needle parallel to the calcaneus and inserted into the plantarolateral joint space just medial to the lateral malleolus. *Source:* © Carolyn Chen, Leah Hixon, Emily Viani.

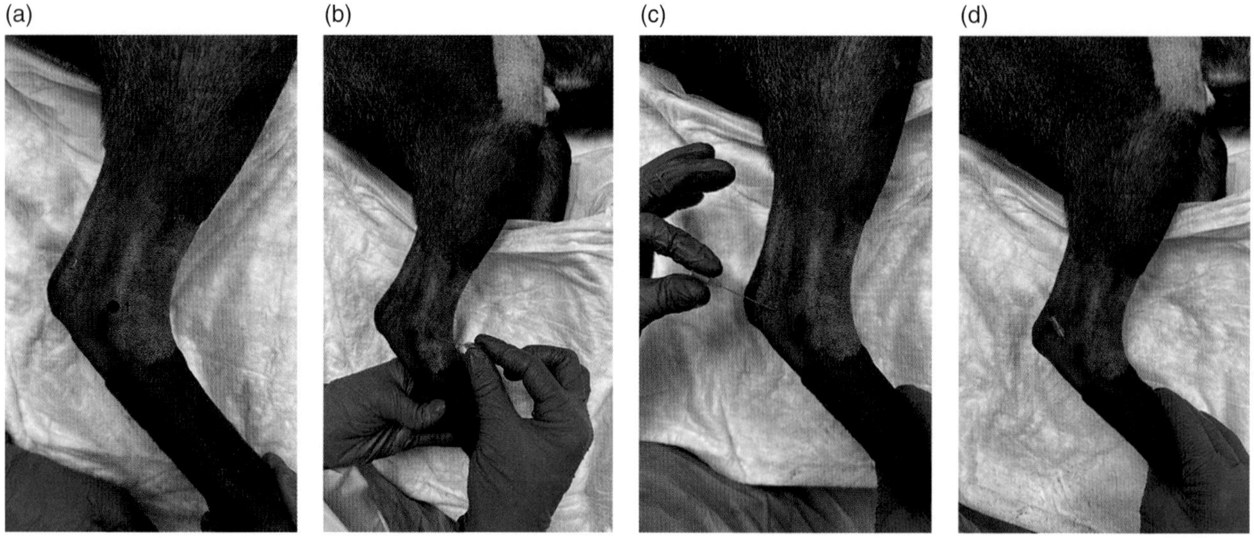

Figure 52.16 (a) Positioning for right tarsal arthrocentesis, lateral aspect. The patient is in left lateral recumbency, and cranial is to the right of the image. 1, lateral malleolus. (b) The needle is inserted just medial to the lateral malleolus on the dorsolateral aspect of the joint in a plantaromedial direction. (c) An alternative approach: the needle is aligned parallel to the calcaneus and inserted into the plantarolateral joint space just medial to the lateral malleolus. (d) The needle is shown fully inserted into the joint. *Source:* © Carolyn Chen, Leah Hixon, Emily Viani.

Though relatively noninvasive, arthrocentesis can be associated with iatrogenic cartilage damage. With increased familiarity of the local anatomy and experience performing arthrocentesis, the amount of damage can be decreased. While no long-term studies have been performed to evaluate the significance of this type of cartilage damage, no clinically significant signs have been documented because of this complication.

Joint sepsis secondary to arthrocentesis is rare but is considered a major complication should it occur. Aseptic technique is extremely important in reducing the risk of contamination of the joint. Provided appropriate aseptic technique is used, the National Research Council classifies arthrocentesis as a clean procedure, and therefore, perioperative antimicrobials are not required unless primary septic arthritis is considered.[39] In immunocompromised patients, perioperative broad-spectrum antibiotics may be considered.[1]

Serial arthrocentesis is often used to accurately monitor treatment efficacy in both immune-mediated polyarthritis and septic arthritis. In one study, nine healthy client-owned dogs underwent four serial arthrocentesis at three-week intervals. One hundred and forty-four samples were evaluated and only mild mononuclear inflammation was detected in 13 samples from 6 dogs. This study concluded that neutrophilic inflammation in healthy dogs does not appear to occur and therefore repeat arthrocentesis is an appropriate method to monitor for resolution of IMPA and septic arthritis without concern for falsely elevated values from serial arthrocentesis.[40]

Post-op Care/Prognosis

Arthrocentesis is considered a relatively noninvasive procedure, so postoperative pain medications related to the procedure itself are not required. Oftentimes, patients undergoing arthrocentesis are likely painful from the underlying disease process, so analgesics appropriate for the condition at hand are recommended. As previously outlined, arthrocentesis is a clean procedure, so perioperative antimicrobials are not required if appropriate sterile technique is performed. Long-term prognosis is generally dependent on the underlying disease process, but the prognosis associated with the procedure is generally considered excellent.[1]

References

1 Clements, D. (2006). Arthrocentesis and synovial fluid analysis in dogs and cats. *In Practice* 28 (5): 256–262.

2 Goldstein, R. (2005). Swollen joints and lameness. In: *Textbook of Veterinary Internal Medicine. 1*, 6e (ed. S.J. Ettinger and E.C. Feldman), 83–87. St. Louis: Elsevier Saunders.

3 Davidson, A. (2017). Immune mediated polyarthritis. In: *Mechanisms of Disease in Small Animal Surgery*, 3e

(ed. M.J. Bojrab and E. Monnet), 743–749. Jackson, WY: Teton NewMedia.
4 Schulz, K., Hayashi, K., and Fossum, T. (2019). Diseases of the joints. In: *Small Animal Surgery*, 5e (ed. T. Fossum), 1134–1279. Philadelphia, PA: Elsevier.
5 Innes, J.F. (2018). Arthritis. In: *Veterinary Surgery: Small Animal. 2*, 2e (ed. S.A. Johnston and K.M. Tobias), 1265–1299. St. Louis, MO: Elsevier.
6 Johnson, M.D., Behar-Horenstein, L.S., MacIver, M.A. et al. (2016). Assessing the effectiveness of a cadaveric teaching model for performing arthrocentesis with veterinary students. *J. Vet. Med. Educ.* 43 (1): 88–94.
7 Lavallee, J.M., Shmon, C., Beaufrere, H. et al. (2020). Influence of clipping on bacterial contamination of canine arthrocentesis sites before and after skin preparation. *Vet. Surg.* 49 (7): 1307–1314.
8 Haseler, L.J., Sibbitt, R.R., Sibbitt, W.L. Jr. et al. (2011). Syringe and needle size, syringe type, vacuum generation, and needle control in aspiration procedures. *Cardiovasc. Intervent. Radiol.* 34 (3): 590–600.
9 Degner, D. (2014). Arthrocentesis in dogs. *Clinician's Brief* 69–74.
10 Barger, A.M. (2016). Musculoskeletal system. In: *Canine and Feline Cytology* (ed. R.E. Raskin and D.J. Meyer), 353–368. Elsevier.
11 Meyer, D.J. (2016). The acquisition and management of cytology specimens. In: *Canine and Feline Cytology*, 3e (ed. R.E. Raskin and D.J. Meyer), 1–15. Elsevier.
12 Medicine CUCoV (n.d.). Animal Health Diagnostic Center 2023. https://www.vet.cornell.edu/animal-health-diagnostic-center/testing/protocols/cytology
13 Font-Vizcarra, L., Garcia, S., Martinez-Pastor, J.C. et al. (2010). Blood culture flasks for culturing synovial fluid in prosthetic joint infections. *Clin. Orthop. Relat. Res.* 468 (8): 2238–2243.
14 Cohen, D., Natshe, A., Ben Chetrit, E. et al. (2020). Synovial fluid culture: agar plates vs. blood culture bottles for microbiological identification. *Clin. Rheumatol.* 39 (1): 275–279.
15 Ling, C.L., Roberts, T., Soeng, S. et al. (2021). Impact of delays to incubation and storage temperature on blood culture results: a multi-centre study. *BMC Infect. Dis.* 21 (1): 173–180.
16 Sautter, R.L., Bills, A.R., Lang, D.L. et al. (2006). Effects of delayed-entry conditions on the recovery and detection of microorganisms from BacT/ALERT and BACTEC blood culture bottles. *J. Clin. Microbiol.* 44 (4): 1245–1249.
17 Kirn, T.J. and Weinstein, M.P. (2013). Update on blood cultures: how to obtain, process, report, and interpret. *Clin. Microbiol. Infect.* 19 (6): 513–520.
18 Hermanson, J. (2013). The muscular system. In: *Miller's Anatomy of the Dog* (ed. H.E. Evans and A. de Lahunta), 185–280. St. Louis: Elsevier Saunders.
19 Kinzel, G.L., Van Sickle, D.C., Hillberry, B.M. et al. (1976). Preliminary study of the in vivo motion in the canine shoulder. *Am. J. Vet. Res.* 37 (12): 1505–1510.
20 Sager, M., Herten, M., Dreiner, L. et al. (2013). Histological variations of the glenoid labrum in dogs. *Anatom. Histol. Embryol.* 42 (6): 438–447.
21 Bardet, J.F. (1998). Diagnosis of shoulder instability in dogs and cats: a retrospective study. *J. Am. Anim. Hosp. Assoc.* 34 (1): 42–54.
22 Sumner-Smith, G. (2009). Shoulder joint. In: *Feline Orthopedic Surgery and Musculoskeletal Disease*, 1e (ed. P.M. Montavon, K. Voss, and S. Langley-Hobbs), 337–342. St. Louis: Saunders Elsevier.
23 Gray, M.J., Lambrechts, N.E., Maritz, N.G. et al. (2005). A biomechanical investigation of the static stabilisers of the glenohumeral joint in the dog. *Vet. Comp. Orthop. Traumatol.* 18 (2): 55–61.
24 Hardy, R.M. and Wallace, L.J. (1974). Arthrocentesis and synovial membrane biopsy. *Vet. Clin. North Am.* 4 (2): 449–462.
25 Pacchiana, P.D., Gilley, R.S., Wallace, L.J. et al. (2004). Absolute and relative cell counts for synovial fluid from clinically normal shoulder and stifle joints in cats. *J. Am. Vet. Med. Assoc.* 225 (12): 1866–1870.
26 Rochat M. Arthrocentesis and arthroscopy. In: Ettinger SJ, Feldman EC, editor. Textbook of Veterinary Internal Medicine. 1. St. Louis: Elsevier Saunders; 2005;1063–1069.
27 Evans, H.E. and de Launta, A. (2013). Arthrology. In: *Miller's Anatomy of the Dog* (ed. H. Evans and A. de Launta), 158–184. St. Louis: Elsevier Saunders.
28 Tokuriki, M. (1974). Electromyographic and joint-mechanical studies in quadrupedal locomotion. 3. Gallop (author's transl). *Nihon Juigaku Zasshi* 36 (2): 121–132.
29 Boulay, J.P. (1998). Fragmented medial coronoid process of the ulna in the dog. *Vet. Clin. North Am. Small Anim. Pract.* 28 (1): 51–74.
30 Constantinescu, G.M. and Constantinescu, I.A. (2009). A clinically oriented comprehensive pictorial review of canine elbow anatomy. *Vet. Surg.* 38 (2): 135–143.
31 Adams, D.R. (2003). Thoracic limb. In: *Canine Anatomy: A Systematic Study*, 4e (ed. D.R. Adams), 35–81. Hoboken, NJ: Wiley-Blackwell.
32 Talcott, K.W., Schulz, K.S., Kass, P.H. et al. (2002). In vitro biomechanical study of rotational stabilizers of the canine elbow joint. *Am. J. Vet. Res.* 63 (11): 1520–1526.
33 Evans, H. and de Launta, A. (2013). *Miller's Anatomy of the Dog*, 4e. St. Louis: Elseiver Saunders.
34 Beale, B.S., Hulse, D.A., Schulz, K.S., and Whitney, W.O. (2003). Arthroscopically assisted surgery of the elbow joint. In: *Small Animal Arthroscopy* (ed. B.S. Beale), 81–95. Philadelphia, PA: Elsevier.
35 Evans, H. and de Lahunta, A. (ed.) (2013). The Skeleton. In: *Miller's Anatomy of the Dog*, 80–157. St. Louis: Elsevier Saunders.

36 Wardlaw, J.L. and McLaughlin, R. (2018). Hip luxation. In: *Veterinary Surgery: Small Animal. 1*, 2e (ed. K.M. Tobias and S.A. Johnston), 956–964. St. Louis, MO: Elsevier.

37 Kowaleski, M.P., Boudrieau, R.J., and Pozzi, A. (2018). Stifle joint. In: *Veterinary Surgery: Small Animal. 1*, 2e (ed. K.M. Tobias and S.A. Johnston), 1071–1168. St. Louis, MO: Elsevier.

38 Carmichael, S. and Marshall, W.G. (2018). Tarsus and metatarsus. In: *Veterinary Surgery: Small Animal. 1*, 2e (ed. K.M. Tobias and S.A. Johnston), 1193–1209. St. Louis, MO: Elsevier.

39 Woods, S. (ed.) (2016). *Arthrocentesis - Why and How to Do It*. World Small Animal Veterinary Association. Midlothian, UK: University of Edinburgh, Roslin.

40 Berg, R.I., Sykes, J.E., Kass, P.H. et al. (2009). Effect of repeated arthrocentesis on cytologic analysis of synovial fluid in dogs. *J. Vet. Intern. Med.* 23 (4): 814–817.

53

Tendon Lacerations

Rebecca J. Webb

VetSurg, Ventura, CA, USA

Key Points
• The most common tendons to experience laceration injuries are the superficial and deep digital flexor tendons and the common calcaneal tendon complex, which is due to the limited overlying soft tissue of these areas. • Repair of tendon lacerations should not be delayed. Following the initial injury, the damaged tendon will slowly retract from the opposite edge, making apposition and definitive repair more difficult than if it was addressed quickly after the injury. • Tendons heal very slowly compared to other tissues of the body, such as bone or skin, which is why post-surgical support of the limb following repair is essential to a successful outcome.

Introduction

Tendon lacerations frequently occur secondary to penetrating wounds. The most common tendons affected are those near the metacarpal and metatarsal regions (superficial and deep digital flexor tendons [SDFTs and DDFTs]) and the common calcaneal tendon (or Achilles tendon) complex. This is due to the limited overlying soft tissue of these areas, which leaves these tendons relatively more exposed to injury. It is not uncommon for wounds in these areas to have a tendon injury that remains unrecognized until the wound is surgically explored. Early diagnosis and apposition of the severed tendon ends is important, as over time, contracture of the severed tendon ends occurs and makes the ends more difficult to appose. For this reason, it is important for clinicians exploring wounds in these areas to be evaluating thoroughly for these tendinous injuries. The clinician should either be adequately prepared to repair these tendons during wound repair themselves or plan for the case to be referred in an expedited manner upon diagnosis of a tendon laceration for repair following initial wound management.

Tendons are composed of dense parallel collagen fibers, proteoglycan matrix, and fibroblasts. The structure of a tendon is similar to a rope with small collagen fibers arranged in bundles. The parallel orientation of these fibers is important for clinicians to be familiar with, as this has implications for suture pattern choice during their repair. Tendons are typically poorly vascularized, and due to this, their healing is slow. The paratenon is a loose connective tissue structure that surrounds individual tendons and is a source of blood supply to these tendons during healing. Tendons with a paratenon are classified as vascular tendons and include the common calcaneal tendon complex and triceps tendon.[1] These tendons gain blood supply from both the paratenon and their intrinsic blood supply during healing. Tendons without a paratenon are classified as avascular tendons and include the digital flexor tendons. These tendons rely only on their intrinsic blood supply for healing, which can lead to more difficulties with their healing process. Maintenance of the anatomic blood supply to the tendon during repair is of vital importance for healing, and therefore, gentle tissue handling of the tendons during the repair is necessary.

Techniques in Small Animal Soft Tissue, Orthopedic, and Ophthalmic Surgery, First Edition. Edited by Kristin A. Coleman.

Companion website: www.wiley.com/go/coleman/surgeries

Apposition of the tendon ends is of paramount importance for adequate healing of a tendon laceration. When the tendon ends are apposed without a gap, the tendon ends heal together without scar tissue. However, when a gap is present, scar tissue forms between the tendon ends, which leads to a biomechanically weaker repair. Overall, the goal of surgical repair is to adequately appose the tendon ends without gap formation while maintaining the blood supply to the tendon. Initially following repair, the tendon will not be able to withstand typical forces and will need to be immobilized and supported. Following the initial recovery period, it is important to progressively allow small amounts of loading of the tendon repair, as this encourages the collagen fibers of the healing tendon to align correctly, giving it long-term strength.[1] This loading should be performed cautiously and gradually, however, as excessive premature overloading of the tendon will lead to repair failure.

In uncomplicated tendon healing, a slow but gradual return of strength of the tendon following injury is expected. At six weeks post-injury, the tendon will have approximately 56% of its original strength, and this increases to a strength of 79% at one-year post-injury.[2] As normal forces strain tendons to 25–33% of their maximal capacity, typically, the strength obtained at six weeks post-surgery is enough to withstand gentle activity.[1]

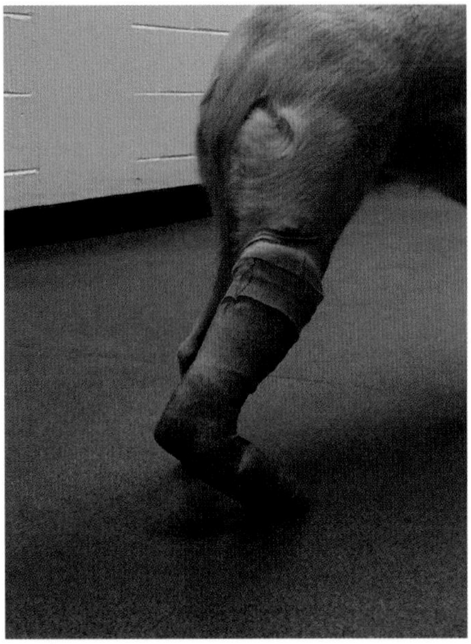

Figure 53.1 Note that even with a support bandage, the right tarsus of this patient displays a plantigrade stance, in which tarsal hyperflexion occurs with concurrent stifle extension. This stance is typically secondary to common calcaneal tendon injury. *Source:* © Rebecca Webb.

Indications/Pre-op Considerations

Most patients with a tendon laceration will present acutely with a laceration or wound and a minimally or non-weight-bearing lameness. In patients who are bearing weight at the time of presentation, characteristic hyperextension or hyperflexion of the affected joints may be noted. For patients with DDFT lacerations, a characteristic hyperextension of the affected digits is noted. Patients suffering from common calcaneal tendon lacerations can present differently depending on which components of the tendon have been affected. Laceration of the complete common calcaneal tendon complex typically presents with hyperflexion of the tarsus during stance (Figure 53.1).

Given these injuries occur secondary to trauma, a full evaluation of the patient's stability prior to anesthesia for surgical repair is indicated. During the time of patient stabilization, the wound should be covered to reduce hemorrhage and reduce the risk of a hospital-acquired infection.

Chronic, untreated tendon lacerations typically present with a chronic lameness and occasionally a palpable defect. Dependent on the tendon involved, dysfunction of the affected joints will be noted. In addition, some patients present with chronic wounds secondary to their altered weight-bearing. Preoperative radiographs of the affected area are recommended to evaluate for both concurrent fractures and radiopaque foreign material. Ultrasound by a skilled ultrasonographer can be useful in cases of common calcaneal lacerations to determine the specific components of the tendon that are damaged and can give information about the extent of this damage.

Surgical Procedure

General Considerations

Patient Preparation

Lacerations should be flushed with sterile isotonic fluids then filled with a sterile lubricant prior to clipping of the fur. The sterile lubricant helps trap clipped fur and prevents it from getting caught in the wound. The lubricant is flushed from the wound once clipping is complete. Dependent on the area of the laceration, the region to be clipped and prepared will vary. However, each patient should have a substantial region clipped, prepared, and draped, as extension of the laceration is commonly needed to allow enough visualization to repair the lacerated tendons.

The patient should be positioned as needed to allow full access to the tendon and wound. In the case of a common calcaneal tendon laceration, this is commonly obtained with the patient in sternal recumbency with the hind limb hanging off the table (Figure 53.2). A hanging limb prep is

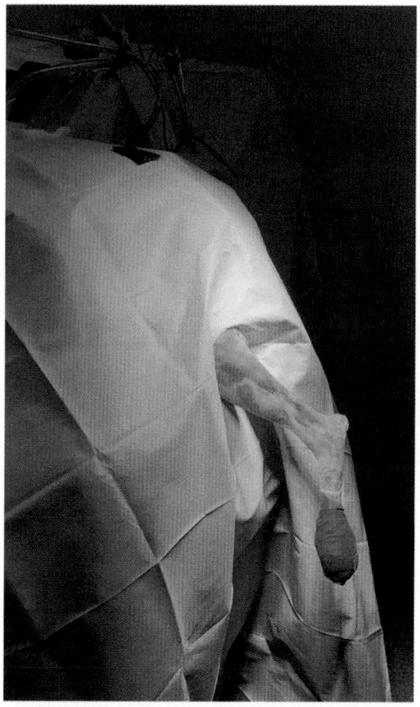

Figure 53.2 This patient with a common calcaneal tendon laceration has been positioned in the surgical suite for repair. The patient is positioned in sternal recumbency with the hind limb outstretched. Note a sterile impervious wrap (impervious drape material) has been placed over the unclipped paw and then covered with sterile Vetrap™ (3M) in this case. *Source:* © Rebecca Webb.

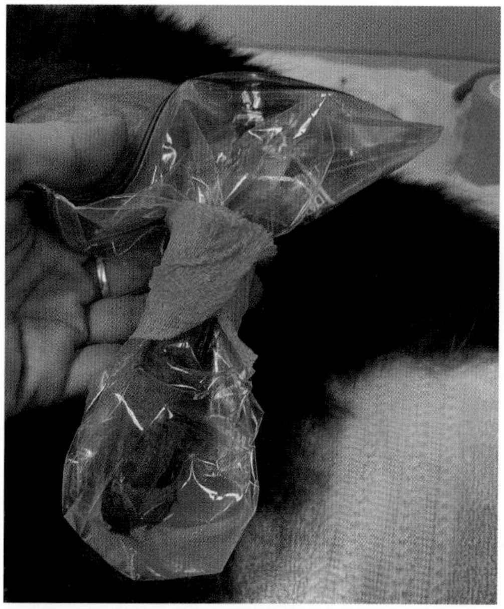

Figure 53.4 Paw soak. This is performed in patients who require the paw to be exposed during surgery. Following clipping of the fur of the digits, the paw is enclosed in a sealable bag or glove containing either dilute betadine or dilute chlorhexidine solution. The top of the bag is taped around the metatarsals/metacarpals to prevent leakage, and the paw is soaked in the solution for five minutes while the patient is moved into the operating room. *Source:* © Rebecca Webb.

performed in these cases, with the hind limb suspended from the ceiling or an IV pole to allow for surgical preparation of the limb (Figure 53.3).

In patients where the paw needs to be exposed for the surgical repair, a paw soak is performed following clipping and prior to moving the patient to the O.R., as surgical preparation of this area can prove challenging with gauze. This is performed by placing the digits and paw in an examination glove or plastic specimen bag with 4% chlorhexidine or 10% povidone-iodine solution for three to five minutes. Porous tape or an elastic adhesive bandage (such as Vetrap™) is used to secure the top of the glove around the distal limb during soaking time to prevent spillage of scrub solution from the glove (Figure 53.4). These patients are then moved to the operating room, and the paw can be suspended for a final surgical preparation and draping using a sterile Backhaus towel clamp in the interdigital space (Figure 53.5).

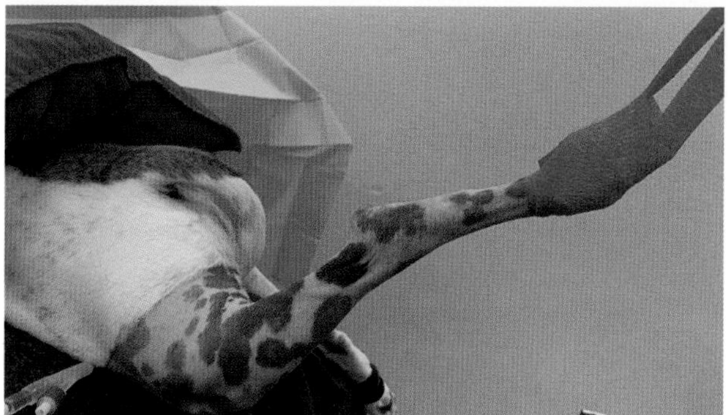

Figure 53.3 The limb is suspended to allow final surgical preparation using a paw wrap of Vetrap™ (3M). Once the patient is draped, the sterile assistant will grasp the paw with an impervious sterile layer (such as sterile disposable drape material or sterilized aluminum foil) and then wrap around the impervious sterile layer with sterile Vetrap™ (3M). In patients where the paw needs to be exposed for surgery, see images 53.4 and 53.5. *Source:* © Rebecca Webb.

Approach

Tendon lacerations can either be treated through the laceration when addressed in the acute phase or through a surgical approach in the chronic phase. In the acute phase, a combination of the two can be utilized, and the laceration can be extended to allow surgical access to the area. When a surgical approach is made, it is important that the approach is made parallel to the tendon fibers. The approach should ideally not be made directly over the tendon to be repaired, as during healing, this can lead to scar tissue extending from the wound to the tendon.

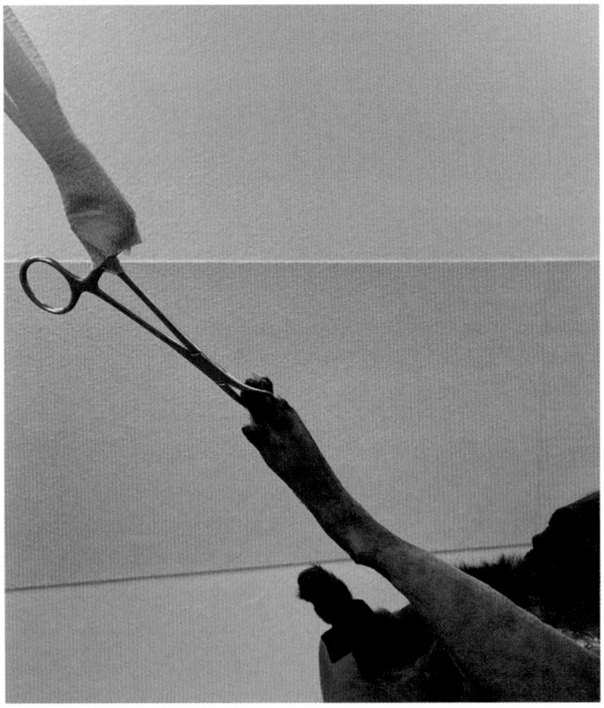

Figure 53.5 For patients in which the surgeon requires the paw to be exposed during surgery, a paw soak is performed (Figure 53.4) prior to moving the patient to the operating room. The paw is suspended from the ceiling or an IV pole using a sterile towel clamp placed in the interdigital space. The towel clamp is then suspended using either tape or Vetrap™ (3M). *Source:* © Rebecca Webb.

Manipulation and Approximation

Gentle manipulation of the tendon ends is required to prevent further damage to the traumatized tendon ends to aid in healing. The use of hypodermic needles or small Kirschner wires can be employed as a handle to manipulate the tendon ends (Figure 53.6). The hypodermic needles (25-22G dependent on tendon size) are inserted perpendicular to the long axis of the tendon, away from the torn tendon ends in grossly healthy tendon. This gives the ability to manipulate the tendons during debridement and approximation with minimal further trauma to the damaged tendon ends.

The ends of damaged tendons can be sharply debrided with a #15 scalpel blade. Debridement should be conservative and restricted to the obviously traumatized tendon. Excessive debridement should be avoided, as tendon tissue is in limited supply and approximation of the tendon ends is required for primary-healing to occur. Approximation of the tendon ends is facilitated by flexion or extension of the underlying joint to relieve pressure on the repair. It is important that the tendon ends can be approximated at this stage prior to suture placement, as suture placement should only be used to maintain approximation of the tendon ends and shouldn't be used to reduce the tendon ends

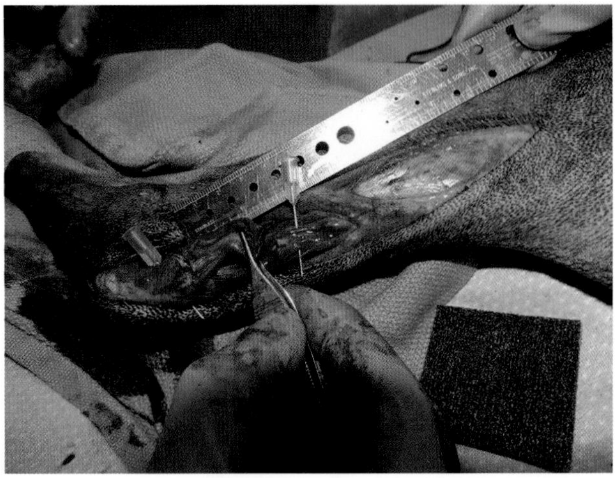

Figure 53.6 Chronic common calcaneal tendon injury repair. Hypodermic needles have been placed in the proximal and distal healthy tendon ends to help with manipulation intraoperatively. The central portion of the tendon was resected, as it was grossly unhealthy. The segment of tissue removed in this case was large due to the chronic nature of the injury. *Source:* © Rebecca Webb.

together. Using the suture pattern to bring the tendon ends together indicates excessive tension on the tendon repair and may increase the risk of suture pull-through and repair failure.

Suture Material

Healing of tendons is a slow process, and for an extended period, the suture repair will need to take almost all the load placed through the tendon. Due to this, the suture material needs to be strong, and due to the slow healing of tendons, the suture is typically made of a non-absorbable material. Given the requirement of the suture to maintain approximation of the tendon ends under high loads, the material of the suture should also be inelastic. Common suture types include polypropylene and nylon. Swaged-on needles are recommended to reduce tendon trauma. Monofilaments are historically preferred to multifilament suture in order to minimize tissue drag, which can cause tissue trauma during placement. Multifilament suture is used in human tendon repairs, as the multifilament suture is stronger and stiffer when compared to monofilament sutures.[3] In repair of canine common calcaneal tendon injuries, there have been successful veterinary reports using multifilament suture for surgical repair.[4] However, careful attention to sterile technique is required when multifilament suture is used for tendon repair due to the proposed increase in risk of infection with a multifilament suture.[5]

Primary Suture Patterns

The orientation of collagen bundles longitudinally within a tendon leads to rapid suture pull-out when traditional suture patterns are utilized in the repair of tendons. This

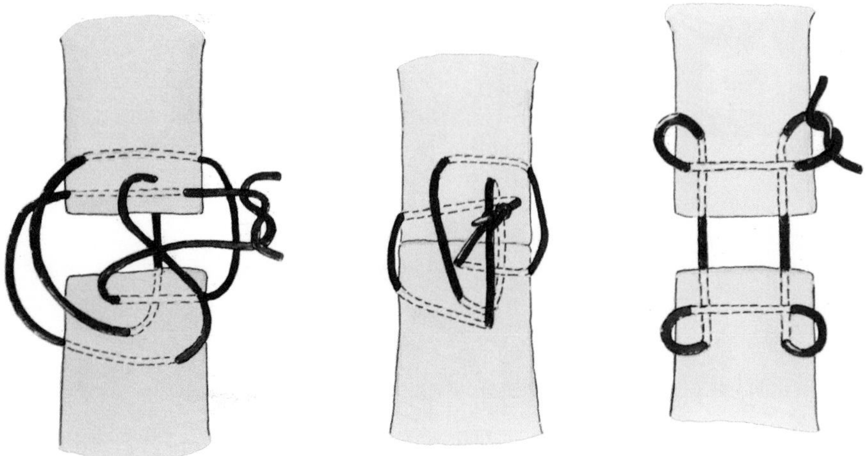

Figure 53.7 The locking-loop (modified Kessler) suture pattern. *Source:* Original artwork by Taylor Bergrud.

has led to the development of specialized suture patterns, which include a suture pass that is oriented perpendicular to the tendon bundles, since this orientation helps prevent suture pull-out and gives strength to the repair. Larger tendons are typically repaired with one or multiple of the below primary tendon patterns, then the repair is then supported with the addition of multiple epitendinous sutures. For the repair of flat and small tendons, such as the SDFT and DDFT, the locking-loop pattern (modified Kessler pattern) (Figure 53.7) is most easily used. This suture pattern encircles two bundles of the tendon in a loop on either side, which gives it strength against suture pull-out. For this suture pattern to be effective, it is important that the transverse component is placed superficial to the longitudinal component, as failure to do so will weaken the construct. Like the locking-loop pattern, the Krakow pattern (Figures 53.8 and 53.9) was also designed for use in flat tendons. It functions in a similar way by grasping a bundle of

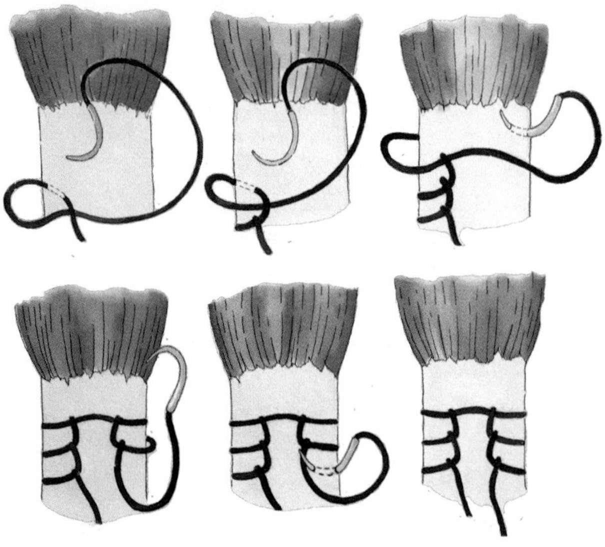

Figure 53.8 The Krakow suture pattern. *Source:* Original artwork by Taylor Bergrud.

tendon on either side to prevent suture pull-out. The three-loop pulley pattern (Figure 53.10) is best suited for round tendons and has been shown experimentally to withstand gap formation more effectively than the locking-loop pattern.[6,7] Ultimately, the choice of suture pattern is dependent upon the size of the tendon to be sutured, the size of the patient, and the surgeon's preference.

Epitendinous Sutures

Epitendinous sutures are sutures placed around the circumference of the tendon repair. Typically used in the repair of larger tendon constructs, the addition of these sutures to the primary repair has been shown to increase its strength and help prevent the formation of a gap between the tendon ends in research models.[6] These sutures are placed after the primary suture pattern has reduced the tendon ends together, and the gap between the two ends has been eliminated. Epitendinous sutures are typically of a finer gauge than the primary suture pattern. Numerous patterns for these sutures have been reported, including horizontal mattress, simple continuous, and interlocking horizontal mattress patterns (Figures 53.11 and 53.9). In research models, it appears the addition of an epitendinous component to the repair is more important to increasing strength than the specific pattern used to place it.[8]

Specific Tendon Lacerations

Digital Flexor Tendons

Injury to the digital flexor tendons occurs most commonly secondary to a laceration at the palmar or plantar aspect of the digits or paw. In patients who are bearing weight, hyperextension of the affected digits is often noted. On palpation of the digits, the clinician should extend each individual digit and feel for the tension of the associated

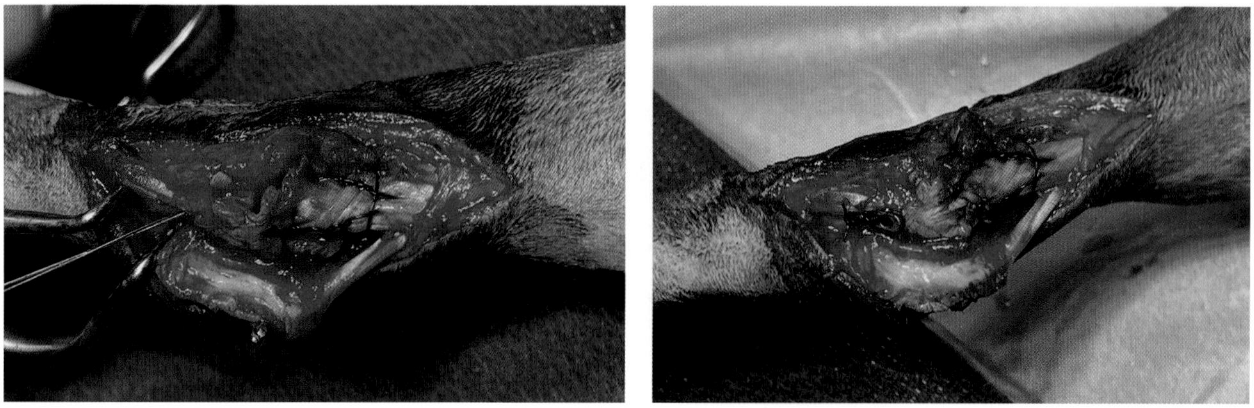

Figure 53.9 A feline patient with a common calcaneal tendon repair. In the left image, the tendon has been reconstructed with a Krakow suture pattern using 0 Novafil™ (Medtronic). In the right image, the previous Krakow suture pattern was adhered to the calcaneus using a bone tunnel and suture button (Arthrex). An epitendinous simple continuous suture pattern has been placed overlying the primary suture pattern using 2-0 Novafil™ (Medtronic). The proximal aspect of the limb is to the right of the image. *Source:* © Rebecca Webb.

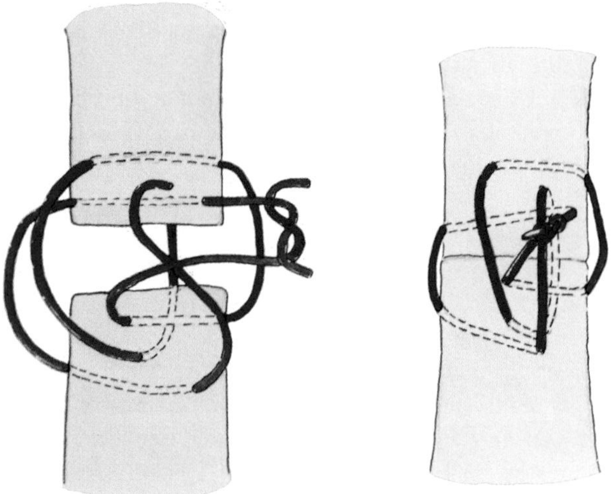

Figure 53.10 The three-loop pulley suture pattern. *Source:* Original artwork by Taylor Bergrud.

flexor tendons on the palmar or plantar surface. A lack of tension is consistent with injury to the associated tendon. Depending on the extent and location of the injury, both the superficial and deep digital flexor tendons can be affected. Both the superficial digital flexor tendons (SDFT) and deep digital flexor tendons (DDFT) run as a common tendon at the caudal aspect of the limbs and then branch to form smaller tendons, which then insert onto the individual digits distally. More commonly, injuries to these tendons occur distal to this branching, and in severe injuries, there can be lacerations to all four deep and superficial digital flexor tendons, leading to eight small flexor tendons that need to be reconstructed. These cases are frequently presented on an emergent basis, as they often have a moderate degree of hemorrhage from the associated wound.

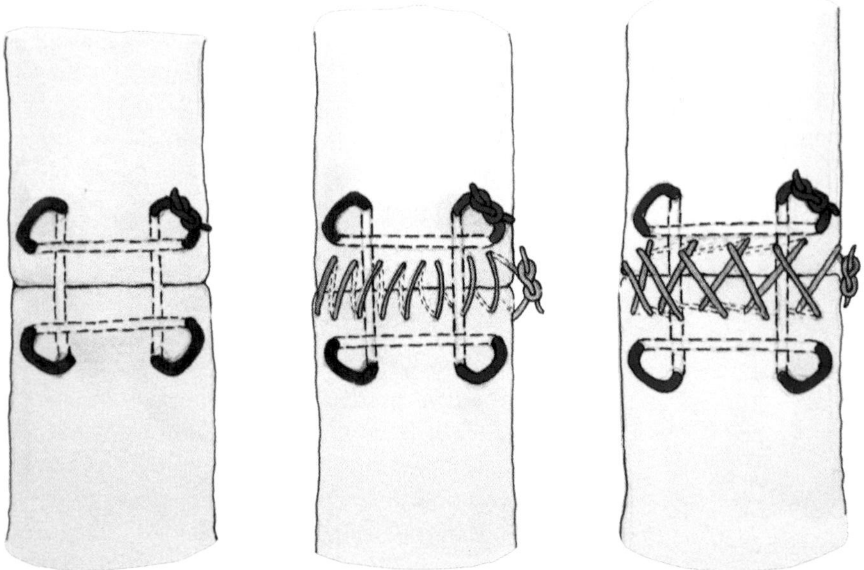

Figure 53.11 Epitendinous sutures have been added to a primary locking-loop suture (modified Kessler pattern). Simple continuous epitendinous sutures in the central image, and the right image shows interlocking horizontal mattress epitendinous sutures. *Source:* Original artwork by Taylor Bergrud.

While timely repair of tendon lacerations is important, because the repair of up to eight individual small tendons is a time-consuming process, when evaluating these cases on an emergent basis, clinicians should exercise their judgment as to whether repair of the tendons can occur during the initial visit or repair should be delayed until time permits appropriate exploration. If tendon repair is delayed, wound management should be performed, a bandage placed to protect the limb, and surgical repair expedited. Once the wound is lavaged and prepped, the clinician will often need to extend the laceration to allow for a complete evaluation of the flexor tendons. Assessment of the tendons is based on both visualization, as well as palpation as above.

While lacerations to the SDFTs are often easily identified, it is important that the DDFTs are thoroughly evaluated, as failure to identify and subsequently repair damage to the DDFT is a common cause of postoperative lameness in these patients. Failure to repair damage to the DDFTs will lead to the patient bearing weight on the palmar or plantar aspect of the metacarpal or metatarsal pad, respectively, the elevation of the affected digits during weight-bearing, and the patient being flat-footed. The abnormal weight-bearing on the pads and digits can lead to pressure wounds and chronic lameness. Given the small size of the tendons in this area, these tendons are often repaired using a locking-loop pattern. It is very important given the small size of these tendons that the suture bites of this pattern are placed accurately. In particular, the transverse pass should be superficial to the longitudinal passes to enable the suture to encircle a bundle of tendon fibers and give it strength. Due to the small size of these tendons, a fine suture (3-0 or 4-0 dependent on tendon size) is required for reconstruction.

Following reconstruction, the paw should be supported, and the tendons should be off-loaded to allow healing. Commonly, this involves placing the paw in a cast or flexion bandage for three weeks, followed by a lateral splint for three weeks, then a soft-padded bandage for the three final weeks. It is important that when the patient is placed in a cast, the cast is constructed to extend past the digits to prevent weight-bearing, as any weight-bearing on the digits will inappropriately load the surgical repair.

Common Calcaneal Tendon Complex

The common calcaneal tendon complex, also called the Achilles tendon complex, is made up of five tendons that are grossly separated into three bundles (paired gastrocnemius tendons, superficial digital flexor tendon, and the combined tendon [gracilis, semitendinosus, biceps femoris]), which may be remembered using the mnemonic, "good sailors build good ships." As discussed, these tendons lie within a paratenon, which can give blood supply to the healing tendon.

Acute or Chronic

A wide range of presentations of common calcaneal tendinopathy can occur from acute lacerations of a healthy tendon to chronic tendinopathy. This chapter will focus on acute laceration, but it is important for clinicians to recognize that some patients with chronic common calcaneal tendinopathy can eventually rupture and present with the typical hyperflexion of the tarsus seen with a complete common calcaneal tear. Radiographs should be evaluated in all cases to evaluate for signs of chronicity, such as calcaneal osseous remodeling and the presence of calcification or osseous remodeling of the calcaneal tendon. Careful palpation of the other hind limb can reveal thickening of the other common calcaneal tendon, which may raise the index of suspicion for underlying chronic tendinopathy. Identification of this subset of cases is important, as these patients often will have a large section of fibrous tissue from the chronic tendinopathy, and a large resection of tissue may need to be planned. Large resections may require further reconstruction options with possible pantarsal arthrodesis, which are outside the scope of this chapter. Failure to identify these cases prior to surgery and failure to remove the fibrous tissue present will lead to a weaker surgical construct, which risks repair failure.

Surgical Repair

The patient is positioned in sternal recumbency and prepared for surgery (Figure 53.2). A surgical approach is made over the common calcaneal tendon. The skin incision is performed laterally or medially to prevent it from being located along the plantar aspect of the tarsus. Once exposed, the paratenon of the common calcaneal tendon is opened and the individual tendons are identified. Surgical repair with a primary suture, such as a three-loop pulley or Krakow pattern, is used to approximate the tendon ends. Secondary epitendinous sutures are placed to complete the repair. Closure of the paratenon is performed if possible.

Complete immobilization of the tarsus for three weeks is performed. Immobilization can be performed in different ways, including a cast, placement of a calcaneotibial screw or plate, or a transarticular external fixator. After approximately three weeks, this support is gradually decreased. In cases where a cast is used, this is typically downgraded to a lateral splint for three weeks. Following this six-week period, the patient is typically downgraded to a soft-padded bandage or custom sports brace for two to three weeks. The added benefit of the sports brace is the ability to gradually decrease support for the patient over time. Some patients will use the brace as a support when they eventually start high-impact activity.

Potential Complications

Failure of the surgical repair can occur leading to hyperextension/hyperflexion of the associated joint and reoccurrence of lameness following repair. The tendon ends in these cases can either be lengthened if they have healed with scar tissue or can be shortened and retracted, depending on the interval from the injury to failure of the repair. Revision of the surgical repair is recommended in these cases, and the surgeon should be prepared to either shorten tendons, which have lengthened or to lengthen shortened tendons to revise the repair. Careful attention to suture placement during the repair and appropriate immobilization are important to prevent construct failure, and if failure occurs, each of these factors should be evaluated and addressed to help prevent repeat surgical failure.

Coaptation/immobilization is required for a number of weeks following tendon repair, and complications associated with this are frequently seen in these cases. The severity of these complications can range from mild bandage-associated dermatitis and wounds to full-thickness pressure ulcers. Adequate restriction of the patient post-surgery is helpful to minimize the occurrence of these complications. However, most of these issues are resolved with the removal of coaptation.

As discussed, failure to address DDFT injury and only suturing the SDFT during initial tendon repair will lead to altered weight-bearing on the metatarsal or metacarpal pads and the digits, leading to chronic lameness and wounds in these regions. Due to this, a thorough evaluation of both the superficial and deep digital flexor tendons at the time of initial repair is of vital importance to prevent injuries to the DDFTs from being undiagnosed and untreated.

References

1 Slatter, D. (2003). *Textbook of Small Animal Surgery*, 3e. Philadelphia: Saunders.

2 Dueland, R. and Quentin, J. (1980). Triceps tenotomy: biomechanical assessment of healing strength. *J. Am. Anim. Hosp. Assoc.* 16: 507.

3 Kim, J.T., Rusly, J.R., and Fruscello, K., et al. (2012). Comparison of Achilles tendon suture repair techniques: Krackow vs. modified Mason-Allen under cyclic loading in an in vitro bovine model. *Proceedings of the Orthopedic Research Society*, San Francisco, CA, 4–7 Feburary 2012.

4 Schulz, K.S., Ash, K.J., and Cook, J.L. (2019). Clinical outcomes after common calcanean tendon rupture repair in dogs with a loop-suture tenorrhaphy technique and autogenous leukoreduced platelet-rich plasma. *Vet. Surg.* 48 (7): 1262–1270.

5 Ahluwalia, R., Zourelidis, C., Guo, S. et al. (2013). Chronic sinus formation using nonabsorbable braided suture following open repair of Achilles tendon. *Foot Ankle Surg.* 19 (2): e7–e9.

6 Putterman, A.B., Duffy, D.J., Kersh, M.E. et al. (2019). Effect of a continuous epitendinous suture as adjunct to three-loop pulley and locking-loop patterns for flexor tendon repair in a canine model. *Vet. Surg.* 48 (7): 1229–1236.

7 Moores, A.P., Owen, M.R., and Tarlton, J.F. (2004). The three-loop pulley suture versus two locking-loop sutures for the repair of canine Achilles tendons. *Vet. Surg.* 33 (2): 131–137.

8 Cocca, C.J., Duffy, D.J., Kersh, M.E. et al. (2019). Biomechanical comparison of three epitendinous suture patterns as adjuncts to a core locking loop suture for repair of canine flexor tendon injuries. *Vet. Surg.* 48 (7): 1245–1252.

54

Bone Grafts

Rebecca J. Webb

VetSurg, Ventura, CA, USA

Key Points

- The four bone grafting properties or tenets of bone regeneration include osteogenesis, osteoinduction, osteoconduction, and osteopromotion.
- Knowing when to apply and how to utilize bone grafts is essential for a successful outcome in challenging cases.
- Bone graft harvesting sites in a canine patient, the proximal craniolateral humerus, proximal medial tibia, and dorsal iliac crest, are chosen based on the known areas of relatively little soft tissue coverage for easy access and of relatively large regions of cancellous bone.

Introduction

Bone grafts are an essential part of veterinary orthopedic surgery. They aid in the healing of acute fractures, joint arthrodeses, and revision of non- or delayed union fractures. Bone grafts can either be categorized depending on their composition (cancellous, cortical, or corticocancellous) or by their origin (autograft, allograft, or xenograft). Autografts are bone grafts harvested from a donor site on the patient and then transferred to another surgical site on the same patient. These are the most used forms of graft in veterinary medicine. Allografts are bone grafts harvested from another patient of the same species, and these grafts are becoming more common with the ongoing development of veterinary transplantation services. Xenografts are grafts from a different species and are the least common in veterinary medicine. Bone grafts enhance bone healing by providing a scaffold for bone regeneration and a source of bone-forming cells, growth factors, and/or minerals that promote new bone formation. Bone regeneration is a complex process, and there are four main tenets of bone regeneration, which are osteogenesis, osteoinduction, osteoconduction, and osteopromotion. Understanding each of the tenets or grafting properties allows the clinician to understand the benefits gained from the various products, so they can choose the graft material that is most appropriate for their case.

1) **Osteogenesis**. Osteogenesis is the formation of new bone tissue by osteoblasts. Osteoblasts synthesize and deposit the extracellular matrix of bone, consisting mainly of collagen and other proteins. Grafts that address this tenet include fresh autogenous bone grafts and bone marrow aspirates.
2) **Osteoinduction**. Osteoinduction is the process by which undifferentiated cells are stimulated to differentiate into osteoblasts, promoting bone formation where otherwise no bone formation would occur. Certain biological substances, such as bone morphogenetic proteins (BMPs), have osteoinductive properties.
3) **Osteoconduction**. Osteoconduction involves providing a scaffold or framework that allows the ingrowth of new blood vessels, cells, and tissues to promote bone regeneration. Osteoconductive materials can be synthetic (such as porous bioceramics) or natural (such as the trabecular network of an allogenic bone graft) that serve as a scaffold for new bone formation.
4) **Osteopromotion**. Osteopromotion involves creating an optimal environment that enhances bone

Techniques in Small Animal Soft Tissue, Orthopedic, and Ophthalmic Surgery, First Edition. Edited by Kristin A. Coleman.

Companion website: www.wiley.com/go/coleman/surgeries

regeneration. It differs from osteogenesis and osteoconduction, as no cells or scaffold are added to the area to stimulate bone regeneration, and differs from osteoinduction, as placement of an osteopromotive substance will not result in bone formation when placed in a region without a healing fracture. Examples include platelet rich plasma (PRP) and biphasic calcium phosphate.[1,2]

The choice of bone graft depends on the procedure being performed, the patient's bone quality, the size and location of the bone defect, and the surgeon's preference. This chapter discusses the benefits of bone grafts, the available types of bone grafts, and the common locations for harvesting bone grafts in canine patients.

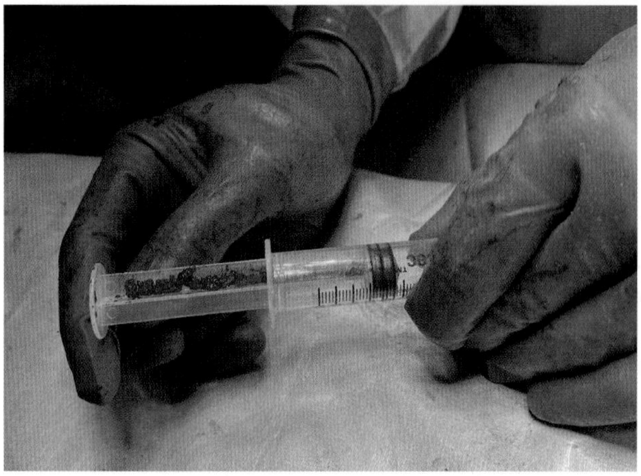

Figure 54.1 Bone graft stored in the barrel of a 12 mL syringe. The plunger is withdrawn, and graft material placed along it. Blood from the harvest of the bone graft can be collected with a 3 mL syringe without an attached needle directly from the harvest site and applied to the bone graft. This helps to keep the bone graft hydrated and prevent desiccation. The plunger can then be closed, and the graft secured within the syringe until use. *Source:* Courtesy of Dr. Joey A. Sapora.

Types of Bone Grafts

Autogenous Cancellous Bone Grafts

Autogenous cancellous bone grafts are pieces of cancellous bone harvested from a donor site on the patient with a reliably large volume of cancellous bone and then transferred to the surgery site. Cancellous autografts are preferred clinically because they have osteogenic, osteoinductive, osteoconductive, and osteopromotion qualities. Cancellous autografts are commonly used in cases when healing will be delayed (e.g., elderly patient), in patients with delayed or nonunions, and in cases where quick healing is of benefit (such as arthrodesis or in patients with expected poor postoperative compliance). In fact, cancellous autograft has been found to increase the rate of bone healing by up to four weeks when used in pancarpal arthrodesis.[3] The most common locations for harvesting cancellous bone grafts in canine patients include the proximal humerus, proximal tibia, and dorsal crest of the ilial wing. The timing of graft collection should be as close to its application to the fracture site to maximize the number of viable cells present within it. The graft should be stored appropriately to prevent necrosis of the viable cells. Options for graft storage between harvest and use include within the barrel of a 5 or 12 mL syringe (Figure 54.1) or, alternatively, within a saline-moistened sterile container (Figure 54.2). The graft should be kept moist with either saline or blood to prevent desiccation of the sample, as desiccation will lead to rapid loss of viable cells within the graft.

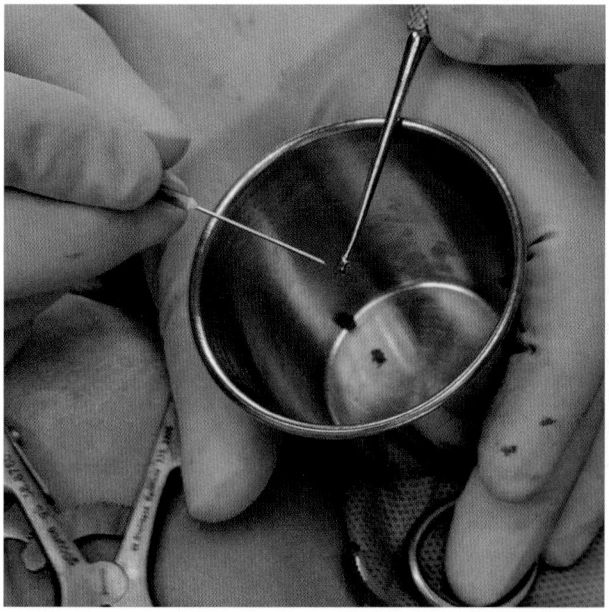

Figure 54.2 Harvested bone graft is being deposited into a sterile metallic container for temporary storage prior to being applied to the patient. When using a small curette, a hypodermic needle is used to remove the bone graft from the curette's concave tip. *Source:* Courtesy of Dr. Nathan Squire.

The clinician should be cautious in cases that are being revised for infection that gloves and instruments are changed between the primary surgery site and graft collection to prevent the seeding of infection to the graft site. Another tip is to remember to copiously lavage the recipient site prior to application of the graft, since flushing after graft placement would be detrimental. Complications following autogenous cancellous bone grafting in small animals are uncommon but have been reported to include bone fracture and early growth plate closure of the graft site.[4,5] Clinicians should be cautious when harvesting bone grafts in immature patients due to this. In addition to the potential for complications from cancellous bone graft harvest, other disadvantages include the increased surgical and anesthesia time to harvest and the low yield from small or geriatric patients.

Common Locations for Harvesting Bone Grafts in Canine Patients

The most common locations for harvesting bone grafts in canine patients are discussed below. Often, the graft site is determined by the volume of graft required (larger volumes can often be harvested from the humerus than other bones) and the location of the fracture to be repaired. The graft site should be able to be accessed at the same time as the fracture site for expedited transfer from the graft site to the recipient site. Generally, the harvest of autogenous bone graft occurs in the same manner for each location. A skin incision is made and overlying soft tissue dissected, a small drill bit or IM pin is used to access the medullary cavity, then a curette is used to harvest the cancellous bone within. The drill bit (or IM pin) and curette used should be sized appropriately for the size of the patient's bone to minimize the risk of donor site morbidity.

Proximal Humerus The proximal humerus is a common site for bone graft harvest, as it tends to produce a large volume of cancellous graft. It is helpful to perform a hanging limb prep or to have the limb available for manipulation, as this can be beneficial during graft collection.

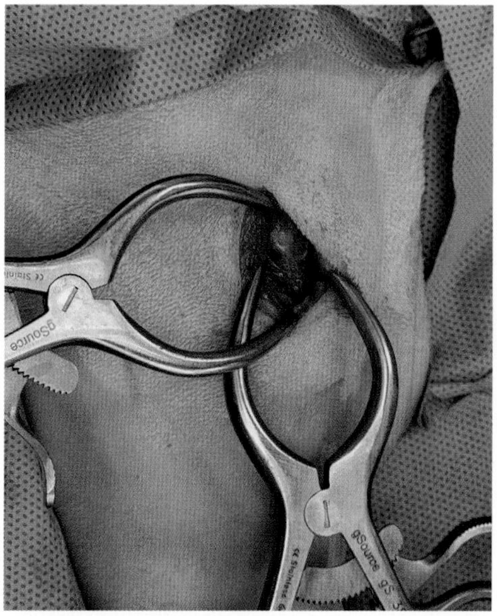

Figure 54.3 Approach to the right craniolateral proximal humerus in a cat. The acromial head of the deltoid is retracted caudally. Note the placement of the two Gelpi retractors at 90° angles to retract the soft tissue in the area. *Source:* Courtesy of Dr. Nathan Squire.

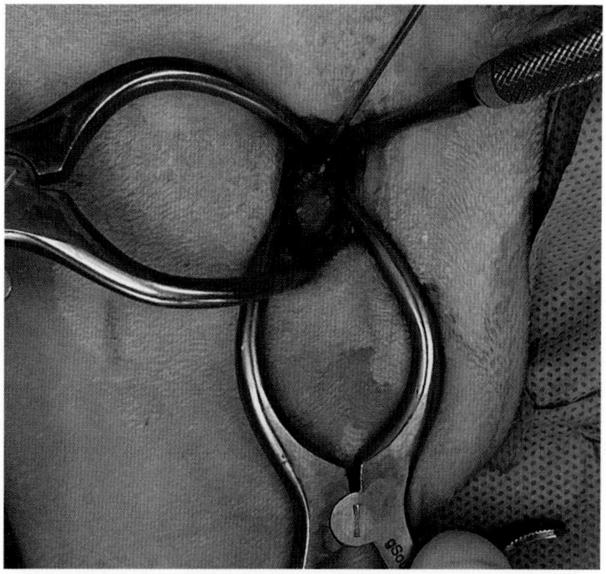

Figure 54.4 A small pin is used in this feline patient to create a cortical defect to access the medullary cavity. *Source:* Courtesy of Dr. Nathan Squire.

With the patient in lateral recumbency and the affected side up, the greater tubercle is palpated, and a craniolateral approach to the humerus is performed in this location. The acromial head of the deltoid is retracted caudally to access the flat aspect of the metaphysis of the humerus. Adequate retraction of the soft tissues is important to prevent graft material from getting lost in the surrounding soft tissues during harvest. Two Gelpi retractors placed at 90° from each other are particularly useful for this (Figure 54.3). The ideal site for bone graft harvest is located just distal to the greater tubercle. In this location, an intramedullary (IM) pin or drill bit is used to create a circular cortical defect in the lateral cortex and allow access to the medullary cavity (Figure 54.4). The size of the cortical defect is determined by the patient's bone size. However, the drill bit or IM pin should be big enough to allow easy insertion of an appropriately-sized curette for the patient. If the cortical defect is not large enough for easy entry of the curette, the clinician will have difficulty retrieving the graft from the medullary canal. Once the curette is inserted, it is used in a single circular scooping motion to harvest the graft, similar to scooping ice cream. Once the scooping motion has been performed, the curette is removed with the harvested graft (Figure 54.5). Avoid multiple scooping actions per curette entry, as this can lead to maceration of the graft material. When using a small curette, removal of the graft from the concave tip can be performed with a hypodermic needle to avoid crushing the graft material (Figure 54.2). It is also helpful to have a 3 mL syringe (no needle) on hand to suction any fluid or blood that accumulates in the cortical defect from the marrow, which is an ideal fluid to then soak the graft in its container prior to transfer. Closure is performed of the subcutaneous and skin layers.

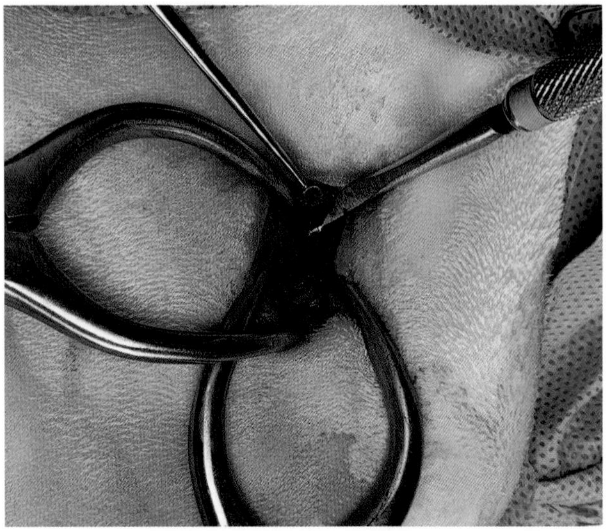

Figure 54.5 A small curette is used to harvest the cancellous bone graft from the proximal humerus in this feline patient. *Source:* Courtesy of Dr. Nathan Squire.

Tibia The proximal tibia can be used to harvest cancellous bone graft. Typically, the volume harvested from this location is less than the humerus, but it can be advantageous for hind limb fractures due to its proximity and ability to include the ipsilateral tibia within the surgical field.

A medial approach to the proximal metaphysis of the tibia is performed. The insertion of the combined tendons of the semitendinosus, caudal belly of sartorius, and gracilis (also referred to as the *pes anserinus*) at the cranial aspect may need to be elevated to access the underlying tibia. During this elevation, the medial collateral ligament (located caudally) should be protected (Figure 54.6). The location for graft harvest is the middle of the bone from the cranial to caudal aspects at approximately the level of the patellar tendon insertion of the tuberosity (Figure 54.7). Radiographs of the area can help guide clinicians in regard to the patient's individual anatomy. Once the tibia is isolated, the soft tissues are retracted as above with Gelpi retractors, and the cortical defect for medullary access proceeds as for the humerus.

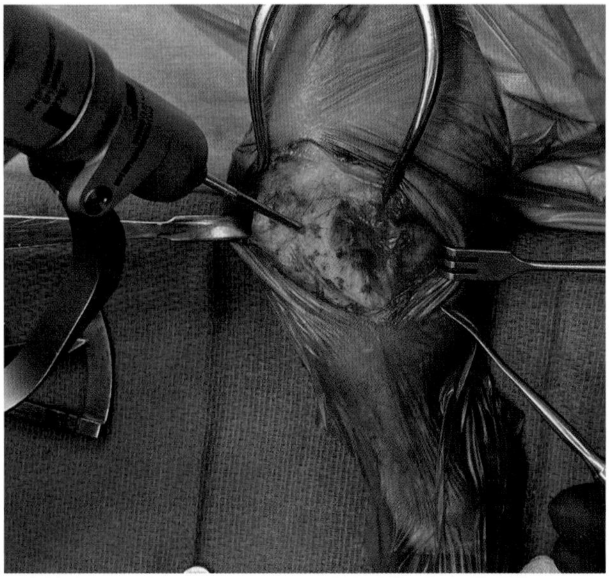

Figure 54.7 The IM pin in this image shows the approximate location for bone graft harvest from the right proximomedial tibia. The pin is placed in the middle of the bone from the cranial to caudal aspect, at approximately the level, or just distal to, the patellar tendon insertion of the tuberosity. Cranial is to the left of the image. *Source:* Courtesy of Dr. Joey A. Sapora.

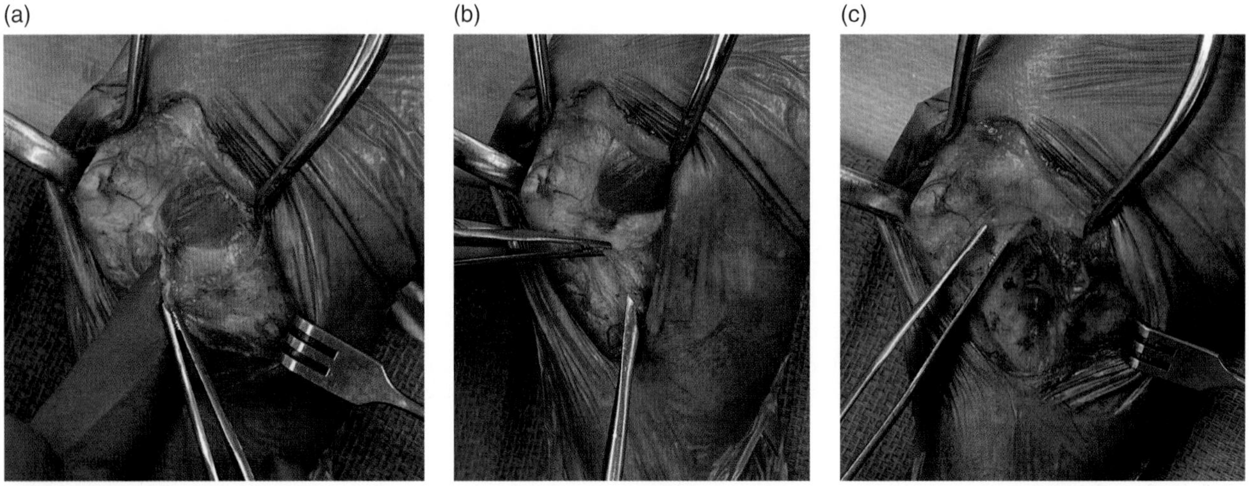

Figure 54.6 Approach to proximal tibial metaphysis in a small breed dog. The combined tendons of the semitendinosus, sartorius, and gracilis muscles (also referred to as the *pes anserinus*) are elevated to access the tibia. During this elevation, the underlying medial collateral ligament is protected by the surgeon's finger (a) or by a periosteal elevator (b). Tips of the thumb forceps denote the underlying medial collateral ligament (c). Cranial is to the left of the images. *Source:* Courtesy of Dr. Joey A. Sapora.

During the closure, the fascia of the pes anserinus is reattached using cruciate mattress sutures with a long-term monofilament absorbable suture, followed by standard subcutaneous and skin closure.

Ilium The ilium can also be used for bone graft harvest. Harvest of cancellous graft through an access hole as above or osteotomy of the iliac crest for a combination of cancellous and corticocancellous bone grafts are described.[6] An approach through the skin is performed over the palpable dorsal iliac crest. The gluteal muscles on the lateral aspect of the crest and the soft tissues on the medial aspect are elevated to expose the iliac crest. Gelpi retractors as described previously are helpful for retraction. An osteotome is used to remove the tip of the crest. A curette is used as previously described to harvest cancellous bone from the remaining iliac crest and wing of the ilium. The removed crest can also be morselized using rongeurs to form corticocancellous graft. Corticocancellous graft, however, has lower osteogenic and osteoinductive qualities compared to cancellous graft alone. Closure is performed of the subcutaneous tissues and skin.

Allografts

Allografts are harvested from another patient of the same species and processed, after which they can be stored for long periods and sold commercially. Allografts typically have osteoinductive and osteoconductive properties but do not have osteogenic properties due to the absence of viable cells present within a cancellous autograft. Allografts are particularly helpful in patients where cancellous autograft is in limited supply (such as small patients or in patients where the yield from cancellous graft harvest was low), as well as in immature patients to avoid trauma to the physis. In small patients where the volume of cancellous autograft from a grafting location is likely to be low, many clinicians will use allografts instead. Alternatively, the low volume of autograft (either from a small patient or from an inadequate yield in an average-sized patient) can be extended by mixing it with a commercial allograft to give an adequate volume for the surgery being performed.

Cancellous Bone Allografts (Cancellous Bone Chips)

Cancellous bone allografts are commercially available in chip form or in combination with demineralized bone matrix (DBM). They provide advantages over an autograft in that they are able to be stored at room temperature within the O.R. and, therefore, can be quickly available when required. Surgical and anesthesia times are reduced, as are the risks of donor site morbidity. However, it is important to note that autogenous cancellous graft is superior to allograft, since it maintains osteogenic properties due to the live cells that are transferred within the autograft. Mixing a cancellous allograft with either cancellous autograft or a bone marrow aspirate can help to overcome the lack of osteogenic properties. Cancellous allograft can be helpful in cases where the harvest of an autograft is undesirable or can be used to extend the autograft to a volume appropriate for the surgery being performed.

Demineralized Bone Matrix (DBM)

This is an allograft that has been processed to remove the mineral component and is ground to a particular particle size. The demineralization process increases the exposure of the native bone morphogenic proteins (BMPs) and other growth factors on the graft material, which in turn accelerates the osteoinductive properties of the DBM. Commonly, DBM is sold as part of a mix with cancellous bone chips, and the two together provide both osteoinductive and osteoconductive properties but lack osteogenic properties. The advantages and uses for DBM are the same as for cancellous allograft. Although the demineralization process increases the native BMPs, products with further surface modifications are becoming commercially available (Fortigen-P™, Veterinary Transplant Services). The manufacturer reports short healing times with the product, but peer-reviewed publications are limited.

Bone Morphogenetic Proteins (BMPs)

Bone morphogenic proteins are growth factors that stimulate bone formation. BMPs can be used alone or in combination with other bone grafts to enhance healing. These substances can be very effective in the regeneration of bone, and there are now multiple reports on their use in canine patients.[7-9] However, the cost is typically prohibitive for widespread veterinary use.

Synthetic Grafts

A number of synthetic grafts are currently under evaluation to determine their value as bone graft substitutes in the veterinary and human markets. The list of synthetic graft options is extensive, however, very few are currently used clinically. Examples of these grafts include bioceramics, calcium phosphates, and coralline hydroxyapatite bone graft substitutes. Each of these grafts typically functions in an osteoconductive manner. Currently, there is limited data to support their use in veterinary patients, however, research is ongoing.[10–12]

References

1 Shuang, Y., Yizhen, L., Zhang, Y. et al. (2016). In vitro characterization of an osteoinductive biphasic calcium phosphate in combination with recombinant BMP2. *BMC Oral Health* 17: 35.

2 Kumar, K.A., Rao, J.B., Pavan Kumar, B. et al. (2013). A prospective study involving the use of platelet rich plasma in enhancing the uptake of bone grafts in the oral and maxillofacial region. *J. Maxillofac. Oral Surg.* 12 (4): 387–394.

3 Johnson, K.A. and Bellenger, C.R. (1980). The effects of autologous bone grafting on bone healing after carpal arthrodesis in the dog. *Vet. Rec.* 107 (6): 126–132.

4 Ferguson, J.F. (1996). Fracture of the humerus after cancellous bone graft harvesting in a dog. *J. Small Anim. Pract.* 37 (5): 232–234.

5 Penwick, R.C., Mosier, D.A., and Clark, D.M. (1991). Healing of canine autogenous cancellous bone graft donor sites. *Vet. Surg.* 20 (4): 229–234.

6 Johnson, A.L. (2013). Fundamentals of orthopedic surgery and fracture management: bone grafting – ilial wing. In: *Small Animal Surgery*, 4e (ed. S.A. Johnston and K.M. Tobias), 1063. Missouri, USA: Elsevier.

7 Massie, A.M., Kapatkin, A.S., Fuller, M.C. et al. (2017). Outcome of nonunion fractures in dogs treated with fixation, compression resistant matrix, and recombinant human bone morphogenetic protein-2. *Vet. Comp. Orthop. Traumatol.* 30 (2): 153–159.

8 Pinel, C.B. and Pluhar, G.E. (2012). Clinical application of recombinant human bone morphogenetic protein in cats and dogs: a review of 13 cases. *Can. Vet. J.* 53 (7): 767–774.

9 Boudrieau, R.J. (2015). Initial experience with rhBMP-2 delivered in a compressive resistant matrix for mandibular reconstruction in 5 dogs. *Vet. Surg.* 44 (4): 443–458.

10 Wheeler, D.L., Eschbach, E.J., Hoellrich, R.G. et al. (2000). Assessment of resorbable bioactive material for grafting of critical-size cancellous defects. *J. Orthop. Res.* 18 (1): 140–148.

11 Hauschild, G., Merten, H.A., Bader, A. et al. (2005). Bioartificial bone grafting: tarsal joint fusion in a dog using a bioartificial composite bone graft consisting of beta-tricalciumphosphate and platelet rich plasma – a case report. *Vet. Comp. Orthop. Traumatol.* 18 (1): 52–54.

12 Franch, J., Diaz-Bertrana, C., Lafuente, P. et al. (2006). Betatricalcium phosphate as a synthetic cancellous bone graft in veterinary orthopedics: a retrospective study of 13 clinical cases. *Vet. Comp. Orthop. Traumatol.* 19 (4): 196–204.

Index

a

Techniques in Small Animal Soft Tissue, Orthopedic, and Ophthalmic Surgery, First Edition. Edited by Kristin A. Coleman.

Companion website: www.wiley.com/go/coleman/surgeries

d

f